ESSENTIAL
CLINICAL
PATHOLOGY

ESSENTIAL CLINICAL PATHOLOGY

Edited by Dinah V. Parums

MA, PhD, BM, BCh, MRCPath
Senior Lecturer and Consultant
Department of Histopathology
Royal Postgraduate Medical School
Hammersmith Hospital
Du Cane Road, London W12 0NN

b

Blackwell
Science

© 1996 by
Blackwell Science Ltd
Editorial Offices:
Osney Mead, Oxford OX2 0EL
25 John Street, London WC1N 2BL
23 Ainslie Place, Edinburgh EH3 6AJ
238 Main Street, Cambridge
    Massachusetts 02142, USA
54 University Street, Carlton
    Victoria 3053, Australia

Other Editorial Offices:
Arnette Blackwell SA
    224, Boulevard Saint Germain
75007 Paris, France

Blackwell Wissenschafts-Verlag GmbH
    Kurfürstendamm 57
    10707 Berlin, Germany

    Zehetnergasse 6, A-1140 Wien
Austria

The Blackwell Science logo is a
trade mark of Blackwell Science Ltd
registered at the United Kingdom
Trade Marks Registry

First published 1996

Set by Excel Typesetters Co., Hong Kong
Printed and bound in Italy by
Vincenzo Bona s.r.l., Turin

A catalogue record for this title
is available from the British Library

ISBN 0-632-03088-7 (BSL)
ISBN 0-86542-751-8 (IE)

Library of Congress
Cataloging-in-Publication Data

Essential clinical pathology / edited by
    Dinah V. Parums.
        p.   cm.
    ISBN 0-632-03088-7
    1. Diagnosis, Laboratory–Handbooks,
manuals, etc.
    I. Parums, Dinah V.
    [DNLM: 1. Pathology, Clinical–
handbooks.   QY 39 E78   1996]
RB37.E68   1996
616.07–dc20
DNLM/DLC
for Library of Congress   95-36944
                                        CIP

DISTRIBUTORS

Marston Book Services Ltd
PO Box 269
Abingdon
Oxon OX14 4YN
(*Orders:* Tel: 01235 465500
            Fax: 01235 465555)

USA
Blackwell Science, Inc.
238 Main Street
Cambridge, MA 02142
(*Orders:* Tel: 800 215-1000
            617 876-7000
            Fax: 617 492-5263)

Canada
Copp Clark, Ltd
2775 Matheson Blvd East
Mississauga, Ontario
Canada, L4W 4P7
(*Orders:* Tel: 800 263-4374
            905 238-6074)

Australia
Blackwell Science Pty Ltd
54 University Street
Carlton, Victoria 3053
(*Orders:* Tel: 03 9347 0300
            Fax: 03 9349 3016)

Contents

4 Haematology and Blood Transfusion, 62
Mark Vickers

5 Chemical Pathology and Toxicology, 73
Paul Holloway

PART 2 ESSENTIAL GENERAL PATHOLOGY

6 Clinical Genetics, 81
Dinah V. Parums

7 Multisystem Diseases, 92
Gavin P. Spickett, Dinah V. Parums, Nicholas G. Ryley, David C. Brown & Paul Holloway

8 Tropical and Imported Infectious Disease, 111
John Paul

9 The Immune System, 131
Gavin P. Spickett

10 Immune Deficiency Disease Including AIDS, 144
Peter R. Millard, Gavin P. Spickett, Dinah V. Parums & Janice Bates

11 Neoplasia, 164
Dinah V. Parums

12 Diseases of Blood and Bone Marrow, 191
Mark Vickers

13 Diseases of Fluid Balance, Sodium, Potassium and Acid–Base Biochemistry, 224
Paul Holloway

PART 3 ESSENTIAL SYSTEMIC PATHOLOGY

14 Endocrine Disease, 237
*Paul Holloway, Dinah V. Parums &
Peter R. Millard*

15 Cardiovascular Disease, 271
Dinah V. Parums & Paul Holloway

16 Diseases of Lymph Nodes, Spleen and Thymus, 340
Kevin C. Gatter, Dinah V. Parums & David C. Brown

17 Diseases of the Ear and Respiratory Tract, 356
Michael S. Dunnill, Dinah V. Parums & Janice Bates

18 Diseases of the Gastrointestinal Tract, 398
Anne P. Campbell, Dinah V. Parums,
Paul Holloway & Stephen J. Gould

19 Diseases of the Liver, Biliary Tract and Exocrine Pancreas, 429
Nicholas G. Ryley, Peter R. Millard &
Paul Holloway

20 Diseases of Bone and Joint, 481
Anne P. Campbell, Dinah V. Parums,
Paul Holloway & Janice Bates

21 Diseases of the Urinary Tract, 503
Michael S. Dunnill, Dinah V. Parums, Paul Holloway & Janice Bates

22 Diseases of the Male Reproductive System, 543
Dinah V. Parums & Janice Bates

23 Diseases of the Female Reproductive System, 554
Brendan McDonald & Janice Bates

24 Breast Disease, 579
Dinah V. Parums

25 Perinatal and Paediatric Disease, 591
Stephen J. Gould, Paul Holloway & Janice Bates

26 Pathology of the Skin and Soft Tissue, 610
Peter R. Millard, Janice Bates & Dinah V. Parums

27 Diseases of the Nervous System, Including the Eye, 639
Brendan McDonald

List of Contributors

Janice Bates PhD, MRCPath, *Consultant Microbiologist, Worthing Hospital, Park Avenue, Worthing, West Sussex, BN11 2DH.* [10, 17, 20, 21, 22, 23, 25, 26]

David C. Brown MD, MRCPath, *Consultant Histopathologist, The Whittington Hospital, Highgate Hill, London N19 5NF.* [7, 16]

Anne P. Campbell MD, MRCPath, *Consultant Histopathologist, Castle Hill Hospital, Royal Hull Hospitals, Castle Road, Cottingham, Hull, North Humberside HU16 5JQ.* [18, 20]

Michael S. Dunnill MD, FRCP, FRCPath, *Emeritus Fellow, Merton College, Oxford OX1 4JD.* [17, 21]

Kevin C. Gatter MA, DPhil, MRCPath, *Head of Department, Department of Cellular Science, John Radcliffe Hospital, Headington, Oxford OX3 9DU.* [16]

Stephen J. Gould BSc, MB, MRCPath, *Consultant Paediatric Pathologist, John Radcliffe Hospital, Headington, Oxford OX3 9DU.* [18, 25]

Ruth M. Hargreaves MRCGP, MRCP, MRCPath, *Consultant Microbiologist, Brighton Public Health Laboratory, Royal Sussex County Hospital, Brighton BN2 5BE.* [2]

Paul Holloway BSc, PhD, BM, BCh, *Department of Clinical Biochemistry, John Radcliffe Hospital, Headington, Oxford OX3 9DU.* [5, 7, 13, 14, 15, 18, 19, 20, 21, 25]

Brendan McDonald BSc, MB, MRCPath, *Department of Neuropathology, Radcliffe Infirmary, Woodstock Road, Oxford OX2 6HE.* [23, 27]

Peter R. Millard MA, MD, FRCPath, *Consultant Histopathologist, Department of Cellular Pathology, John Radcliffe Hospital, Headington, Oxford OX3 9DU.* [1, 10, 14, 19, 26]

Dinah V. Parums MA, PhD, BM, BCh, MRCPath, *Senior Lecturer and Consultant, Department of Histopathology, Royal Postgraduate Medical School, Hammersmith Hospital, Du Cane Road, London W12 0NN.* [1, 2, 6, 7, 10, 11, 14, 15, 16, 17, 18, 20, 21, 22, 24, 26]

John Paul MD, MRCPath, *Consultant Microbiologist, Brighton Public Health Laboratory, Royal Sussex County Hospital, Brighton BN2 5BE.* [8]

Nicholas G. Ryley MA, BM, BCh, MRCPath, *Consultant Histopathologist, King Edward VIIth Hospital Midhurst, West Sussex GU29 0BL.* [7, 19]

Gavin P. Spickett MA, DPhil, BM, BCh, MRCP, MRCPath, *Senior Lecturer and Consultant Clinical Immunologist, Regional Immunology Department, Newcastle General Hospital, Westgate Road, Newcastle upon Tyne NE4 6BE.* [3, 7, 9, 10]

Mark Vickers MD, MRCPath, *Senior Lecturer, Department of Medicine and Therapeutics, Aberdeen Royal Infirmary, Aberdeen.* [4, 12]

Preface

The authors have in common the privilege of teaching a combined 10-week pathology course at Oxford University Medical School during the period 1991–1993. It was during this time that we decided to produce a course textbook, based on our lectures and demonstrations, that would represent the essentials of clinical laboratory medicine as we would wish to distil it to our students. It is in the spirit of the changes in medical education, the new core curriculum and evidence-based medicine, that this book is written.

Part 1 (Chapters 1–5) covers the basic laboratory and diagnostic principles of each pathology specialty; Part 2 (Chapters 6–13) deals with disease processes involving multiple systems; Part 3 (Chapters 14–27) covers the clinical pathology of the systems and integrates the histopathology with the immunology, microbiology and clinical chemistry of these systems. In the systems chapters, we have structured the contents according to the 'pathological sieve', thus:

Normal anatomy, physiology and biochemistry
Congenital disease
Acquired disease
    Clinical presentation
    Infection (microbiology)
    Inflammatory/immune disease
    Vascular/haematological disease
    Drugs/toxins
    Neoplasia
    Traumatic/surgical/degenerative disease

In order to encourage the student to assimilate and to enjoy the information, this book is illustrated with full-colour macroscopic and microscopic figures, with simple diagrams and with cartoons. A glossary is included. A list of recommended texts for further, more specialized reading is included after each chapter and at the end of the book. Throughout, we have assumed a knowledge of the basic principles of pathology as covered in preclinical undergraduate texts.

ACKNOWLEDGEMENTS

I wish to thank the students and staff of Oxford University Medical School and, in particular, the students who helped suggest the contents for the book and who read the first drafts; Anna Donald, Robert Buttery, Robin Choudhury, Graham Ogg, Ashwin Pinto, James Calvert, Ian Crossley, Helen Parsons, Simon Shields, Stuart Williams, James McMorran and Andrew Taylor. I would like to thank Professor James O'D. McGee for the privilege of 3 years spent as Clinical Tutor in the Nuffield Department of Pathology. Dr David Y. Mason provided valuable haematology teaching material and Kingsley Micklem helped with the production of the haematology figures. Thanks go to Dr Rachel Armstrong for her help in providing artwork for teaching purposes and for her figures and cartoons for the book; to Dr Phillip Cox, Dr Catherine Sarraf, Dr Malcolm Alison, Dr Sunil Shaunak and Dr M.J. Mitchinson for reading parts of the manuscript; to Mickie Lennox-Martin for her secretarial skills; to William T. Shaw for Mac-wizardry and continued support; to Andy Robinson for his encouragement and patience, to Peter Saugman who first suggested the project, to Mike Elms, for much of the artwork and to Jody Ball, production editor, at Blackwell Science. Dr David Cassidy and Dr John Keenan provided assistance with the preparation of the Biochemistry teaching material.

DVP

List of Abbreviations

2,3-DPG	2,3-diphosphoglycerate		ATG	antithymocyte globulin
5-HT	5-hydroxytryptamine		ATN	acute tubular necrosis
A1AT	alpha-1-antitrypsin		AVP	arginine vasosuppression
AAA	abdominal aortic aneurysm		AZT	azathioprine
AAT	aspartate aminotransferase		BAL	bronchiolo-alveolar lavage
AB	alcian blue		BALT	bronchus-associated lymphoid tissue
AB/PAS	alcian blue/periodic acid-Schiff		BCC	basal cell carcinoma
ACTH	adrenocorticotrophic hormone		BCG	bacillus Calmette-Guérin
AD	autosomal dominant		BFU-E	burst forming unit-erythrocyte
ADH	antidiuretic hormone		BL	blood level
ADH	atypical ductal hyperplasia		BMT	bone marrow transplantation
ADP	adenosine diphosphate prostaglandin		BNLI	British National Lymphoma Investigation
AFP	α-fetoprotein			
AIDS	acquired immune deficiency syndrome		BPD	bronchopulmonary dysplasia
AIHA	autoimmune haemolytic anaemia		BPH	benign prostatic hyperplasia
ALG	antilymphocyte globulin		BRU	bone remodelling unit
ALH	atypical lobular hyperplasia		BSE	bovine spongiform encephalopathy
ALL	acute lymphblastic leukaemia		BSP	bromsulphthalein
ALP	alkaline phosphatase		BUN	blood urea nitrogen
ALT	alanine aminotransferase		C3b-R	complement receptor C3b
AMA	antimitochondrial antibodies		CABG	coronary artery bypass graft
AML	acute myeloid leukaemia		CAH	chronic active hepatitis
AMP	adenosine monophosphate		CCF	congestive cardiac failure
ANAs	antinuclear antibodies		CD	cluster differentiation
ANCA	antineutrophil cytoplasmic antibody		CDC	Centers for Disease Control
APAAP	alkaline phosphatase-anti-alkaline phosphatase		CE	cholesterol esters
			CEA	carcinoembryonic antigen
apo	apoproteins		CF	cystic fibrosis
APTT	active partial thromboblastin time		CFTR	cystic fibrosis transmembrane conductance regulator
APUD	amine precursor uptake and decarboxylation			
			CFU-E	colony forming unit-erythrocyte
AR	autosomal recessive		CGD	chronic granulomatous disease
ARC	AIDS related complex		CHD	coronary heart disease
ARF	acute renal failure		Chol	cholesterol
ASD	atrial septal defect		CIN	cervical intraepithelial neoplasia
ASO	antistreptolysin O		CK	creatine kinase
AST	aspartate aminotransferase		CK	cytokeratin

CLED	cysteine lactose electrolyte deficient	ERCP	endoscopic retrograde cholangiopancreatography
CLL	chronic lymphocytic leukaemia		
CM	chylomicrons	ERPC	endoscopic retrograde percutaneous cholangiography
CMC	chronic mucocutaneous candidiasis		
CMI	cell-mediated immunity	ESR	erythrocyte sedimentation rate
CMR	chylomicron remnant	ET	embryo transfer
CMV	cytomegalovirus	ETEC	enterotoxigenic *Escherichia coli*
CNS	central nervous system	EVG	elastic van Giesen
CoA	coenzyme A	FA	fatty acids
COAD	chronic obstructive airways disease	FBC	full blood count
CREST	calcinosis, Raynaud's oesophageal dysmotility, syndactyly, telangiectasia	FDC	follicular dendritic cell
		FDP	fibrin degradation product
		FEV	forced expiratory volume
CRF	chronic renal failure	FFP	fresh frozen plasma
CRF	corticotrophin-releasing factor	FH	familial hypercholesterolaemia
CRH	corticotrophine releasing hormone	FIGO	Federation of Obstetrics and Gynaecology
CRP	C-reactive protein		
CSF	cerebrospinal fluid	FNA	fine needle aspiration
CT	computed tomography	FNAC	fine needle aspiration cytology
CUS	catheter urine specimen	FSH	follicle-stimulating hormone
CVA	cerebrospinal fluid	FTA-Abs	fluorescent treponemal antibody absorption test
CVID	common variable immune deficiency		
CVP	central venous pressure	FVC	forced vitality capacity
CVS	chorionic villus sampling	G_6PD	glucose-6-phosphate dehydrogenase
CXR	chest X-ray	GBM	glomerular basement membrane
DAD	diffuse alveolar damage	GC	germinal centre
DCIS	ductal carcinoma-*in-situ*	GCA	giant cell arteritis
DES	dethylstilboestrol	GFAP	glial fibrillary acidic protein
DH	delayed hypersensitivity	GFR	glomerular filtration rate
DHCC	1,25-dihydroxycholecalciferol	GGT	γ-glutamyltransferase
DI	diabetes insipidus	GH	growth hormone
DIC	disseminated intravascular coagulation	GHRH	growth hormone releasing hormone
DIT	diffuse intimal thickening	GI	gastrointestinal
DNA	deoxyribonucleic acid	GIFT	gametic intrafallopian transfer
DPT	diphtheria toxoid	GIT	gastrointestinal tract
dsDNA	double-stranded DNA	GL	germinal layer
DST	dexamethasone suppression test	GLH	germinal layer haemorrhage
DVT	deep venous thrombosis	GvHD	graft-versus-host disease
EBNA	Epstein–Barr virus-associated nuclear antigen	H&E	haematoxylin and eosin
		HAS	human albumin solution
EBV	Epstein–Barr virus	HAV	hepatitis A virus
ECF	eosinophil chemotactic factor	Hb	haemoglobin
ECF	extracellular fluid	HBcAg	hepatitis B core antigen
ECG	electrocardiography	HBeAg	hepatitis B e antigen
EDTA	ethylenediaminetetraacetic acid	HBsAg	hepatitis B surface antigen
EEL	external elastic lamina	HBV	hepatitis B virus
EGF	epidermal growth factor	HCC	hepatocellular carcinoma
EHEC	enterohaemorrhagic *Escherichia coli*	HCG	human chorionic gonadotrophin
EIEC	enteroinvasive *Escherichia coli*	Hct	haematocrit
ELISA	enzyme-linked immunosorbent assay	HCV	hepatitis C virus
EMA	epithelial membrane antigen	HDL	high density lipoprotein
ENT	ear, nose and throat	HDV	hepatitis D virus
EPEC	enteropathogenic *Escherichia coli*	HEV	hepatitis E virus

hGH	human growth hormone	LV	left ventricle
HIV	human immunodefiency virus	M	macrophage
HLA	human leucocyte antigen	MA	membrane antigen
HMD	hyaline membrane disease	MAB	monoclonal antibody
HMFG	human milk fat globule	MAI	*mycobacterium avium-intracellulare*
hMG	human menopausal gonadotrophin	MALT	mucose-associated lymphoid tissue
HPF	high power field	MAP	microtubule associated protein
hPRL	human prolactin	MBC	minimum bacterial concentration
HPV	human papilloma virus	MCH	mean cell haemoglobin
HSP	human serum prealbumin	MCHC	mean cell haemoglobin concentration
HSV	herpes simplex virus	MCTD	mixed connective tissue disease
HTLV	human T-lymphotrophic virus	MCV	mean cell volume
HTS	human thyroid stimulator	MEA	multiple endocrine adenomatosis
HUS	haemolytic–uraemic syndrome	MEN	multiple endocrine neoplasia
HVA	homovanillic acid	MGG	May–Grünwald–Giemsa
HVS	high vaginal swab	MHC	major histocompatibility complex
IAPP	islet amyloid polypeptide	MI	myocardial infarction
IBD	inflammatory bowel disease	MIC	minimum ibitory concentration
ICF	intracellular fluid	MLR	mixed lymphocyte reaction
IDL	intermediate density lipoprotein	MLSO	medical laboratory scientific officer
IEL	internal elastic lamina	MMR	measles, mumps and rubella
IEN	intraendometrial neoplasia	MODY	maturity-onset diabetes of the young
IF	intrinsic factor	MPGN	membranoproliferative
Ig	immunoglobulin		glomerulonephritis
IgE	immunoglobulin E	MRI	magnetic resonance imaging
IGF	insulin-like growth factor	MSAFP	maternal serum α-fetoprotein
IgG	immunoglobulin G	MSH	melanocyte-stimulating hormone
IgM	immunoglobulin M	MSU	midstream urine
IHD	ischaemic heart disease	MTI	malignant teratoma intermediate
IL-2	interleukin 2	MTT	malignant teratoma trophoblastic
INR	international normalized ratio	MTU	malignant teratoma undifferentiated
ISH	*in-situ* hybridization	NA	nuclear antigen
IST	insulin stress test	NADP	nicotine adenine dinucleotide
ITP	idiopathic thrombocytopaenic purpura		phosphate
ITU	intensive therapy unit	NANB	non-A, non-B (hepatitis)
IUCD	intrauterine contraceptive device	NBT	nitroblue tetrazolium
IVC	inferior venae cavae	NCF	neutrophil chemotactic factor
IVF	*in vitro* fertilization	NCI	National Cancer Institute
IVH	intraventricular haemorrhage	NDI	nephrogenic diabetes insipidus
LATS	long-acting thyroid stimulator	NEC	necrotizing enterocolitis
LATS-P	long-acting thyroid stimulator	NEFA	non-esterified fatty acids
	protector	NFPT	non-functioning pituitary tumour
LCA	leucocyte common antigen	NFT	neurofibrillar tangle
LCAT	lecithin cholesteryl acyl transferase	NGU	non-gonococcal urethritis
LCIS	lobular carcinoma-*in-situ*	NHFTR	non-haemolytic febrile transfusion
LCM	lymphocytic choriomeningitis		reaction
LDH	lactate dehydrogenase	NHL	non-Hodgkin's lymphoma
LDL	low density lipoprotein	NPC	nasopharyngeal carcinoma
LFT	liver function test	NSAIDs	non-steroidal anti-inflammatory drugs
LGV	lymphogranuloma venereum	OGTT	oral glucose tolerance test
LH	luteinizing hormone	PA	pernicious anaemia
LPL	lipoprotein lipase	PAN	polyarteritis nodosa
LPS	lipopolysaccharide	Pap	Papanicolaou

PAP	peroxidase anti-peroxidase; prostatic acid phosphatase	RPR	rapid plasma reagin
		RSV	respiratory synctial virus
PAS	periodic-acid Schiff	RTA	renal tubular acidosis; road traffic accident
PBC	primary biliary cirrhosis		
PCNA	proliferating cell nuclear antigen	RTI	respiratory tract infection
PCR	polymerase chain reaction	RV	right ventricle
PDA	patient ductus arteriosus	SAA	serum amyloid A
PDGF	platelet derived growth factor	SCC	squamous cell carcinoma
PECAM	platelet endothelial cell adhesion	SCID	severe combined immunodeficiency
PET	pre-eclamptic toxaemia	SGOT	serum glutamic-oxaloacetic transaminase
PID	pelvic inflammatory disease		
PIE	pulmonary interstitial emphysema	SIDS	serum glutamic-oxaloacetic transaminase
PKU	phenylketonuria		
PL	phospholipids	SLE	systemic lupus erythematosus
PLAP	placental alkaline phosphatase	SNOMED	systematized nomenclature of medicine
plts	platelets		
PMF	progressive massive fibrosis	SPA	suprapubic aspirate
PML	progressive multifocal leucoencephalopathy	SS-A	saline-soluble antigen
		ssNDA	single-stranded DNA
PMR	polymyalgia rheumatica	SSPE	subacute sclerosing panencephalitis
PNET	peripheral neuroectodermal tumour	STDs	sexually transmitted diseases
PNH	paroxysmal nocturnal haemoglobinuria	SVC	superior venae cavae
		T_3	triiodothyromine
PNI	prognostic nutritional index	T_4	thyroxine
PNP	purine nucleoside phosphorylase	TB	tuberculosis
PP	polypeptide	TBG	thyroid binding globulin
PPB	Perl's Prussian blue	TC	transcobalamins
PPF	plasma protein fraction	TCK	total creatine kinase
PRV	polycythaemia rubra vera	TCR	T-cell receptor
PSA	prostate-specific antigen	TD	teratoma differentiated
PSAP	prostatic specific acid phosphatase	TDLU	terminal duct lobular unit
PSC	primary sclerosing cholangitis	TDM	therapeutic drug monitoring
PSS	progressive systemic sclerosis	TG	triglyceride
PT	prothrombin time	TIBC	total iron-bvinding capacity
PTAH	trichome phosphotungstic acid-haematoxylin	TNM	tumour nodes metastases
		TORCH	toxoplasma, rubella, cytomegalovirus
PTH	parathyroid hormone	TPHA	*Treponema pallidum* haemagglutination
PTT	partial thromboblastin time	TPN	total parenteral nutrition
PUJ	pelvi-ureteric junction	TRH	thyrotrophin-releasing hormone
PUO	pyrexia of unknown origin	TSH	thyroid-stimulating hormone
PVC	polyvinyl chloride	TSS	toxic shock syndrome
RA	rheumatoid arthritis	TTC	transitional cell carcinoma
RAST	radioallergosorbent test	TTP	thrombotic thrombocytopenia purpura
RBC	red blood cell	TURP	transurethral prostatectomy
RBCC	red blood cell concentration	UC	ulcerative colitis
RDS	respiratory distress syndrome	UFC	urinary free cortisol
REAL	revised European-American lymphoma	URT	upper respiratory tract
		URTI	upper respiratory tract infection
RER	rough endoplasmic reticulum	UTI	urinary tract infection
Retics	reticulocyte concentration	VAIN	vaginal intraepithelial neoplasia
RhA	rheumatoid arthritis	VDRL	Veneral Disease Research Laboratory
RNA	ribonucleic acid	VIN	vulval intraepithelial neoplasia
RNP	ribonucleoprotein	VIP	vasoactive intestinal peptide

VLDL	very low density lipoprotein	WBCC	white blood cell concentration
VMA	vanillylmandelic acid	WHO	World Health Organization
VSD	ventricular septal defect	XLA	X-linked agammaglobulinaemia
vWF	von Willebrand factor	XLPS	X-linked lymphoproliferative
WBC	white blood cell		syndrome

PART 1

ESSENTIALS OF LABORATORY MEDICINE

Histopathology, Cytopathology and Morbid Anatomy

INTRODUCTION TO LABORATORY MEDICINE

Understanding the range of available laboratory diagnostic techniques and their applications may present quite a confusing and daunting challenge to the medical student during his or her training (Fig. 1.1). It is for this reason that we have chosen to discuss the role of the main laboratory specialities in this first section of the book.

HISTOPATHOLOGY

Introduction

Traditionally, the histopathologist has been involved in the **tissue diagnosis** of disease processes using **light microscopy** (Fig. 1.2). The specialty of **surgical pathology**, as it is called in the USA, embraces this concept and even defines the specialty (or subspecialty) of the

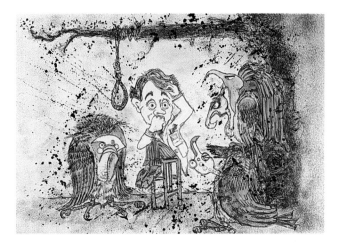

Fig. 1.1 Which laboratory test to request? Contact the clinical pathologist for advice (from an original, courtesy of Dr R. Armstrong).

histopathologist's diagnostic remit. Increasingly, one may encounter cardiovascular or even cardiac pathologists, haematopathologists, dermatopathologists and so

There are a variety of services available in departments of histopathology (sometimes called cellular pathology or surgical pathology). Students must become familiar with these services in order to be able to **communicate** most effectively with their pathologist, with other clinicians and with their patients.

The diagnostic process in histopathology

Figure 1.3 illustrates how a histopathological diagnosis is achieved. Each stage of the process entails an appreciation of **health and safety** requirements, **accuracy** in specimen **identification** and an appreciation of the optimum **fixation**, **staining** and **analysis** of the specimen. The process begins with an **adequate clinical history** from the surgeon and ends with the pathologist providing all the **diagnostic information** that the surgeon needs to carry out the **most appropriate clinical management** of the patient. Often a tissue diagnosis will precede a major line of clinical management, such as further surgery or medical treatment.

Evaluation of diagnostic methods
The **accuracy** of any diagnostic procedure, including technical and interpretative aspects, can be assessed in terms of:

$$\text{Specificity} = \frac{\text{true negative}}{\text{true negative} + \text{false positive}}$$

i.e. how successful was the technique at identifying no abnormality?

$$\text{Sensitivity} = \frac{\text{true positive}}{\text{true positive} + \text{false negative}}$$

i.e. how successful was the technique at identifying an abnormality? (See p. 75.)

Sources of diagnostic errors
Histological diagnosis is considered the definitive method of evaluating tumours (neoplasms). Although histopathology and cytopathology represent the 'gold standard' for diagnosis of many diseases, the student must be aware that errors can occur at each of the following stages in the diagnostic process:
- sampling the patient;
- sampling the biopsy or resection;
- misreading or misinformation about the clinical context;
- technical processing;
- perception of the abnormalities present;
- interpretation of the abnormalities perceived;

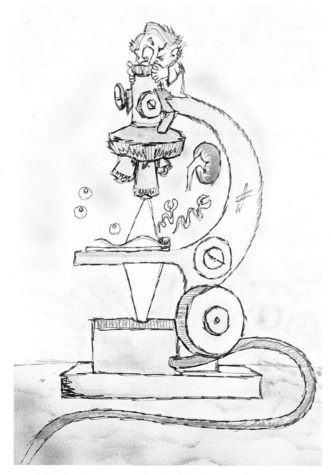

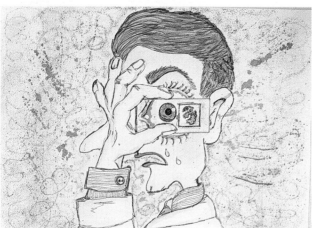

Fig. 1.2 (Top and bottom.) The role of the histopathologist (from an original, courtesy of Dr R. Armstrong).

on. In teaching hospitals, there is an increasing trend for this **subspecialization**. In a small district hospital, the histopathologist will diagnose a range of general diseases, perform cytopathology and provide an autopsy service.

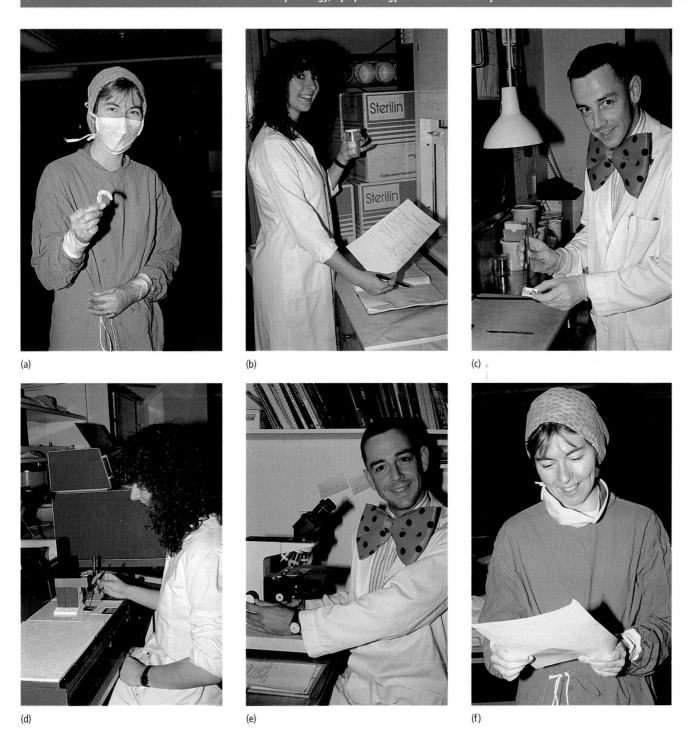

Fig. 1.3 The histopathological diagnostic process. (a) The surgeon will decide whether the specimen needs to be examined fresh (possibly for frozen section or for electronmicroscopical examination or sampling for tumour markers) or fixed in formalin. The surgeon will ensure correct labelling of the specimen, fills in a detailed clinical form and sends the specimen to the laboratory. (b) The medical laboratory scientific officer (MLSO) 'books in' the specimen on arrival in the laboratory. The name on the pot and on the form are checked. The specimen is given its own unique identification number. (c) The Histopathologist notes that the specimen and form identification are correct, notes the clinical information, describes and measures the specimen and samples the specimen appropriately. The tissue pieces are placed in a plastic cassette or block and further fixed in formalin. (d) The MLSO embeds the fixed and processed tissue in paraffin wax, cuts 3–5 µm sections on the microtome, mounts the sections on to glass slides and stains the tissue sections with the appropriate histochemical technique. (e) The Histopathologist examines the tissue under the microscope, dictates the histology report, checks the typed report before signature. (f) The Surgeon receives the written and signed report. This whole process will take a minimum of 24 hours for a routine, paraffin section (acknowledgements to Miss J. Clarke, Dr D.C. Brown and Miss F. Heblich).

- communication of the diagnosis;
- transcription of the written diagnosis.

Tissue processing in histopathology

Paraffin sections

Small blocks of formalin-fixed tissue are dehydrated and embedded in paraffin wax to provide a rigid substance for cutting sections. This process takes about 24 hours. Such permanent sections provide the **best material** for histological diagnosis.

Frozen sections

Tissue sections may be cut from tissue quickly **frozen at the time of surgery**. This technique has the advantage of providing information while the patient is still on the operating table (often within 15–20 minutes). The technique is used when rapid information is required and is seen in the following cases:

- the diagnosis of a tumour;
- the diagnosis of malignancy;
- the extent of lymph node involvement;
- the extent of tumour spread;
- involvement of resection margins by tumour.

The major disadvantage of this method is that the **cell morphology** in frozen sections can be **poor**.

In some instances, the histological features alone do not permit conclusive diagnosis, and **ancillary techniques** such as immunohistology, special stains and electron-microscopy are necessary.

Histochemistry

The haematoxylin and eosin (H&E) stain is the standard stain for tissue sections. **Haematoxylin** stains the **nuclei blue**, and the **eosin** stains **cytoplasm** and **extracellular** (**proteinaceous**) material **pink**.

Special histochemical stains rely upon chemical differences in various tissues (Table 1.1). They include silver stains to display the reticulin framework of the tissue or to stain melanin (in a melanoma); the periodic acid–Schiff (PAS) stiff stain to test for mucin, such as might be found in an adenocarcinoma; elastin and connective tissue stains for integrity of elastic fibres, normal and abnormal connective tissue; stains for micro-organisms; the integrity of basement membranes; soluble and insoluble lipids; fibrin; depositions such as calcium, amyloid and endogenous pigments such as iron and lipofuscin (Fig. 1.4).

The methodologies for performing these techniques may be consulted in standard texts such as Bancroft and Cook (1984).

Immunohistochemistry

The concept of using **labelled antibodies** to **localize antigens** in histological **tissue sections** was pioneered in the early 1940s using fluorescein-labelled antibodies. Since then, the concept has been modified and expanded and today, immunolabelling techniques have enabled the localization of cells and tissues with improved **diversity**, **sensitivity** and **specificity** of staining reactions.

Table 1.1 Histochemical stains in diagnostic histopathology.

Histochemical stain	Material demonstrated	Uses
Elastic van Giesen (EVG)	Elastic tissue	Appreciation of vascular structure, e.g. distinguishing arteries from veins
Reticulin stain	Reticulin framework	Pattern in carcinoma differs from that of lymphoma or sarcoma
Oil-red-O	Lipid	Adrenal cortical adenoma, atheroma (ceroid)
Gram stain	Bacteria	Bacterial infection
Grocott	Fungi	Fungi and *Pneumocystis carinii* in AIDS
Congo red	Amyloid	Diagnosis of amyloidosis
Perl's Prussian blue (PPB)	Iron	Haemochromatosis, old haemorrhage
Fontana stain	Melanin	Melanomas
Trichrome phosphotungstic acid–haematoxylin (PTAH)	Myofibres, glial fibres	Tumours of muscle origin, glial neoplasms
Periodic acid–Schiff (PAS) after diastase digestion	Epithelial mucin	Adenocarcinomas are positive, fungi are positive
von Kossa	Calcium	Mammographically localized breast lesions
Grimelius silver stain	Argentaffin granules	Carcinoid tumours are positive

AIDS, Acquired immune deficiency syndrome.

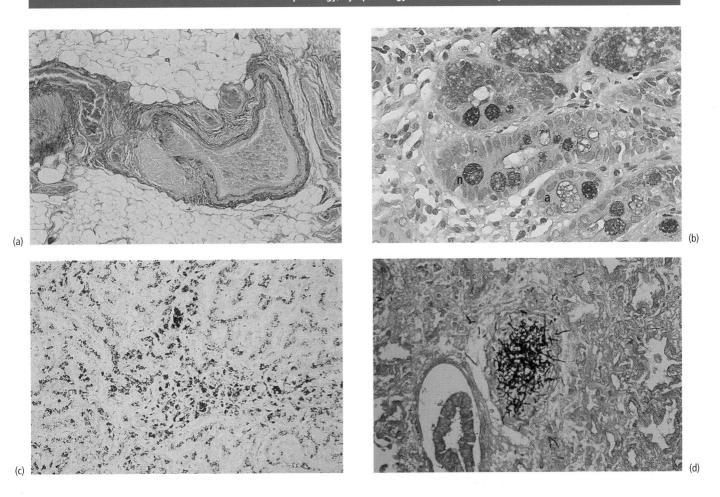

Fig. 1.4 Histochemical stains in diagnostic histopathology. (a) EVG shows collagen (red) and elastin (black) and demonstrates the abnormal vessels in this arteriovenous malformation. (b) Alcian-blue/PAS demonstrates neutral (red/purple) and acidic (blue) mucins in this small bowel biopsy. (c) PPB for iron (blue) demonstrates a case of haemochromatosis in the liver. (d) Grocott's silver stain for fungal organisms (black) demonstrates a mycotic embolus in a small blood vessel.

Of the many types of label available to denote the site of antibody binding, fluorescence- and **enzyme-conjugated** antibodies have been most widely used for light microscopy. Although with immunofluorescence the method is simple and requires no inhibition of endogenous enzyme or incubation in substrate, the technique suffers from the disadvantage that the preparations are not permanent because the fluorescence label eventually fades.

Antibodies can be raised to a wide range of molecular entities; cell structural components, cell products (cytokines, enzymes, peptides, immunoglobulins) and cell surface receptors. Most antibodies are raised against components and products of normal cells, but some are directed against antigens derived from malignant cells.

The technique of immunohistochemistry using monoclonal antibodies has brought precision to diagnostic histopathology (Table 1.2).

Immunoperoxidase techniques

Immunohistochemical stains are a more recent innovation. They use specific labelled antibodies–usually horseradish peroxidase–to identify marker antigens in cells and tissues (Fig. 1.5). When the peroxidase reacts with a substrate, it produces a coloured product that identifies the location of the antigen in the tissues. This method is analogous to the use of fluorescent-labelled antibody method but gives better results on paraffin sections (Fig. 1.6).

Electronmicroscopy

Electronmicroscopy can be performed on paraffin sections, but results are poor. Special fixation (in **glutaraldehyde**) and processing are required for optimal results. Ultrastructural features visible on electronmicroscopy are useful in recognizing infectious agents (Fig. 1.7) and

Table 1.2 Antibodies used in diagnostic immunohistochemistry.

Antibody clone	CD designation	Main specificity/cell association
3D4	CD3	T cells, TCR-associated
T3-10	CD4	T helper/inducer cells, some Mø
Tü102	CD8	T cytotoxic/suppressor cells
UCHL1*	CD45R0	T primed/memory cells, some Mø
SS2/36	CD10	B cells, GC
L26*	CD20	B cell subpopulation
RFD6		RER, plasma cells
21A5	CD21	C3d-R, mature B cells, FDC, GC
bcl-2-100		B and T cell, apoptotic involvement, not in GC
KP1*	CD68	Most Mø, monocytes
PD7/26*	CD45RB	Leukocyte common antigen
JC70*	CD31	PECAM, endothelial cells, some T, B, Mø
F8/86*		Factor VIII, most endothelial cells, von Willebrand factor
Ki-67		Proliferation-associated nuclear antigen for cells in G1, S, G2 and M (not G0) of cycle
PC10		PCNA, cyclin-proliferating cells in G1 and S phase of cell cycle
CIV22		Type IV collagen on basement membrane
1A4		α-Smooth-muscle actin for smooth-muscle cells
Cytokeratin (CK)		Intermediated filaments present in epithelial cells only, including carcinomas
Vimentin		Vimentin intermediate filaments present in mesenchymal cells, including sarcomas
Carcinoembryonic antigen (CEA)		Present in many carcinomas, especially of colon and gastrointestinal tract
α-Fetoprotein (AFP)		Most hepatomas and some germ cell tumours are positive
Prostatic acid phosphatase		Stains only prostatic epithelium, including metastatic prostatic cancer
Glial fibrillary acidic protein (GFAP)		Intermediate filament in astrocytes, ependymal cells and their tumours
Human chorionic gonadotrophins (hCG)		Trophoblastic neoplasms, germ cell neoplasms, some lung cancers
Thyroglobulin		Well-differentiated thyroid carcinoma is positive
Chromogranin		Marker for neuroendocrine neoplasms, some lung cancers
Desmin		Intermediate filament in muscle cells
S100 protein		Present in melanoma, cells of neural origin, and chondrocytes

* Monoclonal antibody that bind antigens on formalin-fixed paraffin embedded tissue.

TCR, T-cell receptor; Mø, macrophage; GC, germinal centre; RER, rough endoplasmic reticulum; C3b-R, complement receptor C3b; FDC, follicular dendritic cell; PCNA, proliferating cell nuclear antigen; PECAM, platelet endothelial cell adhesion.

The CD (cluster designation) terminology for leucocyte antigens has been recommended by the World Health Organization following a series of international workshops.

many types of neoplasms, for example, anaplastic squamous carcinoma, malignant mesothelioma (Fig. 1.8), melanoma, endocrine tumours and soft-tissue tumours.

Figure 1.8 illustrates how the aforementioned techniques may be of value in the diagnosis of a high-grade, anaplastic or poorly differentiated malignancy.

CYTOPATHOLOGY

Introduction

Clinical cytopathology is concerned with the diagnosis of diseases and in the prevention of cancer by screening the population to detect premalignant changes.

Clinical cytology is based on the morphological examination of cells: the features of interest are specific reactive changes and the changes of malignancy. During recent years, diagnostic cytopathology has been one of the most rapidly developing areas in the field of pathology, so much so that it forms a subspecialty of pathology in its own right.

The diagnostic process in cytopathology

The major role of cytology in non-gynaecological sites is to establish proof of the existence of cancer where there is suspicion. Specific diagnoses of tumour types can now be

(a) Direct and indirect techniques

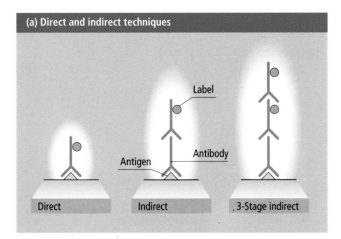

(b) PAP and APAAP technique

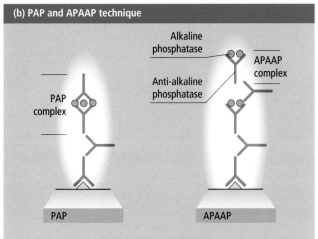

(c) Avidin–biotin techniques

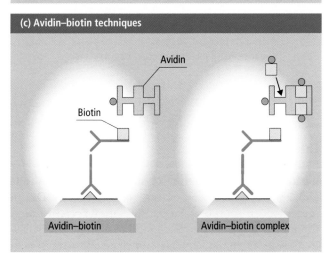

Fig. 1.5 Immunohistochemical methods in diagnostic histopathology.
(a) Direct and indirect techniques. (b) PAP and APAAP techniques.
(c) Avidin–biotin techniques.

Table 1.3 Cytological changes in malignancy.

High nucleus to cytoplasmic ratio
Nuclear pleomorphism
Hyperchromasia
Uneven distribution of chromatin
Irregularity of the nuclear membrane
Abnormal nucleoli
Abnormal mitoses

made with a high degree of accuracy. **Negative results do not exclude the presence of cancer**. Samples for cytological examination may be obtained by a variety of techniques.

Experience is required to distinguish between malignant cells and cells showing cytolytic abnormalities associated with regeneration, repair, metaplasia or inflammation (Table 1.3). The increasing use of immunoperoxidase techniques has improved the reliability of cell and tumour identification. The general rule that cytological diagnosis must be confirmed by histological diagnosis before radical treatment is undertaken has been modified as confidence in cytological and immunohistochemical techniques has grown. In many centres, radical surgery is undertaken on the basis of positive results of fine-needle aspiration for carcinomas such as those of the breast, pancreas and thyroid.

Specimen preparation in cytopathology

Cytological preparations are prepared by smearing the material directly, or after centrifugation, on to a glass slide.

The smear can be **air-dried** and stained with **May–Grünwald–Giemsa (MGG)** stain or be immediately **fixed in alcohol** and stained with **Papanicolaou (Pap)** stain.

With Giemsa the cell appears large and the cytoplasm is well-defined and stains pale blue. The nucleus stains dark blue. Mucus and other ground substances are also well-stained. With Pap the details of nuclear chromatin and nucleoli are enhanced. The cytoplasm is less well-defined except where it contains keratin (e.g. squamous cell carcinoma) which stains orange.

Pap alone is routinely used in gynaecological cytology, sputum, bronchial brushings and urine cytology. All other cytological preparations are stained by both methods, thus providing optimal results.

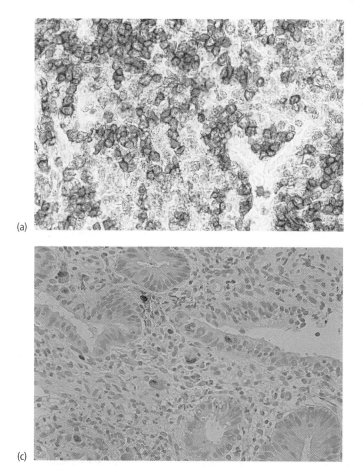

(a)

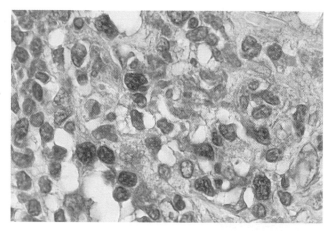

(b)

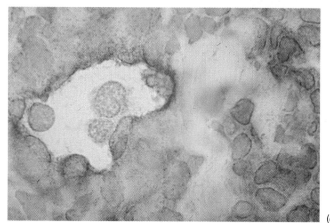

(c)

(d)

Fig. 1.6 Immunohistochemical stains in diagnostic histopathology.
(a) Suspected lymphoma of the retroperitoneum. Staining with CD20 (brown)
for B lymphocytes shows a mixed population of B lymphocytes and T
lymphocytes supporting a diagnosis of an inflammatory process. (b) Staining
of tumour cell nuclei with antibodies to PCNA (red) enables assessment of
cell proliferation and is of prognostic value. (c) Staining with antibody to
(cytomegalovirus) CMV (brown) shows infection of the large bowel in patient
with AIDS. (d) Double immunostaining with antibody to endothelial cells
(CD31) (red) and T lymphocytes, CD3 (brown) shows the close relationship
between these two cell types in an inflamed aorta.

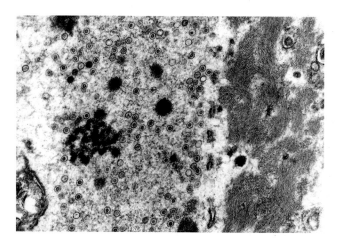

Fig. 1.7 The value of electronmicroscopy in diagnostic histopathology.
Herpes virus is present in a skin biopsy from a young child with immune
deficiency (×42 000).

Types of specimen submitted (Table 1.4)

Exfoliated cells

Exfoliated cells (Fig. 1.9(a)) arise from a contiguous malignant neoplasm—e.g. lung and bladder cancer and
leukaemic involvement of the meninges—and can be
identified in samples of sputum, urine, cerebrospinal
fluid and body fluids. Recognition of malignant cells
in blood (as in leukaemias) or bone marrow smears
(leukaemias, myeloma, metastatic carcinoma) is based
upon similar cytological principles.

Brushing or scraping of epithelium

A lesion that has been visualized by endoscopy (bron-
choscopy, gastroscopy, colposcopy) may be brushed or
scraped to obtain cells for examination (Fig. 1.9(b) and
(c)). Pap smears of the cervix are included in this group.

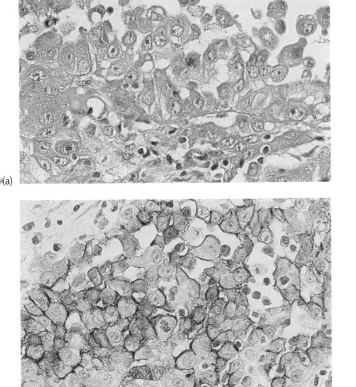

(a)

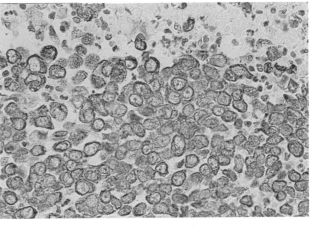

(b)

(c)

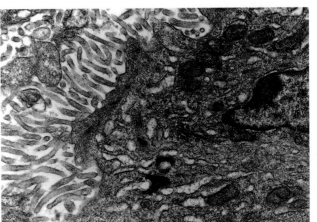

(d)

Fig. 1.8 Special techniques in the diagnostic process. A 64-year-old female patient presented with shortness of breath. CT scan showed an infiltrating tumour encasing the right lung. A biopsy of the tumour was taken. (a) Routine light microscopy (H&E) shows a **poorly differentiated malignant tumour**. Note the pleomorphic cell nuclei, prominent nucleoli, lack of recognizable architecture, mitoses and eosinophilic cytoplasm. The differential diagnosis includes:

• carcinoma;
• lymphoma;
• malignant mesothelioma;
• malignant melanoma;
• sarcoma.

Histochemical studies showed lack of staining for mucin, melanin or bile. A panel of immunohistochemical markers were used including antibodies to:

• cytokeratin (CK) and human milk fat globule (HMFG) I and II (epithelial membrane antigen–EMA) for cells of epithelial and mesothelial origin;
• carcinoembryonic antigen (CEA) for adenocarcinoma;
• leucocyte common antigen (LCA) for leucocytes;
• S100 and melanoma-specific antigen;
• vimentin for cells of mesenchymal origin.

Immunostaining for CEA, S100 and melanoma markers and vimentin is negative. (b) Cytokeratin marker is positive (brown)–note the accentuation around the cell nucleus (typical of mesothelial cells). (c) HMFG II marker is positive (brown)–note the accentuation along the cell membrane (typical of mesothelial cells). (d) Electronmicroscopy shows that the tumour cells possess irregular, long microvilli, consistent with cells of mesothelial origin (× 23 250). These findings distinguish this **malignant mesothelioma** from a lung adenocarcinoma.

Washings are obtained via saline injected via a broncho-scope, re-aspirated and placed in transport medium. It is useful for lesions which are hard to view.

Brushings are obtained by direct vision or by radiologi-cal screening. The brush is rotated on the slide and fixed immediately in ethanol for Pap staining. Cytology often precedes biopsy.

Sputum

Three consecutive morning specimens of sputum sent promptly to the laboratory will diagnose 80% of primary lung malignancies (one specimen 40%, five specimens 87%). The sputum should not consist of saliva or nasal secretions but should be a deep cough specimen. Sputum specimens are routinely Pap stained. Special stains for micro-organisms and eosinophils may be used.

Fine-needle aspiration cytology (FNAC)

A fine (22-gauge) needle can be passed into virtually any location to **aspirate** material directly from a **mass lesion**

Table 1.4 Specimens evaluated in cytopathology.

Spontaneously exfoliated	
Sputum, urine, cerebrospinal fluid	
Effusions in body cavities—pleural, pericardial, peritoneal and joint fluids, cervix	
Cells forcibly removed by:	
Brushing	Bronchial, oesophageal, gastric, colonic, pancreatic, biliary
Scraping	Skin lesions
Imprint	Nipple discharge, rapid assessment of lymph node involvement at operation
Lavage	Bronchoalveolar, gastric

(fine-needle aspiration; Fig. 1.9(d)). Cells obtained are smeared on slides for cytological examination. Radiological techniques such as computed tomography (CT) scan and ultrasonography may help guide the needle into the mass. Tumours are probed with a fine needle attached to a syringe and small amounts of cell suspension are aspirated and then spread on to a slide. Superficial palpable lesions are readily aspirated. Deeply placed lesions can be aspirated under radiological guidance (ultrasound or CT scan).

Aspiration cytology is closely related to histopathology except that sampling is obtained by a fine needle leaving the lesion intact. Seeding of tumour cells into the needle tract is an extremely rare complication and even then usually not of clinical significance.

An obvious disadvantage of aspiration cytology is that tissue architecture is lost and therefore interpretation

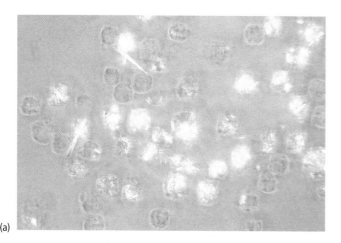

(a)

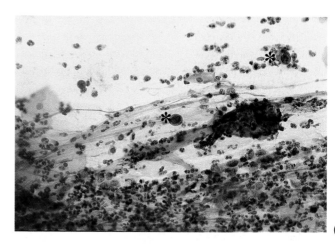

(b)

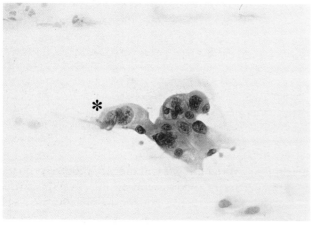

(c)

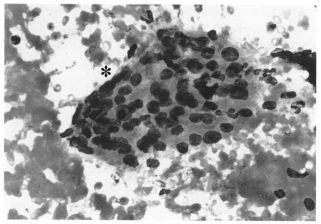

(d)

Fig. 1.9 Cytopathology diagnosis. (a) **Synovial fluid.** A combination of polarized light microscopy and phase contrast microscopy shows neutrophil polymorphs associated with urate crystals in a patient with a knee effusion due to gout. (b) **Exfoliative cytology.** PAP staining of a cervical smear shows inflammatory cell debris and severely dyskaryotic squamous epithelial cells (✱), consistent with CIN3. (c) **Gastric brushing.** PAP staining shows large, atypical glandular cells (✱) showing an increased nuclear to cytoplasmic ratio and pleomorphic cell nuclei, consistent with an adenocarcinoma. (d) **Thyroid FNA.** A cluster of benign follicle cells (✱) consistent with a benign thyroid neoplasm in a patient presenting with a solitary thyroid nodule (MGG).

rests on the recognition of changes in the appearances of single cells or small groups of cells (Table 1.5).

Advantages over conventional biopsy are minimal trauma to the patient, speed and the avoidance of an operation.

Tables 1.6–1.9 list the role of FNAC in the diagnosis of diseases of specific systems.

Table 1.5 Advantages and limitations of cytology.

Advantages
Rapid and simple
    No need for the processing of the specimen required for paraffin
    embedding and sectioning in histopathology

Minimal/no trauma to the patient
    Allows repeated examination of urine cytology in the follow-up of
    carcinoma of the bladder

Can sample wide areas
    For example, bronchial brushing

Can sample areas inaccessible to biopsy
    For example, urine from renal pelvices

Limitations
Interpretation can be difficult

False-positive and false-negative rates generally slightly higher than in
histopathology

Subtyping and grading tumours, which can be prognostically important,
may be difficult to predict by the examination of single cells

In situ and invasive lesions can be difficult or impossible to distinguish,
e.g. breast fine-needle aspiration

The precise site of a lesion, on rare occasions, may be in some doubt,
e.g. a sputum sample may contain malignant squamous cells from a
nasopharyngeal carcinoma; these cells may be misinterpreted as arising
from the bronchus

Table 1.6 The role of fine-needle aspiration cytology (FNAC) in breast pathology.

Diagnosis and treatment of simple cysts
Diagnosis of benign conditions and the avoidance of surgery
Diagnosis of malignancy
    Avoidance of surgery
    Planning of definitive treatment
    Planned use of hospital facilities
Monitoring of known malignancies
Obtaining material for special studies
Breast screening

False-negative rate approximately 10% and false-positive rate of the order of 0.5%.

Table 1.7 The role of lymph node fine-needle aspiration cytology.

The standard management of lymphadenopathy is to observe for a few months and then biopsy.

The role of fine-needle aspiration is to:
• diagnose 'reactive' lymphadenopathy with the possiblity of recognizing some specific conditions and then recommend further observation for 3 months followed by biopsy if it has not resolved. This allows for the diagnosis of clinically important persistent 'reactive' conditions and for the possibility of false-negative diagnosis, particularly of lymphocyte-predominant Hodgkin's disease and low-grade non-Hodgkin's lymphoma
• diagnose metastatic malignancy and to indicate the possible primary site(s), hence avoiding unnecessary biopsy and directing subsequent investigations appropriately
• diagnose lymphoid malignancy, usually followed by biopsy for accurate subtyping unless the patient is unfit for surgery
• monitor malignancy
• diagnose infectious disease (see Fig. 1.10)

Table 1.8 The role of fine-needle aspiration cytology in thyroid disease.

Diagnosis of the solitary thyroid nodule
Diagnosis of the diffuse non-toxic goitre
Confirmation of clinically obvious malignancy

Table 1.9 The role of fine-needle aspiration cytology in prostate disease.

Diagnosis of prostatic carcinoma preoperatively allowing treatment
    planning and staging
Exclusion of malignancy prior to retropubic prostatectomy for benign
    prostatic hyperplasia
Exclusion of malignancy in cases of prostatitis

Screening

Medical education tends to emphasize the importance of not missing an important diagnosis. The move towards a greater interest in preventive medicine has led to enthusiasm for screening tests. National screening programmes in cervical cytology (see Chapter 23) and in breast cytology (see Chapter 24) are presently in progress.

Students become familiar with the idea therefore that a valuable screening method is to ensure that the first stage will pick up almost everyone who may have the disease. At this stage the **false-negative rate** should be low at the expense of a **high false-positive rate**. The next stage should involve a more specific test which ensures that the false-positive rate is low. Thus, a large number of people who go through to the second stage are reassured that nothing is wrong at the second stage.

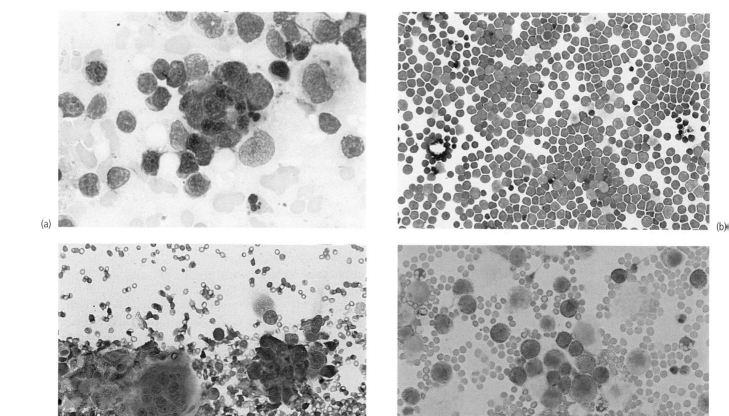

(a)

(b)

(c)

(d)

Fig. 1.10 Cytopathology diagnosis in lymph node pathology. (a) **Imprint cytology,** MGG. Haemophagocytosis in a reactive lymph node. (b) **Cerebrospinal fluid (CSF).** MGG. Low grade non-Hodgkin's lymphoma. (c) **Lymph node FNA.** MGG. Cohesive clusters of large malignant cells which show negative immunostaining for lymphoid markers. (d) **Lymph node FNA.** The cells shown in (c) stain positvely (red) for S100 and other melanoma markers confirming a diagnosis of metastatic malignant melanoma.

An example is cervical screening. Women are encouraged to have a smear, for example, every 3 years. A proportion are informed that their smear is essentially

normal **but** it should be repeated in, say, 3 months just to make sure. These are women where the smear is classified as cervical intraepithelial neoplasia type 1 (CIN 1), or as showing inflammation. When the smear is repeated, a large proportion of these women will be told that the smear is now normal (Table 1.10).

Most patients experience considerable anxiety during the 3 months, and many are not totally reassured by the subsequent 'normal' smear. Such women remain anxious that they may develop cancer, an anxiety which they did not have before the first smear result.

Table 1.10 The possible outcome of a cervical smear.

Normal smear – repeat in 3 years
Inadequate smear – repeat in 6 months
Inflammatory changes – repeat in 6 months (± Rx)
Borderline smear – repeat in 6 months
Mild dyskaryosis (CIN 1) – repeat in 6 months
Moderate dyskaryosis (CIN 2) – refer for colposcopic biopsy
Severe dyskaryosis (CIN 3) – refer for colposcopic biopsy

CIN, Cervical intraepithelial neoplasia; Rx, treatment.

MORBID ANATOMY – THE AUTOPSY

Introduction

Autopsy literally means **to see for oneself** and even in today's world of molecular biology the results of an autopsy are accepted as **the ultimate audit**. The autopsy can be augmented by **microscopic examination** of tissues including **electronmicroscopy, immunocytochemistry** and **molecular biology** as well as all forms of **micro-biological, toxicological** and **biochemical** studies (Fig. 1.11).

Where foul play is suspected, a wide range of forensic investigations are used, involving identification of the origin and type of body fluids as well as the recognition of substances that define the environment in which death occurred.

Autopsies are performed either at the direction of HM Coroner or following permission from the next of kin; any **autopsy without authorization** from either of these sources is **illegal**. Coroners' autopsies are performed by histopathologists, some specialists in forensic pathology who are nominated by the Coroner and if ordered cannot be refused by the relatives, next of kin or others on any grounds including religion (Table 1.11).

Autopsies

The Coroner

The Coroner is either a **legally or medically trained** person of more than 5 years' standing and may be qualified in either law or medicine or both. The Coroner's function is to investigate any death for which a doctor cannot issue a death certificate and to decide **who the deceased was, where, when** and **how** death occurred and to issue a death certificate with a **cause of death**. A further function is to reach a verdict on the cause of death.

About one-third of all deaths are reported to the Coroner. In 80% of these a post-mortem examination is carried out. There are about 150 coroners in England and Wales. Most are solicitors who act as coroner part-time. In Scotland there is no office of coroner. Similar duties are carried out by the Procurator-fiscal.

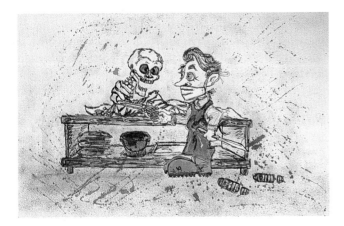

Fig. 1.11 The role of the autopsy in diagnosis, medical education, clinical audit, research, epidemiology and the law (from an original, courtesy of Dr R. Armstrong).

Table 1.11 The routes to post-mortem examination.

Initiated by the Coroner
Initiated by the doctors, for example to establish the exact nature of the final disease or for the purpose of teaching and research

Death certificates

Death certificates must by law be provided for **every person** who dies and given to the Registrar of Births and Deaths for the subdistrict in which the death occurred. A body cannot be disposed of by burial, cremation or the scattering of ashes until the death certificate is accepted by the Registrar. Death certificates were introduced to prevent the concealing of a crime and to provide statistical information on the causes of deaths and patterns of disease. They may be issued by any qualified medical practitioner registered with the General Medical Council or by the Coroner.

Death

Death has **no legal definition** but is for the purposes of certification separated into **natural** and **unnatural**. Qualified medical practitioners can issue death certificates associated with natural death but only the Coroner has the power to issue certificates for an unnatural death. Should the Registrar receive a certificate giving an unnatural cause of death from a medical practitioner the death will then be reported by the Registrar to the Coroner.

Deaths must be reported to the Coroner through the Coroner's officer when the medical practitioner cannot issue a death certificate. This in practice is when:
- death is unnatural;
- the medical practitioner did not attend the deceased during the last illness;
- the medical practitioner did not see the deceased within 14 days of death;
- the medical practitioner did not see the body after death (Table 1.12).

Deaths can also be reported to the Coroner by lay persons, most usually undertakers, but should not be reported by medical practitioners in order to obtain an autopsy.

Unnatural deaths are clearly defined on the back of the death certificate. They are violent deaths including accidents, deaths where the cause is not apparent (a person living alone and being found dead unexpectedly) and those in which drugs, medicine, abortion or poison may have contributed. Deaths during an operation or general anaesthesia and those contributed to by employment are also unnatural, although some of the diseases attributed

Table 1.12 When should a doctor notify the Coroner of a death?

Where the deceased was not seen by a doctor within the 14 days prior to death (this is relevant in general practice)
Where the cause of death is unknown or unexplained
Where the death may have been unnatural, or caused by violence or neglect or was under suspicious circumstances. This would include where accidents such as road and domestic accidents have contributed to cause of death
Where the death may have been due to industrial disease or poisoning. Deaths due to alcohol excess should be reported if following, for example, a binge (e.g. a student dying following ingestion of a bottle of brandy). Deaths due, for example, to liver disease in someone with long-standing excess alcohol intake should not be reported
Where the death has occurred during a medical or surgical procedure, for example, during an operation or before recovery from the anaesthetic, or during a radiological procedure
When a mother dies as a result of termination of pregnancy
Sudden and unexplained infant deaths (e.g. cot deaths)
Suicide
Death of a person whilst in custody
Stillbirths where there was any possibility of the child being born alive

It is considered the duty and the responsiblity of doctors to report the above deaths even though this is not a statutory duty.

to industrial causes may also arise from non-industrial sources, e.g. tuberculosis.

Natural deaths are deaths other than unnatural deaths and must be recorded as a named disease and/or its complications and may be given as a sequence of events but not as the manner of dying, such as coma.

Deaths referred to the Coroner

These generally result in a coroner's autopsy, the finding of death as natural and the Coroner issuing a death certificate. This course of events may be simplified if on discussion with a medical practitioner the Coroner accepts a cause of death as natural and so avoids an autopsy. When death is due to unnatural causes the Coroner will order an **inquest**.

The inquest

The inquest is a public inquiry to establish who the deceased was, where, when and how the person died and to reach a medical cause of death and a verdict. The **verdict**

may be that death was from **natural causes**, **accident**, **misadventure**, **unlawful killing** or left **open** because of insufficient evidence. Any practitioner invited to attend an inquest cannot refuse and should this occur will be subpoenaed. The practitioner may also be asked to provide a written statement which can be referred to with any other records during the inquest.

Hospital autopsies

Hospital autopsies can occur only with the **consent of the relatives** or next of kin and this must be in **writing** and **may be limited** to only certain parts of the body such as the abdomen. The consent must be obtained by the medical practitioner but in large hospitals is often obtained at the request of the practitioner by the hospital Bereavement Officer.

The **signed consent form** should accompany a **summary** of the clinical course, a statement of any **special reason** for an autopsy and the patient's clinical notes, including the results of all **investigations**.

These autopsies can provide information on the effectiveness of treatment, particularly any new approaches; objective data for epidemiological studies; evidence on the emergence of new diseases and their natural course; data for audit studies within a wide range of clinical practices and material for teaching and research as well as support for the clinical diagnosis or evidence of misdiagnosis.

In general, the doctor must obtain permission for the post mortem to be carried out from the closest relatives after the person's death. Close relatives have the legal right to veto this, even if the deceased had made it clear that he or she would be happy for post-mortem examination to be carried out on the body. Conversely, even if the close relatives do not object, a post mortem should not be carried out if there is reason to believe that: 'the deceased had expressed an objection to his body being so dealt with after his death, and had not withdrawn it' (**Human Tissues Act 1961**).

The guidelines given above seem to be a reasonable interpretation of the law, although it should be stated that the law is not absolutely clear. The Human Tissues Act 1961 is the most important piece of legislation in this area. This act is concerned with the use of parts of bodies of deceased persons for therapeutic purposes and purposes of medical education and research, as well as with the circumstances in which post-mortem examinations can be carried out. It is not relevant to organ transplantation with **live** donors.

In English law no one owns a dead body. It is the person or institution which is in '**lawful possession**' of the body who has the legal duty to arrange burial and who can give permission for post-mortem examination to be carried out and parts of the body to be removed. A hospital authority is in lawful possession until someone with better right claims it. The executors or close relatives would have a better right. The person in legal possession can authorize the post mortem and removal of parts of the body if: 'he has no reason to believe:

- that the deceased has expressed an objection to his body being so dealt with after his death;
- that the surviving spouse or any surviving relative of the deceased has reason to believe the deceased objects to the body being so dealt with.'

The person in lawful possession of the body must make **'such reasonable enquiry as may be practicable'** to determine these points.

Some of the issues which are therefore not entirely clear are: what is reasonable practicable enquiry? and, how many, and which relatives need to be asked? It is not even clearly stated who is to count as being 'lawfully in possession' of the body. It does, however, seem widely agreed that where there is no urgency (i.e. where it is not a question of using, say, a kidney for transplant) it is the close relatives who need to be asked for permission to carry out a post-mortem examination, but that there is then no need to seek out more distant relatives.

Asking relatives for permission for post-mortem examination

As house officers and general practitioners you will sometimes ask the relatives of a dead patient for permission for a post-mortem examination to be carried out. This is a sensitive matter to talk about at a particularly distressing time. The way in which you do it may make all the difference between its being experienced by the relatives as positive or negative. It will also affect how you feel.

As house officers, particularly, you may find that the circumstances of your asking for permission are particularly difficult. You may be short of time, you may have the feeling that your job is to ensure that the relatives give permission and that you will have failed if they refuse permission, and you may never have met the relatives before. Furthermore, the relatives may feel that the hospital is to blame for the death.

Table 1.13 gives some guidance as to how this delicate issue might be approached. On those occasions when asking for permission ends up with everyone upset it is usually because of a failure of **communication**.

Take any opportunity you have of seeing experienced people ask relatives for such permission.

Table 1.13 Requesting permission for a hospital autopsy.

Introduce yourself to the family
For example: 'My name is . . . I am one of the team of doctors who have been looking after your mother'

Sit down
Bereaved people feel small. It can feel very uncomfortable to have the doctor towering over you
Sitting down also conveys the feeling that you are giving them your time

Explain the death briefly
For example: 'Your mother woke from sleep at about 1 o'clock this morning and called the nurse. She said that she had some pain in her chest. She then quite suddenly died. The cause of death was almost certainly another heart attack'

Ask for permission for the post-mortem examination
This should be done clearly and concisely but not brutally. For example: 'My consultant (Dr X, who is your mother's consultant) has asked me to ask you if you would be prepared for us to carry out a further examination – a post-mortem examination. This is because we like to verify our practice. We hope that by doing this we will be able to add to our medical knowledge. If this examination were carried out, your general practitioner would be sent a copy of the results. What are your thoughts/feelings about this?'

Be ready to answer the questions likely to be asked
Common questions are:
- Why do you want to do the post mortem?
- What will my mother look like after it?
- Who pays for it to be done?
- Can I go away and discuss it with my daughter? When do you have to know what we decide?
- What exactly does a post mortem involve?
- Do they remove bits of the body?

Pitfalls
Saying that you want to find out what her mother died of, when you have already signed the death certificate (giving a cause of death)

Saying that you want to see whether you should have done anything else in treating her mother. (It would normally be very upsetting to relatives at this point for it to be suggested that the deceased person had not received the right care)

Bereaved people will probably want to talk to you for a long time, but you are unlikely to be able to spend very long with them. When the relatives bring up what is a side-issue to your main purpose, you should briefly acknowledge what they have said and return to the issues you need to cover

Tissues for transplantation

These can only be removed from dead bodies with the permission of either the next of kin or the Coroner, depending upon the cause of death.

Cremation

Cremation can only occur if a **cremation form** is completed and this can only take place following the issuing of a death certificate. The cremation form is in **two parts** and each part must be completed by a **medical practitioner** who has seen the body after death.

The person signing the **first part** must be the same as that completing the death certificate but the person involved with the **second part** must have been qualified for at least 5 years and should not be associated directly with the signatory of the first part, thus a house officer and registrar on the same firm cannot together complete a cremation form. Once completed the cremation certificate is submitted to the Cremation Officer of the local crematorium.

The method of the autopsy

Mortuaries

Mortuaries are included in most large hospitals and many of these provide facilities for both hospital and Coroner's autopsies, in the latter capacity serving as a public mortuary. Their minimum facilities include a table or tables for the autopsy which are easily cleaned, ventilation, adequate lighting, running water and a drainage system. An area restricted for special autopsies is necessary. These involve autopsies on known infected bodies, particularly with *Mycobacterium tuberculosis*, hepatitis

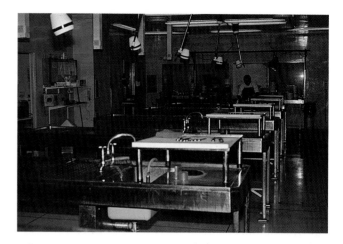

Fig. 1.12 Health and safety in the modern mortuary. Possibly the cleanest part of the hospital.

viruses, human immunodeficiency virus (HIV) and slow-release viruses. Other basic requirements for mortuaries are body storage areas, an area for relatives to view and identify bodies, and in large mortuaries a viewing gallery for clinicians, students, police officers and others.

Health and safety regulations

These are detailed in the Health Services Advisory Committee report of 1991 and apply to all mortuaries and to those who use them (Figs 1.12 and 1.13). These regulations, involving the design and functioning of mortuaries, are to protect the staff from infection and injury and to prevent the spread of infection from the mortuary to out-

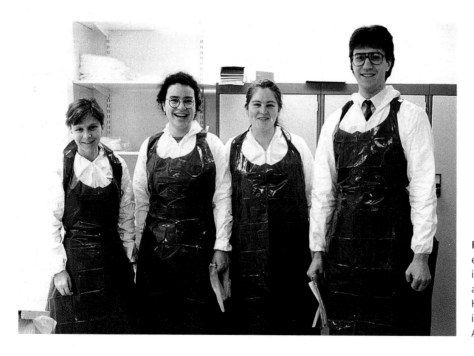

Fig. 1.13 The role of the autopsy in medical education. Dr C.S. Herrington and Dr J. Newby instruct medical students (Miriam Taegtmeyer and Helen Swannie) at the John Radcliffe Hospital, Oxford on health and safety regulations in the mortuary. (Photography courtesy of Dr Adrian Tang).

side areas. The provisions are especially proscriptive for known high-risk infective autopsies. As a part of these, observers are prohibited and the body must be identified to all those who come into contact with it as one with a high risk of infection, a procedure satisfied by clearly labelling the body as infected.

Identification of the body

Identification of the body and permission for an autopsy are essential before an autopsy begins. Identification of a body from hospital sources is provided from the attached name-tag but without this will have to be made by the medical personnel involved or unusually by the next of kin. The Coroner's Officer provides identification of the body in Coroner's autopsies but if the body is severely traumatized or burnt ancillary means of identification such as the matching of dentition and dental records may have to be used.

Autopsy examination

This involves examination of the external and internal appearances and can vary in its thoroughness depending on the interests of the examining histopathologist and the nature of the disease process. Osteoarticular histopathologists will routinely examine joints and bones which are regions rarely dissected in most autopsies and similarly the extent of the examination of the nervous system will be more extensive when this system is clinically involved.

External examination

This is the most important skill of the forensic histopathologist. Recognition of major and minor change is involved and this may help to decide the position of the body at the time of death as well as the environment of the body at that time and the involvement of others with the death. Meticulous attention to patterns of injury can enable weapons associated with injuries to be identified as well as bullet entry and exit sites and their angle in relation to the body at the moment of death. Other features looked for are the same as those reported by clinicians and include such changes as clubbing, cynaosis and jaundice.

Hypostasis is the gravitational drainage of blood into the dependent areas of the body, seen externally as a blotchy red discoloration to the skin. It will reflect the position of the body during the immediate period after death and in most bodies is found on the back of the trunk and limbs within 4–12 hours after death.

Putrefaction is a process which begins immediately death occurs and is naturally completed within 48–72 hours. It alters the external appearance of the body by leading to bloating, most notably of the face, abdomen and scrotum, and produces desquamation as well as a greenish discoloration to the skin, especially of the abdomen. The parallel effect on the internal organs is **autolysis** which results in softening and eventual liquefaction as well as melting of fat and haemolysis of the blood. The process involves the release of intracellular enzymes and bacterial products and will be accentuated by disease, especially infectious, as well as temperature and humidity. Refrigeration is an important and effective way of impairing these processes.

Rigor mortis involves a stiffening of the body from approximately 4 hours after death and is completed within about 6 hours and lasts for a period of 36–48 hours. Stiffening begins in the head and neck area and gradually involves the trunk and limbs and then reverses in the same pattern. The timing is extremely variable and is affected by the mode of death and the environment. Any circumstance involving a violent death and a struggle hastens the process, although paradoxically hanging does not. Septicaemias and any wasting state as well as cooling and severe haemorrhage delay the process while stretching the affected muscles leads to its prompt reversal.

Dissection of the internal organs inevitably varies amongst histopathologists but the methods used incorporate approaches that differ in the extent to which dissection is done *in situ* and after removal of the organs from the body. A very important component of this examination is the weighing of the individual organs which can then be compared in standard charts with the expected weights for the weight and height of the body. Useful adjuncts to a permanent record of any observation are photography and video taping and a report of the examination.

Autopsy reports

These include the observations made at the time of the autopsy, microscopic findings and the results of other investigations performed and an interpretation of these with a cause of death or sequence of events leading to death. The interpretation given to all of the findings will depend upon the knowledge made available to the histopathologist and the greater this is, potentially the more valuable the report. In this respect, close liaison between histopathologists and clinicians is helpful, including death meetings or similar meetings when discussion can occur. The final diagnosis and also all recognized abnormalities should be indexed, incorporating SNOMED (Systematized Nomenclature of Human and Veterinary Medicine — College of American Pathologists, 1993) or other similar systems, for future reference, evaluation of therapy, epidemiology studies, audit and similar purposes.

Reports on Coroner's autopsies

These reports are generally confined to the macroscopic findings and only concerned with the cause of death but a few may be supported by reports on alcohol, drug and carbon monoxide levels. These reports are to the Coroner and can only be seen and used by others with the Coroner's agreement.

Interpretation of the autopsy findings

The most limiting factor in the contribution of autopsy findings to clinical and research studies is the subjectivity of the investigation. Anything the histopathologist sees is interpreted within the limitations of experience and possible observations beyond this may be missed or even unwittingly suppressed. The other very important limitation is the thoroughness and care of the report on the macroscopic appearances since these observations can never be confirmed by others in exactly the same circumstances, even if a second or subsequent autopsy is performed.

Hospital autopsies are an important component of studies of all types, including audit, and have contributed substantially to the understanding of many diseases, most recently acquired immunodeficiency syndrome (AIDS). Within all studies, missed clinical diagnoses of major and even minor significance, the commonest being pulmonary embolism, come to light despite the armamentarium of modern diagnostic investigative procedures. Equally important is the finding of a wrong clinical diagnosis, an example being clinically evident cancer with no evidence found at autopsy. The cause of these different findings includes the fact that autopsy is the only means of examining many organs, especially those of the nervous and cerebrovascular systems where biopsy can only be applied to parts.

Coroner's autopsies have provided a similar wealth of information, not only about purely forensic matters but also about everyday problems such as child cruelty. They also provide an important basis for a wide range of insurance compensation claims and an insight into design and safety in many different aspects of public life. Their remit is sudden and unexpected death and their range of histopathology is consequently much wider than often appreciated, which means that they are also important sources for epidemiology studies. A distinct limitation is that the Coroner requires the cause of death, which is not always an exact morphological phenomenon and not always easy to define, thereby introducing an element of subjectivity. A further common misconception is that the time of death can be precisely established. The time of death can only be crudely estimated and it is essential if this is to be done to know both the rectal temperature and the temperature of the environment in which death occurred as well as to take into account the amount of clothing, how fat or thin the deceased is and if the body was or was not immersed in water.

REFERENCES

Health Services Advisory Committe (1991) *Safety in Health Services Laboratories: Safe working and the prevention of infection in the mortuary and post-mortem room.* HMSO Publications, London.

Bancroft J.D. & Cook H.C. (1984) *Manual of Histological Techniques.* Churchill Livingstone, London.

FURTHER READING

Atkinson B.F. (1992) *Atlas of Diagnostic Cytopathology.* WB Saunders, Philadelphia.

Bancroft J.D. & Cook H.C. (1984) *Manual of Histopathological Techniques.* Churchill Livingstone, London.

Brazier M. (1987) *Medicine, Patients and the Law.* Penguin, London.

Cotran R.S. *et al.* (1989) *Pathologic Basis of Disease,* 3rd edn. WB Saunders, Philadelphia.

Curran R.C. (1985) *Color Atlas of Histopathology,* 3rd edn. Oxford University Press, New York.

Gresham G.A. & Turner A.F. (1979) *Postmortem Procedures (an Illustrated Textbook).* Wolfe Medical, Holland.

Gresham G.A. (1992) *A Color Atlas of General Pathology,* 2nd edn. Mosby, St Louis.

Knight B. (1983) *The Coroner's Autopsy.* Churchill Livingstone, New York and Edinburgh.

Knight B. (1987) *Legal Aspects of Medical Practice,* 4th edn. Churchill Livingstone, Edinburgh.

Netter F.H. *The Ciba Collection of Medical Illustrations,* 12 books. Ciba Medical, New Jersey.

Polak J., Van Noorden S. (eds) (1986) *Immunocytochemistry. Practical Applications in Pathology and Biology,* 2nd edn. Wright, Bristol.

Rosai J. (1989) *Ackerman's Surgical Pathology,* 7th edn. Mosby, St Louis.

Sandritter T. (1992) *Macropathology: Text and Color Atlas,* 5th edn. Mosby, St Louis.

Sternberg S.S. (1992) *Histology for Pathologists.* Raven Press, New York.

Underwood J.C.E. (1987) *Introduction to Biopsy Interpretation and Surgical Pathology,* 2nd edn. Springer-Verlag, London.

Underwood J.C.E. (1987) *Introduction to Biopsy Interpretation and Surgical Pathology,* 2nd edn. Springer-Verlag, Holland.

Underwood J.C.E. (1992) *General and Systemic Pathology.* Churchill Livingstone, New York.

Young J.A. (ed.) (1993) *Fine Needle Aspiration Cytopathology.* Blackwell Scientific Publications, London.

Microbiology

CONTENTS

INTRODUCTION TO MICROBIOLOGY

This chapter will discuss the clinically important aspects of microbiology with emphasis on the practical role of the microbiology laboratory (Fig. 2.1(a)). A knowledge of basic microbial pathogenicity is assumed and for this

reason, we would recommend that the student refer to the bacteriology chapters (7 and 8) and virology chapters (9–12) in the companion textbook *Essentials of Pathology*.

Further in this book, from Chapters 15 to 27, we will discuss **specific infections** in greater depth as they involve each of the systems. **Tropical and imported infectious disease** will be discussed in Chapter 8 with **opportunistic infections, human immunodeficiency virus (HIV) and the acquired immune deficiency syndrome (AIDS)** in Chapter 10.

CLINICAL ASPECTS OF MICROBIOLOGY

Colonization versus infection

The healthy human host harbours a large variety of micro-organisms, many of which are potentially pathogenic. The body surfaces in contact with the exterior, skin, mouth, gastrointestinal tract, respiratory tract, external genitalia and vagina, all possess a **colonizing flora** of bacteria which are normally harmless to the host. In addition other host defences such as mucus and the com-

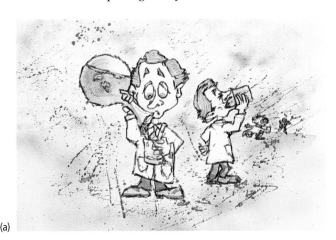

(a)

Fig. 2.1 (a) The microbiological diagnostic process (from an original, courtesy Dr. R. Armstrong).

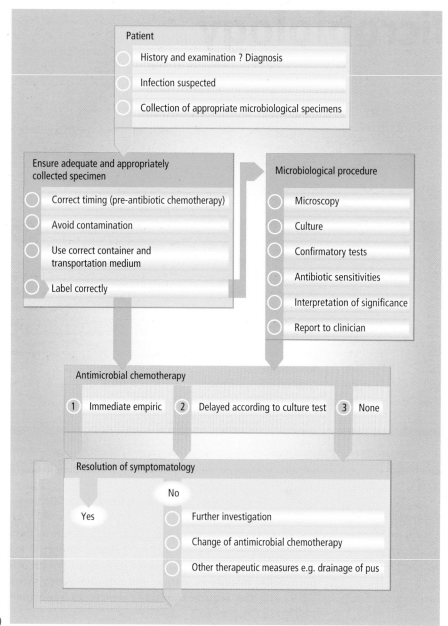

Fig. 2.1 (b) The diagnostic process – flow diagram.

(b)

ponents of the humoral and cellular immune systems interact in protecting the host from invasion by these potentially pathogenic bacteria.

Any insult which disturbs the normal delicate balance between the host and this flora may result in invasion and **infection** by its own **endogenous bacteria**; infection may also arise as a result of introduction of a pathogenic organism from outside, not normally resident in the host's flora – **exogenous infection**. All infections, whether endogenous or exogenous, are preceded by **colonization**; however it can often be difficult to distinguish between colonization and infection when the infecting organism is present in the normal resident bacterial flora. Findings indicating infection include suggestive clinical symptoms and signs, particularly fever and the other cardinal signs of inflammation.

Clinical correlations

Although certain bacterial syndromes may be identified by their characteristic clinical presentation, in the majority of cases it will be necessary to confirm that the suspect organism is indeed the agent responsible, both for management and epidemiological purposes. This process requires the **isolation** of the responsible organism from suitable clinical material (often in the presence of a background of other, contaminating micro-organisms), **confirmation** of its **identity** by special tests and definition of its pattern of susceptibility to antimicrobial agents suitable for the treatment of the disease syndrome produced by that infection in the patient. Further identification tests which define other typeable characters may also be necessary for epidemiological purposes (Fig. 2.1(b)).

Collection of specimens for microbiological testing (Fig. 2.2)

The quality of a specimen for microbiological testing will determine the reliability of the report which is generated on that specimen. Consequently great care must be taken over the following stages.

1 **Choice of the most relevant specimen(s)** in the light of the patient's clinical symptoms (Table 2.1).

2 **Collection of the specimen** (Table 2.2):

(a) From sites with a resident normal flora (e.g. skin, respiratory tract, urogenital tract) **sample the 'infected' area**, e.g. pus or discharge from an abscess, **not** a swab from the surrounding skin or mucous membrane to avoid sampling normal flora (= contaminants) as far as possible.

(b) From normally sterile sites (e.g. blood, cerebrospinal fluid) **avoid contamination** by skin organisms from both the patient and the operator.

(c) **Timing** of specimen collection. Specimens should be collected **before** the start of antimicrobial chemotherapy whenever possible.

(d) Ensure specimens are collected into the correct container (Fig. 2.1(b); Table 2.3) which must be sterile. Special swabs or transport media may be required for certain tests, especially if delay in arrival at the laboratory is likely.

(e) **Correct labelling**. Minimum data on the specimen container include patient name and type of specimen.

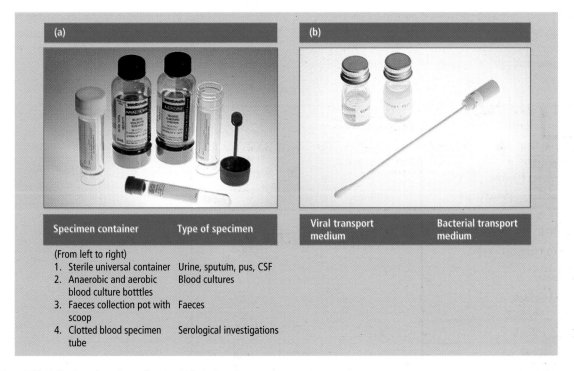

(a)	
Specimen container	**Type of specimen**
(From left to right)	
1. Sterile universal container	Urine, sputum, pus, CSF
2. Anaerobic and aerobic blood culture botttles	Blood cultures
3. Faeces collection pot with scoop	Faeces
4. Clotted blood specimen tube	Serological investigations

(b)	
Viral transport medium	**Bacterial transport medium**

Fig. 2.2(a) and (b) Collection of specimens for microbiological testing.

Table 2.1 Choice of type of specimen by clinical diagnosis.

	Blood culture	Cerebro-spinal fluid	Sputum	Urine	Swab	Other e.g. aspirates, tips, paired sera for viral titres
Pneumonia	+	[+] Pneumococcal	+	–	–	[+] Viral
Meningitis	+	+	[+] Pneumococcal	[+] Coliform	[+] Screening swabs: group B streptococci*	[+] Viral
Septicaemia	+	[+] Meningococcal	[+]	+	[+]	[+] Viral
Pyrexia of unknown origin	+	[+]	[+]	+	[+] Throat	[+] Faeces, viral
Fever in neutropenic patient	+	[+]	[+]	+	[+]	[+] Viral
Neonatal sepsis	+	+	+	+	+ Screen: throat, nose, ear, umbilical	+ Viral

+ Essential specimen; [+] if symptoms are suggestive or a particular clinical syndrome is suspected (organism as indicated).

* Neonatal meningitis.

(f) **Transportation** (Fig. 2.2). Estimate likely delay between collection and processing and whether specimen can be refrigerated and processed routinely or if it requires urgent attention.

3 **Completion of the request form** (Fig. 2.3) to provide as much relevant clinical information as possible, including recent foreign travel, diagnosis, chemotherapy, immune status, to allow the laboratory to assess the most appropriate tests for that clinical picture on the specimen submitted. **Essential information** includes patient name, sex, age, date of birth, date and time of collection, type of specimen, site, sampled address for report, name and contact number of initiating doctor.

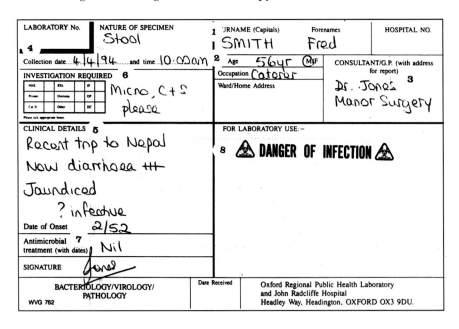

Fig. 2.3 Completed microbiological request form.

Table 2.2 Types of specimen and notes on collection.

Body system affected (symptoms/signs)	Specimen types	Comment	Common pathogens

UROGENITAL TRACT
 	
Urinary tract infection
  Frequency and dysuria
  Offensive urine
  Non-specific (infants and children)
	Urine	Collect in sterile container
		Refrigerate if transport delay
		Screen with dipstick tests
			Escherichia coli
			Proteus spp.
			Klebsiella spp.
			Other coliforms
			Enterococci
			Pseudomonas spp.

	Midstream urine	Most commonly collected Contamination reduced by careful collection	
	Catheter specimen	Reliable if first pass of catheter; if already *in situ*, contamination common Use syringe and needle to collect from tube; do not collect from bag	
	Suprapubic aspirate (SPA)	Most reliable specimen type Requires skill for collection	
	Bag urine	High contamination rate Useful in infants and children where SPA is not applicable	
	Early-morning urine	For pregnancy testing Preferred for TB culture	
Renal abscess Renal angle pain and tenderness	Perinephric pus	Surgical specimen = reliable	

GENITAL TRACT
 	
Discharge from
  Vagina
  Cervix
  Urethra
	Swab of discharge	Contamination by normal flora inevitable	*Neisseria gonorrhoeae*
			Chlamydia trachomatis*
			Candida albicans
			Trichomonas vaginalis
			Anaerobes
			Enterobacteriaceae
			Anaerobes

	Pus from abscess, e.g. Bartholin's	N.B. Presence of anaerobes	
Postop/postpartum infection	Endometrial curettings	Surgical specimen, but usually contaminated by normal vaginal flora	
RESPIRATORY TRACT Pneumonia Chest infection	*Sputum*	Poor-quality specimen due to contamination by normal URT flora Deteriorates rapidly—must be freshly cultured	*Streptococcus pneumoniae* *Haemophilus influenzae* *Moraxella catarrhalis*
Empyema	ENT swab: nose, throat in transport medium	Pernasal swab for suspected *Bordetella pertussis* (whooping cough) Throat swab for diphtheria (rare)	Group A streptococci
Severe pneumonia	Lower respiratory tract Bronchoscopic washings Bronchoalveolar lavage	High-quality specimens, only appropriate in severe pneumonia	Enterobacteriaceae *Pseudomonas* spp.
Pleural effusion	Pleural aspirate	If pleural effusion	
GASTROINTESTINAL TRACT Diarrhoea Food poisoning	*Faeces*—three separately passed specimens	Selective culture required to avoid overgrowth by bacteria Positive findings more likely with liquid stool	*Campylobacter* spp. *Salmonella* spp. *Shigella* spp.

[Continued on p. 26]

Table 2.2 *Continued*

Body system affected (symptoms/signs)	Specimen types	Comment	Common pathogens
Parasite screening		'Concentration' of faeces improves isolation rates for parasites	*Giardia lamblia* cryptosporidia
Abdominal collection/mass; ascites	Other specimens Pus aspirate from abscess Ascitic fluid tap Liver biopsy	Most isolates significant when specimen carefully/surgically collected Culture for TB	Enterobacteriaceae *Staphylococcus aureus* Anaerobes
SUPERFICIAL AND DEEP TISSUE INFECTION	*Swab* of pus in transport medium	Pus or tissue especially more reliable specimens than swabs	*Staphylococcus aureus* Group A (C, G) streptococci
	Pus *Tissue* *Aspirate* from joint	From skin sites with normal flora *S. aureus* may be part of flora Normally sterile; most isolates significant (except skin flora)	Other organisms, e.g. *Pseudomonas* (in special situations, e.g. burns)
BLOOD Septicaemia Pyrexia of unknown origin (PUO) Endocarditis	*Blood cultures*—two sets collected separately Three sets if endocarditis suspected	Blood normally sterile but normal skin flora contamination during collection common; scrupulous attention to sterile technique essential	*All* isolates (including normal flora) must be considered potentially significant and judged according to clinical picture
	Other relevant cultures Intravascular devices, e.g. intravenous catheter tips Heart valves Bone marrow	From suspected/proven endocarditis PUO; suspect tuberculosis	Common normal skin flora may cause infection in patients with indwelling intravenous catheters, neonates and on prosthetic material, e.g. artificial heart valves, joint replacements
	Special tests	Viral titres and other antibody tests in investigation of PUO Antibiotic assays	
NEUROLOGICAL SYSTEM	CSF Lumbar puncture Cisternal puncture Drain/reservoir	CSF is normally acellular and sterile	As for blood, *all* isolates must be considered significant and judged on clinical grounds. Skin flora are common contaminants but may colonize plastic devices
	Pus from cerebral abscess Organism isolated may aid determining source	Direct spread from paranasal sinuses or middle ear Blood stream spread from primary focus elsewhere	*Streptococcus milleri* Anaerobes *Staphylococcus aureus*

TB, Tuberculosis; URT, upper respiratory tract; ENT, ear, nose and throat; CSF, cerebrospinal fluid.
* *Chlamydia trachomatis*: special swab required.

4 Special precautions–'infection risk'–If infection which may be a risk to those handling the specimen is suspected, such as hepatitis or HIV, specimens **must** be appropriately labelled. Specimens from any jaundiced patient or drug addict are examples.

Table 2.3 Types of specimen container, storage and transport.

Specimen	Container	Comment
Urine	Sterile universal container	Refrigerate if transport delay anticipated
Swabs	Cotton-tipped swab broken off into bacterial transport medium	Refrigerate if transport delay anticipated
Genital swabs	Cervical/urethral swab for suspected *Neisseria gonorrhoeae*	Place in bacterial transport medium and transport to laboratory and process as soon as possible. Storage may kill fastidious organisms, e.g. *N. gonorrhoeae*
	Swab in viral transport medium from suspect lesion	For suspected herpes infections
	*Chlamydia** swab from cervix	Use special swabs/transport medium as recommended by laboratory
Pus/tissue/aspirates	Sterile universal container	Refrigerate if transport delay anticipated. Specimen may need urgent processing if clinically indicated
Sputum/lavages etc.	Sterile universal container	Specimen deteriorates if not processed within 4 hours of collection. If delay, refrigerate but note bacterial overgrowth
Faeces	Sterile universal container with scoop	Refrigerate if transport delay anticipated; storage may kill fastidious organisms, e.g. *Shigella*
Blood	Place immediately in aerobic and anaerobic blood culture bottles	Transport immediately to lab and place in incubator using aseptic technique
Cerebrospinal fluid	Sterile plastic container	Most specimens will need immediate processing in view of severity of infection; routine specimens (e.g. myelogram) may be refrigerated

* *Chlamydia*: special swab required.

Hospital infections

Definition
Any infection acquired while in hospital:
- including infections identified after discharge from hospital but acquired while in hospital;
- excluding infections which develop in hospital but were acquired in the community.

Prevalence
The prevalence of hospital-acquired infections in a large UK survey in 1980 was 9.2%, causing 1% of deaths directly.

Monitoring hospital infection rates
Monitoring of infection is done by **surveillance** of microbiology reports together with **investigation of outbreaks**. **Epidemiological** features such as techniques of organism typing (e.g. by antibiotic sensitivity pattern, biotyping, serotyping, phage typing, molecular typing) will allow **'relatedness' of organisms** to be determined in outbreak settings (Tables 2.4–2.8).

Surgical infections
The same general principles apply to surgical infection as to hospital-acquired infection as the majority of surgical infections are hospital-acquired (Table 2.9–2.11).

Pyrexia of unknown origin

Definition
The classical definition of pyrexia of unknown origin (PUO) is of **persistent fever continuing for more than 3 weeks** without definable cause despite appropriate investigations.

Other considerations, not covered by this definition, are the obscure pyrexias which occur in association with hospital-acquired, neutropenic-associated and HIV-associated infection.

Table 2.4 Types and frequency of hospital infection.

Type of infection	Percentage	Mortality rate
UTI	40	Low
Surgical wound infection	25	Low
Lower respiratory tract infection	10	High
Bacteraemia	5	High

(**Source of organism causing bacteraemia:** wound > UTI > respiratory tract > intravenous related > unknown.) UTI, Urinary tract infection.

Table 2.5 Organisms implicated in hospital-acquired infection.

Types of organism causing hospital infection depend on:
- Types of colonizing organism
- Previous antibiotic treatment or prophylaxis
- Geographic location of patient, e.g. burns unit, intensive care units
- Patient host defences
- Age, renal function, diabetes, alcoholism, malignancy
- Specific risk factors—breach in skin, artificial ventilation, neutropenia, prosthetic material/catheters

Common organisms

Escherichia coli	Urinary tract infection
Staphylococcus aureus	Wound infection
Pseudomonas aeruginosa	

Also coagulase-negative staphylococci, Candida spp., enterococci, anaerobes—Bacteroides and other Gram-negative rods

Table 2.6 Prevention of hospital infection.

Reasons
Reduction of serious morbidity and mortality

Reduction of costs:
    To patient: psychological and social
    To hospital: hotel costs, drugs, ?medico-legal aspects

Reduction of resistance: any source or infection, especially in the presence of antibiotics, provides a potential focus for the development of antibiotic resistance

Methods
Exclusion of potential pathogens, e.g. sterility, screened blood, clean linen, wholesome food, removal of staff carriers

Interruption of transmission, e.g. ward and theatre design, isolation policy, aseptic techniques, **hand-washing**

Enhancing host resistance, e.g. immunization, antibiotic prophylaxis, catheter and cannula care

Table 2.7 Routes of spread of hospital infection.

Table 2.8 Source of infection in hospital-acquired infection.

Endogenous (From patient's own flora—may be acquired while in hospital)	Exogenous (From hospital staff, other patients or visitors)
Staphylococcus aureus, Gram-negative rods	Staphylococcus aureus, Gram-negative rods, viruses, tuberculosis
	Environment: fomites, food, water, air, equipment
	Legionella, Aspergillus, Salmonella

Table 2.9 Investigation of fever in a postoperative patient.

Less than 48 hours postop
Procedure-related

More than 48 hours postop
Infection
    Chest infection
        Simple atelectasis
        Early pneumonia
    Wound infection*
    UTI*
    Intravenous cannula-related

Non-infective
    DVT and pulmonary embolus
    Drugs/allergy
    Other

UTI, Urinary tract infection; DVT, deep venous thrombosis.
* Commonest causes.

	Endogenous		Exogenous	
Source	Patient	Patient	Staff	Equipment Environment
Site	Skin Nose	Gastrointestinal tract	Skin Nose	
Main pathogens	Staphylococcus aureus	Gram-negative rods	Staphylococcus aureus Coagulase-negative Staphylococcus	Staphylococcus aureus Pseudomonas Klebsiella Enterobacter Aspergillus Salmonella ⎱ uncommon Legionella ⎰
Mode of spread	Contact from colonized or infected site		Air (skin) Hands	Air Contact

Table 2.10 Features of common surgical infections.

	Urinary tract infection	Wound infection
Aetiology	Catheter-related	Endogenous skin flora
Risk factors	Risk increases with duration of catheterization Approx. 10% of catheterized patients develop infection per day catheterized Commoner in females	Related to inoculum size: commoner with contaminated than with clean surgery Damage to normal host defences, i.e. intact skin, presence of dead/devitalized tissue, presence of prosthetic material, including sutures, which increase infection risk General condition of host Prior antibiotic therapy
Organisms	Enterobacteriaceae, *Escherichia coli*, *Klebsiella*, *Proteus* *Pseudomonas*, enterococci	*Staphylococcus aureus* Group A streptococci Coagulase-negative *Staphylococcus*: prosthetic material
Diagnosis	Catheter urine (CSU) collected with syringe and needle Blood culture	Pus Swab (doubtful significance) Blood culture
Prevention	Avoid catheter use Catheter care policy e.g. minimize system breaks	Good surgical technique Prophylactic antibiotics
Treatment	Remove catheter Antibiotics	Drain pus Antibiotics

Table 2.11 Prophylactic antibiotic use in surgical procedures: general principles.

Operation must have a significant risk of operative site infection
Significant bacterial contamination must occur during surgery
Antibiotics used must be effective against important contaminating micro-organisms
Adequate concentrations of antibiotic must be achieved in the wound at the time of the procedure
Antibiotics should be used for as short a period as possible and be of low toxicity
Different antibiotics should be used for prophylaxis and treatment
The benefits must outweigh the dangers

Although infection is the single most common cause of PUO, other significant non-infectious causes include **neoplasm, collagen vascular disease** and **factitious fever** (Table 2.12).

Approximately **10% of cases remain undiagnosed** despite extensive investigation.

History, examination, investigation and treatment

Important considerations in the **history** when investigating a PUO include:
- recent travel abroad;
- occupation (including animal contact);
- ethnic origin;
- immunization history (bacillus Calmette-Guérin or BCG);

- tuberculosis (TB) contact history and drug history (especially recent antibiotic therapy).

The possibility of PUO as a presenting feature of HIV disease must always be considered.

On **examination** attention should be paid to:
- skin (rashes, other skin lesions, jaundice);
- nails;
- eyes;

Table 2.12 Infective causes of pyrexia of unknown origin.

Bacterial
Common causes
    Tuberculosis, endocarditis, occult abscess (abdominal, pelvic)

Rarer causes
    Enteric fever, osteomyelitis, brucella, lyme/relapsing fever, leptospirosis, rickettsial infection, psittacosis, Q-fever, syphilis

Viral
Epstein–Barr virus (glandular fever), cytomegalovirus, hepatitides (A–E)

Fungal
Cryptococcal infection, histoplasmosis

Parasitic
Common causes
    Malaria

Rarer causes
    Toxoplamosis, amoebiasis, trypanosomiasis etc.

- reticuloendothelial system (enlarged lymph nodes, liver, spleen);
- cardiovascular system (cardiac murmurs);
- character of fever (may be helpful in malaria and brucella).
  Microbiological investigations should include:
- blood cultures;
- serum for viral titres (Cytomegalovirus, Epstein–Barr virus, toxoplasmosis, psittacosis, rickettsial, Q-fever, syphilis and *Borrelia* serology);
- liver, bone marrow or other biopsy specimens (skin, renal, lymph node) for culture (especially TB) may also be required.
  Other **routine investigations**:
- full blood count with film (malarial and other parasites);
- chest X-ray;
- special investigations: computed tomographic scan, gallium scan to localize pus.
  Treatment may include an antipyretic agent to reduce fever or a therapeutic trial of antituberculous chemotherapy, for example.

Use of molecular methods in microbiology/ infectious diseases

Main areas of application
- epidemiological investigations;
- pathogenesis and virulence studies;
- clinical diagnosis;
- identification of unknown agents of clinically presumed infective syndromes.

Epidemiological investigations. Traditional methods of investigation have included simple typing methods:
- antibiotic sensitivity patterns;
- serotyping on the basis of cell surface markers;
- carbohydrate capsule analysis;
- biochemical and enzyme markers;
- phenotypic characteristics.
  The main disadvantage of these methods is that they are not unique to an individual organism, although sufficient for simple investigations in most cases. Genetic-based typing provides a more accurate and unique typing methodology.

Genomic fingerprinting. This allows analysis of either the entire DNA content of a microbe or a small proportion, for example, a series of specific enzymes. DNA is extracted from the organism in question, digested into specific fragments and these are allowed to migrate in a gel, producing a unique pattern which can be compared between isolates for similarity.

Pathogenesis and virulence studies. Virulence factor or antibiotic resistance genes may be coded for on **plasmids** which are extrachromosomal, circular elements of double-stranded DNA present in the cytoplasm of many bacteria, separate from the main chromosomal DNA and can be transferred between bacteria of the same and different species. **Plasmid profile analysis** is used to extract plasmid DNA and run it in a gel, allowing comparisons between strains and species. It is an extremely precise method of defining bacterial strains applicable to both epidemiological and pathogenesis/virulence studies.

Clinical diagnosis. The high sensitivity of molecular methods of identification makes them attractive for routine clinical use. However their drawback is expense, expertise required and lack of ability to quantify organism. There are certain clinical situations when polymerase chain reaction (PCR) can be very useful, for example, in the detection of herpes simplex virus in the cerebrospinal fluid in herpes encephalitis.

Polymerase chain reaction. Fragments of DNA obtained by digestion are denatured by heat and specific primers for the DNA segment under investigation are added and amplified using PCR. Completed reactions are run on gels, allowing visualization of amplified products of the target DNA sequence.
  Other clinical applications of PCR include:
- detection of slow-growing/non-culturable pathogens, e.g. TB, leprosy, rickettsiae, spirochaetes;
- detection of hazardous organisms where culture is dangerous, e.g. plague bacillus;
- organisms which can be difficult to identify;
- mixed cultures, in order to detect organisms of significance from amongst normal flora;
- epidemiological information;
- identification of dead organisms, e.g. formalin-filled specimens;
- research.

CLINICAL BACTERIOLOGY

Introduction

Bacteriology is the study of bacteria; clinical bacteriology is concerned with those bacteria responsible for the major bacterial diseases in humans. The mode of interaction between potentially pathogenic microorganisms and host determines whether or not clinical disease is apparent. Thus both the infecting microorganism and the host's

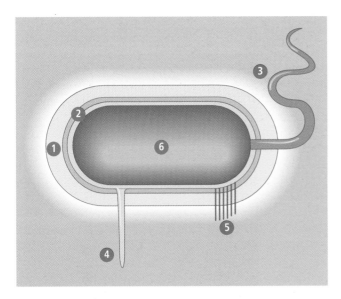

Fig. 2.4 Diagrammatic representation of a bacterium. 1 Capsule, exterior mucopolysaccharide layer; 2 Cell wall, outer lipopolysaccharide membrane [Gram negative only]; 3 Flagellum, external filamentous surface protein ['flagellin'] protuberance concerned with bacterial locomotion and = 'S' or flagellar cx antigen; 4 Pilus, external filamentous surface structures concerned with adhesion between bacteria and transfer of DNA between bacteria during the conjugation process; 5 Fimbriae, filamentous appendages important in adhesion to solid surfaces, e.g. to mucosal surfaces; 6 Cell interior, contains chromosomal DNA, ribosomes, mesosomes. Note that not all the above structures are necessarily present simultaneously.

ability to defend itself against attack are critical components. In order for an organism to produce clinical disease it must be able to: survive and multiply in host tissues and resist host defences for a sufficient period to establish disease.

Laboratory identification of bacteria

Bacterial structure and function

Most pathogenic bacteria must gain access to the body or invade to cause infection. Colonization of mucosal surfaces alone is not sufficient (see above). Bacteria possess a number of specialized features (Fig. 2.4) which aid in their invasiveness and pathogenicity, including the following.

- **Capsule** (Fig. 2.4). Aids in avoidance of phagocytosis by host immune system.
- **Flagellae.** Concerned with locomotion and hence avoidance of host defence mechanisms.
- **Fimbriae, pili.** External structures which aid in attachment to mucosal surfaces.
- **Toxins.** Protein products usually exported from bac-

terial cell which can produce a direct toxic effect on host cells. Disease features may be due to toxin action rather than multiplying bacteria themselves. Specific examples include the **endotoxin** of the Gram-negative cell wall, the **exotoxins** of *Corynebacterium diphtheriae* (diphtheria) and *Clostridium tetani* (tetanus) and the **enterotoxins** of *Vibrio cholerae* (cholera) and food-poisoning strains of *Staphylococcus aureus*.

- **Enzymes.** Wide range of activities from breaking down host tissue, facilitating spread of organism, to breaking open β-lactam ring of antibiotics rendering the bacteria resistant to the action of that group of antibiotics.

Bacteria are not visible individually with the naked eye because of their size–0.5–5 μm. Techniques by which they may be visualized include **staining** in microscopic preparations and **culture** on solid media (usually agar-based), when they appear as distinct colonies with characteristic features which can be used to identify the organism concerned.

Gram staining

This is the most usual method by which bacteria are stained for easy visualization by the light microscope. The staining properties of bacteria form the basis of classification methods and are determined by the composition of their cell wall (Fig. 2.5).

Gram-positive bacteria stain **violet** with Gram's stain (see Fig. 2.3); the stain is taken up by the peptidoglycan in the cell wall and is resistant to decolorization.

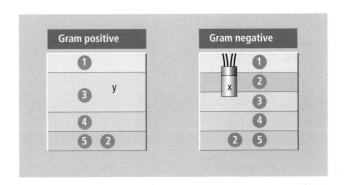

Fig. 2.5 1 Capsule, capsular polysaccharide material exterior to bacterial cell wall. 2 Outer membrane, phospholipid bilayer membrane containing lipopolysaccharide [endotoxin]. Endotoxin is composed of lipid A (x) with a polysaccharide moiety on its external surface and lipoprotein embedded in the peptidoglycan layer (3)ˣ. Present in Gram-negative bacteria only. 3 Peptidoglycan layer, thickness variable; much thicker and contains ʸlipotechoic acid increasing stability in Gram-positive bacteria; less prominent in Gram-negative. 4 Inner membrane, phospholipid bilayer membrane containing proteins, ᶻenzymes etc and maintaining integrity and osmotic pressure of cell interior.

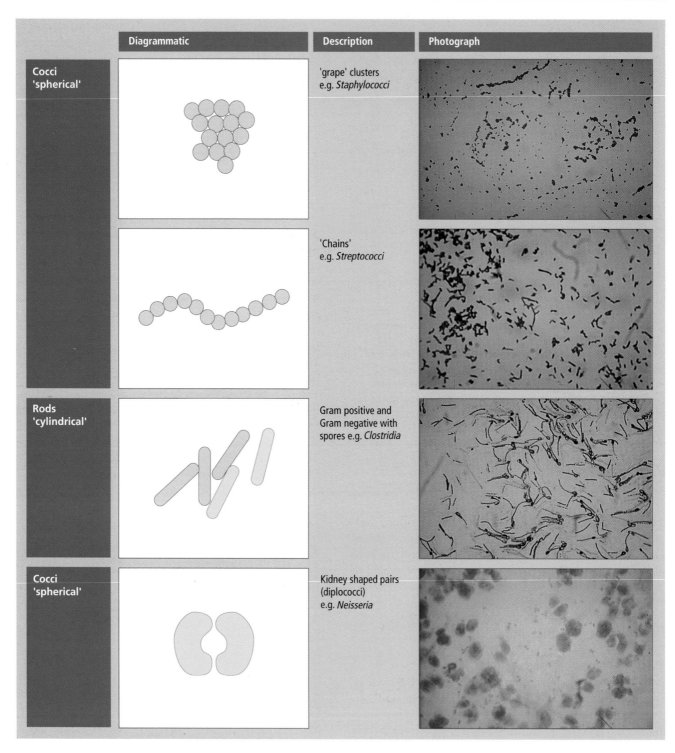

	Diagrammatic	Description	Photograph
Cocci 'spherical'		'grape' clusters e.g. *Staphylococci*	
		'Chains' e.g. *Streptococci*	
Rods 'cylindrical'		Gram positive and Gram negative with spores e.g. *Clostridia*	
Cocci 'spherical'		Kidney shaped pairs (diplococci) e.g. *Neisseria*	

Fig. 2.6 Diagrammatic representation of bacterial morphology.

Gram-negative bacteria stain **red**; the peptidoglycan layer is obscured by an additional outer lipid bilayer membrane which does not retain the methyl violet of Gram's stain; counterstaining with a red stain after decolorization produces the characteristic Gram-negative appearance.

Bacterial morphology is also obvious on light microscopy and individual cells are defined as **cocci**

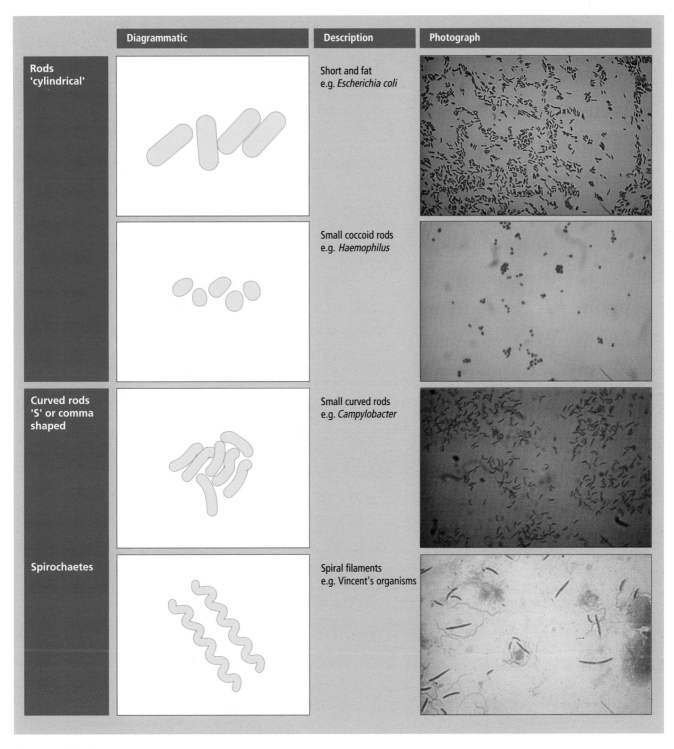

	Diagrammatic	Description	Photograph
Rods 'cylindrical'		Short and fat e.g. *Escherichia coli*	
		Small coccoid rods e.g. *Haemophilus*	
Curved rods 'S' or comma shaped		Small curved rods e.g. *Campylobacter*	
Spirochaetes		Spiral filaments e.g. Vincent's organisms	

Fig. 2.6 *Continued*

(spheres), **bacilli** (rods), **coccobacilli** (short rods), **vibrios** (curved rods) or **spirochaetes** (spiral rods; Fig. 2.6).

Arrangements of groups of bacterial cells are also useful in identification–**pairs**, **clumps**, **chains**, **palisades** or irregular without obvious form.

Other characteristic features such as the presence of **spores**, **capsules** or **flagellae** may be demonstrated with special staining techniques.

Other important microscopic features of clinical specimens include the presence of host cells indicative of an

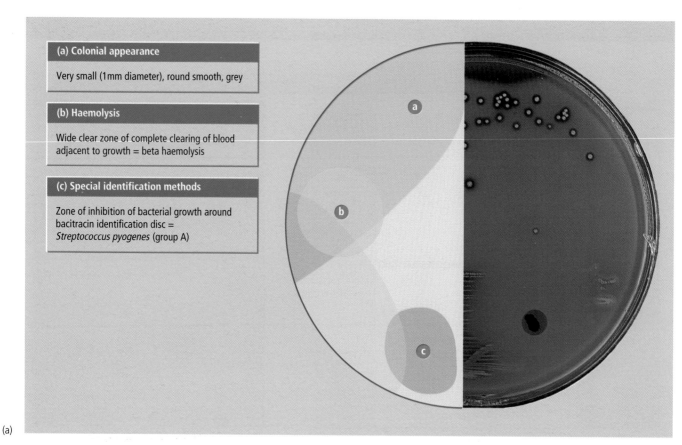

(a) Colonial appearance

Very small (1mm diameter), round smooth, grey

(b) Haemolysis

Wide clear zone of complete clearing of blood adjacent to growth = beta haemolysis

(c) Special identification methods

Zone of inhibition of bacterial growth around bacitracin identification disc = *Streptococcus pyogenes* (group A)

(a)

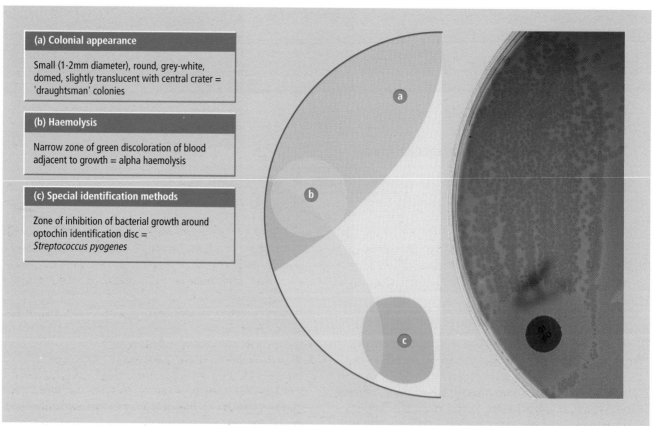

(a) Colonial appearance

Small (1-2mm diameter), round, grey-white, domed, slightly translucent with central crater = 'draughtsman' colonies

(b) Haemolysis

Narrow zone of green discoloration of blood adjacent to growth = alpha haemolysis

(c) Special identification methods

Zone of inhibition of bacterial growth around optochin identification disc = *Streptococcus pyogenes*

(b)

Fig. 2.7 How to look at a microbiology plate. (a) Group A β-haemolytic streptococci on blood agar. (b) *Streptococcus pneumoniae* ['Pneumococcus'] on blood agar

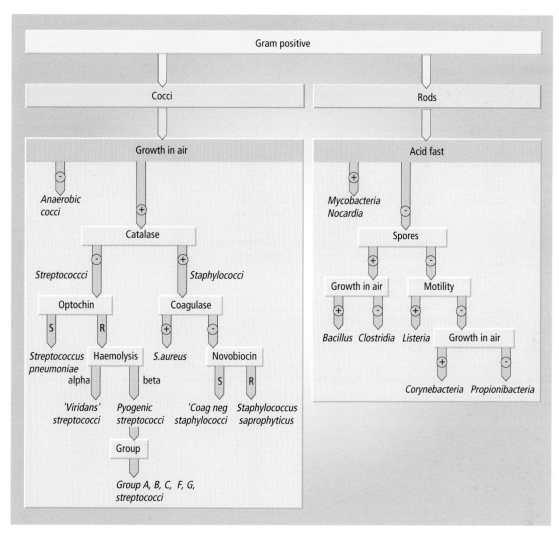

Fig. 2.8 Classification of Gram-positive bacteria.

active inflammatory process, e.g. pus cells (neutrophils) and red cells. Other micro-organisms, for example, yeasts and parasites, may also be visualized in the Gram stain, although they are often more clearly seen using special stains.

Cultural characteristics

The growth of bacteria on solid media results in production of individual colonies (which are visible to the naked eye), each comprising millions of bacteria. The appearance of these colonies on an agar plate is invaluable in the preliminary identification of the bacterial species present in clinical specimens.

The features of importance are illustrated in Fig. 2.7 and include colony size, shape (outline and elevation),

consistency (e.g. mucoid), translucency and colour, smell and whether surrounded by a zone of clearing of blood-based agars (haemolysis). Major factors which influence the growth of bacteria on agar and hence their macroscopic appearance include:

1 the composition of the agar, e.g. nutrients, pH, indicators in agar;

2 the growth rate of the organism;

3 the atmosphere and temperature of incubation.

Figures 2.8 and 2.9 show the classification of medically important bacteria on the basis of their Gram-staining reaction and important cultural characteristics; Table 2.13 shows the Gram-staining features and cultural characteristics of some of the major bacterial groups.

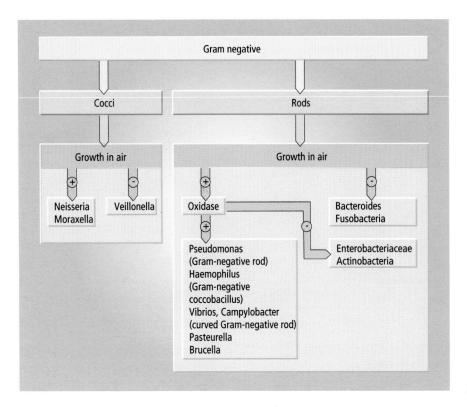

Fig. 2.9 Classification of Gram-negative bacteria.

Antibiotic sensitivity testing

In addition to culture of the responsible organism in suspect infection the laboratory plays an important role in antibiotic sensitivity testing of relevant isolates in order to predict the most appropriate antimicrobial treatment for a particular infection. If empiric antimicrobial therapy is required before these results are available there are recommended empiric regimens which are based on the prevailing sensitivity patterns of common clinical isolates (Table 2.14).

Methods of antimicrobial sensitivity testing

The organism is tested for its ability to grow in the presence of different concentrations of antimicrobial agents.

Disc diffusion method. Antibiotic-impregnated filter paper discs are placed on agar on which the organism under test has been seeded. A zone of inhibition of growth of the organism around the disc indicates sensitivity (Fig. 2.11).

Dilution tests. Antimicrobial agents are added in varying concentrations to liquid broth or incorporated into agar and the organism is added.

The lowest concentration of antibiotic which is capable of inhibiting growth of the organism is defined as the **minimum inhibitory concentration** or **MIC**. Automated methods based on this procedure may be used.

Assays for antibiotic concentrations. In all methods, a control organism of a known sensitivity pattern must be used for comparison. Antibiotic sensitivity patterns can be used for both treatment and epidemiological purposes. Assays for antibiotic concentrations in serum specimens for monitoring the dose of potentially toxic antibiotics, e.g. aminoglycosides and vancomycin, are carried out using automated methods. Clinical serum specimens should be collected as follows:
- do **not** take specimens from the same intravenous line as that being used to administer antibiotics;
- Predose specimen should be taken immediately before the dose is given;

Table 2.13 Classification of bacteria.

Genus	Species	Morphology	Identification	Diseases
GRAM POSITIVE BACTERIA				
Staphylococcus	*Staph. aureus*	Cocci in grape-like clusters	Catalase positive Coagulase positive	Pyogenic infections, e.g. boils, abscesses, wound sepsis, impetigo, osteomyelitis, bacteraemia, bronchopneumonia, toxic shock syndrome, food poisoning
	Staph. epidermidis	Cocci in grape-like clusters	Catalase positive Coagulase negative	Infections of prostheses and implants (e.g. ventriculoatrial shunts, intravascular lines), infective endocarditis, urinary tract infections in elderly males after instrumentation, peritoneal dialysis
	Staph. saprophyticus	Cocci in grape-like clusters	Catalase positive Coagulase negative Novobiocin-resistant	Urinary tract infections in young females
Streptococcus (Lancefield grouping based on poly-saccharide antigen)	*Str. pyogenes* (Group A streptococcus)	Cocci in chains	Catalase negative β-haemolytic Bacitracin-sensitive Lancefield Group A	Pharyngitis, tonsillitis, impetigo, cellulitis, erysipelas, bacteraemia, puerperal sepsis, rheumatic fever acute nephritis
	Str. agalactiae (Group B streptococcus)	In chains	Catalase negative β-haemolytic Lancefield Group B	Neonatal sepsis and meningitis, puerperal sepsis
	Enterococci (*Ent. faecalis*) (Group D streptococcus)	Cocci in short chains	Catalase negative α, β or non-haemolytic Grows in bile Lancefield Group D	Infective endocarditis Urinary tract infections
	Pneumococci (*Str. pneumoniae*)	Cocci in pairs (diplococci)	Catalase negative α haemolytic Optochin sensitive	Otitis media, sinusitis, lobar pneumonia, meningitis, chronic bronchitis.
Actinomyces	*Actino. israelii*	Slender branching bacilli	Microaerophilic or anaerobic	Actinomycosis, chronic sepsis with sinus formation
Clostridia	*Cl. perfringens*	Fat bacilli Spore forming	Obligate anaerobe Nagler positive β-haemolytic	Gas gangrene Wound sepsis Food poisoning
	Cl. tetani	Slender bacilli Round terminal spore (drumstick)	Obligate anaerobe Swarming growth	Tetanus
	Cl. difficile	Bacilli spore-forming	Obligate anaerobe Cytotoxin production	Pseudo-membranous colitis Antibiotic-associated diarrhoea
GRAM-NEGATIVE BACTERIA				
Vibrio	*Campylobacter jejuni*	Slender curved Bacilli	Microaerophilic Thermophilic	Gastro-enteritis
Entero-bacteriacae	*Escherichia coli*	Bacilli	Lactose fermenter Indole + ve O and H antigens	Abdominal sepsis Enteritis UTI Meningitis in neonates

[Continued on p. 38]

Table 2.13 *Continued*

Genus	Species	Morphology	Identification	Diseases
Entero-bacteriacae (*Continued*)	Klebsiella/ Enterobacter	Bacilli		Secondary pathogens especially in hospital acquired infections
	Salmonella	Bacilli	Growth on selective media Non-lactose fermenter O and H antigens	Enteritis Septicaemia Enteric fever
	Shigella	Bacilli	Growth on selective media Non-lactose fermenter O and H antigens	Dysentery
Pseudomonas	*Ps. aeruginosa*	Bacilli	Obligate aerobe Oxidase positive Motile ± pigment	Wound infections, burn infections Urinary tract infections (in catheterized patients) Pneumonia (secondary to ventilation and cystic fibrosis)
Legionella	*L. pneumophila*	Small bacilli or cocco-bacilli, poorly staining	Immunofluorescence Characteristic growth on selective agar (CYE; charcoal yeast extract)	Broncho-pneumonia
Brucella	*Br. abortus*	Small cocco-bacilli	Slow growing on enriched media only	Brucellosis (PUO)
Haemophilus	*H. influenzae*	Small cocco-bacilli (pleomorphic)	Requires X factor (haemin) and V factor (Nicotinamine-adenine dinucleotide; NAD) Growth enhanced on chocolate agar	Meningitis Epiglottitis Bacteraemia Celulitis Osteomyelitis Septic arthritis } <5 years capsulated type b / Otitis media Sinusitis Pneumonia Acute exacerbations of chronic bronchitis } children, adults non-capsulated
Neisseria	*N. meningitidis*	Cocci in pairs	Growth on chocolate agar Ferments glucose and maltose	Meningitis Meningocaemia
	N. gonorrhoeae	Cocci in pairs	Growth on selective medium Ferments glucose	Gonorrhoea Arthritis-dermatitis Syndrome
Bordetella	*Bord. pertussis*	Small cocci-bacilli	Obligate aerobes Slow growth on special media only (e.g. Bordet–Gengou agar)	Pertussis (whooping cough)
Pasteurella	*Past. multocida*	Small	Oxidase positive biochemical tests	Wound infections due to animal bites
Bacteroides	*B. fragilis*	Bacilli	Obligate anaerobe Mastring test	Abdominal sepsis

Table 2.14 Antibiotic prescribing guidelines: empiric antibiotic regimens.

Infection	Common infecting organisms	Empiric regime
Meningitis		
	Neisseria meningitidis Haemophilus influenzae type b Streptococcus pneumoniae	Cefotaxime (penicillin)
Neonates and elderly	Group B streptococci Escherichia coli Listeria	Penicillin + netilmicin in neonate Cefataxime Add in ampicillin if suspected
Pneumonia		
Community-acquired	Streptococcus pneumoniae Atypicals (Mycoplasma, Psittacosis, Legionella)	Ampicillin/cefuroxime + erythromycin
Hospital-acquired	Outside ITU Coliforms ITU	Cefuroxime Rely on sensitivities
Septicaemia		
Unknown source	Escherichia coli Coliforms Staphylococcus aureus	Cefuroxime + gentamicin
GIT source	As above + anaerobes	As above + metronidazole
Immunocompromised	Any	Imipenem + netilmicin (Piperacillin + gentamicin)

Neonatal sepsis
    Within 48 h
    After 48 h
	Group B Streptococcus
	Staphylococcus aureus
		Penicillin + netilmicin
		Flucloxacillin + netilmicin

Prophylactic regimens		

Eradication of carriage	Neisseria meningitidis
	Haemophilus influenzae type b
		Rifampicin
		Note: contacts may already be protected by
		    Hib vaccine (dental procedures) and
		    gentomycin (bowel procedures)

Endocarditis prevention	Viridans streptococci e.g. Strep. sanguis/mitis etc.	Amoxycillin
Surgical prophylaxis	Staphylococcus aureus Enterobacteriaceae ± anaerobes	Cefuroxime + metronidazole
Other miscellaneous		
Antituberculous chemotherapy	Mycobacterium tuberculosis Mycobacterium avium intracellulare	Local policies depend on known prevailing sensitivity patterns
Antifungal and antiviral chemotherapy	Depends on clinical setting	
Special clinical situations requiring attention		
Pregnancy	Some antibiotics contraindicated, especially during first trimester, because of possible teratogenic effects on developing fetus	
Infancy and childhood	Some antibiotics contraindicated Dosage modification required (especially neonates)	
Renal impairment	Reduction in drug dosages and avoidance of nephrotoxic agents	
Drug allergy	Alternative regimens	

ITU, Intensive therapy unit; GIT, gastrointestinal tract.

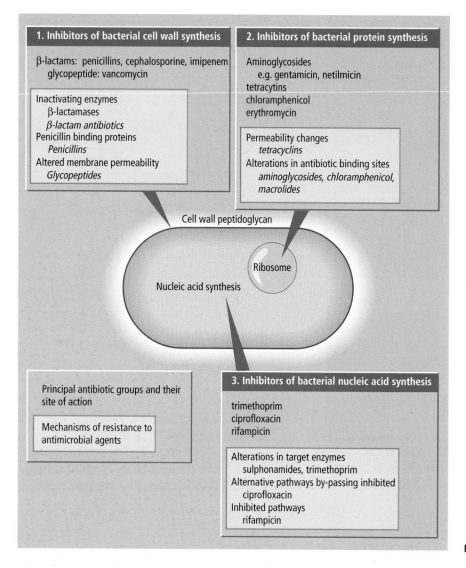

1. Inhibitors of bacterial cell wall synthesis

β-lactams: penicillins, cephalosporine, imipenem
   glycopeptide: vancomycin

Inactivating enzymes
   β-lactamases
   β-lactam antibiotics
Penicillin binding proteins
   Penicillins
Altered membrane permeability
   Glycopeptides

2. Inhibitors of bacterial protein synthesis

Aminoglycosides
   e.g. gentamicin, netilmicin
tetracytins
chloramphenicol
erythromycin

Permeability changes
   tetracyclins
Alterations in antibiotic binding sites
   *aminoglycosides, chloramphenicol,
   macrolides*

Cell wall peptidoglycan

Ribosome

Nucleic acid synthesis

Principal antibiotic groups and their
site of action

Mechanisms of resistance to
antimicrobial agents

3. Inhibitors of bacterial nucleic acid synthesis

trimethoprim
ciprofloxacin
rifampicin

Alterations in target enzymes
   sulphonamides, trimethoprim
Alternative pathways by-passing inhibited
   ciprofloxacin
Inhibited pathways
   rifampicin

Fig. 2.10 The structure of the bacterial cell wall.

- Postdose specimen should be taken 1 hour after a stat dose of aminoglycoside and 2 hours after completion of an intravenous infusion of vancomycin.

It is essential that the request card and specimens are carefully labelled with time of collection of specimens and the time of the dose and dosing regimen being used.

Antimicrobial therapy

Definitions
- **Antibiotic**–**natural** product of micro-organisms able to kill/inhibit growth of other micro-organisms.
- **Antimicrobial agent**–as above but also includes **synthetic** agents.
- **Bacterio*static* agent**–**inhibits** growth of bacteria.
- **Bacter*icidal* agent**–**kills** bacteria.

- **Spectrum of activity**–**broad**-spectrum agent: active against a wide range of Gram-positive and Gram-negative organisms.
- **Narrow**-spectrum agent–active mainly against **either** Gram-positive **or** Gram-negative organisms.

Principal antibiotic groups and their mode of action
Antimicrobial agents can be divided into groups on the basis of their principal site of activity on the target cell (Table 2.15).

Mechanisms of antibiotic resistance
Antibiotic resistance can be classified according to the main site of action of the antibiotic in question (see Fig. 2.10). Resistance mechanisms may be further divided according to the origin of the resistance:

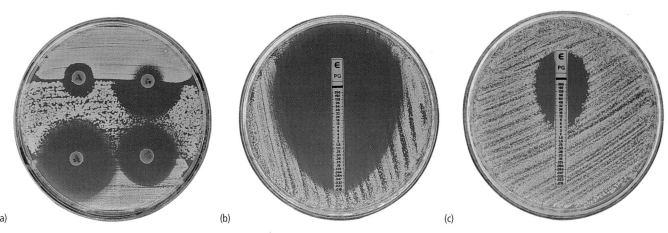

Fig. 2.11 (a) Antibiotic sensitivity plate. *Escherichia coli*-ampicillin and trimethoprim resistant *E. coli* on isosensitest agar compared to sensitive control using 'Stokes' method. Note the different diameters of zones of inhibition of bacterial growth by the antibiotic contained in the discs for the sensitive control *E. coli* organism [inner spread] compared with the trimethoprim (W) and ampicillin (AMP) resistant test *E. coli* [outer spread], both test and control are sensitive to cefuroxime (CXM) and gentamycin (GM). E-strip, (b) penicillin sensitive and (c) penicillin-resistant staphylococci on isosensitest agar. The principle of the E-strip is similar to antibiotic-containing discs except that the dose of antibiotic is graduated along the length of the strip. The MIC (minimum inhibitory concentration) of the organism under test to the antibiotic under test can be read off the strip at the point at which the bacterial growth intersects the strip. (b) Shows a sensitive *Staphylococcus aureus* strain with an MIC to penicillin of 0.02 μg/ml. (c) Shows a resistant *Staph. aureus* strain with an MIC to penicillin of 4.0 μg/ml.

- intrinsic or acquired;
- location: chromosomal mutation or plasmid-mediated;
- expression: constitutive or inducible.

The major mechanisms by which antibiotic resistance occur are as follows.

Enzymatic inhibition, e.g. β-lactamases. β-Lactamases are enzymes which inactivate the β-lactam antibiotics by breaking down their ring structure. They may be chromosomal, or transferable genes carried on plasmids or transposons which are small, extrachromosomal pieces of genetic material which encode for specific functions and can be transferred from one organism to another. They are produced by Gram-positive and Gram-negative bacteria; in the latter they are intrinsic or constitutive and can be induced by exposure to the appropriate antimicrobial agent.

Other enzymes mediating drug resistance include modifying enzymes which result in inactivation of an antibiotic during the process of transport across the cell membrane or acetylation of antibiotic which results in inactivation.

Alterations in bacterial membrane permeability. The passage of antibiotics through the outer membrane in Gram-negative organisms is facilitated by the presence of porins which comprise water-filled protein channels through which they can diffuse. Mutations in these porins can result in increased resistance to β-lactam and some other antibiotics.

Alterations in ribosomal target sites. Failure of an antibiotic may result because it is unable to bind to its target site because of alterations in the target site structure, e.g.

Table 2.15 Principal antibiotic groups and their mode of action.

Site of action	Antibiotics
Cell wall	β-lactams–penicillins, cephalosporins
Cytoplasmic membrane	Amphotericin B (antifungal agent)
Ribosomes	Aminoglycosides, erythromycin, tetracycline
Nucleic acid synthesis	
RNA	Rifampicin
DNA	Quinolones, metronidazole
Microbial enzyme pathways	Trimethoprim

Table 2.16 General principles of antimicrobial chemotherapy.

Collect specimens for culture before starting therapy

Is empiric therapy required immediately?

Factors influencing choice of drug
• Severity of infection
• Site of infection
• Suspected organism and known or predicted sensitivities
• Antibiotic spectrum of activity
• Static/cidal drug
• Drug efficacy versus toxicity
• Ease of administration
• Need for multiple therapy
  Initial empiric treatment
  For synergy, e.g. endocarditis
  To prevent resistance emerging, e.g. in tuberculosis
• Interaction with other drugs
• Known or suspected drug allergies
• Other clinical conditions present, e.g. renal impairment, pregnancy

Administration
• Route: oral/parenteral/topical
  Optimal tissue levels of drug
  Metabolism and excretion (renal and hepatic toxicity especially)
• Dosage interval
• Drug level monitoring

Duration of therapy
• Dependent on severity of infection site and infecting organism

Role of the laboratory
• Bacteriological diagnosis
• Sensitivity testing
  Direct
  Special tests, e.g. MIC and MBC
• Other assays—synergy, serum bactericidal
• Antibiotic peak-and-trough concentrations—aminoglycosides and
  vancomycin

MIC, Minimum inhibitory concentration; MBC, minimum bactericidal concentration.

erythromycin and clindamycin resistance in Gram-positive organisms.

Alterations in target enzymes. Any change in the target site for antibiotic action may result in resistance to the antibiotic activity of that agent. For example, alterations in penicillin-binding proteins result in reduced affinity for β-lactam antibiotics on the bacterial cell surface and hence resistance.

Drug-resistant enzymes may be produced which can effectively bypass the action of antibiotics which block a particular step in a metabolic pathway, e.g. trimethoprim, quinolones.

General principles of antimicrobial chemotherapy
(Table 2.16)

Reasons for failure of antimicrobial chemotherapy
1 **Incorrect diagnosis:**
   (a) incorrect or inadequate specimen examined, e.g. collected after starting antibiotic therapy;
   (b) no bacteriological specimens sent.
2 **Incorrect choice of antibiotic:**
   (a) spectrum of activity inadequate;
   (b) dosage/route/duration of treatment inadequate;
   (c) organism isolated resistant to antibiotic chosen;
   (d) antagonistic drug combination chosen.
3 **Inadequate penetration of antibiotic to affected site**:
   (a) route unsatisfactory for achieving tissue levels needed;
   (b) metabolism/tissue distribution inappropriate for infection being treated.

Table 2.17 Reasons for establishing an antibiotic policy.

• Ensure **appropriate** therapy
• Control levels of antibiotic **resistance** by restricting agents used
• Control use of potentially **toxic** agents
• Control prescribing **costs** by controlling use of expensive agents

Table 2.18 Background to establishing an antibiotic policy.

Sensitivity pattern of current bacterial strains in specified clinical settings
  Staphylococcus aureus, Gram-negative rods in intensive therapy units
    (ITUs), special care baby units, renal and transplant units
  Urinary isolates in general practice

'Reservation' of antibiotics for use in certain clinical settings only—by organism or by specific type of patient
  Imipenem use in ITUs and febrile neutropenic patients
Flexibility is an essential component—antibiotic resistance patterns may change rapidly

Table 2.19 Example of an antibiotic policy.

Antibiotics are divided into five categories with different degrees of accessibility
A Oral and parenteral agents available for prescription by all doctors
B Agents restricted in use to certain units (e.g. intensive therapy units, special care baby units, haematology, renal) or for specific indications
C Prescription limited to senior medical staff (consultants)
D Drug undergoing clinical trial and available only to named doctors involved in trials
E All other antibiotics available in the UK. Not in stock and only ordered via consultants

4 Other therapeutic procedures indicated, for example, drainage of pus.

5 Non-compliance with therapy must always be considered, especially when oral therapy is prescribed.

Adverse drug reactions

The commonest adverse drug reaction is a rash. When most severe, drug reactions can lead to anaphylactic reactions, especially with β-lactam antibiotics.

All antibiotics have general (e.g. rash) and specific reactions (e.g. bone marrow depression secondary to chloramphenicol). A detailed drug history must always be taken from the patient. Some reactions perceived by patients to be allergies may not be and the optimal drug may not be used as a result of such a misconception.

Antibiotic policies

These are written policies usually drawn up by a committee comprising senior clinicians, the control of infection officer (usually a consultant microbiologist) and a senior pharmacist (Tables 2.17–2.19).

Bacteraemia and septicaemia

Definitions

- **Bacteraemia**–bacteria present in blood stream. Usually transient, of low order of magnitude and may be asymptomatic.
- **Septicaemia**–sepsis in blood stream; implies active multiplication of bacteria; usually less transient than bacteraemia and associated with clinical and laboratory signs of sepsis.

The terms may be used interchangeably but bacteraemia is generally regarded as less severe than septicaemia. **Fungaemia**, **viraemia** and **parasitaemia** refer to fungi, viruses or parasites in the blood stream respectively.

Classification

1 Transient–commonly occurs in normal individual, e.g. brushing teeth. Plays an important role in the pathogenesis of septicaemia.

2 Intermittent–represents recurrent transient bacteraemia. Indicative of an established infection outside the blood stream.

3 Sustained–continuous bacteraemia. Indicative of infection within the blood stream, e.g. endocarditis.

Clinical features

Symptoms of bacteraemia and septicaemia include chills, rigor, tachycardia, hypotension resulting in confusion (re-duced cerebral blood flow) and reduced urine output (reduced renal perfusion).

Other clinical presentations include.

1 PUO.

2 Septicaemia associated with primary focus, which can be differentiated into:

(a) **community-acquired**, e.g. urinary tract infection (UTI) and pneumonia;

(b) **hospital-acquired**–UTI, pneumonia, skin sepsis, deep abscess, indwelling intravenous catheters and osteomyelitis.

Mortality rate is in the range of 40–90% and depends on the nature of the infecting organism and underlying host factors (e.g. age, other disease).

Host factors predisposing to infection

Any host factor that is associated with an impaired host immune response will predispose to bacteraemia and septicaemia.

- **Extremes of age.** Increased risk in neonates and elderly.
- **Malignancy.** Especially of reticuloendothelial system or postcytotoxic chemotherapy.
- **Diabetes.**
- **Steroid therapy.**
- **Prosthetic material** *in situ*. Indwelling intravenous lines, urinary catheters, joint implants and central nervous system shunts provide a niche for the organism.
- **Postoperatively**, **posttrauma** or **burns**.
- **Alcohol**, **drug abuse**, **HIV** infection.

Organism factors contributing to infection

Cell wall components of both Gram-positive and Gram-negative organisms play an important role in the pathophysiology of septic shock.

In particular, lipopolysaccharide (LPS), also known as **endotoxin**, of the **Gram-negative** outer membrane is strongly implicated in septic or endotoxic shock. Endotoxin is released in vast quantities on bacterial cell death together with endogenous substances including cytokines, released from host inflammatory cells on exposure to bacteria in the blood stream. These have a profound effect on the host, resulting in a **rapid fall in blood pressure**, **reduced perfusion** of brain and kidneys and widespread **activation of the complement** and blood clotting systems, thereby producing the characteristic features of **septic shock** (Table 2.20).

Microbiological diagnosis

Blood culture. Blood is collected under strictly aseptic conditions to minimize the risk of contamination by normal

Table 2.20 Major causes of septicaemia by organism (%).

Organism	Community acquired	Hospital acquired	Comment
Gram-negative			
Escherichia coli	35	30	UTI–often catheter-related Biliary sepsis, diverticulitis
Other Enterobacteriaceae	5	10	UTI, chest infection
Pseudomonas	5	5	UTI Immunosuppressed
Other Gram-negative rods	2	5	Pneumonia in ventilated patients in ITU
Neisseria meningitidis	3	0	Skin rash, meningitis
Bacteroides	3	1	Bowel and pelvic infections, wounds
Haemophilus influenzae	1	0	Meningitis, pneumonia and epiglottitis in children <5 years
Gram-positive			
Staphylococcus aureus	30	25	Vascular, postoperative wound, skin
Coagulase-negative staphylococci	<1	20	Prosthetic material, intravascular devices
Streptococcus pneumoniae	10	0	Pneumonia, meningitis
Group A streptococci	5	2	Skin, soft tissue
Mixed	10	7	Bowel infections, intensive care units

UTI, Urinary tract infection.

skin organisms. Blood (5–10 ml per bottle) is placed into aerobic and anaerobic liquid culture bottles and incubated at 37°C for 5 days. Bacterial growth is detected automatically; blood is subcultured to solid media (agar) and identity and sensitivity testing carried out in the usual way. Other relevant specimens, e.g. urine, sputum, cerebrospinal fluid, pus, swabs, etc. should be collected as appropriate as the same organism may also be present.

Factors which improve sensitivity include.

- **Number of cultures collected.** Two separately collected cultures 30 minutes apart is optimal;
- **Timing of collection.** Optimal 30 minutes before peak of fever;
- **Volume of blood per culture.** Isolation rate increases with increasing volume.

CLINICAL VIROLOGY

The most important viruses causing disease in humans are listed in Tables 2.21 and 2.22.

CLINICAL MYCOLOGY

Classification of fungal organisms

The identification of pathogenic fungi relies on their morphology in tissue and under a variety of growth conditions such as temperature and growth media. Viewed simply, they are divided into:

- yeasts;
- those capable of being yeasts and moulds;
- moulds (Table 2.23).

Classification of fungal infections
(Tables 2.24 and 2.25)

Dermatophytes
These are fungal infections of keratinous structures of the skin (Chapter 26). Infections are caused by species of the three genera:

Table 2.21 Classification of human viruses.

Nucleic acid	Family	Size (nm)	Viruses	Main disease
DNA-ds	Poxviridae	200 × 300	Ortho-variola	Smallpox
			Vaccinia	Vesicular eruption
			Cowpox	Vesicular eruption
		150 × 200	Para-Orf	Benign epidermal tumours
			Molluscum	Benign epidermal tumours
DNA-ds	Herpesviridae	180–250 enveloped (100 naked)	Herpes simplex	Vesicles/encephalitis
			Varicella	Chickenpox/Shingles
			Cytomegalovirus	Congenital
			Epstein–Barr	Infectious mononucleosis
			Human herpesvirus 6	Roseola infantum
DNA-ds	Adenoviridae	70 naked	Subgeneral A–F	URTI, conjunctivitis
				Haemorrhagic cystitis
				Gastroenteritis
DNA-ds	Papovaviridae	50 naked	Human papillomavirus (>50 types)	Warts, cervical intraepithelial neoplasia (CIN)
		44 naked	Polyomavirus BK, JC	Progressive multifocal leucoencephalopathy
DNA-ds	Heptadnaviridae	42 naked	Hepatitis B	Hepatitis
DNS-ss	Parvoviridae	22 naked	Human parvovirus (B19)	Erythema infectiosum
RNS-ss (+)	Retroviridae	100 enveloped	Onco-HTLV-1	T-cell leukaemia
				Tropical spastic paraparesis
			Lenti-HIV 1,2	AIDS
RNS-ss (+)	Coronaviridae	80–100 enveloped	Coronavirus	URTI
RNS-ss (+)	Togaviridae	42 enveloped	Rubella	Rash, arthralgia
			Ross River	Rash, arthralgia
			Equine enceph.	Encephalitis
RNS-ss (+)	Flaviviridae	42 enveloped	Yellow fever	Hepatitis
			Dengue	Fever ± rash (occasionally haemorrhagic fever)
			Jap. encephalitis	Encephalitis
RNS-ss (+)	Caliciviridae	38 naked	Calicivirus (Norwalk)	Gastroenteritis
RNS-ss (+)	Picornaviridae	27 naked	Rhinovirus	URTI
			Enteroviruses	Meningitis
			Poliovirus	Polio
			Coxsackie B	Bornholm disease
			Hepatitis A	Infectious hepatitis
RNS-ss (−)	Rhabdoviridae	70–180 enveloped	Rabies	Rabies
RNS-ss (−)	Filoviridae	Filamentous enveloped	Marburg	Haemorrhagic fever
			Ebola	
RNS-ss (−)	Paramyxoviridae	150 × 300 enveloped	Measles	Measles
			Mumps	Mumps, meningitis
			Parainfluenza	RTI
			RSV	RTI
8 segments	Orthomyxo-viridae	>100 enveloped	Influenza A, B, C	'Flu'
2 segments	Arenaviridae	100 × 300 enveloped	Lassa	Lassa fever
			L.C.M.	Meningitis
3 segments	Hantaviridae	100 enveloped	Hantaan	HFRS
3 segments	Bunyaviridae	100 enveloped	CCHF	Haemorrhagic fever
			Rift valley	
RNA-ds 11 segments	Reoviridae	70 naked	Rotavirus	Gastroenteritis

ds, double-stranded; ss, single-stranded; +, plus strand; −, minus strand.
URTI, upper respiratory tract infection; RTI, respiratory tract infection; RSV, respiratory synctial virus; LCM, lymphocytic choriomeningitis virus; CCMF, congo-crimean haemorrhagic fever virus; HFRS, haemorrhagic fever with renal syndrome.

Table 2.22 Practical clinical virology.

Features	Causes	Nose throat swab NPA	Urine	CSF	BX	Swab vesicle fluid	Faeces	Serum p	Serum s
Gastroenteritis	Rotavirus, adenovirus						•		
Mesenteric adenitis	Adenovirus				•				
Oesophagitis, colitis	HSV, CMV in immune suppression				•	•			
Tonsillitis	EBV, adenovirus	•							•
Stomatitis, herpangina	HSV, Coxsackie					•	•		
Parotitis, pancreatitis	Mumps, Coxsackie	•						•	
Hepatitis	HepA, B, C, Delta, Yellow fever, EBV, CMV								•
Genital herpes	HSV 2					•			
Genital warts	HPV 6,11,16,18				•	•			
Cervicitis, urethritis	HSV, chlamydia*					•			
Nephropathy	Hantaan							•	
Parotitis, orchitis	Mumps	•						•	
Skin rashes: Maculopapular rashes	Measle, rubella, parvovirus Enteroviruses (EBV, CMV, HepB)	•					•	•	
Vesicular rashes	HSV, orf					•			
Nodular rashes	Papilloma, molluscum contagiosum								
Arthritis	Rubella, parvovirus, arbovirus							•	•
Myositis/myocarditis	Enterovirus, toxoplasma	•		•			•	•	
Meningitis	Enterovirus, mumps, HIV, HSV	•		•				•	
Encephalitis	HSV, mumps, rabies, arbo, HIV, HSV			•	•			•	
Paralysis	Polio	•		•			•	•	
Postinfectious encephalomyositis	Mealses, rubella							•	
Guillain–Barré	Influenza, EBV, CMV							•	
PMLE	Polyoma JC in IS			•	•				•
Spongiform encephalopathy	'Slow viruses'				•				
SSPE	Measles, rubella			•					•
Tropical spastic paraparesis	HTLV-1								•
Conjunctivitis and keratoconjunctivitis	adeno, HSV, chlamydia, enterovirus, Coxsackie A24					•			
Common cold	Rhino, coronavirus	•							
Pharyngitis	Influenza, adeno, HSV, EBV, Coxsackie	•							
Croup	Influenza	•							
	Parainfluenza	•							
Bronchiolitis	RSV	•							
Pneumonia	RSV, flu, paraflu, adenovirus	•						•	
Congenital infection	Rubella, CMV, toxo*, HIV, parvovirus	•	•						•
Perinatal and postnatal infection	HSV, CMV, entero, HepB, HIV	•				•	•	•	
Acute T-cell leukaemia	HTLV-1								•
Lymphoma	EBV in the immune deficient				•				
Immune deficiency	HIV								•
Chorioretinitis	CMV in the immune deficient ⎫								
Travel associated fevers	Arbovirus, Lassa fever ⎭				Discuss with virology laboratory				

NPA, Nasopharyngeal aspirate; Bx, biopsy; P, paired; S, single; PMLE, progressive multifocal; leucoencephalopathy; SSPE, subacute sclerosing panencephalitis; CIN, cervical intraepithelial neoplasia; HIV, human immunodeficiency virus; HSV, herpes simplex virus; EBV, Epstein–Barr virus; CMV, cytomegalovirus.

* Toxoplasma and chlamydia are not viruses but are often classified with viruses.

Table 2.23 Classification of fungal organisms.

YEASTS	
Candida spp.	Speciated by biochemical tests. Rapid identification of *C. albicans* relies on the appearance of pseudomycelia on incubation in serum
Cryptococcus neoformans	Divided into capsular serotypes A–D
Malassezia furfur	A lipophilic fungus—needs oil to grow

DIMORPHIC FUNGI (yeasts in tissue and moulds on media at room temperature)
Histoplasma capsulatum
Sporothrix schenckii
Blastomyces dermatitidis
Coccodioides immitis
Paracoccidioides brasiliensis

MOULDS
Non-septate hyphae

　　　　　　　　Zygomycetes (*Mucor* or bread mould)

Septate hyphae

　　　　　　　　Dermatophytes (*Trichophyton* etc.)
　　　　　　　　Aspergillus spp. (branches at 45°)

Genera (such as *Aspergillus*) are divided into species by the appearances of the reproductive elements:
Asexual spores　　　Macroconidia
Sexual spores　　　Microconidia

- *Trichophyton*;
- *Microsporum*;
- *Epidermophyton*.

Fungi invade through small abrasions in the skin and localize to the keratinized layers of the skin. An inflammatory reaction is produced to the infection. Other keratinized structures (hair and nails) are invaded and degraded.

In the skin, lesions start as a small pruritic papule of scaling skin which advances concentrically, sometimes leaving a healed centre (**ringworm**). The lesions involving different parts of the integument are named as follows:
- tinea corporis—body;
- tinea capitis—scalp and hair; results in alopecia;
- tinea pedis—foot;
- tinea cruris—groin.

The differential diagnosis includes dermatitis, psoriasis, lichen planus and the 'herald patch' of pityriasis rosacea.

Tinea unguium. This is a fungal infection of the nailbed or plate and leads to nail destruction (onycholysis). It is to be differentiated from psoriasis and lichen planus.

Other superficial mycoses

Tinea versicolor. This is an infection of the stratum corneum caused by the lypophilic yeast *Malassezia furfur*. It is distributed worldwide and manifests as perifollicular hypopigmentation which coalesces producing areas of irregular hypopigmentation.

Pityrosporum yeast. Associated with seborrhoeic dermatitis.

Candida spp. (Fig. 2.12)

Candida albicans (80%), *C. tropicalis* (10%), *C. parapsilosis* and *C. guilliermonidii* are associated with human infections. *Candida* is part of the normal microbial flora. The isolation rate is greatly enhanced in people on antibiotics. It is an important cause of disease in the altered host and is associated with the following:
- oral 'thrush'—white plaques of candida on mucous membranes;
- candidal vulvovaginitis (diagnosed on wet preparation or culture of discharge);
- intertrigo;
- nappy rash.

Candida infects prosthetic and other devices such as central venous pressure lines. It is a cause of systemic infections such as in neutropenic patients. In AIDS patients it may present with oropharyngeal candidiasis, osteomyelitis and ophthalmitis.

Aspergillus spp. (Fig. 2.13)

Aspergillus spores are ubiquitous in the environment, which probably explains why it is frequently isolated from specimens. It is not regarded as part of the normal flora. It is associated with three different types of disease.

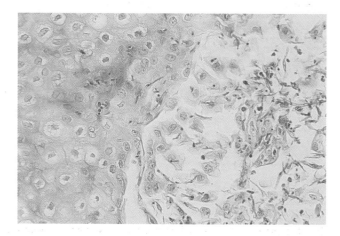

Fig. 2.12 Skin. Candida hyphae and spores, stained dark red with periodic acid–Schiff (PAS).

Table 2.24 Clinical classification of fungal infections.

	Host defences (especially CMI)	
	Normal	**Abnormal**
Systemic (DEEP)		*Candida* spp.
	Histoplasma capsulatum	*Aspergillus* spp.
	Blastomyces dermatitidis	*Cryptococcus neoformans*
	Coccidiodes immitis	*Zygomycetes*
	Paracoccidiodes braziliensis	
Intermediate	*Candida* spp.	
	Eumycetoma (in contrast to actinomycetoma) (fungal and bacterial Madura foot respectively)	
	Sporothrix schenckii	
Cutaneous	Dermatophytes	
	Malassezia furfur (tinea versicolor)	
	Candida spp. (including mucous membranes)	
	Aspergillus spp.	
Allergic	*Aspergillus* spp.	
	Air conditioners, moulds	
	Hay	
Fungus ball	*Aspergillus* spp.	
	Zygomycetes	
Toxins	Poisonous mushrooms (e.g. *Amanita phalloides*)	
	Ergotism (*Claviceps pupurea*)	
Normal flora	*Candida* spp.	

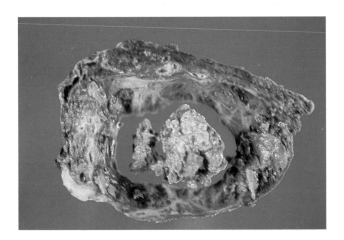

Fig. 2.13(a) Lung. Large, cavitating aspergilloma in an immunosuppressed patient.

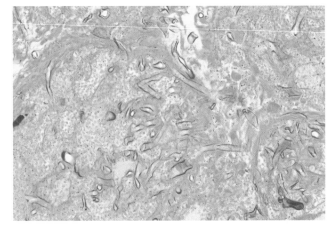

Fig. 2.13(b) Lung histology. Aspergillus hyphae stained with Grocott (black).

Table 2.25 Systems involved (deep infections).

GENERALIZED ACUTE
Candida spp. (80% *albicans*)

	Haematological malignancies
	Line-associated

Aspergillus spp.

	(*flavus* and *fumigatus*)
	Haematological malignancies start in the lung and become overwhelming

SYSTEMIC, SUBACUTE AND CHRONIC
Lungs
Pneumocystis pneumonia†

Histoplasmosis*	Portal of entry
Cryptococcosis	Lobar, nodules and cavities
Coccidioidomycosis	Spread systemically
Blastomycosis	
Paracoccidiodomycosis	Differential diagnosis
Sporotrichosis	Tuberculosis, sarcoid and malignancy

Central nervous system

Cryptococcosis*	Chronic meningitis
Coccidioidomycosis	Differential diagnosis:
Sporotrichosis	Tuberculosis CA, vasculitis, sarcoid
Aspergillus spp.	Acute sinusitis proceeding to invasion
Mucor	of the brain

Bone
Candida spp.

Aspergillus spp.	Chronic osteomyelitis
Soiritrichosis	
Blastomycosis	

Skin
Blastmycosis

Histoplasmosis	Deep ulcers and nodules
Cryptococcoma	
Coccidioidomycosis	

The other organs are less frequently involved

* An opportunistic infection associated with the diagnosis of acquired immune deficiency syndrome (AIDS).
† Of uncertain derivation but most likely to be fungal.

1 Aspergilloma—which colonizes a cavity (e.g. lung cavity).
2 Allergic bronchopulmonary aspergillosis is associated with steroid-dependent asthma. The disease is probably mediated by IgA and IgG antibody antigen reactions.
3 Invasive aspergillosis (especially in neutropenic patients).

Mycetoma

This is a chronic destructive, granulating infection causing destruction of tissue planes with fistulae discharging granules.

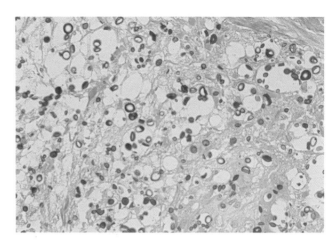

Fig. 2.14 Lung histology. Cryptococcus neoformans stained black with Grocott.

Eumycetoma is caused by many species of fungi, e.g. *Madurella mycetomi*. It is found in the tropical regions of the world and following traumatic inoculation the fungus invades and spreads by contiguity to disorganize the tissues in a limb.

Specimen processing

Skin and appendages
Skin scrapings, hair and nail clippings are obtained and a potassium hydroxide preparation examined microscopically for hyphae. Material is inoculated on to a medium such as Sabouraud's and incubated for up to 6 weeks.

Mycetoma
This is examined by microscopy and inoculated on suitable medium, such as Sabourand's, and the granules examined.

Systemic fungal infections
Potentially contaminated specimens such as sputum are predictive of a systemic fungal infection if fungi other than *Candida* spp. or *Aspergillus* spp. (e.g. *Cryptococcus neoformans*; Fig. 2.14) are isolated. Reliable specimens such as sterile fluids (e.g. blood and cerebrospinal fluid) or biopsy material are highly predictive of a fungal infection if fungal elements are seen on microscopy or a fungus is grown. For many fungi, cultures should be kept for up to 6 weeks (*Candida* spp. and *Aspergillus* spp. are rapid-growers). Special media may be needed for certain fungal species, therefore the laboratory should be warned of the likely fungal pathogen.

Table 2.26 Treatment of fungal infection.

DERMATOPHYTE INFECTIONS
Topical agents
Whitfield's ointment (benzoid acid)
Miconazole and clotrimazole (Azoles)
1% Selenium sulphide—tinea versicolor
Tioconazole solution (fungal infections)

Oral agents
Griseofulvin
Ketoconazole

SYSTEMIC INFECTIONS
Amphotericin B (polyene—macrolide)
Ketoconazole
Fluconazole

TREATMENT FOR SPECIFIC INFECTIONS
Candida *spp.*
Systemic—Amphotericin B/fluconazole
Low-grade invasion—Ketoconazole/fluconazole
Mucous membrane—Nystatin/fluconazole

Aspergillus *spp.*
Systemic—Amphotericin B/itraconazole
Aspergilloma—Surgery
Allergic bronchopulmonary aspergillosis—Corticosteroids

Cryptococcal disease
Pulmonary—Amphotericin B
Central nervous system—Amphotericin B + flucytosine

Sporotrichosis
Skin—Potassium iodide
Systemic—Amphotericin B

Two newer agents
Itraconazole (*Aspergillus*)
Fluconazole (gets into central nervous system—*Cryptococcus*)

Antigen tests

Cryptococcal antigen can be detected with a high degree of sensitivity and specificity in cerebrospinal fluid, urine and serum. Antigen detection assays for the other systemic fungi are being developed.

Serological tests

Antibodies to the fungi which produce systemic infections can be detected, but they are indirect tests of infection and must be interpreted with care. The detection of precipitating antibodies to *Aspergillus* are predictive of allergic bronchopulmonary aspergillosis. DNA probes are being developed.

Treatment of fungal infections (Table 2.26)

FURTHER READING

Mitchinson M.J. *et al.* (1996) *Essentials of Pathology*, Chapters 7–13. Blackwell Science, Oxford.

Young D.W. (1988) Improving laboratory usage: a review. *Postgrad. Med. J.* **64**: 283–289.

Clinical Immunology

Contents

CLINICAL IMMUNOLOGY

What is clinical immunology?

Clinical immunology is a relatively new laboratory specialty that has arisen out of the tremendous strides made in basic immunology (Fig. 3.1).

The clinical immunology laboratory is involved in the diagnosis and monitoring of immunological diseases. The tests performed fall into four categories:

- **immunochemistry**;
- **autoimmunity**;
- **cellular and functional studies**; and
- **tissue typing** for transplantation; these will be discussed in turn.

Basic immunology has far outstripped clinical immunology and it is important to remember that many research tests have not been fully evaluated for routine laboratory use: uncritical use of such tests may be dangerously misleading and there is frequently a need for expert interpretation for immunological tests. Appropriate test selection is critical; immunology, more than most laboratory disciplines, generates significant numbers of irrelevant and useless test requests.

The immunological sections of this book aim to encourage a better understanding of the immunological processes involved in disease and of appropriate test selection.

When performing any test it is appropriate to consider what information you expect to gain from the test and how this information will alter clinical management: the diagnostic process needs to be more structured than a random fishing expedition. Figure 3.2 shows how the diagnostic process might be applied to immunological tests in the diagnosis of systemic lupus erythematosus (SLE).

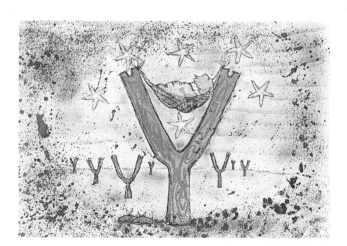

Fig. 3.1 What is clinical immunology? (From an original, courtesy Dr R. Armstrong.)

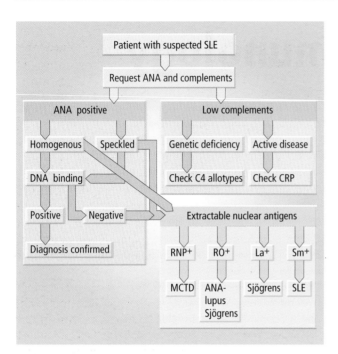

Fig. 3.2 An illustration of how the diagnostic process might be applied to the diagnosis of systemic lupus erythematosus (SLE). CRP, c-reactive protein; MCTD, mixed connective tissue disease; ANA, anti-nuclear antibody; SLE, systemic lupus erythematosus; RNP, nuclear ribonucleic acid; Ro, antibody against a saline soluble antigen or SS-A; La, SS-B; Sm, smooth muscle.

Table 3.1 Serum proteins by electrophoretic mobility.

Region	Protein	Function
α_1	α_1-Acid glycoprotein	Acute phase
	α_1-Antitrypsin	Acute phase/protease inhibitor
	Transcortin	Transport
	α_1-Antichymotrypsin	Protease inhibitor
	α_1-Lipoprotein	Transport
α_1–α_2	Thyroxine-binding globulin	Transport
	Antithrombin III	Protease inhibitor
	Caeruloplasmin	Transport
α_2	Haptoglobin	Transport
	α_2-Glycoprotein	Acute phase
	α_2-Macroglobulin	Acute phase/transport
β	β-Lipoprotein	Transport
	Transferrin	Transport
	C3	Acute phase/immunity
	C4	Acute phase/Immunity
	Fibrinogen	Acute phase/clotting
γ	Immunoglobulins (IgG, IgA, IgM)	Immunity
	C-reactive protein	Acute phase

Immunochemistry

Immunochemistry is the **analysis of substances important in the immune response**. This includes **quantitation of serum proteins, detection of abnormal substances**, such as myeloma proteins, and **functional tests**, such as the total haemolytic activity of the complement pathway.

Table 3.1 lists the **immunologically relevant proteins** for which assays are available. Most of these proteins will be measured by automated instruments, using the interaction of antibody with antigen to generate an immune complex which can be measured by either light scattering or by reduction in light transmission.

Abnormal properties of proteins may be determined by **electrophoresis** or by **direct tests** of function. As most proteins carry a net charge, they will move when placed in an electric field. The way in which proteins will move is determined by the type of buffer and the nature of the medium. Following electrophoresis, the proteins may be visualized by a **protein-binding stain**, by **immunoprecipitation** or **immunofixation**, in which an antiserum specific for the component of interest is allowed to react with the electrophoresed strip: immune complexes are formed in the gel and unreacted proteins are washed away. The immunoprecipitate is then visualized by staining. Functional tests utilize specific properties of the proteins, such as an enzymatic activity. Note in particular the following.

Immunoglobulins

Immunoglobulins (Igs) are proteins intimately involved in specific immune responses. Five isotypes are recognized–IgG, IgM, IgA, IgE and IgD. The first three are the major constituents of the **humoral immune response** to foreign antigens and all are easily measured. **IgE** is involved in **allergic** and **antiparasite** responses. Trace amounts of **IgD** are present in serum but its major role seems to be as a **membrane receptor**; its measurement is of no clinical significance.

Measurement of **IgG, IgM** and **IgA** is important in the investigation of **primary** and **secondary immunodeficiencies** (see Chapter 10). Low levels may be associated with an increased risk of bacterial infections and always warrant further investigation. It is possible to measure the individual **IgG subclasses** and also the specific antibodies. Where **low serum immunoglobulins** are found, it is important to check **urine** for **protein loss (nephrotic syndrome)** and also to consider protein loss from the bowel (**protein-losing enteropathy**). Some **drugs**, such as **phenytoin** and **penicillamine**, have been associated with reduced Ig levels.

Abnormal immunoglobulins (paraproteins) occur in **multiple myeloma** and other lymphoproliferative disor-

Table 3.2 Serum electrophoresis – commonly reported changes.

Decreased α_1	α_1-Antitrypsin deficiency hypoproteinaemia (malabsorption, nephrotic syndrome)
Raised α_2	Increased acute-phase proteins, especially α_2-macroglobulin; infections, arthritis, some connective tissue diseases, burns, some neoplasms, nephrotic syndrome (relative increase only)
Raised β	Iron deficiency (increased transferrin), biliary obstruction, pregnancy and hyperlipidaemias (increased β-lipoprotein)
β–γ bridging	Acute-phase response (increased C-reactive protein), polyclonal increase in immunoglobulin A (liver disease, especially alcoholic)
Polyclonal increase immunoglobulins	See Table 3.3

ders. These are produced by the unrestricted proliferation of single clones of plasma cells and are characterized by restricted mobility on electrophoresis (monoclonal immunoglobulins, **M-bands** or **M-spikes**). The production of monoclonal immunoglobulins is inefficient and **free light chains** are often produced in excess, or some-times alone; these proteins may be detected in the **urine** as **monoclonal bands** on electrophoresis (**Bence-Jones proteins**); thus investigations of myeloma must include analysis of both **urine** and **serum** (Fig. 3.3).

Occasionally more than one paraprotein is present, or the protein may polymerize, giving rise to **multiple bands** on electrophoresis. **Myeloma proteins** may have unusual properties such as **cold precipitability** (a **cryoglobulin**; see below). **Paraproteins** are also associated with increasing age, as the immune system's surveillance decays. **Chronic infection** (e.g. tuberculosis) and **inflammation** (e.g. rheumatoid arthritis) may also give rise to low levels of serum paraproteins but, unlike myeloma, where normal immunoglobulin synthesis is depressed, there is a **polyclonal increase in immunoglobulin**.

The quantity of the paraprotein, as opposed to the total amount of immunoglobulin, may be determined by photometrically scanning the electrophoretic strip and measuring the uptake of protein stain by the band, which is proportional to the amount of protein present. Where high levels of paraproteins, particularly pentameric IgM, are found the **serum viscosity** will be **increased**: this may be clinically significant. Changes in the patterns of immunoglobulins in other conditions are given in Table 3.3.

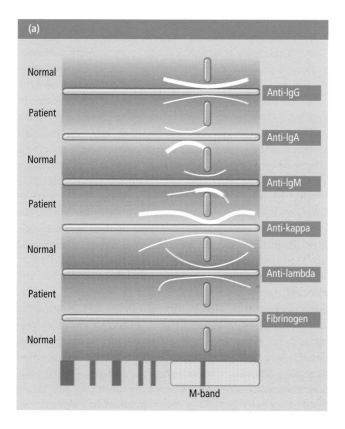

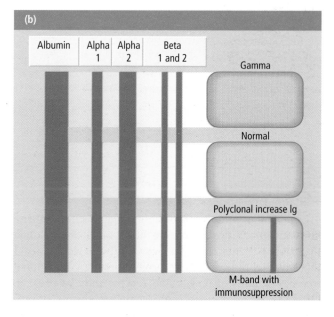

Fig. 3.3 Serum electrophoresis. (a) Shows pattern of IgM kappa paraprotein corresponding to M-band. (b) Shows appearance of normal gamma region (top), polyclonal increase in Igs (middle) and presence of monoclonal Ig (bottom) on serum electrophoresis.

Table 3.3 Factors influencing immunoglobulin (Ig) levels.

Presence of monoclonal immunoglobulins (M-band)	Myeloma, Waldenström's macroglobulinaemia, chronic lymphatic leukaemia, non-Hodgkin's lymphoma, Bence Jones myeloma (M-band in serum only with renal failure, serum Igs reduced), chronic infections (often with polyclonal increase), rheumatoid arthritis, SLE, post-bone marrow transplant, old age
Raised level of an Ig isotype	
Polyclonal increase in IgG	Infections (mainly chronic), infective endocarditis, actinomycosis, hepatitis, HIV, SLE, rheumatoid arthritis, sarcoidosis
Polyclonal increase in IgA	Chronic infections, TB, HIV, chronic liver disease, especially cirrhosis due to alcohol, sarcoidosis
Polyclonal increase in IgM	Infections, SLE, rheumatoid arthritis, Hodgkin's disease, monocytic leukaemia, chronic liver disease, especially primary biliary cirrhosis
Polyclonal increase in IgE	Atopic disease, especially eczema, Hodgkin's disease, chronic liver disease, parasitic infections, immunodeficiency (Job's syndrome)
Reduction of IgG, IgA and IgM	Bence Jones myeloma, burns, acute severe infections (bacterial, viral, e.g. EBV, CMV, HIV), primary immunodeficiency (common variable, immunodeficiency, SCID) immunosuppressive drugs, plasmapheresis
Reduction of IgG and IgA	Nephrotic syndrome, protein-losing enteropathy, Waldenström's macroglobulinaemia (raised IgM), primary immunodeficiency (hyper-IgM syndrome)
Reduction/absence of IgA	Selective IgA deficency (N.B.: IgG subclasses may also be reduced with normal IgG)
Absence of IgG, IgA and IgM	X-linked agammaglobulinaemia

SLE, Systemic lupus erythematosus; HIV, human immunodeficiency virus, TB, tuberculosis; EBV, Epstein–Barr virus; CMV, cytomegalovirus; SCID, severe combined immunodeficiency.

Detection of immunoglobulin light chains in the **urine** does not automatically indicate the presence of myeloma. In elderly patients, those with **renal tubular damage** and those with chronic infections or inflammation, polyclonal free light chains of both κ and λ types may be present. Detection of monoclonal light chains is always significant, and their presence in a myeloma represents a risk factor for renal damage.

Detection of immunoglobulins in the **cerebrospinal fluid (CSF)** has become an important part of the diagnostic process in **multiple sclerosis (MS)**. Examination of CSF and serum in parallel, with measurements of (**IgG**) and **albumin**, enables one to determine whether there is breakdown of the blood–brain barrier and whether there is intrathecal oligoclonal IgG synthesis, which is a feature of MS. The technique is not specific, as other conditions, such as neurosyphilis, neurosarcoidosis, subacute sclerosing panencephalitis (SSPE due to measles virus) and encephalitis are all associated with oligoclonal IgG bands on CSF electrophoresis.

Immunoglobulin E

IgE is the mediator of **type I allergic reactions** (see Chapter 9). Levels of total IgE are highly variable and correlate poorly with symptoms. Very high serum levels are seen in **atopic eczema, parasitic infections, lymphomas** and **liver disease**. Using sensitive techniques it is possible to demonstrate allergen-specific IgE against a wide range of allergens *in vitro* (radioallergosorbent tests or **RAST tests**). However, these tests are **expensive**. **Skin prick testing**, looking for **wheal and flare responses**, is cheaper and gives equivalent information. Skin testing is simple but some experience is required to obtain reproducible results. RAST testing should be restricted to cases where skin testing would be dangerous (e.g. investigation of an anaphylactic response) or difficult to perform (e.g. small children, extensive skin disease or need to continue on antihistamines).

Cryoglobulins

Cryoglobulins are **abnormal immunoglobulins** which **precipitate** from solution as the **temperature is reduced**. The temperature at which this occurs determines whether symptoms result from this. Small quantities of cryoglobulins with very low precipitation temperatures may often be found in healthy persons and are of no significance.

The cryoglobulin may be purified and the purified protein may then be quantitated and analysed. Cryoglobulins are classified into three types depending on the constituents (Table 3.4). To detect a cryoglobulin, a **clotted blood** sample must be transported to the laboratory at body temperature; if the sample cools, the cryoglobulin precipitates out and is lost in the clot. **Cryoglobulins must be distinguished from cold agglutinins.**

Precipitins

Serum precipitins (**IgG antibodies**) are valuable in the diagnosis of **type III reactions** (**immune complex-mediated**; see Chapter 9), such as **farmer's lung** and **bird fancier's lung**. In the former, IgG antibodies are formed against inhaled **thermophilic fungi** (*Aspergillus*, Thermoactinomyces and Micropolyspora); in the latter, antibodies are formed against **avian serum proteins**.

Table 3.4 Classification of cryoglobulins.

Classification	Composition	Associations
Type I	Monoclonal immunoglobulin (IgG, IgA, IgM, rarely Bence Jones proteins–free light chain)	Myeloma Waldenström's macroglobulinaemia, CLL
Type II	Monoclonal immunoglobulin with rheumatoid factor activity binding polyclonal immunoglobulin and complement (C_4 low)	As for type I plus rheumatoid arthritis, Sjögren's syndrome, mixed essential cryoglobulinaemia
Type III	Polyclonal rheumatoid factors (all immunoglobulin isotypes) binding polyclonal immunoglobulin	Autoimmune diseases, viral infections (EBV, CMV, HBV) bacterial infections, chronic (infective endocarditis)

CLL, Chronic lymphocytic leukaemia; EBV, Epstein–Barr virus; CMV, cytomegalovirus; HBV, hepatitis B virus.

Precipitins against *Aspergillus* are also detected in **bronchopulmonary aspergillosis**, often together with specific **IgE** to *Aspergillus*; multiple precipitins against *Aspergillus* will be detected when a mycetoma (fungal ball, usually in an old tuberculous cavity) has formed. Antibodies against *Candida* and *Nocardia* may be helpful diagnostically in immunocompromised patients.

Complement

The complement system is an integral part of the **specific** and **non-specific defence** mechanisms. It comprises the **classical pathway**, involved in complement activation via specific antibody bound to antigen (C_1, C_2, C_4) and the **alternate pathway**, involving activation directly by antigen (factor B, properdin). The pathways converge at the level of C_3 and then use a common lytic pathway (Fig. 3.4). Some of the components are present in sufficient quantities to be easily **measured by automated analysers** (C_{1q}, C_3, C_4 and **factor B**). In practice, sufficient information is usually obtainable from measurement of C_3 and C_4. The integrity of the lytic pathway may be tested by a functional assay of haemolysis of red blood cells; the test may be modified to look at the classical or alternate pathway. The other individual components are usually identified in functional assays, but are not easily measured in mass units.

Complement deficiencies are **rare** and usually present with recurrent infections, particularly recurrent **Neisserial meningitis**, and with atypical connective tissue diseases (see Chapters 7 and 9).

Measurement of C_3 and C_4 is of value in assessing complement activation and consumption. All the complement components are **acute-phase proteins** and their production is increased by infection or inflammation. The measured levels represent the balance between synthesis and consumption. Particular instances where complement measurement is valuable are shown in Table 3.5.

During an immunological reaction **immune complexes** are formed, comprising antibody, antigen and complement. However, measurement of circulating immune complexes is technically unreliable and the tests have no place in routine diagnosis and management. Where complement levels are normal, but a complement-consuming process is thought to be present, measurement of C_3- or C_4-breakdown products, C_{3d} or C_{4a}, is valuable, as these confirm that complement breakdown is occurring. As complement activation may occur after venesection, an ethylenediaminetetraacetic acid (EDTA) sample should be used: the EDTA binds divalent cations, Ca^{2+} and Mg^{2+}, which are required for complement activation.

C_3-**Nephritic factor** is an **autoantibody** with the property of **stabilizing** the alternate pathway C_3-**convertase** ($C_{3b}B_b$–see Fig. 3.4). This allows continuous activation of C_3. This autoantibody has a strong association with partial lipodystrophy and with type II membranoproliferative (mesangiocapillary) glomerulonephritis (**MPGN**). Characteristically, the C_3 is markedly reduced. If a patient with glomerulonephritis has a very low C_3, the **differential diagnosis** is between poststreptococcal GN and type II MPGN. However, the

Width 20 picas

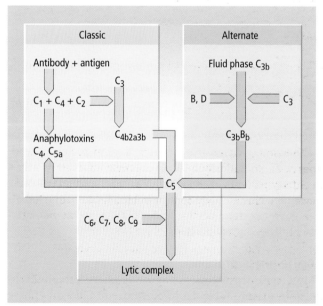

Fig 3.4

Table 3.5 Changes in serum complement levels.

Disease	C_3	C_4	C_{3d}	Measurement useful
SLE–remission	Normal	Normal/low	Normal/raised	Yes
SLE–flare	Normal/low	Normal/low	Raised	Yes
Poststreptococcal glomerulonephritis	Low	Normal	Raised	Yes
C_3-nephritic factor	Low	Normal	Raised	Yes
Infective endocarditis	Low	Low	Raised	Yes
Serious sepsis	Low	Low	Raised	No
Rheumatoid arthritis	Normal/raised	Normal/raised	Normal	No
PAN	Normal/raised	Normal/raised	Normal	No
Wegener's	Normal/raised	Normal/raised	Normal	No
Systemic sclerosis	Normal	Normal	Normal	No
Sjögren's syndrome	Normal	Normal	Normal	No
Type II cryoglobulin	Normal	Low	Normal	No

SLE, systemic lupus erythematosus; PAN, polyarteritis nodosa.

Table 3.6 Interpretation of the acute-phase response (C-reactive protein).

Normal (<0.6 mg/dl)	0.6–10 mg/dl	11–30 mg/dl
Viral infections (most)	Viral infections (especially EBV, CMV)	Moderate bacterial infections
Mild bacterial infections	*Mycoplasma/Legionella* infection	
Active SLE	Active SLE	Active SLE
Inactive Rh.A	Active Rh.A	Active Rh.A.
Inactive GCA/PMR	Active GCA/PMR	Active PMR
		Active GCA
Most tumours	Lymphoma	Lymphoma
Hypernephroma	Hypernephroma	(Rare)

EBV, Epstein–Barr virus; CMV, cytomegalovirus; SLE, Systemic lupus erythematosus; Rh.A, rheumatoid arthritis; GCA, giant cell arteritis; PMR, polymyalgia rheumatica.

C_3 in poststreptococcal GN returns to normal within 6–8 weeks, while the C_3 in MPGN remains low.

The complement control protein, **C_1-esterase inhibitor**, is either **absent** or functionally inactive in the condition of **hereditary angioedema**. Its absence leads to continual activation of the first part of the classical pathway, leading to **C_4** consumption. As C_1-esterase inhibitor is also a control protein for the kinin cascade and the clotting cascade, it is important to use blood taken into ethylenediamine tetra-acetic acid (EDTA) to avoid artefactually reduced levels.

Acute-phase proteins

Most **serum proteins** act as acute-phase proteins to a certain extent (Table 3.6). The nature of the acute-phase response is discussed in Chapter 9.

The most commonly measured acute-phase proteins are **C-reactive protein (CRP)** and **orosomucoid**. As noted above, all the complement proteins respond to acute-phase stimuli. **Fibrinogen** is also increased which contributes to the elevation of the **erythrocyte sedimentation rate (ESR)**. However, fibrinogen is a protein with a long half-life in the circulation (>1 week) and thus the ESR changes only slowly in response to therapeutic manoeuvres.

For regular monitoring, CRP is much better as it has a half-life in circulation of only 8 hours: a reduction of the acute-phase response by a therapeutic intervention will thus be manifest in 24 hours. The dynamic range of the CRP is also much greater than other acute-phase proteins. The CRP is a non-specific marker, and although given levels are associated with particular conditions (Table 3.6), there is very considerable overlap. The ESR and CRP are not interchangeable, and give different results in conditions such as SLE and myeloma (see Chapter 9).

β₂-Microglobulin

This protein is present in low concentrations in serum. It is the **light chain** of the major histocompatibility complex (MHC) class 1 molecule on the **surface** of most cells, but is also **secreted**. Its low molecular weight (c. 19 kDa) means that it is usually cleared through the kidney. In renal failure, serum levels rise dramatically and very high levels are associated with development of **dialysis amyloid**. Less dramatic elevations are seen when there is increased lymphocyte activation and turnover, such as **myeloma** and acquired immunodeficiency syndrome (**AIDS**). In these three conditions regular monitoring is a valuable adjunct to other tests.

Autoimmunity

Autoimmunity denotes the failure of the immune system to distinguish self from non-self. This failure is detectable by the presence of either humoral or cellular immunity against self-components. Mechanisms by which this abnormal response may be generated are discussed in Chapter 9.

It is easier to detect the humoral antiself response: **autoantibodies**. These may be primary (pathogenic) or secondary (not involved directly in causation of disease, but useful as markers). It is important to make this distinction as therapeutic removal of a primary antibody is likely to influence the disease process whereas removal of a secondary antibody will have no effect.

The list of documented autoantibodies is very long and continues to grow; many have not been shown to be useful for diagnosis or management. Conventionally, **autoantibodies** are divided into **organ-specific** and **non-specific**. Autoantibodies may be of any immunoglobulin isotype.

There is little evidence, except in isolated cases, to support a significant role of **IgM** autoantibodies in disease. Many infections, particularly with herpesviruses such as Epstein Barr virus and cytomegalovirus, lead to the transient production of IgM autoantibodies. The role of IgA autoantibodies is also unclear, although there is some evidence that IgA anti-endomysial antibodies are more specific in **coeliac disease** and **dermatitis herpetiformis** than IgG antibodies except where there is IgA deficiency.

In view of the wide range of autoantibody tests available it is important for the clinician to request tests appropriate to the disease being investigated: requests for 'autoantibody screens' are not greeted with much enthusiasm in the laboratory. Try and develop an algorithm of investigations appropriate to the differential diagnoses being considered (see Fig. 3.2).

Non-organ-specific antoantibodies

These are autoantibodies directed against cellular or other constituents which are not unique to one tissue. Table 3.7 lists the most commonly sought antibodies.

As Tables 3.7 and 3.8 show, there are a large number of autoantibodies directed against nuclear constituents. Only some of these have a clear role in diagnosis but others have played a significant role in cell biology in the identification of functional roles of nuclear constituents. Why some antibodies have particular disease associations, such as **anticentromere** antibodies with **CREST** (calcinosis, Raynaud's oesophageal dysmotility, syndactyly, telangiectasia) **syndrome**, is unknown.

Rheumatoid factors. Rheumatoid factors are antibodies directed against the Fc-portion of other antibody molecules. They should not be confused with anti-idiotypic antibodies, which are directed against unique determinants on the **antigen-binding region** of the immunoglobulin

Table 3.7 Non-organ-specific autoantibodies.

Autoantibody	Disease association
Homogenous antinuclear Ab	SLE, drug-induced lupus, autoimmune chronic active hepatitis, juvenile chronic arthritis
Speckled antinuclear Ab	Mixed connective tissue disease, SLE, Sjögren's syndrome, scleroderma, polymyositis
Peripheral antinuclear Ab	SLE
Nucleolar Ab	Systemic sclerosis, scleroderma
Centromere Ab	CREST syndrome (**C**alcinosis, **R**aynaud's **o**esophageal dysmotility, **S**clerodactyly, **T**elangiectasia)
Double-stranded DNA Ab	SLE, autoimmune chronic active hepatitis
Histone Ab	SLE (responsible for LE cell phenomenon) Drug-induced lupus
Ribosomal Ab	SLE
Mitochondrial Ab	Primary biliary cirrhosis, rarely autoimmune hepatitis
Smooth-muscle Ab (antiactin, antimyosin)	Autoimmune chronic active hepatitis
Liver–kidney microsomal Ab	Drug-induced hepatitis
Rheumatoid factor Ab	Rheumatoid arthritis, Sjögren's syndrome, SLE, chronic infections, paraproteins, old age

Ab, Antibody; SLE, systemic lupus erythematosus.

Table 3.8 Extractable nuclear antigens.

Antigen	Associated disease
Sm	SLE
RNP	SLE, mixed connective tissue disease
La (SS-B)	SLE, Sjögren's syndrome
Ro (SS-A)	SLE, discoid LE, neonatal lupus, ANA-negative lupus, Sjögren's syndrome
PCNA (proliferating cell nuclear antigen)	SLE
Scl-70	Systemic sclerosis
Jo-1	Polymyositis

SLE, Systemic lupus erythematosus.

molecule, Rheumatoid factors may be of any isotype, but **IgG** and **IgM** are the important ones. They represent one of the most abused and misunderstood tests in clinical immunology. They are not specific for rheumatoid arthritis but occur in a wide variety of infective and inflammatory conditions. They also occur with increasing frequency and titre in the ageing population without any evidence of involvement in disease; in the over-75s testing for them is of no value whatsoever. They have an association, when present in high titre, in a patient with **rheumatoid arthritis**, with the development of **nodules** and with **systemic rheumatoid vasculitis**. Equally, there is no correlation between disease activity and rheumatoid factor titre. Distinction between an inflammatory arthropathy and a degenerative one is best made by combining clinical acumen with measures of the acute-phase response.

Antinuclear antibodies (ANAs). ANAs are detected by immunofluorescence on frozen sections of rat liver. The pattern of immunofluorescence gives some indication of the actual specificity of the antibodies (see Fig. 3.5 and Table 3.8). As for rheumatoid factors, thee is an increasing incidence of low-titre ANAs in the elderly. Thus, in elderly a significant titre would be >1/160, in a middle-aged adult >1/80 and in a child >1/20. Positive ANAs occur in a wide variety of conditions (see Table 3.7). Where a high-titre ANA is identified, an assay for **DNA-binding antibodies** should be performed. In systemic lupus erythematosus (SLE), there may be high-titre antibodies to double-stranded DNA (dsDNA): such antibodies are found in SLE and rarely in lupoid hepatitis. In contrast, other connective tissue disorders, drug-induced lupus (procainamide, hydralazine) and viral infections all give rise to antibodies directed against single-stranded DNA (ssDNA). As the clinical manifestations may overlap but the prognoses are significantly different, it is important to identify patients with antibodies to dsDNA. Serial

measurements of either ANA or DNA-binding antibodies are not helpful in monitoring disease activity in SLE due to the long circulating half-life of IgG (3 weeks).

Ro antibody. Some patients with clinical SLE are ANA-negative when their serum is tested against rat liver. This is because they have an antibody against a **saline-soluble antigen (SS-A)**, present in the nucleus, called **Ro**. This antigen is lost during processing of the liver. This antibody may be demonstrated by using an alternative tissue substrate for ANA testing. The most versatile substrate is the **HEp-2 cell line**. This has a large nucleus and contains large amounts of Ro antigen. Thus ANA-negative SLE sera often show positive nuclear staining, with a fine speckled pattern against HEp-2 cells. The specificity of the staining may be demonstrated by countercurrent immunoelectrophoresis. In this technique antigen, extracted from a source rich in Ro antigen such as human

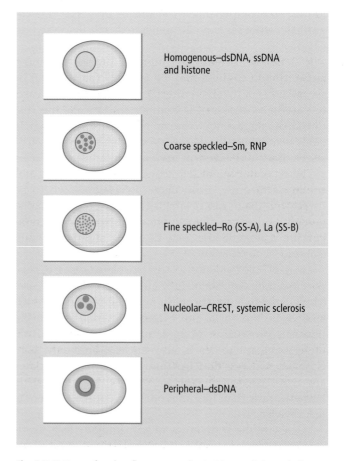

Fig. 3.5 Patterns of nuclear fluorescence. ds, double-stranded; ss, single-stranded; ANA, anti-nuclear antibody; RNP, nuclear ribonucleic acid; Ro, antibody against a saline soluble antigen SS-A; La, SS-B; Sm, Smith; CREST, calcinosis, Raynaud's, oesophageal dysmotility, syndactyly, telangiectasia syndrome.

spleen, is forced towards antibody in sparate well by an electric field. Where antigen and antibody combine a precipitate is formed which can be stained. Using this technique, but substituting a saline extract of rabbit thymus or purified antigens, other autoantibodies can be detected (see Table 3.8). Antibody to Ro is important in pregnancy as the antibody crosses the placenta and may cause **neonatal lupus** or, more seriously, may damage the fetal cardiac conducting system, causing **congenital heart block**.

Anticardiolipin antibodies. Anticardiolipin antibodies have attracted a great deal of attention. These are antibodies directed against phospholipids and were first recognized as **false-positive** Venereal Disease Research Laboratory (VDRLs) in patients with connective tissue diseases, as the antigen in the VDRL test is very similar to **cardiolipin**. These antibodies include the lupus anticoagulant, an antibody that interferes with *in vitro* **clotting** tests. The two tests do not, however, measure the same antibody, as some patients will be positive for one but not the other and vice versa.

Organ-specific autoantibodies

Organ-specific antibodies are autoantibodies directed against specific target organs. They may be **primary**, that is with a functional effect on the tissue, such as thyroid-stimulating or blocking antibodies, or **secondary**, marker antibodies, such as parathyroid antibodies. Table 3.9 covers the most commonly sought autoantibodies, together with an indication of their value in diagnosis and management.

Autoantibodies are most easily detected by immunofluorescence using the appropriate tissue substrate, but some, such as antibodies to thyroid antigens, are detected by **haemagglutination assays**.

Antineutrophil cytoplasmic antibody (ANCA). A new acquisition in the repertoire of organ-specific autoantibodies is antibody directed against neutrophil cytoplasmic granules. This antibody, best detected at present by immunofluorescence on purified human neutrophils, has been shown to be a specific test for Wegener's granulomatosis and microscopic polyarteritis nodosa (see Chapters 7 and 9).

Investigation of cellular and functional immunity

Investigation of cellular and functional immunity is of importance in the diagnosis of primary and secondary immunodeficiencies. While the number of patients with a major primary immune deficiency is small, there is an

Table 3.9 Organ-specific autoantibodies.

Autoantibody	Disease association
Gastric parietal cell Ab	Pernicious anaemia
Intrinsic factor Ab	Pernicious anaemia
Thyroid microsomal Ab	Graves disease, Hashimoto's thyroiditis, autoimmune hypothyroidism
Thyroglobulin Ab	As above
Steroid cell Ab	Addison's disease, primary ovarian failure
Adrenal cell Ab	Addison's disease
Parathyroid Ab	Autoimmune hyperparathyroidism
Pancreatic islet cell Ab	Type I diabetes mellitus
Acetylcholine receptor Ab	Myasthenia gravis
Striated muscle Ab	Myasthenia gravis and thymoma
Cardiac muscle Ab	Cardiomyopathy
Glomerular basement membrane Ab	Goodpasture's syndrome, glomerulonephritis
Neutrophil cytoplasmic granule Ab	Wegener's granulomatosis, microscopic polyarteritis

Ab, Antibody.

increasing realization that larger numbers of patients suffer from less severe and previously uncharacterized reductions in the efficiency of the immune system (see Chapter 10).

The number of primary immune deficiencies are outweighed by secondary immune deficiencies, such as in lymphoproliferative disorders, viral infections (human immunodeficiency virus or HIV) and iatrogenic (immunosuppressive therapy).

Cellular studies

The simplest cellular studies are the enumeration of cell populations. The discovery of the technique for generating monoclonal antibodies of defined specificity by Kohler and Milstein in 1976 revolutionized this aspect of immunology. Monoclonal antibodies against almost any cell are available and can be used on tissue sections, either frozen or paraffin-embedded, or on cell suspensions (see Chapter 1). Another significant technical advance was the development of flow cytometry, a technique for continuous analysis of cells labelled with fluorescent markers.

The combination of these techniques means that routine monitoring of T-cell subpopulations (CD4, T-helper cells and CD8, T-cytotoxic cells) in HIV-infected patients is practicable and sufficiently accurate to be used as a guide to therapy. Present flow cytometers are now accurate enough to be able to identify minimal residual leukaemic cells in bone marrow aspirates. On tissue sections, the use of monoclonal antibodies has significantly increased the diagnostic accuracy of lymphoma typing (see Chapter 16).

Less well-standardized methods are *in vitro* tests of lymphocyte function. In the investigation of patients thought to have **severe combined immune deficiency (SCID**; see Chapter 10), T lymphocytes may be present but non-functional. This may be demonstrated by stimulating the cells with antigen or a **mitogen** (a plant-derived substance reactive with surface components of human cells that causes the cells to multiply) and measuring the degree of cellular proliferation by ^{3}H-thymidine uptake. Similar studies may be undertaken on **B lymphocytes**, measuring the production of immunoglobulin. These tests are difficult to standardize and are therefore performed in specialized centres.

Neutrophils and **monocytes** may equally be functionally inadequate. Tests available include the simple nitroblue tetrazolium (NBT) test. This is a test of the ability of the neutrophil to generate a respiratory burst: the colourless NBT is taken up into neutrophils, which then reduce it to the insoluble blue formazan when stimulated by a mitogen or antigen (zymosan). The blue granules inside the cell may be counted. A negative NBT test is a feature of **chronic granulomatous disease**.

Other investigations include tests of cellular chemotaxis and mobility, of phagocytosis and bactericidal activity. Monoclonal antibodies are available against neutrophil antigens and absence of one antigen (lymphocyte function antigen (LFA)-1, CD11a/CD18, a cellular adhesion molecule) has been associated with a severe immunodeficiency.

Functional studies

In vivo tests of **immune function** provide much useful information. The functional integrity of the humoral immune system may easily be tested by measuring the antibody response to common pathogens and immunizing agents: this requires a comprehensive immunization and infection history. Absence of antibodies to confirmed infections or known immunizations is highly significant and indicates a humoral immune defect. This may be further confirmed by demonstrating the absence of any response to a specific test-immunization. In practice the antibodies most commonly sought are those to tetanus, polio (vaccine strain), diphtheria, measles, rubella, pneumococcal polysaccharide and *Haemophilus influenzae* type b polysaccharide.

Similarly, it is possible to assess cell-mediated immunity by **skin testing**. Antigens used include tuberculin *Candida* and tetanus. As this is testing the cell-mediated response (type IV reaction; see Chapter 9), any immediate

reactions are ignored, and the sites are read at 48–72 hours when the cellular infiltrate is maximum. In a strong reaction this may be felt as a lentil-sized lump under the skin, with erythema.

Similarly, type IV reactions are involved in **contact hypersensitivity**, and these can be documented by **patch testing**. This is performed by placing the test substance on the skin of the back under an occlusive dressing for 48 hours. The site is then inspected for erythema and cellular infiltrate at 96 hours.

Neutrophil function can be assessed *in vivo* using the **Rebuck skin window technique**, although this is rarely done these days. The skin is abraded and a glass cover-slip is taped to the skin. The cover-slip is replaced at intervals and stained for adherent cells. This is a simple test of chemotaxis, motility and adherence.

Tissue typing

Tissue typing has assumed an increasing importance with the expansion of transplantation programmes. Tissue typing is the process of identifying surface antigens involved in self–non-self discrimination.

The surface molecules which play the major (but not exclusive) role in this process are the **MHC antigens**. These are divided into class I antigens, which are encoded by three loci, A–C and class II, encoded by at least three loci, the major ones being DR, DP and DQ (Fig. 3.6).

Class I antigens are expressed on almost every cell in the body, but **class II antigens** are limited to lymphocytes, antigen-presenting cells (macrophages) and certain other tissues when an appropriate cytokine stimulus is applied (this includes vascular endothelium and thyrocytes).

Transplantation of tissue mismatched for MHC antigens will lead to activation of host lymphocytes, with both humoral and a cytotoxic cellular response to the graft. The graft will be destroyed. If a further graft with the same MHC type is given to the host, immunological memory ensures that the rejection is much more rapid (**hyperacute rejection**).

It is therefore important to ensure that grafts are **matched** as far as possible for MHC. For class I antigens this is relatively easy as antisera are readily available and cells may be typed by microcytotoxicity. This process can be automated. Class II antigens have traditionally been identified by using cells cytotoxic for known D antigens, but antisera are now available for most specificities, enabling the **microcytotoxicity** test to be used. Typing for class II antigens is more difficult, as the B lymphocytes must be isolated: this is usually performed by mixing the cells with treated sheep red blood cells to which the T

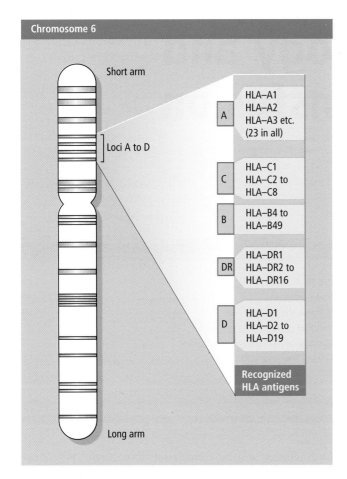

Chromosome 6

Short arm

Loci A to D

| A | HLA–A1
HLA–A2
HLA–A3 etc.
(23 in all) |

| C | HLA–C1
HLA–C2 to
HLA–C8 |

| B | HLA–B4 to
HLA–B49 |

| DR | HLA–DR1
HLA–DR2 to
HLA–DR16 |

| D | HLA–D1
HLA–D2 to
HLA–D19 |

Recognized HLA antigens

Long arm

Fig. 3.6 Chromosome 6. HLA genes and antigens (major histocompatiblity complex–MHC).

cells, but not the B cells, have a receptor. As well as typing donor and recipient cells, the recipient's serum will also be screened for the presence of preformed anti-MHC antibodies. Genetic tests are now beginning to supersede functional assays in HLA typing.

In circumstances where the match between donor and recipient is incomplete or there is a positive mixed lymphocyte reaction (MLR), additional immunosuppression may be required to damp down the host response. In bone marrow transplantation it is the donor cells that are immunologically active, and if there is a mismatch, graft-versus-host disease results. This may be beneficial in leukaemia, as there is a graft-versus-leukaemia effect.

Use of the clinical immunology laboratory

The multiplicity of tests available through the immunology laboratory makes it imperative that tests are selected with care. Many of the tests are not suitable for automation and are performed manually. Tests should be requested with care, considering whether useful information will be obtained from the answer. Nothing irritates laboratory staff more than being presented with requests for 'autoantibodies' (23 easily available in Oxford!) or 'RAST tests' (over 70 tests available!). More than for other specialties, **requests must give sensible clinical details**. Where the immunology laboratory has its own medical immunologists, they will interpret the test results on the basis of the **clinical information** given; if it is wrong, then the interpretation will also be wrong. Do not be afraid to ask the laboratory staff for advice.

Future directions

There is a continual process of technological advance, both in the assays themselves and in the equipment to perform them. We are now able to define more subtle immune defects. New tests such as ANCA have been developed so that we have a marker for a disease that lacked one previously. Tests for **circulating cytokines** and their receptors are now being tested and some will become routine within the next few years.

FURTHER READING

Roitt I. (1994) *Essential Immunology*, 8th edn. Blackwell Scientific Publications, Oxford.

Mitchinson M.J. *et al.* (1996) *Essentials of Pathology*, Chapters 3–5. Blackwell Science, Oxford.

Haematology and Blood Transfusion

C O N T E N T S

INTRODUCTION

The specialty of haematology and blood transfusion concerns itself with the diagnosis and treatment of diseases of the blood and bone marrow. Haematologists will often have postgraduate training in general medicine and will have their own hospital beds to care for their patients (Fig. 4.1).

In this section, the value of the haematology laboratory to clinicians will be considered. Discussion of haematological diseases is deferred to Chapter 12, and many points raised in the present chapter will be discussed in more detail later.

CLINICAL ASPECTS OF HAEMATOLOGY

The full blood count

The indications for the blood count are so wide that they are impossible to list. Suffice it to say the investigation is so cheap (< £5) and can be so informative that virtually all patients who appear ill, including most admissions to hospital, should have one.

The blood count provides information on the numbers and characteristics of circulating blood cells (Fig. 4.2) produced by the bone marrow (Table 4.1).

Anaemia

If the **haemoglobin is low**, the patient is said to be anaemic. Interpretation of an anaemia should be modified in light of the **clinical details**.

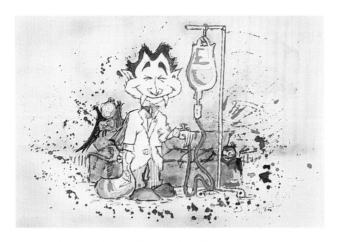

Fig. 4.1 The role of the clinical haematologist (from an original, courtesy Dr Rachel Armstrong).

However, attention should first be directed to the **mean cell volume (MCV)**. If **low**, the patient is said to have a **microcytic anaemia**. Much the commonest cause of this is iron deficiency; in this case the red blood cell concentration (RBC), mean cell haemoglobin (MCH) and mean cell haemoglobin concentration (MCHC) are usually low. It is most commonly caused by chronic blood loss, usually menstruation or pregnancy.

If the RBC is high and the MCHC normal, then thalassaemia (see Chapter 12) should be considered, especially if the patient is not of Northern European extraction. If the MCV is **high** the patient is said to have a **macrocytic anaemia**. The commonest cause of a macrocytosis in Europe is chronic excess alcohol intake or hepatic dysfunction. Other important causes of macrocytosis are vitamin

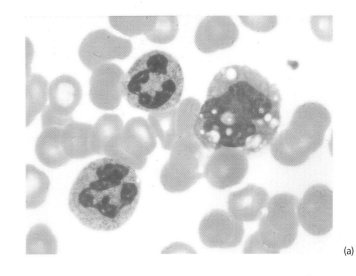

(a)

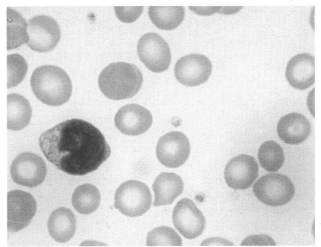

(b)

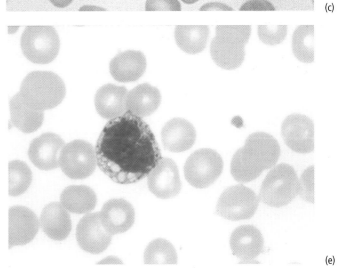

(c)

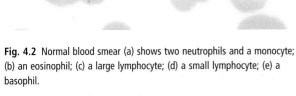

(d)

(e)

Fig. 4.2 Normal blood smear (a) shows two neutrophils and a monocyte; (b) an eosinophil; (c) a large lymphocyte; (d) a small lymphocyte; (e) a basophil.

Table 4.1 The full blood count.

Parameter	Abbreviation	Normal range	Unit
Haemoglobin	Hb	Male 13.0–18.0	g/dl
		Female 11.6–16.4	g/dl
Haematocrit	Hct	Male 0.40–0.54	
		Female 0.37–0.47	
Mean cell volume	MCV	78–100	fl
Mean cell haemoglobin	MCH	27–32	pg
Mean cell haemoglobin concentration	MCHC	31–35	g/dl
Red cell concentration	RBC	Male 4.5–6.5	$10^{12}/l$
		Female 3.8–5.8	$10^{12}/l$
Reticulocyte concentration	Retics	< 2	%
Platelet concentration	plts	150–400	$10^9/l$
White cell concentration	WBC	4–11	$10^9/l$
Neutrophil concentration		2.5–7.5	$10^9/l$
Lymphocyte concentration		1.5–3.5	$10^9/l$
Monocyte concentration		0.2–0.8	$10^9/l$
Eosinophil concentration		0.04–0.4	$10^9/l$
Basophil concentration		0.01–0.1	$10^9/l$

B_{12} or folate deficiency (see Chapter 12), hypothyroidism and some drugs, especially antimetabolites and phenytoin. If all of these causes can be excluded then the patient may well have a primary bone marrow disorder (see Chapter 12).

If the MCV is normal, especially if the MCHC is also normal, then the anaemia of chronic inflammation (e.g. infection, malignancy) or renal failure should be considered. An alternative method of considering anaemia is to request a **reticulocyte count**. These young red cells reflect marrow activity, so if they are few in number, marrow failure is implied. Conversely, if they are numerous then excess red cell destruction (haemolysis), blood loss or a recent response, for example, to iron, is implied. Note that reticulocytes are large cells and so may increase the MCV.

The commonest cause of too many red cells, termed **polycythaemia**, is dehydration. Other causes are considered in Chapter 12.

White cells

Polymorphs

The term **polymorph** is an abbreviation of polymorphonuclear leucocyte and refers to the multiple nuclear lobes characteristic of these cells. 'Granulocyte' is synonymous with 'polymorph'.

The maturation sequence of granulocytes (Fig. 4.3) involves the progressive shrinkage, condensation and folding of the nucleus, resulting in the characteristic lobulated nuclear profile seen in mature granulocytes. Simultaneously, the cytoplasm acquires numerous lysosomal granules, containing microbicidal and other proteins, e.g. myeloperoxidase, lactoferrin, elastase. When granulocytes ingest bacteria or other material, these granules fuse with the wall of the phagocytic vacuoles and release their contents into the lumina of these vacuoles. When challenged with infection, the size and number of granules increase (**toxic granulation**).

Normally only mature polymorphs are seen in the circulation. Under conditions of marrow stress, e.g. severe infection, a few late precursors (**metamyelocytes**) may be seen in the peripheral blood (**left shift**). However, the appearance of large numbers of these cells is abnormal and may indicate **myeloid leukaemia**, as would the finding of early myeloid cells (**myeloblasts**).

The majority of polymorphs are **neutrophils** (their cytoplasmic granules do not stain with either acidic or basic dyes), whose lifespan is about 1 day. Their function is phagocytosis and killing of micro-organisms. **Neutrophilia** is a common finding in bacterial infections, although overwhelming infections, certain non-pyogenic infections (e.g. typhoid) and many viral infections may cause **neutropenia**.

Eosinophils contain prominent granules which stain golden-red with routine haematological stains. Eosinophilia is associated with allergic states, e.g. atopy, drug allergies and parasitic infections.

The frequency of basophils in the peripheral blood is low; changes in the basophil count are rarely significant.

Monocytes

Monocytes leave the marrow, circulate in the blood for a few days, then migrate to the tissues where they mature into tissue histiocytes and macrophages (e.g. Kupffer cells in the liver, alveolar macrophages in the lung, etc.). They have an important role in presentation of antigen to the immune system. Their numbers may be increased in conditions in which histiocytes accumulate, e.g. granulomatous disorders such as sarcoidosis or tuberculosis.

Lymphocytes

Most blood lymphocytes are long-lived cells which appear in the circulation when they migrate from one lymphoid tissue to another. The majority (approximately 75%) are **T cells**, most of the remainder being B cells.

Peripheral T cells can be subdivided into **helper/inducer** (CD4-positive) T cells and **cytotoxic/suppressor** (CD8-positive) populations, which are present in an approximately 2:1 ratio. This ratio may change in some diseases, e.g. acquired immunodeficiency syndrome

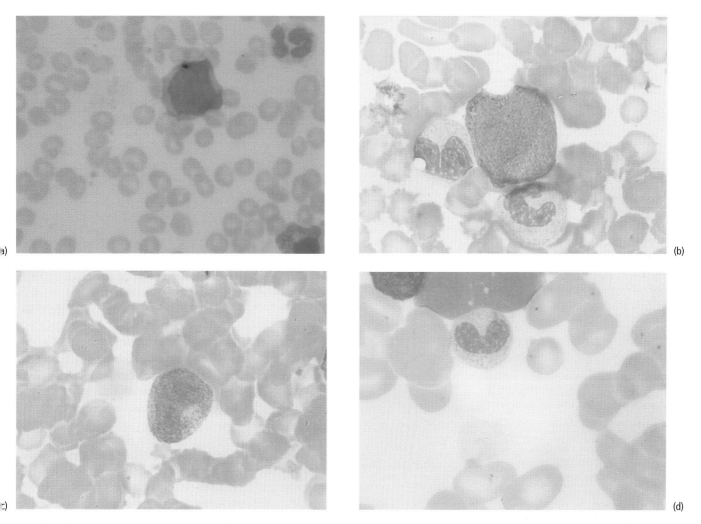

(a)

(b)

(c)

(d)

Fig. 4.3 Myeloid maturation. The maturation sequence is shown as (a centre) blast; (b centre) promyelocyte; (c) myelocyte; (d) metamyelocyte; (a top left) neutrophil.

(AIDS), in which depletion of CD4-positive T cells causes a reversal of the ratio.

One of the commonest disorders of lymphocytes is glandular fever or **infectious mononucleosis**, a primary infection of B lymphocytes by **Epstein–Barr virus** (EBV). This leads to B-cell proliferation and to an exuberant T-cell response. Large numbers of atypical lymphoid T cells (referred to as **mononuclear** cells to distinguish them from polymorphs) appear in the blood (Fig. 4.4). Clinically the patient suffers from severe tonsillitis, generalized lymphadenopathy and some degree of splenomegaly. Agglutinating antibodies specific for animal red cells (heterophile antibodies) appear in the blood and form the basis of the diagnostic **Paul–Bunnell** test (known more commonly by its commercial name, the **Monospot** test).

Platelets

Platelets (see the small cellular fragments in Fig. 4.2(b)&(c)) are produced from **megakaryocytes** in the bone marrow and play an important role in arresting bleeding by the formation of a haemostatic platelet plug. Their lifespan is about 7 days.

The commonest clinical disorder of platelets is **thrombocytopenia**, due either to failure of production or to accelerated destruction. The commonest causes are excess alcohol or an autoantibody (immune thrombocytopenic purpura). A high platelet count is usually caused by an inflammatory response, especially in children, or to an abscess.

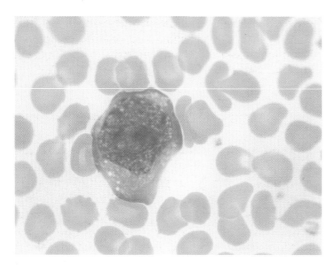

Fig. 4.4 An atypical lymphocyte, note the large size, primitive nucleus, basophilic cytoplasm and stickiness to red cells.

Bone marrow sampling (Table 4.2)

Table 4.2 Indications for bone marrow sampling.

Investigation of pancytopenia (aplasia versus infiltration)
Investigation of unexplained anaemia
Investigation of thrombocytopenia
Diagnosis and monitoring of leukaemia and myeloproliferative disorders
Diagnosis of myeloma or carcinomatous infiltration
Staging of lymphoma

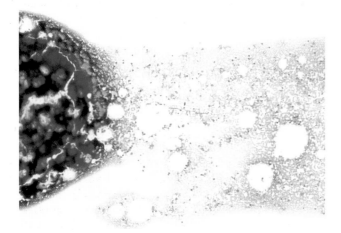

Fig. 4.5 Appearances of a bone marrow aspirate. Note the particle of bone marrow at the end of the smear, the heterogeneous composition of the marrow cells, which spread out behind the particles as the smear is made. Individual cells can be examined in detail.

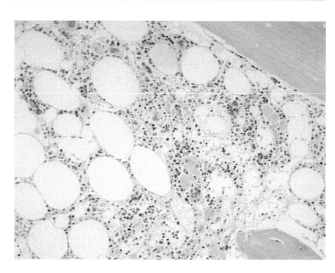

Fig. 4.6 Trephine biopsy of bone marrow. Note the typical mixture of fat spaces and haemopoietic marrow seen in a normal sample. Note the bone trabeculum at the top right of the field. The large cells are megakaryocytes.

Methods of bone marrow sampling

Aspiration. Marrow may be aspirated from a variety of sites, most commonly the **sternum** or **iliac crest**. The marrow is smeared directly on to a microscope slide (in a similar way to the technique for making blood films; Fig. 4.5).

Trephine biopsy. Occasionally attempts to aspirate bone marrow are unsuccessful (**dry tap**). This is most frequently due to **marrow fibrosis**, e.g. myelofibrosis, secondary carcinoma. A marrow sample may then be obtained by taking a core of bone marrow via a trephine needle (usually from the **posterior iliac crest**). This sample is then examined **histologically** (Fig. 4.6).

CLINICAL ASPECTS OF BLOOD TRANSFUSION

Red cell transfusion (Table 4.3)

Table 4.3 Red cell transfusion.

Units of red cells: 450 ml whole blood, 280 ml packed cells

Shelf-life 35 days

With storage, the pH falls, the plasma K^+ increases and the red cell 2,3-diphosphoglycerate falls

In whole blood, the concentration of some clotting factors falls rapidly to almost zero over several days, so fresh frozen plasma may be needed to correct clotting factor deficiencies

This is a commonly used procedure to correct anaemia. Red cell products available from the blood bank include **whole blood**, but the majority of issues are **packed red cells** which may be resuspended in various additive solutions. Some neonatal units prefer not to use additive solutions. The majority of anaemic patients lack only red cells. Therefore, transfuse red cells only and not whole blood.

The plasma removed from these units goes to make fresh frozen plasma (FFP), albumin solution, factor VIII, etc. Whole blood, particularly fresh whole blood, may be useful for actively bleeding patients, and some surgeons (cardiac) like fresh whole blood to use peroperatively. In addition, fresh whole blood is sometimes supplied to neonatal units.

Cross-matching

Most simply means taking a sample of patient serum, incubating it with a sample of red cells from a unit of blood and looking for the presence of red cell clumping (**agglutination**). Of course, the patient's blood group is determined initially and also the patient's serum screened for the presence of **alloantibodies**, i.e. antibodies against red cell antigens not possessed by the patient and which could cause a haemolytic transfusion reaction. The intricacies of blood grouping are beyond the scope of this book. However, one should have a basic understanding of the ABO and rhesus blood group systems (Table 4.4).

Table 4.4 Blood group systems.

Blood group	A	B	AB	O
Antigen on red cells	A	B	A,B	O
Antibody in plasma	Anti-B	Anti-A	O	Anti-A, B
Frequency in UK (%)	42	8	3	47

ABO antibodies are present from a few months after birth, presumably stimulated by bacterial antigens. These antibodies are immunoglobulin M (**IgM**) and fix complement so that only a few millilitres of mismatched blood can be enough to kill. In contrast, most **rhesus antibodies** are caused by exposure to foreign blood (transfusion or pregnancy), are immunoglobulin G (IgG) and usually cause only a less serious delayed haemolytic transfusion reaction. Their main importance lies in their ability to cross the placenta in the 15% of UK women who are rhesus D-negative and cause haemolytic disease of the newborn in rhesus D-positive offspring.

Full grouping, antibody screening and cross-matching take around 1 hour. There is time for this in the majority of patients; emergency use of uncross-matched blood should be kept to a minimum. If possible, a sample of blood for cross-matching should arrive in the laboratory at least 24 hours before blood is required. This helps the laboratory plan its work.

Complications of red cell transfusion

Early (usually during transfusion)

1 Febrile reactions (non-haemolytic febrile transfusion reactions – NHFTR): these are common, particularly in previously transfused or previously pregnant patients. They are due to recipient human leukocyte antigen (HLA) antibodies directed against leukocytes contaminating the transfused red cells. These are usually **mild** reactions and treatment involves administration of **hydrocortisone** and slowing the rate of transfusion. More severe reactions cause **rigors**. Occasionally reactions are severe enough to raise the question of a haemolytic reaction (see later) and in these circumstances the transfusion should be stopped. For patients with NHFTR which cannot be controlled or prevented, even by prophylactic use of hydrocortisone, leukocyte-depleted blood can be given through a filter.

2 Urticaria: this is a common event due to antibodies in recipient plasma against donor plasma proteins. It can usually be treated satisfactorily with antihistamines, e.g. chlorpheniramine.

3 Pulmonary oedema: this is due to an excessive rate of blood transfusion, particularly in the elderly. Treat by slowing or stopping the transfusion and giving diuretics. The usual rate of blood transfusion is 3–4 hours per unit in a euvolaemic patient.

4 Haemolytic transfusion reaction: in contrast to the preceding three complications, which are common and not usually life-threatening, this is rare but may be fatal. It is usually due to a major ABO incompatability (e.g. giving group A blood to a group O recipient). Occasionally, non-ABO antibodies (e.g. rhesus) are implicated. Most severe transfusion reactions are not due to incorrect blood being issued from the laboratory, but are due to an administrative error at some point between taking the blood sample and administering the unit. Remember that **correct labelling** of the sample and the cross-match form is absolutely essential.

A patient given an incompatible transfusion may develop dyspnoea chest and back pain, fever, hypotension and haemoglobinuria. Major complications include **renal failure** and **disseminated intravascular coagulation** (DIC). If you suspect a haemolytic transfusion, the first action is to stop the transfusion. The next thing to do is to ask for help. Then you should promote a diuresis but monitor urine output. Do not pour fluid into a patient already in acute renal failure. Blood can be taken for full blood count (FBC) direct Coombs test to detect antibody on the red cell surface, clotting screen, biochemistry and serology and the suspected unit of blood returned to blood bank. The above investigations will help establish the diagnosis.

Late complications

1 Delayed haemolytic transfusion reaction: this complication is uncommon but may be underdiagnosed. It occurs when a low-titre antibody (e.g. anti-Fy^a) in the serum of a recipient is not detected by the laboratory and red cells carrying the appropriate antigen (Fy^a) are transfused. Five to 14 days posttransfusion, a secondary rise in the antibody titre occurs, haemolysis follows and the patient develops jaundice, fever and a fall in haemoglobin concentration. It is rarely a severe reaction, but if suspected investigation is essential and should be discussed with the hospital blood bank.

2 Posttransfusion purpura: this may **rarely** occur in the 2% of patients who lack the human platelet antigen HPA-1 (old name P1^{A1}). If they are transfused with blood (containing platelets which are HPA-1-positive) an antibody (anti-HPA-1) is formed and severe thrombocytopenia may result analogously to a delayed haemolytic transfusion reaction. The mechanism of thrombocytopenia is unclear as the recipient platelets are, of course, HPA-1-negative. The clinical features are of bruising and petechiae occurring 5–14 days after a transfusion. The thrombocytopenia is short-lived, usually less than a month; treatment with immunoglobulin may hasten recovery.

3 Transmission of infectious agents (human immunodeficiency virus (HIV), hepatitis B and C, cytomegalovirus, etc.) is an uncommon but serious risk of blood transfusion.

4 Iron overload is a complication seen in heavily transfused patients. Each unit of red cells contains approximately 0.2 g of iron.

The normal body stores of iron are 3.0–4.5 g and around 1 mg/day is lost by excretion. In a patient who is not bleeding but receiving regular transfusions, symptoms of iron overload (cardiac failure, endocrine dysfunction, cirrhosis) may develop, usually after 50–100 units have been given. Iron stores can be estimated by measurement of **serum ferritin**. **Iron chelation** (with desferrioxamine) is effective in patients at risk of iron overload.

Massive transfusion

This is loosely defined as the transfusion of a volume of blood greater than the patient's normal blood volume in a short period of time, i.e. minutes or hours.

Complications of massive transfusion include the following.

1 DIC: often caused partly by the underlying process which is responsible for the patient requiring transfusion.

2 Dilutional thrombocytopenia: surprisingly, platelet counts between 50–100 $\times$ 10^9/l are typical and platelet transfusions are usually not needed.

3 Dilution of coagulation factors: FFP may be required but should be given when necessary clinically, as monitored by clotting tests and not as a routine.

4 Fall in 2,3-diphosphoglycerate (2,3-DPG) levels: levels will recover within 24 hours of transfusion. Low 2,3-DPG levels are associated with a left shifted oxygen dissociation curve and relatively poor oxygenation of the tissues. This does not seem to cause clinical problems.

5 Acid–base/electrolyte disturbance: a metabolic alkalosis may occur as a result of massive transfusion. Again, this does not seem to cause clinical problems. **Hypocalcaemia** from citrate anticoagulant sometimes needs correction intravenously.

Plasma transfusion

1 FFP: this is obtained by separating and freezing plasma at −30°C from a donor unit of blood. After thawing, the plasma should be used within 6 hours and preferably within 2 hours to prevent deterioration of the clotting factors. The plasma should be ABO-compatible with the patient blood group, but does not require cross-matching. FFP may be used to correct coagulation deficiencies in patients with liver disease, DIC, after massive red cell transfusion and occasionally in patients with an excess effect from warfarin. FFP may transmit infection.

2 Human albumin solution (HAS): more commonly referred to as albumin or an older name, plasma protein fraction (PPF).

Two preparations are available:
- 4.5% 500 ml 40–50 g albumin/l;
- 20% 100 ml 150–250 g albumin/l.

Albumin is indicated in patients with burns who rapidly lose albumin and in the short-term management of hypoalbuminaemic patients with oedema where diuretics have failed (e.g. liver disease, nephrotic syndrome).

Platelet transfusion

Platelet transfusion is indicated in **thrombocytopenic** patients who have symptoms or signs of bleeding. They may also be appropriate in selected patients with normal platelet, counts but where platelet function is impaired, e.g. myeloproliferative disorders. Platelet transfusion is not usually indicated in patients with immune thrombocytopenia.

HAEMOSTASIS

Normal haemostasis

When a blood vessel wall is injured, the following haemostatic mechanisms are brought into play;
1 local vasoconstriction;
2 local aggregation of platelets to form a haemostatic plug;
3 activation of the clotting cascade to form a local thrombus;
4 activation of the fibrinolytic system to remove unwanted thrombus.

The haemostatic mechanism is in an incompletely understood dynamic equilibrium with a complex series of **antithrombotic** and **fibrinolytic** systems. Failure of the haemostatic mechanism leads to bleeding whilst underactivity of the opposing reactions leads to pathological thrombosis.

Vascular contraction is controlled by **local reflexes**. It is also mediated through **chemical messages**, including prostanoids and nitrogen monoxide, liberated from the vessel wall together with **serotonin** and **thromboxane** A_2 released by platelets. After injury, subendothelial collagen fibres are exposed which interact with platelets to trigger off the complex series of events which result in the formation of **haemostatic plug**. As part of the dynamic process of inhibition of unwanted clotting, the vessel wall is also involved in limiting thrombosis. Endothelial cells synthesize and secrete plasminogen activator (see below). They also secrete a number of potent inhibitors of platelet aggregation, particularly prostacyclin.

Platelet activation
Platelets are anucleate bodies about 2–3 μm in diameter. Platelet function can be considered as follows:
1 **Adhesion.** After injury to a vessel wall, platelets adhere to **subendothelial collagen**. Specific glycoproteins of the platelet membrane and clotting factors, particularly the **von Willebrand factor**, are involved in this process.
2 **Release.** After interacting with collagen, platelets release the contents of their granules in a process called the **release reaction**. Among the many substances released by platelets, **5-hydroxytryptamine** (5-HT), helps to produce local vasoconstriction, while adenosine diphosphate (ADP), prostaglandin endoperoxides and thromboxane A_2 also induce further aggregation and release, thus initiating a self-sustaining process. The release reaction is associated with a change in the shape of platelets from smooth discs to spiny spheres with the formation of **pseudopodia** which interact with other platelets.

3 **Aggregation.** High local concentrations of **agonists** such as ADP, thrombin or thromboxane A_2 produce further platelet aggregation with the formation of a **haemostatic plug**. Changes in the surface **glycoprotein IIb/IIIa** allow binding to fibrinogen, which then acts as a bridge to other platelets.

Local vasoconstriction and platelet aggregation combine to produce temporary haemostasis and may be enough to heal tiny holes in small vessels. However, activation of the clotting system is required to form a thrombus and achieve permanent haemostasis.

The clotting cascade
Blood coagulation comprises a complex series of interactions which involve a number of plasma proteins known collectively as **coagulation factors** which normally circulate in an inactive state. In response to vascular injury, a cascade of proteolytic reactions is set in motion in which factors activate one another, leading to the generation of thrombin that cleaves fibrinogen to form a fibrin clot. The individual factors are designated by Roman numerals I–XII and the activated forms have the suffix a (IXa, Xa and so on).

This is a remarkable amplification system; sufficient thrombin can be generated from the prothrombin in 2 ml of blood to clot the entire circulation. Thus counteractive mechanisms have evolved to ensure that this process does not get out of hand. The cascade of reactions is summarized in Fig. 4.7.

It is not essential to memorize the details of the reactions, which are still not fully understood. The traditional view is that there are two systems, the **intrinsic** and **extrinsic** clotting systems. Although it is useful to understand the intrinsic system in order to understand the active partial thromboblastin time (APTT) test (see below), it is now thought to be an *in vitro* phenomenon.

The intrinsic system is activated when blood comes into contact with a non-endothelial surface. This involves the interaction of factors XI, XII and other blood proteins, including the **kallikrein system**, which combine together to activate **factor IX**.

The tissue factor or extrinsic pathway is more important *in vivo*. Tissue factor, a protein expressed on the surface of non-endothelial cells, binds to and activates factor VII, which activates factor X. This ternary complex is rapidly inactivated by tissue factor pathway inhibitor. Sufficient thrombin is generated to seal small breaks in the circulation. In larger clots, the bulk of thrombin is generated by a second amplification cycle whereby factor VIIa cleaves factor IX, which goes on to activate factor X using factor VIII and phospholipids as cofactors.

Thus deficiencies of factors VIII or IX (the **haemo-**

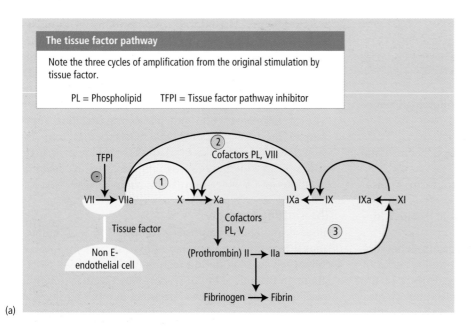

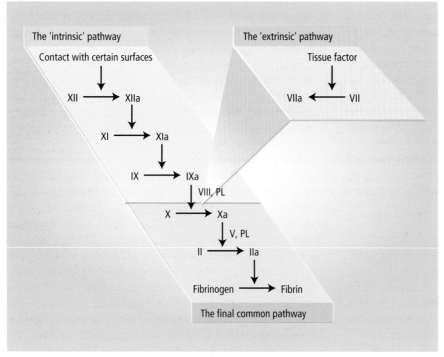

Fig. 4.7 The tissue factor pathway. Note three cycles of amplification after the original stimulation by tissue factor. PL, phospholipid; TFPI, tissue factor pathway inhibitor.

philias) do not result in immediate but delayed bleeding. A further amplification cycle utilizes factor XI and is important in severe haemostatic challenges, especially where the tissues are rich in fibrinolytic enzymes.

Fibrin is formed from the enzymatic cleavage of **fibrinogen** by **thrombin**. Thrombin removes a peptide fragment from the N terminal end of each α and β chain

of fibrin to yield fibrin monomer. Spontaneous polymerization then occurs by end-to-end electrostatic bonding, the result being a fibrin clot. A final clotting factor, XIII, stabilized this clot by covalently cross-linking the γ chains of fibrin.

Inhibition of the clotting cascade is provided by a number of circulating proteins. Most notably **antithrombin III** and **heparin cofactor II** bind to and inhibit thrombin and factor X. Also important are **protein C**, and its cofactor **protein S**, which is activated by thrombin when the latter is bound to thrombomodulin found on normal endothelium. Activated protein C degrades factors V and VIII.

Once fibrin has been formed, it can be degraded by the serine protease plasmin. Plasminogen activators are found in a variety of tissues and body fluids. The most important appear to be associated with endothelial tissues. Other plasminogen activators include **urokinase**, a natural activator synthesized by renal cells and present in the urine, and **streptokinase**, a protein produced by streptococci.

Degradation of fibrinogen and fibrin by plasmin occurs in a series of steps resulting in the formation of a variety of **fibrin degradation products (FDPs)**, which themselves interfere with the action of thrombin and the polymerization of fibrin as well as preventing platelet aggregation. There are a variety of backup proteolytic systems.

Investigation of a bleeding disorder

As in all clinical situations, a careful history and examination can suggest possible diagnoses before any specific laboratory tests are performed. Specifically, the patient should be asked about the nature of the bleeding (e.g. bruising or nose bleeds, excessive menstrual loss, melaena, haematemesis and haematuria). Mucosal bleeding or purpura suggests a defect in platelets. Prolonged oozing after dental extraction, or the need for transfusion in such operations as tonsillectomy need to be documented. A careful family history is particularly relevant to such conditions as haemophilia. The association of other symptoms, such as arthralgia and malaise may suggest an underlying condition (e.g. systemic lupus erythematosus). A complete drug history (including alcohol, oral contraceptives, anti-inflammatory drugs) is particularly important.

Clinical examination may reveal purpura, a swollen joint, telangiectasia on the lips, an enlarged liver, spleen or lymph nodes, or commonly no abnormality.

Investigation of a thrombotic disorder

Thromboses are a common clinical problem. If, however, the thromboses are unusual, for example, multiple, in young people (< 50 years) with no obvious predisposing cause or in unusual sites, the patient should be investigated for deficiencies of antithrombotic proteins.

Tests of haemostatic function

Bleeding time
This is sensitive to platelet number and function and vascular abnormalities. It is performed by inflating a blood pressure cuff to 40 mmHg. A controlled incision with a spring-loaded scalpel is made in the volar surface of the forearm. The resultant blood is absorbed away on filter paper, without touching the incision itself. It is prolonged in platelet deficiencies or von Willebrand's disease.

Prothrombin time
This measures the extrinsic clotting system (factor VII) and common pathway factors (factors X, V, II and fibrinogen). It is extensively used for control of oral anticoagulants and as an index of liver function. Results are usually expressed as the **international normalized ratio (INR)**, which is the ratio of the clotting time of the patient's plasma compared to an internationally defined normal standard.

Active partial thromboblastin time/kaolin-cephalin clotting time (APTT/KCCT)
This measures the intrinsic clotting system (Fig. 4.7), and thus is sensitive to malfunction of many clotting factors including VIII and IX (i.e. haemophilia A and Christmas disease respectively). It is often used for heparin control. It is also sensitive to the lupus anticoagulant. A **clotting screen** usually consists of the prothrombin time (PT) and APTT.

Thrombin time
This measures the final step in the coagulation pathway, the conversion of fibrinogen to fibrin. It is sensitive to hypofibrinogenaemia, congenital or acquired, or dysfibrinogenaemias (most commonly seen in hepatic disease). It is inhibited by heparin and FDPs.

Fibrinogen titre
This is reduced in hepatic failure and consumptive states such as DIC. It is increased in pregnancy and inflammatory conditions, such as rheumatoid arthritis.

Fibrinogen degradation products
These are a measure of fibrinolysis. They are increased in DIC, thrombolytic treatment or renal and liver impairment (the latter two organs help clear FDPs from plasma).

Platelet count
Platelet aggregation studies to ristocetin, ADP, adrenaline and collagen can be performed and are relevant to hereditary platelet disorders, von Willebrand's disease and myeloproliferative conditions.

Antithrombotic proteins

There are specific assays for antithrombin III, protein S, protein C, resistance to protein C and lupus anticoagulant in patients with recurrent thrombotic episodes.

Anticoagulant therapy

Anticoagulant therapy is given to patients with **thrombosis** to prevent extension or to patients with a predisposition to thrombosis or embolization, i.e. curatively or prophylactically. Discussion of the types of thromboses and their individual treatment regimens is beyond the scope of this book. All therapeutic regimens increase the chance of hazardous bleeding, sometimes lethally. The greater the degree of anticoagulation, the greater the risk. It is therefore necessary to make sure the patient can cooperate fully and to monitor the degree of anticoagulation.

Warfarin

Vitamin K antagonists, such as warfarin, inhibit metabolic recycling of the vitamin, so preventing glutamic acid γ carboxylation in factors II, VII, IX, X, and proteins C and S during hepatic synthesis. Warfarin's half-life is about 1 day by mouth. Anticoagulant therapy is common; ~ 0.2% of the UK population takes warfarin.

Generally, the therapeutic INR is 2–3, although patients with metallic heart valves are usually maintained in the range 3–4.5. The warfarin defect may be overcome by vitamin K after ~ 6 hours but subsequent warfarin control may be difficult. In an emergency, FFP or factor concentrates can be used for an immediate effect.

Many drugs interact with warfarin; when the prothrombin time in a previously well-controlled patient suddenly goes out of the desired range, it may be due to a new drug given by an unthinking prescriber, e.g. amiodarone, antibiotics, barbiturates.

Heparin

Heparin must be injected, intravenously or subcutaneously. It potentiates antithrombin III, the main natural coagulation inhibitor of factor Xa and thrombin.

Low-molecular-weight heparins cause antithrombin III to inhibit Xa specifically and not thrombin. They do not significantly prolong the APTT, but their effect is relatively predictable, so their dose does not have to be monitored. Conventional heparin dosage is usually monitored so that a daily APTT (or TT) is maintained between 1.5 and 2.5 times normal.

Its half-life is ~ 3 hours, that of low-molecular-weight heparin is ~ 12 hours. Thus overdosage can be treated quickly by stopping the infusion. In an emergency, protamine can be used as an antidote.

Streptokinase, urokinase and recombinant tissue plasminogen activator

These all activate plasminogen and thereby thrombolysis. They are used intravenously to dissolve clot, mainly after myocardial infarction. Their half-life is a few minutes; they do not usually require laboratory monitoring.

Antiplatelet drugs

Antiplatelet drugs, especially **aspirin**, are used after myocardial infarction and as prophylaxis in high-risk patients. Aspirin's action is irreversible and so lasts the life span of a platelet – 7 days. The action of other non-steroidal anti-inflammatory drugs is reversible.

FURTHER READING

Hoffbrand A.V. & Pettit J.E. (1992) *Essential Haematology*, 3rd edn. Blackwell Scientific Publications, Oxford.

Chemical Pathology and Toxicology

CHEMICAL PATHOLOGY

What is chemical pathology?

Chemical pathology, described once by Professor George Alberti as 'medicine's cuckoo', is often perceived simplistically as the interpretation of results obtained from the clinical biochemistry laboratory (Fig. 5.1). This approach, to what is in reality an extremely broad-based discipline,

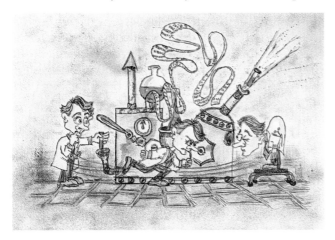

Fig. 5.1 What is chemical pathology? (from an original, courtesy Dr R. Armstrong).

is not only misguided but also a sad reflection on the inadequate effort often applied to teaching this subject.

The term **clinical biochemistry** is often used for the discipline, inferring its confinement to the appliance of biochemistry to the clinical setting. In practice clinical activity in virtually all branches of medicine requires a complete and practical understanding of chemical pathology as the medical practitioner in most routine situations relies on this training to instigate investigations that he or she will then need to interpret and be prepared to act upon. It is clear therefore that the subject needs to be extremely well-covered during the course of medical training and for this training to be updated regularly thereafter. This process requires a good understanding of clinical medicine, physiology, pharmacology, endocrinology, chemistry and biochemistry as well as cellular and molecular biology.

Making a request for a biochemical test

The process of interpretation of a laboratory result begins with the thought processes involved in the instigation of the request and is completed when a clinical decision is taken on the basis of the results provided by the laboratory.

Requests for clinical biochemistry investigations are

required to assist in both diagnosis and follow-up. As most busy laboratories do not have the capacity to provide interpretation for most routine biochemical investigations, in reality virtually every practising clinician needs therefore to be an accomplished chemical pathologist to utilize the information provided by these investigations. The average district general hospital clinical biochemistry laboratory will be able to offer approximately 60 different biochemical plasma analyses as well as analyses on urine, cerebrospinal fluid (CSF), faeces and other body fluids on a routine basis with a vast range also available from specialist laboratories.

Although discretionary testing is encouraged by chemical pathologists purely on scientific and logistical grounds, **financial and legal considerations** will increasingly discipline the use of this laboratory service. Thus, unlike some other branches of pathology, **correct** and **appropriate use** of the clinical biochemistry service requires the medical practitioner to decide not only the type and timing of specimen to collect but also to consider critically the **range of analyses** he or she wishes to be performed on those specimens. The target of teaching this discipline is thus the whole process from begining to end and invariably involves, for convenience and for practical reasons, a considerable amount of pattern recognition.

The initiation of the request for biochemical analysis on a specimen will result from clinical assessment of the patient and in most common usage in general and hospital practice will be aimed at evaluating some biochemical indices of pathology in one or more of the body **systems**. To this aim the laboratory service has developed a reasonably universal set of parameters to assess each system and during clinical training pattern recognition of these profiles should become second nature and considered part of general clinical assessment (Table 5.1).

Table 5.1 Commonly used plasma biochemical profiles.

Renal	Sodium, potassium, urea, creatinine
Liver	Bilirubin, albumin, transaminases, alkaline phosphatase
Bone	Calcium, phosphate, alkaline phosphatase
Cardiac	Creatine kinase, aspartate transaminase, lactate dehydrogenase

In anticipation of making a biochemical request the clinician needs to address the following questions, posed by Asher (1954), in the context of any investigation.
1 Why do I request this test?
2 What will I look for in the result?
3 If I find what I am looking for, will it affect my diagnosis?
4 How will this investigation affect my management of the patient?
5 Will this investigation ultimately benefit the patient?

If such questions are not addressed, particularly in the context of an urgent request which may incur extra cost and inconvenience, inevitably some results indicating significant and treatable pathology may be ignored whilst many other unnecessary analyses may be performed. It is obvious that in order to answer any of these questions an understanding of the processes involved in the development of the profiles under normal conditions needs to be clear before understanding of those in pathology can be interpreted. For many of these, such as plasma concentrations of electrolytes and hormones, an understanding of normal physiological processes will provide this basis. The relationship between abnormal biochemical profiles to underlying cellular and molecular pathology should then become a logical progression and lead to a clearer view to management of that pathology.

The reference interval

The ideal reference interval for a particular analyte is that observed for that analyte obtained when that patient is healthy. This is clearly inappropriate in most instances and every laboratory is thus expected to provide a means whereby a laboratory result can be interpreted with reference to a range of results likely to be found in a healthy population roughly matched for age and sex.

The reference population

In order to obtain such a set of ranges or intervals, samples need to be collected from a large number of people who are considered to be healthy (the **reference population**) and the distribution of results obtained is plotted. If the results obtained are normally distributed it has been acceptable practice to establish the reference interval from those results lying two standard deviations on both sides of the mean value, thus including 95% of the results and excluding 2.5% at both the upper and the lower end from 'healthy' or 'non-diseased' people. In practice the results are often unevenly distributed and thus 95% confidence intervals are established between confidence limits obtained from the calculated geometric mean.

The 'normal value'

The concept of a **normal value** for an analyte is now largely **obsolete**. In some circumstances, such as is the case with plasma cholesterol measurement in certain populations, a significant proportion of the reference population may include those considered to have undesirably 'unhealthy' levels indicating risk of disease and therefore need for therapy.

Sensitivity, specificity and predictive value

An important consideration when evaluating the suitability of a diagnostic parameter is the relationship between the distribution of results for that analyte obtained from **diseased** and **non-diseased** populations.

An ideal analyte in this context would have no overlap between these populations and thus would provide 100% **specificity** and **sensitivity** as **false-positive** and **-negative** rates would be zero. In practice this rarely occurs and so different parameters are compared by their different sensitivities and specificities and, with more power by relating these to the **prevalence** of the disease in that population, by calculating predictive values of a positive and negative test.

In the context of a diagnostic test, sensitivity is defined as the degree of abnormality (or positivity) of that test in disease or the true-positive rate. Thus in a situation where all the positive results of a series of tests occur in patients with disease, with no normal results falling within disease (no false-negatives), the sensitivity is 100%.

The degree of sensitivity of a test demonstrates quantitatively how sensitive that test is for detecting disease. The false-positive rate, the incidence of positive results in patients without the disease, informs of the degree of specificity of the test for that disease. Thus a test with no positives found in patients without disease will have a false-positive rate of 0% and a **specificity** (100 – false-positive rate in %) of 100%.

This information helps to establish the cut-off limits for differentiating health from disease but incorporation of the value for the prevalence of disease in that population provides a more accurate prediction of the value of a test.

Diagnostic sensitivity

$$= \frac{\text{True positives}}{\text{True positives} + \text{false negatives}} \times 100$$

Diagnostic specificity

$$= \frac{\text{True negatives}}{\text{True negatives} + \text{false positives}} \times 100$$

Predictive value of a positive test = % of patients with positive tests that are **diseased**:

$$= \frac{\text{True positives}}{\text{True positives} + \text{false positives}} \times 100$$

Predictive value of a negative test = % of patients with a negative test that are **non-diseased**:

$$= \frac{\text{True negatives}}{\text{True negatives} + \text{false negatives}} \times 100$$

Efficiency of a test = % of patients correctly classified as diseased and non-diseased:

$$= \frac{\text{True positives} + \text{true negatives}}{\text{True positives} + \text{false positives} + \text{true negatives} + \text{false negatives}} \times 100$$

The following is an example to illustrate the appropriate usage of predictive values for a diagnostic test as a function of disease prevalence.

Consider the value of a cardiac enzyme test for the diagnosis of myocardial infarction in two populations– one with a low prevalence of 2% (e.g. from a general practitioner's surgery) and the other with a high prevalence of 50% (e.g. from a coronary care unit). Laboratory tests have established that this test has a diagnostic sensitivity of 95% and a diagnostic specificity of 95%. The sensitivity and specificity have been established on the same population as that for which the prevalence of the disease has been calculated and from these data the predictive value of a positive test in general practice is 27.9% and that in the coronary care unit is 95%. In many situations the predictive power or value of a negative result may be of greater clinical significance (for example, in establishing the ability of a test to exclude the diagnosis of myocardial infarction within certain time limits after the onset of chest pain).

Analytical accuracy and variability

An important component of the interpretation of a diagnostic test is an understanding of the **quality** and **accuracy** of that result and also the **limitations** of the diagnostic process (Table 5.2). Although these components are primarily the responsibility of the clinical and

Table 5.2 Reasons for variation.

Biological
Intraindividual
Interindividual
Age, sex, posture, diet and weight
Analytical
Between assay
Within assay
Between methods

Table 5.3 Commonly requested biochemical tests.

Body fluid	Analyte	Indications	Body fluid	Analyte	Indications
Plasma or serum	Acid phosphatase	Prostatic carcinoma	Plasma or serum	Protein (total)	Hepatic synthetic function, immunoglobulin status
	Albumin	Chronic hepatic synthetic function, renal or gut loss, nutritional and hydration state		Sodium	Hydration state and fluid balance, renal and endocrine disease
	α-Amylase	Acute pancreatitis		Thyroid hormones	Thyroid function
	Alanine transaminase	Hepatocellular damage		Triglycerides	Lipid metabolism
	Alkaline phosphatase	Hepatobiliary disease, bone disease		Urea	Glomerular function, hydration state
	Aspartate transaminase	Hepatocellular disease, skeletal and cardiac muscle disease		Uric acid	Purine metabolism, renal disease
	Bicarbonate	Acid–base status	Urine	Albumin	Renal glomerular and tubular disease
	Bilirubin	Hepatic transport and metabolism		Calcium	Bone, renal and parathyroid function
	Calcium	Bone and renal function, vitamin D and parathyroid activity		Catecholamine metabolites	Adrenomedullary activity
	Chloride	Acid–base status		Cortisol (free)	Adrenocortical activity
	Cholesterol	Lipid metabolism		Creatinine	Glomerular filtration rate
	Cortisol	Pituitary and adrenal function		Glucose	Glomerular permeability
	Creatinine	Glomerular function, hydration state		Hydroxyproline	Bone metabolism
	Creatine kinase	Skeletal and cardiac muscle disease		5-Hydroxyindoleacetic acid	Hydroxytryptamine production
	γ-Glutamyl transferase	Hepatobiliary disease		Phosphate	Renal tubular function
	Glucose	Carbohydrate metabolism		Protein	Glomerular leak
	Glycosylated Haemoglobin	Diabetic control		Osmolality	Fluid balance
	Lactate	Intermediary metabolism		Porphyrins	Haem synthesis
	Lactate dehydrogenase	Skeletal and cardiac muscle disease, haematological malignancies		Potassium	Renal tubular function
				Sodium	Renal tubular activity, fluid balance
	Magnesium	Gastrointestinal absorption, renal disease		Urea	Nitrogen excretion
	Osmolality	Fluid balance		Uric acid	Renal uric acid clearance
	Phosphate (inorganic)	Bone metabolism, renal tubular function	Cerebrospinal fluid	Protein	CNS infections and neoplasms
				Glucose	CNS infections
	Potassium	Renal and endocrine disease		Lactate	Carbohydrate metabolism

CNS, Central nervous system.

scientific staff of the laboratory to which samples are sent for analysis it is nevertheless important for the clinician to have an understanding of the likely **coefficient of variation** of an assay method (Table 5.3).

Thus, for example, an understanding of the overall co-efficient of variation of a sodium result which may be 5% will prevent overinterpretation of a small change of 2 mmol/l from a value of 146 to 144 mmol/l. Current pressure from various sources to encourage near-patient testing in order to attempt to accelerate assay **turnaround time** highlights the importance of these considerations

and, in particular, the paramount need for good **quality control**.

Special investigations

There are many areas of medicine where highly specialized biochemical testing is required. This is most common in areas of medicine where there is limited diagnostic value from clinical investigation alone and thus where there are wide differential diagnoses. These include specialties such as **paediatrics**, **neurology** and **psychiatry**. In these circumstances, and particularly in paediatrics, where repeat sampling is often unacceptable to the patient or relatives, it is important for the clinician to establish a battery of initial investigations whilst being aware of appropriate lines of investigation to follow upon receipt of an abnormal result from this **screen**. Thus, for example, in the case of the diagnosis of one of the glycogen storage diseases, clinical suspicion may lead to a profile of tests including plasma glucose and lactate measurement which, if proven abnormal, may lead to dynamic tests such as a glucagon stimulation test or an ischaemic forearm lactate test as well as liver or skin biopsy for confirmatory evidence and characterization.

Screening in chemical pathology

A significant proportion of the established health screening programmes are based on biochemical testing and there is a strong likelihood that more biochemical programmes will develop over the next few years in advance of much heralded, though still undeveloped, genetic screening for single and polygenic disorders.

Criteria for screening

A fundamental requirement for screening in health is that the condition sought should be a sufficiently important and treatable health problem to warrant the expense involved in a screening programme. The test or procedure for the screening should have proven sensitivity for the condition and be both practical and acceptable to the population to be tested whilst there should be an agreed policy on the criteria for treatment. In order to warrant screening the cost of case-finding should be economically related to the total expenditure on medical care of the condition. Once established, a health screening programme needs to be well-administered and continuity of the programme needs to be ensured.

Examples of successful health screening programmes in the UK involving biochemical testing include neonatal screening of blood to exclude phenylketonuria and hypothyroidism and antenatal screening for neural tube defects and Down's syndrome (see Chapter 25). This is extended in some areas to include screening for cystic fibrosis using a measurement in the neonatal period of serum or whole-blood immunoreactive trypsin. In addition in the clinical biochemistry laboratory there are numerous screening tests used to exclude diseases such as diabetes mellitus (e.g. glycosuria), and for hypercholesterolaemia, some malignancies and toxicology.

TOXICOLOGY

Diagnostic tests in acute poisoning (Table 5.4)

In cases where the nature of the poison is known, the value of the chemical analyses may only be confirmatory, although in many cases it adds prognostic information and provides guidelines for the management.

The most common **drug overdoses** in the UK are with **paracetamol**, **salicylate** and **ethanol**.

In order to allow for the time taken for absorption of the drug, **plasma paracetamol** should not be measured until **4 hours** have elapsed from the time of ingestion. Therapy can then be instituted if the level exceeds a graduated level expected at that time after a dose, although specific therapy is considered largely ineffective from 12 to 16 hours after the overdose.

Raised plasma concentrations of salicylate of greater than 3.6 mmol/l in adults and 2.2 mmol/l in children indicate the need for interventions to increase clearance.

Plasma ethanol can be measured in most laboratories and it is important to be able to distinguish ethanol from methanol as clinical management and outcome are very different. Measurement of **plasma osmolar gap**, the difference between calculated plasma osmolarity (the sum of $2 \times [Na] + 2 \times [K] + [urea] + [glucose]$) and measured

Table 5.4 Acute poisoning.

Common drug overdoses
Benzodiazepines
Tricyclic antidepressants
Paracetamol
Salicylates
Ethanol
Less common drug overdoses
Carbamazepine
Phenobarbitone
Phenytoin
Lithium
Iron
Chloroquine
Quinine
Toxic substances
Carbon monoxide
Methanol
Ethylene glycol
Organophosphorous insecticides
Paraquat

osmolality, is a simple way of estimating elevated plasma alcohol concentrations.

In suspected **carbon monoxide poisoning** blood should be collected as soon as possible as the blood levels will fall rapidly after commencement of oxygen therapy and the symptoms of carbon monoxide poisoning may remain long after blood carbon monoxide levels return to relatively non-toxic levels.

For other acute poisoning **blood** and **urine** should be collected as soon as possible and advice sought from the local laboratory and, when necessary, from a poison centre where a wide range of analyses are available as well as advice on management.

Therapeutic drug monitoring

The efficacy of most drugs used in clinical therapeutics is monitored by their clinical effects (Table 5.5) and toxicity is usually rare.

Some drugs have a narrow therapeutic window and thus the gap between a therapeutic plasma value and a toxic one is relatively narrow and thus potentially problematical. For these drugs it is helpful to monitor plasma levels to ensure that a plasma level in the therapeutic range is achieved.

Other indications for therapeutic drug monitoring are

Table 5.5 Drugs in common use requiring regular monitoring.

Phenytoin
Phenobarbitone
Carbamazepine
Lithium
Digoxin
Theophylline

to test for **compliance**, where symptoms and signs of toxicity may be difficult to diagnose or to distinguish from those of the disease being treated (e.g. **digoxin**) and for when there is a risk of drug **toxicity** from impaired clearance mechanisms such as in liver or renal disease.

REFERENCES

Alberti G. (1976) Chemical Pathology – Medicine's Cuckoo (Inaugural Lecture). University of Southampton Press, Southampton.
Asher R. (1954) Straight and crooked thinking in medicine. *British Medical Journal*; **2**: 460–462.

FURTHER READING

Bryson P.D. (1989) *Comprehensive Review in Toxicology*, 2nd edn. Aspen Publishers, Rockville, Md.

PART 2

ESSENTIAL GENERAL PATHOLOGY

CHAPTER 6

Clinical Genetics

INTRODUCTION

The section of this book from Chapter 6 to 13, represents an overview of general pathological processes that have a wide range of clinicopathological effects.

Medical genetics has developed rapidly from a purely academic discipline into a clinical specialty. Although still largely providing a **regional service**, the clinical cytogenetics and molecular genetics laboratory will be involved in the diagnosis of disease processes that are relevant to every clinical specialty. The diagnosis of classical Mendelian and chromosomal disorders is well-established. The future holds a role for the laboratory in the diagnosis of the commoner disorders of adulthood that show a genetic predisposition, such as athero-sclerosis and cancer.

Molecular genetics techniques are not discussed in this book, and the student is referred to the recommended texts for these techniques and background.

CYTOGENETIC DISEASES

Introduction–cytogenetic notation

Cytogenetic staining techniques produce a unique pattern of transverse bands on each chromosome and each band is numbered. Locations of structural chromosome abnormalities are designated according to the:

- **chromosome** (number);
- **arm** (letter);
- **band** (number).

Standard cytogenetic notation used in reporting results and examples of cytogenetic nomenclature and notation are provided in Tables 6.1 and 6.2.

There are only two normal cytogenetic test results:
1 46,XX: normal female karyotype;
2 46,XY: normal male karyotype.

Small structural chromosomal variations will occur in some normal individuals. These variant chromo-

Table 6.1 Standard cytogenetic notation.

del	Deletion
der	Derivative chromosome
dic	Dicentric
dup	Duplication
f	Fragment
fra	Fragile site
h	Secondary constriction (heterochromatin)
i	Isochromosome
ins	Insertion
inv	Inversion
mar	Marker chromosome
minus (−)	Loss of
p	Short arm of chromosome
parentheses ( )	Used to surround structurally altered chromosome(s) or breakpoint(s)
Ph¹ or Ph	Philadelphia chromosome
plus (+)	Gain of
q	Long arm of chromosome
question mark(?)	Indicates questionable identification of chromosome or chromosome structure
r	Ring chromosome
s	Satellite
semicolon (;)	Separates chromosomes and chromosome regions in structural rearrangements involving more than one chromosome
slant line or solidus (/)	Separates chromosomes and chromosome regions in structural rearrangements involving more than one chromosome
t	Translocation
ter	Terminal (end of chromosome)

Table 6.2 Examples of cytogenetic nomenclature and notation.

Normal	46,XX
	46,XY
Aneuploidy	45,X (monosomy X)
	47,XY,+18 (trisomy 18)
	50,XY,+6,+14,+20,+21 (hyperdiploidy)
Deletion	46,XY,5p−
Terminal	46,XY,del(5)(p14)
Interstitial inversion	46,XY,del(5)(q21q31)
Paracentric	46,XX,inv(3)(q21q26)
Pericentric	46,XX,inv(16)(p13p22)
Isochromosome	46,X,i(Xq)
Translocation	46,XY,t(9;22)(q34;q11)
Interpretation	46,XY,−9,−22.+der(9)+der(22)t(9;22)(q34;q11)
Mosiac	(More than one cell line)
	45,X/46,C,Xp−
	46,XY/46,XY,t(9;22)(q34;q11)/46,XY,t(9;22),−17,+i(17q)

somes may be included in the notation of a normal karyotype.

Chromosomal disease

Chromosome abnormalities are either **constitutional (congenital)** and may be detected pre-/postnatally or **acquired** and associated with tumours.

Patients with constitutional chromosome abnormalities (Table 6.3) are not only seen by paediatricians and obstetricians (see Chapter 25), but are also seen by physicians in virtually every medical specialty.

Chromosome abnormalities are of two basic types: **numerical** (too many or too few chromosomes) and **structural** (the result of chromatin breakage with loss, gain or rearrangement of chromosomal material).

Although the vast majority of cytogenetically abnormal conceptions result in embryonic or fetal death (50% of spontaneous abortions have a chromosome abnormality), constitutional chromosome abnormalities are present in 6 of every 1000 newborns. Diagnosis of a constitutional chromosome abnormality not only suggests appropriate management and accurate prognosis, but is essential for genetic counselling.

Clinical syndromes associated with the more common constitutional chromosome abnormalities are familiar. The phenotypes and natural history are well-described (see below and Table 6.3). The phenotypes of constitutional autosomal cytogenetic abnormalities range from multiple, severe malformations (e.g. trisomy 18) to mild dysmorphisms (e.g. a small deletion). Virtually all include some degree of **mental retardation**. Any unexplained developmental delay is an indication for cytogenetic evaluation (Fig. 6.1).

Chromosome deletions associated with **recognizable syndromes** include 4p− (Wolf syndrome); 5p− (*cri du chat* syndrome); 9p−; 11p− (aniridia/Wilms tumour); 13q− (with or without retinoblastoma); 18p−; and 18q−. Syndromes in which a tiny chromosomal deletion is sometimes but not always found include Prader–Willi syndrome (15q−) and DiGeorge anomaly (22q−). In some of these, a deletion may be too small to detect by cytogenetics and may only be identified by molecular techniques such as fluorescent *in situ* hybridization (FISH).

Table 6.3 Some common constitutional chromosome abnormalities.

Common name	Examples of common karyotype	Incidence	Common phenotypic features
Down syndrome (trisomy 21)	47,XX,+21 46,XY,−14,+t(14q21q)	1/700 birth	Hypotonia, upward-slanted eyes, epicanthal folds, flat face, simian creases, congenital heart defect, mental retardation
Trisomy 18	47,XY,+18 46,XX/47,XX,+18	1/4000–5000 births	Severe growth retardation, micrognathia, congenital heart defect, overlapping fingers, rockerbottom feet, limited survival
Trisomy 13	47,XY,+13 46,XX−14,+t(13q14q)	1/5000 births	Cleft lip/palate, polydactyly, microphthalmia, congenital heart defect, holoprosencephaly, limited survival
Turner syndrome	45,X 46,X,abnormal X 45,X/46,X,abnormal X	1/3000–5000 females	Newborn oedema of hands and feet, webbed neck, short stature, cubitus valgus, absent puberty
Klinefelter syndrome	47,XXY	1/500 males	Hypogonadism, possible gynaecomastia, long legs
Fragile X syndrome	46,fra(X),Y	1/2500 births	Mental retardation, large chin, ears, testes, possible autistic behaviour

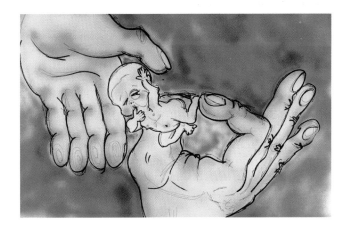

Fig. 6.1 Any unexplained developmental delay is an indication for cytogenetic evaluation. From an original, courtesy Dr R. Armstrong.

INHERITED GENETIC DISEASE

Sex chromosome abnormalities

Turner syndrome (45,XO) is characterized by a phenotypic female with short stature, webbed neck and immature genitalia. The ovaries are small and fibrotic (**streak** ovaries); coarctation of the aorta may be present.

Since only one X chromosome is present, no Barr bodies are observed in nuclei from buccal smears. Patients with mosaic genetics are common and have less pronounced pathological changes.

Klinefelter syndrome (47,XXY) is characterized by a phenotypic male with tall stature, gynaecomastia and small testes that do not produce sperm.

Klinefelter syndrome is the most common sex chromosome abnormality. Variants include mosaics, XXXY, and XXXXY. Increasing numbers of X chromosomes are associated with increasing mental retardation.

Triple X females (47,XXX) are phenotypically normal but have mild mental retardation. **47,XYY** patients are tall, mildly retarded males who have been shown in some studies to have an increased incidence in prison populations. The **fragile X syndrome** (Fra(X)) is usually observed in male patients and is associated with mental retardation, enlarged testes and fragility at the end of the q arm of the X chromosome.

True hermaphrodites are characterized by the presence of both ovarian and testicular tissue, may have either XX or XY genetics, and are rare. **Male pseudohermaphrodites** have normal XX genetics, are phenotypically male, and often have either ovarian or adrenal tumours that produce virilizing hormones.

X-Linked genetic diseases (Table 6.4)

Fewer X-linked genetic diseases have been described than autosomal recessive diseases. In these diseases, affected individuals are usually **homozygote males** who received the gene from their mothers; **heterozygous females** are **carriers** for the gene. Rare homozygous females may have the diseases.

Table 6.4 Common sex-linked disorders.

X-linked recessive
Glucose-6-phosphate dehydrogenase deficiency
Testicular feminization
Duchenne muscular dystrophy
Chronic granulomatous disease
Red-green colour blindness*
Haemophilia A
Christmas disease (haemophilia B)
Bruton's agammaglobulinaemia
X-linked dominant
Hypophosphataemic (vitamin D-resistant) rickets
Y-linked
None known

* Total colour blindness is autosomal recessive and very rare.

Colour blindness is the most common X-linked disease. Glucose-6-phosphate dehydrogenase deficiency is associated with impaired synthesis of the antioxidant glutathione. This deficiency renders erythrocytes vulnerable to oxidant-induced hemolysis by primaquine, infections, fava beans and other drugs.

Both the clotting disorders **classic haemophilia** (see Chapters 4 and 12; haemophilia A, factor VIII deficiency) and **Christmas disease** (haemophilia B, factor IX deficiency) are transmitted in an X-linked fashion and are associated with bleeding into deep tissues and joints.

Duchenne muscular dystrophy produces weakness of heart and proximal skeletal muscle, and usually causes death before age 20.

Syndromes of autosomal disease
(Tables 6.5 and 6.6)

In general, **autosomal** chromosomal abnormalities produce more severe disease than do sex chromosomal abnormalities.

Down syndrome (trisomy 21, mongolism) is the most common autosomal trisomy and occurs in both sexes. It has a significantly increased risk in children of older mothers. The usual cause is non-disjunction of maternal chromosomes. Affected infants tend to have poor motor tone (**floppy** infants); a distinctive face with 'mongoloid' facies, epicanthic folds and a flat nose; single transverse palmar creases and cryptorchidism.

Patients with Down syndrome are mildly to moderately mentally retarded and may also have congenital cardiovascular anomalies and an increased incidence of leukaemia.

Edwards syndrome (18 trisomy) usually causes death in infancy and is more common among female babies. It has a high prevalence of coexisting cardiac and renal abnormalities. Other features include a distinctive face with low-set ears, epicanthic folds, and micrognathia, rockerbottom feet and overlapping second and fifth finger.

Patau syndrome (13 trisomy) affects both sexes. It commonly has cardiovascular anomalies, and may have brain anomalies. Other features include low-set ears, cleft palate and lip and small eyes.

Table 6.5 Features of autosomal dominant and recessive inherited diseases.

Autosomal dominant gene	Autosomal recessive gene
A = abnormal dominant gene	a = Abnormal recessive gene
Patient with disease is Aa heterozygote; AA homozygote is usually not compatible with life	Patient with disease is aa homozygote. AA is normal; Aa is symptomless carrier
Males and females are equally affected	Males and females are equally affected
At least one parent (Aa) shows overt disease.	Both parents are symptomless carriers (Aa); neither parent shows overt disease
Overt disease is present in every generation	Disease skips generations
Higher incidence of overt disease among siblings; 50% chance of disease in children when one parent is affected	Lower incidence of overt disease among siblings; 25% chance of disease in children of two symptomless carriers
Cannot be transmitted by an individual without disease	Can be transmitted by an individual without disease (carrier); offspring of a parent with overt disease (aa) and of a normal individual will all be carriers
No association with consanguinous marriages	Associated with consanguinous marriages

Table 6.6 Common autosomal disorders.

Autosomal dominant	Autosomal recessive
Achondroplasia (dwarfism)	Cystic fibrosis (mucoviscidosis)
Marfan's syndrome	α_1-Antitrypsin deficiency
Neurofibromatosis	Phenylketonuria
Von Willebrand's disease	Wilson's disease
Hereditary haemorrhagic telangiectasia	Tay–Sachs disease
Osteogenesis imperfecta	Sickle-cell anaemia
Acute intermittent porphyria	Glycogen storage diseases
Huntington's chorea	Galactosaemia
Hereditary spherocytosis	
Adult renal polycystic disease	
Hereditary angioedema	
Familiar hypercholesterolaemia	

Approximately 700 autosomal dominant disorders have been described.

Cri du chat **syndrome** (5p–) is a syndrome observed more commonly among females. It is due to deletion of the p arm of chromosome 5. Infants are retarded, have a distinctive cat cry, and are prone to cardiovascular anomalies. Other features include a moonface, micrognathia and a slant to the eyes.

Autosomal dominant disease

Genetic disorders transmitted by autosomal dominant genetics will express in all individuals who carry the gene, and most affected individuals are heterozygotes for the characteristic. Genes coding for structural proteins tend to cause autosomal dominant defects; in contrast, autosomal recessive defects often involve enzymes.

Achondroplasia is a form of dwarfism associated with defective endochondral ossification due to a mutation in the fibroblast growth factor receptor type 3.

Huntington's chorea manifests with dementia, choreic movements, seizures and death.

Marfan syndrome is due to a defect in collagen and elastin synthesis caused by a defect in the **fibrillin gene** that has variable expression. Individuals who express the full disorder tend to be tall, with long extremities and fingers (arachnodactyly), are vulnerable to dissecting aortic aneurysm secondary to cystic medial necrosis and may have subluxation of the lens of the eye.

Gardner syndrome is an example of a genetic syndrome with neoplastic potential that predisposes for skin cysts, osteomas, colonic polyps and colon cancer.

Other autosomal dominant diseases include neurofibromatosis (nerve tumours, pigmented skin lesions), spherocytosis (altered erythrocyte membrane leading to spherical shape), some forms of congenital hyperbilirubinaemia (Dubin–Johnson syndrome, some cases of Rotor and possibly Gilbert syndromes), and hypophosphataemia (abnormal alkaline phosphatase).

Autosomal intermediate disease

The classic description of single-gene autosomal defects involves autosomal dominant and autosomal recessive categories, but some diseases are characterized by mild disease in heterozygotes and severe disease in homozygotes. These conditions can be considered as due to autosomal intermediate abnormalities.

Sickle-cell anaemia is due to an amino acid substitution in the β-chain of haemoglobin A that decreases the solubility of the haemoglobin in a deoxygenated environment. Homozygotes have severe anaemia and frequently die before age 30. Heterozygotes (**sickle-cell trait**) are commonly seen in black populations and have normal longevity, few symptoms and mild anaemia.

The **thalassaemias** are a group of disorders in which decreased amounts of otherwise normal haemoglobin are synthesized. The thalassaemias have complex genetics. Affected individuals may have mild to severe anaemia depending upon the number of affected genes they carry.

Autosomal recessive disease

Autosomal recessive disorders are characterized by phenotypically normal or near-normal heterozygotes and severely affected homozygotes.

Cystic fibrosis

Cystic fibrosis is the most common autosomal recessive disease in the Caucasian population. It is associated with abnormal mucus and sweat production and causes pancreatic insufficiency and bronchiectasis with predisposition for severe pneumonia.

Galactosaemia

Two forms of galactosaemia exist which result from a deficiency in the enzymes involved in the metabolism of galactose from milk lactose. Galactosaemia is characterized by galactosuria, gastrointestinal symptoms, cirrhosis that may progress to liver failure, cataracts and mental retardation.

Wilson's disease

Wilson's disease (see Chapters 7 and 19; hepatolenticular degeneration) is due to a deficiency of the copper-binding protein **caeruloplasmin**. Wilson's disease typically presents in adolescence and leads to accumulation of copper in the deep grey matter of the brain, causing convulsions and ataxia. Copper also accumulates in the liver (cirrhosis), eyes (Kayser–Fleischer rings) and renal tubes.

Glycogen storage diseases (Table 6.7)

The glycogen storage diseases feature glycogen accumulation in tissue cells and are due to autosomal recessive genetic defects.

Type I glycogen storage disease (von Gierke's disease, hepatorenal form) is caused by deficiency in glucose-6-phosphatase, which leads to glycogen accumulation in liver cytoplasm and nuclei. Both liver and kidneys enlarge. Affected infants have difficulty maintaining serum glucose levels and develop hypoglycaemia, hyperlipidaemia, lactic acidosis, ketosis and, later, gout.

Type Ib is a clinical variant due to a defect in the transport membrane protein associated with glucose-6-phosphate.

Type II (Pompe's disease, generalized or cardiac form) is due to deficiency of lysomal acid α_1-4-glucosidase and causes an accumulation of glycogen within striated muscle lysozymes, leading to skeletal muscle hypotonia and massive cardiomegaly that causes heart failure.

Type III (Cori's disease) is due to deficiency of debrancher enzyme (amylo-1,4-to-1,6-glucosidase), leading to glycogen accumulation in liver cells. The clinical course resembles mild type I disease.

Type IV (Andersen's disease, amylopectinosis) is a uniformly fatal disease due to a deficiency of a brancher enzyme (amylo-1,4-to-1,6-transglucosidase), which leads to accumulation in many tissues (liver, heart, skeletal muscle, lymph nodes) of material that resembles amylopectin, rather than glycogen. Hepatosplenomegaly with cirrhosis causes early death.

Type V (McArdle's disease, muscle glycogenesis) is due to a deficiency of myophosphorylase. Glycogen accumulation in muscle is associated with muscle weakness, and sometimes myocytolysis, which may cause renal failure secondary to myoglobinuria.

Lipid storage diseases (Table 6.8)

Lipid storage diseases are predominantly autosomal recessive genetic defects in lysosomal enzymes. Lipids accumulate in reticuloendothelial cells and neurones. Enzymatic analysis of amniotic fluid cells, cultured fibroblasts or blood leukocytes can facilitate the diagnosis of these diseases.

Gaucher's disease is due to deficiency of glucocerebrosidase (β-glucosidase), which leads to the accumulation of glucocerebroside in glia, reticulendothelial cells (Fig. 6.2) and marrow cells. Serum acid phosphatase is usually increased. The chronic form of Gaucher's disease is usually observed in Ashkenazi Jews who slowly develop hepatosplenomegaly, pancytopenia and sometimes a haemopoietic neoplasm. A rare acute infantile form also exists with prominent brainstem involvement and hepatosplenomegaly.

Niemann–Pick disease (sphingomyelin lipidosis) is a fatal disease common in Ashkenazi Jews that is due to a deficiency of sphingomyelin in neurones and reticulendothelial cells. Patients have hepatosplenomegaly and neurological symptoms (infantile psychomotor retardation, blindness, deafness). About one-third of patients have a **cherry-red spot** in the macula.

Table 6.7 Glycogen storage diseases.

Type	Enzyme defect	Severity of disease	Involved tissues
T (von Gierke's disease)	Glucose-6-phosphatase	Severe	Liver, kidney, gut
II (Pompe's disease)	α-1,4-glucosidase	Lethal	Systemic distribution but heart most affected
III (Cori's disease; debranching enzyme)	Amylo-1,6-glucosidase	Mild	Systemic distribution; liver commonly affected
IV (Andersen's disease)	Amylo-1,4→1,6-transglucosidase (branching enzyme)	Lethal	Systemic distribution but liver most affected
V (McArdle's disease)	Muscle phosphorylase	Mild	Skeletal muscle
VI (Hers' disease)	Liver phosphorylase	Mild	Liver
VII–XII	Extremely rare diseases	Variable	Variable

Table 6.8 Inborn errors of lipd metabolism: lysosomal (or lipid) storage diseases.

Disease	Enzyme defect	Accumulated lipid	Tissues involved
Tay–Sachs disease	Hexosaminidase A	G_{M2} ganglioside	Brain, retina
Gaucher's disease	β-Glucosidase	Glucocerebroside	Liver, spleen, bone marrow, brain
Niemann–Pick disease	Sphingomyelinase	Sphingomyelin	Brain, liver, spleen
Metachromatic leukodystrophy	Arylsulphatase A	Sulphatide	Brain, kidney, liver, peripheral nerves
Fabry's disease	α-Galactosidase	Ceramide trihexoside	Skin, kidney
Krabbe's disease	Galactosylceramidase	Galactocerebroside	Brain

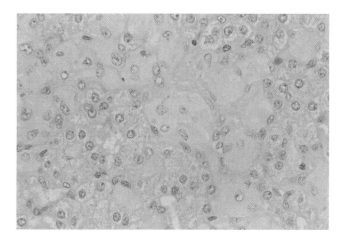

Fig. 6.2 Spleen histology in Gaucher's disease. Note the 'tissue paper' pink granular cytoplasm typical of this storage disease.

Krabbe's disease (globoid cell leukodystrophy) is due to deficiency of β-galactosidase, which leads to accumulation of ceramide galactoside. This material accumulates in multinucleated globoid cells in demyelinating white matter in the cerebral cortex and cerebellum. Patients show infantile psychomotor retardation and die at an early age.

Metachromatic leukodystrophy (sulphatide lipidosis) is due to a deficiency in arylsulphatase A. Sulphatides accumulate in neurones, nerves, kidney and gallbladder. Patients experience psychomotor retardation, weakness, blindness and death.

Fabry's disease (glycosphingolipidosis) differs from other lipid storage diseases by having X-linked rather than autosomal recessive genetics. Fabry's disease is due to a deficiency of α-galactosidase, which leads to accumulation of glycosphingolipids in reticuloendothelial cells, ganglion cells, cornea and vascular endothelium. Patients experience cardiac and renal failure, autonomic instability, skin lesions (angiokeratomas) and impaired vision secondary to corneal opacity.

Tay–Sachs disease is actually a group of diseases characterized by a deficiency of hexosaminidase A, which leads to the accumulation of gangliosides in ballooned neurones and foamy macrophages in the reticuloendothelial system.

By electronmicroscopy, the accumulated ganglioside has a distinctive laminated appearance (laminated bodies). The **classic infantile form (type I)** is seen most often in Ashkenazi Jews, and causes severe psychomotor retardation with convulsions and blindness that progresses to death in early childhood. Similar diseases that present at somewhat later ages are observed in the late infantile (Jansky–Bielschowsky) and juvenile (juvenile amaurotic idiocy of Spielmeyer–Vogt) forms of the disease. **Sandhoff's (type II)** form of Tay–Sachs disease is due to a deficiency of both hexosaminidase A and B, which causes ganglioside and globoside accumulation in kidney, spleen and liver. The **generalized gangliosidoses** are due to deficiency in β-galactosidase. Gangliosides accumulate in neurones, glomeruli (ballooned epithelial cells) and reticuloendothelial cells in liver and bone marrow. Patients experience psychomotor retardation.

Wolman's disease is due to a deficiency of acid lipase, which leads to an accumulation of neutral lipids and xanthoma formation, adrenal involvement and hepatosplenomegaly.

Mucopolysaccharidoses (Table 6.9)

The mucopolysaccharidoses are due to genetic deficiencies of lysosomal enzymes involved in the degradation of acid mucopolysaccharides.

Hurler syndrome (type I mucopolysaccharidosis) is characterized by **'gargoyle' facies** due to accumulation of mucopolysaccharide (dermatan sulphate and heparan

Table 6.9 Mucopolysaccharidoses (MPS syndromes).

Type	Enzyme defect	Accumulated mucopoly-saccharide	Tissue involved	Mode of inheritance	Severity
I (Hurler's syndrome)	α-L-Iduronidase	Heparan sulphate, dermatan sulphate	Skin, cornea, bone, heart, brain, liver, spleen	AR	Severe
II (Hunter's syndrome)	L-Iduronosulphate sulphatase	Heparan sulphate	Skin, bone, heart, ear, retina	XR	Moderate
III (Sanfilippo's syndrome)	Many types	Heparan sulphate	Brain, skin	AR	Moderate
IV (Morquio's syndrome)	N-Acetylgalactosamine 6-sulphatase	Keratan sulphate, chondroitin sulphate	Skin, bone, heart, eye	AR	Mild
V–VII	Rare diseases characterized by many types of enzyme defects		Variable	Variable AR	Mild

AR, Autosomal recessive; XR, X-linked recessive.

sulphate) in chondrocytes, osteocytes and fibroblasts. Other skeletal abnormalities include deformed 'gibbus' back, claw hand and stiff joints. Patients also have hearing loss; visual impairment secondary to corneal clouding; cardiac involvement that often leads to cardiac ischaemia and death before the age of 10 years; and accumulation of mucopolysaccharide in reticuloendothelial cells (hepatosplenomegaly, lymphadenopathy) and glycolipid in neurones (mental retardation).

Hunter syndrome differs from other mucopolysaccharidoses by having X-linked rather than autosomal recessive genetics. Hunter syndrome (type II mucopolysaccharidosis) is due to a deficiency of sulphoiduronate sulphatase, which leads to the accumulation of both dermatan sulphate and heparan sulphate. Hunter syndrome clinically resembles Hurler syndrome but does not show the abnormal back or corneal opacity. Most patients die by mid-adolescence.

Sanfilippo syndrome (type III mucopolysaccharidosis) is due to deficiency of heparin sulphate sulphatase (or N-acetyl-α-γ-glucose amidase). Heparin sulphate accumulates, producing severe mental retardation.

Tyrosine metabolism abnormalities (Table 6.10)
Abnormalities in the metabolism of tyrosine and its derivatives produce a variety of autosomal recessive disease. Tyrosine is synthesized from phenylalanine by the action of phenylalanine hydroxylase. Deficiency of this enzyme produces **phenylketonuria**, which is characterized by phenylketone excretion into (musty-smelling) urine; decreased myelination with mental retardation and convulsions; and fair skin, fair hair and blue eyes. Decreasing dietary phenylalanine hydroxylase can help minimize the mental retardation.

The skin pigment melanin is synthesized from tyrosine (via dopa) by the action of tyrosinase. Deficiency of tyrosinase produces **albinism**, characterized by pale skin, blue irises, red pupils, photophobia and vulnerability to ultraviolet-induced skin cancers.

The thyroid hormones triiodothyronine (T_3) and thyroxine (T_4) are also synthesized from tyrosine, and genetic blocks in this synthesis produce **cretinism**, with hypothyroidism, mental retardation, umbilical hernia and cretin facies. Tyrosine is degraded to homogentisic acid (which is secreted in urine) by the action of *p*-hydroxyphenylpyruvate oxidase. Lack of this oxidase produces **tyrosinosis**, which manifests with acute or chronic liver disease (cirrhosis) and renal tubular disease. Its manifestations can be partially controlled by a diet low in phenylalanine and tyrosine. Homogentisic acid is further degraded to maleilacetoacetic acid by homogentisic acid oxidase. Lack of this oxidase produces **alkaptonuria** (onchronosis), characterized by urine that turns black on standing; blue-black staining of cartilage in ears, nose, and joints; and chronic arthritis.

Genetic counselling

Genetic counselling is now an established part of clinical practice. It is the **communication of information and advice about inherited conditions**. This communication process has five stages:
- examination;
- history and pedigree construction;
- diagnosis;
- counselling;
- follow-up.

Table 6.10 Examples of inherited enzyme deficiency causing abnormal amino acid metabolism.

Disease	Amino acids affected	Enzyme deficiency	Inheritance pattern	Clinical features
Phenylketonuria	Phenylalanine	Phenylalanine hydroxylase	AR	Mental retardation; musty odour; eczema; increased plasma phenylalanine levels
Hereditary tyrosinaemia	Tyrosine	Hydroxyphenylpyruvic acid oxidase	AR	Hepatic cirrhosis, renal tubular dysfunction; elevated plasma tyrosine levels
Histidinaemia	Histidine	Histidase	AR	Mental retardation; speech defect
Maple syrup urine disease	Leucine, valine, isoleucine	Branched-chain ketoacid oxidase (branched-chain ketoaciduria; ketoaminoacidaemia)	AR	Postnatal collapse; mental retardation; 'maple syrup' odour in urine
Homocystinuria	Methionine, homocystine	Cystathionine synthase	AR	Mental retardation; thromboembolic phenomena; ectopia lentis

AR, Autosomal recessive.

Indications for prenatal diagnosis

Prenatal diagnosis of constitutional chromosome abnormalities is possible in most cases and should be **offered to all patients** who are at **increased risk of cytogenetically abnormal progeny**.

Specimens of amniotic fluid, chorionic villus sample or percutaneous umbilical cord blood sample are submitted for the following reasons.

1 Advanced maternal age. Women older than 35 years have three times greater risk than younger women of having a baby with trisomy. For example, the risk of a liveborn trisomy 21 child is about 1 in 1500 below age 30, 1 in 370 at age 35 and 1 in 100 at age 40.

2 Low maternal serum α-fetoprotein (MSAFP). Although most women with low MSAFP have normal fetuses, about one-third of women carrying a fetus with trisomy have low MSAFP.

3 Parental carrier of a balanced chromosome abnormality.

4 Previous child with chromosome abnormality.

5 Carrier of X-linked genetic disorder (to determine fetal sex). Other indications for prenatal diagnosis include a previous child with neural tube defect, high MSAFP and parental carriers of a recessive mutant gene (e.g. Tay–Sachs disease).

6 Abnormalities seen on an **ultrasound** scan.

Indications for postnatal constitutional chromosome analysis

Specimen–blood or solid tissue:

1 multiple congenital anomalies;

2 unexplained mental retardation and/or developmental delay;

3 suspected aneuploidy, for example, trisomy 21 (Down syndrome);

4 suspected unbalanced syndrome, for example, *cri du chat* syndrome;

5 suspected sex chromosome abnormality, for example, Turner syndrome, Klinefelter syndrome;

6 suspected fragile X syndrome;

7 suspected chromosome-breakage syndrome, for example, Fanconi anaemia, xeroderma pigmentosum;

8 infertility–rule out sex chromosome abnormality;

9 multiple spontaneous abortions;

10 relative of a child with chromosome translocation or other structural chromosome abnormality.

ACQUIRED GENETIC DISEASE

Cytogenetic abnormalities are acquired by most tumour cells (see Chapter 11). The abnormalities are present only in the neoplastic cells and not in the non-neoplastic tissues of the patient's body.

Many of these cytogenetic changes are non-random and are specific for a particular type or subtype of neoplasm. In haematological disorders their identification in neoplastic cells provides important independent prognostic information about the patient's disease, and in some instances may be the single most important factor in predicting outcome. In many kinds of leukaemias and some other haematological disorders, cytogenetic analysis of a specimen of bone marrow is a routine part of the diagnostic workup. Establishment of such clinically important associations has begun for cytogenetic changes in chronic lymphoproliferative disorders, lymphomas and solid tumours.

SUBMISSION OF SPECIMENS TO THE CYTOGENETICS LABORATORY

All specimens for chromosome analysis must be collected and handled to preserve living cells capable of cell division. Aseptic technique must be used because cells will be grown in culture medium for days or even weeks. A working diagnosis or pertinent history indicating the reason for cytogenetic evaluation must be provided with the specimen; this information determines which culture systems, staining techniques and methods of analysis will be used. Communication with the local laboratory is advised before specimens are taken.

Blood

Routine cytogenetic studies are performed on blood specimens, specifically the lymphocytes. Special studies that require special culture and staining techniques are done on blood specimens.

Blood (venous, arterial or capillary) must be collected in preservative-free sodium heparin (green-top Vacutainer tube or heparinized syringe or capillary tube).

The specimen should remain at room temperature until delivered to the cytogenetics laboratory. Heart blood (autopsy) or umbilical cord blood (stillborns, perinatal deaths, fetal blood sampling) may be submitted.

Spontaneously dividing cells are not present in normal blood; therefore, static cytogenetic results are not possible from any specimen except bone marrow. Results from blood specimens are routinely available in 5–10 days. In certain cases, preliminary results can be provided in 2.5 days if a rapid result is mandatory and if arranged in advance with the laboratory. Results of special studies may not be available for 2 or more weeks.

Bone marrow

At least 1–2 ml of aspirated marrow is drawn into a preservative-free sodium heparin syringe. The specimen should be transported immediately, at room temperature, to the cytogenetics laboratory. If the specimen must be sent a long distance or overnight, the heparinized bone marrow should be mixed with sterile tissue culture medium as soon as it is collected.

In samples from patients with haematological disorders, dividing cells may be examined directly from the specimen without culture, and/or after overnight and/or 48-hour culture. A direct examination, particularly useful in acute lymphoblastic leukaemia, is usually possible only if the specimen is received in the cytogenetics laboratory before 1 p.m. Preliminary results are telephoned to the physician in 2–4 days; a final report takes about 2 weeks.

Only numerical chromosome abnormalities (aneuploidy) can be reliably detected in neonatal bone marrow specimens. Bone marrow should not be sent for cytogenetic diagnosis if an abnormality of chromosome structure such as translocation, deletion or duplication is suspected. Blood should be used.

Solid tissue

If chromosomal analysis of blood does not yield an unequivocal result, examination of other tissues (cell types) is necessary (e.g. to exclude mosaicism). Culturing of solid tissue (which usually produces fibroblast cultures) is also useful for examination of fetal and autopsy material when blood is not available or usable.

A small piece (e.g. $0.3 \times 0.3 \times 0.3$ cm) of tissue should be obtained aseptically. A 2–3 mm punch biopsy of skin is most commonly submitted for chromosome analysis. Post-mortem organ specimens such as lung or kidney may be used within 48–72 hours of death. Post-mortem samples of placenta may be cultured successfully even when the fetus has been dead for several days *in utero*.

All specimens should be transported to the cytogenetics laboratory as soon as possible in sterile tissue culture medium. Sterile saline can be used when medium is unavailable if the specimen will reach the cytogenetics laboratory within a few hours. Solid tissue specimens should be refrigerated, but not frozen, in tissue culture medium overnight if immediate transport to the cytogenetics laboratory is not possible.

Results from solid tissue specimens are available in 3–5 weeks, dependent on tissue growth in culture flasks.

Chorionic villus sampling

A small biopsy of chorionic villi, obtained transcervically in the first trimester of pregnancy or transabdominally in the first or second trimester, can be cultured and used for prenatal diagnosis.

At least 10 mg of villi (excluding decidua) is required. The specimen should be transported to the cytogenetics laboratory immediately in sterile tissue culture medium at room temperature. Results are available in 1–2 days, but recent data show that direct results are less reliable than those from cultured chorionic villus sample cells.

Amniotic fluid

Cells from amniotic fluid obtained by transabdominal amniocentesis at 14–20 weeks of gestation are grown in culture and used for prenatal diagnosis. About 20 ml of amniotic fluid should be submitted at room temperature in a sterile syringe or other sterile container. Results are available in 10–21 days.

Other specimens

Cytogenetic analysis of specimens such as solid tumours and effusions is also possible in some laboratories. The local cytogenetics laboratory should be contacted for instructions concerning specimen collection and transport.

FURTHER READING

Connor J.M. & Ferguson-Smith M.A. (1993) *Essential Medical Genetics*, 4th edn. Blackwell Scientific Publications, Oxford.

CHAPTER 7

Multisystem Diseases

CONTENTS

INTRODUCTION

There are many pathological processes that have an effect on a wide range of the body's systems. In a traditional way, and because they have not found a complete home in other chapters, this chapter represents a more indepth review of some of these multisystem diseases. They will be discussed, in part, within the systems chapters of this book (Chapters 14–27).

Endocrine disease will be discussed in Chapter 14; the systemic effects of neoplasia in Chapter 11; vasculitis and hypertension in Chapter 15; cystic fibrosis in Chapter 19; immune deficiency disease and acquired immunodeficiency syndrome (AIDS) in Chapter 10. Chromosomal disease and inborn errors of metabolism (storage diseases) have been discussed in Chapter 6.

NUTRITIONAL DISEASES

Nutritional disorders of hospital patients

Little attention is given to the teaching of clinical nutrition in medical school curricula despite the evidence showing that many disease states are altered, exacerbated or directly occur as a result of altered nutritional status.

Protein-energy malnutrition is relatively rare in western general medical practice. It occurs either as a primary condition, such as 'short-gut syndrome', or as a result of deprivational states such as anorexia or self-neglect or it occurs as a secondary phenomenon in other diseases such as hepatic or renal failure or following therapeutic manoeuvres such as chemotherapy or radiotherapy where vulnerable, rapidly turning over cells such as those in the gastrointestinal mucosa are destroyed. It should also be remembered that several drugs, including alcohol, have significant effects on rates of specific nutrient absorption. Amongst hospital inpatients the incidence of protein-energy malnutrition is very dependent on the length of hospital stay. Inadequate nutritional support in the pre- and postoperative patient is recognized as having significant effects on rate of healing, decreasing resistance to infections leading to sepsis and thus delaying recovery and increasing mortality. Despite this there is no sound evidence that preoperative parenteral nutrition has a positive influence on these parameters.

Assessment of nutritional status

Whilst severe malnutrition is relatively easy to diagnose, mild and moderate degrees of malnutrition may be much harder to detect. Assessment of nutritional status not only allows identification and quantitation of a problem but also gives a baseline from which progress of therapy can be monitored.

Measurements based on **clinical examination** and **anthropometric measurements** such as weight, height and skin thickness are more valuable in assessing paediatric nutrition than in adults. Clinical examination is most useful in the diagnosis of specific deficiencies such as those of thiamine (vitamin B₁) and vitamin C deficiency, whilst the anthropometric measurements including skull circumference and growth rates involving centile charts are most useful indicators in children. **Biochemical markers** such as decreased plasma albumin, total protein and transferrin concentrations and creatinine clearance may give the most objective evidence of protein-energy malnutrition in adults, providing that confounding criteria such as liver failure, nephrotic syndrome, the acute-phase response or iron deficiency are recognized. Nitrogen balance, the difference between nitrogen intake and output after correction for losses from skin and faeces, has been used as a means of assessing nitrogen requirements and as a marker of catabolism. Urinary urea measurement has until recently been the mainstay of assessing nitrogen excretion but this assessment needs to be carefully adjusted for plasma urea concentrations in conditions of altered renal function. Other methods such as calorimetry and isotopic measurements of carbon dioxide production can give good indications of rates of energy expenditure but are cumbersome and expensive.

Because of the relative lack of individual objective measures of nutritional status, various **combined indices**, such as the **prognostic nutritional index (PNI)** calculated from serum albumin and transferrin, delayed hypersensitivity reactivity (DHR) and triceps skinfold thickness have been developed to help decide on the need for nutritional support. This latter is restricted by the problems with the DHR test but those with high values are reported to have a significantly increased risk of postoperative complications and mortality.

Some general criteria that have been used for the diagnosis of malnutrition include a 10% recent unintentional loss of weight, body weight of less than 80% of ideal for height, serum albumin of less than $30\,g/l$ and a total lymphocyte count of less than $1.2 \times 10^6/l$.

Obesity

Obesity is due to a **long-term dietary intake that is above that required for maintenance of the body's functions**. It is defined as body weight 20% greater than the ideal weight. In a western population where up to 30% of the population are overweight, defining 'normal' weights from population studies may give a false baseline.

Measurement of skinfold thickness over the triceps is a much better method. Obesity is present if one can 'pinch an inch'. Normal skinfold thickness for males is less than 23 mm.

The mechanisms for increased mortality risk are generally unclear. However, the following are recognized clinical complications. **Hypoventilation syndrome** due to increased fat in the chest wall (**Pickwickian syndrome**) causes decreased alveolar ventilation and chronic carbon dioxide retention and, long-term, will lead to **pulmonary hypertension**.

Many diseases are increased in incidence in obesity. These include adult-onset diabetes mellitus; hypertension; hyperlipidaemia and subsequent atherosclerosis; osteoarthritis and cholelithiasis.

Protein-calorie malnutrition

Malnutrition seen in developing countries is commonly due to deficiency of total calorie and protein intake. Young children are the most affected.

Marasmus represents a compensated phase of protein-calorie malnutrition in which the dietary deficiencies are compensated for by catabolism of the body's expendable tissue (adipose tissue and skeletal muscle). The result is generalized wasting.

Kwashiorkor represents the decompensated phase of protein-calorie malnutrition in which the utilization of endogenous protein through tissue catabolism can no longer compensate for the dietary lack of protein. The result is decreased synthesis of enzymes and structural proteins and decreasing albumin levels. Generalized oedema results with somnolence and malabsorption. A fatty liver develops. Nutritional anaemia will be an associated factor.

DRUGS AND TOXINS

Poisons

There are many chemicals that cause disease. These may be chemicals of abuse (alcohol, cigarettes, cocaine, sedatives), therapeutic drugs (overdoses, interactions, improper prescribing) or industrial and agricultural chemicals (insecticides, heavy metals). The pathologist and the student in training must be aware of these chemicals and their effects.

Alcohol

Many accidents both in the home and on the road are related to alcohol intoxication. Alcohol is a central nervous system depressant and also has a direct irritant or chemical effect on oesophageal and gastric mucosa.

Acute intoxication due to alcohol correlates with the blood alcohol concentration (BAC). Clinical evidence of

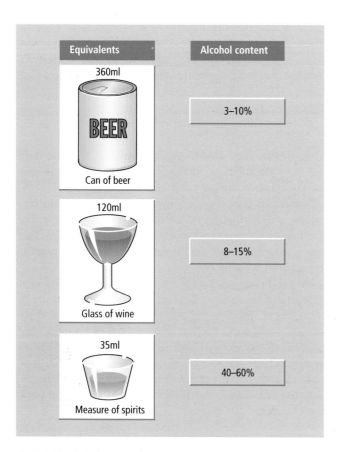

Fig. 7.1 The alcohol content of spirits, wine and beer. A 'measure' of spirits is equivalent to a 'glass' of wine and a 'can' of beer.

intoxication appears at a BAC of 100 mg/dl. However, legally, driving is considered to be affected above a level of 50–80 mg/dl (the legal 'limit'). **Alcoholic coma** will occur when the BAC reaches 300–500 mg/dl.

The effects of alcohol will be enhanced by sedatives and tranquillizers. The alcohol content of different types of beverage varies (Fig. 7.1). The US alcoholic proof is the percentage alcohol content times two (e.g. 100% proof vodka is 50% alcohol); in the UK 87.6 proof equals 100 proof on the US scale.

Rate of **alcohol absorption** varies according to degree of previous alcohol abuse, whether or not alcohol is taken with food and rate of ingestion; rate of **tissue distribution** is related to body weight; rate of **metabolism** depends on the activity of **alcohol dehydrogenase** in the liver and to body weight. An average person metabolizes 150 mg/kg per hour, i.e. 10 g or 20 ml of alcohol per hour for a 70 kg individual, which is the equivalent of a glass of wine (4 oz or 20 ml); the rate of **excretion** in urine or exhaled air is the basis for the alternative tests to blood sampling.

The long-term effects of excess alcohol intake involve almost every organ system. The **hepatic** and **pancreatic** consequences of alcohol are described in Chapter 19. The following concerns the extrahepatic changes.

Heart
A low-output **congestive heart failure** associated with a cardiomyopathy is occasionally seen, although the pathogenesis is unknown. The myocardium also appears more susceptible to **arrhythmias**.

Gastrointestinal tract
Acute **gastritis**, **reflux oesophagitis** and peptic ulceration are common consequences of alcohol intake. In addition, the mucosa of the oesophageal–gastric junction is vulnerable to the vigorous vomiting often accompanying drinking bouts. Tearing of the mucosa and the susequent haematemesis is known as the **Mallory–Weiss syndrome**. Alcohol interferes with the absorption of a number of important nutrients, including amino acids, thiamine and vitamin B$_{12}$.

Haematological effects
Megaloblastic anaemia, partly due to folic acid or vitamin B$_{12}$ deficiency, is frequently seen in chronic alcoholics.

Nervous system
The brain is involved in a number of ways which produce both physical and psychiatric changes. General cortical atrophy is common and particularly in conjunction with thiamine deficiency produces mental confusion, ataxia and polyneuropathy (**Wernicke's encephalopathy**). Cen-

tral pontine myelinolysis is another disorder, probably iatrogenic, and resulting from electrolyte imbalance. It manifests itself as dysphagia and dysarthria leading eventually to coma and respiratory paralysis.

Smoking

Cigarette smoking is the single most important environmental factor contibuting to premature death in the UK and western countries, resulting in a decreased life expectancy for smokers of 6–10 years.

Lung cancer is increased 10 times; ischaemic heart disease (IHD) is doubled in incidence; chronic peptic ulcer is doubled in incidence; carcinoma of the tongue, oral cavity, bladder, larynx and oesophagus have five times the incidence and chronic obstructive airways disease (COAD) has 10 times the incidence in smokers compared with non-smokers.

Most of the associations between smoking and disease have been established by statistical evidence (**epidemiology**). The exact mechanisms by which smoking causes these diseases is not known.

DEGENERATIVE AND METABOLIC DISEASES

Ageing

Ageing is defined as the aggregate of **structural changes that occur with time** and is characterized by progressive inability to sustain vital functions. Life expectancy varies between countries but is generally higher for women than for men. In the UK life expectancy for women is between 75 and 80 years and for men it is between 70 and 75 years.

There are many theories of ageing. A decline in immunological competence accompanies ageing, as does the accumulation of tissue-damaging **free radicals**. It may be that ageing is due to defective DNA repair mechanisms; or that there is **innate programming** in the genome of every cell that determines the mitotic potential of cells. This latter hypothesis is supported by disease processes such as **progeria**, in which the ageing process appears to be accelerated.

Ageing affects every organ system, resulting in atrophy and loss of elasticity of the skin; myocardial fibrosis; pulmonary emphysema; osteoporosis of bone; degeneration of joint cartilage; renal glomerular sclerosis; prostatic hyperplasia; diverticulosis of the colon; pancreatic fibrosis; cortical atrophy of the brain; otosclerosis in the ear and cataract formation in the eye.

Haemochromatosis

Primary haemochromatosis
Definition. Primary/genetic/idiopathic haemochromatosis is an inherited disorder where there is **excess absorption of dietary iron from the gut**.

Epidemiology. It is inherited as a single-gene, **autosomal recessive** disorder, and is one of the three most common genetic disorders with a **gene frequency** of 1 in 10–20 in some populations, and thus a homozygote frequency of approximately 1 in 400. The male to female ratio is 5–7:1; the relative protection of females is due to increased blood (and hence iron) loss due to menstruation and pregnancy.

As the accumulation is progressive, male patients do not usually present until their 40s, and women even later (in their 50s). There are geographical variations due to human leucocyte antigen (HLA) differences between populations (the disease shows HLA linkage).

Aetiology. The disease is closely linked to HLA A3 (75% are A3 as opposed to 28% of the normal population). There are also weaker associations with HLA B7 and B14. The haemochromatosis susceptibility gene would appear to be on **chromosome 6** close to the A locus, and the disease is inherited as an autosomal recessive disorder.

Pathogenesis. The iron overload is due to increased uptake from the gut secondary to abnormal control at the mucosa, but the exact defect is as yet unknown. It is transported around the body by **transferrin** to the various sites which use it (mainly the bone marrow). The liver is the main site of iron storage, containing one-third of the total body iron, mainly in the form of ferritin (Fig. 7.2).

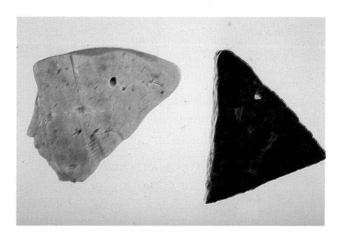

Fig. 7.2 Normal liver (left). Haemochromatosis liver stained with PPB (right).

The increased absorption is from 1 mg/day to 2–4 mg/day, thus the accumulation to pathological levels takes years. The reason for the accumulation is that there is no excretory pathway for iron from the body, normal homeostasis relying on loss via shedding of cells (which contain small amounts of iron) and blood loss.

Iron accumulates in the liver, pancreas, heart, joint linings, other endocrine organs and skin (Fig. 7.3).

The exact mechanism of tissue damage is unknown at a cellular level, but may be due to increased fragility of lysosomes, or to lipid peroxidation and membrane degradation secondary to the formation of free radicals. It results in fibrosis in the liver and pancreas (but not the heart), but the mechanism of the damage in other areas is poorly understood.

Clinical features (Fig. 7.3). Patients present with malaise, weight loss, hepatomegaly, hyperpigmentation of the skin, hypogonadism, diabetes, arthropathy and signs of congestive heart failure (in descending order of frequency). The disease is also known as **bronze diabetes** due to the effects on the skin and pancreas (the characteristic slate-grey colour of the skin is due mainly to increased **melanin** deposition rather than iron).

Patients may be detected at a presymptomatic stage due to abnormalities of blood tests, or because of investigation of relatives of a known haemochromatotic.

Investigations
• Raised serum iron concentration together with decreased serum transferrin, increased transferrin

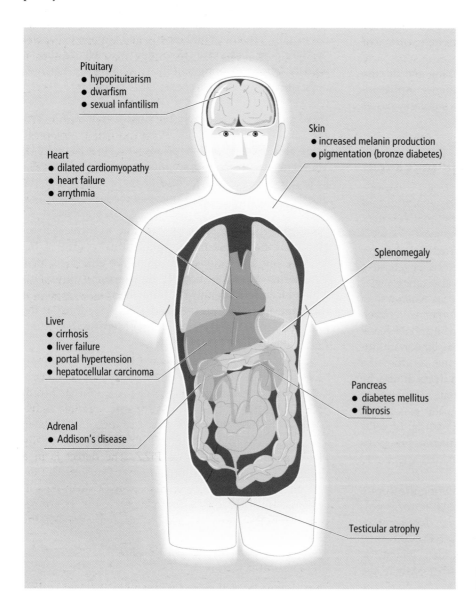

Fig. 7.3 The clinicopathological features of haemochromatosis.

Pituitary
• hypopituitarism
• dwarfism
• sexual infantilism

Skin
• increased melanin production
• pigmentation (bronze diabetes)

Heart
• dilated cardiomyopathy
• heart failure
• arrythmia

Splenomegaly

Liver
• cirrhosis
• liver failure
• portal hypertension
• hepatocellular carcinoma

Pancreas
• diabetes mellitus
• fibrosis

Adrenal
• Addison's disease

Testicular atrophy

saturation and markedly raised serum ferritin is the characteristic pattern.

- Quantitation of iron stores is best done as a chemical measure of iron on liver derived from a biopsy sample.
- Both computed tomography (CT) and, more promisingly nuclear magnetic resonance (NMR), are being used to attempt to assess body iron stores in a non-invasive manner.

Course. Patients are treated by venesection, initially at the rate of 1 unit blood/week, until the serum ferritin drops to 10 mg/ml or the haemoglobin to 10 g/dl (this may take 2 years). Once the iron stores are depleted, 1 unit is removed every 3 months to maintain the normal level of iron stores.

If patients are treated before the advent of cirrhosis, they will have a normal life span. Otherwise death may be due to **hepatocellular carcinoma** developing on top of the cirrhosis, hepatic failure, variceal bleeding secondary to portal hypertension or cardiac failure secondary to the myocardial iron deposition.

Secondary haemochromatosis

Secondary haemochromatosis occurs where there is increased parenchymal deposition of iron due to a number of conditions, including excessive iron ingestion, liver disease with associated iron overload, and various haematological conditions including haemolysis and transfusions. Excess iron deposition in the liver may occur in many other conditions, although not to the level seen in primary haemochromatosis.

It is seen in haematological conditions associated with excessive erythropoiesis, the hyperplastic marrow causing increased absorption of iron despite increasing iron stores. This may be seen in chronic haemolytic states such as β-thalassaemia, sickle-cell anaemia and hereditary spherocytosis. Blood transfusion may also cause increased iron deposition in the liver in patients such as those undergoing long-term therapy for haematological malignancies.

Certain communities ingest vast quantities of iron due to their culinary practices, such as indigenous South Africans who brew their beer in iron pots (**Bantu haemosiderosis**).

Wilson's disease

This disease is due to deposition of **copper** in the liver, basal ganglia of the brain, the cornea and other organs. Presentation is usually between the ages of 5 and 30 years.

Aetiology and pathogenesis

This abnormal copper deposition is due to a rare inborn error of metabolism inherited as an autosomal recessive trait with a homozygote rate of approximately 1 in 100 000. The gene involved is on chromosome 13, but has not been identified yet.

Copper is absorbed from the bowel, carried in the blood by caeruloplasmin, and excreted in the bile. In Wilson's disease there is a low level of caeruloplasmin, decreased biliary and increased urinary copper excretion, and accumulation of ionic copper in various organs.

Clinical features

Patients presenting in childhood usually have **hepatic** manifestations of the disease, those presenting in adulthood usually **neuropsychiatric**. They may present with fulminant hepatitis, chronic active hepatitis or cirrhosis; neurologically with tremor, dystonia and personality deterioration; **Kayser–Fleischer** rings may be seen as a brown deposit at the edge of the **cornea**.

Course

Treatment is by copper chelation with **penicillamine**. The disease is progressive and fatal if untreated. Prognosis depends on the stage of disease at presentation, with those presenting with the acute neurological form of the disease doing particularly badly.

α₁-Antitrypsin (A1AT) deficiency

A1AT is produced by hepatocytes, and is an **acute-phase reactant** and protease inhibitor, most importantly of an elastase from neutrophils which degrades most structural proteins.

Aetiology

A1AT deficiency is an autosomal allelic (codominant) condition with a prevalence of 1 in 3500 in caucasians.

There are 33 different alleles, one being inherited from each parent. Most of the population are described as being PiMM (Pi = protease inhibitor, M = the normal allele); heterozygotes with an abnormal phenotype are usually PiMZ; and homozygotes are PiZZ. The defect is in a single amino acid substitution, different with the different alleles. A1AT is produced in normal quantities in individuals with an abnormal genotype, but is not secreted from the hepatocytes and thus accumulates in the cells.

Clinical features

Patients may present as neonates with **neonatal hepatitis**;

in childhood with **cirrhosis**; and in adults with **cirrhosis** or **emphysema** (although only rarely with the two together).

Course

Pulmonary disease may be treated with **synthetic A1AT**. Cirrhotics may be transplanted, the recipient's phenotype becoming that of the donor so that the disease should not recur.

RADIATION

Burns

A burn is a **localized injury due to heat**. Burns are a major cause of death in the west. They may be evaluated firstly by their depth.

A minor burn will cause erythema and oedema of the epidermis and is termed a **first-degree burn**. They heal rapidly without scarring.

Second-degree burns involve the full thickness of the epidermis but spare the dermal adnexa (hair follicles) and show blister formation in addition to erythema and oedema. These may heal but scarring will occur.

Third-degree burns are full-thickness, including the entire epidermis, dermis and adnexal structures; they result in a protein-rich exudate with fluid loss and risk of infection. These heal very slowly by the ingress of epithelium from the unburned skin edges.

When more than 10% of the body surface is involved, fluid loss will produce hypovolaemia and hypotension unless replaced. Burns of up to 75% of the body surface area are incompatible with survival. A method of calculating the involvement of the body surface area in burns is given in Fig. 7.4.

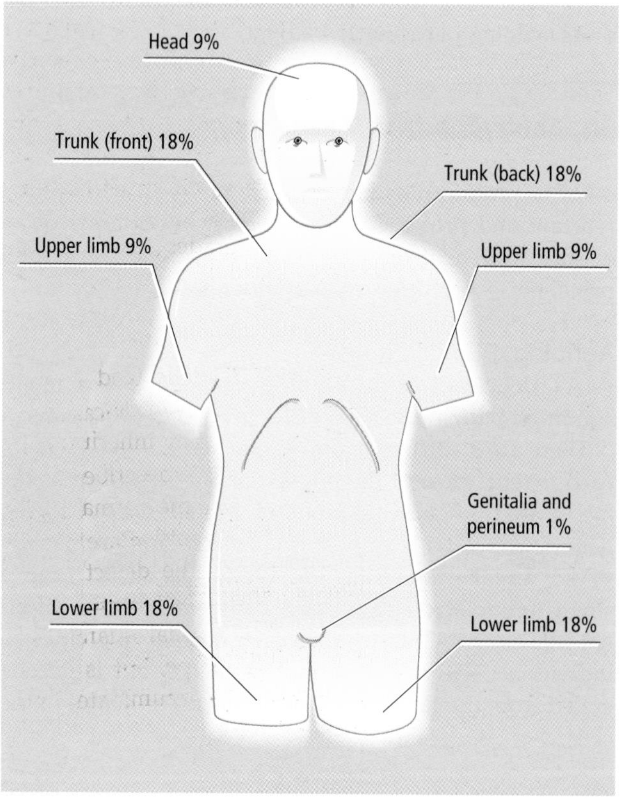

Ionizing radiation (Fig. 7.5)

The effects of radiation are **dose-dependent**. Fortunately, the consequences of exposure to large doses are rarely seen, being restricted to accidents at nuclear reactors such as at Chernobyl or following the use of atomic bombs on Hiroshima and Nagasaki at the end of the Second World War. Much more common, however, are the effects of low-dose radiation, usually as a result of its therapeutic use.

Fig. 7.4 Burns. The rule of '9s' for estimating the percentage of body surface area involved in burns.

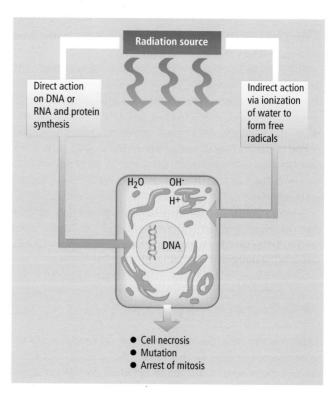

Fig. 7.5 The effects of radiation on cells.

Effects of high-dose radiation exposure

The **lethal dose** of total body irradiation begins around 200 rad. The mode of death is related to three mechanisms, each of which is related to the dosage received.

- **>2000 rad.** Exposure of the whole body to a large dose of radiation (greater than 2000 rad) results in death within 24 hours mainly due to damage of the **central nervous system**. There is direct killing of the neurones and damage to the vascular endothelium produces cerebral oedema and coma.
- **1000–2000 rad.** This dosage will also result in death, although the effects are largely related to the **gastrointestinal system**. The rapidly proliferating intestinal epithelium is particularly vulnerable to the radiation and extensive necrosis and ulceration of the intestinal mucosa result. This breakdown in the mucosal barrier permits the entry of the bowel's bacterial flora into the blood stream and produces septicaemia. In addition there is severe diarrhoea and electrolyte imbalance. Symptoms usually begin a few days after exposure and death occurs within a couple of weeks.
- **200–1000 rad.** This dosage will produce death as a result of damage to the **haematological system**. Since the hematopoietic stem cell is affected, the patients are deficient in white blood cells, erythrocytes and platelets, resulting in lethal infections, anaemia and bleeding problems. Symptoms usually begin within 10 days and death occurs 3 weeks after exposure.

Effects of low-dose radiation exposure

There is probably no safe level of radiation dosage, although those used for investigative medical procedures such as chest X-ray are sufficiently low for their benefits to outweigh by far any possible disadvantages. Therapeutic procedures require the use of higher doses and, although attempts are made to screen and protect normal tissues during treatment, there is inevitable damage to tissues, e.g. the skin, in the path of the radiation beam.

The complications of low-dose radiation can be divided into **neoplastic** and **non-neoplastic**.

Examples of radiation-induced malignancy include **sarcomas** secondary to radiotherapy for breast carcinoma, **lung carcinoma** developing in miners of uranium ore and **osteogenic sarcoma** arising in 'luminous dial' paint workers who licked their brushes to create a fine point and in the process ingested the radium-containing paint. These malignancies usually appear many years after the original exposure.

Non-neoplastic complications of low-dose radiation exposure are often the result of **fibrosis** which follows healing of the damaged tissues. This can take a number of forms depending on which part of the body is irradiated, for example strictures of the oesophagus or small bowel, pulmonary fibrosis or constrictive pericarditis. Cataracts and xerophthalmia may follow irradiation of the eye.

IMMUNE-MEDIATED MULTISYSTEM DISEASES

A number of diseases, often with a major immunological component, affect multiple organ systems (Table 7.1). Some features have been covered in other chapters (particularly Chapter 9), but this chapter aims to give an overview of these conditions and place the organ damage in a more general perspective.

These disorders include almost all the connective tissue diseases and a hotch-potch of other conditions that have defied efforts at classification and whose aetiology is obscure. The diversity of presentations of these diseases means that they are often misdiagnosed or missed altogether. In some cases, there are no specific diagnostic tests available.

Connective tissue diseases

These diseases comprise a family of related conditions. Although there are specific identified syndromes, in practice there is considerable overlap between them and it is best to refer to these cases as undifferentiated connective tissue. Passage of time frequently allows a more precise classification as clinical and laboratory features evolve and fit more clearly into established patterns. All the conditions have evidence for immune involvement, although

Table 7.1 Immune-mediated multisystem disorders.

Connective tissue diseases	Systemic lupus erythematosus
	Sjögren's syndrome
	Systemic sclerosis
	Mixed connective tissue disease
	Polymyositis
	Polychondritis
	Rheumatoid arthritis (see Chapters 9 and 20)
Vasculitis	Polyarteritis
	Wegener's granulomatosis
	Kawasaki disease
	Giant cell arteritis (see Chapter 15)
Miscellaneous	Polyserositis (familial Mediterranean fever)
	Behçet's disease
	Sarcoidosis
	Amyloidosis
	Alcohol poisoning
	Radiation

the connection between the laboratory abnormalities and the pathogenesis of the disease is often obscure (see Chapters 3 and 9).

Systemic lupus erythematosus (SLE)

SLE is the archetypal multisystem disease and no part of the body is spared (Table 7.2). It is not uncommon, with a prevalence of about 1 per 1000. It is predominantly a disease of **young women**, and there is clear evidence from animal models that oestrogens are important in determining disease susceptibility.

There are marked racial differences in susceptibility, with Caribbean blacks having the highest rates. There is a moderately strong association with the **autoimmune** major histocompatibility complex (MHC) haplotype, HLA-A1, B8, DR3, and also with null alleles for complement C4a; some patients are also found to be complement C2-deficient.

The form of presentation is highly variable, but most patients will have symptoms of systemic illness such as malaise, tiredness, weight loss and anorexia. Fevers may

occur, and presentation as a pyrexia of unknown origin is not uncommon.

Investigation of suspected lupus should include the tests listed in Table 7.3. In cases where the first presentation is to a renal unit with renal failure, the diagnosis is frequently made on the renal biopsy (Fig. 7.6; see Chapter 21). Biopsy of other sites is rarely necessary or helpful. Examination of the bone marrow may be valuable where the anaemia is unexpectedly severe, to determine whether there is marrow suppression or an active marrow with excessive peripheral destruction.

Treated patients, on high-dose immunosuppression, are at risk of opportunistic infections (see Chapter 10) especially cytomegalovirus, which may also cause bone marrow suppression and justify bone marrow examination. Under these circumstances, microbiological, virological and serological studies are particularly important. The organ systems involved in SLE will be described (Fig. 7.7).

Brain. Cerebral involvement in SLE is common, and includes severe psychosis, epilepsy, impairment of higher mental function, hemiplegia and migraine. Involvement of peripheral and cranial nerves may occur. Examination of **cerebrospinal fluid** shows elevated cell counts and protein, with a low C4. Autoantibodies have been detected that react with neuronal tissue but their role in disease is uncertain. Small-vessel inflammation probably plays a major role. The anticardiolipin antibody/lupus anticoagulant is associated with cerebral thrombotic events and should always be sought in neurological lupus. Cerebral atrophy occurs.

Lungs. Interstitial lung disease occurs in about a fifth of patients, with pneumonitis and fibrosis ('shrinking lung' syndrome). Biopsy acutely shows an alveolar infiltrate of

Table 7.2 Clinical features in systemic lupus erythematosus (SLE).

Arthritis/arthralgia
Myositis/myasthenia gravis
Pneumonitis/pleurisy/pleural effusions/'shrinking lungs'
Cardiomyopathy/pericarditis/endocarditis (Libman–Sacks)
Hepatosplenomegaly/ascites
Glomerulonephritis
Psychosis/fits/meningitis/migraine
Neuropathy
Anaemia/leukopenia/thrombocytopenia/haemolytic anaemia
Discoid lupus erythematosus/alopecia/livedo reticularis/panniculitis/ vasculitis
Lymphadenopathy
Autoimmune endocrine disease

Table 7.3 Diagnosis of systemic lupus erythematosus (SLE).

Antinuclear antibody (ANA)	May be negative; not useful for monitoring
ds-DNA antibody	Usually positive; titre corresponds poorly with disease activity
Anti-Ro antibody	Present in ANA-negative lupus; neonatal lupus and congenital heart block
Anti-La antibody	Present if there are features of secondary Sjögren's syndrome
Anti-Sm antibody	Specific for SLE; mainly found in West Indians
Anti-RNP antibody	Marker for MCTD but may be found in SLE
Antiribosomal P antibody	Associated with cerebral lupus (not routinely available)
Anticardiolipin antibody	Associated with recurrent thromboses; livedo reticularis; lupus anticoagulant
Complement C4	Low levels may be due to consumption or to presence of null alleles
Complement C3	Low levels during active disease due to consumption
C3 breakdown products (C3d)	Raised levels in active disease
C-reactive protein	May be normal in active disease

MCTD, Mixed connective tissue disease.

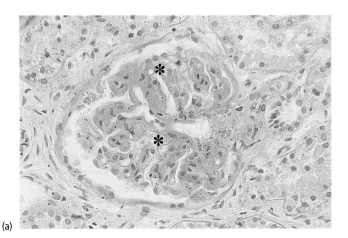

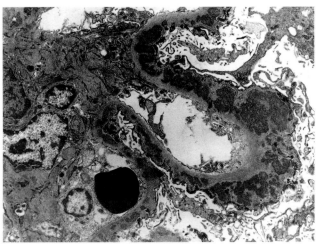

Fig. 7.6 The renal glomerulus in systemic lupus erythmatosus (SLE). (a) Histology. Note the thickened glomerular basement membrane forming the classical 'wire loop' glomerular lesion (✽). (PAS.) (b) Electronmicroscopy. Note the epimembranous glomerular deposits typical of SLE.

mononuclear cells. Pleural involvement, pleurisy and pleural effusions are more common. The effusions have a high protein content (> 30 g/l).

Heart. Pericarditis often accompanies pleural involvement and histologically there is an inflammatory cell infiltrate with fibrin deposition. Chronic constrictive pericarditis appears to be an uncommon sequela. Myocardial involvement is less common but coronary arteritis may lead to myocardial infarction. **Libman–Sacks endocarditis** is commoner as an autopsy finding than a clinical problem. The vegetations comprise degenerating valve tissue with fibrin and platelet thrombi, and immunoglobulin can be detected, suggesting that deposition of immune complexes from the circulation may be the trigger. Peripheral vascular involvement includes **Raynaud's phenomenon**, and small-vessel **vasculitis**, with splinter haemorrhages and digital infarcts. The pres-

ence of the **anticardiolipin antibody** is associated with venous and **arterial thromboses** and **fetal loss** through occlusion of the placental circulation.

Gut. Vasculitis of the bowel blood vessels may lead to perforation. Serositis may occur, as in the chest, and sterile ascites may accumulate. Abnormal liver function tests may be detected, and for reasons that are unclear lupus patients seem prone to develop hepatic dysfunction when treated with high-dose aspirin. Pancreatitis may also occur.

Skin. There is considerable overlap between **discoid lupus** (DLE) and SLE, although not all patients with SLE will have cutaneous manifestations. Typically, there will be a **butterfly rash** across the face. Photosensitivity is particularly associated with the presence of antibodies to Ro (SSA), as this antigen is induced in the skin by sunlight. Skin biopsy in both DLE and SLE often shows deposition of granular immunoglobulin G (IgG) and C3 at the dermoepidermal junction and this is present in uninvolved skin in SLE. Alopecia also occurs in SLE, as well as being a consequence of cyclophosphamide therapy. Livedo reticularis, a small-vessel vasculitis giving rise to a dusky **chicken-wire** pattern on the limbs, is associated with the presence of anticardiolipin/lupus anticoagulant antibodies.

Joints and muscles. Arthralgia is commoner than actual arthritis, although a small number of patients do develop a deforming arthropathy. Often the small joints of the hand are swollen during acute flares of the disease. Myositis and a vacuolar myopathy are also seen.

Blood. Lymphopenia is one of the diagnostic criteria for lupus and lymphocytotoxic antibodies may occur, although they are not sought routinely. Reductions of red cells, platelets and neutrophils may occur either from marrow suppression or from increased destruction due to autoantibodies directed against the cells. Rarely, the first presentation of lupus is with idiopathic thrombocytopenia, and young women presenting with idiopathic thrombocytopenic purpura should have their serology checked for evidence of SLE. During active disease, lymphadenopathy and splenomegaly are common.

Renal. The most feared complication of lupus is **glomerulonephritis**. The biopsy features of lupus are protean (see Chapter 21), and it is invariably possible to demonstrate immunoglobulin and complement (IgG and C3) deposition in the glomeruli. Renal involvement is often found in patients with the highest levels of anti-dsDNA antibodies. Monitoring of serum creatinine, creatinine clearance, protein excretion and regular urine microscopy for the presence of red cells and casts is important. When there is excessive protein loss (nephrotic syndrome), the serum albumin and IgG will be reduced.

Others. Involvement of the lacrimal and salivary glands will lead to a sicca syndrome, similar to that seen in Sjögren's syndrome (see below), and this is associated with the presence of antibodies to Ro (SS-A) and La

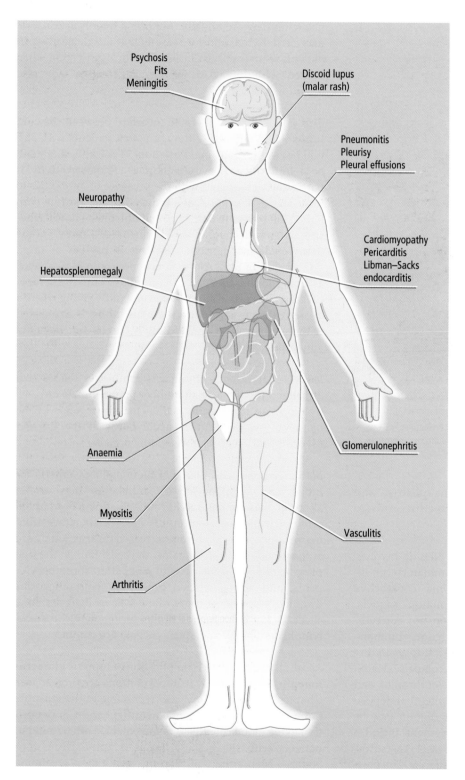

Fig. 7.7 Clinicopathological features of SLE.

(SS-B). SLE patients, presumably because of their immunogenetic background, have a higher incidence of other autoimmune diseases, including thyroid disease and myasthenia gravis. Autoantibodies to thyroid microsomes and to the acetylcholine receptor will be found under these circumstances.

Systemic sclerosis and CREST syndrome

Systemic sclerosis is characterized by induration and thickening of the skin, with excessive collagen deposition (scleroderma).

There is a spectrum of disease ranging from localized scleroderma (morphea) to a disease with multiorgan involvement (progressive systemic sclerosis–PSS).

As with other autoimmune diseases, **females** are more commonly affected than males, and the age of onset is rather older than for SLE. In most cases, the aetiology is completely unknown, although chemicals such as vinyl chloride and aniline derivatives (in Spanish rapeseed oil) can give a very similar picture.

The **CREST syndrome** (calcinosis, **R**aynaud's, o**Eso**phageal dysmotility, sclerodactyly and **t**elangiectasia) appeared at first to be a milder variant of PSS, but significant organ involvement occurs in most patients eventually. The clinical features of PSS are summarized in Table 7.4. **Fibrosing lung disease** is common, with a marked reduction in carbon monoxide transfer factor, and often leads to **cor pulmonale**. Involvement of the oesophagus, with an increase in the fibrous tissue, reduces peristalsis and aspiration into the lungs occurs, further impairing lung function. Similar involvement of the small intestine leads to stasis and bacterial overgrowth, as well as severe malabsorption, particularly of fats and fat-soluble vitamins. Arterial involvement in the kidney leads to renal damage and severe hypertension, which further exacerbates the destruction of the glomeruli. Involvement of blood vessels in the extremities frequently leads to gangrene of the digits and to resorption of the terminal phalanges.

Histological examination of the skin shows **excessive collagen** together with obliteration of the small blood vessels. Calcium, in the form of calcium hydroxyapatite, is deposited in the subcutaneous tissues in the CREST syndrome and may erode through to the surface. Fibrosis is also seen in larger blood vessels and eventually thrombotic occlusion supervenes. These changes involve all organs. The degree of fibrosis is often out of proportion to the inflammatory cell infiltrate.

Antibodies to DNA topoisomerase (Scl-70) are found in 25% of PSS patients and antibodies to nucleolar constituents are often found. CREST is associated with antibodies to the **centromere** and also with **anti-RNP antibodies**. Complement and immunoglobulin changes are not useful diagnostically and the C-reactive protein is usually normal. The clinical features are usually sufficiently striking that routine skin biopsy is unnecessary. The full blood count will give evidence of malabsorption of haematinics, and the prothrombin time and serum calcium will indicate failure of vitamin K and D absorption. As for SLE, a close watch should be kept on renal function.

Sjögren's syndrome

Sjögren's syndrome is an autoimmune disorder of exocrine glands. It may occur alone (primary) or in association with any of the other connective tissue diseases, particularly SLE and rheumatoid arthritis, and with other autoimmune diseases such as primary biliary cirrhosis.

Characteristically there is involvement of the salivary and lacrimal glands, leading to dry eyes and dry mouth with difficulty swallowing (**sicca syndrome**). However, Sjögren's is a multisystem disorder and other organ systems are involved (Table 7.5).

Damage to the mucus-secreting glands lining the **bronchial tree** by infiltrating lymphocytes leads to recurrent infection, due to failure of the mucociliary clearance sytem, and bronchiectasis results. **Renal involvement**

Table 7.4 Clinicopathological features of systemic sclerosis.

Scleroderma/sclerodactyly
Peripheral gangrene
Reduced intestinal motility, malabsorption
Pulmonary hypertension and cor pulmonale
Interstitial lung disease/pleural effusions
Pericarditis
Myositis
Polyarthropathy
Renal failure ('scleroderma kidney')
Peripheral neuropathy

Table 7.5 Clinical features of Sjögren's syndrome.

Keratoconjunctivitis sicca (dry eyes)
Dry mouth
Chronic bronchitis (thickened mucus)
Pneumonitis/pleural effusions
Dysphagia
Gastritis/pancreatitis
Primary biliary cirrhosis/sclerosing cholangitis
Interstitial nephritis/renal tubular acidosis
Myositis
Peripheral neuropathy
Arthralgia/arthritis
Pseudolymphoma/lymphoma
Autoimmune endocrine disease

unusually involves the tubules more than the glomeruli and there is an infiltrate of lymphocytes around the tubules. Renal tubular acidosis, aminoaciduria and renal glycosuria result.

About 10% of patients will have **autoimmune thyroid disease** and a small number will develop **vitiligo**.

Vascular involvement may occur, mainly involving small vessels, and leading to skin ulceration, peripheral nerve damage (to the vasa nervorum) and central nervous system damage (manifest as epilepsy and hemiplegia). Infiltration of the salivary glands by lymphocytes may be massive and mimic lymphoma (pseudolymphoma), although the cells are polyclonal. However, true lymphoma may also occur as a direct development, and is usually B-cell-derived, even though the infiltrates early in the disease include both B cells and activated T cells.

The diagnosis is usually based on a combination of clinical symptoms, the **Schirmer test** to demonstrate reduced tear flow and laboratory tests. Biopsy of the minor submucous salivary glands of the lip is simple and provides evidence of the lymphocytic infiltrate. Needle or open biopsy of a major gland is indicated if there is significant enlargement, to rule out lymphoma, particularly in long-standing disease. The erythrocyte sedimentation rate (ESR) is usually high, but the C-reactive protein is variable; serum immunoglobulins are elevated. The precise pattern of autoantibodies found will depend on the associated conditions, but usually there is a speckled antinuclear antibody, with antibodies to Ro and La but rarely dsDNA (unless SLE is present). Rheumatoid factors are often found, more so in secondary than primary disease. Autoantibodies to thyroid microsomes, smooth muscle and mitochondria may also occur.

Mixed connective tissue disease (MCTD)

Overlap syndromes between all the connective tissue diseases can occur. MCTD has features of several diseases and for many years a debate raged about whether it constituted a separate disease entity. It seems to affect mainly females, usually in the older age range, and does not have any clear racial or familial tendency. The typical features are summarized in Table 7.6.

Raynaud's phenomenon is the commonest feature and most patients also develop mild sclerodermatous changes in the skin of the hands. An erosive arthropathy may occur. Muscle pains and occasionally polymyositis-like symptoms and signs may occur. Changes in the gastrointestinal tract and lungs are similar to systemic sclerosis, though less severe. Originally it was said that renal disease was uncommon in MCTD, but this is clearly not the case: glomerulonephritis is found and may be severe.

Serologically, these patients may be distinguished by having high levels of **anti-RNP** antibodies and a speckled pattern antinuclear antibody without elevated levels of anti-dsDNA antibodies. Complement levels are normal in the majority of patients, but some will show a reduction of C3, as in SLE. Rheumatoid factors are found in about half the patients. Over long periods of time, patients with MCTD frequently progress in a manner similar to PSS or to SLE, and it is incorrect to label MCTD as benign.

Polymyositis/dermatomyositis

This group of diseases is very **heterogeneous** and comprises several distinct syndromes with different associations and clinical features (Table 7.7).

Features of polymyositis commonly accompany other connective tissue diseases such as SLE, PSS and Sjögren's syndrome, or it may occur alone. For these patients there is a female predominance, and family members often have other autoimmune diseases. There is an association with HLA-A1, B8, DR3 haplotype.

Polymyositis and dematomyositis also occur secondary to tumours amongst an older age group and here there is a male predominance. As the skin and muscle changes often precede the diagnosis of malignancy, studies have been done to try and assess the likelihood of a tumour being present. Unfortunately the studies are conflicting, but in patients over the age of 50, 25–50% are likely to have an underlying malignancy. Both conditions occur in childhood but take a rather more aggressive course and have vasculitis as a very prominent feature. The nature of the tissue damage in polymyositis is rather better understood than some of the other connective tissue diseases.

Muscle biopsy reveals evidence of fibre necrosis ac-

Table 7.6 Features of mixed connective tissue disease.

Raynaud's phenomenon
Scleroderma/sclerodactyly
Arthralgia
Interstitial lung disease
Pericarditis
Myositis
Intestinal dysmotility
Glomerulonephritis
Anaemia/leukopenia/thrombocytopenia

Table 7.7 Features of polymyositis.

Primary polymyositis
Primary dermatomyositis
Polymyositis or dermatomyositis associated with malignancy
Juvenile dermatomyositis/polymyositis associated with vasculitis
Dermatomyositis/polymyositis secondary to other connective tissue disease

companied by an inflammatory cell infiltrate of lymphocytes and macrophages, which is most marked around the blood vessels.

Although autoantibodies are detectable in about 30% of cases, they do not seem to be directly involved in tissue damage (secondary antibodies).

Investigation depends on demonstration of muscle damage by measuring the serum **creatine kinase**. The MM isoenzyme is the major skeletal muscle component. However, this is not specific for polymyositis, as elevations are also seen in the primary myopathies and muscular dystrophies. Myoglobin is also detectable in the serum but this is not used routinely as a diagnostic test. **Muscle biopsy** and electrical studies are needed to confirm the diagnosis.

The ESR may be raised, as may the serum immunoglobulins. Antibodies to transfer-ribonucleic acid (RNA) (histidyl and threonyl) and a variety of other nuclear proteins occur. The most useful marker, present in 30% of adult patients, is **anti-Jo-1**, directed against histidyl-transfer-RNA. This seems to identify a group of patients with myositis and interstitial pulmonary fibrosis.

Miscellaneous conditions

Relapsing polychondritis. This is an inflammatory condition of cartilage, which normally affects the auricular cartilage first. Internal structures of the ear may also be involved, leading to deafness, vertigo and ataxia. Involvement of the nasal cartilage leads to a **saddle-nose deformity**. The laryngeal and tracheal cartilage may become involved, with serious embarrassment of the breathing. Other features include **arthritis**, **conjunctivitis**, episcleritis, iritis and keratitis; damage of the aortic root leads to **aortic regurgitation**.

Histological examination of the cartilage shows loss of basophilic staining, indicating loss of the cartilage matrix. There is an inflammatory cell infiltrate, including lymphocytes and plasma cells. Antibodies to type II collagen can be found, but this is not used as a diagnostic test. Antinuclear antibodies may be weakly positive. The ESR is high and the C-reactive protein is substantially elevated (> 20 mg/dl). As well as occurring alone, polychondritis may also occur in patients with established SLE and rheumatoid arthritis.

Familial polyserositis (familial Mediterranean fever). This an unusual inherited condition (**autosomal recessive**) characterized by recurrent bouts of pleurisy, peritonitis and arthritis accompanied by fever. Amyloidosis may occur as a complication. It can occur in any racial group, but has a predilection for the Mediterranean races (hence its name). The pathology of acute attacks is unremarkable: the peritoneal exudate comprises mainly neutro-phils. When amyloid develops, the deposition occurs mainly in arterioles, venules, kidney and spleen. The cause is unknown.

Behçet's disease

This is a multisystem disorder that presents with recurrent oral and genital ulceration, arthritis, uveitis and multiple sclerosis-like symptoms.

The cause is unknown but a viral trigger has been suspected for some time, although never conclusively proven. There is an association with HLA-B51. Three clinical patterns are recognized (Table 7.8).

The histology confirms a vasculitic process with an inflammatory cell infiltrate, endarteritis obliterans, fibrinoid necrosis and thrombosis. Skin involvement includes a folliculitis and erythema nodosum. Minor trauma leads to a florid non-specific inflammatory reaction–so-called **pathergy**. Anterior uveitis is common, but posterior chamber involvement, iritis, retinal vessel occlusion and optic neuritis may all occur and blindness may result. Large-vessel arteritis may occur, with an aortitis and aneurysm formation or with major arterial thrombosis. The arthritis is predominantly of large joints and is non-deforming. There are no specific tests for Behçet's, although the acute-phase proteins and ESR are invariably raised in active disease. The diagnosis is a clinical one.

Sarcoidosis

This is another multisytem disorder of unknown cause. It is characterized by non-caseating granulomas containing predominantly T cells and macrophages (Fig. 7.8).

It is assumed that this is caused by an ineffective immune response to a pathogen, as it resembles the response to *Mycobacterium* and insoluble foreign material. Despite extensive study, no convincing candidate pathogen has been identified. All races and ages and both sexes are affected and there does not appear to be any convincing immunogenetic susceptibility.

The disease may be mild and asymptomatic, with bihilar lymphadenopathy picked up on a routine chest radiograph, or there may be evidence of widespread

Table 7.8 Clinical patterns in Behçet's disease.

Type I	Mucocutaneous (skin, mouth, genitalia)
Type II	Type I with large joint involvement
Type III	Features of type II with neurological and/or ocular involvement

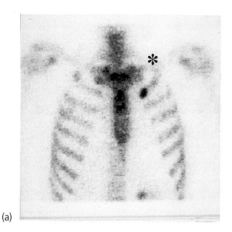

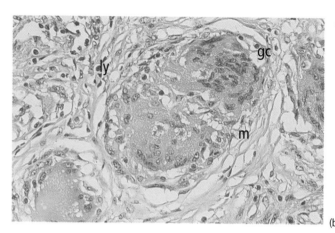

(a)

(b)

Fig. 7.8 (a) Sarcoidosis presenting with hilar lymphadenopathy. This gallium scan shows uptake in enlarged mediastinal lymph nodes (marked with an asterisk). (b) Histology of the enlarged hilar lymph nodes in sarcoidosis. Note the well circumscribed 'naked' granulomas featuring macrophage giant cells (gc), 'epithelioid' macrophages (m) and lymphocytes (ly) without caseous necrosis. (H&E.)

tissue involvement with constitutional symptoms such as weight loss, malaise and anorexia.

Any organ in the body may be affected (Table 7.9 and Fig. 7.9), but typically there is **skin** involvement with erythema nodosum, lymphoid involvement with lymphadenopathy and lung involvement with interstitial disease.

The histology represents the immunological nature of the disease. The typical early lesion comprises aggregates of lymphocytes, mainly activated T cells, and macrophages. This evolves into an organized granuloma with epithelioid cells and multinucleated giant cells becoming prominent; the phagocytic cells occupy the centre and the lymphocytes form the rim of the lesion (Fig. 7.8(b)). A number of different inclusion bodies may be identified within these macrophages, e.g. **Schaumann bodies** are conchoidal, basophilic structures and **asteroid bodies** are star-shaped inclusions present within vacuoles in giant cells. Although these features are distinctive, they are not pathognomonic of sarcoidosis.

If the disease is persistent or untreated then **fibrosis** occurs, with subsequent loss of organ function.

In the peripheral blood, there is marked polyclonal hypergammaglobulinaemia. Hypercalcaemia also occurs and appears to be due to the release of vitamin D metabolites by the activated macrophages in the granuloma. **Angiotensin-converting enzyme** levels are also increased. A positive **Kveim test** results in the development of a granuloma in the skin 4–6 weeks after injec-

tion of a crude extract of sarcoid spleen into the dermis. Both false positives and false negatives occur and there are difficulties in obtaining suitable material: the test is used less often than formerly.

Lymph nodes

Nearly all cases of sarcoidosis show involvement of the lymph nodes, usually in the form of hilar and mediastinal lymphadenopathy.

Table 7.9 Organ involvement in sarcoidosis.

Organ	Features
Lung	Hilar lymphadenopathy; interstitial granulomas; pleural effusions
Lymphoid	Lymphadenopathy, splenomegaly
Bone marrow	Neutropenia, mild anaemia, thrombocytopenia
Liver	Hepatomegaly, granulomatous hepatitis, cholestasis, cirrhosis
Skin	Cutaneous granulomas (lupus pernio), erythema nodosum, clubbing
Eye	Uveitis, iritis, keratoconjunctivitis sicca
Parotid glands	Bilateral enlargement, xerostomia
Bones	Bone cysts
Muscles	Polymyositis; granulomatous myopathy
Heart	Granulomatous involvement of myocardium (left ventricular dysfunction); heart block; pericarditis
Nervous system	Chronic meningitis, space-occupying lesions (rare); pituitary damage; cranial nerve lesions
Kidney	Rarely involved; nephrocalcinosis from hypercalcaemia

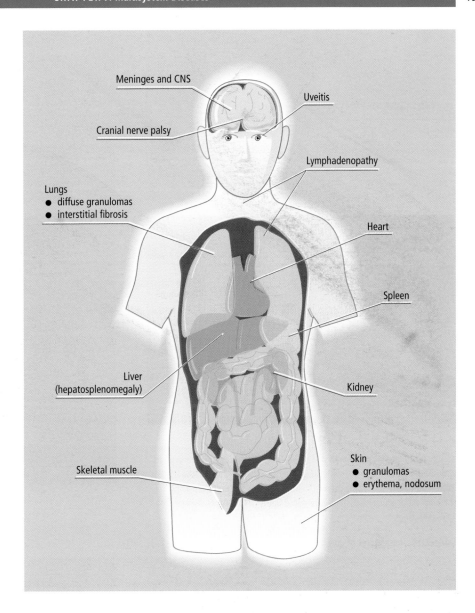

Fig. 7.9 Clinicopathological features of sarcoidosis.

Lungs

These are frequently involved and small discrete nodules, 1–2 cm, are formed. The resulting fibrosis which may occur produces long-term clinical problems. The pleura is also sometimes involved.

Spleen

Although the majority of cases demonstrate splenic involvement histologically, only a minority of cases will exhibit splenomegaly.

Skin

Approximately half the cases of sarcoidosis show skin involvement in the form of small nodules. In addition, some cases are associated with the skin condition ery-

thema nodosum, which is characterized by the presence of painful red raised lesions, usually on the lower leg.

Eyes

Iritis, iridocyclitis and choroiditis may result from ocular involvement.

Salivary glands

These may be enlarged. The combination of eye and salivary gland involvement is known as **Mikulicz's syndrome**.

Others

Involvement of the conducting system of the heart may lead to arrhythmias.

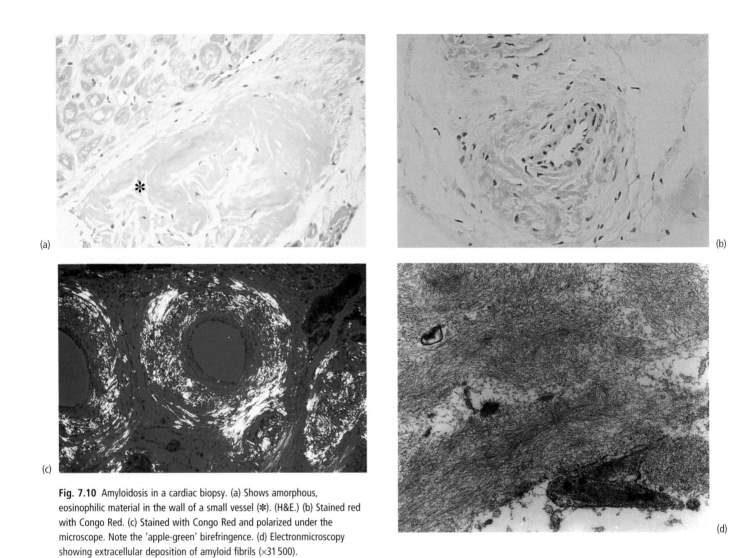

Fig. 7.10 Amyloidosis in a cardiac biopsy. (a) Shows amorphous, eosinophilic material in the wall of a small vessel (✱). (H&E.) (b) Stained red with Congo Red. (c) Stained with Congo Red and polarized under the microscope. Note the 'apple-green' birefringence. (d) Electronmicroscopy showing extracellular deposition of amyloid fibrils (×31 500).

Table 7.10 The features of amyloidosis.

Amyloid protein	Main constituent	Diseases	Distribution
AL	Immunoglobulin light chain	Primary amyloidosis Plasma cell myeloma B-cell malignant lymphoma	Tongue, heart, gastrointestinal tract, liver, spleen, kidney (primary distribution)
AA	Serum A protein (α_1-globulin)	Rheumatoid arthritis Chronic infections (tuberculosis, leprosy, bronchiectasis, osteomyelitis) Hodgkin's disease Inflammatory bowel disease	Tongue, heart, gastrointestinal tract, liver, kidney, spleen
AA	Serum A protein (α_1-globulin)	Familial Mediterranean fever	Liver, kidney, spleen
AF	Prealbumin	Familial amyloidosis (Portuguese, Swedish, etc.)	Peripheral nerves, kidney
AS	Prealbumin	Senile amyloidosis Cardiac amyloidosis Cerebral amyloid angiopathy	Heart, spleen, pancreas Heart Cerebral vessels
AE	Peptide hormone precursors (e.g. calcitonin)	Medullary carcinoma of thyroid Pancreatic islet cell adenomas	Locally in the neoplasm
AD	Unknown	Lichen amyloidosis	Skin (dermis)
Alzheimer	A_4 peptide	Alzheimer's disease	Neurofibrillary tangles, plaques and angiopathy

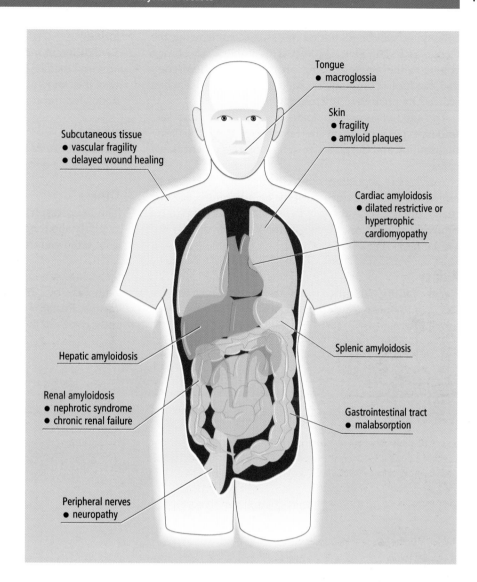

Fig. 7.11 Clinicopathological features of amyloidosis.

The **diagnosis** can be made in a number of ways. Certain **clinical patterns** of this disease are characteristic, for example, the combination of erythema nodosum, arthropathy and bilateral hilar lymphadenopathy is diagnostic. **Histologically** the diagnosis is one of **exclusion** since similar changes may be encountered in a number of other conditions such as mycobacterial or fungal infections, berylliosis and in lymph nodes draining malignant tumours.

Amyloidosis

Amyloidosis is a term which covers a number of diseases which have quite different aetiologies. All these diseases have in common the presence, within a variety of organs,

of **amyloid**, an extracellular proteinaceous substance (Fig. 7.10(a)).

Although there are many types of amyloid, they all have a similar basic physicochemical configuration and an identical electronmicroscopic appearance (Fig. 7.10(d)).

Classification of amyloidosis is complicated because the historical classifications bear no relationship to the chemical structure of the proteins involved (Table 7.10). There are two main types of amyloid, **AL (amyloid light chain)** and **AA (amyloid associated**; see Chapter 3).

AL type is associated with plasma cell disorders which produce free light chains, usually 1 in type. AA type of amyloid is associated with chronic inflammatory suppurative disorders, e.g. osteomyelitis, bronchiectasis and tuberculosis.

Amyloid can be identified in tissue sections using the Congo red stain (Fig. 7.10(b)). This imparts an orange colour to the amyloid using ordinary light microscopy and produces a dramatic apple-green birefringence when viewed by polarizing microscopy (Fig. 7.10(c)).

The subdivision of amyloidosis into **primary** and **secondary** types is based on clinical criteria such as the tissue distribution and the presence or absence of an identifiable cause.

Amyloid is deposited extracellularly and produces its effects through pressure atrophy on adjacent cells. Virtually any organ system can be involved and the pattern of involvement cannot be predicted precisely on an individual basis (Fig. 7.11).

Kidney
Renal failure secondary to renal involvement is the commonest cause of death in patients with amyloidosis.

Spleen
Two different macroscopic patterns are encountered. The amyloid may be confined to the splenic follicles, in which case it is known as a **sago-spleen**, or it may be diffusely deposited, producing a **lardaceous** spleen.

Heart
The heart can be involved as part of a generalized form of amyloidosis or as a localized lesion.

Others
The liver, respiratory system, gastrointestinal tract (particularly the tongue), brain (in Alzheimer's disease) and endocrine glands may all be involved.

The **diagnosis** of amyloidosis must be made on **biopsy** material by **histochemical** or **electronmicroscopic** means. Rectal biopsy and renal biopsy (where clinically indicated) are the most common.

Tropical and Imported Infectious Disease

INTRODUCTION

Many of the important infections that are now virtually confined to the tropics are associated with poor sanitation, limited health care, lack of vector control, inadequate vaccination and overcrowding and are not especially restricted to tropical climates and habitats.

Plague, cholera, leprosy, anthrax and vivax malaria have all caused significant morbidity in northern Europe in the past but have disappeared with improvements in living standards and through deliberate public health measures.

Then there are infectious diseases that are essentially tropical in distribution. The parasite causing falciparum malaria, in its stages outside the human body, requires high temperatures that do not occur consistently outside the tropics, although potential vectors occur well into the temperate zones. Conversely, many geographically localized infectious diseases are restricted in distri-

bution by the ranges of their specific vectors and many zoonoses are confined to the distribution of their reservoir host.

All such infections may be imported as isolated cases and sometimes small epidemics can occur beyond the natural boundaries of the disease. Infectious diseases may also be imported from temperate areas. North America, for example, is the home of several infectious diseases, such as Rocky Mountain spotted fever and coccidioidomycosis, that are not native to Europe.

BACTERIAL DISEASES

Rarer bacterial infections with tropical or restricted geographical distributions are summarized in Table 8.1. The more widespread diseases are reviewed individually. All of them were formerly well-established or have caused outbreaks or epidemics in northern Europe.

Table 8.1 Rarer tropical and imported bacterial infections.

Disease and organism	Geographical distribution	Mode of acquisition	Clinical features	Treatment
Glanders (Gram −ve rod) *Burkholderia mallei*	Asia, Africa	Animal contact	Lymphangitis	Poorly evaluated
Brazilian purpuric fever (Gram −ve rod) *Haemophilus aegyptius*	Brazil	Droplet spread	Conjunctivitis, fever, purpura	Ampicillin Cephalosporin
Tularaemia (Gram −ve rod) *Francisella tularensis*	N. America N. Europe	Animal contact, tick bites	Fever, ulcer, lymphadenopathy	Streptomycin
Plague (Gram −ve rod) *Yersinia pestis*	Asia, Africa N. America	Flea bites, inhalation	Lymphadenopathy (bubo), fever, septicaemia, pneumonia	Streptomycin Tetracycline
Bartonellosis, Oroya fever (Gram −ve) *Bartonella bacilliformis*	S. America	Sandfly bite	Fever, arthralgia, skin nodules	Penicillin Chloramphenicol
Buruli ulcer (Acid-fast) *Mycobacterium ulcerans*	Pantropical	Unknown	Chronic ulcers	Poorly evaluated
Actinomycetoma (Fig. 8.1) *Actinomadura*, actinomycetes *Streptomyces, Nocardia*	Pantropical	Thorns and skin abrasions, especially feet	Granulomatous swellings	Streptomycin Dapsone Co-trimoxazole
Yaws (spirochaete) *Treponema pallidum*	Pantropical	Skin contact	Skin lesions	Penicillin
Pinta (spirochaete) *Treponema carateum*	Neotropics	Skin contact	Skin lesions	Penicillin
Relapsing fever (spirochaetes) *Borrelia* spp.	Worldwide	Louse and tick bites	Recurrent fever	Tetracycline
Endemic typhus (*Rickettsia*) *Rickettsia prowazekii*	Tropical highlands	Louse bite	Rash, fever	Chloramphenicol Tetracycline
Scrub typhus (*Rickettsia*) *Rickettsia tsutsugamushi*	Indo-Australian	Mite bite	Rash, fever	Chloramphenicol Tetracycline
Spotted fevers (*Rickettsia*) *Rickettsia* spp. (Rocky Mountain spotted fever−*R. rickettsiae*; *R. conorii* in Africa and Mediterranean)	Worldwide	Tick bite	Rash, fever	Chloramphenicol Tetracycline

Anthrax

Anthrax is caused by *Bacillus anthracis*, an aerobic, spore-forming, toxin-forming, rectangular, Gram-positive rod. It is a disease of herbivores, which acquire it from contaminated pasture. The disease occurs in Africa and the Middle East. Humans become infected through animal contact and by handling contaminated hides, wool and bone. The bacterium may be imported in such products. Cutaneous contact leads to the formation of an ulcer with a central black eschar, which yields the bacterium when cultured. Inhalation (**wool sorter's disease**) leads to mediastinitis which is usually lethal unless treated. Treatment of anthrax is with **parenteral penicillin**. Vaccination is available for those with high risk of exposure.

Cholera

Vibrio cholerae is an aerobic, Gram-negative, curved rod which occurs naturally in estuarine and other coastal waters. Particular strains are associated with the disease cholera.

The endemic focus of this disease is the Ganges delta from which worldwide pandemics arise. Variation in somatic (O) antigens is used to type strains. Two classic serotypes causing cholera are known as Ogawa and Inaba. The El Tor strain survives better in the environment than classical strains and is less likely to promote disease when carried. O139 is associated with a recent epidemic in India.

Cholera is transmitted by **faecal–oral** route. The organism lives in the gut, is non-invasive and secretes enterotoxin which results in elevation of cyclic adenosine monophosphate in mucosal cells and release of water and salts into the gut. The disease is characterized by dehydration with **rice-water stools** and **shock**. Diagnosis is confirmed by culture on selective media. Treatment is by intravenous or oral fluid and salt replacement and tetracyline or ampicillin. A cholera vaccine is available which is useful for control of epidemics and for travellers to high-risk areas but it is only partly effective.

Mellioidosis

The agent of the disease is a Gram-negative, aerobic rod, formerly known as *Pseudomonas pseudomallei* or **Whitmore's bacillus**. Recently, the name *Burkholderia pseudomallei* has been proposed.

The organism is a soil saprophyte and is especially common in rice paddies in South East Asia but has been reported from Africa, the Americas, Australia and France. Human and animal infections are possibly acquired through skin abrasions or by inhalation. Most cases are reported from South East Asia. There can be a long latent period following exposure and disease has occurred years after leaving an endemic area.

Mellioidosis is characterized by acute, subacute and chronic infection with pneumonia, cavitation, suppurative lymphadenitis, parotitis and septicaemia. The organism forms distinctive colonies on Ashdown's medium. **Ceftazidime** is an effective treatment.

Brucellosis

Brucella spp. are small, aerobic, Gram-negative rods. The generic name honours Sir David Bruce who described the organism as the cause of **Malta fever**. Many mammal species may harbour *Brucella* spp. The *Brucella* spp. causing most human infections are *B. abortus* (mainly from cattle) and *B. melitensis* (mostly from sheep and goats).

Following campaigns involving the testing and vaccination of herds, brucellosis is all but eradicated from the UK and large areas of northern Europe and North America and is mainly an infection of the tropics and subtropics. Infection is acquired through **animal contact** and drinking unpasteurized milk. Farmers, zoologists and slaughterhouse workers are at risk. Microbiology laboratory workers are at risk of infection and cultures must be handled in a safety cabinet.

Brucellosis is protean in its clinical manifestations and may present with vague malaise, fatigue, constant or **undulant fever**, backache and psychological depression. Positive blood culture confirms diagnosis. Serology is useful but not always sensitive or specific. Treatment is with **rifampicin** and **tetracycline**.

Leprosy

The causative agent, *Mycobacterium leprae*, is an acid-fast rod. It is not amenable to *in vitro* culture but will grow in the armadillo, *Dasypus novemcinctus*.

Most cases occur in the tropics but the disease was formerly widespread in Europe and cases are seen in immigrants from endemic areas. Transmission is poorly understood but is possibly spread by skin contact or by droplets from the nasopharynx. The disease may be slow to develop and diagnosed long after leaving an endemic area.

Presentation depends on the host's response to infection and may be tuberculoid, lepromatous or intermediate (see Chapter 26).

Lepromatous leprosy is characterized by widespread skin involvement with erythema, nodules and deformity. There is diffuse nerve involvement with patchy loss of sensation.

Tuberculous leprosy consists of discrete plaques with erythema, hypopigmentation and localized nerve involvement. Anaesthetic areas are prone to injury and secondary infection. Lepromatous patients are prone to develop erythema nodosum, especially in association with treatment. Triple therapy is advised, consisting of **dapsone**, **clofazimine** and **rifampicin**.

Lyme disease

Lyme disease has been reported mainly from northern temperate countries and is especially common in **New England**. Cases acquired in the UK are rare.

Small rodents act as the disease reservoir. The disease is transmitted by ticks (*Ixodes ricinus* in Europe and

I. dammini in New England). The causative agent is a spirochaete, *Borrelia burgdorferi*.

The disease presents with an expanding erythematous lesion (erythema chronicum migrans) at the tick bite site. Patients may develop secondary skin lesions, arthralgia, headache and pain at various sites. A minority of cases have meningoencephalitis and cardiac involvement. Detection of spirochaetes by culture or histology is unreliable. Diagnosis is usually by serology which may be difficult to interpret. Early disease and Lyme arthritis respond to **oral doxycycline**. Intravenous **penicillin** or **cephalosporins** are used for serious infection.

Actinomycosis (Fig. 8.1)

Actinomyces spp. are filamentous bacteria. Infection with these organisms causes a chronic, suppurative inflammation in the lungs, large bowel, jaw and soft tissue, sometimes termed **mycetoma**. Other filamentous bacteria, including *Nocardia* spp. and certain mycelial fungi such as *Madurella* and *Streptomyces* spp. may produce similar clinical patterns of infection and may also involve the soft tissues of the foot (**Madura foot**).

VIRAL DISEASES

A great many viral causes of human infection have been recorded that have tropical or restricted geographical distributions.

Table 8.2 shows some of the important agents and principal clinical features. The diseases are generally **zoonoses**, causing sporadic disease in humans, although urban yellow fever and dengue fever are transmitted from human to human and epidemics of others, such as

o'nyong nyong fever, may occur with human-to-human transmission.

Most of these conditions are transmitted by **biting arthropods (arboviruses)** but some are acquired through direct contact with the host animal, its urine or faeces. Cases of infection may be seen in travellers or contacts of infected imported animals. Diagnosis is by serology and where possible by viral culture.

Vaccination is advised for travellers to areas with a high risk of yellow fever and Japanese encephalitis. Where there has been possible exposure to a rabid animal, courses of antirabies immunoglobulin and vaccine should be given. Persons at risk of rabies, such as zoologists, should be vaccinated. Treatment of viral infection is supportive. Acyclovir should be used in the treatment of *Herpesvirus simiae* infection.

Yellow fever

Silvan yellow fever is a **zoonosis**, being an infection of monkeys, transmitted by forest mosquitoes (*Aedes* spp. and *Haemagogus* spp.). Human cases are sporadic.

Urban yellow fever occurs when a cycle of infection occurs in dense human populations, transmitted by the synanthropic mosquito *A. aegypti*. It occurs in the Neotropics and Afrotropics where famous epidemics have occurred. *A. aegypti*, imported to the UK on ships, has been able to establish temporary colonies in hot weather and there have been yellow fever epidemics at several ports in temperate areas. Severity of infection varies from being almost inapparent to fulminating disease and death. The incubation period is several days, after which the patient becomes febrile with widespread pains. Haemorrhagic illness with jaundice and further deterioration and death may follow. Treatment is supportive.

Dengue fever

Dengue fever has a pantropical distribution and is transmitted by *A. aegypti*. There are several serotypes.

Primary infection is characterized by fever, flushing, aches, nausea and altered sensation. Dengue haemorrhagic fever is a more serious illness associated with subsequent infection by a different serotype. There is thrombocytopenia, bleeding and a mortality rate of several per cent.

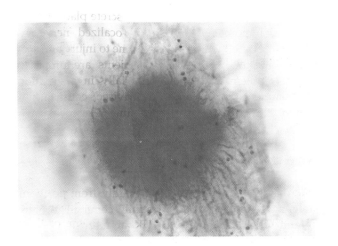

Fig. 8.1 Bacterial disease. Microscopic appearance of an *Actinomyces* colony.

Table 8.2 Simplified account of tropical, imported and geographically restricted viral infections.

Virus family	Virus	Geographical origin	Mode of acquisition of disease	Reservoir	Main features
DNA viruses					
Poxviridae	Monkey pox	Zaire	Monkeys, interpersonal	Monkeys	Variola-like
Herpesviridae	*Herpesvirus simiae*	Asia	Monkey handling	Monkeys	Severe simplex-like
RNA viruses					
Reoviridae	Colorado tick fever	Rocky Mountains	*Dermacentor* tick	Rodents	Fever, meningitis
Togaviridae	O'nyong nyong	Africa	Mosquitoes	Uncertain	Fever, rash
	Sindbis	Africa, Eurasia	Mosquitoes	Birds	Fever, rash
	Chikungunya	Africa, Asia	Mosquitoes	Monkeys, humans	Arthralgia, rash
	Equine encephalitides	Americas	Mosquitoes	Birds	Encephalitis
Flaviviridae	Yellow fever	Africa, S. America	*Aedes* spp. mosquitoes	Humans, primates	Haemorrhagic fever
	Dengue fever	Pantropical	*Aedes aegypti* mosquito	Humans	Haemorrhagic fever
	Japanese encephalitis	Asia	*Culex* sp. mosquito	Birds	Encephalitis
	Murray Valley	Australia	*Culex* sp. mosquito	Birds	Encephalitis
	Tick-borne encephalitis	Europe	*Ixodes* spp. ticks	Birds, rodents	Encephalitis
	Kyasanur Forest	India	Ticks	Mammals	Haemorrhagic fever
	Omsk haemorrhagic	Siberia	*Dermacentro* tick sp.	Rodents	Haemorrhagic fever
Rhabdoviridae	Rabies	Worldwide	Mammal bite	Mammals	Hydrophobia, paralysis
	Duvenhage	S. Africa	Bat bite	Bats	Rabies-like
Filoviridae	Marburg	Africa	Monkey handling	Uncertain	Haemorrhagic fever
	Ebola	Africa	Interpersonal	Unknown	Haemorrhagic fever
Bunyaviridae	Rift Valley fever	Africa	*Aedes* spp. mosquitoes	Mammals	Haemorrhagic fever
	Congo–Crimean	Africa, Asia	Ticks	Birds, mammals	Haemorrhagic fever
	Hantaan group	Asia, N. America	Rodent excreta	Rodents	Haemorrhagic fever
Arenaviridae	Lassa	W. Africa	Rats, interpersonal	*Mastomys* rat	Fever, pharyngitis
	Junin	Argentina	Rodent excreta	Rodents	Haemorrhagic fever
	Machupo	Bolivia	Rodent excreta	Rodents	Haemorrhagic fever

FUNGAL INFECTIONS (Figs 8.2–8.4)

Many species of fungi may cause human disease. Examples of important tropical and North American fungal diseases, seldom seen in Europe, are shown in Table 8.3.

Fungi may be identified by cultures from appropriate specimens. Newer antifungal agents, such as fluconazole, may well be useful in the treatment of some of these conditions but have yet to be evaluated fully.

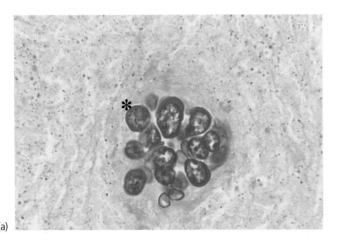

(a)

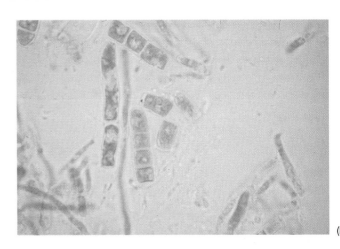

(b)

Fig. 8.2 Fungal disease. (a) Coccidioidomycosis. Lung histology shows the organisms within an area of necrotic lung (✱). (PAS.) (b) *Coccidioides immitis*. A smear shows the morphology of the organism. (Lactophenol blue.)

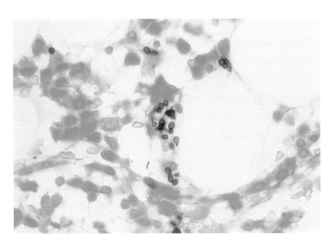

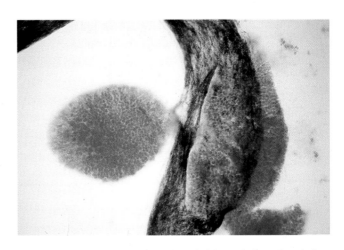

Fig. 8.3 Fungal disease. *Histoplasma capsulatum* seen in this section of lung, stained with Grocott.

Fig. 8.4 Fungal disease. *Trichosporon beigelii* (white pidra) on a hair shaft.

PROTISTAN DISEASES

Malaria

Malaria has a pantropical distribution and was formerly widespread in Europe. Infection is acquired from the bite of *Anopheles* mosquitoes and occasionally from infected blood. Malaria parasites are protists of the genus *Plasmodium* (*P. falciparum*, *P. vivax*, *P. malariae*, *P. ovale*). The infecting stage is the **sporozoite**, which migrates to the liver to form **hepatic schizonts**. These release **merozoites** into the blood which invade erythrocytes to produce **ring forms** and later **trophozoites**.

A cycle of multiplication becomes established in the blood whereby trophozoites produce schizonts which re-

lease merozoites which infect more erythrocytes (Fig. 8.5). Some merozoites produce gametocytes which are infective to mosquitoes. Human disease relates to the erythrocytic stages of the parasite life cycle.

Malaria is characterized by paroxysms of fever and malaise. Physical signs may include anaemia, hepatosplenomegaly and jaundice.

P. falciparum infection is potentially lethal because of overwhelming parasitaemia and possible cerebral malaria or renal failure. *P. vivax* is able to persist in the liver for many months, allowing the parasite to overwinter in temperate climates.

Diagnosis of malaria is confirmed by examination of Giemsa-stained blood smears. The mainstay of malaria prophylaxis is **chloroquine**. In areas of the world where there is chloroquine resistance, mefloquine, Maloprim

Table 8.3 Tropical and imported fungal diseases.

Disease and fungal agents	Geographical distribution	Clinical features	Treatment
Blastomycosis *Blastomyces dermatitidis*	USA	Systemic disease, mainly pulmonary and cutaneous	Amphotericin Ketoconazole
Chromomycosis *Fonsecaea pedrosoi* *Cladosporium carrionii* etc.	Mainly tropical	Cutaneous lesions	Surgery Antifungals
Coccidioidomycosis *Coccidioides immitis* (Fig. 8.2)	Panamerican	Pulmonary, cutaneous and disseminated infection	Amphotericin for severe disease
Histoplasmosis *Histoplasma capsulatum* (Fig. 8.3)	USA Africa	Pulmonary and disseminated infection in immunocompromised	Amphotericin for disseminated infection
Mycetoma (Madura foot) *Madurella* spp. *Pseudallescheria boydii* (see actinomycetoma)	Pantropical	Swelling and deformity of foot and sometimes of other sites	Poorly evaluated
South American blastomycosis *Paracoccidioides brasiliensis*	Neotropics	Pulmonary and cutaneous disease	Sulphonamides Ketoconazole
Sporotrichosis *Sporothrix schenckii*	Mainly neotropical	Cutaneous lesions Lymphatic spread Joint infection	Iodides (amphotericin for serious infection)
White piedra *Trichosporon beigelii* (*T. cutaneum*) (Fig. 8.4)	Mainly tropical	White nodules on hair Systemic infection in immunocompromised	Shaving hair Antifungals

and proguanil may be suitable alternatives. Malaria can be treated with chloroquine. Where there is resistance, quinine and mefloquine may be used. Quinine is the treatment of choice for serious falciparum malaria. It should be noted that resistance patterns change and the latest information should be sought for malaria prophylaxis and treatment.

Leishmaniasis

Leishmaniasis includes a variety of diseases caused by protistan parasites of the genus *Leishmania*, of which there are several ill-defined species and species complexes, each associated with particular natural hosts, vector species, geographical distributions and disease manifestations. Small mammals act as reservoir hosts. Infection is transmitted by **sandflies**, *Phlebotomus* spp. and *Lutzomyia* spp. in the New World. Infection can also be acquired **congenitally** and through **blood** contact.

In the fly, the parasite is of the flagellated, **promasti-**gote form. A granuloma forms at the bite site. The parasites infect macrophages, lymphocytes and other reticuloendothelial cells. In humans, the parasites exist as non-flagellated forms (**amastigotes**). Human disease is classified as cutaneous, diffuse cutaneous, mucosal and visceral.

Geographical distributions and agents of the different forms are shown in Fig. 8.6.

Cutaneous leishmaniasis is manifested by a chronic ulcerating lesion at the bite site. Diagnosis is confirmed from stained smears of ulcer scrapings. Most lesions will heal eventually, leaving a scar, but antimonials may be used for treatment. Diffuse cutaneous leishmaniasis is characterized by chronic disseminated papular lesions.

Antimonials, pentamidine and amphoterecin are used as therapy.

Mucosal leishmaniasis is a progressive mutilating condition of the nose, mouth and throat. Treatment involves antimonials and reconstructive surgery.

In visceral leishmaniasis (kala-azar), there is widespread infection of the reticuloendothelial system,

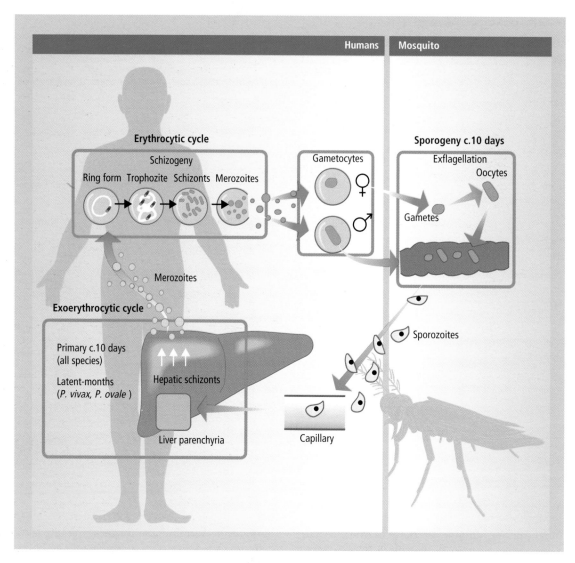

Fig. 8.5 Life cycle of malaria.

resulting in fever, anaemia, immunosuppression, hepatosplenomegaly and secondary infection. Diagnosis is confirmed by examination of bone marrow aspirates. Antimonials are used for treatment.

Trypanosomiasis (Fig. 8.7)

Trypanosomes are protistan flagellates. African trypanosomiasis (sleeping sickness) is transmitted by **tsetse flies**, *Glossina* spp., and is caused by *Trypanosoma brucei gambiense* in West Africa and *T. b. rhodesiense* in East Africa.

At the onset of infection there is a chancre at the bite site from which trypanosomes may be collected for diag-

nosis. The infection spreads to cause regional or widespread lymphadenopathy, anaemia, pancarditis and later meningoencephalitis.

East African disease is the more serious and acute disease. It is a zoonosis, naturally infecting game animals. West African trypanosomes are much better adapted to the human host and may cause asymptomatic or chronic infection. Diagnosis is by Giemsa-stained preparations of blood and cerebrospinal fluid. African trypanosomiasis is treated with **suramin** but meningoencephalitis requires therapy with arsenicals.

South American trypanosomiasis (**Chagas' disease**) is caused by *T. cruzi* and is transmitted by triatomine bugs. A chagoma forms at the bite site and the infection disseminates to regional lymph nodes and via the blood to

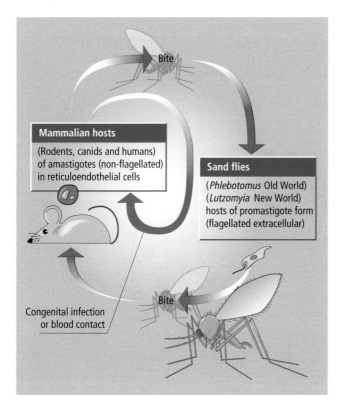

Fig. 8.6 Life cycle of leishmania.

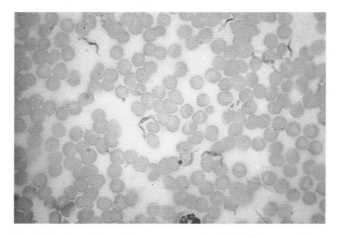

Fig. 8.7 Protistan disease. Trypanosomes seen in a blood film.

muscles. Lesions commonly occur in myocardium, leading to heart failure and digestive tract muscle, leading to dilatation. Chagas disease may be diagnosed by examination of blood smears and serology. Xenodiagnosis is used at specalist centres and employs clean bugs that are fed on the patient and examined later for trypanosomes. Treatment is with Nifurtimox.

HELMINTHS

Worms that parasitize humans are collectively referred to as helminths and belong to two phyla, the **Nematoda** (roundworms and filarial worms) and the **Platyhelminthes** (flatworms) which include the **Cestoda** (tapeworms) and **Trematoda** (flukes). Helminth infections are often associated with **eosinophilia**.

Nematoda

From a medical viewpoint, the nematodes can be conveniently divided into **intestinal nematodes**, whose adult stages reside in the lumen or wall of the gut–roundworms, including hookworms, threadworm and whipworms–and **tissue nematodes**, whose adults occur in the tissues and lymphatic vessels–the filarial worms and the guinea worm.

Toxocara canis, and *Trichinella*, whose adult exists transiently in the ileum, are included with the tissue nematodes because their larvae are destructive to human tissues. Many nematodes have complex life cycles, involving different hosts and vectors and whose larval stages pass through various parts of the human body.

Filarial worms

Four species of filarial worm cause significant morbidity in humans (Table 8.4). They are restricted to the tropics and some adjacent temperate countries. The adult worms reside in the lymphatic vessels or subcutaneous tissues where they reproduce to release larval forms (Fig. 8.8) (microfilariae) into the blood (Fig. 8.9) or tissue fluids. All of them are transmitted by biting flies. Larvae undergo stages of development within the fly.

Diagnosis may be confirmed by finding microfilariae on Giemsa-stained blood smears. Release of microfilariae into the blood is related to the time of day that the vector fly is active. In onchocerciasis, microfilariae may be searched for in skin snip preparations. The adult worms of loaiasis may be seen crossing the conjunctiva or obtained from nodule biopsy (see Fig. 8.8).

Non-filarial tissue nematodes

Three unrelated non-filarial tissue nematodes are important human pathogens (Table 8.5).

Dracunculosis has a wide but patchy distribution in the Old World tropics and is a significant cause of morbidity but seldom life-threatening. **Trichinellosis** and

Table 8.4 Filarial worms and disease.

Species and disease	Features of disease	Geographical distribution	Vector	Location of adult worms	Treatment
Wuchereria bancrofti Bancroftian filariasis	Lymphangitis Lymphoedema Elephantiasis	Pantropical	Mosquitoes (*Anopheles, Aedes*, etc.)	Lymphatics	Diethylcarbamazine (surgery for elephantiasis)
Brugia malayi Malayan filariasis	Lymphangitis Lymphoedema Elephantiasis	S.E. Asia	Mosquitoes (esp. *Mansonia*)	Lymphatics	Diethylcarbamazine
Loa loa Loaiasis (Fig. 8.9)	Swelling	Central and W. Africa	*Chrysops* flies	Migrate through connective tissues including conjunctiva	Diethylcarbamazine (surgical removal)
Onchocerca volvulus Onchocerciasis River blindness	Rash, nodules, blindness	Africa and tropical America	*Simulium* blackflies	Subcutaneous tissues	Ivermectin (surgery)

Table 8.5 Non-filarial tissue nematodes.

Species and disease	Features of disease	Geographical distribution	Mode of acquisition	Location of worm in humans	Treatment
Dracunculus medinensis Dracunculosis (guinea worm)	Subcuataneous inflammation, blister, bacterial infection	Africa, India, Pakistan, Middle East	Water with infected *Cyclops*	Adults migrate through the subcutaneous tissues	Surgery (metronidazole)
Trichinella spiralis Trichinosis	Eosinophilia, muscle pain, orbital oedema	Worldwide	Uncooked pork and carnivores	Adults in larvae encyst in muscles	(Thiabendazole) (Corticosteroids)
Toxocara canis Toxocariasis	Eosinophilia, cough, endophthalmitis	Worldwide	Contact with dog faeces	Larvae migrate through body (visceral larva migrans)	(Corticosteroids)

toxocariasis are worldwide. In both diseases it is the larval worms that damage human tissues.

Very heavy *Trichinella* infection can cause lethal multisystem lesions. Thiabendazole and corticosteroids may be beneficial. The infection is acquired from **undercooked meat**, especially pork, but numerous wild carnivores are potential sources.

Toxocara larvae are ill-suited to life in humans and never mature into adult worms. The migrating larvae are a cause of visceral larva migrans, where larvae wander through the body causing a variety of symptoms. Corticosteroids may be of benefit but toxocariasis is best avoided by worming dogs and avoidance of ground contaminated with dog faeces. Larvae occasionally reach the eye, causing endophthalmitis, retinitis and blindness.

Dracunculosis

The guinea worm, *Dracunculus medinensis*, is acquired by drinking water that contains *Cyclops* (Crustacea), infected with *Dracunculus* larvae.

The larvae penetrate the duodenum and migrate through the body, eventually to mature into adult male and female worms which dwell in the subcutaneous tissues. Fertilized female worms gradually migrate to the extremities (often the foot) and emerge through the skin to release first-stage larvae, especially upon contact with water. The emerging worm causes inflammation, pruritis and the formation of a blister which may become subject to bacterial infection. Larvae need to be ingested by *Cyclops* to continue their development. The whole life

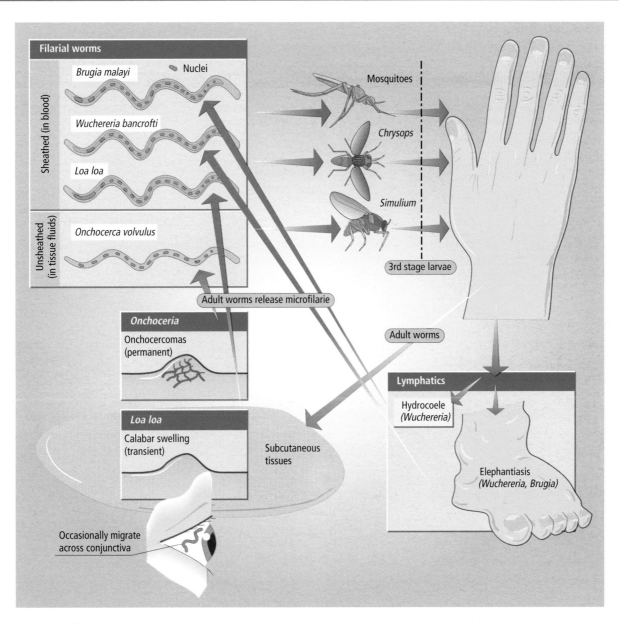

Fig. 8.8 Life cycle of filarial worms.

cycle takes about a year, allowing the guinea worm to survive in arid regions with a short wet season. Worms may be removed surgically or be wound out gradually around a stick. Metronidazole reduces inflammation around the worm. Provision of clean drinking water eliminates *Dracunculus* infestation.

Intestinal nematodes

The intestinal nematodes are parasites whose adults live in the **human gut** (Table 8.6). Infection is often asympto-

matic but worldwide these parasites impose a considerable burden on humanity.

Eggs are passed in the faeces, or in the case of *Enterobius* onto perianal skin and are either directly infective to humans or develop in soil into infective larvae. Therefore, these organisms depend on poor sanitation for transmission and tend to be most abundant in the tropics.

The two species of hookworm *Necator americanus* and *Ancylostoma duodenale* and *Strongyloides stercoralis* (Fig. 8.10) infect humans through the skin as larvae from contaminated soil. Penetration of the skin may result in pruritus. Larvae migrate through the body, pass through

Table 8.6 Intestinal nematodes.

Species and disease	Features of disease	Geographical distribution	Mode of acquisition	Location of adult in humans	Treatment
Strongyloides stercoralis Strongyloidiasis (Fig. 8.10)	Skin rash Pneumonitis Diarrhoea	Pantropical Rare in Europe	Skin contact with soil (autoinfection)	Small intestine	Thiabendazole
Necator americanus Hookworm	Pruritus Cough Enteritis Anaemia	Pantropical N. America	Skin contact	Small intestine	Mebendazole
Ancylostoma duodenale Hookworm	Pruritus Pneumonitis	Pantropical Mediterranean	Skin contact	Small intestine	Mebendazole
Ascaris lumbricoides Roundworm (Fig. 8.11)	Pneumonitis Obstruction Cholangitis	Worldwide	Ingestion of eggs	Small intestine	Mebendazole Piperazine
Enterobius vermicularis Pinworm	Pruritus ani	Worldwide	Ingestion of eggs Autoinfection	Colon	Mebendazole
Trichuris trichiura Whipworm (Fig. 8.12)	Anaemia Rectal prolapse	Worldwide	Ingestion of eggs	Caecum	Mebendazole

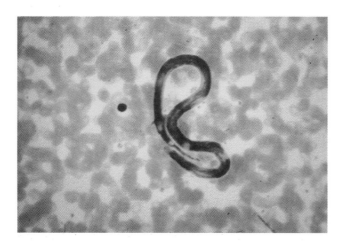

Fig. 8.9 Filarial worms. *Loa loa* in a blood film. (Giemsa.)

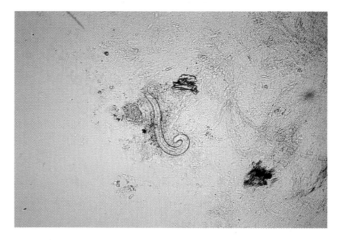

Fig. 8.10 Intestinal nematode. *Strongyloides stercoralis* in a faecal specimen. (Polarized light microscopy.)

the lungs, sometimes causing pneumonitis, and settle as adults in the small intestine.

Ascaris lumbricoides (Fig. 8.11), *Enterobius vermicularis* and *Trichuris trichiuria* (Fig. 8.12) infection is acquired through ingestion of eggs, as might exist on unwashed contaminated raw vegtables, or in the case of *Enterobius*, contaminated bed clothes or hands. On ingestion of *Enterobius* and *Trichuris* ova, larvae emerge which mature in the gut. *Ascaris*, like the hookworms and *Strongyloides*, has a complex life cycle in which the larvae migrate

through the body before returning to the gut to mature into adult worms (Fig. 8.13). On passing through the lungs larvae may cause a Löffler-like syndrome—acute pneumonitis with radiological infiltrates and **blood eosinophilia**.

Diagnosis of infection with all the intestinal nematodes, except for *Strongyloides*, is by detection of eggs in microscopic examination of faecal smears, although occasionally worms are vomited or passed *per rectum*.

Ova of all species are distinctive, except for the two

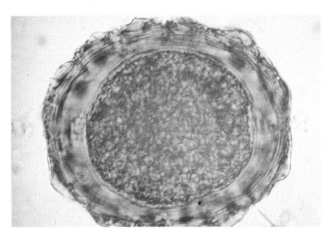

Fig. 8.11 Intestinal nematode. *Ascaris* ovum in a faecal specimen.

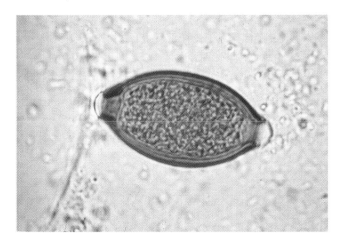

Fig. 8.12 Intestinal nematode. *Trichuris* ovum in a faecal specimen.

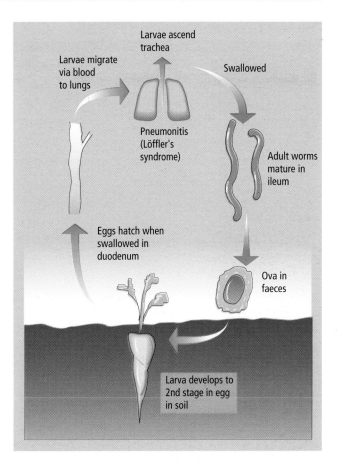

Fig. 8.13 Life cycle of *Ascaris*.

hookworm species, which are indistinguishable. Although eggs of *Enterobius* may be found in faeces, they are more reliably sought by examining sticky tape which has been pressed against the perianal area. *Strongyloides* is unusual in that larvae instead of ova are passed in the faeces. They may be detected by placing a sample of faeces in the centre of a non-nutrient agar Petri dish that has been inoculated with *Escherichia coli*. After a day or two the larvae will have migrated out of the faeces and their tracks may be seen on the *E. coli* lawn. Larvae of *Strongyloides* and eggs of *Enterobius* may directly reinfect the host. In immunocompromised patients, *Strongyloides* hyperinfection may result.

Platyhelminthes (flatworms)

The phylum Platyhelminthes includes free-living flatworms (of no medical significance) and two groups of parasites, the **Trematoda** (flukes) and the **Cestoda** (tapeworms).

Trematodes (flukes)

Many species of trematode have been reported to cause human infection. They can be classified according to the location of the adult fluke in the human body as blood flukes (schistosomes), lung flukes, liver flukes and intestinal flukes.

All of them have complex life cycles in which particular species of **aquatic snail** serve as **intermediate hosts**. Human infection follows direct penetration of skin by larvae, ingestion of cysts on edible water plants or ingestion of an infected second intermediate host, usually a fish or edible crustacean. A few trematodes are widespread and *Fasciola hepatica* is native to the UK but most species have restricted geographical distributions, being limited by the distributions of their intermediate hosts

Table 8.7 Features of *Schistosoma* spp. which infect humans.

Species	Location of adult fluke	Medium of egg release	Features of egg	Geographical distribution
S. mansoni (Fig. 8.16(a))	Mesenteric veins	Faeces	Lateral spine	Africa, Madagascar, Arabia, American tropics
S. japonicum	Mesenteric veins	Faeces	Round, short spine	Japan, China, Indonesia, Phillipines
S. mekongi	Mesenteric veins	Faeces	Round, short spine	Upper Mekong Valley
S. intercalatum	Mesenteric veins	Faeces	Terminal spine	Central Africa
S. haematobium (Fig. 8.16(b) and (c))	Vesical veins	Urine	Terminal spine	Africa, Madagascar, Middle East

and human dietary habits. The treatment of choice for all trematode infections is **praziquantel**.

Schistosomiasis (bilharzia)

Five species of schistosome cause significant morbidity in humans (Table 8.7). All of them use **aquatic snails** as intermediate hosts. Humans become infected through exposure of skin to water which is infested with infected snails (Fig. 8.14). A specialized larval stage, the cercaria, released into the water from the snail penetrates submerged skin. Penetration of the skin may result in dermatitis (Fig. 8.15).

The larvae migrate via peripheral vessels, the lungs and portal vessels to the mesenteric, or in the case of *Schistosoma haematobium*, the vesical veins, maturing on the way to adult flukes. Adults remain as pairs, female flukes being lodged in gynaecophoric canals of the males. Low worm loads may be asymptomatic, severity of disease being related to the host's response to eggs released into the venous plexuses (Fig. 8.16).

S. haematobium infection may result in fibrosis of the ureters and bladder, resulting in dysuria, haematuria, papilloma and transitional cell carcinoma. The other species may cause damage to the colon, fibrosis of the portal tracts (**pipestem fibrosis**), hepatosplenomegaly and pulmonary disease (Fig. 8.16(d)). Diagnosis of schistosomiasis is by examination of faeces or urine for eggs and serology.

Lung, liver and intestinal flukes

All of these flukes may be considered to be **zoonoses**, adult flukes commonly occurring in **animal reservoir** hosts. Humans serve as an alternative host for the fluke. All of them use aquatic snails as intermediate hosts for larval stages, which are passed on to humans via a second intermediate host, or as cysts attached to **edible aquatic plants**. These diseases tend to have rather patchy geographical distributions, depending as they do for their existence on suitable animal host reservoirs, snail species, secondary intermediate hosts and human dietary habits (Table 8.8).

Cestodes (tapeworms)

Adult tapeworms reside in the intestines of vertebrates, attached to the lining by a **scolex** with hooks and suckers, beyond which trails the body of the worm, consisting of a tape-like streamer of proglottids. Most species require two host species of vertebrate to complete their life cycle (Fig. 8.17).

The adult worm lives in the **intestine** of host species of carnivore and releases its eggs in the **host's faeces** to contaminate vegetation. The intermediate host is a herbivore that becomes infected by eating contaminated plants and becomes host to the larval stage that develops in soft tissues such as liver and muscle. The primary host becomes infected by eating larval cysts in the flesh of the intermediate host. Humans serve as a host either for the adult or larval stages of several cestodes.

Tapeworms found in humans are hermaphrodites. The more distal proglottids contain uterine branches with eggs which are released and passed in the faeces. Proglottids may break off and be passed *per rectum*. The dwarf tapeworm, *Hymenolepis nana*, is unusual in that it completes its life cycle within a single host species. Ova passed in human faeces are infectious to humans. Eggs may survive on the skin, clothing and in the environment

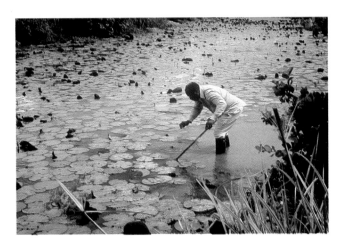

Fig. 8.14 A schistosome-infested pool in Kenya. Examining the lily pads for host snails.

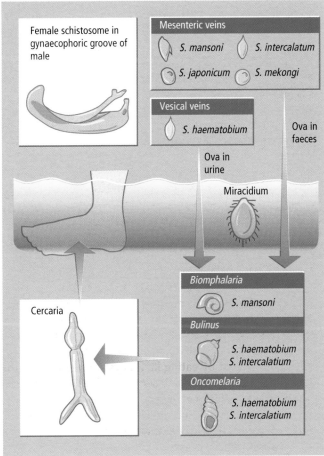

(a)

Fig. 8.15 (a) Life cycle of schistosomiasis. (b) Geographic distribution of schistosomiasis.

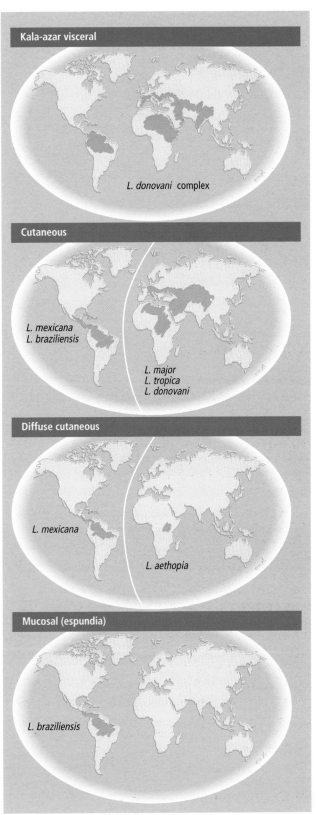

(b)

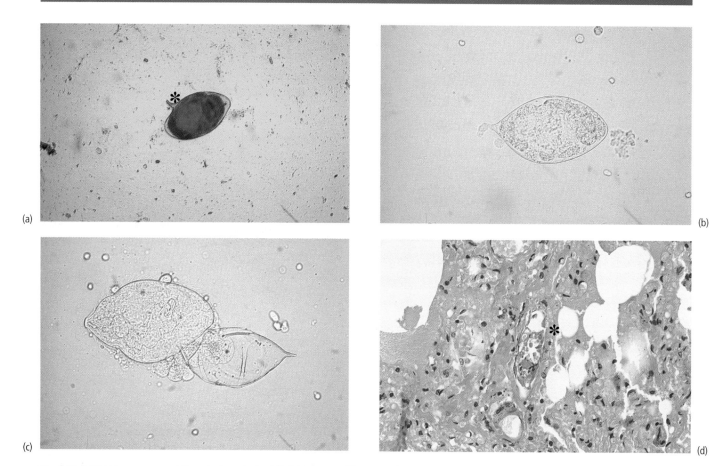

Fig. 8.16 (a) *Schistosoma mansoni*. Note the lateral spine (✱). (b) *S. haematobium*. Note the terminal spine. (c) *S. haematobium* with an emerging miracidium. (d) *S. mansoni* infection in the lung. Histology shows a calcifying egg surrounded by fibrous tissue.

Table 8.8 Features of the more common lung, liver and intestinal trematodes which infect humans.

Species	Geographical distribution	Means of acquistion	Location of adult worm	Clinical features	Medium of egg release	Reservoir host
LUNG FLUKES						
Paragonimus spp.	E. Asia W. Africa S. America	Uncooked crustaceans	Lung	Haemoptysis Lung abscess	Sputum Faeces	Felines
LIVER FLUKES						
Clonorchis sinensis	China, Korea S.E. Asia	Uncooked fish	Bile ducts	Cholangitis	Faeces	Dog
Opisthorchis spp.	E. Europe, Siberia Thailand	Uncooked fish	Bile ducts	Cholangitis	Faeces	Cat Civet cat
Fasciola hepatica	Worldwide	Cysts on watercress	Bile ducts	Fever Eosinophilia	Faeces	Sheep
INTESTINAL FLUKES						
Fasciolopsis buski	S.E. Asia	Cysts on water caltrop, water chestnut	Small intestine	Diarrhoea Malabsorption	Faeces	Pig

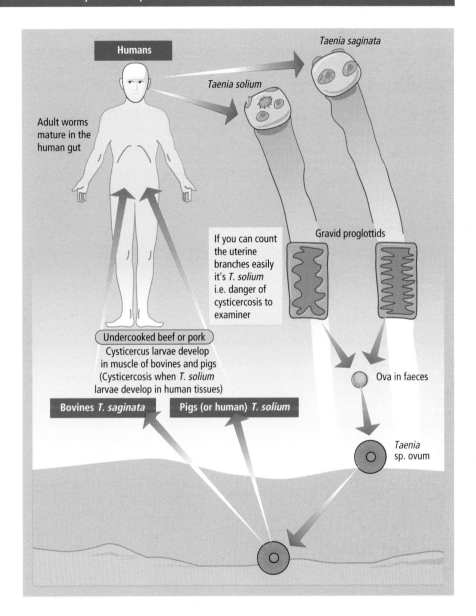

Fig. 8.17 Life cycle of *Taenia* species.

and *Hymenolepis* infection is common amongst institutionalized children in some countries. The main clinical features of infection are intestinal disturbances.

Adult cestodes in humans

Infections with the beef tapeworm, *Taenia saginata*, the pork tapeworm, *T. solium* and the fish tapeworm, *Diphyllobothrium latum*, are acquired by ingesting undercooked flesh of the respective larval host mammals and fish (Table 8.9). The adult worms mature in the human intestine. Clinical features may include vague intestinal upset, pruritus and eosinophilia. *D. latum* competes with the host for vitamin B_{12} to cause macrocytic anaemia. Larvae of *T. saginata* and *D. latum* do not develop in humans. Eggs in the faeces are diagnostic (Fig. 8.18).

Cysticercosis

Ingestion of eggs of the pork tapeworm, *Taenia solium*, results in humans acting as an accidental larval host, a condition called **cysticercosis**, with the formation of larval cysts throughout the body. Cysticercosis may be symptomless, unless occurring in the brain to cause focal neurological phenomena such as epilepsy. Eggs may be ingested on contaminated raw vegetables. Patients who harbour an adult worm are at increased risk of cysticercosis, presumably because of the high probability of ingesting excreted eggs. Diagnosis is by computed tomography and serology.

Echinococcosis (hydatid disease, dog tapeworm)

Hydatid disease occurs worldwide in sheep- and cattle-rearing areas. Other large herbivores, as well as

Table 8.9 Cestode infections of humans.

Species (common name)	Stage in humans	Location in body	Geographical distribution	Mode of acquisition	Treatment
Taenia saginata (beef tapeworm)	Adult	Intestine	Worldwide	Uncooked beef	Niclosamide
Taenia solium (pork tapeworm)	Adult	Intestine	Worldwide	Uncooked pork	Niclosamide
Taenia solium (cysticercosis)	Larva	Throughout body	Worldwide	Ingestion of eggs	Praziquantel
Diphyllobothrium latum and other spp. (fish tapeworm) (Fig. 8.18)	Adult	Intestine	E. Europe N. Asia Americas	Raw fish	Niclosamide
Hymenolepis nana (dwarf tapeworm)	Adult	Intestine	Worldwide	Eggs on hands, clothes, food	Praziquantel
Echinococcus granulosus (hydatid disease, dog tapeworm) (Fig. 8.19)	Larva	Liver, lungs and elsewhere	Worldwide	Exposure to eggs	Surgery Albendazole
Echinococcus multilocularis (alveolar echinococcosis)	Larva	Liver, lungs and elsewhere	Holarctic	Exposure to eggs	Albendazole

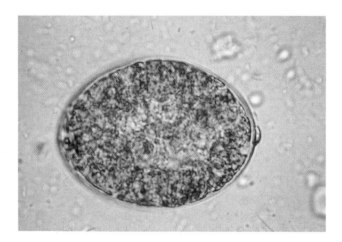

Fig. 8.18 Cestode disease. An ovum of *Diphyllobothrium latum*.

humans, act as larval hosts of *Echinococcus granulosus*.

The primary hosts are dogs and wild canids, which excrete eggs in their faeces (Fig. 8.19). Humans become infected by ingesting eggs. High levels of infection may occur in communities closely associated with dogs, such as the Turkana. Larval cysts develop anywhere in the body but mainly the liver and lungs.

Cysts can become very large and consist of a capsule containing fluid and lined by a germinal layer from which brood capsules, containing **protoscolices** (larval scolices) and **daughter cysts** develop (see Chapter 19). Cysts exert pressure on neighbouring structures and may cause

biliary obstruction and various symptoms depending on site. Rupture of a cyst may be directly fatal due to anaphylaxis or pulmonary oedema. Rupture into the peritoneum results in growth of daughter cysts throughout the abdomen. Diagnosis is by radiology and serology. Treatment consists of surgical removal. To prevent recurrence, the site may be treated with silver nitrate and the patient treated with **praziquantel** or **albendazole**.

E. multilocularis causes alveolar echinococcosis. The parasite has a boreoalpine distribution, human cases being reported from Alaska, Canada, Siberia, Germany and Austria. Foxes act as hosts of the adult worm and the larva develops in small mammals, such as voles. The larva must mature rapidly in such a short-lived host and in humans the parasite infiltrates tissues in the manner of a neoplasm. There is little prospect of surgical removal and most cases are fatal. Albendazole is treatment of choice.

Myiasis

Myiasis is the infestation of human or animal tissues with the larvae of dipterous flies. Many species have been recorded but there are a few that are specialized parasites of humans and these are regularly imported to the UK.

The South American botfly, *Dermatobium hominis* (Fig. 8.20(a)) occurs in the Neotropics. The adult fly lays its

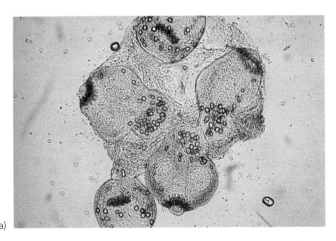

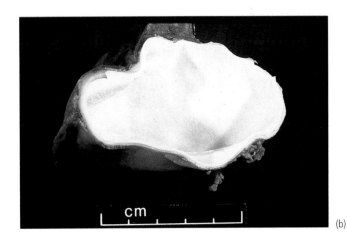

Fig. 8.19 Cestode disease. (a) Protoscolices of *Echinococcus granulosis* from a hydatid cyst. (b) An excised hydatid cyst from the liver contained numerous protoscolices and daughter cysts.

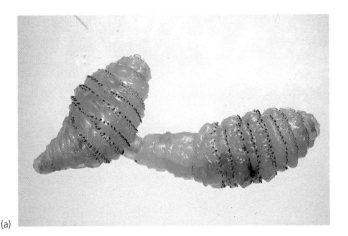

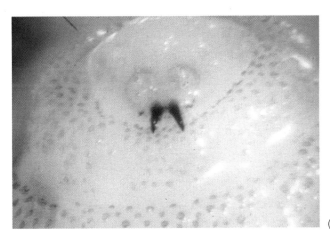

Fig. 8.20 Myiasis. (a) Larvae of the South American botfly, *Dermatobium hominis*, removed from a facial swelling. (b) Larva of the tumbu fly, *Cordylobia anthropophaga*, showing its labial sclerites.

eggs on mosquitoes which transmit the infection when they bite humans. The larva grows in subcutaneous tissues and a boil develops with a breathing hole. Secondary bacterial infection can occur. The **tumbu fly**, *Cordylobia anthropophaga*, is Afrotropical. Eggs are layed on damp clothing and burrow into the subcutaneous tissues on hatching (Fig. 8.20(b)). Ironing of washing prevents infection. Clinically, the infestation resembles that of *Dermatobium*. Both species may be removed through a simple incision. Attempts to squeeze out larvae may destroy them *in situ*, resulting in granulomatous reactions.

Several tropical species of fly cause invasive, poten-tially lethal infestations in humans. These include the New World screw worm, *Cochliomyia hominivorax*, and several Old World Diptera. Such cases require surgical debridement of necrotic tissue and removal of the maggots.

Tungosis

Tungosis is infestation with the gravid female **jigger flea**, *Tunga penetrans*. (Tromboculid mites are sometimes called jiggers, which is confusing.)

The flea occurs in sandy soils in many tropical areas and travellers regularly return with this infection. Fertile females burrow into exposed skin, usually the sole of the foot or under a toenail, where they suck blood and swell with developing eggs. Fleas may be removed through a simple incision. Cases imported to the UK tend to be diagnosed by histological examination of the excised fleas, usually surrounded by a small sample of neighbouring tissue. Repeated infestation with pitting of the feet leads to a risk of bacterial infection and tetanus.

FURTHER READING

Gresham G.A. (1992) *A Color Atlas of General Pathology*, 2nd edn. Mosby Year Book, St. Louis.

Mitchinson M.J. *et al.* (1996) *Essentials of Pathology* (Chapter 13). Blackwell Science, Oxford.

The Immune System

C O N T E N T S

INTRODUCTION

The immune system should be considered in the same way as any other organ system: it has **structure**, **organization** at a series of levels and **function** (Fig. 9.1). It differs in the way its elements are so closely related to other organ systems yet free to move throughout the whole body (Fig. 9.2). Readers who are not familar with the components of the immune system are advised to consult Chapters 3–5 of *Essentials of Pathology* and the other texts recommended at the end of this chapter.

The immune system comprises cellular and humoral components and these may be specific or non-specific. Table 9.1 details the features of an ideal immune response. It is important to remember that non-specific immunity plays a significant role in protection against

Table 9.1 Ideal immune response.

| Removal of foreign antigens |
| Lasting cellular and humoral memory |
| No damage to intrinsic structures |

infection. Defects in this arm, such as chronic granulomatous disease (see Chapter 10), may lead to devastating illness.

Immunological disease may result from:
- **deficiency** of a component of the immune system, e.g. lack of B lymphocytes, as in X-linked agammaglobulinaemia (see Chapter 10);
- production of an **abnormal component** (myeloma proteins);
- normal immune function where the immune system is tricked into becoming **self-reactive** by an invading pathogen.

Immunological disease may be **congenital** or **acquired**. Immunological disease may be **primary** or **secondary**.

Neoplasia of the immune system occurs. By definition, the immune system is involved in all **inflammation** and is thus intimately involved with **organ-specific disease**. The close interrelationship of the immune system with all other systems of the body means that it is hard to discuss it in isolation. This chapter concentrates on the mechanism by which the immune system contributes to disease and details those diseases of immune excess; diseases of immune deficiency will be discussed in Chapter 10. The contribution to specific diseases of the

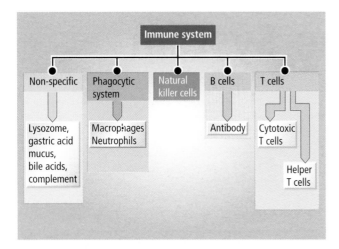

Fig. 9.1 The immune system.

Table 9.2 Classification of immune responses.

Type	Mechanism	Consequences	Diseases
I	IgE/mast cells Basophils, IgG4 Immediate hypersensitivity	Anaphylaxis, vasodilation Increased vascular permeability	Asthma Drug allergy Urticaria, venom Hayfever
II	IgG/IgM cell-bound antibody	Complement activation Lysis, opsonization Neutrophil activation Blocking/stimulating antibodies	Haemolytic anaemia ITP, Goodpasture's Graves disease Myasthenia gravis
III	IgG, IgA, C_3 Immune complexes	Complement activation Anaphylotoxins (C_3a, C_4a, C_5a) Neutrophil activation Phagocytic cell activation	Serum sickness SLE, vasculitis Extrinsic allergic alveolitis
IV	T cells, delayed hypersensitivity	Lymphocyte activation Macrophage activation Lymphokine release Granuloma formation	Tuberculosis GvHD, sarcoidosis Tuberculoid leprosy

IgE, Immunoglobulin E; ITP, Idiopathic thrombocytopenic purpura; SLE, systemic lupus erythematosus; GvHD, graft-versus-host disease.
N.B.: Diseases may involve more than one mechanism at a time.

immunological responses discussed here will be discussed in the appropriate system-based chapters.

TYPES OF IMMUNOLOGICAL REACTIONS

The original classification of Gell and Coombs is still the most valuable scheme for considering the ways in which

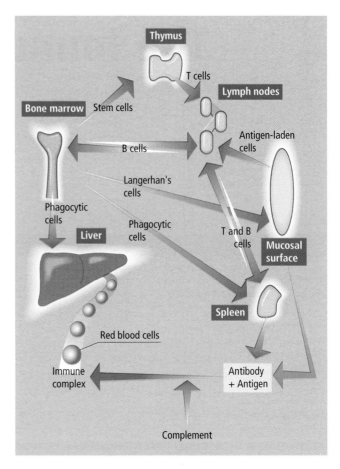

Fig. 9.2 The organization of the immune system.

immunological reactions occur (Table 9.2). It is important to realize that these immunological reactions are not exclusive and that more than one type of reaction may be going on at any one time.

Type I reactions

Type I reactions constitute the basis for **immediate hypersensitivity**. These are mediated by **allergen-specific immunoglobulin E (IgE)**. Figure 9.3 illustrates the process.

Exposure to the allergen, probably in a genetically susceptible individual, leads to an abnormal response with excessive IgE production. This is most probably mediated at the cellular level by an imbalance between the production of the cytokines interleukin (IL-4) and γ-interferon: the former increases IgE synthesis and the latter decreases it. Specific IgE binds to mast cells (Fig. 9.4) in tissue and 'arms' them to respond. When these IgE-coated mast cells encounter the allergen, the binding of allergen to IgE

Table 9.3 Type II immunological reactions.

Cell-bound antibody causing complement and phagocytic cell-mediated cell lysis
Autoimmune haemolytic anaemia
Idiopathic thrombocytopenia

Bound antibodies causing local neutrophil and complement activation with bystander damage
Antiglomerular basement membrane disease (Goodpasture's syndrome)

Receptor-blocking antibodies
Myasthenia gravis (antibody to acetylcholine receptor on muscle)
Myxoedema, rarely (thyroid growth or metabolism-blocking antibodies)
Pernicious anaemia (intrinsic factor antibodies)

Receptor-stimulating antibodies
Graves disease (antibody to thyroid-stimulating hormone receptor on thyrocytes)
Exophthalmos (antibody to receptor on retro-orbital fat cells)
Goitre (thyroid growth-stimulating antibodies)

transmits a signal to the cell which triggers degranulation with the release of preformed mediators. The mediators have the effect of increasing vascular permeability and recruiting other cells. One of the major preformed mediators is **histamine**.

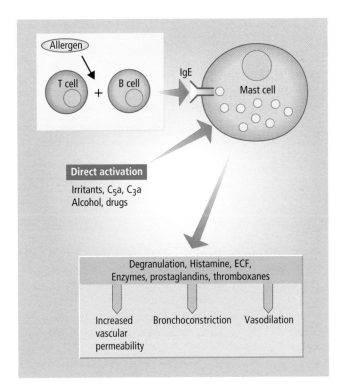

Fig. 9.3 The Type I reaction. ECF, eosinophil chemotactic factor; NCF, neutrophil chemotactic factor.

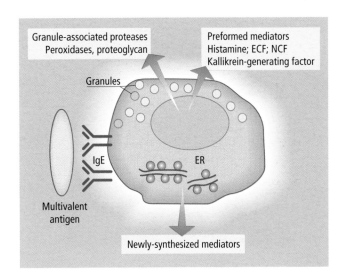

Fig. 9.4 The mast cell.

Simultaneous stimulation of large numbers of mast cells in a highly sensitized individual leads to sytemic reaction (**anaphylaxis**). Where the reaction is more localized, the exact symptoms will depend upon the tissue involved. For example, involvement of the nose and conjunctivae leads to **hayfever** (**allergic rhinoconjunctivitis**), in response to **true food allergy**, in the **bowel** oedema occurs with an eosinophilic infiltrate.

The site at which maximum response occurs will depend on the allergen and the route of sensitization. Some allergen-specific IgE escapes into the circulation and sensitizes distant mast cells. This is detected by **skin prick testing** in which a miniscule amount of purified allergen in introduced into the dermis (Fig. 9.5). If there are sensitized mast cells then histamine will be released, leading to the characteristic **wheal-and-flare reaction**.

Circulating IgE can also be detected in the blood by **radioallergosorbent (RAST) testing**. It is easy to see that if local IgE production is low, then little will escape and both skin prick tests and RAST tests will be negative, even in the presence of definite allergy. Conversely, not all patients with specific IgE to a given allergen will necessarily have symptoms when exposed to the allergen.

As Fig. 9.3 shows, reactions triggered by IgE will lead to activation of other soluble factors such as the **kinin** and **complement cascades**, which are intimately linked and share some regulatory proteins. Agents may therefore activate these cascades directed and mimic the features of a true hypersensitivity reaction. In these cases, specific IgE is not detectable. Such reactions include anaphylactoid reactions to radiographic contrast media and other drugs. Less dramatic responses such as **urticaria**

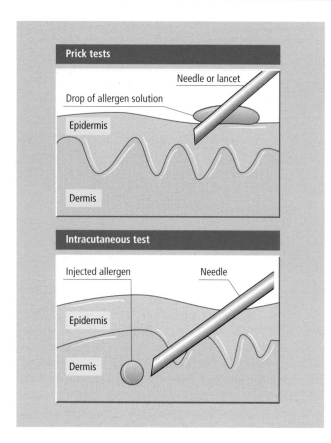

Fig. 9.5 Skin-tests for Type I hypersensitivity.

(histamine-like wheals) and **idiopathic angioedema** (non-itchy swellings, typically involving lips and mucous membranes) can be seen in response to a wide variety of drugs, including **aspirin**, some foods, such as **strawberries** and occasionally without any obvious cause. These responses are often due to direct activation of the kinin system (radiographic dyes), to direct release of histamine from mast cells (strawberries, codeine derivatives) or to other effects such as prostaglandin synthetase inhibition (aspirin). It is important to distinguish these conditions, and also hereditary angioedema due to deficiency of C_1-esterase inhibitor (see Chapter 10), as the treatment will be different.

Atopic eczema always causes some dispute, but there is likely to be a type I component. Total IgE levels are very high, often >1000 ku/l, and there are high levels of allergen-specific IgE, most commonly directed against house dust mite and foods. The chronicity of the condition indicates that there must also be a considerable type IV reaction as well. **Atopic asthma**, in which there is a type I component triggered by IgE to inhaled allergens (animal danders, house dust mite), almost certainly also has a type IV component, particularly in the chronic phase.

Type II reactions

Type II reactions are mediated by antibody. The antibody may be **cytotoxic**, i.e. capable of destroying a cell or structure, usually by binding complement, or it may cause disease by interfering with the function of a cell, for instance by binding to a critical surface receptor. In most cases, type II reactions occur as a result of the formation of **autoantibodies**, but this is not always so.

In the case of an **unmatched blood transfusion**, the ABO-incompatible red cells will be destroyed by the naturally occurring, preformed **IgM antibodies** directed against blood group substances. Another example is the transference to an innocent third party of an abnormal antibody, as in alloimmune neonatal thrombocytopenia. The maternal autoantibody, directed against a platelet antigen (PLA[1]), crosses the placenta and leads to the destruction of the fetal/neonatal platelets if they express the same antigen.

Antibodies may mediate direct functional effects on target cells by binding to surface receptors. There are numerous examples of this. The clearest example is the antiacetylcholine receptor antibody which is found in **myasthenia gravis**. This autoantibody prevents the binding of acetylcholine to the receptor by binding to one of the subunits. **Autoantibodies** directed against the thyroid mediate a variety of effects, including stimulation (**LATS** = long-acting thyroid stimulatory) and inhibition. Where

Table 9.4 Factors controlling type III reactions.

Antibody	Low-affinity antibody is associated with immune complex formation
Genetics	Affinity of antibody is genetically controlled
Complement	Deficiencies of complement components cause abnormal immune complexes, e.g. C2 deficiency and SLE
Complement receptors	Low red cell complement receptors associated with poor immune complex clearance (?acquired deficiency)
Size of immune complex	Small complexes cause little damage (readily solubilized); large complexes readily phagocytosed; medium-sized complexes cause disease
Solubility of immune complexes	Solubility dependent on intact complement pathway
Phagocytes	Carry receptors for IgG and IgG Fc; reduction or blockade reduces immune complex clearance

SLE, Systemic lupus erythematosus; IgG, immunoglobulin G.

an antibody mediates a direct effect, it may be considered to be a primary pathogenic antibody. Table 9.3 summarizes the type II responses that have been documented.

Type III reactions

These are mediated by **immune complexes**. Generation of an immune complex requires the presence of antibody, antigen and complement, although non-specific complexes may be formed by the alternate pathway of complement in the absence of antibody against certain antigens. C-reactive protein also forms complexes with antigens; these have some of the properties of immune complexes and lead to phagocytosis.

Immune complex formation is the immune system's way of packaging garbage for removal to waste disposal unit. Immunological garbage is generated continuously and immune complexes are formed and cleared all the time. This process relies on the intact function of not only the basic constituents of the immune complexes but also the phagocytes (dustmen) and the carriers of the immune complexes (dustcarts) and the liver (the waste tip itself). Failure of any of these components leads to accumulation of immunological garbage with the usual unpleasant effects.

The **size** of the immune complex formed is critical in determining its fate: large complexes are cleared rapidly by direct phagocytosis at the site of production and small complexes, which are readily soluble, are bound by complement receptors on red blood cells and transported to the liver and spleen. However, middle-sized complexes are poorly soluble and poorly phagocytosed. Thus they are cleared slowly and are likely to be deposited in tissues where they excite an inflammatory response.

The size of an immune complex is determined by a number of factors (Table 9.4 and Fig. 9.6). Formation of **low-affinity antibody** frequently leads to pathological immune complexes.

Abnormalities in the complement system are strongly associated with immune complex disease: **inherited deficiencies** of any of the complement components from C1 to C6 have been associated with the development of **systemic lupus erythematosus (SLE)**. The latter condition has also been associated with a reduction in the expression of complement receptors on red blood cells: this leads to poor clearance of complexes from the circulation. It is interesting to note that in SLE the expression of complement receptors on erythrocytes is **reduced**, thus impairing the removal of the already abnormal immune complexes. Equally important are the phagocytic cells: failure to phagocytose complexes occurs when there is reduced or absent expression of receptors for com-

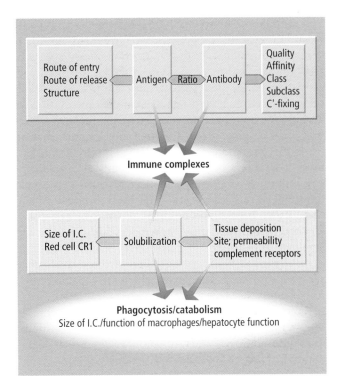

Fig. 9.6 The type III reaction.

ponents of the complexes (IgG Fc receptor, complement receptors).

Other factors important in determining whether immune complexes are formed are:
- the nature of the antigen;
- whether there is continuous or intermittent exposure;
- the quantity of both antigen and antibody, as large excess of either component reduces the formation of complexes;
- the time relationship between exposure to antigen and the production of antibody.

One of the best examples of a type III reaction is **acute serum sickness**. This is usually precipitated by the administration of a **foreign protein**, such as horse antitetanus toxoid serum. The protein is recognized as non-self and an antibody response is mounted. In the immunologically naïve host, the initial response is IgM antibody followed at 14–21 days by IgG. Once IgG antihorse antibody is produced, immune complexes are generated. The clinical features are rash, arthralgia and arthritis, fever (due to stimulation of cytokine production) and glomerulonephritis. As the immune complexes are cleared, the reaction subsides. Re-exposure to the same antigen leads to an accelerated response because the B lymphocytes are already primed to make antihorse antibody.

The difference between a type II reaction and a type III reaction is that the antibody in the former is bound to a surface and may trigger the whole complement pathway with the generation of the lytic complex. In the latter, activation of the first part of the complement cascade occurs in solution with soluble antigen and antibody. Because the immune complexes circulate freely, the reactions may be generalized, although some organs, such as the kidney, are more prone to damage by circulating immune complexes because of their ability to trap them. Once immune complexes have been arrested in a tissue, they will attract phagocytic cells by the release of the chemotactic breakdown products of complement (C4a), and the tissue may suffer 'bystander' damage from the activities of the phagocytic cells so recruited.

As discussed in Chapter 3, there are no satisfactory assays for immune complexes, which are capable of distinguishing the normal continuous production from pathological states. The presence of a type III reaction is inferred from evidence of excess complement consumption (reduced C3, C4 and C1q) and the presence of degradation products (C3 breakdown products, C4a).

Type IV reactions

These are reactions mediated by **T cells**. Recruitment of T cells and their activation leads to the release of large quantities of cytokines (Fig. 9.7). These increase the recruitment of T cells and attract phagocytic cells. The best examples are detailed in Table 9.2.

Because of the time taken for primed T cells to reach a site of antigenic stimulation, type IV reactions develop **slowly**. In the Mantoux test for tuberculin-reactive T cells, the reaction takes 48–72 hours to develop and is characterized by marked induration (Fig. 9.8): this is not oedema but is caused by the infiltrate of cells into the dermis.

Type IV reactions tend to be **chronic**. When antigen is injected into the skin, reactions of several different types may occur sequentially. For instance, intradermal testing with *Candida* antigen may lead to an immediate wheal-and-flare reaction (type I), followed at 6–8 hours by the onset of a type III immune complex reaction. This may last for up to 48 hours, depending on the amount of antigen and the strength of the immune response. At the same time as the immune complex reaction is resolving, the type IV reaction begins, peaking at 60–72 hours. Timing of the final reading of the skin tests must take this sequence into consideration, to avoid falsely identifying an immune complex reaction as evidence of T-cell reactivity.

While antigen persists, there is continuous stimulus to

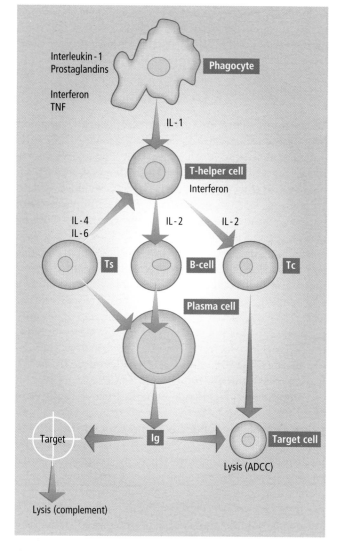

Fig. 9.7 The cell-mediated immune response and the role of cytokines.

recruitment of phagocytic cells and these in turn release cytokines that attract and activate T lymphocytes. T-cell-mediated responses are thus the major type of response to antigens that are inefficiently cleared from the tissues, such as mycobacteria, whose cell wall is relatively resistant to attack by phagocytic cells. In many cases the cause of **granulomatous reactions** is unknown but these clearly represent the immune system's attempt at antigen removal (Fig. 9.9). Although this response is not effective in eliminating the antigen, granuloma formation limits antigen spread. We do not understand the mechanisms that determine persistence or resolution of granulomatous reactions but they are a common immunological response to external insults. Individual examples, such as **sar-**

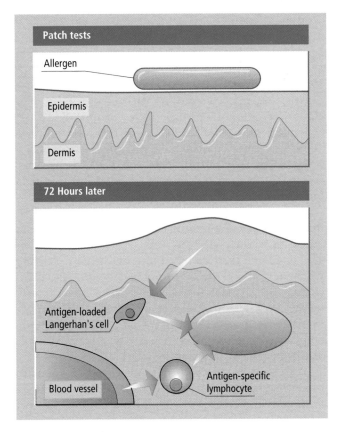

Fig. 9.8 Patch tests for the type IV reaction.

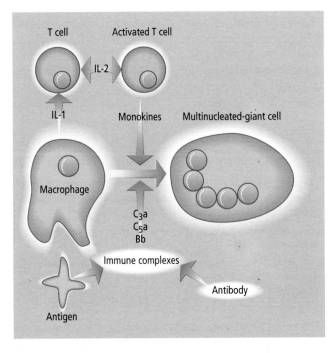

Fig. 9.9 Granuloma formation in the type IV reaction.

coidosis and **mycobacterial disease**, will be discussed further in the relevant chapters.

It is important to remember that each type of immune response is not a unique and independent reaction, but part and parcel of a multifaceted immune response. Different arms of the immune response may occur together or sequentially and this must always be borne in mind when assessing the contribution of the immune system to clinical disease.

Abnormal immunoglobulins

The **normal humoral immune** response is the result of the stimulation by antigen of numerous separate clones of B lymphocytes. While each of these clones of cells produces a single type of immunoglobulin, characterized by a unique genetic rearrangement of the V, D, J and C regions for a specific immunoglobulin isotype, the totality of the response is polyclonal. Ideally, the product of each clone is specific for a single structure (epitope) on a single antigen. The numbers of possible genetic combinations and hence of antibody specificity are colossal, and are further increased by having mutational hotspots in the variable regions.

The system is not foolproof and **cross-reactivity** between different antigens occurs. This has led to a hypothesis for the generation of **autoimmunity** in which exogenous antigens generate an immune response that is cross-reactive with host antigens, such as in the case of cross-reactivity of antibody to *Klebsiella* antigens with human leukocyte antigen (HLA)-B27 antigens.

The exact nature of cellular and humoral immune response generated by any given antigen has a **genetic determinant**: for instance, the cellular response to influenza virus is directed against different antigenic determinants dependent on the HLAs of the host cells.

As **major histocompatibility complex (MHC) antigens** play a key role in the presentation of processed foreign antigens on the surface of cells, it is logical that alterations in the MHC molecules will alter the type of processed antigens that can be presented. B cells also rely on this system for almost all antigens, as antibody production is dependent upon the provision of appropriate singals by antigen-primed T cells. The only exception appears to be complex repeating antigens such as bacterial polysaccharides (e.g. the capsular polysaccharides of *Haemophilus influenzae* and *Streptococcus pneumoniae*), which are capable of stimulating antibody production by B cells directly and without T-cell help.

Monoclonal gammopathies

The clonality of the B-cell response may easily be seen on the serum electrophoretic strip (see Chapter 3). Where there is a **continuous antigenic stimulus** (such as persistent infection, or an autoimmune response), the polycolonal response becomes more marked as **excess antibody** is produced. Occasionally under such extreme stimulation a single clone develops further than others and the unique immunoglobulin becomes visible as a monoclonal band on a background of polyclonal immunoglobulin. Once the antigenic stimulus is removed, this monoclonal immunoglobulin will slowly disappear.

As the immune system ages, there is loss of the normally efficient regulation of antibody production. Clones of B cells then develop and produce monoclonal immunoglobulin in a semiautonomous manner. This is visible as an M-band (paraprotein) on the electrophoresis strip. There is normally no suppression of normal immunoglobulin production, nor other features of myeloma. The incidence of such benign paraprotein bands rises sharply in the elderly, and may reach 15% of over-80-year-olds. However, about 20% of patients with apparently benign paraprotein bands will eventually develop myeloma over a long period (up to 20 years).

Myeloma results from the uncontrolled malignant proliferation of mature immunoglobulin-producing lymphocytes. In contrast to benign paraproteinaemia, there is suppression of normal immunoglobulin production, and of the functional antibody response, increasing susceptibility to infection. All classes of immunoglobulin may be produced, although IgD and IgE are very rare (Table 9.5); in a significant number of cases, there is more than one type of paraprotein. Immunoglobulin production may be unbalanced, with excess free light chains produced. When renal function is normal these are rapidly cleared from serum, and appear in the urine (**Bence Jones proteins**). However, free light chains are toxic to the kidney and renal impairment may occur. If impairment is severe, free light chains may be detectable in the serum.

Table 9.5 Frequency of immunoglobulin (Ig) isotypes in myeloma.

IgG	50%
IgA	25%
Free light chain only	20%
IgD	2%
IgE	<1%
Non-secretory	2%

These figures are approximate.
About 10–20% of patients will have more than one paraprotein band detected.

Structural changes in the paraprotein, in the absence of myeloma, may result in unusual physical properties such as cold insolubility (**cryoglobulin**)–if the temperature at which the protein precipitates out is high (above 30°C), it may precipitate out *in vivo* in cutaneous blood vessels, causing a cutaneous vasculitis. These **monoclonal cryoglobulins** may have rheumatoid factor activity binding to normal IgG (type II cryoglobulin; see Table 3.4). These complexes fix the early components of complement and lead to a low or absent C4, and may precipitate in the renal microvasculature causing renal impairment.

High levels of pentameric IgM paraprotein (**Waldenström's macroglobulinaemia**) lead to a marked increase in **plasma viscosity**: this may lead to vascular sludging, with reduced blood flow and oxygen delivery, which in turn will cause end-organ damage, particularly strokes. The increased workload on the heart engendered by the more viscous blood may lead to cardiac failure. Monoclonal proteins may have autoantibody activity, other than rheumatoid factor activity, and this may be directed against C_1-esterase inhibitor.

Some light chain V-region sequences are particularly prone to deposit in tissues in an insoluble multimeric form (**amyloid**). This form of amyloid (AL) may be primary or secondary (see Chapter 7).

Heavy chain disease

Rare diseases have been identified in which clones of B cells produce only heavy chains, without discernible light chains. α Heavy chain disease is the commonest and is associated with a severe **malabsorption syndrome**, with a lymphocytic infiltrate of the gut. This occurs mainly around the Mediterranean coast, and is also associated with primary bowel lymphoma. μ and γ heavy chain diseases are most usually associated with lymphoproliferative disorders.

Complement abnormalities

The complement deficiencies are strongly associated with autoimmune connective tissue diseases and also with a markedly increased susceptibility to infection, especially meningococcal disease. These will be discussed further in Chapter 10.

Acute-phase response

The acute-phase response is the generic name for a wide-ranging response to infective and inflammatory stimuli. It is identified by the changes in serum protein concentrations. Many such proteins are known to be affected (see Chapter 3) but the range of variation may be as little as 10–20% (complement components) or 100-fold (C-reactive protein; CRP).

C-reactive protein

CRP is a member of the **pentraxin family** of proteins, with a doughnut-shaped structure built up from five monomers. It derives its name from its ability to bind to the C-substance of streptococci. Phylogenetically, it represents an early attempt at a specific immune defence molecule, preceding the immunoglobulins.

It will opsonize certain bacteria, enhancing their phagocytosis, and will also bind to DNA. **Acute bacterial infections** give rise to the highest levels of CRP, usually > 20 mg/dl and often as high 60 mg/dl. **Viral infection**s rarely elevate the CRP, although Epstein–Barr virus and influenza virus infections may lead to a slight elevation (6–10 mg/dl). Inflammatory conditions such as **rheumatoid arthritis** elevate the CRP in the range 2–20 mg/dl.

CRP is the best **indicator** of the degree of inflammation and the response to therapy. Some connective tissues diseases do not cause an elevated CRP. SLE and progressive systemic sclerosis, even when active, usually cause only a trivial increase in CRP (in the range 1–6 mg/dl), although the erythrocyte sedimentation rate (ESR) may be very high. The reason for the discrepancy between ESR and CRP is unknown, but indicates that the two tests are complementary. The insignificant rise in the CRP in active SLE allows it to be used to distinguish intercurrent infection from flaring of disease activity, which is important when patients are on immunosuppression. Certain **malignancies** cause elevation of the CRP, particularly lymphoma (of the order of 10–15 mg/dl).

Proteins involved in the acute-phase response

These are typically proteins involved directly in defence against infection, such as CRP and complement, regulatory proteins, such as **antiproteases**, or carrier proteins, such as α_2-**macroglobulin** (Fig. 9.10). The precise mechanism by which these diverse proteins are regulated is still obscure. The initial trigger is almost certainly cytokine release from phagocytic cells. **Il-6** release is a very early event, and it rises within a couple of hours of a defined insult, such as surgery. It is likely that this cytokine increases gene expression and protein production by hepatocytes. Il-6 binds to α_2-macroglobulin, and this prolongs its half-life in the circulation. Receptors for CRP have been found on phagocytic cells and its ability to bind to DNA may play a role in removing DNA released from dead cells. Other proteins are synthesized more slowly and have a very long half-life, such as **fibrinogen**, with a half-life of approximately 7 days.

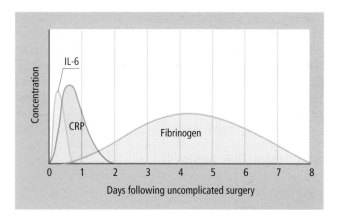

Fig. 9.10 The acute phase response.

The increase in production of antiproteases such as α_1-**antitrypsin** is a response designed to limit the damage to important tissues by proteolytic enzymes released by dying phagocytic cells: impairment of this aspect of the acute-phase response, as occurs in α_1-antitrypsin deficiency, leads to progressive tissue damage.

Other proteins under acute-phase control include the regulatory proteins for the complement cascade (such as C_1-esterase inhibitor), the **clotting cascade** and the **kinin system** of free iron that some micro-organisms require.

The erythrocyte sedimentation rate

The erythrocyte sedimentation rate (ESR) is an old and well-established test for an acute-phase response: the problem is that it is largely determined by fibrinogen, with a long half-life, and is susceptible to influence from red cell mass and morphology and other long-lived serum proteins. Thus it is of little value for monitoring day-to-day changes of the acute-phase response.

It is however cheap and easy to perform. The CRP is much better for monitoring changes in response to therapy, as the half-life is so short. Serum viscosity has also been used, but suffers from drawbacks similar to the ESR.

Orosomucoid

Orosomucoid (α_1-acid glycoprotein) is another acute-phase protein that is often measured. It behaves rather similarly to CRP, although its half-life is rather longer and its dynamic range much smaller. It is said to be a better marker for inflammation in **ulcerative colitis** than the CRP.

Direct measurement of acute-phase proteins is readily performed by autoanalysers and therefore is much less labour-intensive than measurement of the ESR or serum viscosity. The ESR and CRP are not interchangeable and there is a place for both. As for SLE, but for different reasons, myeloma and Waldenström's macroglobulinaemia cause ESRs >100 mm/hr with entirely normal CRPs: this is due in part to the high levels of monoclonal immunoglobulin in the serum in the absence of any inflammatory reponse.

AUTOIMMUNE DISEASE

Introduction

Autoimmunity represents a failure of the immune system to carry out its normal functions: Table 9.1 shows the ideal characteristics of the immune response, while Table 9.6 details ways in which it may fail. Immunodeficiency diseases are covered in Chapter 10 and malignancy of the lymphoid system in Chapter 16.

Autoimmune disease is divided into **organ-specific** and **organ-non-specific** (see Chapter 3). Autoimmunity is most often characterized by the presence of **autoantibodies**, but only in a few cases are the antibodies directly responsible for the disease. More often they are a secondary result of tissue damage initiated by other cellular mechanisms. None the less, they are easy to detect and are thus useful in diagnosis. The long half-life of IgG and their lack of direct pathogenic effect means that in most cases serial measurement of antibody plays only a small role in determining management.

Causes of autoimmune disease

As discussed above, the origin of autoimmune diseases is **obscure**, but the resulting cellular immune response then stimulates antibody production by B cells (Table 9.7).

There is no intrinsic difference between the organ-specific and non-specific diseases: the difference is determined by the distribution of the self-antigens recognized. For instance, in **Graves disease** of the thyroid, there is initially a lymphocytic infiltrate. Antibody is detectable to both thyroglobulin and to thyroid, microsomes. These antigens are specific to the thyroid and do not occur in other tissues. The major thyroid microsomal antigen is thought to be thyroid peroxidase.

In contrast, in **polymyositis**, one of the marker autoantibodies is directed against histidyl transfer-RNA. This moiety occurs in all cells synthesizing protein. Similarly **scleroderma**, **systemic sclerosis** and the **CREST** (**c**alcinosis, **R**aynaud's, **o**eseophageal dysmotility, **s**clerodactyly and **t**elangiectasia) syndrome, are associated with autoantibodies directed against components of the nu-

Table 9.6 Abnormal immune responses.

Failure to respond to extrinsic antigens	
Bacterial	Humoral immunodeficiency
	Combined T- and B-cell immunodeficiency
	Phagocytic cell deficiency
	Complement deficiency
Viral	T-cell deficiency
	Combined T- and B-cell immunodeficiency
Fungal	Phagocytic cell defect
	T-cell deficiency
	Combined T- and B-cell immunodeficiency
Harmful response to extrinsic antigen	Hypersensitivity, allergy
Harmful response to intrinsic antigen	Autoimmunity
Cross-reactive response	Autoimmunity induced by extrinsic antigen
Malignancy of immune system	Lymphoproliferation

Table 9.7 Generation of autoantibodies – putative mechanisms for autoantibody production; more than one mechanism may be operating for any given system.

Release of 'hidden' antigens, e.g. lens protein (unlikely to be a general mechanism)
Virus + self-MHC = neoantigen. Immune response is cross-reactive with self alone
Failure of thymic education: self-reactive T-cells demonstrable – related to production of IgM autoantibodies (common, but clinical disease rare)
Foreign antigens structurally similar to self proteins, e.g. *Mycoplasma* antigens and RBC I antigen: cross-reactive immune response
Drugs + self antigens = neoantigens, e.g. penicillin and red cells, haemolytic anaemia
Interference with immunological control mechanisms, e.g. Epstein–Barr virus B-cell activation, loss of suppression
Immunogenetic background, e.g. association of HLA-A1, B8, DR3 with autoantibody production

MHC, Major histocompatibility complex; IgM, immunoglobulin M; RBC, red blood cells; HLA, human leucocyte antigen.

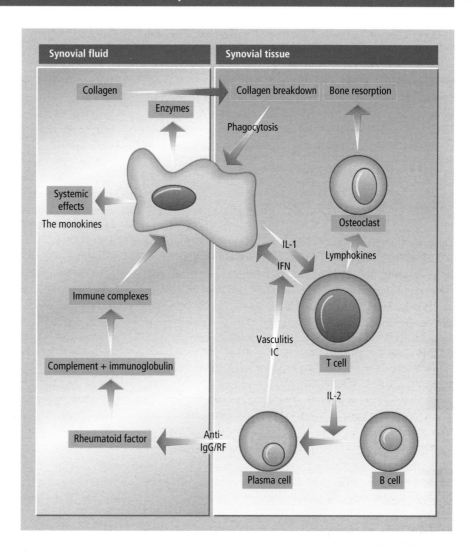

Fig. 9.11 The immunopathogenesis of rheumatoid arthritis. IL, interleukin; IFN, interferon; IC, immune complex; RF, rheumatoid factor.

cleolus, which occur in all cells. These findings raise the question of why autoantibodies against such widely distributed antigens are associated with rather specific clinical disease. There is no answer to this paradox at present.

In other cases, the role of the antibodies, if any, is obscure. Why is SLE characterized by antibodies to double-stranded DNA and other nuclear components? Such antibodies are unlikely to penetrate viable cells to gain access to the antigens in the intact nucleus. Furthermore, some patients may have clinically inactive disease while retaining high levels of anti-ds-DNA antibodies. Similar problems arise in most of the so-called connective tissue diseases. Figure 9.11 shows a rather simplified schema for the immunopathogenesis of rheumatoid arthritis.

TRANSPLANTATION

Introduction

The ability to perform 'spare-part surgery' is constrained by the immune system. Although not its prime evolutionary function, the major role is played by the MHC system.

For renal, cardiac and bone marrow transplants, matching donor and recipient for MHC antigens significantly improves the graft survival.

For **bone marrow transplants** where viable immunocompetent cells are being transferred, the reactivity may be against the recipient rather than the donor, so-called **graft-versus-host disease (GvHD)**.

Liver allografts, on the other hand, are less susceptible to MHC-mediated rejection. This is explained because the vascular endothelial cells in other solid grafts are capable of expressing MHC class II antigens on exposure to cytokines: these antigens will be recognized as foreign by circulating host lymphocytes. The sinusoids of the liver have no endothelial lining and the hepatocytes rarely express MHC class II antigens. There is less stimulation of host lymphocytes.

Tissue typing

In **graft rejection** both T-helper (CD4+) and T-cytotoxic cells (CD8+) play significant roles. Antibody is important in mediating hyperacute rejection: the renal graft will become blue and flabby immediately the arterial clamps are released. Preformed antibody against MHC antigens is present in multiply-transfused patients, multiparous women and those who have previously received mismatched transplants.

As it is exceedingly rare for a patient to have a histocompatible donor available, donors and recipients must be **cross-matched** in rather the same way that blood for transfusion is cross-matched. The complexity of the matching operation is increased by the number of MHC specificities that may occur. All recipients and donors are typed by collecting lymphocytes, either from peripheral blood or lymph node and spleen in the case of cadaveric donors; serum from the recipient will also be tested for preformed antibodies. Typing for class II antigens has led to significant improvement in graft survival when compared to matching only for class I.

Immunosuppression

Despite the improvement in tissue typing, most transplant recipients will receive a graft containing some foreign antigens and will require some form of immunosuppressive therapy. This initially comprised **steroids**, often in heroic doses, and the immunosuppressive drug **azathioprine**. The advent of the fungal metabolite, **cyclosporin**, which is active against T cells, has significantly enhanced the clinician's ability to provide adequate immunosuppression without side-effects from steroids. Unfortunately, cyclosporin is **nephrotoxic** in high doses and plasma levels must be carefully monitored. Newer drugs, such as tacrolimns (FK506) are now being introduced.

Transplant rejection

For reasons that are unclear, pretransfusion of a renal allograft recipient with random or donor-specific blood also has an immunosuppressive effect that improves graft survival; this is less effective since the advent of cyclosporin.

The occurrence of **rejection** in a solid graft may be documented by needle biopsy. More recently, **fine-needle aspiration**, stained to identify invading lymphocytes has proved to be a swift and accurate diagnostic tool. Established rejection may be treated by increasing the steroids and reducing the invading activated lymphocytes. The latter may be achieved using either a complement-fixing polyclonal **antilymphocyte globulin** (usually raised in rabbits against thymocytes = **ATG**) or more recently using monoclonal antibodies directed against specific lymphocyte antigens. As these are foreign proteins, allergic reactions are common.

Rejection of a solid graft is a **cell-mediated response**, involving both helper and cytotoxic T cells. Involvement of antibody is only of significance in the presence of preformed antibody, which leads to **hyperacute rejection**. A rejecting graft will be heavily infiltrated with lymphocytes expressing activation markers. The release of cytokines by these cells will recruit other lymphocytes and phagocytic cells to amplify the response. The key cell is the **CD4+ helper cell**, which has a pivotal role in the immune response and it is this cell which is the primary target of cyclosporin.

Bone marrow transplantation

Bone marrow transplantation presents additional problems related to the presence of the host immune system and the transfer of viable donor cells. As the bone marrow is being transplanted to provide a fresh source of pluripotent stem cells to regenerate all haematopoietic cells, it is possible to purge the bone marrow of mature lymphocytes using monoclonal antibodies. New lymphocytes, developing in the recipient after the transplant, can be maintained in a tolerant state towards host MHC antigens by regular follow-up treatment with monoclonal antibodies directed against T-cell antigens.

If alloreactive T cells do enter the recipient, GvHD will result. In its chronic form this bears many similarities to the autoimmune disease systemic sclerosis, with a chronic inflammatory cell infiltrate and excessive collagen deposition in the skin. It is interesting that in transplants given to treat leukaemic disease, the leukaemic relapse rate is lower in those patients with GvHD than those without.

Immunosuppression in transplant patients

The use of high levels of immunosuppression for solid organ grafts renders the host susceptible to **opportunistic infections**. The reduction in non-specific as well as specific immunity means that the normal signs of infection, such as inflammation and pus formation, may be much reduced. The pyrogenic effect is unimpaired. The most troublesome pathogens are cytomegalovirus, *Pneumocystis*, fungi and *Mycobacteria*.

In bone marrow transplants, the time taken for donor cell engraftment leads to a long cytopenic phase. The absence of neutrophils leads to major bacterial and fungal sepsis. Strenuous efforts are required to reduce the risks of bacterial contamination, by barrier nursing, using prophylactic antibiotics, irradiation of food and the use of cytokines to stimulate early stem cell differentiation.

FURTHER READING

Chapel H.M. & Haeney M. (1993) *Essentials of Clinical Immunology*, 3rd edn. Blackwell Scientific Publications, Oxford.

Mitchinson M.J. *et al.* (1996) *Essentials of Pathology*, (Chapters 3–5). Blackwell Science, Oxford.

Roitt I.M. (1994) *Essential Immunology*, 8th edn. Blackwell Scientific Publications, Oxford.

Immune Deficiency Disease Including AIDS

CONTENTS

INTRODUCTION

In this chapter, the immunology, histopathology and microbiology (opportunistic infections) of immune deficiency disease will be discussed. Causes of immune deficiency are summarized in Table 10.1.

PRIMARY IMMUNE DEFICIENCY

All the primary immune deficiencies are **rare** diseases, with the exception of immunoglobulin A (IgA) deficiency, which occurs with a frequency of between 1 in 400 to 1 in 800 persons. None the less, it is important to recognize these disorders as they are treatable provided that the diagnosis is made early, before structural damage has occurred.

Antibody deficiency

Primary antibody deficiency represents the commonest form of immune deficiency. There are three major forms

of primary antibody deficiency and a number of rarer variants. Table 10.2 outlines their major features. Common to all is the increased susceptibility to bacterial infections.

X-Linked agammaglobulinaemia

X-linked agammaglobulinaemia (XLA) presents in early childhood, usually within the first 3 years of life. The child may present with **recurrent bacterial infections** and often with an **'aseptic' arthritis** that is due to *Mycoplasma* which may mimic juvenile rheumatoid arthritis. **Malabsorption** is also common, often due to infective causes such as *Giardia*.

The primary defect is a failure of marrow pre-B cells to mature into cells capable of making immunoglobulin. As a result, serum immunoglobulins are all low or undetectable, lymphoid tissues lack follicles and B cells are not detectable in the peripheral blood. The gene on the long arm of the X chromosome that is responsible for the disease has been identified as a tyrosine kinase, $G + K$.

Under some circumstances, carrier females can be recognized by the lack of random X inactivation in their B

Table 10.1 Immune deficiency diseases.

	Peripheral blood lymphocytes	Peripheral blood T cells	Peripheral blood B cells	Tissue lymphoid cells	Serum immunoglobulin
Severe combined immunodeficiency (SCID)	↓↓	↓↓	↓↓	Absent	↓↓
Thymic hypoplasia (DiGeorge syndrome)	↓	↓↓	N	T cells depleted in thymus-dependent areas of lymph nodes and spleen	N
T lymphopaenia (Nezelof's syndrome)	↓	↓↓	N	T cells depleted in thymus-dependent areas of lymph nodes	N/↓
Bruton's congenital agamma-globulinaemia	N	N	↓	Absence of follicles and plasma cells in lymph nodes	↓↓
Selective IgA deficiency	N	N	N	N	↓ IgA only
Wiskott–Aldrich syndrome	N/↓	N/↓	N	N	↓ (Especially IgM)
Ataxia-telangiectasia	↓	N/↓	N	Variable	↓ (Especially IgA)
HIV infection (AIDS)	N/↓	↓ (Especially helper T cells)	N	Abnormal follicular hyperplasia or lymphocyte depletion	N

N, Normal.

Table 10.2 Primary immunodeficiency disorders.

B-cell defects	T-cell defects
X-linked agammaglobulinaemia (Bruton's agammaglobulinaemia)	Congenital thymic dysplasia (DiGeorge syndrome)
Common variable immune deficiency	Chronic mucocutaneous candidiasis (± endocrinopathy)
X-linked hyper-IgM syndrome	Purine nucleoside phosphorylase deficiency
Selective IgA deficiency	
IgG subclass/specific antibody deficiency	
X-linked lymphoproliferative syndrome (Duncan's syndrome)	

Ig, Immunoglobulin.

cells, although their humoral immunity is entirely normal. Treatment is by replacement of the missing antibodies by regular infusions of intravenous purified human serum immunoglobulin, prepared from large pools of normal healthy donors.

Common variable immune deficiency

Common variable immune deficiency (CVID) can present at any age, although it is very rare for it present under the age of 3 years. It is a heterogeneous group of conditions, probably with different aetiologies, which manifest themselves by **antibody deficiency**. Unlike XLA, the cellular defects are not confined to the B cells, but include T cells and antigen-presenting cells.

The cause of CVID is not known, but is neither clearly genetic nor obviously secondary to infection. Serum immunoglobulin may be detectable and 85% of patients will have detectable B cells in the peripheral blood. While most patients will present with **recurrent bacterial infections** involving the sinopulmonary system, autoimmune disease is also common, particularly autoimmune thrombocytopenia, haemolytic anaemia and neutropenia.

Lymphadenopathy and **splenomegaly** are also common and a granulomatous condition resembling sarcoidosis may occur. **Malabsorption** also occurs. There appears to be an increase in the incidence of neoplasia, particularly stomach and lymphoma. Treatment is as for XLA.

Selective IgA deficiency

Selective IgA deficiency may be entirely **asymptomatic**. This is presumably because other classes of immunoglobulin can substitute on the mucosal surface. Complete absence of IgA means that the immune system will see exogenous IgA, such as may be infused with a blood transfusion, as foreign and will generate an immune response against it.

IgG subclass deficiency

Some patients lacking IgA do seem to be affected by recurrent infections and in these patients IgG subclass deficiency may be detected, usually IgG_2 and IgG_4. Only in a tiny minority of cases is there an obvious genetic defect (gene deletion), but in most cases the cause of the immune deficiency is unknown.

Sometimes a patient will have normal immunoglobulin levels. Recurrent infections may then indicate an IgG subclass deficiency or a failure to make specific antibodies, for instance against pneumococcal or *Haemophilus influenzae* polysaccharide.

There are four IgG subclasses: IgG_1 is the predominant antibody against protein antigens; IgG_2 is mainly directed against polysaccharide antigens (such as bacterial polysaccharides); IgG_3 is involved in antiviral antibody responses and IgG_4 may play a role in the control of IgE-mediated responses.

Because IgG_1 constitutes the majority of serum IgG, the clinical features of deficiency are those of CVID. IgG_3 deficiency is said to be associated with allergic disease, although the evidence supporting this is not strong. IgG_2 deficiency may be particularly troublesome because antibodies to polysaccharides are of this class. Polysaccharide antigens are associated with the capsules of pathogens such as the pneumococcus, *Haemophilus influenzae* and *Branhamella (Moxarella) catarrhalis*. Failure to generate an adequate response leads to recurrent respiratory infections. Patients have now been identified with normal serum immunoglobulins and normal IgG subclasses, but who cannot respond to capsular polysaccharides.

Defective humoral immune responses

Poor humoral immune responses are a feature of combined B- and T-cell defects such as ataxia telangiectasia, Wiskott–Aldrich syndrome and the DiGeorge syndrome, as well as SCID (see below). However, the degree of impairment is very variable and may not be of obvious clinical significance.

There are a number of other, very rare, antibody deficiency syndromes, including the X-linked lymphoproliferative syndrome (XLPS, Duncan's syndrome). This interesting X-linked condition has been described in a number of families worldwide. Affected males are normal until they encounter Epstein–Barr virus, when they then develop lymphomas and/or severe humoral immune deficiency. The reason for this is unknown, but the gene maps to the same area of the X chromosome as other X-linked immune deficiency disorders.

T-cell deficiencies

T-cell defects are **rare**. The two best known are **chronic mucocutaneous candidiasis (CMC)** and the **DiGeorge syndrome** (or 22q 11 syndrome).

CMC seems to be a very specific defect of T-cell immunity against *Candida*, as immunity to viruses and other organisms is usually normal. Likewise, humoral immunity against pathogens is also normal, and these patients often have high levels of anti-*Candida* antibodies. There is a strong association with an **endocrinopathy**, particularly involving the parathyroids and adrenals and accompanied by organ-specific autoantibodies. However, the endocrinopathy and CMC may occur separately. The nature of this T-cell defect is uncertain. The clinical features are of severe candidal infection of the nails and mucous surfaces. For inexplicable reasons, systemic candidal infection is not a major problem. Other clinical features relate to the endocrinopathy, and CMC patients who do not have the endocrinopathy should have their serum calcium measured at regular intervals.

DiGeorge syndrome is due to **congenital aplasia** or **hypoplasia** of the the **thymus**. The full syndrome includes a characteristic facies, with a fish-shaped mouth and low-set ears, and marked hypocalcaemia from failure of parathyroid gland development. Congenital heart disease also occurs. Presentation of severe cases is soon after birth, with tetany from hypocalcaemia or heart failure.

The defect arises during embryogenesis at 12 weeks' gestation with failure of development of the third and fourth pharyngeal pouches. However, less severe forms may occur, and presentation may be delayed until early childhood. In these cases there is some residual thymic tissue. The thymic defect predisposes to fungal, viral and protozoal infections and there is a marked T-cell lymphocytopenia. This is an autosomal dominant condition; there is often a deletion on chromosome 22.

As B-cell function is critically dependent on T-cell function for the majority of antigens, it is not surprising to find abnormalities of humoral immunity: these defects are overshadowed clinically by the T-cell defects. Infection by bacterial organisms is usually dealt with satisfactorily, probably because bacterial capsular polysaccharides are capable of directly stimulating B cells to produce antibody (T-independent antigens).

Treatment of the immune defect is controversial; both thymic and bone marrow transplants have been attempted. The cardiac abnormalities may require corrective surgery and the hypocalcaemia needs treatment with calcium together with vitamin D.

Combined immune deficiency

Table 10.3 indicates the main combined defects that are of clinical significance. As for other primary immunodeficiencies, these are all rare.

Severe combined immune deficiency (SCID) is the commonest. This may occur as in **X-linked** or **autosomal recessive** forms.

The clinical features, as one would expect, are of recurrent bacterial, viral, fungal and protozoal infections commencing very early in life, often in the neonatal period. There is frequently **hepatosplenomegaly** and also **lymphadenopathy**. Peripheral blood lymphocytes are markedly reduced, more so the T cells than the B cells, and there is an absence of T-cell proliferation to the usual mitogenic stimuli. B-cell function is variable, and serum immunoglobulin and sIg + B cells may both be present. Lymph nodes may show excess histiocytes and granuloma formation.

Urgent treatment is required, as the prognosis without treatment is uniformly fatal. Infections should be treated with appropriate antibiotics while a search is made for a bone marrow donor. The 'take' of donor bone marrow is improved by conditioning the recipient, to deplete residual functional lymphocytes. If a mismatched marrow is used, **graft-versus-host disease** may occur in the recipient.

In patients with T-cell defects, engraftment of foreign lymphocytes occurs readily, and for this reason it is vital that all blood products used for support are irradiated, to prevent transfer of viable lymphoid cells. It is thought that placental transfer of maternal lymphocytes at delivery may engraft and lead to a graft-versus-host disease, due to recognition of paternal antigens, on top of the SCID, accounting for the lymphadenopathy and skin changes seen in some cases.

Live viral immunization is dangerous, as is administration of bacillus Calmette–Guérin (BCG), which is routine practice for Asian neonates in some units, as both may lead to disseminated infection. With a successful transplant the results are good, with early restoration of T-cell function. B-cell function takes longer to reconstitute and prophylactic replacment therapy with intravenous immunoglobulin, as for antibody deficiency, may be required for some time after transplant.

Milder forms of SCID are recognized: 'Nezelof's syndrome', adenosine deaminase deficiency (ADA) and purine nucleoside phosphorylase (PNP) deficiency.

'Nezelof's syndrome' has rather similar clinical features to SCID, but presents much later in childhood with milder T-cell deficiency and poor antibody production. Some cases are due to lack of a component of the T-cell receptor.

ADA deficiency leads to the accumulation of adenosine which is toxic to lymphocytes (Fig. 10.1). There is a progressive lymphopenia and diminishing B- and T-cell function. As a result, clinical symptoms are absent at birth, but appear with the passage of time. ADA also occurs in red cells and repeated red cell transfusions will preserve a degree of lymphocyte function by mopping up excess adenosine; the problem with this therapy is eventual iron overload, and concurrent chelation therapy is required. The gene for the enzyme has been cloned and can be expressed. Purified ADA can be complexed with polyethylene glycol to improve its stability, and this has been injected *in vivo* with good results. As it is a single-gene defect, it is possible that genetic engineering may be able to replace the missing enzyme in stem cells eventually.

PNP deficiency (Fig. 10.1) is rather similar, but the metabolites that accumulate are more toxic to T cells than to B cells, and the resulting immune deficiency is much milder.

Both **Wiskott–Aldrich syndrome** and **ataxia telangiectasia** are accompanied by variable T- and B-cell defects. The immunological aspects of these conditions are overshadowed by the haematological and neurological features respectively.

Table 10.3 Combined T- and B-cell defects.

Severe combined immune deficiency (X-linked, autosomal recessive)
Adenosine deaminase deficiency
Wiskott–Aldrich syndrome (eczema, thrombocytopenia)
Ataxia-telangiectasia

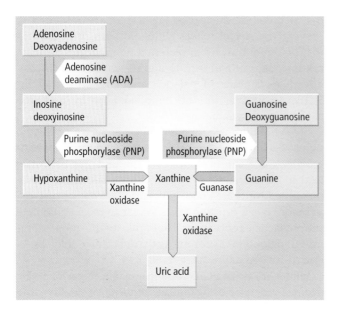

Fig. 10.1 Purine metabolic pathways.

Phagocytic cell defects

Table 10.4 identifies the major phagocytic defects. There is wide variation in the clinical features of phagocytic cell defects, from recurrent skin infections to fatal systemic infections. The usual infecting organisms are bacteria and fungi, while protozoa and viruses are handled normally.

Tests of neutrophil function are complex and require specialized facilities; they are thus not widely available. The attributes most readily tested are chemotaxis, phagocytosis, oxidative metabolism and superoxide generation and bacterial killing.

Chronic granulomatous disease

Chronic granulomatous disease (CGD) may occur as either an X-linked or autosomal recessive disorder. Both affect the cytochrome system of the neutrophils and lead to failure of bacterial killing. Presentation is in early childhood with deep-seated infections, abscesses and osteomyelitis. **Lymphadenitis** and marked **hepatosplenomegaly** occur.

The infecting organisms are often of low virulence in normal individuals, such as *Serratia marescens*, *Staphylococcus epidermidis* and *Aspergillus*. The simplest test to identify CGD is the **nitroblue tetrazolium** (NBT) test, in which the ability of the neutrophils to reduce the colourless NBT to the insoluble blue compound formazan is assessed: patients with CGD are unable to perform this reduction and carriers have an impaired ability, identified by using a quantitative NBT test. Tests of bacterial

Table 10.4 Phagocytic cell defects.

Disease	Underlying defect
Chronic granulomatous disease	Abnormality of cytochrome system X-linked or autosomal recessive (failure of killing and superoxide generation)
Glucose-6-dehydrogenase deficiency	X-linked enzyme deficiency, similar to chronic granulomatous disease
Myeloperoxidase deficiency	Absence of enzyme, poor bacterial killing, superoxide generation normal
Chédiak–Higashi syndrome	Autosomal recessive syndrome, with partial albinism, hepatosplenomegaly, CNS abnormalities and poor neutrophil killing (superoxide production normal)
Hyper-IgE syndrome, Job's syndrome, Buckley's syndrome	Eczema, recurrent bacterial infections, abscesses and high IgE. Abnormal neutrophil chemotaxis
Leucocyte adhesion molecule deficiency	Absence of adhesion molecules from cell surface, poor neutrophil phagocytosis, recurrent abscesses, delayed separation of umbilical stump

CNS, Central nervous system.

cell killing and superoxide generation are also abnormal, while chemotaxis and phagocytosis are normal. Treatment is restricted to prompt therapy with appropriate antifungals and antibiotics; prophylactic antibiotics have a role. As the genes have been identified, this is another condition for which genetic engineering may hold the key to future treatment.

Complement deficiencies

Deficiencies of almost all complement defects have been documented, although most are rare (Table 10.5). There is a strong association of complement deficiency with immune complex disease and recurrent bacterial infection, especially with *Neisseria*. The association with **systemic lupus erythematosus (SLE)** is likely to be caused by the formation of inappropriately sized immune complexes and failure of their normal clearance and breakdown (see Chapter 9).

C2 deficiency typically gives rise to an atypical SLE, in which **vasculitis** predominates. There is an increased susceptibility to infection and **hypogammaglobulinaemia** may occur.

Table 10.5 Complement deficiencies.

Component	Disease
C_1	SLE, vasculitis
C_2	Atypical SLE, antibody deficiency, bacterial infections
C_3	Immune deficiency, SLE, glomerulonephritis
C_4	SLE, poor phagocytic function
C_5	SLE, recurrent neisserial infections
C_6	Neisserial infections
C_7	Autoimmunity, neisserial infections
C_8	Neisserial infections
C_9	Asymptomatic
Properdin (alternate pathway)	Neisserial meningitis (not recurrent), pneumonia

SLE, Systemic lupus erythematosus.

C4 occurs in two forms, C4A and C4B, due to a gene duplication, and null alleles, particularly in C4A, are common and increase the risk of developing lupus. C4A null alleles occur as part of the extended haplotype A1, B8, DR3, which is strongly associated with autoimmune disease for reasons that have not been fully elucidated. As a clinical test, determination of the C4 haplotypes is not useful. Deficiencies of C5, C6, C7 and C8 all give rise to **neisserial** infection due to the failure to develop effective attack complexes capable of puncturing the bacterial cell membrane. Autoimmune phenomena also occur.

C9 deficiency occurs with high frequency in Japanese, but seems to be **asymptomatic**. Attack complexes lacking C9 are still capable of lysing targets, although the rate of lysis is slower.

Deficiency of properdin, in the alternate pathway, leads to recurrent bacterial infections; it is inherited as an X-linked disorder. Deficiencies of complement components are detected by screening for the haemolytic activity of serum in a functional test; individual components may be then assayed immunochemically and functionally.

C1-esterase inhibitor

C1-esterase inhibitor is a control protein, not only for the complement system, but also for the clotting and kinin systems. Two forms of deficiency have been identified – failure of production and production of an immunochemically normal but functionally inactive protein. Both lead to **angioedema** – non-pruritic swellings which typically involve the lips and tongue, upper airway and bowel (Fig. 10.2). Treatment with attenuated **androgens** increases the output of inhibitor and prevents attacks. If attacks occur, they are treated with **purified**

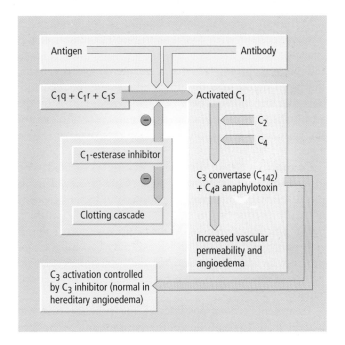

Fig. 10.2 Angioedema.

inhibitor. During attacks, the C4 becomes undetectable due to continued activation of the first part of the classical pathway, but C3 remains normal. Patients with lymphomas and autoimmune diseases may develop autoantibodies directed against the C1-inhibitor which inactivate it and lead to a secondary angioedema.

C3-nephritic factor

An **autoantibody**, C3-nephritic factor, has also been identified that stabilizes the alternate pathway C3 convertase C3bBb. This antibody has been found in patients with partial lipodystrophy, who are susceptible to bacterial infections and nephritis and in patients with type II membranoproliferative glomerulonephritis. The hallmark of this autoantibody is the persistently low serum C3.

SECONDARY IMMUNE DEFICIENCY

Introduction

The secondary immune deficiencies are far more common than the primary immune deficiencies. Immunological abnormalities have been associated with a wide range of disorders, but they are only of clinical significance in a small number of conditions.

Malignancy, particularly lymphoid malignancy, is often associated with poor T- and B-cell function. This is exacerbated by treatment with **drugs** and **radiation**. In the cases of chronic lymphatic leukaemia and myeloma, the B-cell defect may be sufficiently severe for recurrent bacterial infections to be a problem. Treatment is by the administration of replacement immunoglobulin, as for the primary B-cell disorders. **Hodgkin's disease** is also associated with neutrophil chemotactic defects.

Connective tissue disorders may be associated with global immune impairment (see Chapter 7). This is multifactorial. Abnormalities in the complement cascade not only predispose to the initiation of autoimmunity, but impair host defences. Abnormalities in both T and B cells enhance this defect and sepsis may become a major problem in SLE. Treatment for these disorders also involves immunosuppressive treatment that worsens this aspect.

Treatment, where possible, of the primary disorder usually leads to resolution of the symptomatic secondary immune deficiency. Sensitive laboratory testing may continue to demonstrate abnormalities of immune function even when the primary disorder is clinically in remission.

Histopathology

Both primary and secondary immune deficiency states are recognized clinically by repeated infections, mainly respiratory. These infections include not only organisms associated with infection amongst immunocompetent populations but also organisms which rarely cause infection in the general population– **opportunist infections**.

Neoplasia is the other potential penalty for any immunosuppressed patient. Patients with the commonest examples of secondary immunosuppression, such as following corticosteroid therapy, rarely develop tumours, in contrast to those with less frequent but more profound immunosuppression associated with human immunodeficiency virus (HIV) infection. Infections may occur amongst both examples but are commoner, more often in more than one site, and more often involve more than one organism in the HIV-positive patients. A comparable spectrum of neoplasms and infections occurs in the primary immune deficiency patients where the incidence of both is highest amongst the longer survivors and the most severely immunocompromised.

Infections

These are important causes of morbidity and mortality amongst all groups of immune-deficient patients but if recognized their effects can be prevented.

Any organism may be involved and in any patient more than one type and more than one site at a time, with the lungs and the brain as the sites most commonly infected. Few organisms are unique to specific tissues but *Toxoplasma* is virtually confined to the **brain** and **cryptosporidiosis** to the **gastrointestinal tract**.

The organisms largely reflect the immune deficit and the patient's environment (Tables 10.6 and 10.7). Predominantly cellular defects are associated with fungus and viral infections, while impaired humoral responses favour bacterial infections. Specific infections may consequently characterize specific immune deficiencies, for example, capsulate bacterial infections (*Pneumococcus*) in splenectomized patients. Nonetheless, such divisions are not absolute, probably in part because the different facets of the immune system function in concert rather than in isolation, but also because inflammatory responses are involved as well as the organism's own protective mechanisms.

The influence of the **environment** on the type of organism is displayed either by geographical differences, e.g. *Histoplasma* is common amongst **acquired immune deficiency syndrome (AIDS)** sufferers in the USA but rare in the European equivalents, or by local environmental influences, e.g. operation sites permit easy access for fungus (*Candida* and *Aspergillus*) to transplant recipients.

It is not uncommon for a local epidemic of *Pneumocystis carinii* pneumonia to occur in a ward of immunocompromised patients once one patient has this infection. Modern travel nevertheless alters the individual's normal environmental influence by transporting infected individuals to areas unpractised in the diagnosis of certain infections and by providing a new environment in which an organism may develop.

Previous exposure to the organism is also important, not only because established responses may be unimpaired, but also because many latent organisms may be able to express themselves in immune deficiency, a state of affairs seen both with tuberculosis and many herpesvirus infections.

Therapeutic intervention will further influence the pattern of infection: most immunodeficient patients experience patterns of infection changing from bacterial through viral to fungus and protozoal, in part affected by the use of antimicrobial agents either to treat specific infections or, and as importantly, to prevent, i.e. prophy-

Table 10.6 Infections in patients with impaired immunity.

Clinical setting	Pyogenic bacteria	Mycobacteria (atypical)	Fungi Cryptococcus	Viruses Herpes Papovavirus	CMV Pneumocystis	Giardia	Toxoplasma	Cryptosporidia
Severe combined immunodeficiency	+	+	+	+	+	–	–	–
Thymic hypoplasia (DiGeorge syndrome)	–	+	+	–	–	–	–	–
Bruton's congenital agammaglobulinaemia	+	–	–	–	–	+	–	–
Variable common immunodeficiency	+	–	–	–	–	+	–	–
Complement deficiency	+	–	–	–	–	–	–	–
HIV infection (AIDS)	–	+	+	+	+	+	+	+
Immunosuppressive drug therapy	–	+	+	+	+	–	+	–

CMV, Cytomegalovirus.

Table 10.7 Factors governing infection and types of infection.

Immune competence	Primary
Latent organisms	Reinfection
Environment	Reactivated
Local	
Geographical	
Therapeutic intervention	

laxis. All of these therapeutic agents may either facilitate infection by other organisms or modify but not entirely prevent the effects of the organism against which they are intended. Hence, the increasing number of HIV-positive patients with systemic *Pneumocystis carinii* is attributed to prophylactic pentamidine inhalation.

Infection may present as a **pyrexia** or **local lesion**, most commonly an abscess, or remain undetected until autopsy. Infection within the brain is notorious for escaping clinical recognition. At autopsy brain infection may be surprisingly widespread and combined with substantial tissue destruction. **Cytomegalovirus** in the **salivary gland** is also invariably asymptomatic, although not a cause of tissue damage, while within the liver it can produce liver cell destruction and hepatic dysfunction.

To identify an organism as a cause of tissue damage the organism must either be demonstrated within the abnormal tissue or there must have been an appropriate antibody response since few organisms result in tissue changes that are diagnostic and therapy may well have modified the expression of the organism. The occurrence of granulomas in both mycobacterial and fungus infections illustrates these points, as does the effect of even short courses of antituberculous therapy in masking tuberculous organisms.

The immunosuppressed patient is commonly thought to be unable to mount an inflammatory response to infection, but inflammatory responses are certainly found and it is probable that the defect is qualitative rather than predominantly quantitative.

Neoplasms

Kaposi's sarcoma and **non-Hodgkin's lymphoma** are the neoplasms most characteristic of immune deficiency. Hodgkin's disease, leukaemias and carcinomas also occur but their incidence is not much higher than in immunocompetent populations and their behaviour and prognosis are similar. Other sarcomas and soft-tissue tumours are not found in greater numbers than in other groups of patients.

Kaposi's sarcoma

This tumour was first recognized as a complication of

immune deficiency amongst renal transplant recipients, although it had previously been reported sporadically in patients with other forms of secondary immune depression (Table 10.8). The lesion was originally described in the skin of the lower limbs of elderly, predominantly male patients of middle European extraction and also in the indigenous population, mainly male, of parts of central Africa.

African patients either had an indolent, rarely fatal skin tumour similar to those in Europe or a rapidly fatal tumour invariably confined to lymph nodes, a younger age group was involved. It was recognized that a separate lymphoma could be associated with the sarcoma either at the same time or preceding or following the development of Kaposi's sarcoma and that spontaneous remission occurred. Recent studies in these populations reveal a mild T-cell deficit but this may be the consequence of the neoplasm rather than a condition preceding and causing the disease. Kaposi's sarcoma in immunodeficient patients demonstrates many of these features, although it is a neoplasm almost entirely of long-standing organ recipients and patients with AIDS.

This tumour is described in Chapter 26. The tumour in the skin or viscera ranges from a small area of telangiectasia to fairly large, purple lesions (Fig. 10.3(a)). Haemorrhage is apparent on sectioning and it is this haemorrhage which may cause death if the tumour involves the lung or gastrointestinal tract. The histology shows multiple thin-walled vessels, atypical spindle cells featuring mitoses and free red blood cells in the interstitium (Fig. 10.3(b)).

The **cell of origin** of the tumour is disputed but this appears to involve endothelial cells, probably both lymphatic and vascular. An exploratory hypothesis is that an angiogenic stimulus is released by immunosuppression and initiates a lesion which ultimately becomes neoplastic. This concept could explain the propensity to regression and is also important in the argument about

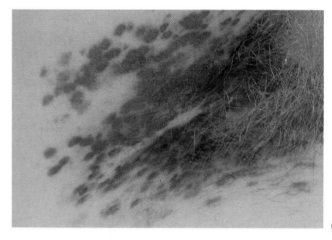

(a)

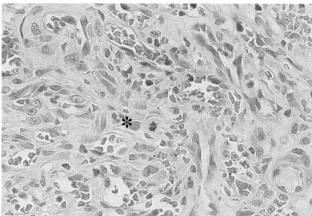

(b)

Fig. 10.3 (a) Kaposi's sarcoma of the groin in a patient with AIDS (courtesy of Dr S. Shaunak). (b) Histology of Kaposi's sarcoma. Note the pleomorphic spindle cells around vascular slits and note the free red cells and mitoses (✳). (H&E.)

whether Kaposi's sarcoma is a true sarcoma or really an endothelial hyperplasia. Possible **angiogenic stimuli** include antigens from grafts and infections, especially viruses. The **cytomegalovirus** was believed to be responsible but molecular biology techniques have failed to sustain this view and the role for a herpes virus or an unidentified **retrovirus** of the **lympholeucosis group** is now proposed.

Non-Hodgkin's lymphoma

Lymphomas amongst immunocompromised populations differ from those in immunocompetent patients. The gross and microscopic features are, however, similar.

Amongst graft recipients a sequence of reactive hyperplasia progresses to non-Hodgkins lymphoma (NHL) with an early polyclonal B-cell response but ultimately a restricted monoclonal response.

The Epstein–Barr virus has been clearly implicated in initiating this reaction and it is very probable that a simi-

Table 10.8 Percentage incidence of Kaposi's sarcoma amongst different populations and main site of involvement.

Population	%	Site
General population	0.6	Skin
Central Africa	9.0	Skin
		Lymph nodes
Primary immune deficiency	0.0	
Transplant recipients	4.9	Skin
AIDS patients (USA)	30.0	Skin

AIDS, Acquired immune deficiency syndrome.

lar sequence and basis is common to the majority of lymphomas in all examples of immune deficiency. The lymphomas can affect any site including lymph nodes but are characteristically extranodal and seen in a high incidence in the brain, an organ otherwise rarely involved by lymphoma. Although B cell in type, these lymphomas are generally high-grade and responsive to therapy but this response is not sustained and the prognosis is consequently poor.

Other tumours

The carcinomas encountered with immune deficiency are those particularly associated with the **papillomaviruses**. Skin, cervical and anal carcinoma are all increased in some groups of patients but the behaviour and thus prognosis of these tumours are otherwise no different from that of similar tumours in immunocompetent patients. The high rate of **gastric carcinoma** in those with the common variable type of sex-linked hypogammaglobulinaemia is an interesting and unexplained exception.

ACQUIRED IMMUNE DEFICIENCY DISEASE

Introduction

AIDS was recognized in the early 1980s from an increase in the USA in patients with *Pneumocystis carinii* **pneumonia** and with **Kaposi's sarcoma**.

It became apparent that these patients were mainly from the cities, particularly of the west coast, and that most were male and homosexual with smaller numbers amongst intravenous drug abusers and haemophiliacs. These observations, together with the rapid rise in the numbers of affected patients, all indicated an infectious basis for the immune deficit.

In the mid 1980s a retrovirus, HIV, was recognized as the cause of the disorder. Serological tests were rapidly developed and those with the disease thereby easily identified as well as the virus within tissues. The affinity of the virus for the lymphocyte CD4 receptor became apparent and thus the role of the virus in inducing immune deficiency. The disease is now recognized worldwide and many of the early observations have been confirmed.

The at-risk populations remain the same in the west (Table 10.9), although worldwide mainly heterosexual individuals, male and female, are affected. Children born to HIV-positive mothers can develop and die from the

Table 10.9 Main HIV positive groups.

Group	%
Homosexuals	59
Intravenous drug abusers	21
Haemophiliacs	1
Via intravenous transfusion	2.9
Heterosexuals, children	3.6

HIV, Human immunodeficiency virus.

disorder and a relentless increase in the disease with an inevitable mortality has occurred. By 1990 over 100000 had died from AIDS within the USA and over 1 million were HIV-positive, but within Africa the numbers are even greater, although accurate figures are unknown.

A patient's life expectancy following a diagnosis of AIDS remains just over 1 year, although the incubation period may extend for up to 9 years. Following infection, there is a spectrum of clinical outcome (Table 10.10).

The virus is transmitted in **all body fluids**, including breast milk, vaginal fluids or semen, and the main routes of disease are via sexual activity and blood. AIDS amongst health care workers has developed but has invariably involved large inoculations of blood rather than close contact. The infectivity to health care workers is approximately 20 times less than infective hepatitis and has involved less than 1% of those at risk. To date there is no effective means of immunization against HIV infection and no method of eradicating the virus once infected. The only proven helpful treatment is for the secondary infections.

The virus

HIV is a retrovirus and replicates via a reverse transcriptase (Fig. 10.4).

The virus occurs as HIV1 and the closely related HIV2 (rare outside West Africa) and binds via a **viral envelope glycoprotein** (gp 120) to CD4 receptors on mainly T cells, most of which are **T-helper cells**. This gradually leads to an ablation of cell-mediated immunity (CMI). AIDS is the most severe manifestation of a clinical spectrum of illness following HIV infection (Table 10.10). It is defined by the development of serious opportunistic infections and neoplasms (Table 10.11).

Table 10.10 Clinical outcome of infection with human immunodeficiency virus (HIV).

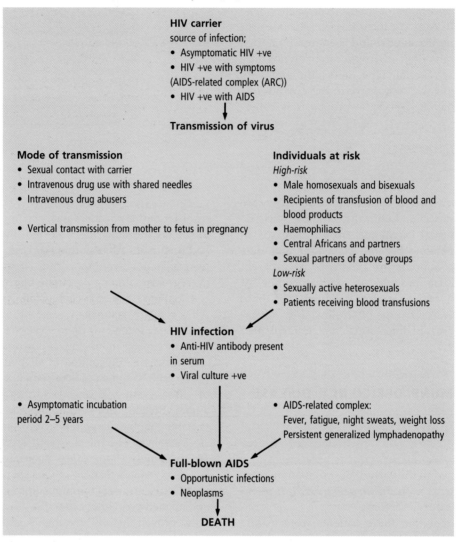

AIDS, Acquired immune deficiency syndrome.

Table 10.11 Classification of stages of human immunodeficiency virus (HIV) infection according to the Centers for Disease Control (CDC) staging.

CDC I	Asymptomatic infection (flu-like illness)
CDC II	Conversion to HIV-positive serology (by ELISA test)
CDC III	Onset of immunological defects, generalized lymphadenopathy (also known as AIDS-related complex or ARC)
CDC IV	Overt AIDS with opportunistic infections and neoplasms

ELISA, Enzyme-linked immunosorbent assay; AIDS, acquired immune deficiency syndrome.

Epidemiology

In the UK up until 1993, there were over 8000 reported AIDS cases, with a male to female ratio of approximately 10 to 1. High-risk groups include:

- homosexual males (anal intercourse is especially associated with transmission);
- intravenous drug abusers (IVDA);
- haemophiliacs from previously infected factor VIII;
- heterosexual partners of the above and promiscuous heterosexuals.

In Africa heterosexual spread is well-established. The mode of transmission is therefore sexual contact, and parenteral exposure to blood products. HIV may also cause congenital infections by transmission of the virus

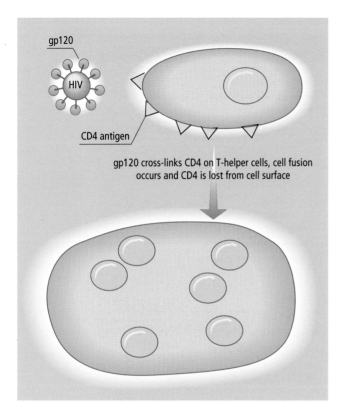

gp120

HIV

CD4 antigen

gp120 cross-links CD4 on T-helper cells, cell fusion occurs and CD4 is lost from cell surface

Fig. 10.4 Syncytium formation by the HIV virus.

from HIV-positive mothers *in utero* or postnatally via breast milk.

Clinical features

After the initial **seroconversion illness** there is a **latent period** with a mean incubation period of 8 years (shorter for congenitally infected infants with an incubation period as little as 2 years). Oral candidosis, persistent lymphadenopathy, weight loss and diarrhoea herald the start of the **AIDS-related complex (ARC)**. With further drops in the lymphocyte counts full-blown AIDS follows (Table 10.10).

Pneumocystis carinii pneumonia is the indicator disease of AIDS in over 40%. AIDS patients are at an increased risk of acquiring:

- well-established pathogens, e.g. pneumococcal disease, *Salmonella* and tuberculosis;
- opportunistic infections (Table 10.12).

Diagnosis of HIV infection

This is done via **antibody detection**. Enzyme-linked immunosorbent assay (ELISA) methods are used for detecting anti-HIV antibodies (HIV1 and 2). These tests are highly sensitive but occasional false-positives occur. The

procedure for all positive results is to retest a second sample and to test using at least two different methods. Antigen detection, detection of p24 antigen, co-cultivating virus or polymerase chain reaction is relatively insensitive and rarely used (Table 10.13).

Prevention

This is important, and as yet, the only way to combat the disease. This is done as follows:

- **health education** targeted at specific groups is the most important step;
- by **screening** of blood products for HIV antibodies;
- **vaccines** are awaited but may prove difficult due to the heterogenicity of the virus.

Treatment

Azathioprine (AZT) in patients with AIDS has proven benefits in terms of raising CD4 counts. Its role in asymptomatic HIV-positive patients to delay the onset of AIDS is debatable. Treatment is of specific diseases, particularly of opportunistic infections.

HIV infection in infants

The serological diagnosis of HIV infection in neonates born to HIV-seropositive mothers is difficult. Maternal HIV antibody of IgG class is passively transferred across the placenta to the fetus in such pregnancies, although only about one-third of neonates are actually infected. Passively transferred anti-HIV can persist for up to 15 months; therefore, the HIV antibody tests are of little use in determining whether an infant is actually infected.

The p24 antigen test may be of some diagnostic help, as may viral culture. However, negative results by these methods do not assure the absence of infection. More specialized tests such as the polymerase chain reaction and tests for IgA or IgM HIV antibody may be most rewarding, but are often not readily available.

Patient consent

Patient consent and counselling for HIV testing are important issues. Because of the unusually prominent social, psychological, financial and legal issues surrounding HIV testing in the UK, USA and Europe, most hospitals have adopted policies defining procurement of patient consent prior to HIV testing. Some countries have passed legislation regarding this issue. In addition, both pretesting and posttesting counselling of patients are advocated by most hospital administrators.

Table 10.12 Opportunistic infections in patients with acquired immune deficiency syndrome (AIDS).

Organism	Typical disease	Treatment
BACTERIA		
Listeria monocytogenes	Septicaemia Meningitis	Ampicillin and gentamicin
Atypical Mycobacterium M. avium-intracellulare	Chronic pneumonia Disseminated disease	Often multiresistant to first-line antimycobacterial drugs
FUNGI		
Candida albicans and spp.	Oral thrush, oesophagitis Disseminated disease	Fluconazole Amphotericin
Pneumocystis carinii	Pneumonitis	Co-trimoxazole, dapsone or clindamycin as alternatives Prophylactic pentamidine
Cryptococcus neoformans	Meningitis Pneumonia	Amphotericin and flucytosine Fluconazole
PROTOZOA		
Toxoplasma gondii	Encephalitis	Pyrimethamine
Cryptosporidium parvum	Chronic diarrhoea	No treatment
VIRUSES		
Herpes simplex	Disseminated disease Encephalitis	Acyclovir
Cytomegalovirus	Retinitis, pneumonitis Colitis, meningoencephalitis	Ganciclovir
Varicella-zoster	Recurrent zoster Disseminated disease	Acyclovir
JC virus	Progressive multifocal leukoencephalopathy	No treatment

Table 10.13 Laboratory tests for human immunodeficiency virus (HIV) infection.

ELISA test	Tests for presence of antibodies to HIV proteins Sensitivity: high (99%) Specificity: high (99.5%) Predictive value: limited (because of low prevalence of HIV infection in the population)
Western blot	Detects HIV proteins Specificity: very high (test is, however, difficult to interpret) Use: as a confirmatory test when ELISA is positive
HIV culture	Difficult and time-consuming; requires special test facilities because result is production of live virus
p24 antigen assay	Detects viral antigen; not available for clinical use
Polymerase chain reaction for HIV nucleic acid	Amplifies viral nucleic acid sequences up to 1 millionfold, at which point they are readily detectable. Highly specific and extremely sensitive

ELISA, Enzyme-linked immunosorbent assay; HIV, human immunodeficiency virus.

Immunology of HIV infection

The immunology of HIV infection is complex, and despite intensive study is not fully understood. The principal immunological manifestations are the progressive reduction of the CD4+ T cells, the rise in the CD8+ T cells and polyclonal hypergammaglobulinaemia. The remaining lymphocytes have a high level of activation and the elevation of serum β_2-microglobulin mirrors this.

In the early stages of disease, specific cytotoxic T cells, directed against HIV-infected target cells can be demonstrated. Serum antibodies directed against viral proteins are also detectable. At the time of initial infection, during the seroconversion illness, very marked cellular immunological abnormalities are present, but antibody will be absent. The cellular abnormalities return to normal and antibody appears. There is then a prolonged asymptomatic phase, during which time there is little detectable derangement of the immune system.

HIV is not truly a latent virus, as there is a detectable but very low level of viral production during this period.

For reasons that are not understood, the end of the asymptomatic phase is heralded by the gradual decline of absolute CD4+ T-cell numbers. Viral replication increases.

It has been assumed that the CD4+ T-cell tropism of the virus and its ability to destroy these cells by multicellular syncytium formation (Fig. 10.4) is responsible for the lowering of the peripheral T-cell count, but this is certainly an oversimplification.

Where the virus is integrated into the host cell genome, activation of the lymphocyte, say by another infection, leads to viral replication. The immune system becomes compromised when the CD4+ T-cell count falls below 400 cells/mm^3, leading to opportunistic infections. The polyclonal increase in immunoglobulins is due to the increase in non-specific T-cell activation: evidence that HIV directly activates B cells is inconclusive. Recurrent bacterial infections are a rare problem in AIDS, but occasional patients, particularly in Africa, are prone to septicaemia.

Macrophages also express the CD4 antigen and are infectable *in vivo* and *in vitro*. These cells may represent a primary reservoir of HIV infection, in the same way that occurs for the closely related Maedi-Visna virus in sheep and goats. Certain neural cells have also been shown to express an antigen closely related to CD4, and infection of these cells by neurotropic strains of HIV may explain the neurological syndromes (**AIDS dementia**) that occur.

Monitoring HIV infection in the laboratory

Single measurements of cell counts, immunoglobulins and β$_2$-microglobulin are not helpful. Abnormalities of CD4+ and CD8+ T cells are not unique to HIV and quite alarming drops in the CD4+ cell count may be seen transiently in otherwise trivial viral infections.

Cell marker analysis should not therefore be seen as a surrogate for proper serological and virological testing (with appropriate informed consent). Sequential monitoring in known HIV-positive patients is valuable and will predict quite accurately when therapeutic interventions such as AZT administration will become necessary. The lymphocyte count undergoes a marked diurnal variation and it is important to take sequential samples at approximately the same time of day. The diurnal variation disappears with progression of HIV disease and so the problem diminishes as the accuracy of the count becomes more critical.

HIV is inactivated by β-propriolactone and this can be used to treat blood samples and render them safe for laboratory assays. Most laboratory assays are unaffected by this treatment, but there is some damage to proteins, such that it is no longer possible to perform electrophoresis satisfactorily.

Development of a vaccine against HIV

The obvious lack of protection against progressive disease conferred by anti-HIV antibody indicates that immunization strategies directed at generating high levels of antibody are unlikely to be successful. In contrast, the presence of cytotoxic T cells does seem to relate to a degree of protection and vaccination with HIV antigens chosen for their ability to stimulate the development of specific cytotoxic T cells may prove valuable.

Pathology of AIDS

Without knowledge of the HIV status the histopathologist cannot, in most tissues, make a diagnosis of HIV-positivity. The most notable exception is the nervous system and particularly the brain, where fairly specific changes develop. The features in other tissues are predominantly the results of the coincident immunodepression and consequent infection and tumour formation. For example, the changes within lymph nodes both early and late include no unique features separating them from other causes of hyperplasia, as seen in early HIV infection, and lymphoid atrophy, the feature of end-stage HIV infection.

The spectrum of infections and tumours does include differences amongst the affected populations, such as the absence of Kaposi's sarcoma amongst HIV-positive haemophiliacs, but few are diagnostic. The differences in infection are substantially influenced by the patient's environment—hence tuberculosis, widespread in Africa and Haiti, is consequently common in HIV-positive patients in these areas. Cytomegalovirus infection, however, is invariably present amongst homosexuals and an important cause of morbidity if these men become HIV-positive.

Tumours
Kaposi's sarcoma (Fig. 10.3). Once this is recognized the patient has AIDS. A biopsy diagnosis in the early stages of the tumour can be extremely difficult to interpret and the lesion needs to be distinguished from other vascular lesions and in particular **bacillary angiomatosis**, a condition due to the cat scratch bacillus and curable with antibiotics.

Amongst HIV-positive patients with Kaposi's sarcoma, homosexuals are the most widely affected group while haemophiliacs never develop this tumour. Rarely, the tumour precedes HIV antigenaemia, but most often it is the patient's presenting feature or recognized at a later date. Amongst homosexuals the incidence of Kaposi's sarcoma has dropped since the inception of the AIDS epidemic, an observation attributed to, but not demonstrated as being due to, a reduction in promiscuity and the use of recreational drugs by these patients. The tumour is recognized usually in the skin, particularly the face and upper trunk, but other organs can be involved even in the absence of cutaneous lesions. Fatal haemorrhage has resulted, particularly with mucosal lesions of the respiratory and gastrointestinal tracts.

Other tumours

- **Lymphoma:** Both NHL and Hodgkin's disease occur amongst all types of HIV-positive patients. The incidence of NHL is 60 times greater than amongst HIV-negative populations but any increase in Hodgkin's disease is less clear-cut and has to be distinguished from the usual rate found amongst young men. Haemophiliac patients are particularly affected and common sites are extranodal, especially the brain.
- **Anal and oral squamous cell carcinoma:** This is a hazard for the HIV-negative and HIV-positive homosexual. The tumours may be preceded by *in situ* stage and an association with the **human papillomavirus** has been recognized.

Infections

Pneumocystis carinii (Fig. 10.5). *Pneumocystis carinii* infection first attracted attention to the AIDS epidemic and this pneumonia still forms an essential part of the clinical diagnosis of AIDS. It occurs in over 60% of AIDS sufferers at some time and despite therapy reinfection is common.

The organism formally grouped with the protozoa and responding to antiprotozoal agents is now regarded as a **fungus**. Specific species types exist but infection across species is unknown. The organism's origin is obscure but the focal epidemics experienced by AIDS patients suggest infection is directly from one patient to another and that infection is air-borne. Reinfection rather than reactivation of latent infection following childhood exposure is therefore probably the cause of the pneumonia in HIV-positive patients and this is almost inevitable once the peripheral lymphocyte count has dropped below 200 cells per cubic millimetre.

The organism is unique to the lung where **trophozoite** and **cyst forms** are recognized but how it damages the lung and produces hypoxia and eventually severe respiratory distress is unknown. Prior to medical treatment, and notably prophylactic aerosol therapy, infected lung included no specific features other than the organism. AIDS patients may now develop a spectrum of pulmonary changes largely attributable to the use of this therapy (Table 10.14).

Protozoa (Table 10.15)

- *Toxoplasma gondii.* **Cerebral infection** is the main manifestation of this protozoal infection in AIDS, although **heart** and **skeletal muscle** and **lymph nodes** as well as other less common sites have all been involved. Within the brain there is invariably more than one focus of infection and the effects vary from **cysts** in otherwise normal brain to **abscesses** associated with granulomas in which

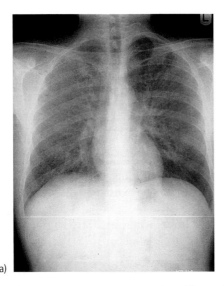

(a)

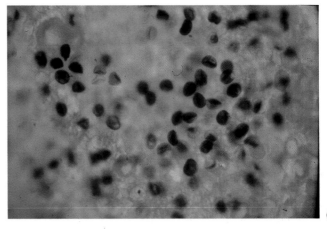

(b)

Fig. 10.5 (a) Pneumocystic *carinii* pneumonia in a patient with AIDS. (Chest radiograph.) Note the bilateral diffuse pulmonary shadowing and the cavitation in the left upper zone (courtesy of Dr S. Shaunak). (b) Pneumocystic *carinii* pneumonia in a broncho–alveolar lavage specimen. The organisms are stained black with Grocott.

Table 10.14 Changes in the manifestations of *Pneumocystis carinii* infection in the lung that have appeared with the use of therapy.

Granulomas
Miliary dissemination
Nodules
Cavity formation
Pneumothorax
Extrapulmonary spread

Table 10.15 Common protozoal infections found in patients with acquired immunodeficiency syndrome (AIDS).

INTESTINAL
Cryptosporidium
Isospora belli
Microsporidiosis
Giardia
Amoebiasis

BRAIN
Toxoplasma gondii

VISCERA/SKIN
Leishmania

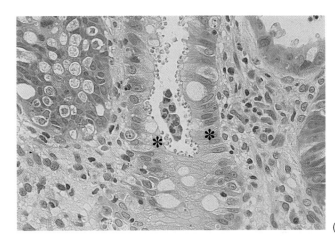
(a)

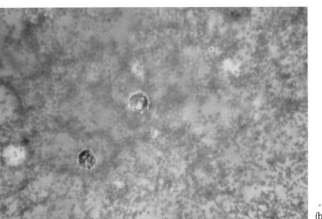
(b)

Fig. 10.6 (a) Cryptosporidium (✱) in a large bowel biopsy from a patient with AIDS (H&E). (b) Crytosporidium in a stool smear stained by modified Ziehl–Neelsen's method showing Crytosporidium cysts (courtesy Mr M. Crow).

there are cysts and tachyzoite forms. Since many adults are seropositive, cats providing the source of infection, infection in HIV-positive patients is invariably due to reactivation. Serum antibody levels are not helpful in diagnosis in HIV-positive patients and a confident diagnosis can only be made from brain smears or biopsies. At autopsy the infection is almost always more widespread than realized clinically.

• *Cryptosporidium* (Fig. 10.6). This organism can cause a profound chronic greenish diarrhoea in HIV-positive patients and most notably those in Africa. Diarrhoea may also result in immunocompetent individuals but in these patients the disorder is self-limiting. However, in either group the organism may be present without symptoms. Infection is acquired from contaminated meat and water and the natural reservoir is young domestic animals, including calves, goats, lambs and pigs. The organism is recognized either in the stools or in biopsies from any part of the gastrointestinal tract.

Isospora belli, *Giardia* and amoeba are other intestinal protozoa, each capable of producing diarrhoea but also found in the absence of symptoms in HIV-positive patients. Their incidence is highest amongst homosexuals.

Viruses (Table 10.16). **Cytomegalovirus** (Fig. 10.7). This herpesvirus is virtually endemic in homosexuals and

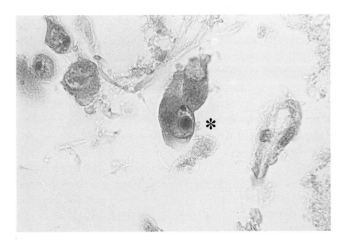

Fig. 10.7 CMV infected oesophageal epithelial cells in a patient with AIDS (✱). These have been exfoliated and the cytology shows the large 'owl's eye' nuclear inclusions. (H&E.)

many HIV-positive patients have characteristic **owl's eye intranuclear inclusions** within their tissues. Amongst all HIV-positive patients all tissues including the nervous system have been involved, although the retina, lung and gastrointestinal tract are those most affected.

Infection in some instances is due to **activated latent virus** but also arises from reinfection since different subtypes can be identified. Latent virus can reside in endothelial cells, macrophages and lymphocytes and transmission of the virus can occur via blood and other body fluids, including breast milk and semen.

The role of the virus as a cause of symptoms and tissue damage is difficult to assess, although a number of potential cytopathic mechanisms are recognized. Any role in neoplasia, notably Kaposi's sarcoma, is however unsubstantiated. The virus may also play a synergic role with other viruses, including HIV, thereby enhancing any potential effects of either virus including T-cell destruction and immunodepression.

Other **herpes viruses**, such as herpes simplex and herpes zoster, produce tissue damage in patterns similar to those experienced by immunocompetent populations, although in the HIV-positive individuals these infections are often more indolent and more subject to recurrence (Fig. 10.8). The infections may precede the clinical recognition of the HIV state.

Epstein–Barr virus and **human papillomaviruses** are important because of their relationship with the NHLs and squamous epithelial tumours that occur in AIDS.

Bacteria. Bacterial infections of all types occur in HIV-positive and AIDS patients but they are usually responsive to antibiotic therapy. Septicaemias are particularly prone to occur amongst African patients and IVDAs and in either group these may prove fatal.

Mycobacterial infection, due to both *Mycobacterium tuberculosis* and atypical *Mycobacterium*, is increased, the former particularly amongst African AIDS patients where infection may precede the recognition of AIDS. Infection is often restricted to the lung but miliary dissemination is usual with the atypical mycobacteria. The commonest of the atypical forms is *M. avium intracellulare* (Fig. 10.9). Clinically mycobacterial infection contributes quite substantially to the profound terminal wasting characteristic of AIDS, **slim disease** in Africa.

Fungus (Table 10.17). Oral *Candida* can be a presenting feature of HIV infection (Fig. 10.10) and may develop and recur at any time subsequently. Spread into the pharynx and oesophagus may follow but widespread systemic infection is uncommon. The condition clears with therapy but may reappear.

Cryptococcus, predominantly an infection of the lungs,

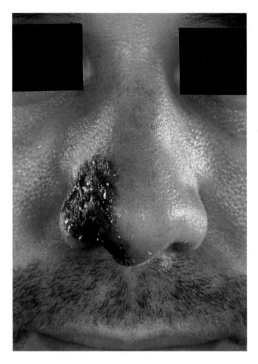

Fig. 10.8 Herpes simplex infection of the nose in a patient with AIDS (courtesy of Dr S. Shaunak).

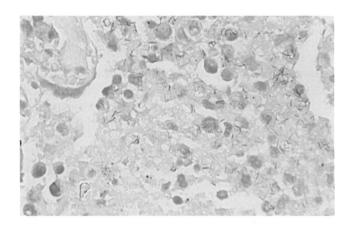

Fig. 10.9 Lymph node biopsy from a patient with AIDS showing foamy macrophages containing *Mycobacterium avium* intracellulare (red). Ziehl–Neelsen's method.

menginges and brain (Fig. 10.11) and *Histoplasma*, primarily confined to the lungs but often disseminated in AIDS (Fig. 10.12), are uncommon fungus infections in AIDS in the UK.

In Africa cryptococcal meningitis is a very significant cause of death amongst AIDS patients and in the USA *Histoplasma* contributes to morbidity in HIV-positive individuals. Recognition of either fungus may herald the onset of AIDS.

Table 10.16 Examples of viruses prevalent in human immunodeficiency virus-positive patients.

> Herpes simplex
> Herpes zoster
> Hepatitis viruses
> Molluscum contagiosum
> Cytomegalovirus
> Papavovirus
> Epstein–Barr virus
> Human papillomavirus

Table 10.17 Fungus infections recognized in patients with acquired immunodeficiency syndrome (AIDS).

> *Candida*
> *Cryptococcus*
> *Histoplasma*
> *Nocardia*
> *Penicillium*
> *Aspergillus*
> Botryomycosis
> Sporotrichosis

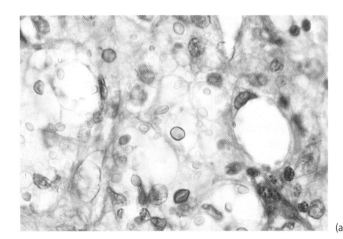

(a)

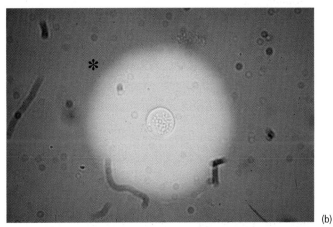

(b)

Fig. 10.11 (a) Cryptococcus neoformans in the lung in a patient with AIDS. Note the intramacrophage location and the capsule stained with PAS. (b) *Cryptococcus neoformans* in an Indian ink preparation of cerebrospinal fluid (✳). The stain demonstrates the large capsule.

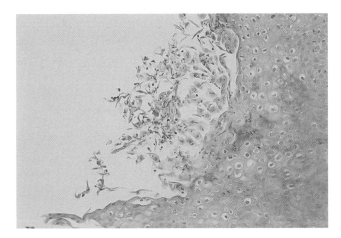

Fig. 10.10 Histology of the oesophagus in an AIDS patient showing Candida hyphae. (H&E.)

In contrast, *Aspergillus* infection appears at the end-stage of the disease and most commonly in patients who have survived for some years. This infection is nevertheless uncommon and, although usually confined to the lungs, may via infected emboli spread to other sites. Other fungus infections are even more unusual but generally and more obviously reflect the patient's environment.

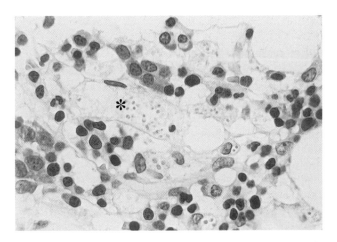

Fig. 10.12 Histoplasmosis in the liver in a patient with AIDS. Note the organisms within macrophages in portal tracts. (Giemsa.)

Nervous system involvement

Lesions affecting any part of the nervous system occur in AIDS patients with and without symptoms and are not clearly related to the period of HIV-positivity (Table 10.18). Their symptomatic effects were initially overlooked because they were either masked or attributed to coexistent infection or neoplastic lesions. Similarly, the potential diversity of the nervous system involvement was also not appreciated because of the clinical dominance of the cerebral features.

An **encephalopathy** (or encephalitis) is present in at least 20–30% of AIDS patients (Fig. 10.13), often with a **myelopathy** and invariably with a **neuropathy**. Within the nervous system HIV can be demonstrated in macrophages, microglia and macrophage-derived multinucleate giant cells, but how myelin damage is

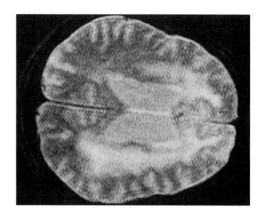

Fig. 10.13 A magnetic resonance imaging (MRI) scan showing periventricular enhancement in a patient with HIV encephalitis (courtesy of Dr S. Shaunak).

Table 10.18 Human immunodeficiency virus (HIV) and the nervous system.

Pathological lesions	Anatomical location	Clinical effects
Encephalopathy	>Frontal/temporal lobes	AIDS dementia
Myelopathy	>Upper cervical spinal cord	Progressive spastic paraparesis; impaired position and vibration sense
Peripheral neuropathy	Cranial and peripheral nerves	Painful sensory, mixed sensory and motor polyneuropathy
Autonomic neuropathy	Sympathetic and parasympathetic	Effects uncertain

AIDS, Acquired immune deficiency syndrome.

effected is unclear. Direct damage by HIV and damage via products released from infected macrophages are currently being investigated. The histopathological results are manifest primarily by microscopy but involve white and grey matter, sometimes with a fairly characteristic vacuolar change in the myelin.

Other systems

A wide variety of clinical features and associated or independent histopathological features occur amongst AIDS sufferers (Table 10.19). In the absence of any infective or neoplastic disorder there is a temptation to ascribe these findings to HIV, although the effects of the patient's lifestyle, especially the usage of intravenous drugs, and of therapy, must also be discounted.

However, with experience, it invariably becomes apparent that explanations other than HIV underlie these observations–any infected HIV-positive patient with or without malignancy can develop the **nephrotic syndrome** associated with an immune complex glomerulonephritis and a wide range of **rashes** can be

Table 10.19 Lesions possibly due to human immunodeficiency virus.

Skin	*Biliary tract*
Macular-papular rashes	Biliary stenosis
Seborrhoeic dermatitis	Sclerosing cholangitis
Folliculitis	
Ichthyosis	*Pancreas*
	Diabetes mellitus
Heart and vessels	Pancreatitis
Pericardial effusion	Atrophy
Lymphocytic myocarditis	
Cardiomyopathy	*Salivary gland*
Vascular fibrocalcification	Lymphocytic sialadenitis
	Cysts
Gastrointestinal tract	
Villous atrophy	*Kidney*
Colitis	Segmental nephritis
	Mesangial proliferative nephritis
Liver	
Non-caseating granulomas	
Focal hepatitis	
Kupffer cell hyperplasia	

anticipated amongst any group of patients receiving the drugs administered to AIDS patients. Similarly, pancreatitis has many causes and in insulin-dependent diabetes mellitus many viruses can damage insulin-secreting cells.

Nevertheless, there is the possibility that HIV is directly responsible for any of these lesions, all of which can develop with HIV infection, either directly or via the release of cytokines from HIV-infected macrophages. Macrophages populate, and circulate, in almost all organs and HIV may be inoculated on to or carried in tissue fluids directly to epithelial cells. HIV-infected macrophages may for these reasons underlie the lymphocytic sialadenitis seen in the parotid glands and the lymphocytic myocarditis while virus, either free within body fluids or released from macrophages, may contribute to the **villous atrophy** of the small intestine and the **apoptosis** in the large intestine, liver and some skin lesions.

Neoplasia

CONTENTS

INTRODUCTION

The terms **tumour**, **new growth** and **neoplasia** are used interchangeably. The word **cancer** implies a malignant neoplasm, usually, but not always, of epithelial origin. Neoplasia represents a defect in cellular differentiation, maturation and control of growth.

Neoplasms are **benign** or **malignant** depending on several features, chiefly the ability of malignant neoplasms to spread from the site of origin. Benign neoplasms grow but remain localized.

The definition of neoplasm proposed in the early 1950s by Rupert Willis remains the best: 'A neoplasm is an abnormal mass of tissue, the growth of which exceeds and is uncoordinated with that of the surrounding normal tissues and persists in the same excessive manner after cessation of the stimuli that evoked the change'.

In this chapter, clinical aspects of neoplasia will be discussed. The student is referred to the recommended texts for a more indepth review of basic mechanisms of oncogenesis.

ONCOGENESIS

Many aspects of neoplasia remain poorly understood. There have been many theories of oncogenesis and these will be reviewed.

Theories of oncogenesis

Multifactorial origin
More than one step is required to produce a neoplasm.

The action of an **initiator** will produce the first steps in neoplasia, followed by the prolonged action of one or more **promoters** to cause neoplastic growth (promotion). The requirement of multiple successive insults (the **multiple-hit** theory) explains the long **latent period** between initiation of the disease and the appearance of the neoplasm.

The role of genetic mutation

Changes in the cell's genome may result from **spontaneous mutation** or the action of external agents (**carcinogens**). Neoplasia will result if the genes involved are **growth-regulating genes**.

Consistant genetic abnormalities are found in some neoplasms. Examples include retinoblastoma (partial deletion of the long arm of chromosome 13) and chronic granulocytic leukaemia (Philadelphia chromosome, Ph[1]).

Chromosomal instability is associated with xeroderma pigmentosum, Fanconi's anaemia and Bloom's syndrome. Ageing results in an increasing incidence of many of the most common neoplasms, implying faulty deoxyribonucleic acid (DNA) repair with ageing.

The viral oncogene theory (Table 11.1)

Neoplastic transformation may occur as a result of activation (or depression) of specific DNA sequences (**cellular oncogenes**; c-*onc*) in cells. Cellular oncogenes are inherited as part of the cell genome and are identified in cells by the use of complementary DNA (or ribonucleic acid (RNA)) probes (manufactured nucleotide sequences that show a reciprocal fit with segments of the oncogene). Cellular oncogenes are believed to control productions of growth factors and may be important in normal growth regulation. Activation may be effected by various carcinogens, including viruses, radiation and chemicals.

Certain RNA oncogenic viruses contain nucleic acid sequences, called **viral oncogenes** (v-*onc*), that are mutated forms of cellular genes. Such sequences have been found in certain animal neoplasms.

Many oncogenes have been recognized in human cancer cells. Their role in the genesis of neoplasia remains unclear, particularly since similar genes (**proto-oncogenes**) have also been found in normal cells. For many oncogenes tested to date, the gene product is a protein kinase, tyrosine phosphorylase with growth-regulating properties. In other instances, the oncogene product serves as a cellular receptor for known growth factors (e.g. epidermal growth factor).

DNA oncogenic viruses also appear to contain oncogene segments, which are inserted directly into the host cell genome; normal non-infected host cells do not appear to contain intrinsic DNA sequences (cellular oncogenes) analogous to viral oncogenes of DNA viruses.

The oncogene hypothesis unifies these causes (Fig. 11.1).

Epigenetic theory

In this theory, the fundamental cellular alteration occurs not in the genetic apparatus of the cell but in the **gene products**, specifically the protein products of growth-regulating genes.

Immune surveillance theory

This theory proposes that neoplastic cells produce new

Table 11.1 Viral oncogenesis.

Oncogene	Species origin	Tumour type	Viral-determined DNA in host cell
V-*src*	Chicken	Sarcoma	Yes
N-*yes*	Chicken	Sarcoma	Yes
V-*myc*	Chicken	Carcinoma, sarcoma, leukaemia	Yes
V-*myb*	Chicken	Leukaemia	Yes
V-*abl*	Mouse	Leukaemia	Yes
V-*mos*	Mouse	Sarcoma	Yes
V-*ras*	Rat	Sarcoma, leukaemia	Yes
V-*fes*	Cat	Sarcoma	Yes
Y-*sis*	Monkey	Sarcoma	Yes

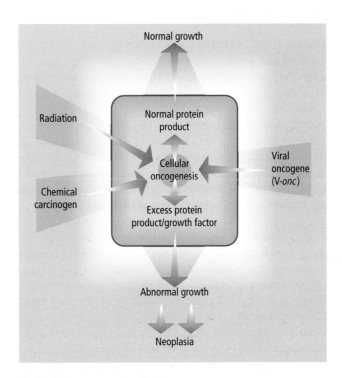

Fig. 11.1 The oncogene hypothesis.

molecules (neoantigens, **tumour-associated antigens**). The immune system of the body recognizes these neoantigens as foreign and mounts a cytotoxic immune response that destroys the neoplastic cells expressing the neoantigen (Fig. 11.2). Neoplastic cells produce clinically detectable neoplasms only if they escape recognition and destruction by the immune system.

Apoptosis (programmed cell death)

Apoptosis or programmed cell death refers to individual cell dropout. It is seen in tissue growth, morphogenesis and remodelling. It plays an important role in regulating the size of a cell population.

It can be seen in actively dividing cell populations, in tissues following chemotherapy or radiotherapy and is seen in benign and malignant tumours. The appearances are those of round, membrane-bound bodies which ultimately undergo phagocytosis (Fig. 11.3(a)). The occurrence of apoptosis in slow-growing tumours with a high mitotic count implies an important role in tumour prognosis. Apoptosis differs from necrosis in the following ways:

- it involves single cells;
- it occurs due to biochemical activation of endogenous endonuclease which digests DNA;
- ultrastructurally, the cell shows condensation of the cell nucleus (Fig. 11.3(b)).

Known oncogenic agents

Chemical carcinogens (Table 11.2)

Carcinogens are substances that are known to cause an increased incidence of cancer. Most chemical carcinogens act by producing changes in DNA. A small number act by **epigenetic** mechanisms.

Chemical carcinogens that act **locally** at the site of application without having to undergo metabolic change in the body are called **proximate** or direct-acting carcinogens. Other chemicals produce cancer only after they are converted into metabolically active compounds within the body; these are termed **ultimate carcinogens**.

Cigarette smoking. Cigarette smoking is responsible for more human cancer than all of the other listed chemicals combined and is associated with an increased risk of cancer of the lung, bladder, oropharynx and oesophagus (Chapter 7). There is evidence that the risk of cancer associated with smoking is not limited to the smoker but may extend to others in close physical proximity to the smoke for long periods. It has been estimated that smoking alone accounts for more cancer deaths than all other known carcinogens combined.

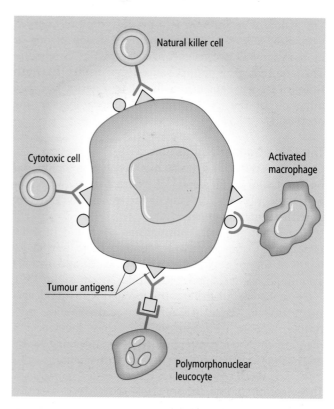

Fig. 11.2 Immune mediated cytotoxicity.

Numerous carcinogens are present in cigarette smoke but the most important are probably **polycyclic hydrocarbons** (tars). These are **direct-acting** carcinogens in the skin; they act as **procarcinogens** in producing lung and bladder cancer. Inhaled tars are converted in the liver to an epoxide by a microsomal enzyme, aryl hydrocarbon hydroxylase. This **ultimate** carcinogen is an active compound that combines with guanine in DNA, leading to neoplastic change.

The risk of developing cancer is about 10 times higher in someone who smokes a pack of cigarettes a day for 10 years (10 **pack years**) than in a non-smoker. The risk drops almost to that of a non-smoker after about 10 years of abstinence.

Aromatic amines. Exposure to aromatic amines such as **benzidene** and **naphthylamine** is associated with an increased incidence of bladder cancer. Aromatic amines are **procarcinogens** that enter the body through the skin, lungs, or intestine. In the body they are converted to carcinogenic metabolites that are excreted in the urine.

Aflatoxin. Aflatoxin is a toxic metabolite produced by the fungus *Aspergillus flavus* and is thought to be an important cause of liver cancer in humans. This fungus grows on

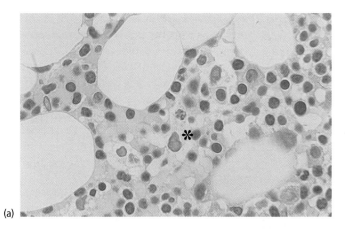

(a)

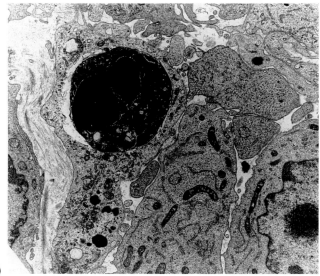

(b)

Fig. 11.3 Apoptosis. (a) Bone marrow in a patient given chemotherapy for acute leukaemia. Note the apoptotic cells (✱) showing condensation of the nuclear chromatin. (H&E) (b) Electronmicrograph of mouse tumour showing an apoptotic body. Note the characteristic condensation of nuclear chromatin, ×7800 (courtesy, Dr C. Sarraf).

Table 11.2 Chemical carcinogens.

Chemical	Types of cancer
Polycyclic hydrocarbons	
Soot (benzo[a]pyrene, dibenzanthracene)	Skin, scrotal cancer in chimney sweeps
Inhalation or chewing of tobacco products (mainly cigarettes)	Lung, bladder, oral cavity, larynx, oesophagus
Aromatic amines	
Benzidine, 2-naphthylamine	Bladder
Aflatoxins	Liver
Nitrosamines	Oesophagus, stomach
Chemotherapeutic agents	Leukaemias
Cyclophosphamide, chlorambucil, thiotepa, busulphan	
Asbestos	Lung cancer, mesothelioma
Heavy metals	
Nickel, chromium, cadmium	Lung
Arsenic	Skin
Vinyl chloride	Liver (angiosarcoma)

improperly stored food, particularly grain and nuts. In Africa, large amounts of aflatoxin ingestion have been shown to correlate with a high incidence of **hepatocellular carcinoma**.

Nitrosamines. Nitrosamines are derived mainly from conversion of nitrites in the stomach. Nitrites are found in preservatives, particularly those associated with tinned meat. The local action of nitrosamines is thought to be an important cause of oesophageal and gastric cancer.

Betel leaf. In parts of India and Sri Lanka chewing of betel leaf is responsible for a high incidence of squamous carcinoma of the oral cavity.

Chemotherapeutic drugs. Alkylating agents, such as cyclophosphamide, chlorambucil and busulphan alter nucleic acid synthesis in cancer cells and interfere with DNA synthesis in normally dividing cells, particularly those in the bone marrow. They may thus cause oncogenic mutations, particularly leukaemia.

Asbestos. Asbestos has been widely used as an insulating material and fire retardant and is found in many buildings built before 1950.

Asbestos is inhaled into the lung, where it produces fibrosis and chronic lung disease (Chapter 17). Asbestosis also leads to fibrous proliferation in the pleura, where it results in fibrous plaques that are a reliable radiological indicator of previous asbestos exposure. Asbestos is associated with two types of cancer:

1 Malignant mesothelioma. This uncommon neoplasm is derived from mesothelial cells, mainly in the **pleura** but also in the **peritoneum** and **pericardium**. Malignant mesothelioma is the most specific cancer associated with asbestos exposure.

2 Bronchogenic carcinoma. The most common form of lung cancer is bronchogenic carcinoma. Patients with asbestos exposure have a risk of lung cancer about twice that of the general population; this risk is greatly magnified by smoking. It is not as specifically associated with asbestosis as is mesothelioma but lung cancer is the commonest malignant neoplasm in patients with a history of asbestos exposure.

Other industrial carcinogens. Miners exposed to **heavy metals** such as nickel, chromium and cadmium show an increased incidence of lung cancer.

Agricultural workers exposed to **arsenic**-containing pesticides show a high incidence of skin cancer.

Vinyl chloride used in the manufacture of polyvinyl chloride (PVC), is associated with angiosarcoma of the liver, mainly in experimental animals.

Radiation

Several different types of radiation cause cancer, most probably by direct effects on DNA or possibly by activation of cellular proto-oncogenes.

All radiation derived from X-rays, therapeutic isotopes and nuclear power plants accounts for less than 1% of the total radiation exposure of the population; the remainder comes from radioactive rocks, the earth and cosmic rays.

Ultraviolet radiation. Ultraviolet radiation is associated with different kinds of skin cancer, including squamous carcinoma, basal cell carcinoma and malignant melanoma (Chapter 26). Skin cancer is the most common type of cancer in the UK and the USA, being common in fair-skinned individuals exposed to sunlight and sunbeds.

Ultraviolet light is believed to induce formation of linkages between pyrimidine bases on the DNA molecule. Normally, these defects will undergo repair. Skin cancer due to exposure to sunlight is thus a disorder seen most often in those with faulty DNA repair mechanisms, in the **elderly** and in people with **xeroderma pigmentosum**.

X-ray radiation. **Radiotherapy** for cancer can be associated with radiation-induced malignant neoplasms, commonly **sarcomas**, that appear 10–30 years after radiation therapy.

Diagnostic X-rays use such small doses of radiation that no increased risk of cancer is believed to be associated with their use. A possible exception is that abdominal X-rays during pregnancy may slightly increase the incidence of leukaemia in the fetus. Radiation doses are increasing with newer forms of radiology such as mammography and computed tomography (CT) scans and the question of carcinogenic risk again arises.

Radioisotopes. Radioactive **radium** is metabolized in the body in the same way as calcium and is therefore deposited in bone, where it induces **osteosarcoma**. Occupational exposure to radioactive minerals in the mines of central Europe and the western USA is associated with an increased incidence of lung cancer.

Thorotrast, a dye containing radioactive **thorium**, was used in diagnostic radiology between 1930 and 1955. Thorotrast increases the risk of several types of liver cancer, including angiosarcoma, liver cell carcinoma and cholangiocarcioma (Chapter 19).

Radioactive **iodine**, which is used to treat thyroid disease, is associated with an increased risk of cancer developing 15–25 years after treatment; the risk is weighed against the nature of the primary disease and the therapeutic benefits.

Nuclear fallout. The Japanese in Hiroshima and Nagasaki who survived the atomic bomb blasts, inhabitants of the Marshall Islands who were accidentally exposed to fallout during atmospheric testing of nuclear devices in the southern Pacific Ocean and survivors of the accident at the Chernobyl nuclear power plant in the USSR in 1986 have shown a greatly increased incidence of cancer, including **leukaemia** and **carcinoma of the breast, lung** and **thyroid**.

Viral oncogenesis

Both DNA viruses and RNA viruses can cause neoplasia (Table 11.3). DNA viruses insert their nucleic acid directly into the genome of the host cell. RNA viruses require RNA-directed DNA polymerase (**reverse transcriptase**), an enzyme that causes the production of a DNA copy of the RNA viral genome; this DNA copy (**provirus**) can then be inserted in the host genome.

Some RNA viruses contain a 'built-in' **oncogene** that directly activates the cell; others insert nucleic acid adjacent to an endogenous cellular proto-oncogene, which is thereby activated.

The presence of a viral genome in a cell can be demonstrated in the following ways:
- reciprocal hybridization studies using DNA probes;
- recognition of virus-specific antigens on infected cells;
- detection of virus-specific messenger RNA (Fig. 11.4).

Oncogenic RNA viruses (retroviruses) (Table 11.3). Formerly called oncornaviruses, these cause many neoplasms in experimental animals, including leukaemia and lymphoma in mice, cats and birds; various sarcomas in birds (Rous sarcoma virus) and primates; and breast carcinoma in mice (Bittner milk factor, or mouse mammary tumour virus).

Table 11.3 Oncogenic viruses.

Group	Virus	Host	Tumour
RNA viruses (retroviruses)			
	Avian leukaemia–sarcoma	Chicken	Leukosis, Rous sarcoma
	Murine leukaemia–sarcoma	Mouse, rat, hamster	Leukaemia, sarcoma
	Feline leukaemia–sarcoma	Cat/dog	Leukaemia, sarcoma
	Murine mammary tumour virus (Bittner milk factor)	Mouse	Breast cancer
	HTLV-I	Human	T-cell leukaemia
	Human immunodeficiency virus (AIDS virus)	Human	AIDS-related lymphomas
DNA viruses			
Papovavirus	Papillomavirus	Human, rabbit, cow, dog	Papilloma (laryngeal), condylomata acuminata, verruca vulgaris, carcinoma of cervix
	Polyomavirus	Mouse	Many tumours in newborn hamsters
	SV40	Monkey	Tumours in hamsters only
	Herpesvirus	Herpes simplex type 2	Human ?carcinoma of cervix
	Epstein–Barr virus	Human	Carcinoma of nasopharynx, Burkitt's lymphoma
	Avian	Chicken	Marek's disease
	Rabbit	Rabbit	Lymphoma
Poxvirus	Fibroma–myxoma	Rabbit	Fibromyxoma
	Molluscum contagiosum	Human	Molluscum contagiosum
Hepatadnavirus	Hepatitis B	Human, rodent, duck	Hepatocellular carcinoma

HTLV-I, Human T-lymphotropic virus I; AIDS, acquired immune deficiency syndrome.

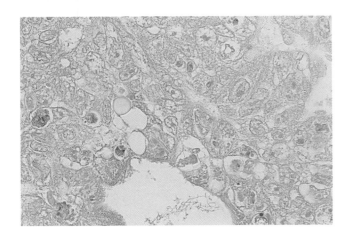

Fig. 11.4 Cervical biopsy. *In situ* hybridization for human papilloma virus (HPV). RNA shows localization of viral nucleic acid in the cervical epithelial cell.

Retroviruses have been implicated in only a few human neoplasms.

- **Japanese T-cell leukaemia.** This form of leukaemia was first described in Japan. A retrovirus (human T lymphocyte virus type I; HTLV-I) has been cultured from tumour cells in this disease and the virus is believed to play a direct causative role.
- **Infection with HIV.** Human immunodeficiency virus (HIV) is a retrovirus that infects human lymphocytes and causes acquired immune deficiency syndrome (AIDS; Chapter 10). The malignant B-cell lymphomas associated with AIDS may result from HIV oncogenesis.
- **Leukaemias and lymphomas.** There is evidence to suggest that haematological cancers may have a viral origin. Tissue samples taken from many patients with leukaemias and lymphomas contain viral reverse transcriptase, and there have been reports of isolation of virus in cultures or identification of viral nucleic acid by DNA probes in human leukaemia cells. Epidemiological case clustering in some patients with Hodgkin's disease suggests that the cause is a transmissible virus.

Oncogenic DNA viruses. Several groups of DNA viruses have been implicated as the cause of human neoplasms:

- **Papillomaviruses.** These viruses cause benign squamous epithelial cell neoplasms including the **common wart** (verruca vulgaris), the venereal wart (**condy-**

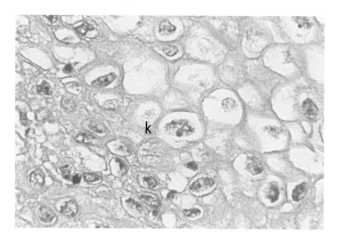

Fig. 11.5 Cervical biopsy. Note the koilocytes (k) indicating HPV infection with enlarged, irregular nuclei showing a peri-nuclear halo. (H&E.)

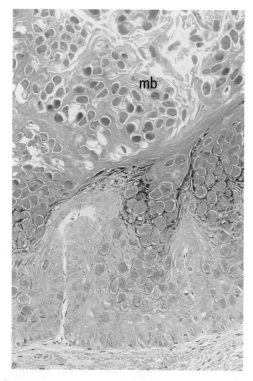

Fig. 11.6 Skin biopsy. *Molluscum contagiosum*. Note the molluscum bodies (mb) or viral inclusions. (H&E.)

loma acuminatum; Fig. 11.5) and recurrent laryngeal papillomas in children (**laryngeal papillomatosis**).

DNA hybridization studies have revealed **papillomavirus types 6 and 11** in most cases of condyloma acuminata, whereas severe dysplasia and invasive carcinoma of the uterine **cervix** are associated with **types 16, 18, 31 and 33**. Papilloma viral DNA appears to be present in

extrachromosomal episomes in the condylomas but is in an integrated form in severe dysplasia and carcinoma.

- **Molluscum contagiosum.** Molluscum contagiosum is a poxvirus that causes wart-like squamous epithelial cell tumours in the skin (Fig. 11.6). These are self-limited and probably not true neoplasms.
- **Epstein–Barr virus (EBV).** This herpesvirus causes **infectious mononucleosis**, an acute infectious disease that occurs worldwide. EBV is also thought to cause **Burkitt's lymphoma** in Africa and **nasopharyngeal carcinoma** in the Far East.
- **Herpes simplex virus (HSV) type 2.** Epidemiological evidence has previously implicated HSV type 2 as a cause of **cancer** of the uterine **cervix**. DNA probe studies have identified the HSV type 2 genome in cervical cancer cells but the association is not as strong as that for human papillomavirus (HPV).
- **Cytomegalovirus (CMV).** The nucleic acid of this herpesvirus is commonly present in cells of the lesions associated with **Kaposi's sarcoma**, a disorder most commonly found in immunodeficient patients.
- **Hepatitis B virus.** This is an important cause of **hepatocellular carcinoma**, which is common in Africa and the Far East (Chapter 19).

Nutritional oncogenesis

There is little hard evidence linking cancer to diet, despite much media reporting. The exception is the possible presence in the diet of known chemical carcinogens. A diet high in animal fat has been associated statistically with an increased incidence of cancer of the colon and with breast cancer; this observation remains unexplained.

The relationship between **dietary fibre** and **colonic carcinoma** represents the best evidence for the role of diet in oncogenesis. Burkitt, recognizing that Africans had a low incidence of colon cancer compared with people in western countries, suggested that this was due to the high fibre content of the African diet, which produces bulky stools that pass rapidly through the intestine. Low-fibre western diets produce a small, hard stool with a long transit time.

Hormonal oncogenesis
Induction of neoplasms by hormones

- **Oestrogens.** Patients with oestrogen-producing tumours of the ovary (**granulosa cell tumour**) or with persistent failure of ovulation (resulting in high levels of oestrogen) have a high risk of **endometrial cancer**. Oestrogen causes endometrial hyperplasia.
- **Diethylstilboestrol.** This is a synthetic oestrogen that was used in high doses between 1950 and 1960 to treat threatened abortion. Female children who were exposed to diethylstilboestrol *in utero* have a greatly in-

creased incidence of clear-cell adenocarcinoma, a rare vaginal cancer that develops in young women between 15 and 25 years of age.

- **Steroid hormones.** Use of oral contraceptives and anabolic steroids is rarely associated with development of benign **liver cell adenomas**. Less commonly, liver cell carcinoma has been reported.

Hormonal dependence of neoplasms. Some neoplasms that are not caused by hormones are dependent on hormone for optimal growth. The cells of such neoplasms are thought to have **hormone receptors** on their cell membranes for binding hormones. Treatment of some common human neoplasms takes advantage of the property of controlling cell proliferation by removal of the hormone.

- **Breast cancer.** Breast cancer can be dependent on oestrogen and, less frequently, on progesterone. Hormone dependence correlates strongly with the presence of oestrogen and progesterone receptors in the cell. Verifying the presence or absence of these receptors through biochemical and immunological techniques is part of the diagnosis of breast cancer. **Oophorectomy** or treatment with the oestrogen-blocking drug **tamoxifen** causes regression of most receptor-positive breast cancers. This regression is usually temporary.
- **Prostatic cancer.** This is almost always dependent on androgens. Removal of both testes or the administration of oestrogen may result in regression of the tumour.
- **Thyroid cancer.** Well-differentiated thyroid tumour may be dependent on thyroid-stimulating hormone (TSH). Administration of thyroid hormone to suppress TSH secretion is part of the treatment.

Inherited neoplasia

Many animal strains show a genetic susceptibility for development of neoplasms due to the presence of one or more cellular oncogenes inherited as part of the genome. No hereditary human neoplasm has been shown to be due to oncogenes, although the possibility cannot be ignored.

Neoplasms with single-gene inheritance. Cancer-causing genes may act in a **dominant** or **recessive** manner. If dominant, they may produce a molecule that directly causes neoplasia. If recessive, lack of both normal genes may lead to failure of production of a factor necessary for maintaining control of normal growth.

- **Retinoblastoma.** This is an uncommon malignant neoplasm of the retina that occurs in children (Fig. 11.7),

and 40% of cases are inherited. The morphological appearance of familial retinoblastoma is the same as that of the non-inherited form (Chapter 25).

The familial form displays other distinguishing features:
1 It is commonly bilateral.
2 Chromosomal analysis consistently shows deletion of part of the long arm of chromosome 13.
3 Spontaneous **regression** is common.

- **Wilms tumour (nephroblastoma).** This is a malignant neoplasm of the kidney that occurs mainly in children (Fig. 11.8). Many cases are associated with deletion of part of chromosome 11. Both sporadic and familial cases occur.
- **Neurofibromatosis (von Recklinghausen's disease)** is characterized by multiple neurofibromas (Fig. 11.9) and pigmented skin patches known as *café au lait* spots. Expressivity and penetrance are variable and the clinical severity varies.
- **Multiple endocrine neoplasia (MEN)** is manifested by

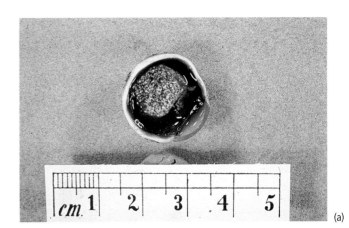
(a)

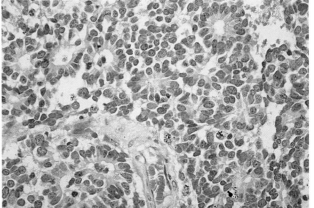
(b)

Fig. 11.7 The eye. (a) Congenital retinoblastoma. (b) Histology of congenital retinoblastoma. Note the small, blue cells forming rosettes (Homer–Wright rosettes). (H&E.)

benign neoplasms in the thyroid, parathyroid, pituitary and adrenal medulla (Chapter 14).

- **Familial polyposis coli.** This is characterized by numerous adenomatous polyps in the colon (Fig. 11.10). Cancer eventually develops in all patients unless they undergo colectomy (Chapter 18). **Gardner's syndrome** is a variant in which colonic polyps are associated with benign neoplasms and cysts in bone, soft tissue and skin.
- **Naevoid basal cell carcinoma syndrome.** This is char-

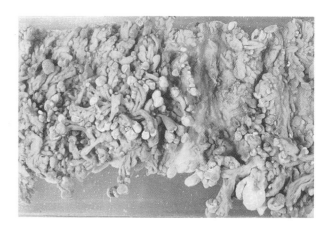

Fig. 11.10 Large bowel in familial adenomatous polyposis coli. There are hundreds of adenomatous polyps.

acterized by dysplastic melanocytic naevi and basal cell carcinomas in the skin.
- **Turcot's syndrome.** This is a very rare disease in which multiple adenomatous polyps of the colon are associated with malignant tumours (gliomas) of the nervous system. It is thought to have **autosomal recessive** inheritance pattern.

Neoplasms with polygenic inheritance. Many common human neoplasms are familial. They occur in a group of related individuals more often than would be expected on the basis of chance alone.
- **Breast cancer.** First-degree female relatives (mother, sisters, daughters) of a premenopausal woman with breast cancer have a risk of developing breast cancer that is five times higher than that of the general population. The risk is even greater if the patient has bilateral breast cancer.
- **Colon cancer.** Cancer of the colon tends to occur in families both as a complication of inherited familial polyposis coli and independently of familial polyposis coli. A few families exist with a reported predisposition for development of colon cancer. Some of the 'cancer families' also have other cancers, notably of the endometrium and breast.

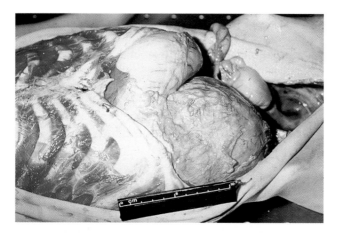

Fig. 11.8 Post mortem photograph. An infant with Wilms tumour.

Neoplasms occurring more frequently in inherited diseases. Many inherited diseases are associated with a high risk of neoplasia. These include:
- **syndromes characterized by increased chromosomal fragility:** xeroderma pigmentosum, Bloom's sydnrome, Fanconi's syndrome and ataxia telangiectasia), in which neoplasia is due to frequent DNA abnormalities;
- **syndromes of immunodeficiency,** in which failure of immune surveillance or inappropriate immune stimulation of any remaining lymphoid cells predisposes to

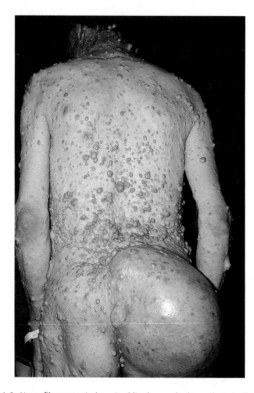

Fig. 11.9 Neurofibromatosis (von Recklinghausen's disease). Note the multiple large and small skin and soft tissue tumours. They are well circumscribed but have grown at variable rates.

neoplasia. In these disorders, it is not the neoplasm itself that is inherited but rather some susceptibility to neoplasia.

HISTOGENESIS AND CLASSIFICATION OF NEOPLASMS

Introduction

Although all neoplasms possess certain characteristics in common, particularly the capacity for deregulated continuous growth, they vary enormously in their gross and microscopic features, their behaviour and their response to treatment. It is important that the student has an understanding of the classification of these neoplasms because of the major implications for prognosis and therapy.

Chapter 1 discusses the approach to histopathology diagnosis, including the role of histochemistry and immunohistochemistry.

Table 11.4 lists the classification of the common neoplasms.

Table 11.4 Classification of neoplasms.

Cell type	Site	Benign neoplasm	Malignant neoplasm
Totipotential cells	Germ cell	Teratoma (mature)	Teratoma (immature), seminoma (dysgerminoma), embryonal carcinoma, yolk sac carcinoma, choriocarcinoma
Pluripotential cells (embryonic blast cells of organ anlage)	Retinal anlage		Retinoblastoma
	Renal anlage		Nephroblastoma (Wilms tumour, neuroblastoma)
	Primitive (peripheral) nerve cells		
	Primitive neuroectodermal cells		Medulloblastoma
Differentiated cells			
Epithelial cells			
Squamous	Skin, oesophagus, mouth	Squamous papilloma	Squamous carcinoma
			Basal cell carcinoma
Glandular	Gut, respiratory tract, secretory glands, bile ducts, ovary, endometrium	Adenoma	Adenocarcinoma
Transitional	Urothelium	Papilloma	Transitional cell carcinoma
Hepatic	Liver cell	Adenoma	Hepatocellular carcinoma (hepatoma)
Renal	Tubular epithelium	Adenoma	Adenocarcinoma
Endocrine	Thyroid	Adenoma	Adenocarcinoma
Mesothelium	Mesothelial cells	Benign mesothelioma	Malignant mesothelioma
Placenta	Trophoblast cells		Hydatidiform mole
			Choriocarcinoma
Mesenchymal cells			
Fibrous tissue	Fibroblast	Fibroma	Fibrosarcoma
Cartilage	Chondrocyte	Chondroma	Chondrosarcoma
Nerve	Schwann cell	Schwannoma	Malignant peripheral nerve sheath tumour
	Neural fibroblast	Neurofibroma	Malignant peripheral nerve sheath tumour
Bone	Osteoblast	Osteoma	Osteosarcoma
Fat	Lipocyte	Lipoma	Liposarcoma
Notochord	Primitive mesenchyme		Chordoma
Vessels	Endothelial cells	Haemangioma	Angiosarcoma
		Lymphangioma	Kaposi's sarcoma
Pia and arachnoid	Meningeal cells	Meningioma	Malignant meningioma
Muscle	Smooth muscle	Leiomyoma	Leiomyosarcoma
	Striated muscle	Rhabdomyoma	Rhabdomyosarcoma
Melanocytes	Melanocytes	Naevi (various types)	Melanoma (malignant)
Glial cells	Astrocytes		Astroyctomas
	Ependymal cells		Ependymoma
	Oligodendroglial cells		Oligodendroglioma

Neoplasms of totipotential cells

The totipotential cell is capable of differentiating (maturing) into any cell type in the body. The prototype is the **zygote**, which gives rise to the fetus. In postnatal life, the only totipotential cells in the body are the **germ cells**. These are most commonly found in the **gonads** (ovary and testis) but also occur in the retroperitoneum, mediastinum and pineal region.

Germ cell neoplasms (Fig. 11.11) may show minimal differentiation and appear in the form of malignant primitive germ cells (seminoma and embryonal carcinoma; Fig. 11.12), yolk sac (yolk sac carcinoma) or somatic structures (teratoma; Table 11.5). Mixtures of different tissues frequently coexist in a single neoplasm.

Teratomas show somatic differentiation and contain elements of all three germ layers: endoderm, ectoderm and mesoderm. Thus, brain, respiratory and intestinal mucosa, cartilage, bone, skin, teeth or hair may be seen in the neoplasm (Fig. 11.13). Teratomas are further classified as **mature** (well-differentiated and composed of adult-type tissues) or **immature** (made up of fetal-type tissues). Immature teratomas are malignant, whereas mature teratomas vary in their biological

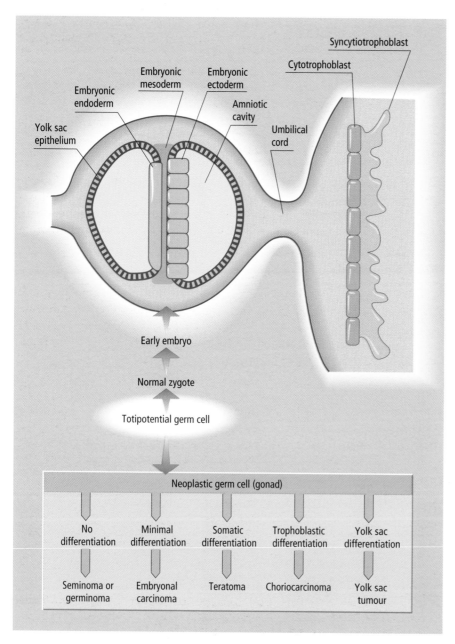

Fig. 11.11 Neoplasms arising from totipotential cells of the zygote (germ cell neoplasms).

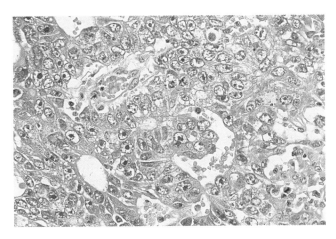

Fig. 11.12 Testicular biopsy. Embryonal carcinoma. Note the large, primitive cells without any discernible differentiation. (H&E.)

Table 11.5 The histogenesis of human neoplasms.

Cell type	Normal occurrence	Derived neoplasms
Totipotential cell	Zygote Germ cells in the gonad (or extragonadal)	May develop into any cell type
Pluripotential cell	Primitive cells of the organ anlage	Multiple cell types including two germ layers
Differentiated cell	Adult labile and stable cell	Most neoplasms arise from these cells and are usually of one cell type
End-cell	Permanent (postmitotic) cell of the epithelia, muscle and brain	Do not produce neoplasms

potential. Most mature teratomas are benign when they occur in childhood but are usually malignant in adult testes.

Neoplasms of embryonic pluripotential cells (blastomas)

Pluripotential cells can mature into several different cell types, and the corresponding neoplasms have the potential for formation of diverse structural elements, for example, neoplasms of the renal anlage cells (**nephroblastoma**) commonly differentiate into structures resembling renal tubules and less often into rudiments of muscle, cartilage and bone. These neoplasms are generally called **embryomas** or **blastomas**. Embryonic pluripotential cells are found only in the fetal period and during the first few years of postnatal life. The corresponding neoplasms usually occur in early childhood and only rarely in adults.

Neoplasms of differentiated cells

Differentiated, adult-type cells make up most of the cells in the body in postnatal life. They show a restricted potential for differentiation, as seen when they undergo **metaplasia**. Most human neoplasms are derived from differentiated cells.

Nomenclature

Epithelial neoplasms. A benign epithelial neoplasm is called an **adenoma** if it arises from glandular epithelium (e.g. thyroid adenoma, colonic adenoma; Fig. 11.14) and a papilloma if it has a papillary architecture. Papil-

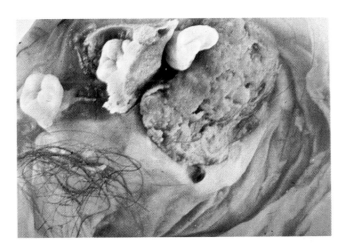

Fig. 11.13 Mature cystic teratoma (benign dermoid) of the ovary. Note the hair and teeth.

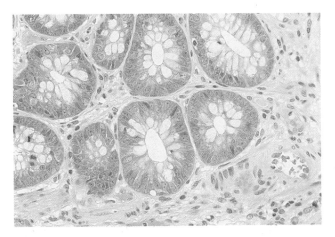

Fig. 11.14 Large bowel biopsy from the case shown in Fig. 11.10. A benign adenoma in which the glandular epithelial cells resemble those of the glandular cells of origin. (H&E.)

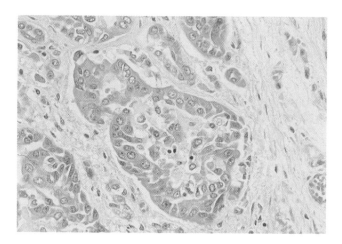

Fig. 11.15 Large bowel biopsy from the case shown in Fig. 11.10. A moderately differentiated adenocarcinoma is present with discernible gland formation but featuring cells with dissimilar features to the cells of origin. (H&E.)

lomas may arise from squamous, glandular or transitional epithelium (e.g. squamous papilloma, intraductal papilloma of the breast and transitional cell papilloma, respectively).

Malignant epithelial neoplasms are called carcinomas (adenocarcinomas if derived from glandular epithelium; Fig. 11.15); squamous carcinoma, transitional cell carcinoma and so on). Names may also include the organ of origin and descriptive adjectives, e.g. papillary adenocarcinoma of the thyroid, cystic and solid papillary carcinoma of the pancreas.

The recognition of **intermediate filaments** may be of value in the diagnosis of poorly differentiated carcinomas. They tend to be cell-type-specific even after neoplastic transformation. Using immunohistochemistry (Chapter 1), they may distinguish between epithelial, mesenchymal and neural neoplasms. Five distinct classes are recognized:

1 cytokeratins comprise a multigene family of proteins characteristic of epithelial cells and carcinomas (including mesothelial cells);
2 vimentin, found in mesenchymal cells and sarcomas;
3 desmin, found in smooth muscle and striated muscle neoplasms;
4 glial fibrillary acidic protein (GFAP) typical of glial cells and gliomas;
5 neurofilament proteins are specific for neurones and paraganglia.

Figure 11.16 illustrates the use of intermediate filaments and other markers in the diagnosis of anaplastic malignant tumours.

Mesenchymal neoplasms. Benign mesenchymal neoplasms are named after the cell of origin (a Greek or Latin word

is used) followed by the suffix **-oma** (Table 11.4). The names of these tumours may contain the organ of origin and a descriptive adjective, e.g. pleomorphic liposarcoma of the retroperitoneum.

Other neoplasms

Neoplasms that 'sound benign' but are really malignant. The names of some malignant neoplasms are formed by adding the suffix -oma to the cell of origin, e.g. lymphoma (lymphocyte), plasmacytoma (plasma cell), melanoma (melanocyte), glioma (glial cell) and astrocytoma (astrocyte). These neoplasms are assumed to be malignant because there is no benign lymphoma, melanoma, glioma, etc. If possible, the adjective 'malignant' should be used–malignant lymphoma, malignant melanoma.

Neoplasms that 'sound malignant' but are really benign. Two rare bone neoplasms, **osteoblastoma** and **chondroblastoma**, may sound malignant because of the suffix -blastoma but are in fact benign neoplasms derived from osteoblast and chondroblasts present in adult bone.

Leukaemias. Neoplasms of blood-forming organs are called leukaemias (Chapter 12). These disorders are all considered malignant although they have a variable clinical course and may be classified as **acute** or **chronic** and by their cell of origin as lymphocytic, myeloid or monocytic.

Mixed tumours. Neoplasms composed of more than one neoplastic cell type are called mixed tumours. Malignant mixed tumours may have two epithelial components, as in **adenosquamous carcinoma**; two mesenchymal components, as in **malignant fibrous histiocytoma**; or an epithelial and a mesenchymal component, as in **carcinosarcoma** of the lung.

In the case of benign mixed tumours such as **fibroadenoma** of the breast, only the epithelial (adenoma) component is neoplastic; the fibrous tissue represents a reaction to the adenoma cells.

Neoplasms of unknown histogenesis (eponymical). When the cell of origin is unknown, the name of the person who first described the neoplasm is commonly used to name the tumour (Table 11.6). As the histogenesis of these neoplasms is clarified, the name is often changed: Wilms tumour is now called **nephroblastoma**, and Grawitz's tumour is better known as **renal adenocarcinoma**. Some neoplasms of uncertain histogenesis are named descriptively, e.g. alveolar soft-part sarcoma.

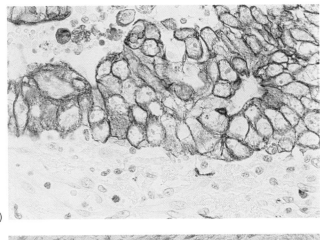

(a)

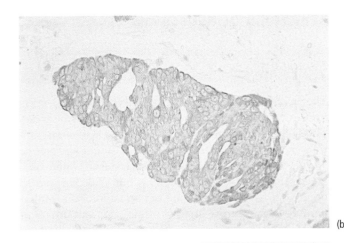

(b)

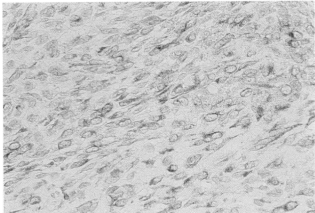

(c)

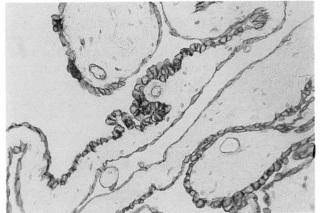

(d)

Fig. 11.16 Anaplastic carcinomas. The role of immunohistochemistry. (a) Lymph node biopsy. Poorly differentiated cells show cytokeratin positivity confirming the diagnosis of **metastatic carcinoma**. (b) Biopsy of a testicular tumour. Positive HCG immunostaining shows areas of **choriocarcinoma** associated with areas of haemorrhage. (c) Soft tissue tumour biopsy from patient shown in Fig. 11.9. Poorly differentiated tumour cells show positivity for S100 consistent with a **malignant peripheral nerve sheath tumour**. (d) Peritoneal biopsy in a patient with previous radiotherapy for lymphoma. A provisional diagnosis of mesothelial proliferation is not confirmed with cytokeratin staining. Staining for endothelial cells (using CD31) is positive supporting a diagnosis of radiation-induced **angiosarcoma**.

Table 11.6 Eponymical terms for neoplasms.

Eponym	Cell of origin
Neoplasms of uncertain histogenesis	
Ewing's sarcoma	Primitive neuroectodermal cell
Hodgkin's lymphoma	B cell/T cell or macrophage
Brenner tumour	Probably coelomic epithelium covering ovary
Neoplasms of known histogenesis	
Burkitt's lymphoma	B lymphocyte
Kaposi's sarcoma	Vascular endothelial cell
Krukenberg tumour	Metastatic adenocarcinoma cell involving ovary
Wilms tumour	Pluripotential embryonic renal cell (nephroblastoma)
Grawitz's tumour	Renal tubular cell (renal adenocarcinoma)
Hürthle cell tumour	Thyroid follicular cell

Hamartomas

A hamartoma is composed of tissues that are normally present in the organ in which it arises. For example, a hamartoma of the breast consists of a disorganized mass of glandular epithelium, adipose tissue and fibrous tissue. Hamartomas grow with the patient.

A **choristoma** resembles a hamartoma but contains tissues that are not normally present in the organ in which it arises. A disorderly mass of smooth muscle and pancreatic acini and ducts in the wall of the stomach is properly called a choristoma.

Hamartomas and choristomas are not true neoplasms.

BEHAVIOUR OF NEOPLASMS

Introduction

The biological behaviour of neoplasms constitutes a spectrum with two extremes. A **benign** neoplasm grows slowly and is encapsulated (Fig. 11.17). There is no infiltration or active destruction of surrounding tissue and no spread to distant sites (i.e. **no metastasis**). Such neoplasms are rarely life-threatening but may become so because of hormone secretion or critical location. **Malignant** neoplasms grow rapidly, infiltrate and destroy surrounding tissues and metastasize throughout the body. If left untreated, malignant neoplasms kill the host (Fig. 11.18).

Between these two extremes is a smaller third group of neoplasms that are locally invasive but have low metastatic potential, sometimes called low-grade malignant neoplasms; an example is basal cell carcinoma.

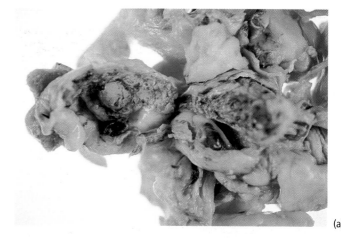

(a)

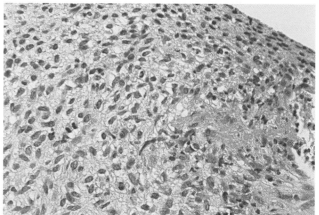

(b)

Fig. 11.18 Neurofibromatosis (von Recklinghausen's disease). (a) Same patient as in Fig. 11.9. Biopsy of one of the large, deep tumour masses. The tumour is irregular and infiltrative and on section shows areas of necrosis and haemorrhage. (b) Histology shows a cellular tumour featuring pleomorphic cells unlike those seen in Fig. 11.15(a) with enlarged, hyperchromatic nuclei and abundant mitoses together with areas of necrosis and haemorrhage. This is a **malignant peripheral nerve sheath tumour (malignant schwannoma)**. (H&E.)

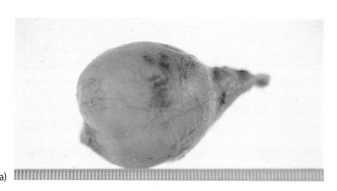

(a)

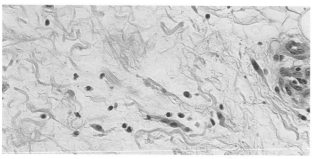

(b)

Fig. 11.17 Neurofibromatosis (von Recklinghausen's disease). (a) Same patient as in Fig. 11.9. Biopsy of one of the small subcutaneous nodules. A well circumscribed, encapsulated benign neurofibroma is removed along with its attached nerve. (b) Histology shows a benign neurofibroma with bland spindle cells. (H&E.)

Biological behaviour of neoplasms

The pathologist usually classifies a neoplasm as benign or malignant on the basis of **histological** and **cytological** features in association with the cumulative clinicopathological experience gained with various types of neoplasms. There are no absolute criteria for distinguishing benign from malignant neoplasms. The characteristics listed in Table 11.7 serve as general guidelines only.

Rate of growth

Malignant neoplasms generally grow more rapidly than benign ones. Assessment of the growth rate is based upon

Table 11.7 Features of benign and malignant neoplasms.

Benign	Malignant
Gross features	
Smooth surface with a fibrotic capsule; compressed surrounding tissues	Irregular, infiltrative margin
Small to large, sometimes very large	Small to large
Slow rate of growth	Rapid rate of growth
Rarely fatal (except in central nervous system) even if untreated	Usually fatal if untreated
Microscopic features	
Growth by compression of surrounding tissue	Growth by invasion of surrounding tissue
Highly differentiated, resembling normal tissue of origin microscopically	Well or poorly differentiated. Most malignant neoplasms do not resemble the normal tissue of origin (**anaplasia**)
Cells similar to normal	Cytological abnormalities including enlarged, hyperchromatic, irregular nuclei with large nucleoli; marked variation in size and shape of cells (**pleomorphism**)
Few mitoses	Increased mitotic activity; abnormal, bizarre mitotic figures often present
Well-formed blood vessels	Blood vessels numerous but poorly formed
Necrosis unusual common	Necrosis and haemorrhage
Distant spread (metastasis) does not occur	Metastasis to distant sites
Investigative techniques: DNA content usually normal	DNA content of cells increased, additional chromosomes commonly present
Karyotype usually normal	Karyotypic abnormalities, including aneuploidy and polyploidy, are common

are important indicators of tumour aggression and a prognostic marker in soft-tissue tumours.

Size

Many benign neoplasms become very large and, conversely, highly malignant neoplasms may be lethal by virtue of extensive dissemination even though the original primary tumour is still small. An example is breast cancer which can disseminate before being palpable.

In a few neoplasms, however, size is the deciding factor in distinguishing benign from malignant growths. An **adrenal cortical adenoma** is considered benign unless it is larger than 5 cm, in which case it is regarded as malignant; this distinction is based on the observation that the risk of metastasis increases with increasing size of the primary neoplasm.

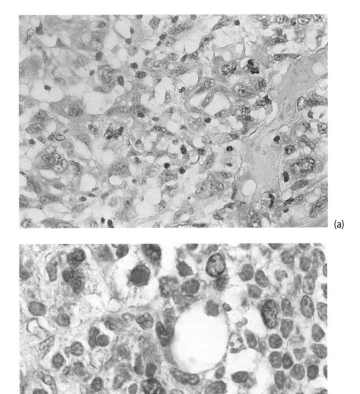

(a)

(b)

Fig. 11.19 (a) Biopsy from a metastatic, anaplastic carcinoma in a lymph node. Note the numerous mitoses, many of which are atypical with tripolar mitotic figures. (H&E.) (b) Biopsy from a metastatic, anaplastic lymphoma in a lymph node. PCNA staining highlights the high proliferation index.

clinical information and on microscopic examination (Fig. 11.19). The number of mitotic figures and the metabolically active appearance of nuclei (enlarged, dispersed chromatin, large nucleoli) correlate positively with the growth rate of the neoplasm. **Necrosis** and **haemorrhage**

Degree of differentiation

Differentiation denotes the degree to which a neoplastic cell resembles the normal cell of origin (Fig. 11.20). Benign neoplasms are usually fully differentiated and resemble normal adult tissue. Malignant neoplasms show variable degrees of differentiation and frequently demonstrate little resemblance to normal tissue (i.e. they are poorly differentiated). **Anaplastic** tumours show no morphological resemblance to the cell of origin and pose a diagnostic challenge.

Premalignant changes

Premalignant conditions are listed in Table 11.8 and they are important to recognize because surgical excision is curative.

Metaplasia implies a major switch in tissue differentiation (e.g. squamous metaplasia of bronchial and endocervical glandular epithelium). In isolation, it is not a

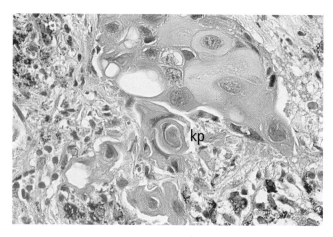

Fig. 11.20 Skin biopsy. Well differentiated squamous carcinoma showing keratin 'pearl' formation (kp).

premalignant change but it is the prerequisite for malignant change (squamous carcinoma) at certain sites such as the bronchus and the uterine cervix.

Occult cancer

Occult cancers remain small and may not become manifest clinically during life. Small prostatic cancers are found incidentally at autopsy, in patients who die of other causes, in about 30% of men over age 60 years. This figure rises to 90% of men over age 90 years.

Delayed metastatic disease (**occult metastasis**) may develop 15–20 years following removal of a primary lesion such as breast cancer.

Characteristics of neoplastic cells

Surface alterations (Fig. 11.21)

Surface membrane changes include alteration in level of activity of membrane enzymes, decrease in glycoprotein and fibronectin content, abnormalities in electrical charge, and alterations in the microtubular and microfilamentous cytoskeleton.

Cancer cells in culture grow as disorganized, multilayered masses that pile up on one another. This loss of contact inhibition is characteristic. Failure of contact inhibition, coupled with lack of adhesiveness among individual tumour cells, may partially explain the ability of malignant neoplastic cells to **invade** and **metastasize**.

Table 11.8 Precancerous (premalignant) lesions.

Precancerous lesion	Cancer
Hyperplasia	
Endometrial hyperplasia	Endometrial carcinoma
Breast-lobular and ductal hyperplasia	Breast carcinoma
Liver–cirrhosis of the liver	Hepatocellular carcinoma
Dysplasia	
Cervix	Squamous carcinoma
Skin	Squamous carcinoma
Bladder	Transitional carcinoma
Bronchial epithelium	Lung carcinoma
Metaplasia	
Glandular metaplasia of oesophagus	Adenocarcinoma of the oesophagus
Intestinal metaplasia of the stomach	Adenocarcinoma of the stomach
Squamous metaplasia of the bronchus	Lung carcinoma
Inflammatory lesions	
Ulcerative colitis	Adenocarcinoma of the colon
Atrophic gastritis	Adenocarcinoma/lymphoma of the stomach
Autoimmune (Hashimoto's thyroiditis)	Malignant lymphoma/thyroid carcinoma
Benign neoplasms	
Neurofibroma	Malignant schwannoma (malignant peripheral nerve sheath tumour)
Colonic adenoma	Adenocarcinoma of the colon

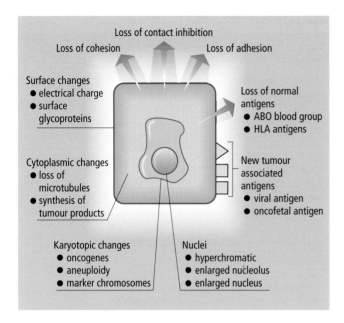

Fig. 11.21 Tumour cells. Note the cell membrane, cytoplasmic and nuclear changes associated with neoplasia.

Changes in DNA

Neoplasms are associated with abnormalities in their DNA content which increase with the degree of malignancy. Malignant cells are **hyperchromatic** (showing increased staining of the nucleus). **Cytogenetic** studies demonstrating aneuploidy and polyploidy are also indicative of malignancy. When measured by **flow cytometry**, the DNA content of malignant cells correlates well with the degree of malignancy.

Immunological alterations

Tumour-associated antigens. Most neoplastic cells express new antigens (neoantigens, tumour-associated antigens) on their surfaces. These antigens probably represent expression of the altered genome but they are not entirely limited to cancer cells.

Viral antigens. In viral-induced neoplasms, new antigens are coded by the virus and all neoplasms caused by a particular virus will show the same new antigen.

Unique antigens. Neoplasms induced by chemicals or radiation manifest new antigens that are distinctive for each different neoplasm induced. Separate neoplasms occurring in the same tissue in the same individual will produce different antigens, which reflects the random genomic alterations produced by radiation and most chemicals.

Oncofetal antigens. These include carcinoembryonic anti-

gen (CEA) and α-fetoprotein (AFP). These antigens result from depression of genes that normally are active only in fetal life. They have diagnostic value.

Tumour-associated antigens are often weakly immunogenic and may evoke humoral and cellular immune responses, as demonstrated by antibody production and a lymphocytic infiltrate surrounding the neoplastic cells. Although lymphocytes are commonly present in neoplasms, evidence that they may play a role in controlling tumour growth is limited to a small number of neoplasms.

Loss of antigens normally present. Neoplastic cells also frequently lack antigens that are present in normal cells and loss of antigens may correlate with the biological behaviour of the neoplasm. In bladder neoplasms loss of ABO blood group antigens tends to be associated with a propensity for invasion and metastasis.

Karyotypic abnormalities

Increasing numbers of chromosomal abnormalities are being identified in neoplastic cells (Table 11.9). Many malignant cells show major non-specific chromosomal abnormalities such as aneuploidy and polyploidy. Of greater importance are specific chromosomal abnormalities.

Tumour cell products (Table 11.10)

The production of various tumour cell products are important for two reasons: they act as tumour markers and they may produce clinical effects (**paraneoplastic syndromes**) unrelated to the direct effect of the tumour.

Oncofetal antigens. These are antigens that are normally expressed only in fetal life but that may be produced by tumour cells. Detection of these oncofetal antigens in adults can be of clinical value.

CEA is found in most malignant neoplasms arising from tissues that develop from the **embryonic endoderm**, e.g. colon and gastric cancer. About 30% of breast cancers also produce the antigen, which may be directly detected in tumour tissues by immunohistological methods and may be measured in serum. CEA is not specific for cancer since slight increases in serum levels also occur in nonneoplastic diseases, e.g. cirrhosis of the liver. The value of CEA as a tumour marker lies in monitoring the response to therapy and in the early diagnosis of recurrence after treatment in patients with colon cancer.

AFP is synthesized by normal yolk sac and fetal liver cells as well as by embryonal or yolk sac tumour and liver cell carcinoma. As with CEA, elevated levels of AFP may occur in other diseases.

Enzymes. Elevated serum levels of prostate-specific acid

Table 11.9 Chromosomal abnormalities in neoplasms.

Abnormality	Neoplasm
Aneuploidy, tetraploidy, polyploidy	Many malignant neoplasms, especially poorly differentiated and anaplastic types
Translocations	
9 = 22 t(9;22) (Philadelphia chromosome)	Chronic myeloid leukaemia (90%) Acute myeloid leukaemia Acute lymphocytic leukaemia (FAB type L$_1$ and L$_2$)
8 = 14 t(8;14)	Burkitt's lymphoma Acute lymphoctyic leukaemia (FAB type L$_3$) Immunoblastic B-cell lymphoma
15 = 17 t(15;17)	Promyelocytic leukaemia
4 = 11 t(4;11)	Acute lymphocytic leukaemia (FAB type L$_2$)
11 = 14 t(11;14)	Chronic lymphocytic leukaemia
14 = 18 t(14;18)	Some B-cell lymphomas
6 = 14 t(6;14)	Cystadenocarcinoma of ovary
3 = 8 t(3;8)	Renal adenocarcinoma Mixed parotid tumour (benign)
Deletions	
Deletion of 8 and 17	Blast crisis of chronic myeloid leukaemia
5q– and 7q–	Acute myeloid leukaemia Acute monocytic leukaemia
3p–	Small cell carcinoma of lung
1p–	Neuroblastoma
13q–	Retinoblastoma
11p–	Nephroblastoma
–22	Meningioma
Trisomy	
Trisomy 12	Chronic lymphocytic leukaemia

Table 11.10 Tumour cell products.

Product	Commonly associated neoplasms
Oncofetal antigens	
Carcinoembryonic antigen (CEA)	Carcinoma of colon, pancreas, stomach, lung, breast
α-Fetoprotein (AFP)	Hepatocellular carcinoma, some germ cell neoplasms
Enzymes	
Prostatic acid phosphatase	Prostatic carcinoma
Alkaline phosphatase	Carcinoma of pancreas
Lactate dehydrogenase	Many malignant neoplasms
Immunoglobulin (monoclonal)	B-cell lymphomas, plasma cell myeloma
Hormones (from endocrine neoplasms)	
Growth hormone, prolactin, ACTH	Pituitary adenoma
Insulin, glucagon, gastrin	Pancreatic islet cell neoplasms
Parathyroid hormone	Parathyroid neoplasms
Cortisol, aldosterone	Adrenocortical neoplasms
Catecholamines	Phaeochromocytoma
Calcitonin	Medullary (C-cell) carcinoma of thyroid
Serotonin (5-HT)	Carcinoid (neuroendocrine) neoplasms of gut, lung
Histamine	Mast cell neoplasms
Human chorionic gonadotrophin (hCG)	Choriocarcinoma, some germ cell neoplasms
Androgens, oestrogens	Testicular and ovarian neoplasms
Osteoclast-activating factor	Plasma cell myeloma

ACTH, Adrenocorticotrophic hormone.

phosphatase occur in prostate cancer, usually associated with invasion which has occurred beyond the capsule of the gland. High levels of **Regan isoenzyme** (an isoenzyme of alkaline phosphatase) are noted in some cases of pancreatic cancer. Levels of common cytoplasmic enzymes such as **lactate dehydrogenase** are elevated in many neoplasms.

Immunoglobulins. Some B-cell lymphomas and myeloma frequently synthesize immunoglobulins. Since these neoplasms are **monoclonal**, only one type of immunoglobulin is produced which may be of diagnostic value (producing a monoclonal band on serum protein electrophoresis).

Excessive hormone secretion. Well-differentiated neoplasms of endocrine cells are frequently associated with excessive production of hormones identical to that produced by the corresponding normal cell. Overproduction is due to the increased number of cells in the tumour and to a failure of normal control mechanisms. The clinical course and prognosis depend more on the biological behaviour of the neoplasm than on the hormone it produces.

Ectopic hormone production (Table 11.11). Abnormal synthesis of hormones (so-called ectopic hormone production) may occur in malignant neoplasms derived from cells that normally do not secrete hormones. This phenomenon represents derepression of genes associated with the neoplastic process.

Table 11.11 Ectopic hormone production by neoplasms.

Hormone	Commonly associated neoplasms
Human chorionic gonadotropin	Carcinoma of lung (30%), breast carcinoma
Parathyroid hormone	Squamous carcinoma of lung, renal adenocarcinoma, other squamous carcinomas
Adrenocorticotropic hormone	Small-cell carcinoma of lung, pancreatic islet cell neoplasms
Antidiuretic hormone	Small-cell carcinoma of lung
Insulin	Hepatocellular carcinoma, retroperitoneal sarcomas
Erythropoietin	Renal adenocarcinoma, cerebellar haemangioblastoma, hepatocellular carcinoma

Growth pattern of neoplastic cells

The appreciation of the cellular growth abnormality associated with neoplasia by the histopathologist serves to distinguish benign from malignant neoplasms.

Cell proliferation

Neoplastic cells generally multiply more rapidly than their normal counterparts. The rate of proliferation of neoplastic cells varies greatly. Some neoplasms grow so slowly that growth is measured in years. Other tumours proliferate so rapidly that an increase in size can be observed in days. The degree of malignancy of a neoplasm tends to correlate with its rate of growth; however, important exceptions exist, e.g. keratoacanthoma, a benign neoplasm of epidermal cells in the skin, initially grows more rapidly than does squamous carcinoma of the skin.

Clinically, the rate of growth of a neoplasm can be measured by the time needed for it to double in size. This **doubling time** varies. A histopathological assessment of the growth rate is the mitotic count, which is usually expressed as the number of mitotic figures counted in 10 consecutive high-power fields in the most active area of the neoplasm (Fig. 11.19).

Differentiation

Slow-growing malignant neoplasms tend to be well-differentiated, resembling the cell and tissue of origin. Thus well-differentiated squamous carcinomas may show keratin production (Fig. 11.20) and well differentiated adenocarcinomas will form glands (Fig. 11.15).

Structural abnormalities appear both in the cytoplasm and in the nuclei of neoplastic cells, including:
- pleomorphism (variation in appearance of cells);
- increased nuclear size;
- increased nuclear:cytoplasmic ratio;
- hyperchromatism;
- prominent nucleoli;
- abnormal chromatin distribution in the nucleus;
- nuclear membrane abnormalities;
- failure of cytoplasmic differentiation.

The severity of these cytological abnormalities increases as the degree of malignancy increases. When the cell of origin cannot be recognized on microscopic examination, the neoplasm is said to be **undifferentiated** or **anaplastic**.

In situ malignancy

In epithelium, particularly squamous epithelium of the skin, bronchus, larynx and uterine cervix, there exists a spectrum of preinvasive or premalignant change called **dysplasia**. The epithelial cells show all the cytological characteristics listed above which increasingly fill the full thickness of the epithelial layer. These changes are described as mild, moderate and finally, severe dysplasia or carcinoma-*in-situ* (Fig. 11.22).

These premalignant changes form the basis for exfoliative cytological diagnosis of, in particular, cervical carcinoma. The equivalent exfoliated cells, in a cytological preparation, are referred to as mildly, moderately or severely **dyskaryotic** (Fig. 11.22b).

Invasion

Benign neoplasms do not invade adjacent tissue but tend to expand centrifugally, forming a capsule of compressed normal tissue and collagen. Malignant neoplasms invade normal tissue. Malignant neoplasms usually do not form a capsule.

Carcinomas and sarcomas demonstrate similar patterns of invasion and metastasis. Invasion of the basement membrane by carcinoma distinguishes invasive cancer from intraepithelial (or *in situ*) cancer. Having penetrated the basement membrane, malignant cells invade the lymphatics and blood vessels, which is the first step towards metastasis.

The mechanisms whereby neoplastic cells invade and destroy tissues are poorly understood but surface membrane abnormalities, loss of contact inhibition and decreased cell adhesiveness are believed to play a part.

Assessment of the extent of invasion by gross examination at the time of surgery may be difficult and appropriate surgical treatment of malignant neoplasms involves a wide **margin of excision** of apparently normal tissue surrounding the tumour.

Metastasis

Metastasis is the establishment of a second tumour mass

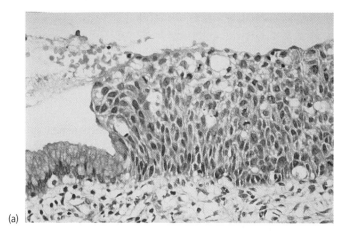

(a)

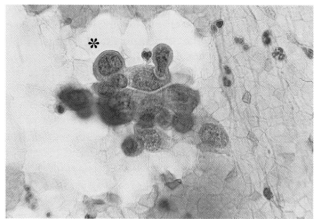

(b)

Fig. 11.22 (a) Cervical biopsy. The transformation zone. A site for squamous metaplasia (right) of the endocervical glandular epithelium (left). Here the metaplastic epithelium has undergone severe dysplasia (cervical intra-epithelial neoplasia grade III – CIN III or carcinoma-*in situ*). There is no invasion. (H&E.) (b) Cervical smear from the same patient, stained with Papanicolau stain. Note the severely dyskaryotic cells showing hyperchromatic, enlarged cell nuclei occupying most of the cell (✱), consistent with CIN III.

through transfer of neoplastic cells, via a fluid medium, from the primary site to a secondary location separate from the original tumour. Metastasis occurs only in malignant neoplasms and explains why they may ultimately kill the host.

Lymphatic metastasis. Metastasis via the lymphatics occurs early in carcinomas and melanomas (Fig. 11.23). Most sarcomas spread via the blood stream.

Malignant cells are first carried by the lymphatics to the regional lymph nodes. Removal of lymph nodes at surgery is performed only for those neoplasms in which lymphatic metastasis is common, such as carcinoma and melanoma. Knowledge of the lymphatic drainage of various tissues enables the clinician to predict the sites of lymph node involvement.

Blood-borne metastasis. Blood-borne metastasis (Fig. 11.24) can only succeed if enough tumour cells survive transit in the blood to become established and proliferate at a second site (Fig. 11.25). Survival at the primary site and site of metastasis depends on successful establishment of a new vascular microenvironment. The production of **tumour angiogenesis factors** by the tumour cells stimulates growth of new capillaries in the vicinity of tumour cells and encourages vascularization of the growing metastasis.

The first site of a metastasis is most commonly the first capillary bed encountered by blood draining the primary site. Some types of cancer apparently favour particular metastatic sites, through unknown mechanisms; bone metastases are common in cancer of the prostate, thyroid, lung, breast and kidney.

Coelomic spread. Entry of malignant cells into the

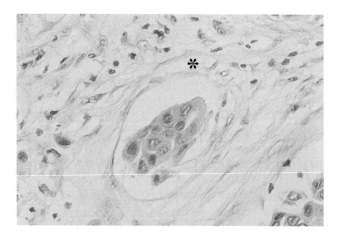

Fig. 11.23 Biopsy from a malignant ductal carcinoma of the breast showing invasion of malignant cells into lymphatics. This patient has lymph node metastases (✱). (H&E.)

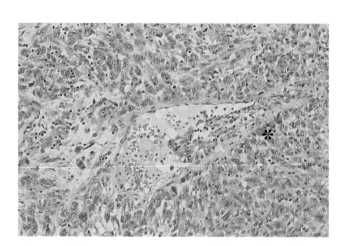

Fig. 11.24 Biopsy from a malignant adenocarcinoma of the colon showing invasion of malignant cells into blood vessels (H&E.)

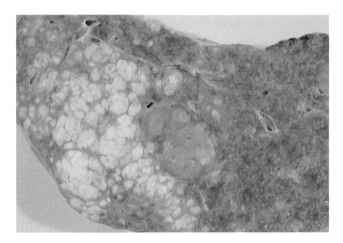

Fig. 11.25 Liver metastases from the colonic adenocarcinoma shown in Fig. 11.24.

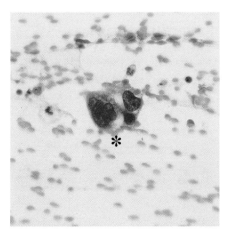

Fig. 11.26 Cytology of ascitic fluid in a patient with known adenocarcinoma of the ovary 5 years previously. Note the poorly cohesive clusters of cells showing vacuolated cytoplasm (✳). (PAP.)

coelomic cavities of the pleura, peritoneum or pericardium or the subarachnoid space may be followed by transcoelomic spread.

Cytological examination of the fluid from these body cavities may confirm the diagnosis of metastasis (Fig. 11.26).

In conclusion, development of **occult metastases** makes it difficult confidently to pronounce a patient as cured. Five-year survival after treatment is considered a sign of cure for most cancers. However, 10- and 20-year survival rates are usually lower than the 5-year survival rates. This suggests that many patients experience **late metastases**.

Disseminated metastases are usually **incurable**. Recent advances in anticancer therapy raise hopes of cure in certain types of disseminated cancer, including leukae-mias, high-grade malignant lymphoma, germ cell neoplasms of the testis and choriocarcinoma.

DISTRIBUTION AND INCIDENCE

Incidence and mortality rates

Cancer is the second commonest cause of death (after ischaemic heart disease) in the west. The incidence of cancer varies in different populations and in different areas.

Epidemiological study of cancer distribution often sheds light on the causes of cancer. Thorough knowledge of the incidence and pattern of cancer in the local population is important for the clinician evaluating the possibility of cancer in a given patient.

Both the **incidence** and the **death rate** of cancer must be considered. The latter reflects both the incidence and the success of diagnosis and treatment. Skin cancer is the commonest cancer in the UK and the USA but it is usually diagnosed early and cured by excision which results in a low death rate from skin cancer in the overall cancer death rate statistics.

Factors affecting incidence

The presence or absence of any of the many factors previously discussed in this chapter which are known to influence the incidence of cancer must be established during history-taking and physical examination of the patient.

Sex
Prostate cancer in men and cervical cancer and breast cancer in women are obviously sex-specific. In other types of cancer, the reasons for the difference in incidence between the sexes are less evident. For example, stomach cancer is more common in men and thyroid cancer is more common in women. Both bladder and lung cancer are more common in men, possibly because of greater occupational exposure (dye and rubber industries for bladder cancer; mining and asbestos for lung cancer) and smoking habits. Recent figures show that the rate of lung cancer in women is fast approaching that in men as smoking habits of women match those of men.

Age
The frequency of occurrence of most types of cancer varies greatly at different ages.

Carcinoma is rare in children, but leukaemias, blastomas, tumours of the brain and kidney and some types of connective tissue tumours are relatively common (Table 11.12). Most of these childhood neoplasms grow rapidly and are composed of small, very primitive cells with large, hyperchromatic nuclei, scant cytoplasm and a high mitotic rate.

In adults, carcinomas make up the largest group of malignant tumours; sarcomas occur in adults but are less common than carcinomas.

Neoplasms of the haematopoietic and lymphoid cells (leukaemias and lymphomas) occur at all ages. The incidence of different types of these neoplasms varies with age; acute lymphoblastic leukaemia is common in children, whereas chronic lymphocytic leukaemia occurs more often in the elderly.

Occupational, social and geographic factors

An occupational history is an essential part of a full medical examination as there are many malignancies associated with occupational chemical carcinogen exposure (Table 11.2).

Social habits such as cigarette smoking represent risk factors for development of several types of cancer.

Epidemiological studies also show that a patient's sexual and child-bearing histories are important. Women who have had several children and have breast-fed them have a significantly lower incidence of breast cancer. (Nuns have a high incidence of breast cancer.) Conversely, nuns have a lower incidence of cervical cancer, which appears to be most common among women who begin sexual activity early, particularly those with multiple partners.

Circumcised men have a much lower incidence of car-

cinoma of the penis than their uncircumcised counterparts, and some studies have suggested that carcinoma of the uterine cervix is more common in women whose sexual partners have not been circumcised.

Geographical variations in the overall incidence of cancer and in the incidence of specific types of cancer also occur from one country to another, from one city to another and from urban to rural areas.

Family history

Certain cancers have a pattern of genetic inheritance and are so striking that they warrant careful study of relatives of known cases (e.g. retinoblastoma, polyposis coli and carcinoma of the colon). 'Cancer families' with a high incidence of cancer have also been described. Cancer in such families may skip generations, suggesting the possible interplay both of recessive genetic mechanisms and of environmental factors.

History of associated diseases

The most important finding in the history of a patient with suspected cancer is a record of diagnosis or treatment of previous cancer. In certain disorders that in themselves are non-neoplastic carry an associated higher risk of neoplastic diseases. These diseases are uncommon, but

Table 11.13 Diseases associated with an increased risk of neoplasia.

Non-neoplastic disease	Neoplasm
Mongolism (trisomy 21)	Acute myeloid leukaemia
Xeroderma pigmentosum (plus sun exposure)	Squamous cancer of skin
Gastric atrophy (pernicious anaemia)	Gastric cancer
Tuberous sclerosis	Cerebral gliomas
Café au lait skin patches	Neurofibromatosis (dominant inheritance); acoustic neuroma, phaeochromocytoma
Actinic dermatitis	Squamous carcinoma of skin; malignant melanoma
Glandular metaplasia of oesophagus (Barrett's oesophagus)	Adenocarcinoma of oesophagus
Dysphagia and anaemia (Plummer–Vinson syndrome)	Oesophageal cancer
Cirrhosis (alcoholic, hepatitis B)	Hepatocellular carcinoma
Ulcerative colitis	Colonic cancer
Paget's disease of bone	Osteosarcoma
Immunodeficiency states	Lymphomas
AIDS	Lymphoma, Kaposi's sarcoma
Autoimmune disease (e.g. Hashimoto's thyroiditis)	Lymphoma (e.g. thyroid lymphoma)
Dysplasias (e.g. cervical dysplasia)	Cancer

AIDS, Acquired immune deficiency syndrome.

Table 11.12 Childhood neoplasms.

Neoplasm	Site	Proposed progenitor cell
Acute lymphocytic leukaemia	Blood or marrow	Embryonic lymphoblasts
Lymphoblastic lymphoma	Lymph nodes or lymphoid tissue	Embryonic T lymphoblasts
Burkitt's lymphoma (B cell)	Lymph nodes or lymphoid tissue	Embryonic B lymphoblasts
Medulloblastoma	Cerebellum	Embryonic cerebellar neuroectodermal cells
Retinoblastoma	Retina	Embryonic retinal blast cells
Neuroblastoma	Adrenal medulla; sympathetic ganglia	Embryonic neuroblasts
Nephroblastoma (Wilms tumour)	Kidney	Embryonic metanephric cells
Hepatoblastoma	Liver	Embryonic liver cells
Osteosarcoma	Bone	Osteoblasts

together they constitute a significant group of risk factors (Table 11.13).

EFFECTS OF NEOPLASIA ON THE HOST

Neoplasia may be the underlying cause of almost any sign or symptom anywhere in the body. Recognizing the ways in which neoplasms produce symptoms and signs is an important part of diagnosis.

Direct effects of primary tumours

Signs and symptoms arising from local growth of a benign neoplasm or a primary malignant neoplasm vary with the site of the lesion, the nature of the surrounding anatomical structures and the growth rate of the neoplasm. The growing tumour may compress or destroy adjacent structures, cause inflammation, pain, vascular changes and varying degrees of functional deficit (Tables 11.14 and 11.15). If the tumour is growing near a vital structure (e.g. the brainstem) these local effects may be lethal, whether the neoplasm is benign or malignant.

Metastases

Metastatic deposits will produce the same local effects as primary tumours but these effects will be multiplied by the number of metastases.

Paraneoplastic syndromes

Systemic effects of a malignant neoplasm, other than those due directly to the tumour or its metastases, may occur and are known as paraneoplastic syndromes. They may be of clinical relevance as the first indication that a malignancy is present and permit early diagnosis and treatment, although this is not a common occurrence. Table 11.16 lists some examples of well-recognized paraneoplastic syndromes. In most cases, other than those involving ectopic hormone secretion, the underlying mechanism is unknown.

CANCER DIAGNOSIS

Clinical suspicion

From the previous discussion in this chapter, it is clear

Table 11.14 Properties of neoplasms.

Usually produce mass lesions
Grow steadily, though rate varies with different neoplasms
Display variable degree of autonomy
Mimic structure of cell or tissue of origin
Mimic function of cell or tissue of origin
Mimic antigenic properties of progenitor cell
May induce immune response
Induce growth of supporting stroma and blood vessels
Invade and metastasize (malignant neoplasms only)
Cause disease through compression, destruction and distant effects

Table 11.15 Local effect of neoplasms.

Local effect	Result
Mass	Presentation as tissue lump or tumour
Ulcer (non-healing)	Destruction of epithelial surfaces (e.g. stomach, colon, mouth, bronchus)
Haemorrhage	From ulcerated area or eroded vessel
Pain	Any site with sensory nerve endings; tumours in brain and many viscera are initially painless
Seizures	Tumour mass in brain; seizure pattern often localizes the tumour
Cerebral dysfunction	Wide variety of deficits depending on site of tumour
Obstruction	Of hollow viscera by tumour in the wall
Perforation	Of viscera
Bone destruction	Pathological fracture, collapse of bone
Inflammation	Of serosal surface
Effusions	Pleural effusion, pericardial effusion, ascites
Space-occupying lesion	Raised intracranial pressure in brain neoplasms; anaemia due to displacement of haematopoietic cells by metastases to the bone marrow
Loss of sensory or motor function	Compression or destruction of nerve or nerve trunk
Oedema	Due to venous or lymphatic obstruction

that a thorough clinical history is the essential first step in cancer diagnosis. This includes:
- a family history (for genetic predisposition or disorders associated with a high cancer rate);
- social history (e.g. smoking);
- occupational history (e.g. shipyard worker, miner);
- diet and geographic origin (e.g. aflatoxin, high incidence of hepatitis B);
- sexual and child-bearing history.

A complete history takes into account all of the possible **causative factors** as well as all of the possible **effects of neoplasia** for a particular patient.

Table 11.16 The paraneoplastic syndromes and their major associated malignancies.

Syndrome	Associated malignancy
Acanthosis nigricans	Carcinoma of the stomach, lung
Fleeting thrombophlebitis (Trousseau's phenomenon)	Carcinoma of the pancreas
Nephrotic syndrome	A variety of malignancies including lymphomas
Finger clubbing and hypertrophic pulmonary osteoarthropathy	Carcinoma of the lung
Eaton–Lambert syndrome (myasthenia-like symptoms)	Oat cell carcinoma of lung
Peripheral neuropathy Central nervous system effects	Carcinoma of the lung
Endocrinopathies Cushing's syndrome Hypercalcaemia Hypoglycaemia Polycythaemia	Oat cell carcinoma of lung Squamous cell carcinoma of lung Fibrosarcoma Renal cell carcinoma Cerebellar haemangioma

Physical examination is directed toward finding localizing symptoms or signs and thereby discovering a mass lesion that may be sampled by biopsy or aspiration for a **histological diagnosis**.

Early diagnosis—the role of screening

Symptoms and signs associated with cancer mean that the disease is usually already at a fairly advanced stage. In order to maximize the chance of cure, routine (**screening**) examinations of **asymptomatic individuals** may be performed.

Routine cytological screening in the form of **annual cervical smears** (Papanicolaou smears) in all sexually active women is the best example of this screening technique (Fig. 11.22b). Mammographic screening for breast cancer is routinely employed in the UK for women over 50 years. The establishment of routine health checks (and 'well-women' clinics) and increased public awareness about skin cancer and the risks of smoking make it more likely that patients will present with a suspicion of malignancy based on their own observations which may include the following:

• haemorrhage (rectal bleeding, haematuria);
• lump (breast lump, a 'mole' that changes in size or colour);
• a wound that fails to heal;
• an unexplained feeling of ill health.

These symptoms must all be investigated with the possiblity of cancer in mind.

Histopathological diagnosis (Table 11.17)

The information, obtained from histopathological diagnosis, will include:

• **the type of neoplasm:** the name of the neoplasm will be given in the pathology report;
• **biological behaviour:** the pathology report will state whether the neoplasm is **benign** or **malignant**, if that information is not implicit in the type of the neoplasm;
• **histological grade:** the histological grade of a malignant neoplasm describes the **degree of differentiation** of the neoplasm, expressed either in words (e.g. well,

Table 11.17 Prognostic indices in neoplasia.

Tissues sampling for prognostic indices
Tumour typing, grading and staging
Sampling and sample size
Tissue fixation and processing

Identification of tumour subtypes of prognostic importance
Receptors for steroids and growth factors
  (ER, PR, AR, cathepsin D, EGFR)
Oncogene and tumour suppressor gene expression
  (c-erbB-2/HER2/neu, c-myc, ras, p53)
Lectin binding (PNA)
Polymorphic epithelial mucins (HMFG1 and 2)

Nuclear features and tumour grading
Proliferative fraction = proportion of cells in S-phase
DNA ploidy
Estimation of cell proliferation
  (^{3}H-thymidine uptake, BrdU uptake, proliferation antigens
  (Ki-67, PCNA, DNA polymerase α))
Nucleolar organizer regions in interphase nuclei
Nuclear morphometry

Refinements in tumour staging
Basement membrane integrity
Vascular and lymphatic invasion
Micrometastases
Type IV collagen
Angiogenesis (using endothelial markers such as CD31)

ER, oestrogen receptor; PR, progesterone receptor; AR, androgen receptor; EGFR, epidermal growth factor receptor; PNA, peanut agglutinin; HMFG, human milk fat globule; PCNA, proliferating cell nuclear antigen.

moderately or poorly differentiated adenocarcinoma) or in numbers (e.g. grades I, II or III – grade I being the least and III the most malignant). Specific criteria exist for histological grading of many tumours. The histological grade has significant implications for prognosis, metastasis and survival;

- **invasion and spread:** this information is vital in planning treatment of many neoplasms;
- **stage:** the pathological stage describes the extent of spread of a neoplasm. Staging is important because it determines what further treatment a patient may be given, and it is a valuable guide to prognosis. Criteria for pathological staging vary with different neoplasms and different organs. An attempt to standardize pathological staining is the so-called **TNM classification**, which classifies neoplasms on the basis of **size** of the primary **tumour** (T), lymph **node** in volvement (N) and distant **metastases** (M).

Other methods of diagnosis

Serological diagnosis
Cancer cell products may be detected in the serum, and there are tests which are of value for certain tumours (Table 11.18).

Radiological diagnosis
CT and magnetic resonance imaging scans are invaluable for localizing masses as part of the primary diagnosis or for staging tumours. Radiological findings suggestive of cancer must be confirmed by either cytological or histological examination of biopsy material before treatment can be started.

Table 11.18 Serological assays for cancer diagnosis or follow-up.

Substance in serum	Cancer type
Carcinoembryonic antigen (CEA)	Gastrointestinal tract cancer (especially colon), breast and lung cancer; elevated levels in some non-cancerous states
α-Fetoprotein (AFP)	Hepatoma, yolk sac tumours
Human chorionic gonadotrophin (HCG)	Greatly elevated in choriocarcinoma; rarely elevated in other neoplasms
Prostatic acidphosphatase; prostate-specific epithelial antigen	Levels of both are elevated in metastatic prostatic cancer
Monoclonal immunoglobulin	Myeloma, some B-cell lymphomas
Specific hormones	Endocrine neoplasms and 'ectopic' hormone-producing tumours
CA 125	Ovarian carcinoma; other neoplasms

MANAGEMENT OF NEOPLASMS

The purpose of accurate diagnosis of the specific tumour type is to enable the clinician to select an appropriate mode of therapy. Even with the best treatment, survival rates vary greatly for different types of neoplasm (Fig. 11.27).

Surgery

Benign neoplasms
Surgical removal is curative. In a few cases, surgical removal may be difficult because of the locations, e.g. cerebellar medulloblastoma.

Malignant neoplasms
Wide local excision. Malignant neoplasms infiltrate tissues, which makes excision difficult. Local excision requires careful pathological examination of the margins of resection to ensure complete removal. This may involve marking of the margins with ink by the histopathologist and careful sampling of the resection margins for histology. A frozen-section histology assessment of adequacy of

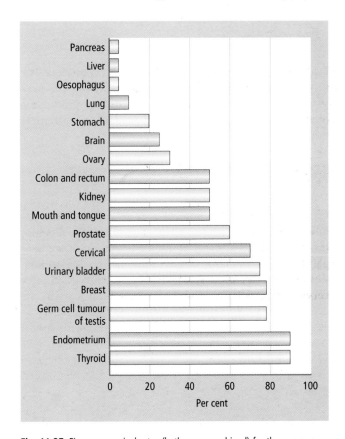

Fig. 11.27 Five year survival rates (both sexes combined) for the common malignancies by site.

excision margins may be made while the patient is on the surgical table. For low-grade malignant neoplasms, wide local excision is frequently sufficient for cure. Incomplete removal will lead to local recurrence.

Lymph node removal. Malignant neoplasms with a high risk of early lymphatic metastasis are often treated by excision of the primary tumour together with removal of the lymph node group of primary drainage (**radical surgery**).

Surgery for metastatic disease. Removal of solitary or limited numbers of metastases in the lung and the liver from many neoplasms can improve survival rates if combined with effective chemotherapy. Removal of metastases reduces tumour bulk, which will enhance the effect of chemotherapy and amplify any residual immune response.

Palliative surgery. Surgery also plays an important role in palliation of symptoms by relieving pain and restoring function in patients with incurable cancer, particularly when the tumour is associated with obstructive effects.

Radiation therapy

Malignant neoplasms may be sensitive to radiation. The more primitive and the more rapidly growing the neoplasm (the more poorly differentiated or high-grade), the more likely it is to be radiosensitive. Radiosensitivity is not synonymous with cure.

Chemotherapy

Choriocarcinoma and **testicular germ cell tumours** are now successfully treated with chemotherapy. Chemotherapy is the treatment of choice for many other neoplasms, such as **malignant lymphoma** and **leukaemia**. Chemotherapy improves survival rates when used with surgery in breast and lung carcinoma.

Anticancer drugs act in one of several ways:
- by interfering with DNA and RNA synthesis (**antimetabolites**);
- by blocking DNA replication and mitotic division (**antimitotic agents**);
- by exerting **hormonal** effects, e.g. oestrogens in prostate carcinoma and antioestrogenic agents such as tamoxifen in breast carcinoma.

Immunotherapy

This is the least successful area of tumour therapy. Specific immunotherapy using monoclonal antibodies developed against tumour-associated antigens has been used in the treatment of malignant melanoma, lymphoma and some carcinomas, but is still largely experimental.

Antibodies may be used to carry cytotoxic drugs, toxins or radioisotopes to the tumour site.

Stimulation of the immune system in melanoma patients with adjuvants such as bacillus Calmette-Guérin (BCG) have met with limited success. Interferon and interleukin-2 are under investigation for the treatment of Kaposi's sarcoma, malignant melanoma and lymphoma.

REFERENCE

Willis R.A. (1952) *The Spread of Tumours in the Human Body.* Butterworths, London.

FURTHER READING

Curran R.C. (1985) *Color Atlas of Histopathology*, 3rd edn. Oxford University Press, New York.
Mitchinson M.J. *et al.* (1996) *Essentials of Pathology* (Chapters 16–18). Blackwell Science, Oxford.
Royal College of Surgeons of Edinburgh (1983) *Color Atlas of Demonstrations in Surgical Pathology.* Williams & Wilkins, Baltimore.
Skarin A.T. (1991) *Atlas of Diagnostic Oncology.* JB Lippincott, Philadelphia.

Diseases of Blood and Bone Marrow

C O N T E N T S

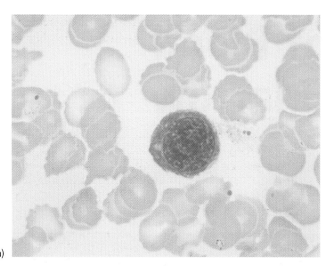

(a)

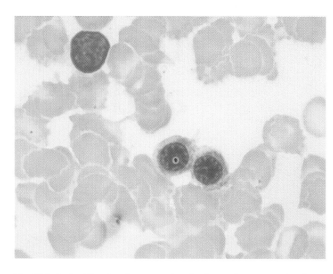

(b)

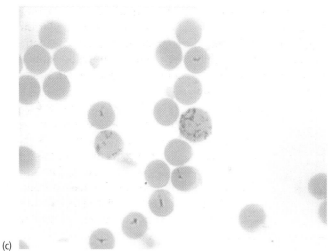

(c)

Fig. 12.1 Erythroid maturation; examples of cells are shown, maturing from (a) to (c). Erythroblast–normoblast–reticulocytes. The final cell is stained with methylene blue.

Pathology of the blood

The initial half of this chapter considers abnormalities that mainly affect red cells, while the second half considers disorders of white cells.

ERYTHROPOIESIS

Introduction

Red cell precursors are derived from **pluripotential stem cells** (Fig. 12.1). Different populations of erythroid precursors have been defined which form the early committed erythroid population but which cannot be recognized as such under the microscope. The maturation of red cells starts from colony forming units-stem cell (CFU-S) to burst forming units erythroid (BFU-E) and to colony forming units-erythroid (CFU-E).

It is believed that the BFU-E form an amplification compartment which can respond to requirements for erythropoiesis by rapid contraction or expansion. The CFU-E give rise to the first recognizable red cell precursors in the marrow, the basophilic **pronormoblasts** (erythroblasts; Fig. 12.1(a)).

The pronormoblasts give rise to approximately 16 daughter cells by a series of cell divisions. During this time there is gradual accumulation of haemoglobin in the cytoplasm of the red cell precursors. By the fourth division the cells are uniformly pink-staining (orthochromatic normoblasts) and the nuclear chromatin is highly condensed. The nucleus is then lost from the cell which becomes a reticulocyte, i.e. a cell which contains some residual RNA and other organelles which, on supravital staining, clump and produce a characteristic appearance on light microscopy. Reticulocytes spend approximately 24 hours in the marrow before they are released into the peripheral blood.

Nucleated red cells are only seen in the circulation when the marrow architecture is abnormal, for example, when there is carcinomatous infiltration or when the marrow is severely stressed, e.g. by hypoxia. This peripheral blood picture is usually termed **leukoerythroblastic** anaemia (since a few white cell precursors also enter the circulation; Fig. 12.2).

The whole process of red cell maturation takes about a week; the first 3 or 4 days are spent in cell division and the remainder in maturation and haemoglobin synthesis. Approximately 1% of the red cells are lost from the peripheral circulation each day.

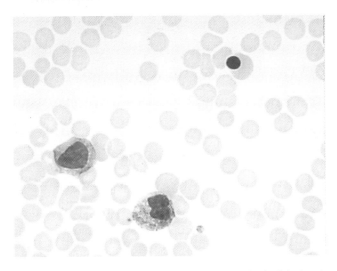

Fig. 12.2 Leucoerythroblastic anaemia; note the nucleated red cell (top) and immature myeloid cells.

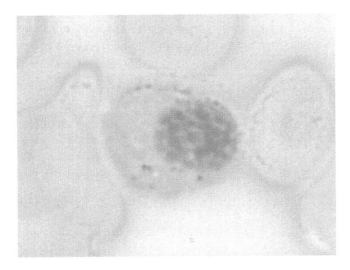

Fig. 12.3 A ringed sideroblast, the blue granules are iron loaded mitochondria. (PPB.)

Cytoplasm

Haemoglobin is the major cytoplasmic constituent of red cells and consists of a four-chain protein, **globin**, each chain of which nurses a molecule of **haem**. Haem consists of a flat tetrapyrrole **protoporphyrin** ring in the centre of which an atom of iron is held. All of the elements (globin, protoporphyrin, iron) must be available to the maturing red cell in equal amounts for normal haemoglobin synthesis.

Protoporphyrin production is rarely abnormal; the most frequently encountered defect is sideroblastic anaemia, a condition in which a block in synthesis of the tetrapyrrole ring leads to deposits of unusable iron in the cytoplasm of the developing red cells (**sideroblasts**; Fig. 12.3).

Red cell regulation

The major regulator of erythropoiesis is a hormone called **erythropoietin** which is synthesized mainly in the **kidney**, although there are extrarenal sites of production; in the **fetus** it is synthesized in the **liver**. Erythropoietin is produced in response to reduced oxygenation of the tissues and stimulates erythropoiesis until the oxygen-carrying capacity of the blood is restored. The precise mechanism of action of erythropoietin is still not known, although its receptor is cloned; it increases the rate of erythroid precursor cell division and their transit time through the marrow. The hormone works mainly at the level of the CFU-E and the later stages of erythroid maturation. Genetically engineered human erythropoietin is given to patients with anaemia who cannot synthesize their own due to renal disease.

Red cells survive an average of 120 days in the circulation and at the end of this time are destroyed by **histiocytic cells** (macrophages), predominantly in the **spleen**. Haem is then separated from the globin molecule and split into iron and the protoporphyrin ring. The iron is efficiently recycled, being carried by the plasma transport protein transferrin to marrow red cell precursors, whilst the protoporphyrin ring is converted to bilirubin and then taken up by the liver for conjugation with glucuronic acid (see Chapter 19). This water-soluble glucuronide is then excreted in **bile**.

Clinical features of anaemia

Anaemia, from whatever cause, induces a series of compensatory changes. In mild cases there is a shift to the right in the oxygen dissociation curve due to an increased production of 2,3-diphosphoglycerate in the red cells. As anaemia becomes worse there is an increase in cardiac output. A hyperkinetic circulation ultimately develops, characterized by tachycardia, a wide pulse pressure and flow murmurs.

These adaptive changes explain why patients who have become anaemic slowly may be **asymptomatic**. Much depends on their age and general condition; those with coronary artery disease, for example, may develop angina as the first symptom. As anaemia progresses, the characteristic symptoms and signs appear. These include tiredness, exertional dyspnoea, pallor, tachycardia, palpitations and a variety of cardiac murmurs. Ultimately, a state of high-output cardiac failure may develop with basal crepitations, peripheral oedema and ascites. Such patients are at risk if transfused too rapidly.

Classification of anaemia

The anaemias may be classified into two broad groups, reduced red cell production and increased loss or rate of destruction of red cells. The two groups can be distinguished with a reticulocyte count, which should be low and high respectively. The latter is caused by bleeding or haemolysis (see later). Reduced production may be due to reduced proliferation of red cell precursors (Table 12.1) or defective maturation of red cell precursors (Table 12.2) associated with a hyperplastic marrow due to increased erythropoietin production in response to anaemia. However, many of the precursors are destroyed in the marrow and hence there is a poor reticulocyte response. These are the hallmarks of ineffective erythropoiesis.

Table 12.1 Reduced proliferation of red cell precursors.

Causes
Iron deficiency

Anaemia of chronic inflammation (infection, cancer, etc.)

Reduced erythropoietin production (renal disease)

Primary disease of the marrow
  Aplastic anaemia
  Infiltrative disorders—leukaemia, myelofibrosis, cancer

Pure red cell aplasia (rare—congenital or associated with thymic tumours and myelodysplastic syndrome)

Table 12.2 Defective maturation of red cell precursors.

Causes
Defective nuclear maturation (megaloblastic anaemia)
Vitamin B_{12} deficiency
Folic acid deficiency
Defective cytoplasmic maturation
Iron deficiency
Disorders of globin synthesis—thalassaemia
Disorders of haem metabolism—sideroblastic anaemia

Note that some disorders are associated with both reduced proliferation and ineffective haemopoiesis.

As a practical screening test for the cause of anaemia, estimation of cell size and degree of haemoglobinization by an electronic cell counter, together with examination of the blood film, allows anaemias to be classified as outlined in Chapter 4.

HAEMOLYSIS

Introduction

Normal red cells survive for approximately 120 days in the circulation before being removed, mainly in the spleen. In haemolytic anaemia, the haemoglobin level falls because of a rapid rate of red cell destruction (Table 12.3). The bone marrow compensates with increased red cell production by increasing the volume of erythropoietic tissue, both by resorption of fat spaces and by spreading into unused areas within the bone. However, the marrow cannot produce red cells at more than ~8 times the normal rate.

A characteristic of almost all haemolytic anaemias is an increase in the number of immature red cells in the circulation. These are recognized by their blue staining (polychromatic) appearance on routine blood smears, and they can be counted accurately by using a special stain which reveals these young cells (reticulocytes) (see Fig. 12.1). In normal subjects reticulocytes account for less than 2% of circulating red cells.

Table 12.3 Classification of haemolytic anaemias.

Defect	Disease
Hereditary	
Membrane	Hereditary spherocytosis, hereditary elliptocytosis
Metabolism	Glucose-6-phosphate dehydrogenase deficiency, pyruvate kinase deficiency
Haemoglobin	Abnormal (HbS, HbC)
	Defective synthesis (thalassaemia)
Acquired	
Immune	
Autoimmune haemolytic anaemia	
Isoimmune, e.g. haemolytic transfusion reaction	
Haemolytic disease of the newborn	
Chemical or drug-induced haemolytic anaemia	
Red cell fragmentation syndrome	
Hypersplenism	

Hb, Haemoglobin.

Common features of haemolysis

Clinical

Apart from the usual symptoms and signs of anaemia, the hallmark of haemolysis is **jaundice**, representing an increase in the rate of bilirubin production from lysed red cells and the inability of the liver to conjugate this material rapidly enough. Since this bilirubin is largely unconjugated (i.e. is not water-soluble) bile is not present in the urine, as occurs when the lesion occurs further 'downstream' in the bile excretion pathway. However, the urine may turn dark on standing because of the presence of excess urobilinogen (see Chapter 19).

Occasionally patients suffering from chronic haemolysis suffer a dramatic fall in haemoglobin level (**aplastic crisis**) which is due to the marrow temporarily failing to compensate for the high rate of red cell turnover. Infection of red cell precursors with **parvovirus** has been shown to cause most such episodes.

Laboratory

The **peripheral blood** will show an increased reticulocyte count and a **marrow aspirate** will show a marked increase in the number of red cell precursors. When the bone marrow is under particularly severe stress, nucleated red cells are seen in the circulation (Fig. 12.4). Serum bilirubin will be raised. If serum **haptoglobins** are measured, they will be **absent** or **low**. This protein scavenges free haemoglobin from plasma and once the complex is formed it is removed from the circulation.

The peripheral blood may give a clue as to the cause of haemolysis–fragmented cells suggest direct mechanical damage, while spherocytic cells are seen in hereditary spherocytosis and also in antibody-mediated haemolytic anaemia. Agglutination of red cells may sometimes be seen on the blood film due to anti-red cell antibodies. **Haemoglobinopathies** should also be considered,

although anaemia in these patients is due as much to destruction within the marrow of biochemically abnormal cells (ineffective erythropoiesis) as to shortened red cell survival. Possible visible abnormalities include **sickle cells** and the characteristic cells seen in **thalassaemias** (e.g. target cells).

Hereditary haemolytic anaemias

Hereditary spherocytosis

This is due to defects in the **cytoskeleton**, which gives structural rigidity to the red cell membrane. The underlying abnormality may lie in the genes for the major constituent of the cytoskeleton, **spectrin** or **ankyrin**, a protein involved in fixing spectrin to the cell membrane. Membrane is then lost from red cells, which become increasingly spherical and liable to be trapped and destroyed in the spleen.

The disease varies markedly from one patient to another and rarely causes severe anaemia. Because of the long-standing nature of the haemolytic process, **pigment gallstones** frequently occur. The disorder usually shows an **autosomal dominant** inheritance pattern.

The disease is diagnosed both by showing spherocytic cells on a blood film and also by demonstrating excessive osmotic fragility of red cells (Fig. 12.5). Treatment is often not necessary; should it be needed, splenectomy is effective.

Red cell metabolic disorders

The circulating red cell, having lost its nucleus and containing little in the cytoplasm other than haemoglobin, is stripped down to bare biochemical essentials. One requirement is the maintenance of a reducing environment within the cell, so that sulphydryl groups are not oxidized, leading to cross-linking of haemoglobin and membrane proteins, and the appearance of denatured haemoglobin inclusions (**Heinz bodies**). This environment is maintained by an excess of the tripeptide glutathione, in which a sulphydryl group is available for oxidation, thus protecting sulphadryl groups on proteins. Reduced glutathione is promptly regenerated by reduced nicotine adenine dinucleotide phosphate (NADP). A crucial enzyme in this pathway is glucose-6-phosphate dehydrogenase (G6PD), deficiency of which constitutes the commonest type of haemolytic anaemia due to an intrinsic red cell enzyme defect.

Glucose-6-phosphate dehydrogenase deficiency

The clinical features of this deficiency vary, reflecting different genetic abnormalities which can affect the enzyme (e.g. low levels, reduced stability). The disorder is

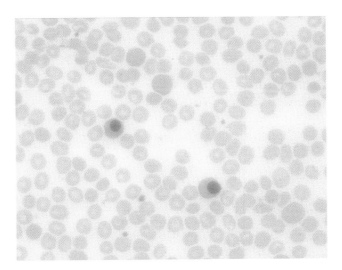

Fig. 12.4 From a patient with an immune haemolytic anaemia showing a high reticulocyte count and nucleated red cells, polychromasia and spherocytes.

commonest in the Mediterranean, the Middle East, South east Asia and West Africa; it is found only rarely in northern Europeans. It is **X-linked** and probably provides protection against malaria when in the heterozygote form, i.e. females.

Patients suffer from acute episodes of **intravascular haemolysis** precipitated by exposure to drugs, infection or other acute illness. The drugs include antimalarials, analgesics and antibacterial agents (e.g. sulphonamides). Exacerbation of haemolysis may also follow ingestion of fava or broad beans—hence the old name **favism**.

During one of these crises, the blood film shows Heinz bodies within red cells when appropiately stained, and red cells may appear distorted due to removal of Heinz bodies in the spleen (Fig. 12.6).

Between haemolytic episodes the blood count is normal, except in very severe cases. The level of G6PD in red cells can be assayed directly when enzyme deficiency is suspected.

Glycolytic enzyme defects

The red cell is entirely dependent on anaerobic glycolysis for adenosine triphosphate production. Deficiencies in glycolytic enzymes may cause chronic haemolysis and sometimes abnormalities in skeletal muscle and nervous tissue. The commonest of these is lack of pyruvate kinase.

Acquired haemolytic anaemia

Autoimmune haemolytic anaemia

There are two basic types of autoimmune haemolytic anaemia (AIHA), the distinction depending on whether the autoantibody is of immunoglobulin G (IgG) or IgM type.

IgG-mediated haemolysis (warm AIHA). IgG antibodies react best at body temperature. Consequently antibody can be found on the red cell surface in freshly drawn blood. The **Coombs** (antiglobulin) test provides a simple means of demonstrating this: when red cells from the patient are washed and suspended in an antiserum raised against human immunoglobulin they promptly agglutinate.

The blood film shows, in addition to evidence of increased red cell turnover, spherocytic cells from which part of the surface membrane has been removed by splenic macrophages (Fig. 12.7).

In some patients no obvious predisposing cause for the haemolysis is evident. In others, it is secondary to drug

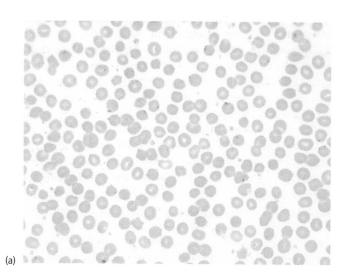

(a)

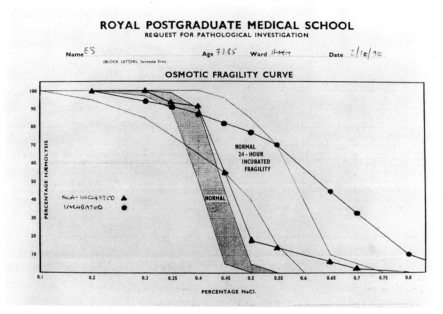

(b)

Fig. 12.5 Hereditary spherocytosis. (a) Blood film. (b) Osmotic fragility curve; osmotic pressure plotted against percentage lysis.

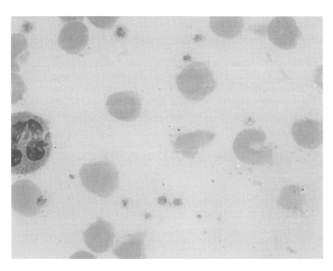

Fig. 12.6 Haemolysis in G6PD deficiency; note some of the cells appear to have chunks removed from them ('bite cells'), many cells have clumps of oxidized haemoglobin which have retracted from the membrane.

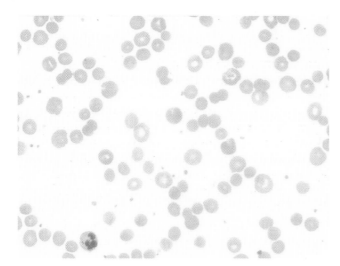

Fig. 12.7 Autoimmune haemolytic anaemia; note the many spherocytes.

therapy (most commonly **methyldopa**), to an underlying lymphoid neoplasm (e.g. chronic lymphocytic leukaemia) or to another autoimmune disease (e.g. systemic lupus erythematosus; SLE).

When treatment is required, **prednisolone** is tried at a high initial dose (e.g. 80 mg/day) which is then tapered off as the response allows. In some patients, **splenectomy** may be necessary. Treatment with immunosuppressive drugs is occasionally of value.

IgM-mediated haemolysis ('cold' AIHA). IgM antibodies bind best to red cells at low temperatures, so that much of the antibody in a sample from the patient will be in the serum. It is therefore demonstrated by testing for **cold**

agglutinins, i.e. antibody that agglutinates red cells at room temperature or below (Fig. 12.8).

Circulating red cells carry little or no antibody (unless the sample is cooled), although a direct Coombs test (see above) will sometimes be positive with an antiserum directed against complement components. The tendency of an IgM autoantibody to bind in the cold means that some patients who suffer symptoms due to red cells agglutinating in the peripheral cooler circulation, e.g. **Raynaud's phenomenon**, have cold-induced haemolytic episodes.

There is often no obvious predisposing cause for haemolytic anaemia of this type. It may transiently occur in association with infection, most commonly *Mycoplasma pneumoniae* and **infectious mononucleosis** in younger patients, or with a lymphoproliferative disorder in the elderly.

Isoimmune haemolysis

The most common setting in which this type of haemolytic anaemia is seen is in a rhesus-positive child born to a rhesus-negative mother. Antibodies in the maternal circulation against rhesus antigen (anti-D), usually stimulated by previous pregnancies, are actively transported across the placenta (being of IgG type) and cause **intrauterine haemolysis**.

This disease is rarer than in the past, since the administration of human antirhesus antibodies to most rhesus-negative mothers at the time of delivery (if the baby is rhesus-positive) effectively prevents immunization, by coating fetal red cells with antibody and causing their rapid clearance by splenic macrophages without presentation to antigen-responsive lymphoid cells. However, the disease has now reached a relatively constant plateau level and for some of these pregnancies intrauterine

Fig. 12.8 Cold agglutinins; note the clumps of red cells.

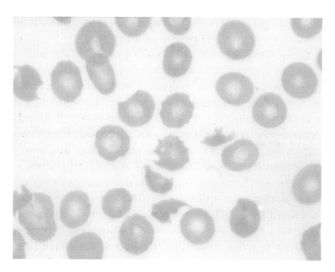

Fig. 12.9 Red cells exhibiting damage secondary to disseminated intravascular coagulation (DIC).

Table 12.4 Iron-binding proteins.

Protein	Properties	Amount in body
Haemoglobin	Oxygen transport	3 g
Ferritin	Intracellular store of iron, especially reticuloendothelial cells and liver	2 g in normal males Stores = 4000 atoms per ferritin molecule
Haemosiderin	Insoluble store of iron; stains with Prussian blue	
Transferrin	High-affinity serum protein–binds two atoms of iron per molecule. Serum transport protein	4 mg
Lactoferrin	Iron-binding protein in milk, secretions and neutrophils; bacteriostatic protein	Trace
Cytochromes	Electron tansfer and redox enzymes	Trace

transfusion of rhesus-negative blood to the baby may be needed. An increasing proportion of disease is caused by antigens lying outside the rhesus system.

Red cell fragmentation

Occasionally red cells are **mechanically damaged** in the circulation. This may be due to abnormalities of flow introduced by **prosthetic materials** (e.g. heart valves, vascular grafts). In **disseminated intravascular coagulation (DIC)**, strands of fibrin in small vessels can damage the red cells (Fig. 12.9).

A rare cause of mechanical damage to red cells occurs in **march haemoglobinuria**, in which red cells travelling through the vessels in the feet are mechanically damaged during prolonged running. A similar, but presumably even rarer, cause of haemolysis has been seen in karate aficionados following repeated striking of hard surfaces with the hand.

Hypersplenism. A large spleen from a variety of causes may increase the rate of destruction of, as well as produce excessive pooling of blood cells, and so result in pancytopenia.

IRON

Biochemistry and metabolism

Although 4% of the earth's crust is iron, **iron deficiency** is the commonest cause of anaemia worldwide. This paradox occurs because iron in its usual **oxidized (ferric)** form is **insoluble** and the soluble ferrous form is toxic. Thus iron-binding proteins are required to render iron soluble but safe. Examples of iron-binding proteins are listed in Table 12.4.

Iron absorption

The amount of iron in food and the percentage absorption varies widely, but a normal diet contains approximately 15 mg of iron daily, of which about 5–10% (1 mg) is absorbed. Iron as haem, the form of iron present in meat, is better absorbed than iron in vegetables (including spinach). Absorption takes place mainly in the duodenum and is helped by acid, which tends to keep it in the ferrous (Fe^{2+}) state. The exact mechanisms which control iron absorption are still not clear. Nevertheless, one factor is the body's requirement for iron; in iron deficiency uptake increases.

Iron transport

Recycling of iron in the body is so efficient that little iron absorption is usually necessary. Iron is released when red cells die and are taken up by macrophages, and transferred to plasma transferrin to be transported back to the bone marrow for erythropoiesis. Transferrin can bind two atoms of iron per molecule. In normal serum about a third of the iron binding sites are occupied. Specific **transferrin receptors** are required by cells in order to obtain iron from transferrin. Erythroblasts and hepatocytes are particularly rich in transferrin receptors. Excess iron is stored in **ferritin**, some of which leaks out to serum. **Haemosiderin** is probably a metabolically inaccessible breakdown product of ferritin.

Assessment of iron stores

The 'gold standard' for assessing the iron status of

patients is to visualize iron in bone marrow and liver by microscopic examination of a sample stained for iron with **Prussian blue**. Iron-deficient patients have no visible iron in the bone marrow; in contrast, in iron-overloaded patients, the liver shows excess iron deposition.

It is more convenient to infer the iron status from testing serum; iron-deficient patients have low serum ferritin and reduced serum iron and transferrin saturation.

In contrast, iron-loaded patients have raised serum ferritin, normal serum iron but lowered **total iron-binding capacity** (TIBC; therefore increased iron saturation). Serum ferritin is also raised in liver disease and by an inflammatory response. The latter may also cause a fall in the serum iron and TIBC.

Iron deficiency

Before iron deficiency causes anaemia the iron stores in the reticuloendothelial system must be depleted. Many women in the reproductive age group have low storage of iron due to menstrual blood loss. As iron deficiency develops, symptoms arise from anaemia.

The classic features of chronic iron deficiency are only rarely seen in the UK: glossitis, spoon-nails (koilonychia), dysphagia due to pharyngeal webs (Plummer–Vinson syndrome) and unusual dietary cravings (pica).

The causes of iron deficiency are summarized in Table 12.5. The major cause of iron deficiency in western countries is chronic blood loss. Do not forget that iron deficiency must not be considered a trivial diagnosis but a sign of possible gastrointestinal neoplasm. In the tropics the high prevalence of iron deficiency is related to **dietary deficiency** and blood loss from **hookworm infestation**.

The increased demands during infancy, adolescence, pregnancy, lactation and in menstruating women account for the high prevalence of latent iron deficiency (absent iron stores without anaemia) and consequent high risk of

anaemia in these groups. Similarly, **malabsorption** may predispose to iron deficiency but only rarely is the chief cause of a marked deficiency state.

Diagnosis

The blood film shows microcytic hypochromic red cells with occasional target cells and pencil-shaped poikilocytes (Fig. 12.10). The haemoglobin, mean cell volume (MCV), mean cell haemoglobin (MCH) and mean cell haemoglobin concentration (MCHC) fall progressively as the anaemia worsens. The platelet count may often be above the upper limit of the normal range if there is bleeding. The serum iron falls and the TIBC rises so that the saturation may fall to less than 10%. A good proof that an anaemia is due to iron is reversal by the administration of iron (Table 12.6).

Treatment

The underlying cause of the iron deficiency should be rectified if possible.

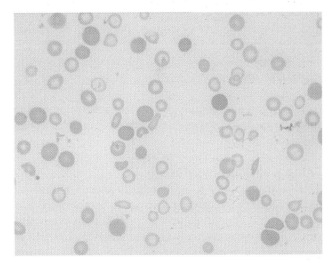

Fig. 12.10 An iron-deficient film showing pale hypochromic red cells and characteristic elongated 'pencil cells'.

Table 12.5 Causes of iron deficiency.

Blood loss
Uterine
Gastrointestinal
Increased demands
Prematurity
Growth
Pregnancy
Malabsorption
Gastrectomy
Coeliac disease

Table 12.6 Factors influencing serum iron, total iron-binding capacity (TIBC) and ferritin values.

Measurement	Elevated in	Decreased in
Serum iron (10–30 µmol/l)	Iron poisoning	Iron deficiency; inflammation
Serum TIBC (45–70 µmol/l)	Iron deficiency; Pregnancy	Iron overload; protein loss; inflammation
Serum ferritin (20–300 µg/l but age- and sex-dependent)	Iron overload; liver disease; inflammation	Iron deficiency

The simplest way to correct iron deficiency is by **oral iron**. In general, blood tranfusions should not be given, even in severe anaemia caused by chronic iron deficiency. **Ferrous sulphate** is the standard preparation, usually prescribed as 200 mg up to three times a day. Side-effects such as abdominal pain or diarrhoea are often reported and may sometimes be avoided by reducing the dose or changing to a different iron preparation. Therapy should be continued in order to correct the anaemia and to replenish the iron stores, which generally requires a further 6 months of therapy. As a rough guide, the haemoglobin should rise by about 1 g/dl per week.

A common problem is failure to respond to oral iron. The possible causes are:
- continuing haemorrhage;
- failure to take tablets;
- incorrect diagnosis–especially thalassaemia trait.

Parenteral iron may be given as **intramuscular injections** in situations where oral iron is ineffective (e.g. severe malabsorption). Parenteral iron does not act more quickly than oral iron. Iron may also be given intravenously but may result in severe anaphylactoid reactions and should not be given except in special circumstances.

Iron overload

Iron overload may be due to increased absorption of iron from the gut or excess parenteral administration of iron or blood.

Primary haemochromatosis

This is an uncommon and underdiagnosed autosomal recessive condition causing increased absorption of iron from the gut. Patients present in midlife with symptoms caused by increased iron loading of parenchymal cells of liver, heart or endocrine organs. Their clinical features include pigmented skin, diabetes mellitus ('bronzed diabetes'), early osteoarthritis, cardiac failure or cirrhosis of the liver (see Chapter 7).

The diagnosis of haemochromatosis is made by showing a raised serum ferritin, a near-saturated TIBC and measuring the amount of hepatic iron with a biopsy or magnetic resonance imaging (MRI).

A diagnosis of primary haemochromatosis requires exclusion of secondary causes by examination of the blood film and, if necessary, the bone marrow. The patient's siblings should be screened by measurement of serum ferritin, iron and TIBC. Regular **venesection** is required until the serum ferritin returns to normal.

Iron-loading anaemias

Many congenital haemolytic anaemias are associated with a degree of iron loading. In chronic refractory anaemias, severe iron overload may result from regular blood transfusions.

Cardiac iron loading is inevitable in patients who have received more than 100 units of blood (20 g of iron).

MEGALOBLASTIC ANAEMIA

Introduction

Megaloblastic anaemia refers to a group of disorders resulting in distinctive dyserythropoietic abnormalities in the bone marrow associated with abnormally large red cells in the peripheral blood (Table 12.7).

Megaloblasts are larger than their normal equivalents. The early precursors have a large **primitive nucleus** with lacy **open chromatin** and seem to develop more slowly than the surrounding cytoplasm, resulting in **maturation asynchrony**. Late megaloblasts, and even peripheral blood red cells, may retain their nucleus. Double or multiple nuclei are seen in some cells; abnormal nuclear bridging occurs between others. White cell and platelet precursors are also affected causing, for example, **giant metamyelocytes** (Fig. 12.11).

Function of vitamin B$_{12}$ and folate

Both vitamins act as **cofactors** for various **enzymes**.

Folate circulates as **methyltetrahydrofolate**, is translocated across the plasma membrane and must be turned into **tetrahydrofolate** (FH$_4$) before further metabolism takes place. The latter reaction also turns homocysteine into methionine and uses **methylcobalamin**, a form of B$_{12}$, as a cofactor.

Table 12.7 Some causes of megaloblastic anaemia.

Vitamin B$_{12}$ or folate deficiency (much the commonest)
Congenital abnormalities of B$_{12}$/folate metabolism
Other abnormalities of DNA synthesis Congenital DNA synthetic abnormalities, e.g. orotic aciduria Congenital dyserythropoietic anaemia Erythroleukaemia (AML-M6) Myelodysplastic syndromes, especially sideroblastic anaemia Drugs: antimetabolite cytotoxic agents, e.g. azathioprine,   6-mercaptopurine, hydroxyurea

AML, Acute myeloid leukaemia.

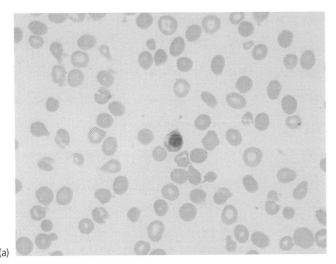

(a)

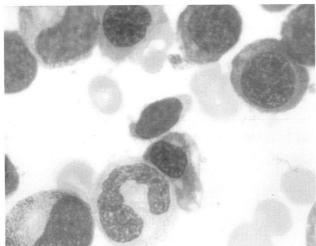

(b)

Fig. 12.11 Megaloblastic anaemia. Note the bizarrely shaped red cells (poikilocytes), and (a) the nucleated red cells in the peripheral circulation. (b) In the marrow, note the nuclei of the red cells are immature relative to cytoplasm and the chromatin appears to be pin pricked. The nucleus of the metamyelocyte appears to have been blown up like a balloon.

B_{12} is known to be involved in only one other reaction in humans; adenylcobalamin is needed in the isomerization of methylmalonyl coenzyme A (CoA) to succinyl CoA. Tetrahydrofolate acts as recipient/donor in reactions involving the transfer of single carbon groups and is involved in numerous biochemical reactions. Three of these are concerned in the synthesis of **purines** and **pyrimidines**. Its role in deoxythymidine monophosphate synthesis, a rate-limiting step in DNA synthesis, is the most important in causing megaloblastic anaemia.

When B_{12} or folate is deficient, red cell production is predominantly affected, resulting in anaemia, although white cell and platelet production may also be impaired. Non-haematopoietic tissue may also suffer, resulting in glossitis, malabsorption and melanin pigmentation.

The clinical effects of severe B_{12} or folate deficiency (Fig. 12.12) are indistinguishable except that folate deficiency is often of more rapid onset and the unique effects of B_{12} on the nervous system (Table 12.8). The underlying reason for this is unclear, but a **demyelinating neuropathy** affects the peripheral sensory nerves and posterior and lateral columns. If severe, **optic atrophy** and **psychiatric symptoms** may result. Anaemia is usually present, but the neurological symptoms may present before the peripheral blood count is affected.

B_{12} absorption

Vitamin B_{12} exists in a number of different chemical forms called **cobalamins**. The main dietary form is

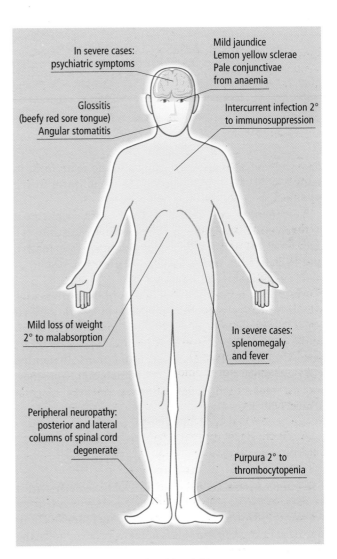

Fig. 12.12 The clinical effects of B_{12}/folate deficiency.

Table 12.8 The clinical effects of B$_{12}$ or folate deficiency.

Organ	Defect	Clinical effect
Blood	Macrocytic anaemia	Anaemia, jaundice (lemon yellow)
	Neutropenia	Infection
	Thrombocytopenia	Bleeding
Skin	Angular cheilosis	Sore mouth
	Glossitis	'Beefy red' tongue
		Pigmentation, alopecia
Gut	Epithelial abnormalities of stomach and small bowel (subtotal villous atrophy)	Anorexia, weight loss, altered bowel habit, malabsorption
Genital tract	Epithelial abnormalities	Infertility
CNS	Mental abnormalities	Dementia
Clinical effects unique to B$_{12}$ deficiency		
CNS	Peripheral neuropathy, subacute combined degeneration of the cord	Paraesthesia, numbness, difficulty walking, weakness
Eyes	Retrobulbar neuritis	Poor vision
	Optic atrophy	Blindness

CNS, Central nervous system.

Table 12.9 Some causes of vitamin B$_{12}$ deficiency.

Nutritional	Vegans
Malabsorption	Pernicious anaemia
	Congenital intrinsic factor deficiency
	Gastrectomy
Abnormal ileum	Surgical resection
	Crohn's disease
	Congenital selective malabsorption with proteinuria
Intestinal organisms	Blind loop syndromes (excess B$_{12}$ consumption)
	Fish tapeworm

deoxyadenylcobalamin, which is also the main form in human liver. Methylcobalamin is the main form in the plasma.

B$_{12}$ is found only in animal products. As a coenzyme it is regenerated, there are no known catabolic pathways and losses are small. Stores (liver/kidney) are extensive and will last for up to 4 years, so that the results of deficiency are slow to develop.

Absorption occurs in the distal ileum but requires **intrinsic factor**, a glycoprotein produced by gastric parietal cells. This binds to B$_{12}$ and facilitates uptake in the ileum in the presence of calcium and a neutral pH. B$_{12}$ is transported in plasma tightly bound to the **transcobalamins** (TC), of which TC II is the most important. The commonest cause of B$_{12}$ deficiency is pernicious anaemia (Table 12.9).

Pernicious anaemia

Pernicious anaemia (PA) is a disease of the elderly with a peak age of onset of 60 years. It has been said to be commoner, with an annual incidence of 120:100000, in northern Europeans but this is not now believed to be the case.

PA occurs more commonly than by chance in close

relatives, in those of blood group A and supposedly in those with prematurely grey hair and blue eyes. Adult PA is an **autoimmune** disorder. Symptoms are preceded by an autoimmune **gastritis** which results in asymptomatic **atrophy** of the **body** and **fundus** of the **stomach**. Intestinal metaplasia may be seen and there is an increased risk of carcinoma of the stomach. Loss of gastric parietal cells results in **reduced intrinsic factor** (IF) production and consequent B$_{12}$ malabsorption.

Serum autoantibodies to gastric parietal cells are present in 90% of cases, although this is not diagnostic since they are also found in other autoimmune disorders, in normal relatives of those with PA and in 15% of normal women over 60 years. Antibodies to IF are more specific, are found in the serum of 55% of cases and in gastric juice in 80%. The latter antibodies may be important in pathogenesis.

There are associations with other autoimmune disorders; especially of the thyroid, parathyroid and adrenal glands in patients and family members. A rarer association is with late-onset IgA deficiency or hypogammaglobulinaemia. Steroid therapy has been shown to improve the gastric mucosa with regeneration of glandular elements and renewed IF production, but effects are short-lived and steroids are not used under normal circumstances.

Diagnosis depends upon a macrocytic anaemia, low serum B$_{12}$ and abnormal B$_{12}$ absorption which can be corrected by the addition of IF (**Schilling test** – see Chapter 18) and/or the demonstration of autoantibodies to IF.

Treatment of PA is with replacement vitamin B$_{12}$; there is no specific treatment for the gastritis. Hydroxocobalamin is given by intramuscular injection every 3 months or larger daily oral doses, for life. Other than the effects of subacute combined degeneration of the cord, which may persist after treatment, all other features of deficiency recover. Life expectancy is normal unless carcinoma of the stomach develops. Endoscopic surveillance is probably not justified, but clinical suspicion should be maintained.

Establishing the cause of B$_{12}$ deficiency

If antibodies to IF are demonstrable, further investigation is probably unjustified. Otherwise, **absorption tests** should be considered – many patients on lifelong B$_{12}$ do not, in fact, have PA. Reduced absorption of a single oral dose of radiolabelled B$_{12}$ indicates malabsorption of B$_{12}$ which will correct to near normal levels with addition of IF if malabsorption is due to PA. Absorption of B$_{12}$ is not corrected by IF if it is due to ileal disease.

Absorption of oral radiolabelled B$_{12}$ is measured by whole-body counting or excretion in the urine (Schilling test). A parenteral loading dose of unlabelled B$_{12}$ is given; any of the oral dose subsequently absorbed will then be excreted in the urine. Malabsorption is diagnosed if less than 10% of the administered radiolabelled B$_{12}$ appears in a 24-hour urine collection.

Childhood B$_{12}$ deficiency

B$_{12}$ deficiency developing in children aged 2–3 years may be due to congenital abnormalities of IF production. The picture resembles adult PA but the gastric mucosa appears normal and autoantibodies are not found.

Megaloblastic anaemia occurring in the first few weeks of life may be due to congenital TC II deficiency. Serum B$_{12}$ levels may be normal, since TC I is not affected. The anaemia responds to very large doses of B$_{12}$.

Folic acid absorption

Pteroylglutamic acid is the parent compound of a large family known as the folates. Naturally occurring folates exist as polyglutamates, with three or more glutamic acid residues. Unlike B$_{12}$, folate is present in most foods, especially green vegetables, but it may be destroyed by cooking. The normal western diet supplies about six times the daily requirement.

During metabolic reactions, folate is not completely reutilized and daily requirements are greater than measurable losses in skin, faeces and urine. Deficiency is more likely in conditions where there is increased cell turnover and DNA synthesis, e.g. pregnancy, infection, malignancy (Table 12.10). Hepatic stores contain sufficient folate for only about 4 months, but less when demands are increased.

Folates are absorbed rapidly and efficiently (50–100% of an oral dose) in the duodenum and jejunum.

Table 12.10 Causes of folate deficiency.

Nutritional	Poverty, elderly, alcoholism, anorexia
Malabsorption	Gluten-induced enteropathy, tropical sprue, congenital specific malabsorption
Abnormal utilization	Folate antagonist drugs, e.g. methotrexate Congenital enzyme deficiencies Other drugs; anticonvulsants
Increased requirements	Physiological, e.g. pregnancy, prematurity Pathological, e.g. malignancy, haemolysis, myeloproliferative disorders
Increased losses	Dialysis

Polyglutamate forms of folate are deconjugated to monoglutamates, completely reduced to tetrahydrofolate and methylated to the active coenzyme form, which passes to the portal circulation. Methyltetrahydrofolate is carried either free or loosely bound to albumin (one-third).

There is a significant **enterohepatic circulation**. Folate is filtered by the glomerulus but mostly reabsorbed in the renal tubules. It is also removed from plasma in those on chronic haemodialysis.

Folate deficiency is often multifactorial. A poor intake is common and may compound other causes of deficiency. Drugs affecting folate metabolism, e.g. **methotrexate** in malignancy and **Septrin** in infections, are used at a time when demands for folate are high. People in institutional care may become folate-deficient through a combination of over-boiled vegetables and **anticonvulsant** or **barbiturate** therapy.

Folate deficiency occurs commonly in neonates, pregnant women (in whom it contributes towards neonatal spina bifida), alcoholics, the elderly and those unwell from a variety of causes, especially gastrointestinal or haematological. Macrocytic anaemia, especially in association with the features of hyposplenism on the blood film, may be the presenting feature of coeliac disease.

The diagnosis rests on measurement of folate levels and treatment consists of oral replacement therapy (folic acid 5 mg/day). Serum folate levels fluctuate and, although they may reflect acute folate deficiency, red cell folate levels reflect stores better. It is important to investigate and treat the cause of any deficiency. Prophylactic folic acid is sometimes given to pregnant women, those with proliferative haematological disorders and those with chronic malabsorption.

Folinic acid (formyltetrahydrofolate) bypasses dihydrofolate reductase inhibition and is used as an 'antidote' to the side-effects of methotrexate therapy.

If the cause of folate deficiency is not apparent from

clinical history, examination and preliminary laboratory tests, tests for malabsorption should be performed (see Chapter 18).

Treatment of B₁₂ and folate deficiency

Blood transfusion is rarely indicated except in severe anaemia or where other causes of anaemia, e.g. bleeding, coexist. **Vitamin B₁₂**, as hydroxocobalamin, is usually given **parenterally** (except in supplementation of a vegan diet) and **folic acid orally**.

Whilst waiting for the results of blood levels both vitamins are given together because of the risk of exacerbating the neurological lesions of B₁₂ deficiency if folate treatment is instituted without B₁₂. In severe anaemias, potassium or iron deficiency may occur in the recovery phase of exuberant haemopoiesis, and supplements should be considered.

Patients generally feel better within 24–48 hours of starting treatment. The blood reticulocyte count rises after 2 days, peaking at 7 days, paralleled by the platelet count (which may rebound temporarily to abnormally high levels). The haemoglobin rises by 1 g/dl per week, unless there are additional causes of anaemia.

Failure to respond to vitamin replacement therapy should suggest that either there is more than one cause of anaemia or that the macrocytic anaemia is due to another cause, e.g. myelodysplasia.

HAEMOGLOBINOPATHIES

The genetic disorders of haemoglobin are the commonest single-gene disorders in the world; the World Health Organization suggests that 5% are carriers for a serious haemoglobin disorder. Their prevalence is explained by conferment of resistance to severe malaria.

Genetic control of human haemoglobin

Different haemoglobins are synthesized in the embryo, fetus and adult. Each haemoglobin is adapted to particular oxygen requirements. All haemoglobins have a **tetrameric structure** made up of two pairs of globin chains; each chain is attached to one haem molecule.

Fetal and adult haemoglobins (Hb) have α- (alpha) chains combined with γ- (gamma) chains (Hb F, $\alpha_2\gamma_2$) or β- (beta) chains (Hb A, $\alpha_2\beta_2$) and δ- (delta) chains (Hb A₂, $\alpha_2\delta_2$, a minor variant) respectively. In embryos, α-like chains called ζ- (zeta) chains combine with ε- (epsilon) chains to make the definitive embryonic haemoglobin $\zeta_2\varepsilon_2$.

The α- and ζ-chains are produced from a gene cluster on chromosome 16; the ε, γ, δ and β globin chains are directed by another cluster on chromosome 11. During normal human development the ζ and ε genes are switched on in embryonic life, α genes and γ genes during fetal life, and δ and β together with α genes during adult life. The normal switch from fetal to adult haemoglobin production starts at about 32 weeks' gestation and is complete by about 6 months after birth.

Classification of haemoglobin disorders

Haemoglobin disorders can be classified as follows.
- **Structural haemoglobin variants.** Most result from single amino acid substitutions in the α- or β-chains. The most important are haemoglobins S, C and E. Rare variants may interfere with oxygen transport and produce hereditary polycythaemia or cyanosis. Another rare group of mutations produces unstable haemoglobin molecules and hence chronic haemolytic anaemia.
- **The thalassaemias.** These disorders are characterized by a reduced rate of production of one or more pairs of globin chains. This leads to imbalanced globin chain synthesis and resultant anaemia.
- **Hereditary persistence of fetal haemoglobin.** These are usually clinically innocuous conditions characterized by genetic defects in the switch from fetal to adult haemoglobin synthesis such that fetal haemoglobin production persists into adult life.

The sickling disorders

The sickling disorders consist of the usually asymptomatic heterozygous state for haemoglobin S or the sickle-cell trait (A S), the homozygous state or sickle-cell disease (S S), and the compound heterozygous state for haemoglobin S together with haemoglobins C, D, E or other structural variants, or different forms of β-thalassaemia.

The sickling disorders are found most frequently in Black Africans, although they also occur in certain Mediterranean, Middle Eastern and Indian populations.

Pathogenesis
Haemoglobin S differs from haemoglobin A by the substitution of valine for glutamic acid at position 6 in the β-chain. When **deoxygenated**, haemoglobin S aggregates into parallel, helical, rod-like structures. They are the basis for the **sickle deformity** of the red cell which occurs during deoxygenation of the blood (Fig. 12.13).

The effect of sickling in the circulation is to shorten the survival of red cells, leading to a **haemolytic anaemia**. In

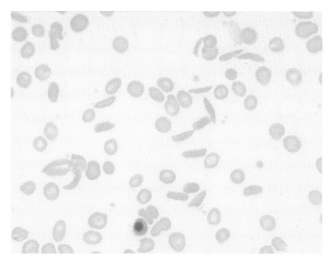

Fig. 12.13 Sickle cell anaemia; note the sickled cells and a nucleated red cell.

addition, aggregation of sickled erythrocytes in the microcirculation leads to **vascular stasis** with possible **infarction**. Large vessels may also, for ill-understood reasons, infarct. Furthermore, intravascular aggregation of sickled cells may cause their **sequestration** in organs such as the liver and spleen with the production of sudden and profound anaemia.

Clinical features

Because of the shortened red cell survival, patients with sickle-cell anaemia run a low haemoglobin level, usually 8–9 g/dl, with a **persistent reticulocytosis** and other features of **chronic haemolysis**. As the oxygen dissociation curve of sickle haemoglobin is shifted to the right, they compensate well and usually lead normal lives. However, the disorder is complicated by acute exacerbations, called **crises**.

Sickle-cell crises are classified as follows:
- **Painful.** Much the commonest type, these are acute exacerbations characterized by severe bone pain. A common presenting symptom is the so-called **hand-and-foot syndrome** which occurs early in infancy and is characterized by a painful **dactylitis**. Later in life the bone pain is particularly marked in the back and limbs. The abdomen is also a common site of pain. These episodes may be set off by infection or cold, although often no precipitating cause can be found.
- **Aplastic.** Occasionally red cell production ceases in the bone marrow; the causative agent is **Parvovirus B19**. Because of the shortened red cell survival, profound anaemia may result.
- **Sequestration.** In infancy these crises are characterized by massive enlargement of the spleen which is full of

sequestered sickled cells; similar episodes may occur in the liver in adults.
- **Lung.** These crises are characterized by chest pain, pulmonary infiltrates seen on chest X-ray and hypoxia due to ventilation–perfusion mismatch. They may be fatal.
- **Haemolytic.** These crises may not be a distinct entity but in many patients with painful crises or infection there is an increased rate of haemolysis and a worsening of anaemia.

As well as these acute episodes, patients with sickle-cell anaemia have **chronic complications** due to tissue damage.

Most patients with sickle-cell anaemia have **splenomegaly** in early childhood, but the spleen atrophies later due to recurrent sickling. These patients are functionally hyposplenic and therefore prone to infection with encapsulated bacteria; prophylactic antibiotics have been shown to prevent death in childhood.

Aseptic necrosis of the femoral or humeral heads may lead to their destruction and renal damage may occur. Recurrent attacks of priapism may lead to permanent deformity of the penis. Repeated infarction may also lead to chronic fibrosis of the liver. Recurrent neurological crises may lead to permanent **brain damage. Retinal damage** may cause blindness. In some parts of the world, leg ulcers are common.

Sickle-cell disease is very variable in its outlook. In rural parts of Africa children rarely survive beyond the first year. On the other hand, in western countries many patients with sickle-cell anaemia survive well into adult life. The commonest cause of death is infection. Many factors modify the condition: elevated levels of fetal haemoglobin and the coexistence of α-thalassaemia ameliorate the condition.

Although the **sickle-cell trait** is harmless it may produce tissue infarction in conditions of **severe hypoxia**. All patients of appropriate racial groups should have a screening test for sickling before anaesthesia.

Sickle-cell crises are managed by rest, analgesia, supplementation with oxygen, transfusion where necessary and appropriate treatment of infection. Couples who have the sickle-cell trait should be offered genetic advice because prenatal diagnosis can be carried out in the first trimester.

Haemoglobin SC disease

This is an important variant of the sickling disorders seen in **West Africans**. Such patients are not as anaemic as those with sickle-cell anaemia but there is a particular tendency for small **microvascular complications** which include aseptic necrosis of the femoral heads, proliferative retinal disease and blindness, and pulmonary infarction, particularly in the postpartum period.

The thalassaemias

The thalassaemias are the commonest genetic disorders in the world and occur at high frequency in a belt extending from Africa through the Mediterranean region, the Middle East, the Indian subcontinent and throughout South-East Aisa.

Pathogenesis

The defect in thalassaemia is a reduced rate of production of either the α or β globin chains of haemoglobin, causing the α- and β-thalassaemias respectively.

The **α-thalassaemias** tend to result from a **gene deletion**. Many different point mutations have been found in the β globin genes of patients with β-**thalassaemia**; premature stop codons, frameshift mutations, defects in the splicing of exons and defects in the regulatory regions outside the structural genes have all been described.

It is useful to divide the thalassaemias into the α^0- and β^0-thalassaemias, in which no gene product is produced, and the α^+- and β^+-thalassaemias, in which some α- and β-chains are produced but at a reduced rate.

β-thalassaemia

Defective β-chain production results in excess α-chain synthesis. The excessive α-chains are unstable and accumulate in the red cell precursors, causing their destruction in the bone marrow. The resulting anaemia leads to increased erythropoietin production and massive proliferation of the marrow. Precursors that do get into the circulation are damaged in the microvasculature of the spleen and liver because they contain α-chain inclusions. Thus the anaemia is primarily **dyserythropoietic**, but with a haemolytic element. There is progressive **splenomegaly** due to bombardment of the spleen with abnormal red cells. The massive expansion of the marrow leads to serious bone deformities with a typical facies, bossing of the skull and thinning and trabeculation of the long bones and bones of the hands and feet.

In **thalassaemia major** there is profound anaemia from about the third month of life, after fetal haemoglobin disappears. If not transfused, patients usually die in the first year of life. If they are transfused the hyperplastic marrow is switched off and growth and development are normal but iron accumulation may cause death at the end of the second decade from myocardial, hepatic and endocrine dysfunction. Regular infusions of the chelating agent desferrioxamine relieve the overload. Encouraging results have been reported for bone marrow transplantation.

The haematological changes are characterized by gross hypochromia and variation in shape and size of the red

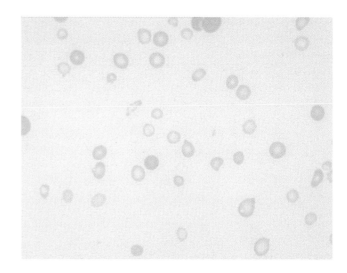

Fig. 12.14 β-thalassaemic cells.

cells (Fig. 12.14) together with a variable increase in fetal haemoglobin. **Heterozygous carriers** have microcytic, hypochromic red cells and mild anaemia with an elevated level of haemoglobin A_2. Cases of **thalassaemia intermedia** have a more severe anaemia but are not, by definition, transfusion-dependent. The disease can be identified prenatally and genetic counselling offered.

α-Thalassaemia

The **normal α-genotype** can be written α α/α α since we receive two α-globin genes from each parent. α^0-Thalassaemia usually results from the deletion of both pairs of α-genes and so a carrier has the genotype $--/\alpha$ α. α^+-Thalassaemia usually results from the deletion of a single α globin gene and so the carrier state can be written $-\alpha/\alpha$ α.

The **homozygous state** for α^0-thalassaemia (genotype $--/--$) is associated with perinatal death at about 38 weeks' gestation or immediately after birth (**hydrops fetalis**). The problem is mainly confined to South-east Asia.

Complete absence of α-globin chains leads to an excess of γ-chains which form γ_4 tetramers (haemoglobin Bart's). This has a very high oxygen affinity and therefore is physiologically useless. Thus these fetuses have severe anaemia due to defective haemoglobin production. The swollen oedematous fetus is a reflection of severe intrauterine hypoxia. Enormously **hypertrophied placentas** make the birth of these stillborn fetuses extremely difficult and there is also a high incidence of **maternal toxaemia** of pregnancy.

When an α^0-thalassaemia determinant is inherited with an α^+-thalassaemia (genotype $--/-\alpha$), **haemoglobin H** disease results. Haemoglobin H is a β_4 tetramer which occurs because of the excess β-chains produced. Patients are moderately anaemic with splenomegaly. Haemoglobin H has a high oxygen affinity and is also unstable and precipitates in the circulation, giving rise to **intracellular inclusions** (Fig. 12.15), which damage the red cells in their passage through the microvasculature. Transfusion may be necessary.

The heterozygous carrier states for α-thalassaemia have microcytic, hypochromic red cells with a normal level of haemoglobin A$_2$ (compare β-thalassaemia). They often cannot be distinguished from normal except by gene mapping.

Pathology of the bone marrow

HAEMOPOIESIS

Figure 12.16 illustrates the developmental relationships between the different types of blood cells. Although lymphoid cells originate from the same stem cell as do the other cell types, their maturation and physiological activities take place mainly outside the bone marrow. As a result, diseases affecting the bone marrow influence the red cell, platelet and myeloid cells rather than the lymphocytes.

All peripheral blood cells arise from **pluripotent haemopoietic stem cells**. An important property of pluripotent cells is **self-renewal**. When required, a stem cell begins to divide and differentiate, losing the capacity for self-renewal. Each pluripotent cell is thus capable of producing an individual clone consisting of a number of red cells, granulocytes, platelets and lymphocytes. Indeed, in mice, normal haemopoiesis has been reconstituted from a single stem cell. Whether and how each stem cell differentiates depends upon a large number of haemopoietic regulatory proteins and their receptors.

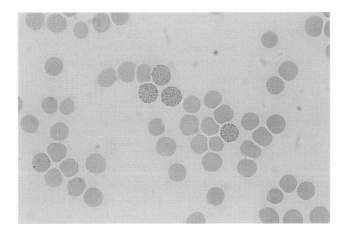

Fig. 12.15 Brilliant cresyl blue stain showing HbH inclusion bodies. The red cells resemble 'golf balls'.

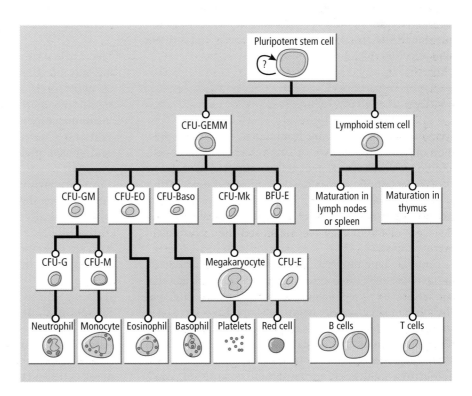

Fig. 12.16 Differentiation pathways of haemopoietic cells.

They seem to form a hierarchy of molecules with increasing levels of specificity for the regulation of all stages of haemopoiesis. However, partly because their effects overlap so much, we are still far from a full understanding of the process.

Recombinant DNA technology has allowed the isolation of many of these proteins and their genes. Each has a varying degree of specificity. For example one protein, granulocyte–macrophage colony-stimulating factor (GM-CSF), is active in stimulating granulocyte and macrophage colonies. More specific proteins, G-CSF and M-CSF, have a higher degree of specificity for granulocytes or macrophages respectively. In addition, some regulatory molecules have more general stimulatory effects on haemopoiesis. These include **interleukins 2** and **3** (IL-2 and IL-3) and **stem cell factor**. Some of these purified proteins are given to patients to stimulate specific aspects of haemopoiesis.

BONE MARROW FAILURE

The normal adult marrow produces about 2×10^{11} red cells (20 ml), 1.0×10^{11} neutrophils and 2×10^{11} platelets each day, and can substantially increase output on demand.

Failure of haemopoiesis results in anaemia, neutropenia, thrombocytopenia, or combinations of these; reduction of all three is termed **pancytopenia**.

Mild impairment of marrow function may become apparent only during times of increased demand, for example due to bleeding or infection. More severe impairment will affect the blood count in the steady state.

Causes of marrow failure

Marrow failure may result from damage to, or suppression of, either pluripotent or committed progenitor cells (Table 12.11). Destruction of cells committed to each line of differentiation, as produced by most cytotoxic drugs used in the treatment of malignant disease, results in general marrow hypoplasia and pancytopenia; but recovery is possible by regeneration from the pluripotent compartment.

Damage to committed, and sometimes to pluripotent, progenitors may also occur in patients taking drugs that are not primarily cytotoxic. Such reactions are rare, and the mechanism is usually obscure. Many drugs have been implicated in blood dyscrasias of this sort. Neutropenia is the most common manifestation, but thrombocytopenia or aplastic anaemia may also occur.

Marrow failure is an important feature of acute leukaemias, the later stages of the chronic leukaemias and myeloproliferative disorders, and the **myelodysplasias**. Again, the mechanism of marrow failure is unclear, but active suppression of normal stem cell clones is probably involved.

Table 12.11 Types and causes of marrow failure.

Types
Aplastic anaemia
Pure red cell aplasia
Selective neutropenia
Selective thrombocytopenia

Primary causes
Acquired aplastic anaemia
Congenital (e.g. Blackfan–Diamond and Fanconi's anaemias, Kostmann's neutropenia)

Secondary causes
Radiation
Cytotoxic drugs
Drug idiosyncracy (especially chloramphenicol, sulphonamides, anti-inflammatories, antimalarials, antithyroids, antiepileptics, phenothiazines and antidepressants)
Chemicals (e.g. benzene)
Autoimmune
Marrow infiltration
Infections

Clinical features

The cardinal signs of marrow failure are anaemia, bleeding and infection. Red cells survive longer than platelets or neutrophils; anaemia thus develops slowly, unless significant bleeding intervenes. Bleeding is typically **thrombocytopenic**, with petechial haemorrhages in skin and mucous membranes. Infection is usually with **commensal organisms** of the skin or gastrointestinal tract.

An early manifestation of developing marrow failure is often a sore throat, or a chest or soft-tissue infection which typically does not respond completely to antibiotics. A blood count should always be performed in such circumstances, or at the first sign of infection in any patient taking drugs known to cause marrow failure.

Investigations

A **full blood count** will detect anaemia, neutropenia or thrombocytopenia. The anaemia is normocytic or macrocytic, and reticulocytes are markedly reduced. Blast cells may be evident in patients with leukaemia, and morphological changes in neutrophils may suggest myelodyplasia.

Severe marrow failure is indicated by a platelet count below $10 \times 10^9/l$ and a neutrophil count below $1.0 \times 10^9/l$. Such patients are at risk from overwhelming septicaemia or severe spontaneous bleeds. The former may occur without signs of focal infection, and the only clinical features may be malaise and fever.

Marrow examination is often necessary to exclude leukaemia or other malignant infiltration. **Trephine biopsies** should be obtained as well as **aspirates**. The marrow is hypocellular or acellular in aplastic anaemia (Fig. 12.17).

Management

Management of patients with marrow failure involves identification and reversal of the underlying cause with supportive care until marrow function is restored. Bleeding and infection due to marrow failure are medical emergencies.

- **Anaemia** is corrected by **transfusion** of packed red cells. The haemoglobin level should be maintained above 8–9 g/dl; haemorrhage is likely at lower levels.
- **Thrombocytopenia**: active bleeding, or platelet counts less than $10 \times 10^9/l$, should be treated with **platelet concentrates**.
- **Neutropenia**: suspected infection should be treated promptly with **broad-spectrum antibiotics**, probably intravenously. A suitable initial choice would be an aminoglycoside and a broad spectrum penicillin.

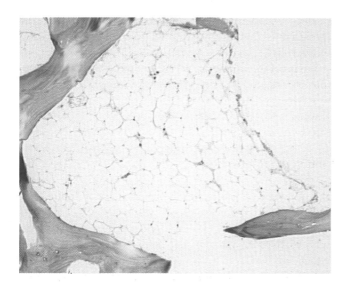

Fig. 12.17 Aplastic anaemia. The marrow has been almost completely replaced by fat cells.

More controversial areas of management include the use of **reverse barrier isolation** and **granulocyte transfusions**. Strict isolation in a sterile environment together with skin and gastrointestinal decontamination has been shown to reduce the risk of acquiring infection, but usually has little impact on the eventual outcome of the underlying disorder. Granulocyte transfusions are now confined to the relatively rare situations in which a proven infection does not respond to appropriate antibiotic therapy.

APLASTIC ANAEMIA

Aplastic anaemia is a rare condition characterized by anaemia, thrombocytopenia and neutropenia with a hypocellular bone marrow (Fig. 12.17). It comprises a heterogeneous group of disorders.

Aetiology and pathogenesis

Aplastic anaemia is usually an acquired disorder, though congenital forms also occur. Many underlying factors have been implicated in the aetiology of aplastic anaemia (see below). However, an underlying cause can be identified in only ~20% of patients, the remainder being **idiopathic**. The disease might result from a defect in either the haemopoietic stem cells (the 'seed') or the marrow microenvironment (the 'soil'). The ability of bone marrow transplantation (BMT) to correct the abnormality suggests that stem cell defects are the commonest causes.

The following are causes of aplastic anaemia:
- **Drugs**: aplastic anaemia may result from an unpredictable idiosyncratic reaction to a drug such as phenylbutazone or chloramphenicol. Aplasia may occur weeks or months after starting treatment. Genetic predisposition probably plays an important role. Some drugs or their metabolites are toxic to haemopoietic precursor cells, while immune-mediated mechanisms may also be important.
- **Chemicals**: benzene and other aromatic hydrocarbons have long been associated with aplastic anaemia. The effect appears idiosyncratic and the mechanism is unknown.
- **Ionizing radiation** is cytotoxic to the marrow in a dose-related fashion. Reversible depletion of stem cells occurs after single doses of 10 Gy or less. Higher doses damage the marrow microenvironment irreversibly, leaving the irradiated areas unable to support haemopoiesis as seen after therapeutic irradiation for malignancy.

- **Infection**: aplastic anaemia may develop concurrently with, or following, a variety of **viral infections**. Most notably, **hepatitis C infection** often precedes marrow aplasia by a few months. This probably accounts for the high rates of aplastic anaemia in the Far East. There is usually accompanying lymphocytopenia and cellular immune deficiency; the virus has been shown to infect lymphocytes. **Parvovirus** infects red cell precursors, causing a transient red cell aplasia which may be serious in chronic haemolytic states. Many infections cause a non-specific depression of haemopoiesis, which is usually not severe.
- **Autoimmune**: the mechanism may be either humoral or cellular. Autoantibodies to haemopoietic stem cells have occasionally been detected; T cells have been occasionally shown to produce suppression *in vitro* of autologous marrow. Several clinical observations support the role of autoimmunity in the pathogenesis of aplastic anaemia. Both pan- and selective cytopenias may occur in association with **SLE** and **thymomas**. Only 50% of those treated by transplantation of bone marrow from identical twin donors recover normal haemopoiesis without intensive immunosuppression. Furthermore, approximately 50% of patients treated with antithymocyte globulin (ATG) or antilymphocyte globulin (ALG) recover without marrow transplantation.
- **Suppressor clones**: it is thought that about 20% of idiopathic cases are explained by the emergence of a suppressor clone. The evidence for this arises from demonstrations that residual haemopoiesis arises from a single, presumably abnormal, clone in about this proportion. Furthermore, about this proportion eventually develop acute myeloid leukaemia after a number of years.

Treatment

The treatment of aplastic anaemia has three major aims:
1 identification and withdrawal of suspected aetiological factors;
2 supportive care with blood products and prompt treatment of infection;
3 specific therapy to restore normal haemopoiesis.

The distinction between severe and less severe forms of the disorder is important in determining **prognosis** and **treatment**. Aplastic anaemia is said to be severe in patients with a hypocellular marrow and two or more of the following:
- a neutrophil count below $0.5 \times 10^9/l$;
- a platelet count below $20 \times 10^9/l$;
- a reticulocyte count below $20 \times 10^9/l$.

Many patients with **mild to moderate aplasia** will re-

cover spontaneously, and others can be successfully supported with transfusions and antibiotics for years. Androgens, such as oxymetholone, improve marrow function in a small proportion of patients with mild or moderate aplastic anaemia, but are ineffective in severe aplasia. Fewer than 10% of patients with **severe aplasia** with recover spontaneously; most of the remainder will die within months without specific therapy. Two forms of effective treatment are marrow transplantation and immunosuppression.

Bone marrow transplantation

BMT restores haemopoiesis by transplantation of stem cells from a normal donor. Results of BMT in aplastic anaemia have improved, with 5-year survival exceeding 80%. The major causes of failure are **graft rejection**, **graft-versus-host disease** (**GvHD**; see Chapter 9), and infections, siuch as interstitial pneumonia, which are related to posttransplant immunodeficiency. Patients with aplastic anaemia require intensive immunosuppressive conditioning prior to transplantation in order to prevent graft rejection.

Most deaths are caused by GvHD, where the donor lymphocytes mediate damage and possible destruction of host skin, gut, liver and lung. It is treated by immunosuppression (e.g. methotrexate, cyclosporin, ATG), but acute GvHD develops in 45% and chronic GvHD in 25–60% of transplant recipients.

Patients who have previously received blood transfusions may be sensitized to antigens present on donor cells and have a higher risk of rejection than other patients. Transfusions should therefore be withheld, if possible, prior to transplant conditioning. If they are necessary, the transfusions should be filtered to remove sensitizing white cells.

Survival in patients undergoing BMT for aplastic anaemia correlates strongly with age; younger patients do much better. Patients over 50 years of age have very poor results.

Immunosuppression

Randomized controlled trials report haematological improvement and prolonged survival in 40–70% of patients treated with ATG, ATG or cyclosporin. Combinations with **corticosteroids** may also be useful. Substantial side-effects to ATG or ALG occur in most patients. These include fever, chills, erythematous or urticarial rashes, hypertension, and a temporary worsening of thrombocytopenia. A few patients exhibit **anaphylaxis**. Serum sickness may occur 6–18 days after the start of therapy.

These adverse effects are controlled with antihistamines and steroids.

Some 1–3 months usually elapse before haematological improvement is detected. Recovery of one or more cell lines may then be observed, but many patients never attain normal blood counts.

Recently, several human haemopoietic growth factors have been used. Granulocyte-macrophage colony-stimulating factor (GM-CSF) and erythropoietin have achieved encouraging results. Early reports have, however, demonstrated the possibility of early transformation to acute leukaemia.

MYELOPROLIFERATIVE DISORDERS

Each of these disorders is probably due to transformation of a marrow progenitor cell, although the proliferative process which follows is often only slowly progressive. Figure 12.18 illustrates the diseases which may arise.

The transforming event, although appearing to affect a committed stem cell (e.g. the red cell lineage in polycythaemia) often occurs at an earlier stage of development, with the consequence that other marrow cell lineages, whilst appearing superficially normal, may also be involved. This has been shown by demonstrating the clonality of the different lineages. Clonality was originally analysed using lyonization or G6PD variants but is now demonstrated using karyotypes or DNA polymorphisms on the X chromosome.

The different **myeloproliferative disorders** thus have more in common with each other than might appear at first sight, and this is illustrated by the existence of intermediate forms and the tendency of one disease to transform to another.

In most clonal disorders of haemopoiesis the abnormal clone appears to outstrip or suppress the normal haemopoietic clones. This is fairly self-evident in the acute leukaemias, where the marrow appears completely replaced by leukaemic blast cells, but is often the case in the myeloproliferative disorders.

Chronic granulocytic leukaemia

Clinical features
The disease occurs only rarely below the age of 20 and slowly increases in incidence thereafter. It affects about 1 per 100 000 adults per year.

Symptoms are often non-specific (e.g. weight loss, lassitude, symptoms of anaemia) and in almost 20% of cases the diagnosis is made by chance. **Splenomegaly** is frequent, so that some patients present with abdominal discomfort or digestive symptoms, or occasionally with pain of pleuritic nature due to splenic infarction. Occasionally **abnormal bleeding** (e.g. menorrhagia, cutaneous haemorrhage) occurs, possibly due to abnormal function of the neoplastic platelets.

Laboratory features
The **granulocyte count** is **elevated**, often markedly. These cells are at all stages of myeloid maturation and include precursors which are normally confined to the bone marrow. There is usually a moderate degree of anaemia but the platelet count is frequently normal or increased (Fig. 12.19). The leucocyte alkaline phosphatase level is low.

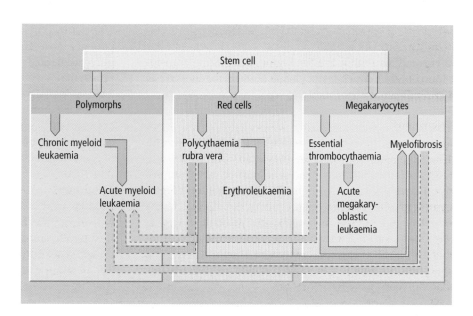

Fig. 12.18 Plan of the myeloproliferative disorders arising from different marrow cells.

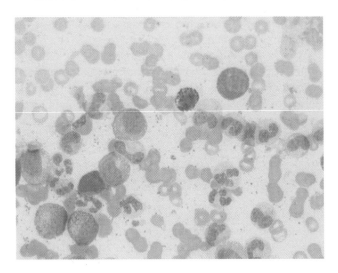

Fig. 12.19 Chronic myeloid leukaemia peripheral blood.

Analysis of blood or bone marrow cells reveals a unique chromosomal abnormality in 95% of cases–the Philadelphia or Ph chromosome (t9;22(q34;q11)). This was the first specific association between a cytogenetic marker and a human malignancy to be discovered. The 9;22 translocation has been studied in considerable detail and shown to cause juxtaposition of most of the *c-abl* proto-oncogene on chromosome 9 with another gene (*bcr*) on chromosome 22. The hybrid *bcr/abl* product has greatly enhanced protein kinase activity and plays a direct role in the abnormal proliferation of the neoplastic clone, switching on the ras pathway.

In almost every case of Ph-positive chronic granulocytic leukaemia, nearly all haemopoietic cells are Ph-positive at the time of diagnosis and usually remain so even during periods of clinical remission. A few clinically typical cases of chronic granulocytic leukaemias are Ph-negative but molecular analysis has shown similar abnormalities within the *bcr* region, suggesting translocation of DNA which is not visible to the cytogeneticist as a chromosomal abnormality.

Treatment

The ribonucleotide reductase inhibitor **hydroxyurea** and alkylating agent **busulphan** (**Myleran**) are commonly used during the chronic phase and reduce the white cell count and produce symptomatic improvement. Treatment with α-**interferon** often controls the disease, to the extent of making the malignant cells difficult to detect, and gives a survival advantage over conventional chemotherapy. BMT is the only treatment shown to cure the condition. Its role is generally confined to patients less than 50 years for whom a suitable donor can be found.

The acute transformation may be treatable with aggressive chemotherapy but the prognosis is poor.

Clinical course

Despite the initially indolent behaviour of this disease, the median survival of patients is about 4 years, due to the transformation in about 20% of cases per year from the chronic phase to an aggressive accelerated phase or to frank **blast crisis**. Only two-thirds of these acute leukaemias are of myeloid type, the remainder being of lymphoblastic origin, providing further evidence that the neoplastic transforming event occurs in a primitive marrow cell.

Polycythaemia rubra vera (primary proliferative polycythaemia)

Clinical features

The disease occurs most frequently in patients over the age of 50. They usually appear **red-faced**, but the skin is often rather dusky and **cyanotic** in hue. Non-specific symptoms (e.g. night sweats, headaches) may be reported and skin itching, especially after a bath, is common. The increased haematocrit may cause neurological symptoms such as headache, dizziness, vertigo and tinnitus. There is an increased risk of thrombosis and also of haemorrhage, probably due to abnormal platelet function exacerbated by the high haematocrit. Other features include splenomegaly and hyperuricaemia leading, in some cases, to **gout**.

Laboratory features

The most important feature is an elevated red cell mass, which is reflected in an increased haemoglobin and haematocrit. A concomitant **iron deficiency** is common. The neutrophil and platelet counts are raised in most patients and this may be helpful in distinguishing polycythaemia rubra vera (PRV) from other causes of polycythaemia. The **leucocyte alkaline phosphatase** level is usually high. Other causes of polycythaemia should be considered. These can be categorized into appropriate causes of high erythropoietin levels (e.g. chronic hypoxia) or inappropriate ectopic production (e.g. renal tumours).

Treatment

Regular venesection (removing a pint of blood at a time) will lower the haemoglobin level, reducing the risk of thrombotic complications. Longer-term therapy may be achieved by administering gentle **oral chemotherapy** or ^{32}P, an isotope which irradiates and suppresses the marrow. Response to this isotope lasts several years.

Clinical course

The disease is only slowly progressive and survival for 10–20 years is not unusual. However, patients remain at risk from thrombosis and haemorrhage unless the haemoglobin level is reduced. The relationship of the disease to other myeloproliferative disorders is evidenced by the tendency to transform, after a period, to **acute leukaemia** (10–20% of patients) or to **myelofibrosis** (about a third of patients)

Myelofibrosis

The striking feature of this disorder is progressive accumulation of fibrous tissue in the bone marrow, replacing normal marrow. Haemopoietic function is taken over by the spleen and liver, both of which show marked enlargement. Initially thought to be a disorder of fibroblasts, it is now believed to be **secondary** to fibroblast-stimulating growth factors released by abnormal megakaryocytic cells. The disease is thus related to essential thrombocythaemia (see below) and to the megakaryoblastic form of acute leukaemia.

Clinical features

Patients are usually elderly and present with symptoms of anaemia. The spleen is frequently massively enlarged and this may be directly responsible for symptoms.

Laboratory features

The patient is usually anaemic, and white cell and platelet counts are normal or high. A characteristic finding is a **leukoerythroblastic anaemia**, in which the peripheral blood contains immature erythroid cells (**normoblasts**) and myeloid cells (**metamyelocytes** and **myelocytes**). In addition, red cell morphology is abnormal, with marked variation in size and shape and the presence of 'tear-drop' cells (Fig. 12.20). Attempts to aspirate marrow are usually unsuccessful ('dry tap'); a trephine biopsy will reveal marked **fibrosis**.

Treatment

Blood transfusions will maintain the haemoglobin level. **Splenectomy** may be considered if transfusion demands become excessive, if there are symptoms due to the large spleen, or if the platelet count is greatly reduced. When the spleen becomes very large it tends to lower the haemoglobin, white cells and platelets because of splenic pooling and red cell destruction (**hypersplenism**). However, the spleen may also be contributing substantially to the production of red cells. The loss of its haemopoietic function must be balanced against the benefits of its removal.

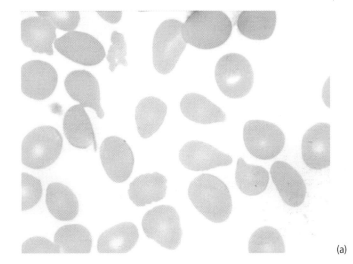

(a)

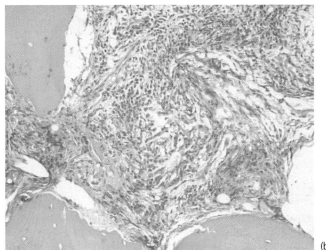

(b)

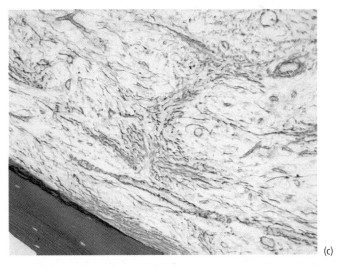

(c)

Fig. 12.20 Myelofibrosis showing: (a) tear drop poikilocytes in peripheral blood; (b) fibrosis in the bone marrow as seen by the whorled appearance; and (c) increased reticulin staining.

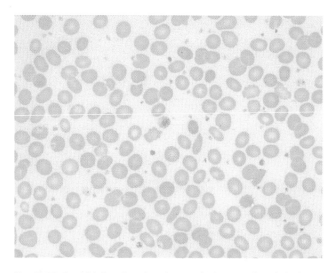

Fig. 12.21 Essential thrombocythaemia; note the large number of platelets and their varied sizes.

Clinical course

Median survival is ~3 years, but many patients may live much longer. Occasional patients transform to an acute leukaemia.

Essential thrombocythaemia

In this disorder the platelet count is high and may exceed $1000 \times 10^9/1$ (Fig. 12.21). There is a risk both of **thrombosis** and also of **haemorrhage** (probably due to abnormal platelet function). Presentation is as a result of these phenomena, by chance or through the symptom of strange aches in the extremities. The white cell count is normal or increased and the haemoglobin level is either increased, indicating the relationship of this disorder to polycythaemia rubra vera, or reduced due to gastrointestinal haemorrhage. Treatment is with aspirin, ^{32}P or gentle oral chemotherapy. The disease tends to progress to **myelofibrosis**.

BONE MARROW MALIGNANCIES

Myelodysplasia

This is a group of disorders characterized by ineffective production of one or more haemopoietic cell lines, due to a haemopoietic clone which shows abnormal differentiation and maturation characteristics.

Clinical features

These conditions affect predominantly the elderly. They may present with symptoms of anaemia or bleeding, but are not infrequently discovered as a result of investigation of some other problem. The spleen may be palpable, but is never grossly enlarged. The leucocyte count is usually normal or low, with **neutropenia** and sometimes **monocytosis**. Neutrophils may be **hyposegmented** or show **defective granulation** (Fig. 12.22).

Thrombocytopenia is often a feature and there may be atypical giant platelets present. The marrow is usually hyperplastic with **dyserythropoiesis**, i.e. many of the nucleated red cells may have multiple nuclei or resemble megaloblasts (Fig. 12.23).

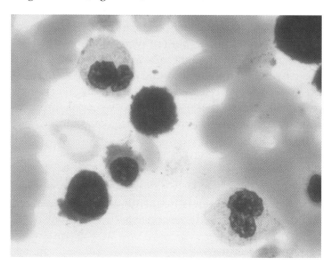

Fig. 12.22 Myelodysplasia. Hypogranular and hyposegmented neutrophils are termed Pelger–Huet forms. In the marrow, both dysplastic myeloid and erythroid cells are seen.

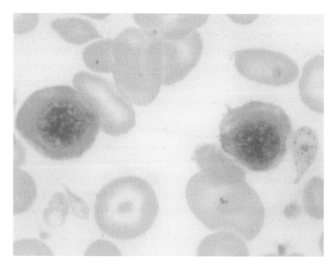

Fig. 12.23 Megalobastic change and dyserythropoiesis in myelodysplasia. Note the basophilic stippling in one red cell and the thin interchromatin bridge.

Ring sideroblasts (Fig. 12.3) (i.e. red cell precursors containing granular deposits of iron caused by defective haem synthesis) are found in about 20% of cases. There may be some increase in blast cells but not sufficient to make the diagnosis of overt leukaemia.

The myelodysplastic syndromes evolve into frank **acute myeloid leukaemia** over a period of a few years. Leukaemic progression occurs more commonly in patients having a high proportion of blasts in the marrow at presentation, and in those with cytogenetic abnormalities.

ACUTE LEUKAEMIA

Acute leukaemias are characterized by the accumulation of malignant haemopoietic cells in the bone marrow and, to a variable degree, in the peripheral blood. Acute leukaemias differ from chronic leukaemias in that they are more rapidly progressive and the neoplastic cells are immature white cells (**blast** cells), in contrast to the mature white cells which predominate in chronic leukaemias.

Causes

Acute leukaemias are due to an abnormality (e.g. a base mutation, a chromosomal translocation) in the **genome** of a **white cell precursor**, leading to its uncontrolled proliferation as a clone of neoplastic cells which tend to replace and suppress other marrow cells. Many specific abnormalities have now been described – indeed, far too many to list. More than one genetic event is necessary in **leukaemogenesis**.

The risk of such neoplastic or preneoplastic chromosomal events may be increased by a variety of factors, such as **radiation**, certain **chemicals** (e.g. benzene), and **drugs** (particularly cytotoxic). Although leukaemias caused by viruses have been widely studied in animals, they are uncommon as a predisposing element in leukaemia in most parts of the world. However, the retrovirus **human T-lymphotrophic virus I (HTLV-I)** appears to predispose to T-cell leukaemia/lymphoma in Southern Japan and the Caribbean.

Classification

The important distinction is between myeloid and lymphoid leukaemia. Both of these types of acute leukaemia can be subclassified as shown in Table 12.12.

Table 12.12 Classification of acute leukaemia.

Acute myeloid leukaemia (AML; Fig. 12.24, p. 217)	
M0	Undifferentiated
M1	Myeloblastic without maturation
M2	Myeloblastic with maturation to neutrophils
M3	Promyelocytic, hypergranular
M4	Myelomonocytic
M5a	Monocytic–poorly differentiated
M5b	Monocytic–well-differentiated
M6	Erythroleukaemia
M7	Megakaryocytic leukaemia

Acute lymphoblastic leukaemia (ALL; Fig. 12.25, p. 217)
A classification based on morphology (L1, L2, L3) has been replaced by a lineage-based system:
CALLA (CD10) positive. 70% of cases. These are early B-lineage cells as demonstrated by antigen expression and Ig gene rearrangement; best prognosis
T cell. 20% of cases. Often associated with mediastinal disease and a high WBC
Late B cell. Uncommon, e.g. Burkitt's lymphoma
Null cell. 9% of cases. No specific lineage markers expressed

Ig, Immunoglobulin; WBC, white blood cell count; CALLA, common ALL antigen.

Clinical features

Acute lymphoblastic leukaemia (ALL) is commonest in children, with a peak around 3 years. Its frequency then declines sharply with age, although there is a second smaller peak in adult life.

AML is seen most commonly in adults, its frequency rising with increasing age.

Presentation is usually as a result of marrow failure (see previously). Bone pain, in contrast to multiple myeloma, occurs only infrequently. Childhood ALL may present with joint and bone pain, and a misdiagnosis of viral arthralgia, septic arthritis or seronegative arthritis may initially be made.

Acute leukaemia cells may infiltrate extramedullary tissues, more commonly in ALL than in AML; the tissues most frequently involved are lymph nodes, spleen, liver and meninges. AML-M5 type shows a tendency to infiltrate **gums**. AML-M3 type may present with **DIC**. T-cell ALL may sometimes present with superior vena caval obstruction and mediastinal compression due to massive enlargement of the thymus.

Laboratory features

The peripheral white count is usually markedly elevated,

most of the cells being primitive blast cells. Occasionally, leukaemic cells are almost undetectable in peripheral blood ('aleukaemic leukaemia'). However, in such cases the marrow is heavily infiltrated with malignant cells.

Because of the differing clinical behaviour of the two sorts of leukaemia it is important to distinguish ALL from AML. Although there are some morphological differences, it is usually necessary to use immunological and cytochemical markers, as shown below.

Treatment

The aim of cytotoxic therapy in acute leukaemia is to destroy all detectable leukaemic cells in the bone marrow, blood and elsewhere. If the patient enters **remission**, consolidation or maintenance treatment is then given, with the aim of killing off residual leukaemic cells and preventing subsequent **relapse**.

Acute myeloid leukaemia

The treatment of AML typically involves about four monthly cycles of therapy. Details of treatment regimens are not important; the standard drugs are an Anthracycline (e.g. Daunorubicin), cytosine arabinoside and a third variable agent. Each cycle renders the patient severely pancytopenic, which requires extensive support, as outlined earlier. Approximately 75% of patients will obtain a complete remission of treatment, although relapse is frequent and the 5-year survival is less than 30%. The chances of success diminish with age and careful consideration should be given before treating patients over the age of 70 years.

BMT is an option for selected young patients for whom a human leucocyte antigen (HLA)-matched donor is available, usually a sibling. Transplants from HLA-mismatched family members or from HLA-matched unrelated donors are performed but remain risky experimental procedures.

Acute promyelocytic leukaemia (M3) can enter remission with oral *all-trans* retinoic acid, without the risks of DIC that otherwise characterize M3 leukaemia treatment. The drug has been shown to bind to, and normalize the function of, the aberrant protein produced at the t(15;17) breakpoint. Unfortunately, without additional conventional chemotherapy all cases relapse.

Acute lymphoblastic leukaemia

Treatment has three components:
1 induction chemotherapy to obtain remission;
2 maintenance (outpatient) chemotherapy to maintain remission – this treament continues for around 2 years;

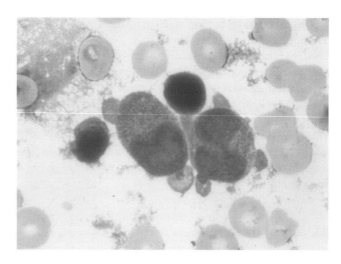

Fig. 12.24 Acute myeloid leukaemia; blast cells typical of type M3 are shown.

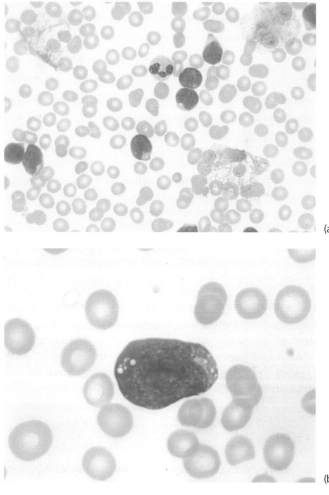

Fig. 12.25 Acute lymphoblastic leukaemia: (a) typical blast cells; and (b) cells of Burkitt's type are shown.

3 central nervous system treatment with radiotherapy and intrathecal methotrexate.

As with AML, the details of the treatment protocols are not important to you. However, vincristine, prednisolone and 6-mercaptopurine remain the backbone of treatment.

The majority of patients (> 90%) will obtain a complete remission and approximately 50% can expect to be cured. Adults have a much worse prognosis than children, the reasons for which are not clear.

Side-effects. Bone marrow failure is an integral part of treatment. Other complications include alopecia; nausea and vomiting; diarrhoea; oral ulceration; and infertility. A specific common side-effect of vincristine is neurotoxicity, which presents with both numbness in the fingers and toes and constipation.

Acute leukaemia is an unpleasant disease requiring unpleasant treatment. A great deal of support needs to be given to the patient and his or her family. Patients who die usually do so with relapsed or resistant leukaemia and the cause of death is often infection and/or bleeding. It should not be painful.

CHRONIC LEUKAEMIAS

Introduction

In this condition, neoplastic mature small lymphoid cells accumulate relatively slowly. They are usually a type of B cell. Patients, usually elderly, frequently present incidentally with a high lymphocyte count. Alternatively, they may complain of painless lymphadenopathy, which has often developed over a period of months or years. On examination the **spleen** is often **enlarged**, and hepatomegaly may also be present.

The accumulation of lymphoid cells interferes with normal lymphoid function, resulting in **hypogamma-globulinaemia** and a **susceptibility to infections**, most commonly in the chest and sinuses. Occasionally, by a mechanism which is not understood, **autoantibodies** against the patient's own blood cells are produced, causing an **autoimmune haemolytic anaemia** or **thrombocytopenia**.

Chronic lymphocytic leukaemia

In most cases the bone marrow is infiltrated, but this is often not sufficient to cause more than mild anaemia. Only in more advanced disease is severe marrow depression observed.

The disease can be staged – patients can be categorized in terms of how extensive the disease is at the time of presentation. This classification (often referred to as the **Rai staging**, after its originator) is made as shown in Table 12.13.

Table 12.13 Rai staging of chronic lymphocytic leukaemia.

Stage	Characteristics	Median survival
0	Absolute lymphocytosis >15 × 10⁹/l	>10 years
I	As stage 0 plus enlarged lymph nodes	>8 years
II	As stage 0 plus enlarged liver and/or spleen	<7 years
III	As stage 0 plus anaemia (Hb < 11 g/dl)	2–5 years
IV	As stage 0 plus thrombocytopenia (platelets <100 × 10⁹/l)	<2 years

Hb, Haemoglobin.

Treatment is often unnecessary because of the benign nature of the disease. When therapy is required, because of the volume of neoplastic lymph nodes or because of marrow suppression, steroids and/or oral alkylating agents (**chlorambucil** or **cyclophosphamide**) are given. This treatment is relatively non-toxic and patients are usually followed as outpatients. **Radiotherapy** may be given to large local masses. Patients often die from unrelated conditions.

Laboratory features

There is an increased lymphocyte count, with the blood film showing numerous small lymphocytes, some of which are disrupted to form characteristic **smear** cells (Fig. 12.26). If anaemia is present, it is usually of **normochromic normocytic** type. On the rare occasions

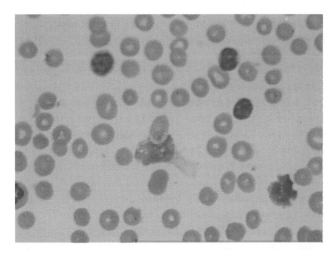

Fig. 12.26 Chronic lymphocytic leukaemia; the cells are mature and fragile.

that lymph node biopsy is performed (the diagnosis usually being evident from peripheral blood examination) diffuse replacement of normal tissue architecture by small lymphocytes is seen.

On immunological analysis with monoclonal antibodies, most cases are shown to be of B-cell type (subtype CD5+). These cells carry surface membrane immunoglobulin of a single light chain class (in contrast to normal B cells which are a heterogeneous mixture of κ- and λ-bearing cells). Occasional atypical cases of chronic lymphocytic leukaemia are of mature T-cell type.

Myeloma

Pathogenesis

A mutant B lymphoid clone is present from which many of the cells differentiate to the plasma cell stage. The proliferating cells diffusely infiltrate the bone marrow (Fig. 12.27).

Myeloma cells may secrete an osteoclast-stimulating factor (probably tumour necrosis factor) leading to characteristic punched-out bony erosions (Fig. 12.28).

The main sites of myeloma involvement in the skeleton mirror the normal distribution of normal marrow—the skull, vertebral column, thoracic cage, pelvis and proximal long bones.

Myeloma cells synthesize and release immunoglobulin. However, in contrast to normal polyclonal immunoglobulin, all the molecules produced by a myeloma clone are identical; a sharply defined band (**M-band** or **paraprotein**) is seen on **protein electrophoresis** of plasma.

In at least half of myeloma cases, an excess of light immunoglobulin chains is synthesized by the neoplastic plasma cells (in about 20% of myeloma cases, this is the only immunoglobulin product). Free light chains in the serum are filtered by the kidney and partially reabsorbed. Severe damage ensues; renal failure is an important cause of death in myeloma.

Clinical features

Patients are usually over the age of 50. The principal symptom is usually **bone pain**, almost always in bones which bear weight or are subjected to stress (e.g. vertebrae). Other clinical features include **infection** (due to suppresssion of normal antibody production), most frequently respiratory; anaemia; renal failure and **pathological fractures**. On clinical examination, bony tenderness is often present.

Occasionally, **solitary masses** are formed that may be extramedullary (the more usual type of myeloma is often called **multiple myeloma**). In contrast to most other

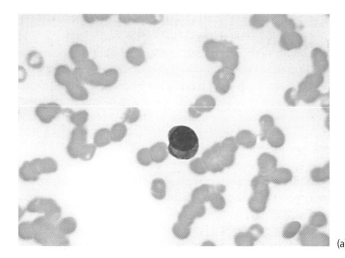

(a)

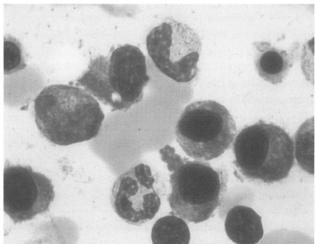

(b)

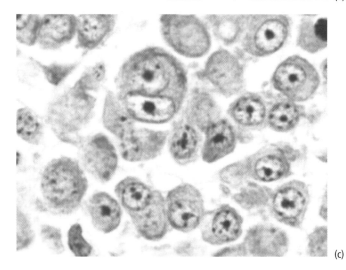

(c)

Fig. 12.27 Myeloma: (a) Gross rouleaux formation in the peripheral blood with a circulating plasma cell; numerous and dysplastic plasma cells are seen in: (b) a marrow aspirate; and (c) a trephine.

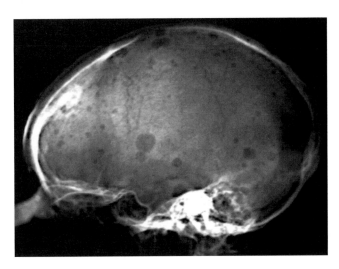

Fig. 12.28 'Pepperpot' skull showing numerous punched out lesions typical of myeloma.

lymphoproliferative disorders, lymphadenopathy and splenomegaly are exceptional. High levels of a paraprotein may cause a hyperviscosity syndrome with cardiac failure, confusion, haemorrhage (e.g. epistaxis) and engorged retinal veins.

Investigations

- **Haematology.** There is mild to moderate anaemia. White blood cell count and platelets are usually normal. There is a high erythrocyte sedimentation rate and rouleaux formation, both due to the paraprotein. The bone marrow is infiltrated by neoplastic plasma cells.
- **Biochemistry.** Blood urea and creatinine may be raised. Hypercalcaemia is frequent but alkaline phosphatase levels remain low, in contrast to other cases of malignant hypercalcaemia.

 A **monoclonal M-band** is almost always found by electrophoresis from serum and/or urine. Rare examples of non-secretory myeloma are seen. About two-thirds of serum paraproteins are of IgG class, the remainder almost all IgA. Suppression of background normal immunoglobulin is usually present (**immune paresis**).
- **Radiology.** Punched-out erosive lesions are often seen. Fractures and vertebral collapse are common.

Treatment

In younger patients aggressive combination chemotherapy is increasingly used, sometimes followed by some form of **transplantation**. The cure rate is still <10%. In the much commoner form in elderly patients, oral alkylating agents, e.g. melphalan, often accompanied by prednisolone, induce clinical remission in 60–70% of cases. The disease then enters a quiescent plateau phase; however, remission tends to be of limited duration and relapse, often drug-resistant, usually occurs within a few years.

Waldenström's macroglobulinaemia

In this rare lymphoid neoplasm the tumour cells secrete IgM and have the **lymphoplasmacytoid** morphology of plasma cell precursors. Clinically the picture varies widely, some cases being aggressive, others benign. IgM paraprotein may cause symptoms due to **increased serum viscosity**.

Benign paraproteinaemia

Monoclonal imunoglobulins can occasionally be found in the serum of healthy individuals, the frequency increasing with age (Fig. 12.29). Such patients should not be given an inappropriate diagnosis of myeloma. Correct diagnosis involves showing the absence of classical features of myeloma, e.g. marrow plasma cell infiltration, bony destruction and immune paresis. Over many years, some benign paraproteinaemias evolve into myeloma.

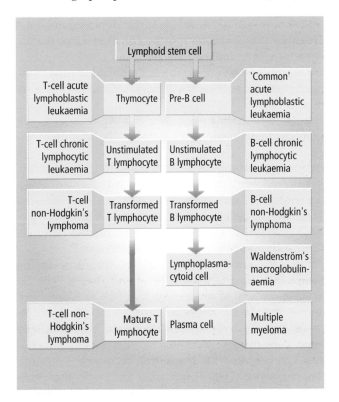

Fig. 12.29 A simplified scheme of lymphoid cells and their neoplastic counterparts.

Bleeding disorders

Defects in the vascular and platelet phases of haemostasis result in spontaneous subcutaneous (purpura) and mucous membrane bleeding. On the other hand defects in the coagulation pathway usually require some form of **trauma** to produce bleeding and, because of the relatively normal reaction of the platelets and vessel wall, the bleeding is often delayed. If there is breakdown of both platelet and coagulation mechanisms, a state of **generalized haemostatic failure** occurs with spontaneous bleeding from a wide variety of sites.

The purpuras

Purpuras may be divided into **vascular** and **thrombocytopenic** purpuras. The vascular purpuras result from damage to the vessel wall and may occur in infection, allergic states including drugs or Henoch–Schönlein purpura, vitamin C deficiency, as part of the process of ageing (senile purpura) or where there is local increased venous pressure.

Thrombocytopenic purpuras can be divided into **immune** and **non-immune** forms. The former are usually **autoimmune** conditions, often associated with disorders such as SLE. **Drugs** may also produce a genuine immune thrombocytopenia. The non-immune thrombocytopenias are either congenital or due to conditions in which there is bone marrow failure (see above).

Thrombocytopenic purpura is, in general, related to the level of the platelet count; spontaneous bleeding is common when the platelet count falls below $10 \times 10^9/l$. Life-threatening bleeding may occur intracranially or in the gastrointestinal tract.

Idiopathic thrombocytopenic purpura
In **children** this is usually an **acute self-limiting** disorder occurring after viral illnesses such as rubella or measles. The child is usually purpuric with a platelet count of $10 \times 10^9/l$ or less. No specific treatment is usually required. Corticosteroids may be used for severe cases.

In **adults**, however, it is classically a **chronic relapsing** illness. It is important in the older age group to look for evidence of related diseases such as **SLE** or **lymphoma**, and a history of relevant drugs (thiazides, quinine, ranitidine). The few platelets in the blood film are usually large. Bone marrow aspiration reveals a large number of small megakaryocytes, suggesting peripheral consumption of platelets. Platelet antibodies are usually present in idiopathic thrombocytopenic purpura (ITP). The clinical presentation is often **insidious** with haemorrhage and bruising.

If the platelet count is only moderately reduced (e.g. $50–100 \times 10^9/l$) treatment is usually not warranted unless there is a special indication such as pregnancy or operation. However, treatment is needed if the patient is symptomatic or the count is dangerously low. **Corticosteroids** are the normal first-line therapy; other steroid-sparing immunosuppressives such as azathioprine and cyclophosphamide are also used in conjunction with prednisolone.

Recurrent episodes of thrombocytopenia, or the need to give unacceptably high levels of steroids to maintain remission, may necessitate a **splenectomy**. This is curative in some patients, while in others the disease persists, though hopefully with a higher platelet count than before splenectomy.

Treatment by intravenous infusion of **human gammaglobulin** is nearly always effective, but its effect only lasts a few weeks. The mechanism behind this therapy is presumed to be reticuloendothelial blockade preventing uptake of antibody-coated platelets. The roles of this expensive therapy are in emergencies and preparation for operation.

Thrombotic thrombocytopenic purpura
This rare syndrome, more common in women, is characterized by the triad of fluctuating neurological dysfunction, renal impairment and thrombocytopenia.

Haematologically, a microangiopathic haemolytic anaemia (Fig. 12.30) is present, characterized by fragmented red cells which have been physically sheared by passage through vessels which contain multiple small thrombi. The platelet count is low, because of consumption in the microthrombi. Haemolysis causes an el-

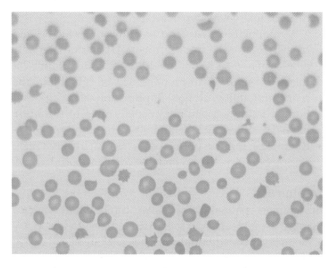

Fig. 12.30 Microangiopathic haemolytic anaemia, note the fragmentation of red cells and absence of platelets.

evated lactate dehydrogenase (LDH) and bilirubin, but clotting tests are usually normal. The disease is probably caused by endothelial cell damage.

Management depends upon **plasmapheresis** using **fresh frozen plasma**, together with **corticosteroids** and **aspirin**. The nature of the inhibitor/activator in fresh frozen plasma is as yet undetermined.

Haemolytic–uraemic syndrome

Haemolytic–uraemic syndrome (HUS) is a condition similar to thrombotic thrombocytopenic purpura (TTP) but is found in children after a viral infection or gastroenteritis caused by a verotoxin-producing pathogen, usually *Escherichia coli*. It is manifested by a microangiopathic haemolytic anaemia, thrombocytopenia and deteriorating renal function. Specific bacterial toxins damage endothelial cells, promoting thrombosis, especially in the kidney. The treatment is **dialysis** for severe cases until renal function improves.

INHERITED BLEEDING DISORDERS

The haemophilias

Haemophilia A or classical haemophilia is an X-linked recessive bleeding disorder and is due to a deficiency of factor VIII in the blood.

Haemophilia B or **Christmas disease** is a related bleeding disorder due to deficiency of factor IX, also X-linked. The genes responsible for synthesis of factors VIII and IX have been cloned: the factor VIII gene is 180 kb long and encodes a protein comprising 2332 amino acids. The factor IX gene is 34 kb long and encodes a protein comprising 415 amino acids.

Haemophilia breeds true in a family, so that in some families all affected members are severely affected whereas in other families all affected members are mildly affected. However, one-third of cases arise from new mutations in families without a previous family history.

It is usually possible to detect the carrier state using clotting factor assays for factor VIII or IX and molecular genetic methods to detect the mutations or genomic polymorphisms. Antenatal diagnosis can therefore be offered.

Incidence

Although uncommon, both disorders are relatively common compared to most other single-gene disorders. This is explained by the X-linkage and and complexity of the underlying genes. Thus the prevalence of haemophilia A in the UK is approximately 90 per million of the population while that of haemophilia B is 16 per million. There are approximately 5000 haemophilia A patients and 1000 haemophilia B patients in the UK.

Clinical features

Because the first-line haemostatic mechanisms are intact, haemophiliac bleeding is often delayed and follows trauma. The severity of bleeding in the haemophilias is related to the level of factor VIII or factor IX in the blood.

Approximately half of all haemophiliacs in the UK are severely affected with no detectable factor VIII or IX in their blood. The principal bleeding symptoms include prolonged bleeding following accidental injury or surgery and repeated, often spontaneous, bleeding into joints and muscles. The latter type of bleeding is the main feature of severe haemophilia and can occur two to three times per week and, if not treated effectively quickly, leads to severe crippling deformities, local nerve damage and the formation of large cysts. Bleeding from the gut and the renal tract occurs less frequently but may be serious, while bleeding in the region round the mouth may track and cause asphyxiation. Cerebral haemorrhage is uncommon but was the commonest cause of death before the advent of acquired immunodeficiency syndrome (AIDS).

Treatment

Bleeding is treated by giving **transfusions** of material rich in **factor VIII** or **IX**. In the past cryoprecipitate was used, but now freeze-dried lyophilized concentrates prepared from large pools of 1500–5000 donations are used; **recombinant product** is also available. Mild haemophiliacs may respond to DDAVP (see later).

The usual practice in the UK is to give factor VIII (or IX) on demand as soon as possible after onset of bleeding. Regular **long-term prophylaxis** is useful in Christmas disease but is not so commonly used in haemophilia A.

Because of the need for early transfusion therapy, most severely affected patients receive treatment at home. In the case of children aged about 5 years or more, the mother is trained to reconstitute the dose, to carry out venepuncture and adminster the dose. Older patients adminster the dose to themselves.

Complications

Coagulation factor replacement may be accompanied by undesirable side-effects. These include development of antibodies to factor VIII: 5% of severely affected patients are affected. As a consequence the patient becomes resistant to standard therapy, and requires larger doses of factor VIII. Porcine factor VIII may also be useful in such cases.

Hepatitis B and C transmission has now been virtually eliminated since routine screening for the viruses. In addition, all haemophiliacs are vaccinated against hepatitis B. However, many haemophiliacs have been infected with hepatitis C. Some of these patients develop **cirrhosis**. Heat-treated concentrates carry no apparent risk of transmission of hepatitis. For those patients with chronic liver disease, interferon has proved useful in reducing hepatic inflammation and may even eradicate the virus.

Approximately one-third of all haemophiliacs in the UK were infected with **human immunodeficiency virus (HIV)** between 1979 and 1985. Following the introdution of **heat-treated concentrate** in 1985 there is now no detectable risk of transmission of HIV to those patients free of infection. AIDS is now the commonest cause of death amongst haemophiliacs in the UK. Cohort studies have shown that some 40% of infected patients progress to AIDS after a 10-year period. HIV may be transmitted to the sexual partners of infected patients: approximately 5% of female sexual partners have been infected.

Other inherited bleeding disorders

Von Willebrand's disease

This disease usually has an **autosomal dominant** pattern of inheritance. Von Willebrand factor (vWF) acts as the main plasma carrier for factor VIII and so the latter's level is also reduced. It is characterized clinically by prolonged skin bleeding times, bleeding from mucous membranes and superficial cuts. There is reduced aggregation of platelets by ristocetin. The disease may be treated by giving transfusion of cryoprecipitate to raise the level of vWF–factor VIII complex. More easily, infusion of **DDAVP** (a synthetic derivative of desmopressin) may cause release of sufficient endothelial vWF–factor VIII to normalize the abnormalities.

It is possible to classify von Willebrand's disease into subtypes by studying the multimer pattern of vWF following electrophoresis and platelet responsiveness to ristocetin.

Deficiencies of factors I (fibrinogen), II, V, VII, X, XI and XIII

These disorders are very uncommon. Bleeding is usually less severe than in haemophilia and follows injury; bleeding into joints is not common.

Factor XIII deficiency probably causes the most severe bleeding. Delayed wound healing with scarring occurs. **Cerebral haemorrhage** occurs in 25–30% of cases. The deficiency is therefore treated prophylactically by giving factor XIII concentrate every month.

Acquired clotting factor deficiencies

These are common. **Vitamin K deficiency** may occur in **neonates** or in adults with **malabsorption**. It results in impaired carboxylation of factors II, VII, IX and X. Oral **anticoagulants** of the coumarin group (e.g. warfarin) interfere with the vitamin K cycle and produce effects identical to those seen with deficiency of the vitamin.

Liver disease plays a complex role in blood coagulation, being the site responsible for the synthesis of many clotting factors. A wide variety of coagulation abnormalities is seen in patients with liver disease and, in addition, thrombocytopenia is common.

Generalized haemostatic failure

The most common cause is triggering of the entire coagulation system leading to the syndrome of **DIC**. Production of thrombin leads to formation of **intravascular fibrin** with secondary activation of the fibrinolytic system. These, in turn, lead to consumption of many of the clotting factors and platelets. Spontaneous bleeding often occurs from the skin and gastrointestinal tract; dry venepuncture sites may start to bleed again even after several days.

The main triggers are **obstetric disease** such as septic abortions, amniotic fluid embolism, intrauterine death; **septicaemias**, **malignancy** (especially disseminated carcinoma and promyelocytic leukaemia) and **shock**. Laboratory investigations usually reveal a prolongation of all clotting tests with low fibrinogen and elevated fibrin degradation products, accompanied by a low platelet count. There may also be some red cell fragmentation seen (Fig. 12.9), but this is not always present.

The treatment of DIC involves treatment or removal of the underlying cause, e.g. removal of a dead fetus, treatment of septicaemia with intravenous antibiotics, resuscitation of the shocked patient. It is also conventional to compensate for the consumption of haemostatic factors (e.g. with fresh frozen plasma, cryoprecipitate and platelets) until the underlying cause has been effectively treated.

The stimulus for fibrin deposition in the circulation may be **thromboplastins** released from the placenta, **endotoxin** from a Gram-negative septicaemia causing vascular endothelial damage or **aberrant expression of tissue factor** by stimulated monocytes. The fibrinolytic enzyme system is also activated; conditions such as carcinoma of the prostate and colon have hyperplasminaemia as the main feature. Release of plasminogen activators when surgery is performed on these organs can cause hyperplasminaemic haemorrhage.

DIC has been treated in the past with heparin or a fibrinolytic inhibitor (ε-aminocaproic acid), but there is little evidence for their beneficial value in most cases. It is important to realize that laboratory results apparently indicative of haemostatic failure can be due to iatrogenic reasons, such as overdosage with heparin (often contamination from indwelling lines used to sample blood) or warfarin, or to massive blood transfusion causing dilution of clotting factors and platelets. Further laboratory tests and the clinical setting should distinguish these from DIC (though the treatment may be similar).

Thrombophilia

Inherited abnormalities of the clotting inhibitory pathways are not believed to underlie most cases of thrombosis occurring in clinical practice. When, however, unusual features are observed, a high proportion of patients have such an abnormality. Thus, patients less than 45 years old with no obvious environmental determinants, recurrent thromboses, a family history of thrombophilia, thrombosis in unusual sites or other unusual factors should be investigated. In such patients ~5% each will turn out to be **heterozygotes** for **proteins C** or **S** or **antithrombin III deficiency**.

The **homozygous state** is either incompatible with life or presents with severe necrotizing infarctions neonatally. Recently, it has been shown that about half of high-risk patients are heterozygotes for resistance to protein C, a mutation at a cleavage site of protein C in factor V. Five per cent of northern Europeans carry this mutation and it is turning out to be an important risk factor for venous thrombosis secondary to, for example, pregnancy or the oral contraceptive. A further 5% will turn out to have the **lupus anticoagulant**. This is an **autoantibody** with a specificity against phospholipids complexed with other clotting proteins. Usually, these are **anticardiolipin antibodies** and so cause a **false-positive Wassermann reaction**. The antibody can be detected by its interference with the phospholipids used in the activated partial thromboplastin time assay and subsequent prolongation of the latter (hence the paradoxical 'anticoagulant' term). Thrombosis is probably caued by interference with endothelial phospholipids. It was initially found in patients with SLE, hence 'lupus' anticoagulant, but there is an increasing group of patients who do not have classic SLE syndrome or its serology, who have its clinical features. It is a cause of recurrent abortion.

FURTHER READING

Hoffbrand A.V. & Pettit J.E. (1992) *Essential Haematology*, 3rd edn. Blackwell Scientific Publications, Oxford.

CHAPTER 13

Diseases of Fluid Balance, Sodium, Potassium and Acid–Base Biochemistry

CONTENTS

INTRODUCTION – DISEASES OF BIOCHEMISTRY

In this chapter, normal and abnormal biochemistry of fluid balance, sodium, potassium and acid–base biochemistry will be discussed. These topics are not covered in any depth in other chapters; however, they affect all the systems of the body. It is particularly fitting to consider these biochemical processes in association with diseases of the endocrine (Chapter 14), respiratory (Chapter 17) and renal (Chapter 21) systems.

FLUID BALANCE

Body water

In a 70 kg adult, the total body water is about 42 litres (60% of body weight) (Tables 13.1 and 13.2).

Osmolality/osmolarity

- **Osmolality.** A colligative property proportional to the number of particles per kilogram of solvent (i.e. in plasma, per kilogram of plasma water). Osmolality is directly measured in an osmometer (e.g. by measuring freezing point depression or vapour pressure).

  Units = mmol/kg

- **Osmolarity.** A colligative property proportional to the number of particles per litre of solution (i.e. in plasma, per litre of whole plasma. Plasma or serum osmolarity can be calculated from the formula:

$$\text{Plasma osmolarity} = 2 \times [\text{Na}] + 2 \times [\text{K}] + [\text{Urea}] + [\text{Glucose}] - \text{units in mmol/l}$$

Table 13.1 Body water.

Intracellular fluid (ICF)	~28 litres
Extracellular fluid (ECF)	
Interstitial fluid	~12 litres
Intravascular fluid (plasma water)	~3 litres

These values will differ significantly with differing body weight.

Table 13.2 Water balance.

Intake (~2500 ml/24 h)
Oral intake, controlled by thirst
Intravenous administration of fluids

Output (~2500 ml/24 h)
Renal – controlled by antidiuretic hormone (ADH)

Insensible losses – loss in breath, sweating
~500 ml/day but increased in hot environment, fever and
    hyperventilation

Abnormal losses

Water excretion

The ratio of urinary osmolality (U_{osm}) to plasma osmolality (P_{osm}), the osmotic gradient achieved by the kidney, is 1 when they are iso-osmolar and increases to values in excess of 4 under the influence of antidiuretic hormone (ADH; $U_{osm} \sim 1400$ mosmol/kg; Table 13.3).

Conversely the ratio may fall to <0.2 in conditions of **marked diuresis**. An increase of 1 mosmol/kg of plasma osmolality results in an increase of ~100 mosmol/kg in urine osmolality in normal circumstances.

The **osmolar clearance** (C_{osm}) is the volume of water needed to excrete urinary solutes at the equivalent plasma osmolality. Extra water excreted in hypo-osmolar urine in diuresis is termed the free water clearance and is calculated thus;

Table 13.3 Normal control of renal water output.

Loss of water
Increased ECF osmolality
Shrinkage of osmoreceptor cells
Increased ADH release
Reduction of water output by kidneys

ECF, Extracellular fluid; ADH, antidiuretic hormone.

$$\text{Free water clearance} \left(CH_2O\right) = \text{Volume} \left(V\right) - C_{osm}$$
$$= V\, U_{osm}/P_{osm}$$

Free water clearance can be as much as 18 ml/min in extreme diuresis whilst the figure becomes negative when extra water is absorbed by the collecting ducts to give a hyperosmolar urine.

ADH (arginine vasopressin – AVP; see Chapter 14) secretion is controlled almost entirely by plasma osmolality via **osmoreceptors** in the anterior hypothalamus. The highly sensitive response of these cells, probably by an alteration in cell volume, is determined by changes in extracellular osmolality and thus is not affected by solutes that distribute readily into cells (such as urea). An approximate 1% increase in plasma osmolality stimulates ADH release. There is also a far less sensitive and physiologically significant non-osmotic stimulus to ADH secretion by changes in blood volume, physical pain, emotional stress, hypoxia, liver disease, adrenal insufficiency and cardiac failure, probably mediated by autonomic tone. A fall in blood volume of ~10% is needed before there is a stimulus to ADH secretion and is thus only a response in life-threatening situations. ADH secretion may be modified by some drugs.

SODIUM BIOCHEMISTRY

This is essentially a chemical marker of the osmotic gradient across cell membranes and hence also of the cellular hydration state of the patient.

Control mechanisms for plasma sodium

Whilst glomerular filtration rate and renal tubular reabsorption of sodium occurring at four sites along the nephron are significant components of plasma sodium homeostasis, the main control mechanism of plasma sodium is via the effects of ADH on water permeability and reabsorption. There are also significant contributions from the **renin–angiotensin–aldosterone** system on renal sodium handling (Fig. 13.1) and possibly from **atrial natriuretic peptide.**

There are several possible approaches to understand fluid balance but one convenient way is to consider if the patient has depletion or overload of either water or saline.

Water depletion rarely occurs on its own and is usually accompanied by a degree of saline depletion. As water is lost from the extracellular fluid, the extracellular fluid osmolality will rise, causing water to be drawn from cells, leading to cell shrinkage. This mechanism means that quite a large volume of fluid can be lost before there is a

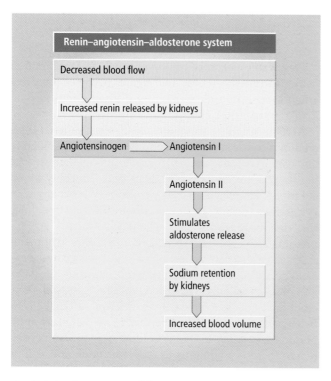

Fig. 13.1 A major component of the control of blood volume is the renin–angiotensin–aldosterone system.

significant degree of hypovolaemia and the appearance of features of true dehydration. Severe water depletion leads to hypernatraemia.

Water overload, caused either by excessive intake or excessive retention by the kidneys, is common and causes the syndrome of water intoxication (see Hyponatraemia, below).

Saline depletion infers loss of both sodium and water as sodium depletion by itself does not occur. Loss of isotonic saline from extracellular fluid does not lead to fluid loss from the intracellular fluid and so loss of only a small amount of saline will lead to hypovolaemia. This leads to the clinical features of saline depletion of '**dehydration**' (really '**desalination**') of reduced skin turgor, dry tongue and reduced intraocular tension as well as tachycardia and hypotension. Saline depletion will only give rise to hyponatraemia when sufficient hypovolaemia has occurred (~10%) to stimulate ADH secretion.

Saline overload results in expansion of the ECF and hence to hypertension and/or oedema. Sodium overload is usually accompanied by an equivalent water overload and so in most cases plasma sodium remains within the reference interval. When water overload exceeds sodium overload, as may occur in severe oedema states, a dilutional hyponatraemia may occur. Saline overload is usually caused by decreased output.

Hyponatraemia

Hyponatraemia, defined as a plasma sodium concentration of <130 mmol/l, is a common finding in hospital practice (prevalence ≤5%) with a high mortality when symptomatic. The clinical effects of hyponatraemia occur as a result of the osmotic difference across cell membranes resulting in brain oedema but the morbidity of this condition appears not to be related either to the rate of fall or the magnitude of the hyponatraemia (Table 13.4). Recent evidence suggests that children and menstruant women are at greatest risk from symptomatic hyponatraemia.

Cerebral cellular overhydration with brain swelling >5% of brain volume may lead to sudden apnoea, bradycardia, unequal pupils, dilated pupils, hypoventilation, cardiovascular instability, impaired temperature regulation, urinary and/or faecal incontinence and respiratory arrest (Table 13.5). If sodium depletion is present reduced skin turgor and postural hypotension ± evidence of circulatory deficiency with cold extremities, tachycardia and venoconstriction may be present.

Causes of hyponatraemia

It is most helpful in the management of a patient with hyponatraemia to establish the underlying relationship between body water and sodium content. The clinical history will usually reveal the likely cause of the hyponatraemia and treatment of the cause should effect a correction of the electrolyte disturbance. Management of the symptomatic hyponatraemic patient is complicated and controversial but there is universal agreement that correction should not be too rapid (i.e. not >12 mmol/l per day).

In normal conditions of loss of sodium from the extracellular fluid there is a fall in ADH secretion and an increase in free water clearance (Table 13.6). Thus extracellular osmolality is preserved at the expense of volume, which decreases. When the sodium deficit becomes more severe there is a fall in renal perfusion and glomerular filtration, increased tubular salt reabsorption and impaired urinary dilution. Eventually the need for maintenance of extracellular volume overcomes the mechanisms controlling osmolality and hyponatraemia develops.

Table 13.4 Symptoms of hyponatraemia.

Headache
Nausea
Vomiting
Confusion
Fits leading to coma and death

Table 13.5 Saline depletion and overload and water overload.

Conditions of saline depletion – deficiency of both total body water and sodium ('dehydration')	
Renal losses	Excessive diuretic therapy
	Salt-losing nephropathy
	Mineralocorticoid deficiency
	Polycystic kidneys
Gastrointestinal losses	Vomiting
	Diarrhoea
	Fistula
Skin losses	Febrile states and hot climate
	Severe burns
	Excessive exertion
Conditions of saline overload – increased total body sodium with water retention (overhydration) with oedema	
Hypoproteinaemia	Nephrotic syndrome
	Protein-losing nephropathy
Decreased GFR	Acute renal failure
	Severe chronic renal failure
Secondary hyperaldosteronism	Cardiac failure
	Liver failure
Conditions of water overload – retention of water with normal total body sodium	
Inappropriate ADH secretion	CNS lesions
	Lung carcinoma (oat cell)
	Drugs
Hypothyroidism	
Hyperglycaemia	Diabetes mellitus
Overhydration	Stress
	Physical pain
	Postoperative
	(Iatrogenic)
	Psychogenic polydipsia
	Beer drinkers
	(Potomania)
Artefactual	Drip arm dilution
	Hyperlipidaemia
	Hyperproteinaemia

GFR, Glomerular filtration rate; ADH, antidiuretic hormone; CNS, central nervous system.

Table 13.6 Syndrome of inappropriate antidiuretic hormone (ADH) secretion – SIADH.

ADH secretion despite hypotonicity and normal or increased ECF volume is inappropriate

High ADH + continuing water intake → *Hyponatraemia*

There may in some patients be increased thirst

Most important causes:
  Malignancy
  Chest infections
  CNS disturbances

Oat cell carcinoma of lung most common carcinoma to secrete ADH

Most important and common drug causes of SIADH are:
  Chlorpropamide
  Carbamazepine
  Vincristine
  Cyclophosphamide

ECF, Extracellular fluid; CNS, central nervous system.

Hypernatraemia

Hypernatraemia (Table 13.7), defined as a plasma sodium of >148 mmol/l, is less common but can be dangerous, with symptoms ranging from **thirst** to **mental confusion** and eventually **coma**.

Hyperosmolality in hypernatraemia is usually caused by loss of water (with hypovolaemia) and rarely by excess sodium (with hypervolaemia). The most common cause of increased sodium + water (salt gain) is from overadministration of sodium-containing fluids such as hypertonic saline or sodium bicarbonate. Hypernatraemia may occur due to increased renal sodium excretion in conditions of mineralocorticoid excess, although often this situation is offset by ADH secretion which decreases water loss.

Causes of hypernatraemia (Table 13.7)

POTASSIUM BIOCHEMISTRY

Potassium is the predominant intracellular cation with only 2% of total body potassium existing in the extracellular fluid and so the plasma potassium level is only a poor indicator of total body potassium. Indeed, plasma potassium concentration can be positively misleading if there is a disturbance of the normal mechanism controlling the

During treatment for hyponatraemia it may be helpful to estimate the degree of water excess which should be excreted. Assuming that 60% of body weight is water, the excess water can be calculated using the following equation:

Excess water
= calculated body water vol
$$-\left(\frac{\text{Serum [sodium]}}{\text{Normal serum [sodium]}} - \text{calculated body water vol}\right)$$

Table 13.7 Hypernatraemia.

Loss of hypotonic fluid (sodium and water)
Extrarenal
Vomiting/diarrhoea
Excess sweating
Dialysis
Renal
Osmotic diuresis (glucose, urea, mannitol)
Normal sodium but loss of water
Extrarenal
Decreased water intake + normal or increased loss
Unconscious
Thirst centre dysfunction (hypodipsia)
Mechanical obstruction
Inadequate intravenous therapy
Increased water loss + normal or decreased intake of water
Fever
Thyrotoxicosis
Hot dry environment
Non-humidified ventilators
Renal
Diabetes insipidus: nephrogenic and neurogenic
Increased sodium + increased water (salt gain)
Increased sodium intake
Accidental or iatrogenic (hypertonic saline, sodium bicarbonate)
Low sodium output
Mineralocorticoid excess

balance between intracellular versus extracellular potassium, e.g. with acid–base disturbances – thus in diabetic ketoacidosis there is usually a total body potassium deficit but the plasma potassium may be high before treatment.

Control mechanisms for plasma potassium

Dietary potassium intake varies from 20 to 100 mmol/day and there is an equivalent urine excretion with only small quantities lost in faeces. Control of renal potassium excretion occurs in the distal tubule as most of the potassium filtered at the glomerulus is reabsorbed in the proximal tubule. Control of distal tubular potassium excretion is complex and relates directly to sodium reabsorption, tubular cell potassium concentration and urine flow rate and is influenced significantly by mineralocorticoid activity and acid–base status.

Relationship between acid–base disturbances and potassium

Normally, alkalosis causes hypokalaemia and vice versa. The mechanism for this is twofold:

1 In the distal renal tubule, sodium is reabsorbed in exchange for either potassium or hydrogen ions. If one is deficient, more of the other is lost into the urine.

2 The intracellular/extracellular balance of potassium and hydrogen ion is similarly affected.

Acidosis and hyperkalaemia bear a similar relationship to each other. However, the combination of hypokalaemia with acidosis is rather unusual and points to a simultaneous loss of potassium and bicarbonate, e.g. a renal tubular disorder like renal tubular acidosis.

Hypokalaemia (Tables 13.8 and 13.9)

This is defined as plasma potassium <3.5 mmol/l.

Hyperkalaemia (Table 13.10)

This is defined as plasma potassium >5.5 mmol/l.

The most important clinical features are tall tented T-waves on electrocardiograph and the potential for cardiac arrest. The higher the plasma potassium, the greater is the risk.

ACID–BASE BIOCHEMISTRY

Hydrogen ion activity plays a major role in the body's metabolic functions and defects in its homeostasis can

Table 13.8 Clinical features of hypokalaemia.

Cardiac
ECG abnormalities (flattened T waves)
Cardiac arrhythmias
Potentiates the toxic effects of digoxin
Renal
Prolonged hypokalaemia impairs the ability of the tubule to reabsorb water → polyuria
Muscle
Skeletal muscle weakness
Impaired recovery from postoperative paralytic ileus

ECG, Electrocardiogram.

Table 13.9 Causes of hypokalaemia.

Decreased intake or absorption – rare, e.g. malabsorption syndrome
Increased losses
Urinary
Hyperaldosteronism
Diuretics
Alkalosis
Cushing's syndrome
GI tract
Vomiting
Diarrhoea
Laxative abuse
Nasogastric tube losses, fistulae, etc.
Transfer from ECF to ICF
Treatment of diabetic coma
Alkalosis
Stress (e.g. surgery, myocardial infarction) almost certainly related to increased catecholamine levels
Familial periodic paralysis (*rare*)

GI, Gastrointestinal; ECF, extracellular fluid; ICF, intracellular fluid.

Table 13.10 Causes of hyperkalaemia.

Factitious pseudohyperkalaemia	Improper collecting / handling
↑ Input	Oral, intravenous therapy (not usually a problem with normal renal function)
Altered distribution	Acidaemia Insulin deficiency Hyperkalaemic periodic paralysis (rare)
Decreased excretion	Renal failure Mineralocorticoid deficiency Renal tubule transport defect
Drugs	Spironolactone Triamterene Amiloride Captopril Prostaglandin inhibitors (e.g. indomethacin)

lead to significant and life-threatening pathology. The most significant elements of this role include the charge and conformation of proteins which thus modulate enzyme activity, membrane transporters of metabolites and ions and affinity of ligand binding, such as haemoglobin for oxygen and albumin for calcium. H^+ gradients drive critical reactions such as many involved in oxidative phosphorylation and hydrogen ion activity will deter-

mine the dissociation of weak acids and bases (both physiological and pharmacological), therefore affecting distribution across cell membranes.

There is considerable variability in hydrogen ion activity within tissues (Tables 13.11–13.14).

Control mechanisms for acid–base balance

In clinical practice the physiological control mechanisms of the lungs and kidneys are of paramount importance as defects of respiratory function leading to either retention or excessive excretion will lead to a metabolic compensatory mechanism to correct the subsequent acid–base de-

Table 13.11 Hydrogen ion activity within tissues.

	pH	H^+
Extracellular fluid	7.35–7.45	36–44 nmol/l
Cytosol	6.7–7.2	~100
Mitochondria	Slightly more alkaline than cytosol	
Liposomes, endosomes and Golgi	5.0 (essential for their function)	

Table 13.12 Control of acid–base homeostasis.

Buffering systems	Instant
Physiological mechanisms	Lungs (minutes) Kidneys (hours/days) Liver (hours/days)

Table 13.13 Buffers.

Bicarbonate	50%	$H_2O + CO_2/H_2CO_3/H^+ + HCO_3^-$
Protein		
Hb	38%	
Plasma protein	6%	
Phosphate		
Ammonia		

Hb, Haemoglobin.

Table 13.14 Physiological control of acid–base.

Lungs	Important for eliminating greatest source of acid–carbonic acid – ~25 000 mmol H^+/day as carbon dioxide
Kidneys	~40–80 mmol H^+/day – mainly non-volatile acids Tubular regeneration of bicarbonate
Liver	H^+ production from NH_4 and bicarbonate consumption in urea cycle

fect, and vice versa with a metabolic defect. The principal source of proton generation and removal is the metabolism of substrates, either endogenous or derived from the diet, which contributes approximately 80 mol/day, a figure matched by the excretion rate.

Carbon dioxide generated from aerobic respiration is the major vehicle both for hydrogen ion production via condensation in erythrocytes to carbonic acid by means of carbonate dehydratase and thus to H^+ and HCO_3^- and of hydrogen ion excretion via carbon dioxide loss from the lungs. If excretion via the lungs becomes impaired or deficient a signficant quantity of carbon dioxide is hydrated to form H_2CO_3 with subsequent dissociation to H^+ and HCO_3^-. At a resting rate of carbon dioxide production if respiratory excretion ceased, pH would fall to < 7 within 20–30 minutes.

The role of the liver in acid–base balance

Recent evidence suggests that there is a link between **hepatic protein metabolism** and proton balance. Atkinson and Bourke (1984) suggested that the primary determinant of the rate of ureagenesis is the need to dispose of HCO_3^- derived from the carbon skeletons of amino acids rather than the need to dispose of NH_4, as thought hitherto.

The average protein contains an amino acid mixture in which oxidation produces a small excess (few %) of NH_4 which either is excreted in the urine or produces H^+ via the urea cycle. Whilst maintaining proton balance is a multiorgan process, urea synthesis is exclusive to the liver. The liver also metabolizes NH_4 to glutamine, a process itself affected by pH, and glutamine is metabolized in kidney to produce NH_4. The liver is also the main site of clearance of **lactic acid** via **gluconeogenesis** (Table 13.15).

Table 13.15 Reference intervals for arterial blood gas values.

	Mean	Reference intervals
pH	7.4	7.35–7.45
[H^+]	40 nmol/l	36–44
Pco_2	5.3 kPa	4.5–6.1 (35–45 mmHg)
Po_2	12 kPa	11.3–12.6 (85–95 mmHg)
Bicarbonate	25 mmol/l	21–27.5
Base excess	0	−2.5–+2.5
Anion gap	16 mmol/l	15–20
Standard bicarbonate	24 mmol/l	22–26
Total CO_2	27	24–30

Some definitions

- **Base excess** – Amount of strong acid required to titrate 1 litre of fully oxygenated blood to pH 7.4 at 37°C and Pco_2 5.3.
- **Standard bicarbonate** – Bicarbonate measured at 37°C at Pco_2 5.3; originally easier to measure as non-physiological.
- **Total CO_2** – CO_2 released from plasma by strong acid, mainly from HCO_3 (95%) but also H_2CO_3, dissolved CO_2, CO_3^{2-} and carbamino compounds.
- **Acidaemia** (hyperacidaemia) – A blood pH below reference interval.
- **Alkalaemia** (hypoacidaemia) – A blood pH above reference interval.

Blood sampling

An arterial sample is usually considered most valuable as a reflection of the respiratory component and a radial or brachial stab is most commonly used, although a femoral stab is usually easier and quicker. Venous samples will give extra information on the metabolic component, although this may vary at different sites of the body.

Conventional training in physical chemistry teaches the use of pH units to quantify hydrogen ion activity as this allows one to compact the large scale conveniently (Table 13.15). This is perhaps now considered too compact for practical clinical purposes, as the physiological range in blood ranges from pH 6.5 to 7.8 and modern analysers are accurate enough to allow for more sensitive measurement. Thus H^+ activity is becoming widely used in clinical practice and this allows reference and use of Henderson's original equation, derived from the equation used to calculate the ionization constant for carbonic acid.

The Henderson equation

$$[H^+] = K \times \frac{[H_2CO_3]}{[HCO_3]}$$

K = first ionization constant of carbonic acid = 7.94×10^{-7}

$[H_2CO_3]$ can be replaced by $S. Pco_2$ (S = solubility coefficient of CO_2 = 0.23 mmol/l)

Thus: $$[H^+] = 7.94 \times \frac{0.23 Pco_2}{[HCO_3^-]} \times 10^{-7}$$

The Henderson–Hasselbalch equation

$$pH = pK + \log_{10} \frac{\left[HCO_3^-\right]}{\left[H_2CO_3\right]} \quad (\text{or } S\,P_{CO_2})\,(S = 0.03)$$

$$\text{Thus}: \quad pH = 6.10 + \log_{10} \frac{\left[HCO_3^-\right]}{0.03 P_{CO_2}}$$

$$pH \; \mu \; \log \frac{\left(\text{metabolic or non-respiratory parameter}\right)}{\left(\text{respiratory parameter}\right)}$$

Conventionally, acid–base defects are classified into broad categories of respiratory and metabolic acidoses or alkaloses. In practice there is often considerable overlap, which leaves this classification misleading and confusing.

Respiratory acidosis (Table 13.16)

Causes
The cause is CO_2 retention usually due to impaired alveolar ventilation (Table 13.17).

Table 13.16 Respiratory acidosis – features.

Decreased pH
Raised [H$^+$]
Raised P_{CO_2}
Raised HCO_3^-

Table 13.17 Causes of respiratory acidosis.

Acute respiratory failure
Bronchopneumonia
Status asthmaticus
Chronic respiratory failure
COAD (pH may be normal)
Renal bicarbonate production
Essential for compensation

COAD, Chronic obstructive airways disease.

Metabolic acidosis (Table 13.18)

Causes
The causes are bicarbonate lost in urine or gastro-intestinal tract or bicarbonate generation impaired or H$^+$ production exceeding buffering capacity (Table 13.19).

Table 13.18 Metabolic acidosis – features.

Decreased pH
Raised [H$^+$]
Decreased P_{CO_2}
Decreased HCO_3^-

Table 13.19 Causes of metabolic acidosis.

Raised bicarbonate loss	Severe diarrhoea
	Fistulae
Decreased bicarbonate generation	Proximal renal tubular acidosis (carbonate-inhibited)
Raised H$^+$ production	Ketosis in diabetes and starvation
	Lactic acidosis (shock, diabetes)
	Drug-induced

Respiratory alkalosis (Table 13.20)

Causes
Primary fall in P_{CO_2} due to abnormally rapid or deep respiration when transport capacity of the pulmonary alveoli is relatively normal (Table 13.21).

Table 13.20 Respiratory alkalosis – features.

Raised pH
Decreased [H$^+$]
Decreased P_{CO_2}
Decreased HCO_3^-

Table 13.21 Causes of respiratory alkalosis.

Hysterical overbreathing
Raised intracranial pressure or brainstem lesions
Hypoxia
Pulmonary oedema
Lobar pneumonia
Pulmonary collapse or fibrosis
Excessive artificial ventilation
Salicylate overdosage

Table 13.22 Metabolic alkalosis – features.

Raised pH
Decreased [H$^+$]
Raised Pco_2
Raised HCO$_3^-$

Table 13.23 Causes of metabolic alkalosis.

Raised renal HCO$_3^-$ produced in K$^+$ depletion (e.g. hyperaldosteronism)
HCO$_3^-$ administration
HCO$_3^-$ generation by gastric mucosa (hypochloraemic alkalosis)
Pyloric stenosis or gastric aspiration

Metabolic alkalosis (Table 13.22)

Causes

Primary rise in plasma bicarbonate concentration (Tables 13.23–13.25). In general, metabolic acid–base defects are corrected by respiratory compensation and vice versa.

RENAL TUBULAR ACIDOSIS

These comprise functional disorders, due to primary or systemic renal diseases, characterized by inadequate H$^+$ secretion despite preservation of normal or adequate glomerular filtration (Table 13.26).

There are three types:

1 type 1 (distal or classical);
2 type 2 (proximal);
3 type 4 (hyperkalaemic).

Types 1 and 2 are characterized by acidosis, low plasma HCO$_3^-$ and K$^+$ and high chloride, together with inability to produce minimum urinary pH in systemic acidosis.

Type 1 may present with:

• acidosis (and hyperventilatory compensation);

Table 13.24 General effects of metabolic acidosis.

Respiration	Hyperventilation and Kussmaul breathing
	Eventually decreased CSF pH may lead to direct central respiratory depression
	'Shock lung'
Cardiovascular	Heart-decreased cardiac contractility
	Peripheral arteriolar dilatation
	Venous constriction
Intermediary metabolism	↓ Glycolysis (PFK inhibition)
	↓ Hepatic gluconeogenesis (PC inhibition)
Oxygen uptake and delivery	Right shift of oxygen dissociation curve
	↑ Tissue unloading
	↓ Pulmonary uptake (↓ 2,3-DPG causes return to left after several hours)
CNS	Impaired consciousness
	Degree of disturbance not closely related to pH
Electrolyte homeostasis	Potassium out of cells → ECF
	↑ Renal K$^+$ loss → decreased body K$^+$ stores
Kidney	↑ Renal gluconeogenesis (↑ PEPCK act)
	↑ Ammoniagenesis from glutamine
	↑ H$^+$ excretion (~ fivefold)
Bone	In chronic metabolic acidosis – loss calcium carbonate

CSF, Cerebrospinal fluid; CNS, central nervous system; 2,3-DPG, 2,3-diphosphoglycerate; ECF, extracellular fluid; PFK, phosphofructokinase; PC, pyruvate carboxylase; PEPCK, phosphorenal pyruvate carboxykinase.

Table 13.25 Differential diagnosis of metabolic acidosis.

Normal anion gap (hyperchloraemic)	Increased anion gap
Gastrointestinal loss of HCO_3^-	Increased acid production
Diarrhoea	Diabetic ketoacidosis
Small bowel or pancreatic fistula	Lactic acidosis
Ureterosigmoidostomy or obstructed ileal conduit	Starvation
Anion exchange resins	Alcoholic ketoacidosis
	Inborn errors of metabolism
Renal loss of HCO_3^-	Ingestion of toxic substances
Carbonic anhydrase inhibitors	Salicylate overdosage
Renal tubular acidosis	Methanol ingestion
Hyperparathyroidism	Ethylene glycol ingestion
Hypoaldosteronism	Solvent inhalation
Miscellaneous	Failure of acid excretion
Recovery from ketoacidosis	Acute renal failure
Dilutional acidosis	Chronic renal failure

Table 13.26 Causes of renal tubular acidosis.

Distal	Proximal
Hypokalaemic	
Primary (inherited)	Primary (inherited)
Hypercalcaemia	Cystinosis
Nephrocalcinosis	Wilson's disease
Multiple myeloma	Lead toxicity
Hepatic cirrhosis	Cadmium toxicity
Lupus erythematosus	Mercury toxicity
Amphotericin B	Amyloidosis
Lithium	Multiple myeloma
Toluene	Nephrotic syndrome
Renal transplant rejection	Medullary cystic disease
Medullary sponge kidney	Outdated tetracycline
Hyperkalaemic	
Hypoaldosteronism	
Obstructive nephropathy	
Sickle-cell nephropathy	
Lupus erythematosus	
Cyclosporin nephrotoxicity	

- muscle weakness (secondary to hypokalaemia);
- nephrocalcinosis and renal calculi;
- ricketts and growth retardation in childhood.

Urine pH fails to become acid at any stage of systemic acidosis.

Type 2 may present with:
- acidosis (and hyperventilatory compensation);
- muscle weakness (secondary to hyperkalaemia);
- osteomalacia and ricketts;

- polyuria and thirst;
- Fanconi syndrome (other proximal tubular leaks).

Nephrocalcinosis and renal calculi are virtually never seen. Urine pH will acidify in severe systemic acidosis.

Hyperkalaemic acidosis is the main feature of type 4 renal tubular acidasis (RTA). Usually there is hyporeninaemic hypoaldosteronism.

Anion gap

This is the difference between unmeasured anions and unmeasured cations.

$$= \left(\left[Na^+ \right] + \left[K^+ \right] \right) - \left(\left[Cl^- \right] + \left[HCO_3^- \right] \right)$$

Normal anion gap

$$= (142 + 4) - (103 + 27) = 146 - 130 = 16 \, \text{mmol ion charge/l}$$

Unmeasured cations (mmol/l)

- (K^+) (4);
- Ca^{2+} (2);
- Mg^{2+} (2);
- Others (1).

Table 13.27 Causes of lactic acidosis.

Type A
Hypovolaemic shock
Cardiogenic shock
Septic shock
Mesenteric vascular insufficiency
Hypoxaemia
Type B
Muscular hyperactivity
Seizures
Marathon running
Systemic conditions
Diabetes mellitus
Liver failure
Malignancy
Renal failure
Infections
Falciparum malaria
Toxic conditions
Ethanol and methanol
Phenformin
Carbon monoxide

Lactic acidosis is serious condition with a >50% mortality and there is little effective specific treatment.

Unmeasured anions (mmol/l)

- Phosphate (2);
- Sulphate (1);
- Organic anions, e.g. lactate (5); protein (16).

Lactic acidosis

This is defined as, an **acidosis in the presence of a raised plasma lactate concentration** (e.g. $> 5\,\text{mmol/l}$) and is caused by either overproduction or underutilization of lactate or both (Table 13.27). There are two types:

- type A – with tissue underperfusion;
- type B – without tissue underperfusion.

REFERENCE

Atkinson D.E. & Bourke E. (1984) The role of ureagenesis in pH homeostasis. *Trends in Biomedical Science*, **9**:297–300.

PART 3

ESSENTIAL SYSTEMIC PATHOLOGY

Endocrine Disease

CONTENTS

INTRODUCTION

Diseases of the endocrine system are relatively uncommon. As they are characterized by diseases of **hyper-** and **hypoproduction**, this is the approach we have taken in the discussion of the endocrine pathology of each organ system in this chapter.

It is important for the student to have an understanding of the normal physiology and biochemistry of the endocrine system in order to interpret the **functional tests** received from the laboratory. On the basis of these results, the appropriate diagnosis can then be rationally sought and the patient managed appropriately.

This chapter discusses the main endocrine glands which include the hypothalamus and pituitary, the thyroid, the parathyroid, the adrenal, the multiple endocrine neoplasias (MEN), the diffuse neuroendocrine or amine precursor uptake and decarboxylation (APUD) system and the endocrine pancreas.

The pathology of the exocrine pancreas is discussed in Chapter 19. The detailed biochemistry of bone and calcium is discussed in Chapter 20. Tumours of the central nervous system (CNS) not covered here are discussed in Chapter 27.

Endocrine hyperfunction

Excessive secretion of hormones may be due to:
- **primary hyperfunction**, due to increased numbers of hormone-secreting cells, which may occur due to **hyperplasia** or **neoplasia** of the hormone-secreting cells;
- **secondary hyperfunction** due to increased stimulation by increased levels of trophic hormones or decreased feedback inhibition;
- **ectopic hormone production** by cells that do not usually produce the hormone.

Endocrine hypofunction

Decreased secretion of hormones may be due to:

- **primary hypofunction**, due to decreased numbers of hormone-secreting cells, which may occur due to:
  - (a) congenital absence or hypoplasia of the gland;
  - (b) destruction of the gland by infection, surgery, immunological mechanisms, ischaemia or tumour;
  - (c) deficiency of enzymes required to produce the hormone;
- **secondary hypofunction** due to decreased stimulation by absence of tropic hormones, which is always associated with atrophy of the hormone-secreting cells;
- **pseudohypofunction**, where normal hormone levels are present but there are defective target organ receptors (usually congenital).

Secretion of abnormal hormones by endocrine glands is usually due to **enzyme deficiency**.

THE HYPOTHALAMUS

Hypothalamic control of the pituitary gland is effected by releasing and inhibiting hormones carried to the anterior and posterior pituitary by the portal venous system (Fig. 14.1).

Diseases of the hypothalamus

Symptoms and signs of hypothalamic disease include polyphagia, disruption of physiological temperature control mechanisms, somnolence, loss of control of blood pressure and hypopituitarism (Table 14.1). These may represent or be present in a variety of disease states which may be associated with hypothalamic disease, although the pathophysiological mechanisms for most of these are poorly understood.

Biochemical diagnosis or confirmation of hypothalamic disease is sometimes reached by inference from dynamic tests of pituitary function such as **corticotrophin-releasing hormone (CRH)** deficiency following an impaired **adrenocorticotrophic hormone (ACTH)** response to an

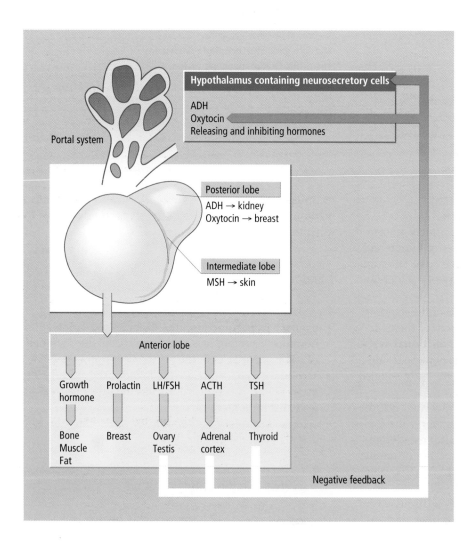

Fig. 14.1 The pituitary and hypothalamus.

Table 14.1 Some conditions which may be associated with hypothalamic disease.

Anorexia nervosa
Fröhlich's disease (obesity and hypopituitarism)
Precocious puberty
Hypogonadotrophic hypogonadism (Kallmann syndrome with anosmia)
Infertility when GnRH responsive—clomiphene-unresponsive
Functional infertility—responsive to clomiphene
Idiopathic growth hormone deficiency
CRH deficiency
Pituitary Cushing's disease without an adenoma
Idiopathic diabetes insipidus

GnRH, Gonadotrophin-releasing hormone; CRH, corticotrophin-releasing hormone.

insulin stress test with normal response to CRH administration.

Arginine vasopressin (AVP; antidiuretic hormone—ADH) is the only hypothalamic hormone which has analytical methods routinely available but deficiency is best established by the use of either a **water deprivation test** or following administration of **hypertonic saline**. Structural lesions of the hypothalamus may be detectable by various imaging techniques.

THE PITUITARY

The pituitary (**hypophysis**) is a small gland weighing 350–900 mg, lying in the sella turcica in the base of the skull. Up to 75% of the pituitary comprises the anterior lobe (**adenohypophysis**), and 25% the posterior lobe (**neurohypophysis**) with a vestigial intermediate lobe.

Although pituitary disease is usually caused by a tumour of one of the cell types of the pituitary gland many other disease states may affect the pituitary, leading to decreased release of either one or, much more commonly, all of the pituitary hormones. These include the conditions listed in Table 14.2.

Table 14.2 Conditions associated with hypopituitarism.

Hypothalamic disease
Congenital defects
Cysts
Abscesses
Granulomas
Vascular accidents
Fractures of the base of the skull
Hypophysectomy
Tumours

Clinically, the picture of pituitary disease may include a combination of **panhypopituitarism** with underproduction of some, if not all, of the pituitary hormones. For example, a mass lesion may cause pressure atrophy on the trophic cells, blindness or give overproduction of a specific hormone (e.g. prolactin). Very rarely, congenital absence of a specific hormone may exist. Panhypopituitarism may be associated with hypothalamic disease if the pathological process extends into the hypothalamus (e.g. craniopharyngiomas, which are locally invasive tumours, may cause diabetes insipidus—DI).

Anterior pituitary (adenohypophysis; Table 14.3)

Tests of pituitary function

Anterior pituitary function has, in the past, been assessed by the use of complex, expensive, time-consuming and often dangerous stimulation tests such as the **triple stimulation test**, described below (Table 14.4).

However, evidence is emerging that these do not give much more information than basal serum levels of hormones. Indeed, in certain disease states stress tests may give conflicting results and false-positive and negative results are not uncommonly seen. They are included in this discussion as they are still in use.

The advent of improved imaging techniques, computed tomography (CT) and magnetic resonance imaging (MRI) would seem to be largely responsible for the decline in the importance of stimulation tests in the investigation of adult pituitary disease. Stimulation tests may, however, be required in assessing human growth hormone (hGH) release in children with short stature (see below).

Table 14.3 Cell types of the anterior pituitary (adenohypophysis).

Immunocytochemistry and electronmicroscopy (granule structure) have shown that the following cell types exist:	
GH cells	50%
PL cells	20%
ACTH cells	20%
TSH cells	5%
LH/FSH cells	5%
The following is old terminology which should be disregarded:	
Chromophobes	50% (PL and ACTH)
Acidophils	40% (GH and PL)
Basophils	10%

GH, Growth hormone; PL, prolactin; ACTH, adrenocorticotrophic hormone; TSH, thyroid-stimulating hormone; LH, luteinizing hormone; FSH, follicle-stimulating hormore.

Table 14.4 Anterior pituitary–triple stimulation test.

Stimulus	Hormone to be assessed	Hormone measured after stimulus	Samples taken (minutes)
Soluble insulin	hGH	hGH	BL, +30, +60, +90, +120
0.15 u/kg	ACTH	Cortisol	BL, +30, +60, +90, +120
i.v.		(Glucose)	BL, +10, +20, +30, +60, +90, +120
		(ACTH)	BL, +15, +30, +45, +60
TRH	TSH	TSH	BL, +20, +60
200 µg i.v.	hPRL	hPRL	BL (+20, +60)
GnRH	LH	LH	BL, +20, +60
100 µg i.v.	FSH	FSH	BL, +20, +60

hGH, Human growth hormone; ACTH, adrenocorticotrophic hormone; BL, blood level; TRH, thyrotrophin-releasing hormone; TSH thyroid-stimulating hormone; hPRL, human prolactin; GnRH, gonadotrophin-releasing hormone; LH, luteinizing hormone; FSH, follicle-stimulating hormone.

Insulin stress tests (ISTs). These are rarely indicated and should probably only be carried out in specialist centres. Senior cover, i.e. the consultant in charge of the patient or the senior registrar, should be available. The conditions are as follows.

- The patient should be **fasting**.
- **Cortisol levels** can be used as indirect measurements of ACTH production only if the adrenal cortex is normally responsive to ACTH. If the patient has been on steroids or has had hypopituitarism for a long time, the adrenals may atrophy. Their responsiveness can be checked by a **Synacthen test** (see below) if atrophy is suspected.
- **Blood glucose** must be followed to assess adequacy of hypoglycaemia. (If blood glucose is followed by 'stick' tests, samples should subsequently be sent to the laboratory to document the hypoglycaemia properly.)
- **Prolactin** response to thyrotrophin-releasing hormone (TRH) is not helpful.
- The calculation of the dose of **insulin** should be checked by another person. The dose is about 10 µg for a 70-kg patient; this gives a rough check on the calculation. The patient should be supervised at the bedside throughout the test by a doctor. If the patient becomes clinically hypoglycaemic, i.e. unable to converse, 25 ml of 50% glucose should be given intravenously; if the patient does not respond to this, a further 25 ml of 50% glucose should be given. The test should be continued as planned. If the patient does not respond to the second dose of 50% glucose, call for senior cover and give hydrocotisone 100 mg. Overadministration of 50% glucose leading to hyperosmolar brain damage is a more common cause of death during ISTs than the hypoglycaemia.

- ISTs are **contraindicated** in **epileptics** and in patients with **ischaemic heart disease**. Reduced doses of insulin should be given to patients with evidence of or symptoms of hypoglycaemia if the test is really required in this situation.
- **Increased doses** of insulin may be required in patients with **insulin resistance**, i.e. patients with Cushing's and acromegaly.
- A number of safer stimuli of hGH and ACTH release can be used, particularly in children, i.e. exercise, glucagon, clonidine, etc.

A satisfactory hypoglycaemic response is indicated by the development of symptoms of hypoglycaemia or by the blood sugar falling to less than 2.2 mmol/l for two consecutive samples.

The TRH response. Pituitary hypothyroidism shows an absent or impaired response with low normal baseline levels and an inadequate +20 minutes rise of less than 4 mu/l. This test is now rarely indicated and not helpful in studying pituitary disease.

High-sensitivity thyroid-stimulating hormone (TSH) levels. This technique can achieve sensitivity of 0.08 mU/l or less and hence can measure 'low' levels of serum TSH. The reference range for TSH is about 0.5–5.0 mU/l. Levels of less than 0.5 mU/l may be seen in situations when there is an absent or impaired TRH response, i.e. hypopituitarism, sick euthyroid patients, patients on thyroxine (T_4) therapy, thyrotoxicosis and as a normal variant. This assay has largely replaced the TRH response in the management of thyroid disease (Table 14.5).

A third-generation TSH assay is now available with a sensitivity of <0.001 mU/l and even greater sensitivity is

Table 14.5 Normal reponse of pituitary function tests.

Test	Hormone	Baseline	Peak	Increment	Units
IST	hGH	<10	>20		mu/l
IST	Cortisol	>140	>500	>200	nmol/l
TRH	TSH	<5.0	<20*	(see text)	mu/l
GnRH†	FSH:				
	female	0.5–5.0	2–25*		U/l
	male	0.5–5.0	2–7*		U/l
	LH:				
	female	3–16	12–42*		U/l
	male	3–10	13–58*		U/l

IST, Insulin stress test; hGH, human growth hormone; TRH, thyrotrophin-releasing hormone; TSH, thyroid-stimulating hormone; GnRH, gonadotrophin-releasing hormone; FSH, follicle-stimulating hormone; LH, luteinizing hormone.

* TSH peak at ~+20 minutes.

† GnRH responses are very variable in puberty.

anticipated with the development of a fourth-generation assay, although the added benefit of this degree of sensitivity is questionable.

However, the following **basal levels** of hormones in serum are probably all that are required in assessing the majority of disorders of the pituitary taken in conjunction with the CT scans and/or in puberty MRI findings.

- **cortisol** taken at 9 am this reflects the action of ACTH on the normal adrenal;
- **short** or **depot Synacthen test** may also be useful in assessing prolonged ACTH deficiency;
- T_4;
- free fT_4;
- **thyroid-binding globulin (TBG)**;
- **TSH**;
- **FSH** (follicle-stimulating hormone);
- **LH** (luteinizing hormone);
- **testosterone** or **oestradiol**;
- **hGH**;
- **hPRL** (prolactin) levels.

Disorders of hyperpituitarism

The majority of cases of anterior pituitary hypersecretion are due to benign pituitary adenomas (Fig. 14.2). Hyperplasia of pituitary cells is extremely rare.

Pituitary adenomas are uncommon and constitute approximately 10% of all **primary intracranial neoplasms**. They occur at all ages but are most common in the age group 20–50 years. Their frequency in men is slightly more than in women.

Thirty per cent are non-functional, causing destruction of the gland and presenting with selective or generalized hypopituitarism or compression of the optic nerve; 30%

secrete prolactin; 25% secrete growth hormone and 10% secrete ACTH. The remainder secrete thyrotrophin or gonadotrophins.

Occasionally, pituitary adenoma is seen as part of the syndrome of **MEN type I** – Werner's syndrome.

Acromegaly. Acromegaly is caused by overproduction of hGH by pituitary adenomas or rarely abnormal growth hormone-releasing hormone (GHRH) production.

The soft tissues, bones and organs are increased in size, with resultant clinical complications such as deafness and cardiac failure (Fig. 14.3). Glucose tolerance is decreased and 10% of patients present with diabetes. Twenty per cent of GH-secreting adenomas produce prolactin, leading to galactorrhoea.

The diagnosis is made on the following grounds:
- clinical (Fig. 14.3);
- radiological;
- biochemical (see below).

Treatment is with **bromocriptine, radiotherapy** or by surgery to remove the adenoma via **transsphenoidal hypophysectomy**.

Laboratory diagnosis of acromegaly
- Measurement of **hGH levels** suppress to 2 mu/l or less in normal subjects during an oral glucose tolerance test (OGTT). The serum hGH levels in acromegalic patients do not suppress following oral glucose and usually show a paradoxical rise. The normal basal resting fasting hGH is <10 mu/l; random levels are very labile.
- **Insulin-like growth factor 1** (IGF 1; somatomedin C). This protein-bound plasma peptide correlates well with hGH production. It probably exerts a negative feedback on pituitary hGH production, and is raised in

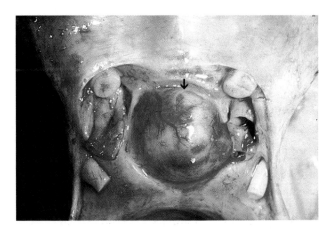

Fig. 14.2 Pituitary adenoma. This photograph is taken in the post mortem room and shows a pink, fleshy tumour mass occupying the sella turcica (arrowed).

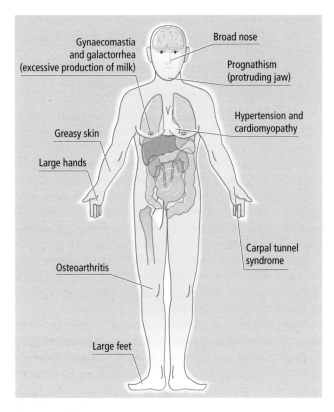

Fig. 14.3 Clinicopathology of acromegaly.

Table 14.6 Causes of hyperprolactinaemia.

Hypothalamic lesions
Craniopharyngiomas
Metastatic tumours
Head trauma, sarcoidosis, encephalitis

Pituitary lesions
Prolactin-producing tumours
Acromegaly
Cushing's disease

Endocrine disorders
Hypothyroidism (~50%)
Addison's disease
Diabetes mellitus
Nelson's disease
Sheehan syndrome
Hyperthyroidism

Drugs
Dopaminergic blocking agents
    Phenothiazines
    Metoclopramide
Dopamine-lowering agents
    Methyldopa
    Reserpine
Tricyclic antidepressants
    Amitriptyline
Oestrogens
Androgens

Other
Pregnancy
Chronic renal failure
Adrenocarcinoma
Chest disease
Breast disease
Ectopic prolactin-producing tumours

acromegaly, when it can be used as a tumour marker for active disease.

- **TRH administration** to normal subjects and 50% of acromegalics does not stimulate the release of hGH; other acromegalics show a rise in the serum levels of hGH, which can be used diagnostically and as a tumour marker for successful treatment or to demonstrate a recurrence after surgery.
- **Urinary hGH** may be increased in acromegaly but is not used as a test routinely.

Hyperprolactinaemia (Table 14.6). Hyperprolactinaemia may be seen in many forms of pituitary disease, particularly in patients with adenomas of the lactotrophs, **prolactinomas**, which produce large quantities of hPRL resulting in very high serum levels.

Prolactinomas in males are often asymptomatic but may present with low libido and impotence. Females may present with amenorrhoea, sterility or galactorrhoea. The diagnosis may show a low FSH/LH and raised PRL. Treatment is with bromocriptine, radiotherapy or surgery.

Laboratory diagnosis of hyperprolactinaemia. The normal serum prolactin (hPRL) level is <450 mU/l but up to 600 mU/l may be normal in some patients. The hPRL may occasionally rise to 1000 mU/l as a result of the stress of venepuncture or 'seeing a doctor', and collecting a repeat sample after resting may bring the level into the normal range. Values over 1000 mU/l are nearly always pathological and may result in amenorrhoea, infertility, impotence and gynaecomastia and/or galactorrhoea and visual symptoms in the presence of some tumours.

Microprolactinomas may have hPRL levels less than 8000 mU/l and may be stable for years without treatment, usually when the hPRL is less than 3000 mU/l or may require bromocriptine.

Macroprolactinomas are associated with levels over 7000 mU/l and are large tumours which may or may not have suprasellar extensions. If the latter damages the optic chiasma causing blindness, emergency decompression is required to prevent permanent blindness. The differential diagnosis in this situation is usually between a macroprolactinoma and a **non-functioning pituitary tumour (NFPT)**. A preoperative course of bromocriptine will shrink macroprolactinomas, but not NFPTs. Preoperative bromocriptine treatment in macroprolactinomas makes subsequent surgery easier and results in fewer complications. If the hPRL is < 7000 mU/l, presumably due to a NFPT, emergency pituitary surgery is indicated. The decision to operate before or after bromocriptine therapy is made on the serum prolactin concentration which is measured as an emergency.

Investigations for male and female infertility are discussed in Chapters 22 and 23 respectively.

Cushing's disease. This will be discussed in the adrenal section, below.

Nelson's syndrome. Adenomas of the pituitary producing **ACTH** and **melanocyte-stimulating hormone** (MSH) may occur in patients who have had **bilateral adrenalectomies**, usually for Cushing's. The serum ACTH levels are high, over 1000 ng/l, and may be resistant to steroid suppression. Isolated deficiency of ACTH, TSH and hPRL has been described but is very rare.

Table 14.7 Causes of hypopituitarism.

Pituitary adenoma
Pituitary carcinoma
Pituitary metastasis
Hypothalamic tumours
Craniopharyngioma
Chordoma
Glioma
Pineal teratoma
Metastasis
Infarction
Pre-existing adenoma
Sheehan's syndrome
Sickle-cell disease
Diabetes
Empty sella syndrome
Granulomas
TB, sarcoid, syphilis, Hand–Schueller–Christian disease
Trauma
Metabolic
Haemochromatosis, Tay–Sachs disease

TB, Tuberculosis.
There are also isolated hormone deficiencies, e.g. pituitary dwarfism.

Table 14.8 Effects of hypopituitarism.

Secondary hypoadrenalism – Hypotension, debility, pale skin
Secondary hypothyroidism – Sensitive to cold
Secondary hypogonadism – absent axillary and pubic hair
Growth hormone deficiency – Small stature if prepubertal, prone to hypoglycaemia

Disorders of hypopituitarism (Tables 14.7 and 14.8)

Pituitary dwarfism. Short stature may be associated with impaired (7–20 mU/l) or absent (<7 mU/l) hGH production in response to the stress of exercise, glucagon, clonidine, or during a sleeping hGH profile, or the less safe IST which may be used as a last resort to demonstrate hGH deficiency. Pituitary dwarfism may be sporadic or familial, or may be associated with **panhypopituitarism**. There are many other causes of short stature (see Chapter 25).

IGF 1 levels are low in hGH deficiency, although there may be some overlap with the nomal range. Normal IGF 1 levels in a dwarfed child probably exclude hGH deficiency. Urinary hGh levels are also low in pituitary dwarfism.

Growth and weight velocity curves are of great importance in managing this problem and assessing response to treatment with recombinant hGH.

Isolated gonadotrophin deficiency. **Hypogonadism**, or impaired sexual development, which in this case is due to inadequate gonadotophin production by the hypothalamopituitary axis, may be demonstrated by failure of most cases to respond normally to the exhibition of gonadotrophin-releasing hormone (GnRH), although some cases may achieve a normal response. The disorder is probably hypothalamic in origin.

Kallmann syndrome consists of hypogonadotrophic hypogonadism associated with anosmia.

Investigation of delayed puberty. Puberty is the event of sexual maturity and fertility which is associated with a period of changing patterns of hormone secretion. Altered hypothalamic pituitary sensitivity to circulating steroids is the first manifestation together with increased adrenal androgen output (Tables 14.9 and 14.10).

Posterior pituitary (neurohypophysis)

ADH, vasopressin, is an octapeptide produced by the hypothalamus, transported to the posterior pituitary by the portal system, and released from the latter into the general circulation, usually under the influence of

Table 14.9 Causes of delayed puberty.

Constitutional
Malabsorption
Primary gonadal failure
Girls
45,X Turner's sydrome
46,XY Androgen insensitivity due to 5α-reductase deficiency
46,XX/XY Pure gonadal dysgenesis
Autoimmune ovarian failure
Resistant ovary syndrome
Boys
Undescended testes
Congenital anorchia
Klinefelter's syndrome
Noonan's syndrome
Secondary gonadal failure
Congenital isolated gonadotrophin deficiency
Tumours (pituitary, hypothalamic)
Chronic disease in childhood associated with CNS disease
Kallmann syndrome
Spinocerebellar syndromes, e.g. Prader–Willi syndrome
Iatrogenic
Radiotherapy, chemotherapy
Psychological
Anorexia nervosa
Thyroid disease
Adrenal disease
Cushing's
Rare syndromes

CNS, Central nervous system.

Table 14.10 Combined pituitary function testing for delayed puberty.

Basal concentrations of
Luteinizing hormone (LH)
Follicle-stimulating hormone (FSH)
Growth hormone (GH)
Cortisol; thyroxine; oestradiol; testosterone; prolactin
Response to
Intravenous insulin 0.15 U/kg (effect of GH and cortisol)
Intravenous thyrotrophin-stimulating hormone (TRH) 200 μm (effect on TSH)
Intravenous gonadotrophin-releasing hormone (GnRH) 100 μg (effect on LH/FSH)

TSH, Thyroid-stimulating hormone.

changes in plasma osmolality and to a lesser degree volume.

Its deficiency results in **DI**, the lack of ADH resulting in the inability of the kidneys to conserve water; this is one of several causes of **polyuria** and **polydipsia**. DI should be suspected in a patient with these symptoms, no other obvious cause such as diabetes mellitus or renal failure, and also with a low urine osmolality.

Tests of pituitary function

Water deprivation test. The diagnosis of DI is usually made by the use of a water deprivation test where the patient is deprived of water for 8 hours or until 3% of the patient's body weight is lost, a potentially hazardous state. Before the test the patient is hydrated and a sample of urine collected for osmolality and of plasma for osmolality and electrolytes. Samples of urine passed during the test are collected hourly for volume and osmolality. Plasma osmolality and sodium are measured 2-hourly. Patient weight is also measured hourly (Table 14.11).

During this test, normal subjects achieve a urinary osmolality of over 800 mosmol/kg with little change in the plasma Na⁺ or osmolality. In DI the urinary osmolality remains at ~200 mosmol/kg whilst the plasma osmolality and serum Na⁺ rise. An alternative to the water deprivation test is to infuse saline and follow the response of plasma and urine osmolality and also that of the plasma ADH concentration.

Disorders of hypopituitarism

Diabetes insipidus. **Cranial** (central) **diabetes insipidus** (CDI) may be caused by a large range of **acquired** cerebral conditions and there is also a **familial** cause. In all of these there is impaired or absent release of ADH from the posterior pituitary (Table 14.12).

Nephrogenic diabetes insipidus (NDI) may be caused by a large number of acquired renal and metabolic conditions (Table 14.13) and there is also a congenital X-linked recessive disorder, probably involving an abnormal gene for the V2 ADH receptor. The condition is associated with a lack of end-organ (i.e. the kidney) sensitivity to ADH. The patient presents with DI but fails to respond to desmopressin given parenterally or intranasally at the end of the water deprivation test. The differential diagnosis of DI includes other causes of polydipsia, i.e. diabetes mellitus, diuretic administration, chronic renal failure, hypercalcaemia, hysterical (psychogenic) polydipsia).

Hysterical (psychogenic) polydypsia. This is a psychiatric disorder in which patients drink hypotonic fluids to ex-

Table 14.11 Water deprivation test.

	Urine osmolality (mosmol/l)		
	Pre*	Post†	Post-DDAVP
Normal	< 200	> 800	
Cranial diabetes insipidus (CDI)	< 200	< 200	> 200
Nephrogenic diabetes insipidus	< 200	< 200	< 200
Partial diabetes insipidus or psychogenic polydipsia	< 200	< 600	Minimum change except in partial CDI

* Pre-water deprivation
† Post-water deprivation

Table 14.12 Causes of cranial diabetes insipidus.

Familial (rare)
Idiopathic
Cranial lesions
    Head trauma
    Tumours
    Neurosurgery
    Cerebral ischaemia or hypoxia
    Cerebral aneurysms
    Infections (meningitis, encephalitis)
Miscellaneous
    Other tumours
    Sarcoidosis

Table 14.13 Causes of nephrogenic diabetes insipidus.

Congenital
Drugs
    Lithium
    Demeclocycline
    Loop diuretics
    Osmotic diuretics
Renal failure
Hypercalcaemia
Hypokalaemia
Pregnancy
Amyloidosis
Sjögren's syndrome

cess, resulting in **haemodilution**, even to a point of **coma**. The diagnosis is made by water deprivation, when the patient will show some renal concentration of the urine but does not acheive normal levels of osmolality; likewise their kidneys respond to desmopressin but not usually as well as normal. The water deprivation test is hard to perform in these individuals as they will usually go to extreme lengths to satisfy their thirst.

THE THYROID GLAND

Normal structure and function

Anatomy

The thyroid develops from a tubular invagination of the embryonic pharynx (the **thyroglossal duct**), which during embryogenesis migrates downwards into the neck. Arrest of migration at any site along this pathway will lead to **ectopic thyroid** in adult life (Table 14.14). Arrest at a proximal site along descent may result in **lingual thyroid**, seen at the base of the tongue; migration which proceeds too far may result in a mediastinal location of the gland (**plunging thyroid**). Epithelial remnants of the thyroglossal duct may persist into adult life as **thryoglossal duct cysts**.

The adult thyroid gland weighs 20–25 g and is composed of two lateral lobes joined across the midline by the **thyroid isthmus**. A pyramidal lobe of varying size extends upwards from the isthmus and represents the attachment of the thyroglossal duct.

Histologically, the thyroid gland is composed of tightly packed **follicles** containing **colloid** (a proteinaceous material containing **thyroglobulin** and stored **thyroid hormones**). Parafollicular **C cells** that secrete **calcitonin** are seen between the thyroid follicles.

Table 14.14 Developmental anomalies of the thyroid.

Aplasia and hypoplasia
Abnormalities of descent
    Lingual thyroid
    Subhyoid thyroid
    Retrosternal thyroid
    Thyroglossal duct, cysts and sinuses

Biochemistry of the thyroid gland

The thyroid gland synthesizes and secretes predominantly T_4, as well as lesser amounts of **triiodothyronine** **(T_3)** and reverse T_3 (rT_3; Table 14.15).

Table 14.15 Biological actions of thyroid hormones.

> Increased calorigenesis
> Increased protein synthesis
> Effects on carbohydrate metabolism
>   Modification of effects of catecholamines and insulin
>   Enhancement of intestinal glucose uptake
>   Increased supply of substrates for gluconeogenesis
> Effects on lipid metabolism
>   Mobilization of lipid stores
>   Effects on apolipoprotein metabolism
>   Increased hepatic triglyceride synthesis
> Increased requirements for vitamins
> Mimicking of sympathetic nervous system activity

T_4 is best considered as a **prohormone** as the physiological actions are in the main promoted by its product, T_3. Conversion of T_4 to T_3 by **monodeiodination** occurs in all tissues but most of its metabolism occurs in liver, kidney and muscle. T_4 and T_3 have, probably as a result of a single common mechanism of action at the cellular or molecular level, a variety of biological actions to a certain extent dependent on the site of tissue action.

Thyroid function tests

Few tissues are likely to escape some metabolic disturbance from either over- or undersecretion of the thyroid hormones.

The most compelling theory for a single initiating component of thyroid hormone action is via its nuclear receptor-mediated effects on protein synthesis. Regulation of gene transcription of a variety of different proteins with hormone or enzyme activity is thus likely to be the major component responsible for thyroid hormone action with a small component derived from effects at the cell membrane via specific receptors. Overall degree of activity would thus be controlled by differential expression of cell membrane and nuclear receptors and also rates of activity of deiodinases converting T_4 to the far more bioactive T_3.

Thyroid dysfunction may be suggested by the manifestation of recognized symptoms of either over- or underproduction of T_4, as described earlier. The extent of clinical expression is highly variable and differing signs and symptoms may confuse the clinician, particularly in elderly patients. The relative frequency of thyroid dysfunction means that the clinician should be prepared to consider the diagnosis when there may be only limited indication and instigate a biochemical screen of **thyroid function tests** (Fig. 14.4).

Most laboratories will offer assays of plasma or serum T_4 (total and 'free'; fT_4), T_3 (total and 'free'; fT_3) and TSH. Many laboratories now, largely for financial savings, will structure the process of thyroid hormone measurement by selecting a single front-line investigation, examples of which include TSH, total T_4 or free T_4, followed when necessary by selected tests depending on the result of the first and also on the clinical details.

Other tests that should be available are serum TBG, thyroid autoantibodies and thyroglobulin. There is no consensus on these algorithms used in practice and the most suitable process may be determined by the sensitivity and relative costs of the assays in use.

There are rare situations where alternative diagnoses should be considered, such as with T_4 autoantibodies, variant albumins or T_3 toxicosis, where low TSH values may be associated with normal free T_4 levels.

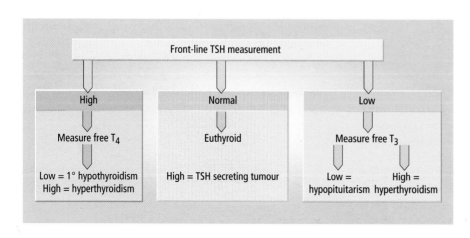

Fig. 14.4 An example of a simple thyroid diagnostic cascade.

Thyroid hormones in non-thyroid illness

In many illnesses there may be abnormalities in plasma thyroid hormone concentrations in the absence of any thyroid gland disease, a situation often described as the **euthyroid sick syndrome**. The condition may also be caused by a range of **drugs**.

Local and systemic release of inhibitors of TSH release, changes in plasma TBG hormone concentrations and binding affinity, decreases in peripheral uptake and metabolism of thyroid hormones and alteration in end-organ T_3 receptors may all play a part in this process, which characteristically leads to lowered T_3, elevated rT_3 and low total T_4 with low free T_4 and TSH levels in severe cases. Correct timing and choice of biochemical markers of thyroid status are essential in any ill patient, particularly in those who are symptomatic of thyroid disease and in the elderly.

Elevated total thyroid hormone levels are encountered in euthyroid patients in whom there is an elevation of thyroid-binding protein, the classic example being during **pregnancy**, when markedly **elevated circulating oestrogens** are responsible. This situation also occurs in patients taking the oral contraceptive pill, although this is less marked in low-oestrogen preparations.

The pathology of hyperthyroidism

A variety of causes of hyperthyroidism need to be considered (Table 14.16).

Table 14.16 Causes of hyperthyroidism.

Common (99%)
Diffuse toxic goitre (Graves disease)
Toxic multinodular goitre
Toxic adenoma
Acute phase of thyroiditis
Hyperfunctioning thyroid carcinoma
Choriocarcinoma, hydatidiform mole (TSH-like activity)
TSH-secreting pituitary tumour
Neonatal thyrotoxicosis (mother with Graves disease)
Struma ovarii (teratomatous)
Iatrogenic (exogenous)

TSH, Thyroid-stimulating hormone.

Thyroid function tests in hyperthyroidism

Except in the rare cases of pituitary-induced hyperthyroidism, plasma levels of TSH are very low and usually undetectable in hyperthyroidism. New assays for TSH claim sufficient sensitivity to allow diagnosis of hyperthyroidism by this test alone but there is considered to be some overlap with euthyroid patients and so, even if TSH is used as a front-line test, total or free T_3 should be measured to confirm the diagnosis.

Thyroid hormone release increased in all forms of hyperthyroidism, with plasma T_3 concentrations usually greater than T_4. Occasionally plasma T_4 is normal (T_3 toxicosis) and so plasma T_3 or free T_3 is most reliable.

The value of the highly sensitive TSH assay is mostly in confirming the diagnosis of hyperthyroidism where T_3 concentrations are borderline. Monitoring of therapy is best achieved by clinical criteria and plasma T_3, T_4 and TSH concentrations.

Immunological/inflammatory diseases

Graves disease. Graves disease is the commonest cause of hyperthyroidism. It is a relatively common disease in women (female:male ratio is 5:1) in the 15–40-year age group. There is a familial tendency and an association with the histocompatibility antigen human leucocyte antigen (HLA) DR3. It is associated with a wide range of autoimmune conditions (see Chapter 9).

Graves disease is an **autoimmune disease** characterized by the presence of a variety of TSHs including long-acting thyroid stimulator (LATS), human thyroid stimulator (HTS) and LATS protector (LATS-P) in the serum. The eye changes are dependent on a separate autoantibody causing a chronic inflammatory process in the eye muscles and retro-orbital connective tissue. The immunology of this disease is discussed in Chapter 9. The clinical manifestations of Graves thyrotoxicosis are illustrated in Fig. 14.5.

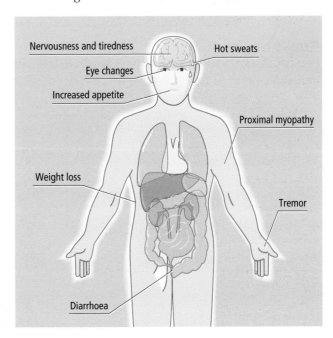

Fig. 14.5 Clinical manifestations of Graves' thyrotoxicosis.

Macroscopically, the thyroid gland is diffusely enlarged. **Histology** shows hyperplastic small thyroid follicles containing scanty colloid and occasional lymphocytes.

Benign thyroid tumours

Goitres (Table 14.17). The thyroid gland (Fig. 14.6) may show diffuse enlargement (goitre). The commonest cause in the west is diffuse, non-toxic and multinodular thyroid goitre (Fig. 14.7). This represents the culmination of mild deficiency of thyroid hormone production followed by feedback increase in TSH secretion by the pituitary, which results in hyperplasia. Hyperplasia of the gland corrects the hormonal deficiency and maintains the **euthyroid** state.

The condition may be **endemic**, associated with regions of low iodine deficiency away from coastal waters (such as the Alps) and **sporadic**, usually at times of physiological demand such as pregnancy and puberty (**physiological goitre**).

Figure 14.8 illustrates the diagnostic approach to the clinical investigation of thyroid enlargement.

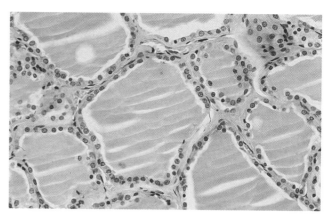

Fig. 14.6 Histology of the normal thyroid follicle. Note the pink colloid in the centre of the follicles. (H&E.)

Table 14.17 Causes of thyroid goitre.

Simple non-toxic goitre
Physiological, including endemic
Goitrogens
Dyshormonogenetic
Nodular goitre
Toxic goitre
Thyroiditis

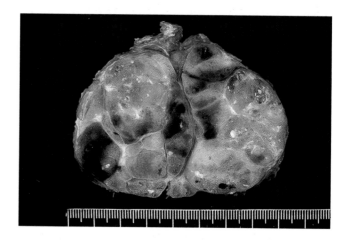

Fig. 14.7 Thyroid. Multinodular goitre. Note the brown haemorrhage and yellow colloid.

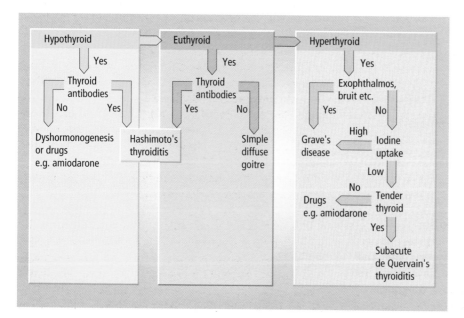

Fig. 14.8 Investigation of thyroid goitre.

Table 14.18 Thyroid neoplasms.

Primary tumours
Benign
    Adenoma
    Atypical adenoma (lipomas, haemangiomas, dermoid cysts, teratomas)
Malignant
    Angioinvasive encapsulated follicular carcinoma
    Papillary carcinoma
    Follicular carcinoma
    Medullary carcinoma
    Anaplastic carcinoma
    Lymphoma, sarcomas

Secondary tumours

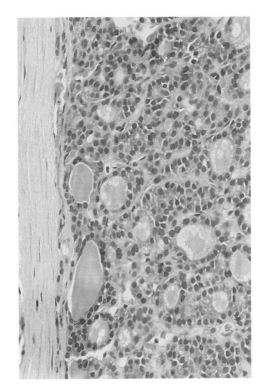

Fig. 14.9 Thyroid histology. Follicular adenoma. Note the intact capsule (left) and lack of invasion beyond the capsule or in to vessels. This distinguishes the tumour from follicular adenocarcinoma. (H&E.)

Solitary thyroid nodule. This is a common clinical problem. Autopsy studies have shown that solitary nodules of the thyroid are present in up to 10% of patients.

A solitary nodule will be malignant in fewer than 5% of cases; 30% or more are **benign adenomas**; the remainder are non-neoplastic conditions such as haemorrhagic cysts, Hashimoto's thyroiditis, early nodular goitre (**colloid nodule**) or normal thyroid (Table 14.18).

Fine-needle aspiration cytology (see Chapter 1) plays an important role in diagnosis of the solitary thyroid nodule. Thyroid scan is less reliable (20% of so-called 'cold' nodules turn out to be carcinomas).

Follicular adenoma. This may occur at any age but has a female:male ratio of 4:1. Patients are clinically **euthyroid**, although rare **toxic adenomas** occur.

Macroscopically, they appear as encapsulated, firm grey or red nodules up to 5cm in diameter. They may show cystic change, haemorrhage, calcification or fibrosis.

Microscopically they show follicles of varying size (described as embryonal, microfollicular or macrofollicular; Fig. 14.9). Other adenomas are composed of bright pink oncocytic cells (Hürthle cell adenoma). Capsular invasion and vascular invasion are the criteria for the diagnosis of malignancy.

Malignant thyroid tumours

These represent 0.5% of all cancer deaths. There is a female predominance (M/F = 2.5:1). Death occurs mainly by local invasion.

Predisposing factors include irradiation, nodular goitre, adenomas, dyshormonogenetic goitres (Hashimoto's disease and lymphomas). The histological type determines behaviour and prognosis. Thyroid carcinomas are euthyroid but the well-differentiated tumours may present with hyperthyroidism. Follicular and papil-

lary carcinomas are positive for thyroglobulin, which may be used as a tumour marker; medullary carcinoma secretes calcitonin.

Papillary carcinoma. This is the most common thyroid carcinoma. There is a female predominance with a peak age of 30–40 years but it may present in patients in their teens. It has a good prognosis with mainly local lymph node spread.

These tumours may be microscopic or present as large masses over 10cm in diameter. They are **locally infiltrative**. Microscopically, they have a **papillary architecture**, large, clear cell nuclei (Fig. 14.10), **intranuclear inclusions** caused by cytoplasmic invaginations into the nucleus and 40% show **psammoma bodies** (round laminated calcified bodies).

Treatment is surgical by hemithyroidectomy. Papillary carcinoma has an 80% 10-year survival.

Follicular carcinoma. Follicular carcinoma accounts for 20% of thyroid carcinomas. This tumour may be indistinguishable macroscopically from adenoma. Histology will show invasion of the capsule or blood vessels. This is a slow-growing tumour which may show early blood stream spread with metastases to the lung and bone. The

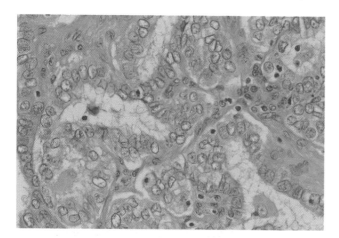

Fig. 14.10 Thyroid histology. Papillary carcinoma. Note the pale cells with large open nuclei that line the papillary cores. (H&E.)

5-year survival is 70%. There is a female predominance with a peak age of 40–50 years. Treatment is surgical or using radioactive iodine-131. T_4 therapy may be of value in disseminated disease.

Medullary carcinoma. Medullary carcinoma represents 5% of thyroid carcinomas. It presents in a range of age groups from teenagers to 30 years of age. Eighty per cent of cases are sporadic and 20% are associated with MEN syndrome type II (concurrence of thyroid medullary carcinoma, adrenal phaeochromocytoma and parathyroid adenoma).

Macroscopically they are firm and grey-white. Derived from parafollicular C cells, microscopically they consist of small polygonal and spindle cells arranged in nests, often showing **amyloid** in the stroma (Fig. 14.11). They grow slowly but with an infiltrative pattern and blood stream and lymphatic spread is seen. Treatment is surgical.

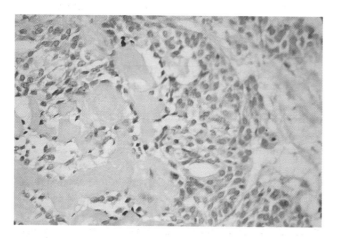

Fig. 14.11 Thyroid histology. Medullary carcinoma. Note the small, round cells and the deposits of amyloid (pink) in the interstitium. (H&E.)

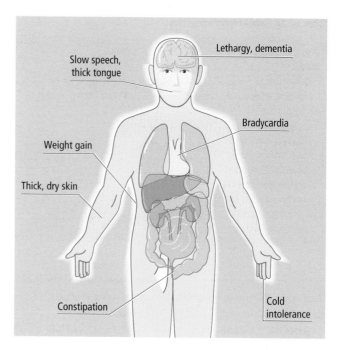

Fig. 14.12 Clinical manifestations of myxoedema in Hashimoto's thyroiditis.

Anaplastic carcinoma. This is a rare tumour representing 5% of thyroid carcinomas. It occurs most commonly in patients over 50 years. Macroscopically, it may be hard and gritty and it is highly infiltrative. The histology shows spindle cells which are poorly differentiated with frequent mitoses. Death occurs rapidly usually due to local invasion of neck structures.

Lymphoma. Primary malignant lymphoma of the thyroid gland (B-cell immunoblastic lymphoma) is extemely rare and is seen in patients with a history of Hashimoto's thyroiditis (Fig. 14.12).

The pathology of hypothyroidism (Table 14.19)

Thyroid function tests in hypothyroidism

Hypothyroidism from all causes will result in a decrease in secretion of thyroid hormones and in **primary hypothyroidism** the fall in serum T_4, and later in T_3, may be preceded by an increase in serum TSH concentrations as a result of the decrease in feedback inhibition. A decrease in serum T_4 is a more reliable indication of hypothyroidism than that of T_3, as peripheral conversion of T_4 to T_3 may be decreased in many conditions of nonthyroidal illness and also T_3 production by the thyroid may continue under the influence of the serum TSH levels.

Neonatal hypothyroidism is detected by screening

Table 14.19 Causes of hypothyroidism.

Deficiency of thyroid parenchyma
No goitre
Surgical or radiation ablation postthyrotoxicosis or carcinoma treatment
Primary autoimmune myxoedema
Agenesis or hypoplasia

Goitrous hypothroidism
Hashimoto's thyroiditis
Endemic iodine deficiency
Exogenous goitrogens, e.g. cassava, lithium, brassicas, antithyroid drugs
Dyshormonogenetic–congenital biosynthetic defects

Suprathyroidal lesions
Hypopituitarism and hypothalamic lesions

Peripheral resistance to thyroid hormones

Thyroiditis
Autoimmune throiditis
  Hashimoto's
  Primary myxoedema
  Focal thyroiditis

blood in the neonatal period for TSH measurement, with significantly elevated levels requiring confirmation by quantitative TSH and T_4 estimations prior to commencement of T_4 therapy. Borderline rises in TSH should be monitored. Current practice is to maintain T_4 replacement until the age of 5 years and then undergo a trial of withdrawal.

In **secondary hypothyroidism** plasma TSH levels are usually low but the condition may be confirmed by an absent or weak response in plasma TSH to injected TRH (Table 14.20).

Biochemical monitoring of hypothyroidism

Measurement of free and total thyroid hormone concentrations in the plasma of patients on replacement therapy is not helpful in establishing adequacy of replacement or

Table 14.20 Thyroid function tests in disease.

Condition	T_4	fT_4	T_3	TSH
Primary hypothyroidism	↓	↓	↓	↑
Thyrotoxicosis	↑	↑	↑	↓
Euthyroid sick	↓	↓	↓	N/↓
Amiodarone	N/↑	N/↑	N	N/↑
Lithium	↓	↓	↓	N/↑

T_4, Thyroxine; fT_4, free thyroxine; T_3, triiodothyronine; TSH, thyroid-stimulating hormone; N, normal.

compliance as the levels will be variable and are likely to fluctuate. Monitoring is important as undertreatment can lead to recurrence of hypothyroid symptoms whilst chronic overtreatment may cause symptomatic hyperthyroidism and osteoporosis. The most reliable indicator for this is plasma TSH with the aim of maintaining levels within the reference intervals. The slow rate of response of TSH makes it a valuable marker of **compliance**.

Inflammatory thyroid disease

Hashimoto's thyroiditis. This is an **organ-specific auto-immune** disease (Chapter 9) seen in middle-aged women. There is an association with the histocompatability antigen human leucocyte antigen (HLA) DR5. It is associated with other immune diseases, including Graves disease. Thyroid antibodies are present, including those to thyroglobulin, microsomal antibody and to colloid. Titres of these immunoglobulin G (IgG) antibodies do not correlate with severity of the disease and thus T-cell-mediated immunity may also play a part in its pathology.

In the early stages, the thyroid is diffusely enlarged, firm and 'rubbery'. As the disease progresses, it becomes smaller and finally **atrophic** and **fibrosed**.

Microscopically, there is destruction of thyroid follicles with lymphocytic infiltrates and lymphoid follicle formation.

Clinical features are variable as the patients may be euthyroid or mildly hypothyroid. Rarely, they may present with hyperthyroidism.

Without treatment these patients progress to primary hypothyroidism and 5% develop malignancy of the thyroid, either papillary carcinoma or malignant B-cell lymphoma.

Subacute/(granulomatous/DeQuervain's) thyroiditis. This condition is uncommon and affects both sexes equally and all ages. It is thought to have a viral aetiology (including mumps and coxsackievirus) and presents with **pain** and **enlargement** of the thyroid with **fever**.

It is self-limiting but it sometimes leads on to myxoedema. It has no relationship with Graves or Hashimoto's disease. Histology shows focal acute inflammation with a foreign-body granulomatous reaction to damaged follicles and colloid.

Riedel's thyroiditis. This rare disease can be confused with malignancy as it is a fibrosing process which destroys the gland and extends through the capsule. The resulting fixed, 'woody' mass may cause obstructive symptoms. It may represent a form of **fibromatosis** (see Chapter 26).

THE PARATHYROID GLANDS

Normal structure and function

Normally, there are four parathyroid glands, situated in two pairs on the posterior aspect of the thyroid gland.

In approximately 10% of patients, the number of glands is increased. The inferior glands arise from the same brachial arch as the thymus and they may occasionally have a mediastinum location.

Each parathyroid is encapsulated, brown-yellow in colour and has a maximum diameter of 5mm and maximum weight of 40mg.

Microscopically, the parathyroid gland contains three types of cell: water clear cells, chief cells and oxyphil cells. There is abundant fat within the intervening parenchyma. Each cell type produces **parathyroid hormone (PTH)**. The biochemistry and clinicopathology of calcium and bone are discussed in Chapter 20.

The pathology of hyperparathyroidism

Hyperparathyroidism is defined as elevated serum PTH due to increased secretion.

Primary hyperparathyroidism

This is due to intrinsic abnormality of the parathyroid gland (Table 14.21). The incidence is 42/100000 of population, increasing after the age of 50 years with a female/male ratio of 3:1.

Secondary hyperparathyroidism

This is commonly due to raised PTH **secondary** to **persistent hypocalcaemia**. This most commonly occurs in patients with **chronic renal failure**, the low renal mass and hyperphosphataemia-induced decrease in mitochondrial 1 alpha hydroxylase activity leading to a decrease in vitamin D-induced calcium absorption and subsequent PTH overstimulation.

Secondary hyperparathyroidism may also occur in patients with chronic **intestinal malabsorption**. This process induces **hyperplasia**–usually of all four parathyroids.

Tertiary hyperparathyroidism

This is commonly due to **autonomous adenoma** of parathyroid as a complication of secondary hyperparathyroidism or hypoparathyroidism.

Parathyroid adenoma

This is a **benign**, **solitary** tumour that involves one gland. Rarely there may be multiple adenomas. They are commonly between 1 and 2cm in diameter, and weigh 1–2g. They are well-encapsulated. Their size and location make them difficult to find.

Microscopically parathyroid adenomas are composed of a mixed population of chief cells, oxyphil cells and water clear cells arranged in sheets (Fig. 14.13).

Adenoma may be differentiated from normal or hyperplastic gland by the absence of fat in the tumour, size and the finding of a compressed rim of normal parathyroid at one edge. When a solitary adenoma is present, the remaining three glands are of normal size and microscopic appearance.

Parathyroid hyperplasia

Primary hyperplasia. The most accurate method of diagnosing primary parathyroid hyperplasia is by demon-

Table 14.21 Causes of primary hyperparathyroidism.

Single adenoma	83%
Multiple adenoma	4.3%
Carcinoma	1.7%
Hyperplasia	
Clear cell	7.6%
Chief cell	3.6% (associated with MEN 1)

MEN 1, Multiple endocrine neoplasia type 1.

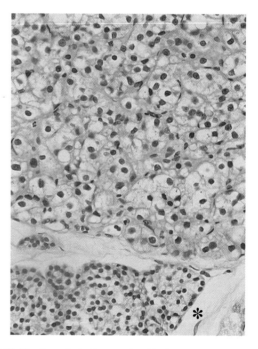

Fig. 14.13 Histology of a benign parathyroid adenoma. Note the compressed rim of normal parathyroid containing clear cells (✱). (H&E.)

strating increased weight of all four glands of above 40 mg each. Histologically there is proliferation of all three cell types at the expense of glandular fat.

Microscopic examination of a single enlarged gland does not permit differentiation from adenoma unless a rim of normal tissue is seen.

Secondary hyperplasia. The pathology in secondary parathyroid hyperplasia is identical to that seen in primary hyperplasia.

Parathyroid carcinoma

Parathyroid carcinoma is very rare. Patients tend to have a higher serum calcium and PTH than patients with adenoma.

The diagnosis of malignancy is made histologically by the findings of local infiltration of tumour cells beyond the capsule, high mitotic rate and fibrosis within the tumour.

Carcinoma of the parathyroid has a high rate of local recurrence. Metastases tend to occur to regional lymph nodes.

The pathology of hypoparathyroidism

Major causes (Table 14.22)

Table 14.22 Causes of hypoparathyroidism.

Inadequate secretion of PTH
Surgical—following thyroid, parathyroid and radical neck surgery
Familial
Sporadic
Di George syndrome
Suppression of PTH secretion from normal parathyroids
Neonatal—from maternal hypercalcaemia
Severe magnesium depletion
Defective end-organ response to PTH
Pseudohypoparathyroidism types I and II
(pseudopseudohypoparathyroidism)

PTH, Parathyroid hormone.

THE ADRENAL GLAND

Normal structure and function

The two adrenal glands occupy a retroperitoneal position above the kidneys. The normal weight is up to 4 g each.

The adrenal **cortex** is derived from the mesoderm of the **urogenital ridge** and has an origin independent from the **medulla**, which is of **neural crest** origin.

The cortex is composed of the **zona glomerulosa** (10–15%), the **zona fasciculata** (80%) and the **zona reticularis** (5–10%; Fig. 14.14).

The pathology of hyper- and hypoplasia of the adrenal gland is highly variable and depends upon the anatomical location of the disease process.

Diseases of the adrenal cortex

Congenital adrenal hyperplasia

This is a common inborn error of metabolism, with an incidence of about 1:6000 births. It is due to a **congenital deficiency** of one or more of the **enzymes** required for the intermediary synthesis of steroids. The result is an inability to synthesize **cortisol**, and in some instances **aldosterone**. These usually present in early childhood but milder forms may present in adulthood.

The most common form is complete 21-hydroxylase deficiency which accounts for about 95% of patients with congenital adrenal hyperplasia (CAH). The severe form has an incidence of about 1 in 12000 while a milder form is more common at 1 in 100–1000. The gene defect has been localized to the cytochrome p450c21 gene in the midst of the HLA locus on chromosome 6. A great number of different defects have been found and the disease is usually in compound heterozygotes with a high incidence of defective alleles rather than a specific gene defect. The severity is determined by the activity of the less severely affected of the two alleles. Abundant extra-adrenal 21-hydroxylase activity mediated by enzymes other than p450c21 (as yet unknown) probably explains why the severity of the disease is usually lessened with time.

Clinical forms of CAH. There are three clinical forms—salt-wasting, simple virilizing and non-classical. These probably represent points on a continuous spectrum of disease severity.

The **salt-wasting** form manifests as hyponatraemia, hyperkalaemia and metabolic acidosis in the first 2 weeks of life with a profound fall in aldosterone and cortisol synthesis. The condition is easier to diagnose in affected females as they have severe genital virilization but males are often missed and may present in severe salt-losing crisis.

The **simple virilizing** form has no salt-wasting and is diagnosed in virilized newborn babies or rapidly growing virilized boys. They do have some defective mineralocorticoid synthesis but it is not sufficient to cause significant salt loss.

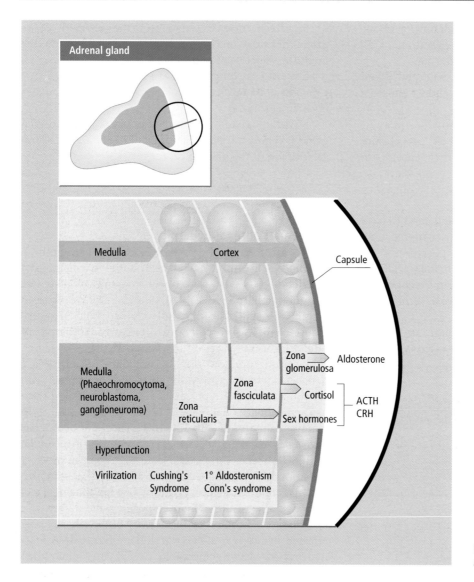

Fig. 14.14(a) Structure and function of the adrenal gland.

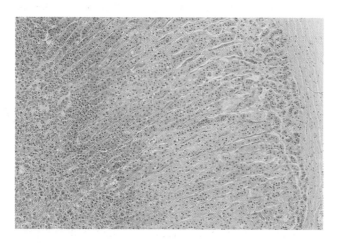

Fig. 14.14(b) Low power photomicrograph of the normal adrenal gland. (From left to right, zona reticularis, zona fascitulata, zona glomerulosa and the capsule.)

Diagnosis of CAH. Affected males are at greatest risk, presenting with hyponatraemia, hyperkalaemia, acidosis, dehydration, vomiting and diarrhoea. Viral diseases are in the differential diagnosis.

Basal 17-hydroxyprogesterone (in the morning) will be greatly increased and a sample for that as well as a urine sample for a urinary steroid profile should be collected prior to steroid replacement therapy. An intravenous Synacthen test has been advocated. Affected individuals are hyperresponsive to ACTH and the test helps to distinguish it from other forms of CAH and other disorders causing genital ambiguity.

Antenatal genetic diagnosis is available from **chorionic villus sampling (CVS)** to allow maternal treatment with **dexamethasone** to prevent androgenization of affected females. The success of this practice is still to be established.

Other causes of CAH are 11-hydroxylase deficiency, 17-hydroxylase and isomerase deficiency and 18-hydroxylase deficiency.

The pathology of hyperadrenalism (Table 14.23)

Cushing's disease and Cushing's syndrome. **Cushing's disease** is the clinical picture resulting from the overactivity of the adrenal cortex due to a functional disorder in the hypothalamus or a pituitary tumour.

Cushing's disease may be secondary to ectopic ACTH-like peptide-producing tumours. A modest **hypertension** is seen in 70–80% of patients. There is no correlation between severity of hypertension and biochemical changes. Blood pressure usually falls after appropriate surgery. The aetiology of the hypertension is unknown but it is not thought to be due to **sodium retention**.

Cushing's syndrome is the term used to describe the same set of clinical signs and symptoms resulting from an excess of glucocorticoids in the circulation (Table 14.24) but includes that involving a pathological process in the adrenal itself, from ectopic or inappropriate production of ACTH or from excessive administration of glucocorticoids (Fig. 14.15).

The most productive first-line investigations for adrenocortical hyperfunction following a clinical suspicion of Cushing's syndrome are biochemical screening tests to establish excessive production of glucorticoids which may include or be followed by biochemical tests to help establish the primary pathology. In addition to a range of specific tests, routine biochemical investigations may detect hypokalaemic alkalosis secondary to increased mineralocorticoid activity. Random plasma cortisol estimations are of little or no value as there is a

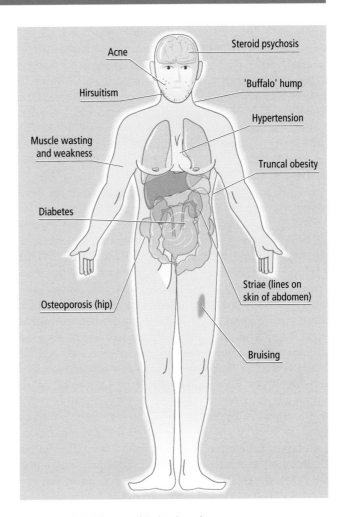

Fig. 14.15 Clinical features of Cushing's syndrome.

Table 14.23 Causes of adrenocortical hyperfunction.

Cushing's syndrome (hypercortisolism)
Conn's syndrome (hyperaldosteronism; adenomas and carcinomas)
Adrenogenital syndrome

Table 14.24 Causes of Cushing's syndrome.

Primary pituitary basophil adenoma
Bilateral adrenal hyperplasia – ? defective negative feedback of steroids on hypothalamus
Exogenous ACTH, e.g. oat cell carcinoma
Benign and malignant adrenocortical tumours (N.B.: children)
Iatrogenic

ACTH, Adrenocorticotrophic hormone.

marked diurnal variation in the production rate of cortisol, due to the nychthemeral rhythm in secretion of ACTH, with a peak in the early morning and a nadir at about midnight and most laboratories will only quote reference intervals for these times.

The following tests are recommended to establish the existence of Cushing's disease or syndrome.

1 Diurnal variation of plasma cortisol is abolished in Cushing's and a value for a midnight cortisol (2300 hours is acceptable) of >280 nmol/l (10 µg/dl) is highly suggestive of Cushing's disease. High levels may also be encountered in severely ill patients and in some psychotic state due to 'stress'.

2 Dexamethasone suppression test (DST). Dexamethasone is a very potent synthetic glucocorticoid and when 2 mg is given before retiring at night will suppress ACTH production in normal individuals sufficiently to suppress the rise in morning plasma cortisol levels to <140 nmol/l (5 µg/dl). Failure to suppress to this level is again highly suggestive of Cushing's, with the same exceptions as for the midnight cortisol test. Administration of a low dose (1 mg) will give a higher sensitivity at the expense of specificity, whilst extension of this test for 48 hours (with 0.5 mg given 6-hourly from 0900 hours on the first day and measurement of plasma cortisol at 0900 hours after 48 hours) will yield the best results but may be difficult to perform as an outpatient. This latter test is preferable.

3 Urinary free cortisol (UFC). Although most plasma cortisol is protein-bound and is metabolized in the liver mainly to metabolically inctive conjugates that are excreted by the kidneys, a small amount of free plasma cortisol is excreted intact and its measurement in urine provides a good indication of production rate. Whilst plasma total cortisol concentrations are affected by circulating oestrogens (raised in, for example, pregnancy, oestrogen therapy and the oral contraceptive pill) which affect cortisol-binding protein concentrations, oestrogens have little effect on urinary free cortisol levels. Thus an excretion rate of free cortisol of greater than 280 nmol/24 hours is a very effective screening test for adrenocortical hyperfunction. This test can easily be performed as an outpatient.

4 The **insulin hypoglycaemia (stress) test**, normally used as part of the assessment of the hypothalamic–pituitary–adrenal axis, can be used to help distinguish between stress-related increased cortisol production and that caused by Cushing's from whatever cause. The test (see biochemical investigations of pituitary disease) will be normal in stress-related conditions, obesity and depression whilst in Cushing's (when hypoglycaemia may be difficult to induce) there will be no rise in plasma cortisol during the test.

Other tests such as measurement of plasma ACTH levels are not indicated as screening tests for adrenocortical hyperfunction.

Establishing the site of an adrenocortical hyperfunctional lesion. The differentiation between **pituitary-dependent** (Cushing's disease) and **adrenal** (Cushing's syndrome) may be distinguished on the basis of the following.

1 Serum ACTH levels. In lesions with excess production of ACTH from either pituitary or ectopic tissue leading to adrenal hyperplasia, serum ACTH levels are usually greater than 10 ng/l (may reach 250 ng/l). In patients with adrenal tumours the ACTH level may be undetectable but will be <10 ng/l. Samples for serum ACTH levels should be collected into plastic tubes (ACTH is absorbed on to glass) and rapidly separated and frozen.

2 Radiological investigations such as abdominal CT/ultrasound or MRI scanning should be able to detect an enlarged adrenal due to a tumour with a contralateral atrophic or absent gland as well as detecting bilateral hyperplasia. Results of radiological investigations of the pituitary fossa do not correlate well with operative findings and are thus not very reliable in detecting pituitary-dependent Cushing's disease.

3 The **prolonged DST**, when the 48 hours of dexamethasone 0.5 mg q.d.s. is followed by a further 48 hours at 2 mg q.d.s., is also a useful discriminator for pituitary disease. The plasma cortisol level by day 4 of this test will be suppressed to 50% of basal levels in approximately 80% of patients with pituitary disease. Patients with adrenal tumours do not usually show suppression of cortisol production on either dose but some patients with ectopic ACTH syndrome may suppress.

In most cases the underlying pathology will be detected by the preceding tests but two others may play a role in localizing the pathology:

4 The **corticotrophin-releasing factor-41 (CRF-41) test.** CRF-41 is a 41 amino acid peptide, originally isolated from bovine hypothalami but which can now be synthesized, which has the physiological action of the native hormone in inducing ACTH release and synthesis from the anterior pituitary.

CRF-41 (100 μg) is given intravenously after basal samples are taken for plasma cortisol and ACTH. Further samples are collected at 15, 30, 45, 60, 90 and 120 minutes for cortisol and ACTH. The normal response to this test is a rise in plasma cortisol to 430–820 nmol/l at 60 minutes and a rise of plasma ACTH to 28–231 ng/l after 15–30 minutes. Most (at least 75%) patients with Cushing's disease show an exaggerated response (i.e. >820 nmol/l of cortisol and >231 ng ACTH/dl) whilst no change occurs with adrenal Cushing's or ectopic ACTH syndrome. This test is currently the most useful biochemical discriminator between pituitary and ectopically produced ACTH in Cushing's.

5 The **metyrapone test**. Metyrapone is an inhibitor of 11-hydroxylase and its administration to a normal individual will result in a decrease in cortisol production, leading to unopposed ACTH production and release with a concomitant rise in adrenal cortisol presursors. After basal collections of plasma for measurement of 11-deoxycortisol (±ACTH and urine for oxogenic steroids), metyrapone (750 mg) is given orally 4-hourly for 24 hours and further samples collected over the next 2 days. Patients with Cushing's disease show a rise in 11-deoxycortisol (from 24 to 36 nmol/l) to >600 nmol/l whilst in adrenal Cushing's there may be only a slight rise from an elevated baseline. There is also an approximate threefold rise in urinary oxogenic steroids in Cushing's disease with only a 50% rise in adrenal Cushing's. This test is now rarely performed but metyrapone is a useful medical treatment for Cushing's, particularly prior to pituitary or adrenal surgery.

Other tests for adrenocortical hyperfunction may include analysis of the urinary steroid profile as the concentrations of some of these may be significantly raised in adrenal and gonadal carcinoma. Dehydroepiandrosterone sulphate (DHEAS) in the serum and urine may be useful as a tumour marker in adrenal carcinoma.

Primary aldosteronism (Conn's syndrome; Table 14.25 and 14.26). There are three forms of primary aldosteronism—aldosterone-producing adenoma or carcinoma, idiopathic hyperaldosteronism and glucocorticoid-remediable hyperaldosteronism (rare).

All result in **excessive** and relatively **autonomous** aldosterone production. Bilateral adrenal hyperplasia is found in most cases of idiopathic disease. Hyperaldosteronism in this condition is almost always associated with lowered plasma renin activity, due to hypervolaemia, and lowered plasma potassium with no rise in serum ACTH.

Such a mechanism may possibly be responsible for part of a spectrum of **essential hypertension**. Thirty per cent of patients with essential hypertension have lowered plasma renin activity (Table 14.27).

Table 14.25 Causes of Conn's syndrome.

80% adenomas
Histology resembles adrenal hyperplasia
20% Multinodular adrenal hyperplasia
Very occasionally, pure hyperaldosteronism due to carcinoma

Table 14.26 Clinical features of Conn's syndrome.

Hypertension
Polyuria, nocturia, polydipsia
Neuromuscular signs, periodic muscle weakness, spontaneous tetany, cramps
Hypokalaemic alkalosis, low renin and angiotensin, high aldosterone

Table 14.27 Other causes of hypokalaemia.

Diuretic therapy
Aldosterone secondary to raised renin from renal disease or severe essential hypertension
Cushing's syndrome
Hypokalaemia secondary to liquorice or carbenoxolone
Renin-secreting tumours
Chronic active hepatitis

Classical presenting features of primary hyperaldosteronism include hypokalaemia, alkalosis and hypertension. It is rare for this disorder to result in malignant hypertension.

Diagnosis of primary aldosteronism. Hypokalaemic alkalosis is usual at presentation and plasma sodium is usually raised or at the top of the normal range (compared to secondary hyperaldosteronism and lowered sodium). Raised aldosterone secretion, unsuppressed by high salt intake, is found and suppression of plasma renin activity leads to a plasma aldosterone:renin ratio of greater than 1000 (units are pmol/l and pmol/ml angiotensin per hour).

A failure of plasma aldosterone to rise upon change from a recumbant to an erect posture or sodium depletion is suggestive of an adenoma and there is also no rise in plasma renin activity. An adenoma also tends to produce more severe biochemical changes. Plasma/salivary aldosterone or 18-hydroxycorticosterone rises at midday or after about 30 minutes of erect posture in normal patients and those with idiopathic hyperaldosteronism. The finding of raised plasma aldosterone and lowered plasma renin activity should then, together with ultrasonography and radioimaging, be followed by bilateral adrenal vein catheterization and sampling for aldosterone, renin and cortisol secretion. This is the most useful diagnostic procedure in the work-up to surgery, although the technique is difficult.

Dexamethasone treatment may be helpful in the diagnosis of the rare glucocorticoid-remediable hyperaldosteronism but should not be carried out unless there is a very strong suspicion of that diagnosis.

Adrenal cortical hyperplasia. Once thought to be a primary disorder of the adrenal gland, bilateral adrenal hyperplasia is now believed to be secondary to increased ACTH production, either from a pituitary adenoma or a malignant non-pituitary tumour.

Both adrenal glands are found to be enlarged and may have a nodular or diffuse appearance with visible widening of the zona fasciculata and zona reticularis.

Adrenal cortical adenoma. These are well-encapsulated tumours usually less than 5cm in diameter (Fig. 14.16). They are yellow in colour due to their high lipid content, or occasionally black (lipofuscin).

On microscopy, the cells resemble compact cells of zona reticularis with foci of clear cells (Fig. 14.17).

Adrenal cortical adenocarcinoma. These are large, weighing >60g and measuring >50g with areas of haemorrhage

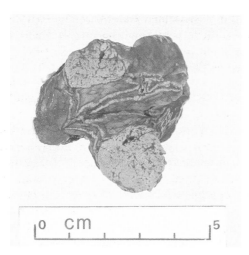

Fig. 14.16 Adrenal. Cortical adenoma. Note the striking yellow colour due to fat within the cells.

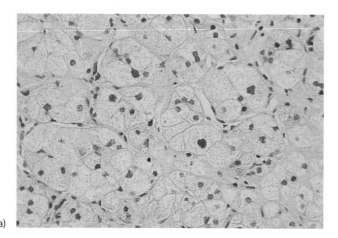

(a)

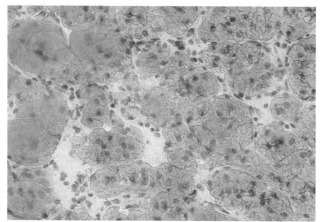

(b)

Fig. 14.17 Adrenal histology. (a) Cortical adenoma. Note the pale, foamy, regular cells with small nuclei. (H&E.) (b) Oil-red O stain for lipid in a frozen section shows the abundant orange–red-staining fat.

and necrosis. A capsule may be present but is often infiltrated by tumour which may involve the kidney.

At microscopy it may be difficult to distinguish benign from malignant tumours. The latter tend to have larger and more pleomorphic cells, more mitotic figures and blood vessel invasion.

The pathology of hypoadrenalism

Adrenocortical hypofunction (Addison's disese). Addison's disease is more common in females and can occur at any age. The clinical features include weakness, hypoglycaemia, weight loss, hyperpigmentation, vitiligo, anorexia, nausea, salt and water depletion (Table 14.28). Adrenal crisis may occur; this features circulatory collapse, vomiting and abdominal pain.

Adrenocortical hypofunction may be caused by **primary**, local pathological processes, **secondary** to pituitary disease or **tertiary** to hypothalamic failure of CRH or other ACTH secretagogues. This latter type is the most common cause of adrenal hypofunction and is usually caused by chronic administration of glucocorticoids (steroids). A total of 75% of cases of primary adrenal insufficiency are caused by an **autoimmune adrenalitis** and approximately 50% of these are associated with at least one other autoimmune disorder (Chapter 9).

The biochemical consequences of **adrenocortical failure** can be severely life-threatening and are often valuable pointers to the diagnosis, so an understanding of the physiological mechanisms of the failure leading to the metabolic disturbance is essential. In **primary adrenocortical insufficiency** failure of adrenal aldosterone production disturbs the balance of the renin–angiotensin–aldosterone regulatory system, decreasing renal tubular sodium reabsorption and enhancing potassium reabsorption and leading to a profound decrease in intravascular volume and **hypotension**. All three zones of the adrenal cortex are affected and so decreased cortisol production commonly leads to **hypoglycaemia** due to unopposed action of insulin (Table 14.29). In **acute adrenal crisis**, often triggered by

Table 14.28 Causes of Addison's disease.

Primary pituitary or hypothalamic
Primary adrenal – only manifest when 90% of the gland is destroyed
80% adrenal atrophy–autoimmune
Tuberculous
Congenital adrenal hypoplasia
Adrenal haemorrhage: Waterhouse–Friderichsen syndrome
Others – amyloidosis, sarcoidosis, haemochromatosis, metastatic carcinoma, surgical

Table 14.29 Causes of adrenocortical insufficiency.

> *Primary adrenocortical insufficiency*
> Autoimmune adrenalitis
> Infections (e.g. TB, CMV, meningococcal, HIV)
> Metastatic tumour deposits
> Congenital adrenal hypo- and hyperplasia
> Adrenoleukodystrophy
> Drugs (e.g. aminoglutethamide, ketoconazole, suramin)
>
> *Secondary adrenocortical Insufficiency*
> Panhypopituitarism
>   Tumours
>   Infections
>   Trauma
>   Metastases
>   Postpartum pituitary infarction (Sheehan's syndrome)
> Isolated ACTH deficiency
>
> *Tertiary adrenocortial insufficiency*
> Chronic glucocorticoid administration
> Postsurgery for Cushing's

TB, Tuberculosis; CMV, cytomegalovirus; HIV, human immunodeficiency virus; ACTH, adrenocorticotrophic hormone.

the metabolic stresses of an infection, the lack of mineralocorticoid secretion predominates in the clinical picture. In **chronic adrenal insufficiency**, androgen deficiency may also be symptomatic in women with loss of libido and of pubic hair. In **primary adrenal insufficiency** the excess ACTH production is commonly accompanied by **excess MSH production** and characteristic **hyperpigmentation**.

Diagnosis of adrenocortical insufficiency. Classical symptoms and signs of hypoadrenalism, such as hyperpigmentation, hypotension and salt craving, are usually preceded by many non-specific features such as weight loss, weakness, fatigue and gastrointestinal symptoms and so the diagnosis should be considered and investigated far more often.

Basal plasma cortisol estimations, particularly in the early morning or when the patient is stressed, are often informative but rarely can they be considered diagnostic. A value of less than 140 nmol/l (< 5 μg/dl) in stress allows a presumptive diagnosis of adrenocortical insufficiency and < 275 nmol/l (< 10 μg/dl) is also strongly suggestive, whilst a value of > 1000 nmol/l (< 35 μg/dl) excludes the diagnosis.

Basal serum ACTH can be measured and will be significantly elevated in primary adrenocortical insufficiency but this is seldom necessary to make an initial diagnosis.

- **The short Synacthen test.** Synacthen (tetracosactrin) is a synthetic peptide of the first 24 amino acids of the human ACTH peptide (synACTHen). Injected intramuscularly, this peptide stimulates in normal individuals a rise in plasma cortisol concentration to at least 430 nmol/l (15 μg/dl) at 30 minutes and 580 nmol/l (21 μg/dl) at 60 minutes. There is usually at least a doubling of the basal level during the test. Failure to reach these values confirms the diagnosis of adrenal insufficiency in most cases. This test can be performed after commencement of steroid therapy after making a presumptive diagnosis but patients should have their therapy changed to dexamethasone on the day of the test to prevent cross-reactivity of other preparations with the cortisol assay.
- **The long Synacthen test.** Long-acting (depot) Synacthen may be given by intramuscular injection twice daily for up to 5 days in order to attempt to stimulate some adrenal cortisol production in chronically suppressed adrenals from secondary or tertiary causes. A rise in plasma cortisol of > 1100 nmol/l (40 μg/dl) 6 hours after the last injection would be expected in normal subjects and in secondary and tertiary adrenocortical insufficiency but no rise will occur in primary disease.

Isolated mineralocorticoid deficiency–hyporeninaemic hypoaldosteronism. This is a relatively common condition where persistently decreased renin secretion by the renal juxtaglomerular apparatus leads to hypoaldosteronism.

About 50% of cases are in **diabetics** but other conditions associated with this condition include amyloidosis, cirrhosis, acquired immune deficiency syndrome (AIDS), systemic lupus erythematosus and myeloma. It is characterized by a **hyperkalaemic acidosis** (type 4 renal tubular acidosis) with **low plasma aldosterone** levels, even under stimulatory conditions such as low salt diet and low plasma renin activity.

Diseases of the adrenal medulla (Table 14.30)

Table 14.30 Tumours of the adrenal medulla.

> Phaeochromocytoma
> Ganglioneuroma–benign tumour of nerve cells
> Neuroblastoma–malignant tumour of childhood
> Secondary malignancies

Phaeochromocytoma

This tumour is a **paraganglioma** of the adrenal medulla (Table 14.31). It is a catecholamine-secreting tumour,

Table 14.31 Clinical presentation of phaeochromocytoma.

	Affected (%)	
	Paroxysmal	Persistent
Headache	92	72
Sweating	65	69
Palpitation	73	51
Anxiety, fear	60	28
Tremor	51	26
Pain in chest, abdomen	48	28
Nausea ± vomiting	43	26
Prostration	38	15
Severe weight loss	14	15

Symptoms from local effects may present, such as dysphagia.
In general, physical signs suggesting a specific diagnosis are rare.

Table 14.32 Some features of phaeochromocytomas.

99% are in abdomen or pelvis
10% are outside the adrenal medulla
10% are bilateral (more so in familial cases)
10% are malignant (more so in familial cases)

Table 14.33 Differential diagnosis of phaeochromocytoma.

Anxiety states
Hyperventilation
Thyrotoxicosis
Recurrent hypoglycaemia

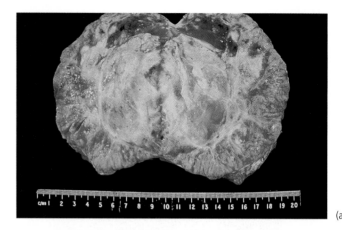
(a)

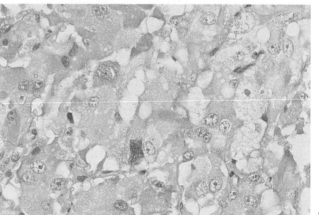
(b)

Fig. 14.18 Adrenal medulla. (a) Phaeochromocytoma with a characteristic yellow–brown colour. (b) Histology of the phaeochromocytoma shows large, glassy, pink cells with large, irregular nuclei. (H&E.)

found in < 0.5% of hypertensives. It may secrete noradrenaline, adrenaline or both.

Phaeochromocytoma is known as the **10% tumour**– 10% malignant, 10% bilateral, 10% extra-adrenal and 10% in children (Table 14.32).

Phaeochromocytomas arise in **chromaffin cells** of neuroectodermal origin and may be found anywhere in the sympathoadrenal system from neck to bladder. Familial tumours are well-recognized (MEN II) and nearly always found in the adrenal medulla. Both adrenals are involved in 70% of familial cases (Table 14.33).

Macroscopically, it is an encapsulated **yellow-brown** vascular tumour often with areas of haemorrhage and necrosis (Fig. 14.18(a)). Microscopically it consists of **pleomorphic** pink cells (Fig. 14.18(b)) with occasional ganglion cells. The only reliable marker of malignancy is the presence of metastasis.

Investigation of phaeochromocytoma. A demonstration of overproduction of catecholamines is needed and one nor-

mal measurement alone may not exclude the diagnosis so three urine collections are recommended, preferably collected when the patient is symptomatic. The 24-hour urine collection should be into acid to prevent catecholamine metabolism. Laboratories will offer the following assays:
- vanillylmandelic acid;
- metadrenaline (more reliable index–quantitative);
- normetadrenaline;
- methoxytyramine (dopamine metabolite);
- noradrenaline (also reliable index but very low concentrations);
- adrenaline.

Plasma noradrenaline and adrenaline can be measured but sample collection procedures have to be stringent to prevent false positives and the assays are difficult, and difficult to interpret. Selective venous sampling for plasma catecholamines is the ideal method if other tests are equivocal.

Dynamic tests for phaeochromocytoma. These include **pentolinium** and **clonidine** tests where serum cate-

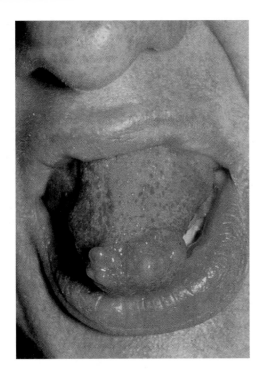

Fig. 14.19 MEN IIb. This patient presented with a neuroma of the tongue and was known to have von Recklinghausen's disease. He also had thyroid and adrenal adenomas.

Table 14.34 Multiple endocrine neoplasia (MEN) syndromes.

Type I – Werner's syndrome
Pituitary adenomas
Parathyroid hyperplasia
Pancreatic islet cell tumours (including gastrinoma)
Peptic ulceration (Zollinger–Ellison syndrome)
  (Adrenocortical adenomas rarely)

Type IIa – Sipple syndrome
Phaeochromocytoma (often bilateral) or adrenal medullary hyperplasia
Medullary carcinoma of thyroid
Multiple mucosal neuromas
Marfanoid appearance
Ganglioneuromas of bowel
  (Parathyroid hyperplasia/adenoma occasionally)

Type IIb (Fig. 14.19)
Mucocutaneous neuromas (tongue, lips, eyelids, mouth, gut)
  (von Recklinghausen's disease)
Thyroid adenoma/carcinoma
Adrenal adenoma/carcinoma

Inheritance: autosomal dominant, incomplete penetrance

Occasional spontaneous forms

Within an individual, tumour may be synchronous or asynchronous

cholamine excretion continues despite presynaptic blockade in patients with the disease.

Neuroblastoma

This is an **adrenal medulla** tumour of **primitive neuroblasts** (Chapter 11). Seventy per cent occur in children aged under 4 years. This tumour is associated with **neurofibromatosis** and other congenital syndromes.

Macroscopically, they are large grey soft tumours made up of small uniform cells with rosetting ('small, blue cell tumours of childhood'; see Chapter 25).

Catecholamines and **precursors** can be found in urine but hypertension is rare. Seventy per cent have metastases at diagnosis. Prognosis is age-, stage- and grade-dependent.

MULTIPLE ENDOCRINE NEOPLASIA SYNDROMES

The MEN syndromes or multiple endocrine adenomatosis (MEA) syndromes are characterized by the association of neoplasms of endocrine glands, inherited as an autosomal dominant trait with incomplete penetrance.

Three types of MEN syndrome are described (Table 14.34).

THE DIFFUSE NEUROENDOCRINE SYSTEM

The occurrence of multiple familial tumours of the endocrine system indicates that these cells are related in some way. The term neuroendocrine system or APUD system has been applied to these interrelated cells. These cells are believed to be derived from neuroectodermal cells of the neural crest (Table 14.35).

The effects of neuroendocrine tumours depend on several factors, including the site, size, peptide production and malignant features (Table 14.36).

Histology of these tumours shows round or polygonal cells with clear or eosinophilic granular cytoplasm (Fig. 14.20). Nuclei are round, small and uniform. Mitoses are uncommon, as are necrosis and haemorrhage. Connective tissue strands and vascular spaces separate nests and strands of cells.

The behaviour is difficult to predict from histology alone. Even when malignant, these tumours are often **well-differentiated** and **slow-growing**. Most morbidity and mortality is related to **peptide production**, rather than to the tumour mass. Most tumours can be demonstrated to produce several peptides, not all of which are biologically active. The predominant peptide can change with time. The peptides produced are not restricted to those normally produced by the cells from which the tumour has arisen.

Table 14.35 The diffuse neuroendocrine system.

Definitions	
Diffuse	Not organized into discrete glandular structures
Neuroendocrine	Both endocrine and nerve cells seem to share similar characteristics
System	Irrespective of site, the cells share similar microscopic features, appear to work in similar ways, producing similar substances— *regulatory peptides*
Synonyms	Amine precursor uptake and decarboxylation (APUD) cells; chromaffin cells Other names refer to these cells when found in specific sites, e.g. Kulchitsky cells in the stomach, Fehrter cells in the bronchus
Features	
Origin	Once thought to be entirely of neuroectodermal origin, now some known to be of endodermal origin
Distribution	Most organ systems, including gastrointestinal tract, genitourinary tract, skin, respiratory tract, thyroid gland, adrenal medulla, pituitary gland
Light microscopy	Pear-shaped cells, cytoplasm clear and granular, small round and uniform nuclei. Cells poorly stained on haematoxylin and eosin
Histochemistry	Masked metachromasia, lead haematoxylin, silver impregnation techniques (argentaffin, argyrophil)
Electronmicroscopy	Electron-dense secretory granules, specialized microvilli
Immunocytochemistry	Chromogranin; cytokeratin (dot-positivity); neurone-specific enolase; neurofilaments; specific peptides, e.g. vasoactive intestinal peptide, substance P

Diagnosis is confirmed by direct serum/urine assay or by stimulation/suppression tests for specific peptide, tumour-selective venous sampling, radioisotope-labelled specific antibodies, MRI scans, angiography, ultrasound, CT scans or specific antibodies.

Metastases should be sought clinically, particularly to the liver.

THE ENDOCRINE PANCREAS

Normal structure and function

The **islets** are distributed throughout the pancreas, although most are found in the head. Each islet is invested by a thin pseudocapsule and has a substantial sinusoidal blood supply arising from a single afferent arteriole and draining into numerous efferent arterioles.

The **endocrine cells** at light microscopy appear similar but immunocytochemically and at electronmicroscopy there are four main types: A, B, D and PP (Table 14.37), each characterized by its hormone content. The four cell types are not randomly arranged within islets but have strict relationships compatible with a paracrine function. The B cells lie mainly in the centre of islets and maintain contact primarily with other B cells while A and D cells are always closely apposed and lie predominantly at the edges of the islets.

Insulin is released from the β **cells** into the lumen of the vascular sinusoids by exocytosis and a similar secretory process probably occurs with the other cell types (Figs 14.21 and 14.22). Although serum hormone levels as well as blood glucose levels are important factors governing secretion, sympathetic, parasympathetic and hormones of the extrapancreatic gastrointestinal neuroendocrine system are also involved.

Diabetes mellitus

This disorder involves a number of factors and clinically separates into two main primary types and a number of secondary types (Table 14.38), all with the common denominator of an absolute or relative deficiency of insulin.

The disorder affects two in every 100 people in the UK and 60 000 new sufferers are recognized annually, 3000 of whom are children. The disease is a major cause of blindness, end-stage renal disease and limb amputation and its importance is principally this morbidity as well as an important contributor to death in young adults (Table 14.39). The aim of clinicians is clearly to lower the incidence of these and other complications and ideally to prevent them altogether, which logically should arise from strict control of the diabetes, an association that has not been unequivocally proven.

Biochemistry of diabetes mellitus

Diabetes mellitus is conventionally classified, from both clinical and pathological criteria, into **type 1** (insulin-dependent—IDDM: hitherto juvenile-onset—JOD) and **type**

Table 14.36 Neuroendocrine tumours (APUDomas).

Site	Tumour	Secretory product
Bronchus	Carcinoid, small cell (oat cell) carcinoma	5-HT, ADH, ACTH, PTH
Gastrointestinal tract	Carcinoid	Gastrin, VIP, 5-HT
Pancreas	Islet cell tumour	Insulin, glucagon, VIP, PP somatostatin 5-HT, ACTH, bombesin
Thyroid	Medullary carcinoma	Calcitonin
Parathyroid	Adenoma/carcinoma	PTH
Adrenal medulla	Phaeochromocytoma	Catecholamines
Skin	Merkel cell tumour	Calcitonin, PTH

5-HT, 5-Hydroxytryptamine; ADH, antidiuretic hormone; ACTH, adrenocorticotrophic hormone; PTH, parathyroid hormone; VIP, vasoactive intestinal peptide; PP, pancreatic polypeptide.

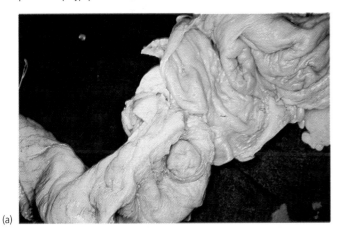

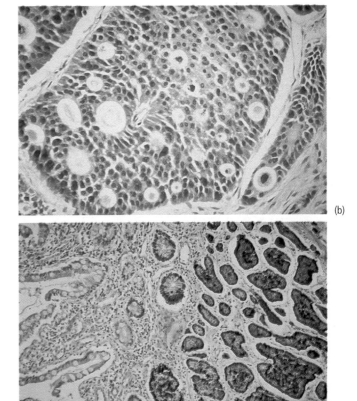

Fig. 14.20 Ileal carcinoid tumour. (a) Note how well-circumscribed the tumour is. This patient presented with small bowel obstruction. (b) Histology shows small dark blue cells arranged in trabeculae with a well-circumscribed border. (H&E.) (c) Positively stained with Grimelius (dark brown–black granules), indicating a neuroendocrine origin.

2 (non-insulin-dependent–NIDDM: hitherto maturity-onset–MOD).

The clinical condition of diabetes may occur transiently in pregnancy (gestational diabetes), as a result of malnutrition, as a secondary phenomenon in pancreatic disease or in endocrine diseases such as acromegaly, hypercortisolism (Cushing's syndrome) or phaeochromocytoma (increased catecholamine production).

Drugs such as thiazide diuretics, oestrogen-containing oral contraceptives and catecholaminergic drugs such as

salbutamol can induce impairment of glucose tolerance or diabetes.

Immunogenetics

Type 1. A familial tendency of approximately 10% in parents and also in siblings together with a concordance rate in identical twins of only 50% suggests that there is no consistent genetic element in type 1 diabetes mellitus. There is however an established association between certain HLA types and autoimmune type 1 diabetes with

Table 14.37 Hormone-producing cells in the pancreas.

Designation	% of islet	Location	Granule	Hormone
α	15–20	Mainly body and tail	Round with dense centre and paler rim	Glucagon (gastric inhibitory peptide, cholecystokinin, endorphin)
β	75–80	Uniformly	Variably shaped, including rectangular and hexagonal	Insulin (C peptide, pro-insulin, islet amyloid)
σ	5–15	Uniformly	Moderately dense and large	Somatostatin
PP	1	Mainly uncinate lobe	Large round to angular granules of varying density	Pancreatic polypeptide

These cells may be demonstrated by immunocytochemistry using the appropriate antibody.

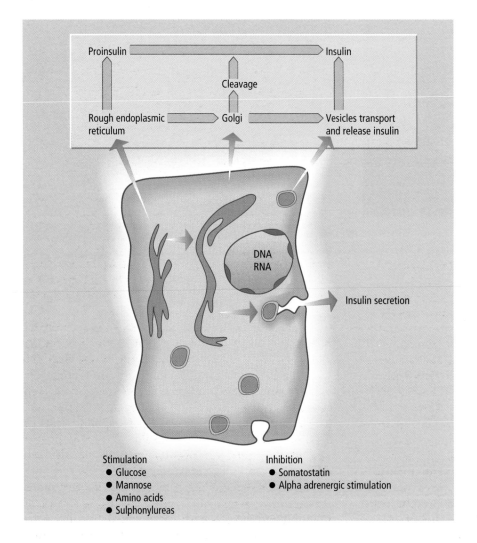

Fig. 14.21 Insulin synthesis and secretion by the pancreatic islet cell.

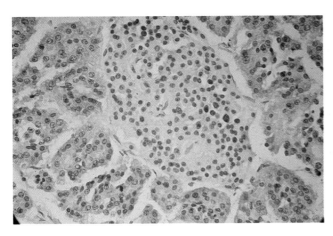

Fig. 14.22 Pancreas histology. The normal pancreatic islet. (H&E.)

Table 14.38 A classification of diabetes mellitus.

Primary
Type I—insulin-dependent islet cell antibodies
Type II—insulin-independent

Secondary
Pancreatic resection
Pancreatitis
Haemochromatosis
Mucoviscidosis
Endocrine disorders

Table 14.39 Clinical complications of diabetes mellitus.

Infection
(Skin infections)
Localized
Pneumonia (treatable)

Renal disease
Diabetic glomerulosclerosis
Renal impairment (Kimmelstiel–Wilson kidneys)
Pyelonephritis
Papillary necrosis
Hypertension
Glomerulonephritis

Vascular disease
Small vessels (microangiopathy)
   Blindness
   Strokes
   Neuropathy
   Myocardial ischaemia
Large vessels (macroangiopathy/arteriosclerosis)
   Peripheral vascular disease
   Myocardial infarction

Neuropathy
Sensory nerves
Autonomic systems

Polyneuropathy
Diarrhoea

approximately 95% of white type 1 diabetes having either DR3 or DR4 and 55–60% having both.

It is now thought that alleles of HLA-DQ β-chain are responsible for determining a susceptibility or resistance to the autoimmune destruction that is known to occur in type 1 diabetes. Full susceptibility to autoimmune β-cell destruction is conferred if both DQ β-chain alleles have an aspartate missing at position 57, whilst this is reduced to 10% with only one of these (DQw8) alleles present. There may be a further HLA relationship to distinguish between primary autoimmune destruction and environmental risk that is followed by autoimmune events.

The autoimmune destruction of pancreatic islet β-cells may occur as a result of repeated environmental exposure to a variety of possible stimuli, including viruses occurring over several years and this eventually leads to insulin deficiency. Islet cell autoantibodies, thought to be against glutamate decarboxylase, are present in the serum in 60–90% of patients at the time of diagnosis and have gone within 2 years.

Type 2. In the common form, no HLA association has been noted but it is thought there is a **strong genetic element** as the concordance rate in identical twins is virtually 100% within 5 years of onset in the first twin. It is likely that **environmental factors** also contribute significantly to the aetiology.

There is a greater risk of type 2 diabetes if the proband is a sibling as opposed to a parent. There may be an additional relationship with low birth weight and also with a rise in standard of living from previous deprivation. Patients with type 2 diabetes have a high incidence of pancreatic islet amyloid deposits and it is thought that islet amyloid polypeptide (IAPP or amylin) is cosecreted with insulin and may play a role in the metabolic disturbance and on islet cell destruction.

Insulin resistance is common in type 2 diabetes and is enhanced by obesity, which itself may also be a cause of insulin resistance. There is a continuing debate about the cause of the hyperglycaemia in type 2 diabetes, centred on whether the primary defect is a decrease in hepatic glucose production or a decrease in glucose uptake by skeletal muscle. Recent data support more strongly the latter site of decreased insulin action. There are several **candidate genes** for the impaired glucose-induced β-cell insulin response, including genes for the enzymes **glucokinase** and **glucose-6-phosphatase** and for **glucose transporters**. It is likely that the genetics of type 2 diabetes is considerably **heterogeneous**.

Maturity-onset diabetes of the young (MODY) is a form of type 2 diabetes in which mutations in the gene for glucokinase in hepatocytes and pancreatic β cells have been found in about 55% of familial cases. The gene defect leads to an impairment of glucose-induced insulin release and to a decrease in hepatic glucose uptake.

It has been estimated that defects in the glucokinase gene may contribute approximately 10% of familial type 2 diabetics, although this represents a small fraction of the total type 2 diabetes of white populations.

Clinical presentation of diabetes

Symptoms of thirst and polyuria, caused by the osmotic diuresis induced by hyperglycaemia, together with weight loss and wasting are common together with recurrent skin and urinary tract infections. Symptoms of the microvascular complications of diabetes include visual disturbances secondary to retinopathy and cataracts, leg ulcers and gangrene, pruritus and a sensory peripheral neuropathy.

Diagnosis of diabetes mellitus

Random blood glucose sample together with **urine testing** for glycosuria may be adequate in a new case with clear history. A random venous blood glucose of >11.1 mmol/l is diagnostic and no further assays are needed.

Ideally, a fasting blood glucose should be taken together with a urine test for glucose and ketones. Fasting venous blood glucose of greater than 7.8 mmol/l is diagnostic of diabetes but if marginal or if you suspect another cause for the raised blood glucose, then an oral glucose tolerance test should be performed.

Oral glucose tolerance test. The test should be carried out in the morning following an overnight fast (ideally 14 hours). The patient has blood taken at the start of the test and again at 1 and 2 hours (the 2-hour sample is the most important). The patient is given 75 g of glucose as a drink (or 300 ml of Lucozade) if adult or 1.75 g/kg up to a maximum of 75 g if a child.

A diagnosis of **impaired glucose tolerance** carries an overall risk of progression to overt diabetes of approximately 2% per year. It is important to understand that results of glucose tolerance tests vary considerably in an individual and so borderline tests should be repeated at least once and preferably on two occasions (Table 14.40).

Table 14.40 World Health Organization criteria for the diagnosis of diabetes mellitus.

	Glucose concentration (mmol/l)		
	Venous whole blood	Capillary whole blood	Venous plasma
Diabetes mellitus			
Fasting	> 6.7	> 6.7	> 7.8
2 hours after glucose	> 10.0	> 11.0	> 11.1
Impaired glucose tolerance			
Fasting	< 6.7	< 6.7	< 7.8
2 hours after glucose	> 6.7–≤ 10	> 7.8–≤ 11.1	> 7.8–≤ 11.1

Pathology of diabetes mellitus

Type II diabetes. This pattern of the disorder accounts for 75% of patients with diabetes mellitus, most of whom are elderly and most of whom do not require insulin therapy.

Macroscopically the pancreas is reduced in size and has an increased fat content and hence is similar to that of many elderly patients. Histopathological changes are mild and lack any consistent feature.

Amyloid, lying extracellularly, is the change within the pancreas that is nearest to being characteristic of type II diabetes. This is found in the **islets** in variable amounts, sometimes as distinct amorphous eosinophilic globules, but not uniformly distributed. The amyloid, islet-amyloid polypeptide, is synthesized within the B cells of the islets and may produce diabetes mellitus simply by obstructing the secretion of insulin into the islet sinusoids or by replacing islets. Amyloid can also be found in pancreases from elderly patients without type II diabetes mellitus and is not universal amongst all those with this form of diabetes mellitus.

Morphometric studies show a reduction by about half of the volume of islet B cells and this inevitably produces an alteration in the ratio of these cells with the other islet cells, which is further affected by an increase in the number of A cells. The numerical changes in B and A cells in themselves are not sufficient to produce diabetes mellitus but the changed ratios and the potential effects these may have on the paracrine control of their secretions may be important.

Fibrosis is evident between and around acini and islets and is the most frequent finding in affected pancreases but it is also seen in those patients without diabetes mellitus. The change may in part be aggravated by the diabetes since it progresses with the duration of the disease and partly correlates with the worsening arteriosclerosis.

Arteriosclerosis is a feature of many of the patients of the age group involved and this change is invariably found in the large vessels supplying the pancreas as well as in their smaller branches.

Fatty replacement of the exocrine components of the pancreas occurs with increasing age and consequently is seen in diabetes mellitus. Surviving islets may be encased by the fat cells.

There is currently no satisfactory or universally accepted explanation of the development of this form of diabetes mellitus. The role of amyloid is currently receiving widespread investigation but its absence in some patients clearly shows that its deposition is not essential for the appearance of the disorder. The possible role of a wide number of other agencies, including genetic, infectious and immunological, has been exhaustively studied but no association has emerged. Similar comments apply to hypotheses based on the concepts of overstretching the insulin demand from obesity, loss of peripheral insulin receptors or the blocking of insulin.

Type I diabetes. This is the form of diabetes mellitus that is best known to the general public, largely because of the necessity for **insulin injections**. Nevertheless, it is much less common than type II diabetes mellitus, although because of the younger age group involved it carries a higher morbidity and mortality rate and is in many countries the main cause of end-stage renal disease. Unlike type II diabetes mellitus, much is known about its cause, which includes a **genetic predisposition** and involves immunological and viral agencies acting in some patients singly and in others in concert. The end-result is a loss of B cells, amounting to over 20% at the inception of the clinical disorder, and consequently altered relationships between the islet cells, conspiring to decrease available insulin.

Histopathology. The **pancreas** ultimately is **smaller** than normal but the extent of this will be affected by the duration of the disorder. Atrophy, predominantly but not solely of the endocrine component, underlies this change.

Islets are smaller than normal and may be difficult to distinguish from the surrounding exocrine cells with which they merge. A cells predominate with smaller numbers of D cells and few or no B cells, except in the very early phases when B cells may be plentiful and large. Throughout the pancreas there is no uniformity amongst these changes in the islets.

Insulitis is a feature confined to early type I diabetes mellitus in which some and usually a minority of islets are surrounded and mildly infiltrated by lymphocytes and a few eosinophil polymorphs. In contrast with

autoimmune disorders, plasma cells do not form part of this infiltrate and there is no follicle formation.

Fibrosis and **amyloid deposition** in islets are extremely rare occurrences.

Interstitial changes probably promote gradual exocrine atrophy and these are similar to those found in type II diabetes mellitus and include fibrosis, arteriosclerosis and fatty replacement. Their extent and degree will reflect the duration of the disorder, the age of the patient and, in some patients, the severity of the disorder.

Complications of diabetes mellitus

The range of complications is common to both type I and type II diabetes mellitus, although the consequences to the type I diabetic are greater, mainly because they appear and are fully developed at a younger age. Infections (Table 14.41), vascular lesions (Table 14.42) and renal disorders (Table 14.43; Fig. 14.23) form the basis of these complications and consequently provide the potential for

Table 14.41 Common organisms causing infection amongst diabetics.

Organisms	Pathogenetic factors
Yeast	Altered chemotaxis
Fungus	Impaired polymorph adhesion
Staphylococci	Lowered bactericidal activity
Escherichia coli	Depressed phagocytosis
Mycobacterium tuberculosis	Depressed phagocytosis

Table 14.42 Vessel changes in diabetes mellitus.

Lesions	Pathogenetic factors
Vessel wall hyalinization	Endothelial cell damage
Intimal fibrosis	Impaired prostaglandin formation
Atherosclerosis	Platelet aggregation
Medial calcification	Impaired platelet formation
	Increased fibrinogen breakdown products

Table 14.43 Diabetic glomerulosclerosis.

Glomerular lesions	Pathogenetic factors
Mesangial nodules	Increased glomerular filtration
Basement membrane thickening	Renal hypertrophy
Capsular drops	Accumulated mesangial protein
Fibrin caps	Accelerated ageing of type IV collagen
Arteriolar hyalinization	Intrarenal vascular disease

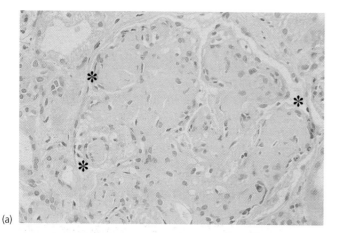

(a)

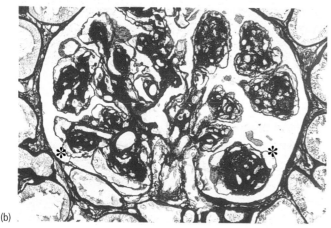

(b)

Fig. 14.23 Renal histology in diabetes mellitus, Kimmelstiel–Wilson lesions of the renal glomerulus (✱). (a) H&E, (b) silver stain.

major vital organ derangements involving the brain, heart, kidneys and eyes.

It would seem logical that the extent and severity of the complications should reflect the adequacy of the control of the metabolic effects of diabetes and that good control should equate with few complications. These beliefs in practice are not always sustained, probably because it is not entirely clear which factor is accountable for any one complication and because more than one factor may be instrumental in producing more than one form of complication. **Hyperglycaemia** emerges as the most important factor with its secondary effects on phagocytosis, complement function, platelets, endothelium and clotting. The effects of **ketosis**, once believed the fundamental cause of many diabetic complications, are now largely **discounted**.

The impact of hyperglycaemia is readily demonstrated during **pregnancy** when poor control clearly has an adverse effect upon the **fetus**. High glucose levels during the first 8 weeks of pregnancy are largely instrumental in producing **congenital abnormalities** in the fetus at a rate

three times greater than that in the fetus of non-diabetic mothers. These abnormalities partly explain the number of **spontaneous abortions** amongst pregnant diabetics since both can be substantially reduced by careful control of the maternal blood glucose during the very early phases of pregnancy. A similar approach has lowered perinatal mortality to 30%, which is in part due to prevention of **hyperinsulinaemia**. Insulin secretion is stimulated in the fetal pancreas where islet hypertrophy and hyperplasia occur and its effect is to produce selective organomegaly and an increase in fat in the fetus which both reverse after birth. Additionally there are decreased levels of surfactant in the lungs and raised levels of circulating **erythropoietin**. The changes contribute to difficulties during delivery, respiratory distress, polycythaemia, hyperbilirubinaemia and renal vein thrombosis, any of which may be fatal.

Endocrine tumours of the pancreas

The terminology of these tumours is confusing since many are associated with hormones not usually native to the pancreas, a phenomenon explained by the concept of a multipotential endocrine stem cell that has undergone inappropriate or incomplete differentiation. The term **islet cell tumour** (Fig. 14.24) is consequently a poor one and they are best distinguished according to the hormone they produce, although some are still referred to by eponyms (Table 14.44).

Tumours within the pancreas that secrete hormones have been known of for many years but only following the use of **immunocytochemistry** has their range been appreciated and their categorization become possible. Even so, precise recognition also requires **endocrinological investigation** of the patient and **biochemical analysis** of the tissues, since hormones may be formed but not secreted; also the hormones may vary physically and functionally from their normal counterparts and the tumours may be part of a **multiple endocrine syndrome**. Surprisingly, none of these procedures nor even histopathological examination can distinguish benign from malignant variants, which ultimately hinges upon the appearance of **metastatic lesions**. **Malignant tumours**, fortunately, are **rare** and generally low-grade and slow-growing.

Endocrine tumours invariably produce more than one hormone, although the functional effects can generally be attributed to only one of those formed. These effects in part depend upon the balance produced by stimulating and inhibitory receptors as well as interrelationships between other hormones produced by the tumour and the hormones normally secreted. These opposing forces un-

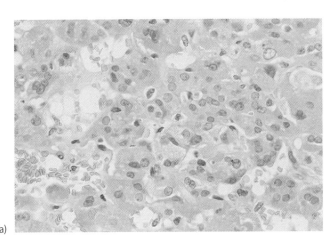

(a)

Fig. 14.24 (a) Pancreas histology. Islet cell tumour. Note the regular round cells with pink granular cytoplasm. This patient presented with hypoglycaemia. (b) Electronmicrograph of the islet cell tumour shown in Fig. 14.23(a). The neurosecretory granules are round with dense centre and pale rim, consistent with alpha granules of a glucagonoma (×31 500) (courtesy of Dr M. Allison).

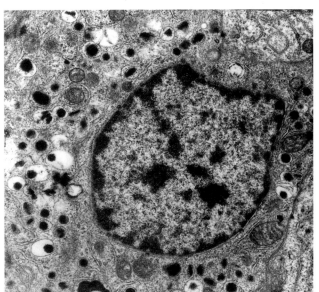

(b)

Table 14.44 Examples of pancreatic endocrine tumours.

Main hormone	Subsidiary hormones	Eponym	Clinical features	Malignancy rate
Gastrin	Insulin Pancreatic polypeptide	Gastrinoma Zollinger–Ellison syndrome	Peptic ulceration Hypersecretion of acid gastric juice Hypergastrinaemia	>90%
Insulin	Pancreatic polypeptide Glucagon	Insulinoma	Transient hypoglycaemia CNS features	<10%
Vasoactive intestinal polypeptide (VIP)	Pancreatic polypeptide Glucagon	VIPoma Verner–Morrison syndrome	Watery diarrhoea Hypokalaemia Achlorhydria	>75%
Glucagon	Pancreatic polypeptide Insulin Somatostatin	Glucagonoma	Necrolytic migratory erythema Diabetes mellitus Anaemia	>50%
Somatostatin	Pancreatic polypeptide Calcitonin Insulin	Somatostatinoma	Mild diabetes Dyspepsia Cholelithiasis	>50%
Pancreatic polypeptide (PP)	None	PPoma	Abdominal pain Weight loss Diarrhoea GIT bleeding	Occurs rarely

CNS, Central nervous system; GIT, gastrointestinal tract.

doubtedly contribute to the many non-specific clinical features produced and, in turn, to the substantial delay in diagnosis that occurs—on average 2 years. Tumours over 0.5g are more likely to have **functional effects** than smaller examples but histologically the tumour cells associated with a particular hormone cannot be distinguished without resort to immunocytochemistry with either light or electronmicroscopy.

A single tumour or multiple tumours may be present. Localization usually requires invasive procedures such as selective angiography with and without venous sampling for hormone levels, but may be achieved in many patients by ultrasound.

FURTHER READING

Cotran R.S., Kumar V. & Robbins S.L. (1989) *Pathologic Basis of Disease*, 4th edn. W.B. Saunders, Philadelphia, Pa.

Trainer P.J. & Besser M. (1995) *The Bart's Endocrine Protocols*. Churchill Livingstone, Edinburgh.

Watts N.B. & Keffer J.H. (1989) *Practical Endocrinology*, 4th edn. Lea & Febiger, Philadelphia.

Cardiovascular Disease

Cardiovascular disease accounts for much of the morbidity and mortality affecting western society. Although many of these diseases are often regarded as degenerative and therefore inevitable, great progress is being made in the understanding of their causation, genetics and management. An understanding of the pathology of these disease processes is important before appropriate treatment can be undertaken.

Because these diseases are so common, the clinical medical student should be familiar with the terminology used. For this reason, definitions are given throughout the text.

This chapter is divided into two parts. The first deals with vascular disease – arterial, venous and lymphatic; here, the single most important disease process affecting our society, namely atherosclerosis, will be discussed. The second part covers cardiac disease – myocardial, endocardial (valvular) and pericardial disease. Vascular tumours are covered in the soft-tissue tumour section of Chapter 26. Pulmonary vascular disease is included here including its effects on the heart.

Vascular disease

Table 15.1 provides a classification for the most important of the vascular diseases. In this first section, the normal structure and function of the vasculture will be described, followed by congenital and acquired vascular disease including infections and neoplasms. Under the category of degenerative vascular disease we have included arteriosclerosis (which includes atherosclerosis and vasculitis) and vascular aneurysms.

THE VASCULAR CIRCULATION

The systemic circulation

The systemic circulation supplies the arterial blood to the tissues. It starts at the aortic valve and ends with the openings or the superior (SVC) and inferior (IVC) venae cavae at the right atrium of the heart. It consists of the following areas.

Elastic arteries

These include the aorta and its main branches, which convert the pulsatile left ventricular output to a more continuous distal flow. Large elastic arteries like the aorta possess a media which contains numerous parallel elastic fibres (Fig. 15.1).

Table 15.1 Classification of the major vascular diseases.

Congenital disease
Coarctation of the aorta
Marfan's syndrome
Congenital (berry) aneurysm
Acquired diseases
Neoplasms
Haemangioma
Glomus tumour
Angiosarcoma
Kaposi's sarcoma
Inflammatory diseases
Syphilis
Giant cell arteritis
Polyarteritis nodosa
Wegener's granulomatosis
Small vessel vasculitis
Degenerative diseases (overlaps with inflammatory)
Atherosclerosis
Diabetes mellitus
Hypertension
Cystic medial necrosis

Fig. 15.1 The elastic fibres of the adult aorta and of large musculo–elastic arteries are arranged in parallel bundles. (H&E.)

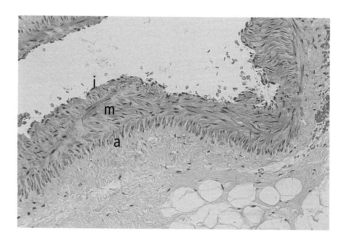

Fig. 15.2 Histology of a muscular renal artery. (H&E.) a, adventitia; i, intima; m, media.

Muscular arteries

The internal carotid, coronary, brachial, femoral, renal (Fig. 15.2) and mesenteric arteries are concerned with distribution of blood to the main peripheral tissues.

Arterioles

These are arteries less than 100 μm in diameter (Fig. 15.3). They have muscular walls. Sympathetic innervation controls luminal size. Thus they regulate the pressure decrease from aortic to capillary levels. Adjustment of arteriolar resistance is a major factor determining systemic blood pressure and distribution of flow.

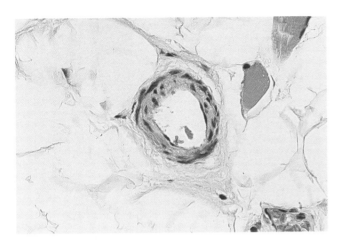

Fig. 15.3 Histology of an arteriole. Note the thin media. (H&E.)

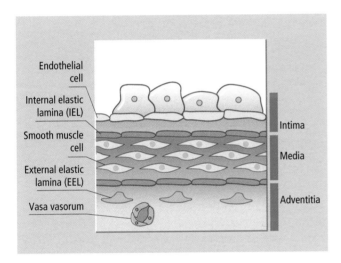

Fig. 15.4 The structure of the arterial wall.

The microcirculation

This consists of capillaries and postcapillary venules. This is the site of exchange between the blood and tissue fluids.

Veins

These are low-pressure capacity vessels that return blood to the heart. Veins contain valves derived from the endothelium. Valves facilitate forward blood flow.

The pulmonary circulation

The pulmonary circulation begins at the pulmonary valve and ends in the left atrium. The main function of the pulmonary circulation is to effect respiratory gas exchange in the pulmonary capillary bed.

The pulmonary circulation is at **low pressure** (25/10 mmHg) which is lower than plasma oncotic pressure. This means that there is normally no fluid movement out of the alveolar capillaries. This permits the alveoli to remain dry for optimal gas exchange.

The portal circulations

The portal circulations provide a specialized second capillary bed within the systemic circulation:
- The **hepatic portal circulation** delivers intestinal and splenic blood to the liver (Chapter 19).
- A minor portal circulation in the **pituitary stalk** transports releasing hormone from the hypothalamus to the anterior pituitary gland (Chapter 14).

The lymphatic circulation

Lymphatics originate in the interstitial tissues and end in the thoracic duct, which drains into the internal jugular vein. The function of the lymphatics is to transport large molecules and excess fluid from the interstitium back into the blood. Lymphatic vessels have thin walls and possess endothelial valves. This system operates at very **low pressure**.

DISEASES OF ARTERIES

Normal arterial anatomy

Arteries are compliant, distensible structures with a flat internal surface. They consist of three layers; the intima, the media and the adventitia (Fig. 15.4).

At birth, the **intima** consists of a single layer of endothelial cells that rests on the basement membrane. The intima is separated from the media by the internal elastic lamina (IEL).

The **media** consists of interconnected smooth-muscle cells. In muscular arteries the media is separated from the adventitia by the external elastic lamina (EEL).

Pericytes are modified smooth-muscle cells that surround the vessel wall. Their function is largely unknown.

Glomus cells are derived from the neuromyoarterial glomus and are temperature-sensitive and are involved in the regulation of arteriolar blood flow.

Vasa vasorum (literally 'vessel of the vessel') are found in the **adventitia** of larger arteries. They provide oxygenation and nutrition to the outer layers of the artery.

Normal arterial physiology

Endothelial cells

Vascular endothelium consists of a single layer of cells that line the entire internal surface of the vascular system (Fig. 15.5). They possess intercellular junctions that act as pores to allow water and small molecules in and out under hydrostatic and osmotic pressure (Table 15.2); the ultrastructural hallmark of the endothelial cell is the

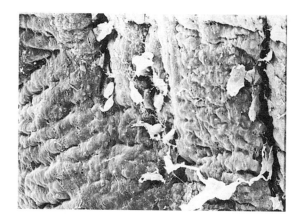

Fig. 15.7 Scanning electronmicrograph of recently denuded vascular endothelium showing adherence of leucocytes and platelets in response to exposed collagen and basement membrane.

Table 15.2 Endothelial cell function.

Permeability barrier
Non-thrombogenic and antithrombogenic (factor VIII – von Willebrand factor, cyclo-oxygenase, prostacyclin, heparan sulphate)
Metabolism of vasoactive substances (endothelium-derived relaxing factor – now known to be nitric oxide, angiotensin-converting enzyme
Production of growth factors and growth inhibitors (e.g. interleukin-1)
Connective tissue production
Oxidation of low-density lipoprotein

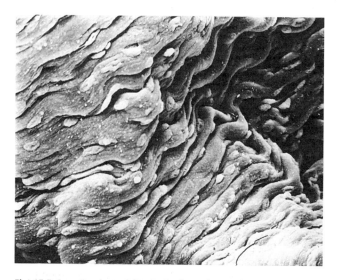

Fig. 15.5 Scanning electronmicrograph of vascular endothelium at a vessel branch point.

Weibel–Palade body, a site for storage of von Willebrand factor (vWF) (Fig. 15.6).

Any loss of endothelial integrity will lead to the accumulation of leucocytes and platelets (Fig. 15.7), followed by intimal proliferative and inflammatory reactions. This forms the basis for atherogenesis, according to the response to injury hypothesis (see below).

Smooth-muscle cells

Blood vessels can be characterized by the amount of muscle in their walls; the aorta has the most and capillaries and lymphatics have none at all. Smooth-muscle cells act in concert with endothelial cells to perform a variety of contractile, thrombotic and antithrombotic, secretory and proliferative functions (Fig. 15.8; Table 15.3). The importance of the integrity of the media in muscular and musculoelastic arteries is demonstrated by disease processes such as vasculitis and aneurysm (see below) where loss of medial integrity may have fatal consequences.

Lipids, lipoproteins and hyperlipidaemia

Lipids are ubiquitous in distribution and play a vital role

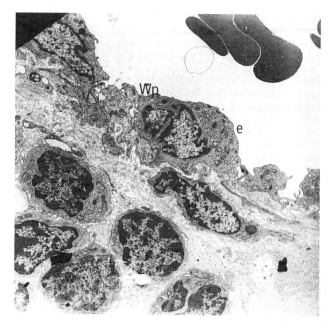

Fig. 15.6 Transmission electronmicrograph of vascular endothelial cell. The endothelial cells (e) contain dense, round Weibel–Palade bodies (Wp). (×7800).

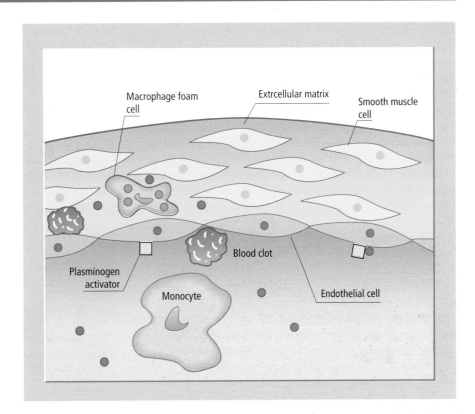

Fig. 15.8 The role of endothelial and smooth muscle cells in arterial physiology.

Table 15.3 Smooth-muscle cell function.

Contractility
Connective tissue production
Lipid metabolism (LDL, cholesterol, prostaglandin)
Proliferation is induced by platelet-derived growth factor, monocyte-derived growth factor, endothelial cell-derived growth factor, LDL and prostacyclin

LDL, Low-density lipoprotein.

in virtually all aspects of biological life. Some of these functions include:

- hormones and hormone precursors;
- digestion;
- energy storage and metabolism;
- functional and structural components in biomembranes;
- insulation, nerve conduction and heat conservation.

Lipids

Plasma lipids comprise:

- triglycerides;
- cholesterol;
- phospholipids;
- cholesteryl esters;
- free fatty acids (non-esterified fatty acids).

Triglycerides (triacylglycerols, TG). These are the most important dietary energy source and during adequate feeding, after intestinal metabolism to constituent monoglycerides, fatty acid and glycerol, TG are resynthesized in the body and stored, providing an energy source for periods of starvation. Mobilization of TG from adipose tissue, via the activity of the rate-limiting enzyme triacylglycerol lipase (a hormone-sensitive lipase) is mainly controlled by the balance of insulin and some prostaglandins (antilipolytic) and catecholamines (lipolytic). Lipolysis releases fatty acids and glycerol which enter the circulation and are available for oxidation and for gluconeogenesis.

Cholesterol (Chol). This is an important component of plasma membranes and a precursor of bile acids, steroids, hormones and vitamin D. Dietary intake of Chol is low and most derives from hepatic synthesis from acetate and mevalonic acid under negative feedback control of the rate-limiting enzyme hydroxy methyl glutaryl coenzyme A reductase (HMG CoA). Most circulating cholesterol is esterified with fatty acids forming cholesterol esters (CE).

Phospholipids (PL). PL are important components of cell membranes and of lipoproteins.

Lipoproteins

TG, Chol, PL and CE are insoluble in plasma. These lipids combine with special proteins called apoproteins (apo-lipoproteins) to form lipoproteins and this process solubilizes lipids in plasma. The lipoproteins therefore provide a transport system for lipids. Apoproteins are important not only in maintaining the structural integrity of lipoproteins and thereby facilitating the solubilization of lipids, but they also play an important role in lipoprotein receptor recognition and regulation of certain enzymes in lipoprotein metabolism (Tables 15.4 and 15.5).

Five classes of apoproteins have been identified:

- A;
- B–B48, B100;
- C–CII;
- D;
- E.

Lipoprotein metabolism (Fig. 15.9)

Fate of exogenous (dietary) lipid. After digestion and absorption of dietary lipids, TG and Chol (as esters) combine with PL and specific apoproteins (apo) to form chylomicrons (CM; rich in TG). CM are secreted into the lymphatic system where they acquire apoC and E from high-density lipoproteins (HDL). The CM enters the systemic circulation in the jugular vein.

Within the circulation TG is removed from the CM by

Table 15.5 Classification of lipoproteins. Traditionally, lipoproteins have been classified in order of increasing density.

> 1 Chylomicrons: produced in intestinal mucosal cells; major lipid is TG, major apoprotein is B48; responsible for transport of dietary TG
> 2 Very-low-density lipoproteins (VLDL): produced in liver; major lipid is TG, major apoproteins are B100, CII, E; responsible for transport of endogenous TG
> 3 Intermediate-density lipoproteins (IDL): derived from breakdown of VLDL after removal of some TG
>   Contains both TG and cholesterol and B100 and E apoproteins
>   Some is taken up by specific receptors in the liver, some forms LDL
> 4 Chylomicron remnants (CMR): derived from breakdown of CM after removal of TG
>   Major lipid is cholesterol; major apoprotein is B48. Taken up by specific receptors in the liver
>   Therefore delivers dietary cholesterol to the liver
> 5 Low-density lipoproteins (LDL): derived from IDL after further removal of TG
>   Major lipid is cholesterol, major apoprotein is B100
>   Taken up by specific receptors in the liver and peripheral tissues
>   Therefore delivers endogenous cholesterol to liver and peripheral cells
> 6 High-density lipoproteins (HDL): produced in liver and intestinal mucosal cells
>   Major lipid is PL, major apoproteins are A, D—also provides apo CII to CM and VLDL to activate LPL and facilitate TG removal
>   Important in transport of cholesterol from peripheral tissues to liver

TG, Triglycerides; PL, phospholipids; LPL, lipoprotein lipase.

the action of lipoprotein lipase (LPL) which is found on the endothelial surface of cells and is activated by apo CII. LPL is also stimulated by insulin (this enzyme is distinct from hormone-sensitive lipase which is found within cells, especially adipose tissue, and breaks down stored TG in cells and which is inhibited by insulin). TG from CM is converted to glycerol and non-esterified fatty acids (NEFA). NEFA provide a major energy source for aerobic metabolism.

As TG is removed the remnant particle (CMR) becomes smaller and some of the more water-soluble components become redundant: PL, apo CII which transfer to HDL. The CMR is cholesterol-rich and is removed from the circulation by hepatic receptors via apo B48 and E recognition. Dietary free cholesterol therefore is delivered to the liver.

Fate of endogenous lipid. Very low-density lipoprotein (VLDL) is a TG-rich lipoprotein synthesized in the liver; it also contains cholesterol. TG are produced from glycerol and fatty acids (FA), which reach the liver from fat stores or by synthesis from glucose. Hepatic cholesterol may be synthesized locally or be derived from lipoproteins, e.g. CMR.

Table 15.4 Functions of individual apoproteins.

A–A1	Binds PL in lipoproteins Activates lecithin cholesterin acyltransferase (esterified cholesterol in plasma)
B–B48	Produced in intestinal mucosal cells An important component of chylomicrons (CM): contributes to hepatic uptake of CM remnant by receptor recognition
B–B100	Produced in liver; component of very-low-density lipoprotein (VLDL), intermediate-density lipoprotein (IDL) and low-density lipoproteins (LDL): contributes to hepatic and peripheral tissue uptake of LDL by receptor recognition
C–CII	Component of high-density lipoprotein (HDL) After transfer to CM and VLDL it activates the enzyme lipoprotein lipase (situated on the endothelium) which removes TG from CM and VLDL
D	Component of HDL
E	Involved in receptor recognition of IDL and CM remnant by the liver

PL, Phospholipids; TG, triglycerides.

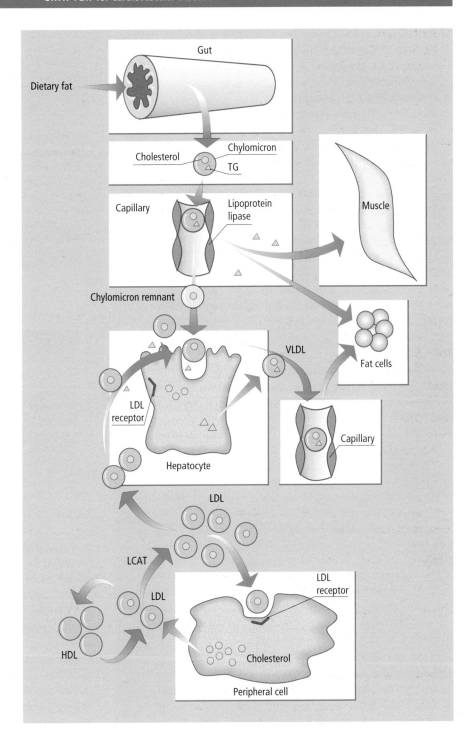

Fig. 15.9 Exogenous and endogenous lipid pathways.

VLDL is secreted from the liver and when in the blood acquires apo CII from HDL. The TG of VLDL is removed by the successive action of apo CII-activated LPL, producing intermediate-density lipoproteins (IDL; VLDL remnants). Some IDL is taken up directly by specific receptors in liver. Receptor recognition is facilitated by apo B100.

Some IDL is converted to LDL after further removal of TG by the action of LPL. The loss of TG produces a smaller lipoprotein which is cholesterol-rich: LDL.

LDL is removed from circulation via two routes.

- **High-affinity LDL receptor** – liver and peripheral cells; recognition of the receptor is via apo B100. LDL within the cell is degraded to amino acids and cholesterol. An increase in the intracellular pool of cholesterol inhibits endogenous synthesis of cholesterol and suppresses the synthesis of LDL receptors.

- **Low-affinity LDL receptors**, which become increasingly important when the plasma concentration of LDL is raised. This pathway is believed to be important in the development of atherosclerosis. The level of LDL in blood is directly related to the risk of coronary heart disease (CHD).

HDL plays an important role in lipoprotein metabolism; apo CII is transferred from HDL to VLDL and CM and then activates LPL; after TG removal apo CII and other redundant components are transferred back to HDL. It is also important in the transport of peripheral cholesterol (as cholesteryl esters via the action of LCAT– lecithin cholesteryl acyl transferase) to the liver. The level of HDL in blood is inversely related to the risk of CHD.

Hyperlipidaemias

These conditions reflect an increase in blood lipoprotein levels which is either derived from increased synthesis due to a diet high in saturated fat and/or a genetically determined reduction in removal from blood.

- An increase in CM or VLDL leads to increase in plasma TG.
- An increase in LDL or IDL leads to increase in plasma Chol.

Hypercholesterolaemia is associated with an increased risk of CHD. Hypertriglyceridaemia is associated with an increased risk of pancreatitis (mechanism and relative risk not understood) and may also be associated with CHD.

Secondary hyperlipidaemias (Tables 15.6 and 15.7). These should be excluded in all cases before consideration of the, usually rarer, primary hyperlipidaemias.

Primary hyperlipidaemia

- **Familial hypercholesterolaemia (FH).** 1:500 people are affected. There is an **autosomal dominant** inheritance. FH is associated with high cholesterol levels due to gene defect leading to a reduced number of high-affinity LDL receptors, resulting in an increase in LDL. FH is associated with an increased risk of premature CHD; tendon xanthomas are common. Cholesterol levels are usually > 7.5 mmol/l.
- **Familial hypertriglyceridaemia.** A high TG level > 5 mmol/l is associated with eruptive xanthomas (elbows, back, buttocks), lipaemic retinalis, abdominal pain, hepatosplenomegaly and an increased risk of acute pancreatitis (with TG > 10 mmol/l). It is uncom-

Table 15.6 Secondary hyperlipidaemias.

Hormonal factors	*Nutritional factors*
Pregnancy	Obesity
Diabetes mellitus	Anorexia nervosa
Hypothyroidism	Alcohol abuse
Renal dysfunction	*Iatrogenic*
Nephrotic syndrome	High-dose steroids
Chronic renal failure	β-Blockers
	Exogenous sex steroids
	Retinoids
Liver disease	
Primary biliary cirrhosis	
Extrahepatic biliary obstruction	

Table 15.7 Secondary hyperlipidaemias.

	Cholesterol	Triglycerides
Diabetes mellitus	(↑)	↑↑
Hypothyroidism	↑↑	↑
Alcoholism	↑	↑↑
Obesity	↑	↑
Nephrotic syndrome	↑↑	(↑)
Stress	↑	↑

mon. Associated features include impaired glucose tolerance or overt diabetes, hyperinsulinism, hyperuricaemia and obesity.

Familial hypertriglyceridaemia may be due to increased VLDL synthesis (TG 5–500 mmol/l) or LPL or apo CII deficiency–inability to clear dietary lipid: (CM.TG 20–100 mmol/l).

- **Familial combined hyperlipidaemia.** These patients suffer from premature CHD associated with ↑TG and ↑Chol. There is a family history of CHD but not xanthomas with a variable, mild lipoprotein and therefore lipid abnormality. There may be predominantly ↑TG whilst some predominantly ↑Chol. This is possibly due to a **single-gene defect**.
- **Remnant hyperlipoproteinaemia.** Raised IDL and some CMR is associated with ↑TG and ↑Chol due to apo E abnormality, which prevents normal uptake of these lipoproteins via liver receptors. This condition is associated with an increased risk of premature CHD, tuboeruptive xanthomas (e.g. elbows) and palmar crease xanthomas.
- **Common polygenic hyperlipidaemia.** This multifactorial (i.e. genetic + environment) condition is as-

Table 15.8 Hyperlipidaemia.

	WHO phenotype	Inheritance	Typical lipid levels (mmol/l)		Lipoproteins	Clinical signs
			Cholesterol	Triglycerides		
Lipoprotein lipase deficiency	I	AR	<6.5	10–30	Chylomicrons ↑	Eruptive xanthoma, xanthelasma, lipaemia retinalis, hepatosplenomegaly
Polygenic hypercholesterolaemia	IIa	Polygenic	6.5–9	<2.3	LDL ↑	Xanthelasma, corneal arcus
Familial hypercholesterolaemia	IIa	AD	7.5–16	<2.3	LDL ↑	Tendon xanthomas, corneal arcus, xanthelasma
Familial defective apoprotein B 100	IIa	AD	7.5–16	<2.3	LDL ↑	Tendon xanthomas, corneal arcus, xanthelasma
Familial combined hyperlipidaemia	IIa, IIb, IV or V	?AD	6.5–10	2.3–12	LDL ↑, VLDL ↑ HDL ↓	Arcus, xanthelasma
Remnant particle disease	III	Polygenic (AD, other + environmental)	9–14	9–14	IDL ↑	Palmar striae, tuberoeruptive xanthomas
Familial hypertriglyceridaemia	IV, V	AD	6.5–12	10–30	VLDL ↑	Eruptive xanthelasma, lipaemia retinalis
					Chylomicrons ↑	Hepatosplenomegaly
Primary HDL abnormalities						
Hyperalphalipoproteinaemia		AD	HDL cholesterol > 2.0		HDL ↑	
Hypoalphalipoproteinaemia		?AD	HDL cholesterol < 0.9		HDL ↓	

WHO, World Health Organization; AR, autosomal recessive; AD, autosomal dominant; LDL, low-density lipoproteins; VLDL, very-low-density lipoproteins; HDL, high-density lipoproteins.

sociated with hypercholesterolaemia (LDL) and premature CHD. This is the commonest cause of hypercholesterolaemia.

Table 15.8 summarizes the clinical and laboratory findings in the hyperlipidaemias.

Hypolipidaemias

Hypocholesterolaemia may occur as a secondary phenomenon in end-stage liver failure, some malabsorption syndromes and protein-losing enteropathies and in kwashiorkor. It also occurs in hypo- and abetalipoproteinaemia and in familial alphalipoprotein deficiency (Tangier disease) where HDL is deficient.

Treatment of hyperlipidaemias

For secondary hyperlipidaemia the underlying cause is treated; for primary hyperlipidaemia the cornerstone of treatment is dietary modification (Tables 15.9 and 15.10) with a modified fat diet (reduced total fat). If this fails, drugs are recommended:

• hypercholesterolaemia–bile acid sequestrant (e.g.

cholestyramine) HMG CoA reductase inhibitors (inhibits synthesis of cholesterol; simvastatin);
• hypertriglyceridaemia or combined hyperlipidaemia– weight loss; fibrates–nicotinic acid; fish oils.

Table 15.9 Some basic guidelines for measuring plasma lipids.

Patient should be starved (~14 hours) especially if triglyceride measurement is required

If postmyocardial infarction, sample should be taken either within only a few hours of the onset of symptoms and/or >3 months later

There is rarely any indication for measurement of lipids in the very elderly (>80 years)

Remember that there are inter- and intra-assay variations in the cholesterol results from the laboratory as well as interindividual variations. These may give up to a 20% overall variation in results between samples

If borderline, take another sample

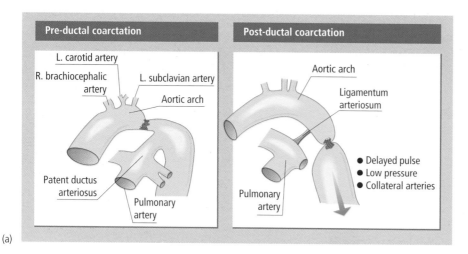

(a)

Fig. 15.10(a) Coarctation of the aorta.

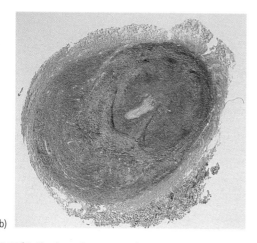

(b)

Fig. 15.10(b) Histology of a segment of coarctation of the aorta, shows black elastic tissue and fibrous tissue stenosing the lumen. (EVG.)

Congenital arterial disease

Coarctation of the aorta

Coarctation of the aorta is a congenital malformation characterized by focal narrowing of the vessel lumen. There are two recognized types (Fig. 15.10).

Infantile (preductal) coarctation. This is a rare defect characterized by extreme narrowing of a segment of aorta proximal to the ductus arteriosus. This means that the upper half of the body is supplied by the aorta proximal to the coarctation; the lower half is supplied from the pulmonary artery through a patent ductus arteriousus. This produces **cyanosis** confined to the lower half of the body (as blood from the pulmonary artery is deoxygenated venous blood). This defect is usually fatal unless corrected early in life.

Adult coarctation. This is a more common defect. It is seen more commonly in males than in females. It is associated with bicuspid aortic valve and in females there is an association with Turner's syndrome. It is characterized by extreme narrowing of a segment of aorta immediately distal to the closed ductus arteriosus. The lower half of the body may receive an adequate blood supply from well-developed collaterals. Thus it may be asymptomatic. These collateral vessels are found around the shoulder girdle. In severe cases, the following clinical signs may be present:

• collaterals may be very pronounced and visible clinically and on X-ray;

Table 15.10 Interpretation of lipid biochemistry results.

Normal ranges based on 95% of population	
Total cholesterol	3.9–7.8 mmol/l
Fasting triglycerides	0.55–1.9 mmol/l
Optimum upper limit of cholesterol adopted as 6.5 mmol/l	
Age 25–34 years	10–12% >6.5 mmol/l
Age >55 years	30–40% >6.5 mmol/l
If total cholesterol is between 6.5 and 8.0 mmol/l (and triglycerides < 2.0 mmol/l and patient < 65 years), there is an indication for measuring the HDL cholesterol fraction	
If HDL < 1.0 mmol/l, there is cause for concern. LDL cholesterol can be estimated using the Freidewald equation (LDL cholesterol = total cholesterol – HDL cholesterol – 0.46 × triglycerides)	
If HDL > 1.0 mmol/l, the patient is considered less at risk	
If total cholesterol > 8.0 mmol/l and/or triglycerides > 2.0 mmol/l, exclude diabetes, jaundice, myxoedema, nephrotic syndrome	

HDL, High-density lipoprotein; LDL, low-density lipoprotein.

- there may be ischaemia in the lower half of the body with intermittent claudication in the legs;
- hypertension may be present (due to a decrease in renal blood flow which stimulates the renin–angiotensin–aldosterone mechanism);
- the femoral pulse may be delayed (due to the circuitous passage of blood to the lower aorta via collaterals);
- the blood pressure in the legs may be lower than that in the arms.

Congenital (berry) aneurysm (Fig. 15.11)

Berry aneurysms feature replacement of the muscular wall of small arteries by fibrous tissue. These are most commonly found at bifurcations of vessels, particularly in the **circle of Willis**. They are associated with hypertension in young patients and their rupture leads to **subarachnoid haemorrhage**. The aneurysms are not present at birth and so may not be classified as truly congenital.

Haemangioma

Haemangiomas are common. Approximately 70% are present at birth. They should be considered to be hamartomas (developmental abnormalities) rather than neoplasms.

Any organ may be involved but the most common sites are skin, liver, lung and brain. The histology shows well-formed vascular spaces lined by endothelial cells.

Haemangiomas are classified as **capillary** haemangiomas, composed of vessels of capillary size and **cavernous** haemangiomas (Fig. 15.12), composed of large, thin-walled vascular spaces.

Capillary haemangioma. These are usually found in the skin and mucous membranes. They are small, usually less than 1 cm in diameter. They grow slowly. The exception to this is the 'strawberry' haemangioma which grows rapidly during the first few months of life. Eighty per cent of 'strawberry' haemangiomas regress completely by 5 years.

Cavernous haemangioma. These occur in the skin and the viscera (Fig. 15.12). They may reach 2–3 cm in size. They grow slowly. Haemangiomas may occur in deep subcutaneous tissues and in muscle (intramuscular haemangiomas). These may be ill-defined and require wide excision as they are prone to recur but they do not metastasize.

Arteriovenous malformation

These are complex malformations containing elements of **arterial, venous** and **capillary structures** (Fig. 15.13). They may be acquired secondary to trauma, but are more commonly congenital. They are seen in skin and dermis,

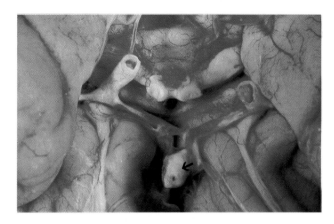

Fig. 15.11 A berry aneurysm (arrowed) in the posterior communicating cerebral artery.

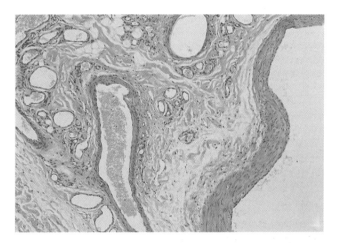

Fig. 15.12 Histology of skin. Cavernous haemangioma. Note the thick- and thin-walled, large and small vascular channels. (H&E.)

liver and lung. They may reach an enormous size and the shunting of blood between the arterial and venous systems may lead to heart failure. These malformations may also be associated with erosion or pressure effects. In women, they increase in size during pregnancy and are thus thought to be oestrogen-dependent.

Hereditary haemorrhagic telangiectasia (Osler–Weber–Rendu)

This is inherited as an **autosomal dominant** and consists of multiple capillary microaneurysms in the skin and mucous membranes. These vessels are exceedingly fragile and become more conspicuous with age. They predispose to acute and chronic bleeding. When they occur in the gastrointestinal tract, the condition is associated with chronic iron deficiency.

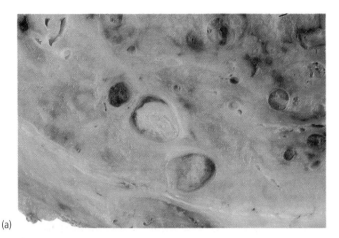

(a)

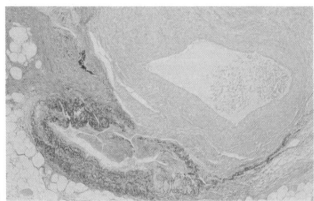

(b)

Fig. 15.13 (a) An arteriovenous malformation of deep muscle of the leg. Note the large and small vessels. (b) Histology. Note the large and small vessels with irregular thick and thin walls and variable (black) elastin. (EVG.)

Sturge–Weber syndrome

This is a rare disease, characterized by a large, unilateral cutaneous angioma of the face (**portwine stain**) associated with a venous malformation involving the ipsilateral cerebral hemisphere and meninges. The cerebral angioma leads to cortical atrophy and epilepsy. The angioma may be visible radiologically due to its characteristic linear calcification.

Von Hippel–Lindau disease

This is transmitted as an **autosomal dominant** disease. It is charaterized by **multiple haemangiomas** of the retina and brain, a benign neoplasm of the cerebellum called a **haemangioblastoma** and **cysts** in the kidney and pancreas. There is an increased incidence of renal adenocarcinoma and phaeochromocytoma in this disease. Cerebellar haemangioblastoma is associated with erythropoietin production which may lead to **polycythaemia**.

Inherited disorders of connective tissue

Rare inherited connective tissue disorders exist in which there is defective connective tissue formation. These diseases have in common aortic medial degeneration and weakening with predisposition to aneurysm formation, aortic dilatation and rupture.

Marfan's syndrome

Originally described in 1896 by the paediatrician A.B. Marfan as a 'congenital malformation of the four limbs', this syndrome is now known to have a complex and varied phenotype. This is a single-gene, **autosomal dominant** abnormality with a variable degree of expression. Mutation of the **fibrillin gene** (fib-15), located on chromosome 15, represents the primary defect in Marfan syndrome. Over 20 mutations of the fibrillin gene have been described. However, some patients with a Marfan-like syndrome have no alterations in known fibrillin genes and so abnormalities of elastin gene, located at chromosome 7, have been implicated.

Connective tissues at all sites are involved, with myxomatous tissue deposits. The most significant changes are listed in Table 15.11.

Ehlers–Danlos syndrome

This disease is due to **defective type III collagen** production which affects the vascular, dermal and pulmonary tissues. Patients have hypermobile joints. These patients have folds of loose skin which heal poorly if traumatized. Ten groups have been described according to clinical features and inheritance. The most common types have an **autosomal dominant** inheritance.

Pseudoxanthoma elasticum

This is a rare, **recessively inherited** disorder of elastic fibres that produces soft yellowish plaques in the skin. There is progressive calcification of elastic tissues. The arteries and ocular fundi may also be affected. The underlying biochemical abnormality remains unknown.

Table 15.11 Marfan's syndrome.

Cystic medial necrosis of the aortic media with premature aortic dissection and rupture and aortic valve incompetence
Mirtal valve prolapse
Arachnodactyly ('spider fingers')
Increased height
Hypermobile joints
High arched palate
Optic lens subluxation

Vasculitis

Vasculitis is interesting for several reasons. First, there is often **overlap** between local vascular and systemic **hypersensitivity** and possibly with **autoimmune** disease processes.

Second, there is, sometimes violent, **controversy** over nomenclature and classification (so much so, that some of the vasculitides that will be described in the following pages are not thought to exist by some clinicians, so beware!).

Third, the **diagnosis** is not always made on the pathology alone. More often the clinical information and presentation is the only way to arrive at the final diagnosis (so give your pathologist all the clinical information on your patient).

Finally, **rational approaches** to diagnosis and to the pathogenesis of the vasculitides are starting to emerge, based on **serological markers**. Some of these diseases occur in the collective group of **collagen vascular diseases** (carditis/arthritis/vasculitis) and some in the group of connective tissue diseases and are discussed in Chapters 7, 9, 20 and 21.

The pathological and clinical effects of vasculitis are varied and depend upon:

- the **size and type** of the vessels involved: medium-sized muscular vessels versus arterioles; arteries versus veins;
- the **number and distribution** of the vessels involved: variable distribution throughout the body tends to produce a highly variable and often bizarre clinical picture; circulation of vital organs (brain, heart, kidneys) may be affected;
- the **chronicity** of the lesions: acute forms may run a rapid course with all the lesions at the same stage of development; chronic forms show a more prolonged course with lesions in various stages of development and periods of remissions and exacerbations;
- **complications**: thrombosis; rupture of vessels with haemorrhage; aneurysm formation.

Definition

'Inflammation and structural damage of vessel walls.'

Remember that the following terms all mean the same thing;

vasculitis = arteritis = angiitis.

Inflammation and structural damage of vessels may be produced by **infections** with micro-organisms, by many **chemical** and **physical agents** and by **hypersensitivity** phenomena.

Raynaud's disease is a process of unknown cause char-

acterized by small vessel spasm without structural vascular abnormality.

Raynaud's phenomenon occurs as a secondary manifestation of many diseases in which small vessel vasculitis occurs.

Both Raynaud's disease and Raynaud's phenomenon are characterized by **numbness**, **pallor** or **cyanosis** of the hands and feet in response to **cold**.

Classification

The classification of the vasculitides is one of the most controversial areas in clinical pathology. A system is needed that is understandable, memorable and that can be used clinically. Two classification systems are given in Tables 15.12 and 15.13. The former classification (based on aetiology) is used more commonly by physicians and the second (based on size of the vessel involved) is more commonly used by surgeons.

In almost all the vasculitides, with the exception of Buerger's disease, there is strong evidence of an inflammatory response, with elevation of the **acute-phase proteins** and the **erythrocyte sedimentation rate (ESR)**. Wegener's granulomatosis and polyartertis nodosa (PAN) patients often have a high-titre **autoantibody** directed against **neutrophil cytoplasmic granules (ANCA)** at presentation. The level falls with successful treatment and a subsequent rise often heralds relapse. The antigen recognized is probably proteinase 3. Other forms of vasculitis may give a different pattern of staining, directed against other cytoplasmic antigens, including myeloperoxidase and lactoferrin, called **p-ANCA**. This is the perinuclear pattern, which is in fact induced by the fixation technique—an example of a useful technical artefact! The ANCA-positive and ANCA-negative vasculitides form another method of classification (Table 15.14).

Table 15.12 Aetiological classification of vasculitis.

Infectious
Non-infectious
Hypersensitivity (type II hypersensitivity)
Acute (leukocytoclastic)
Chronic (polyarteritis)
Granulomatous (type IV hypersensitivity)
Giant cell arteritis
Wegener's granulomatosis
Thromboangiitis obliterans
Takayasu's disease
Rheumatoid arthritis
Churg–Strauss
Kawasaki's disease

Table 15.13 Clinicopathological classification of vasculitis (Zeek, 1952).

Infectious

Non-Infectious
Involving large, medium and small vessels
   Idiopathic (Takayasu's)
   Granulomatous
   Vasculitis of rheumatic disease

Involving medium-sized and small vessels
   Thromboangiitis obliterans
   Polyarteritis (PAN, Kawasaki disease)
   Allergic granulomatosis and vasculitis (Wegener's, Churg–Strauss, sarcoid)
   Vasculitis of collagen vascular disease (Rf, RA, SLE, Behçet's, systemic sclerosis, Sjögren's)

Involving small blood vessels
   Serum sickness, HSP, drug-induced, malignancy-associated, mixed cryogobulinaemia, hypocomplementaemia, IBD, PBC, Goodpasture's, transplant vasculitis

PAN, Polyarteritis nodosa; Rf, rheumatic fever; RA, rheumatoid arthritis; SLE, systemic lupus erythematosus; HSP, Henoch–Schönlein purpura; IBD, inflammatory bowel disease; PBC, primary biliary cirrhosis.

Table 15.14 Subtypes of antineutrophil cytoplasmic antibodies (ANCA) in the 'ANCA-associated vasculitides'.

ANCA	Target antigen	Associated diseases
cANCA (cytoplasmic)	Proteinase 3 (CAP 57) (Wegener's autoantigen)	Wegener's granulomatosis (90%), occasionally in microscopic polyarterities, Churg–Strauss syndrome, classic polyarteritis nodosa
pANCA (perinuclear)	Myeloperoxidase, elastase, cathepsin G, lysozyme, elastase	Renal vasculitis (microscopic polyarterities, rheumatic disease, collagen vascular disease)
Atypical (x)ANCA or pANCA	Lactoferrin, lysozyme, β-glucoronidase, cathepsin G	Ulcerative colitis, autoimmune hepatitis, primary sclerosing cholangitis

Aetiological classification

Infectious. Many infectious agents cause a vasculitis as part of their mechanism for invading and colonizing the host. Pyogenic bacteria and *Pseudomonas* sp. have a particular preference for blood vessel walls; fungi, particu-

larly *Mucor* (Fig. 15.14a) and viruses, particularly cytomegalovirus (CMV; Fig. 15.14b) will also involve blood vessels.

- **Syphilis**. Syphilis remains a common disease worldwide, but syphilitic aortitis is uncommon because of the successful treatment of the early disease.

  Syphilitic aortitis occurs at the tertiary stage of the disease, often many decades after the primary infection. As the spirochaete cannot be detected in the lesions, it is likely that hypersensitivity is responsible for the pathogenesis of the disease.

  The key histological lesion is endarteritis obliterans or luminal narrowing due to intimal fibrosis of the adventitial vasa vasorum. This leads to ischaemia and fibrosis of the outer two-thirds of the aortic media which gives the aorta a macroscopically irregular or 'tree bark' appearance.

  Weakening of the aortic wall causes aneurysmal

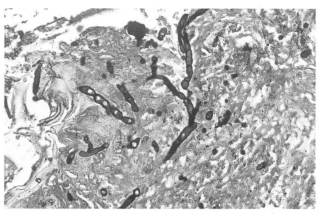

(a)

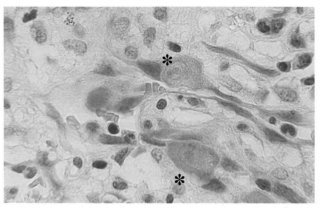

(b)

Fig. 15.14 Infective vasculitis. (a) Histology shows mucor fungal hyphae in the vessel wall, stained black with Grocott. (b) Histology shows cytomegalovirus nuclear inclusions (✱) in the endothelial cells. (H&E.)

dilatation of the aorta (see below); dilatation of the aortic root and aortic incompetence; narrowing of the ostia of the coronary arteries, which results in myocardial ischaemia.

Non-infectious

- **Hypersensitivity:** A number of conditions characterized by inflammation and segmental necrosis of small vessels is attributed to immunological injury and often grouped under the generic term **necrotizing vasculitis**. Necrotic regions often contain considerable amounts of fibrin (**fibrinoid necrosis**).

The model for these forms of vasculitis is the experimentally induced vasculitis found in the Arthus reaction of serum sickness. Immune complexes may also lodge in the glomerular basement membranes, producing an acute necrotizing glomerulonephritis.

(a) **Acute (hypersensitivity (leukocytoclastic) vasculitis):** There may be a history of hypersensitivity to drugs or foreign proteins. This is a disease of short duration (weeks); small veins, arteries and capillaries are affected. Lesions may be self-limited and regress, may cause death or may progress to chronic forms. Renal glomeruli may be involved.

Most of these diseases are mediated by type III immune complex hypersensitivity. Fibrinoid necrosis may be present in the walls of small-calibre vessels, particularly arterioles. Intense neutrophilic infiltration of vessels is seen together with lysis of neutrophils (leukocytoclasia; Fig. 15.15). Thrombosis and haemorrhage are common. Immunoglobulin and complement can be demonstrated in these lesions.

These diseases are characterized by involvement of multiple organs. Skin involvement leads to raised purpuric patches. Renal involvement is associated with glomerulonephritis.

(b) **Chronic–polyarteritis (PAN) group:** produced experimentally by repeated exposure to an antigen. In humans, it is thought be be due to a type II (immune complex)-mediated phenomenon. Hypertension is often present but a causal relation is not established.

The condition has a long duration (months to years) with remissions, exacerbations and eventual death (two-thirds die within 1 year).

Lesions may be seen in various stages of development, even in the same vessel. The more common form, PAN, involves both arteries and veins, mainly in the kidneys, skin, heart, liver, gastrointestinal tract, pancreas, skeletal muscle, peripheral and central nervous system, but does not involve the lungs.

- **Polyarteritis nodosa:** this is an uncommon disease that presents in young adults. Males are more frequently af-

fected than females. Hepatitis B surface antigen is present in immune complexes in 40% of patients but the antigen involved in other cases is unknown.

Medium-sized and small arteries throughout the body show characteristic **segmental lesions** consisting of nodular reddish swellings and multiple microaneurysms. In the acute phase, arterial rupture with haemorrhages and thrombosis may occur. In the chronic phase, the involved artery is thickened by fibrosis.

Histologically, the key feature in the acute phase is **fibrinoid necrosis** of the media and acute inflammation of all layers of the vessel (Fig. 15.16). In the chronic phase, the artery shows concentric fibrosis. Commonly, acute and chronic phases may exist in close proximity in the same vessel. The usual course is progressive, with remissions and exacerbations. Without treatment, the 5-year survival rate is 20%; with steroid therapy, 50% of patients

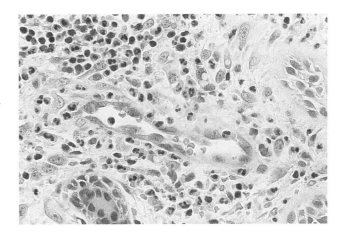

Fig. 15.15 Small vessel leucocytoclastic vasculitis. Note the neutrophil polymorphs emigrating through the vessel wall. (H&E.)

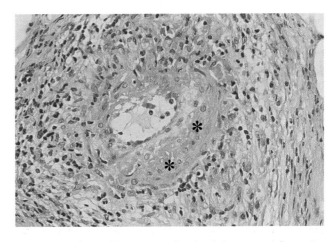

Fig. 15.16 Histology of polyarteritis nodosa (PAN) shows acute inflammation with areas of fibrinoid necrosis (✻). (H&E.)

are alive after 5 years. In the acute phase, patients develop fever with variable symptoms and signs depending on the affected organ. Diagnosis of PAN is clinical, with biopsy of the affected tissue providing histological confirmation.

Granulomatous disease

1 Giant cell arteritis (temporal arteritis; cranial arteritis). This is a focal, granulomatous inflammation of medium and small arteries (especially cranial vessels) of the elderly. There is a female to male ratio of 3:1. The cause is uncertain but is likely to be mediated by a type IV hypersensitivity reaction to vessel wall components. The histology is dominated by the formation of granulomatous chronic inflammation associated with giant cells.

Fragmentation of the internal elastic lamina is followed by fibrosis (Fig. 15.17). There may be occlusive thrombosis in the acute stages. The disease affects medium-sized arteries with a predilection for the superficial temporal artery and intracranial arteries, including those supplying the retina. Patients present with headache, throbbing temporal pain and tenderness. It may have a benign course over 6–12 months but may result in blindness and death. This disease may also present with fever and malaise. There is a dramatic response to steroids.

2 Wegener's granulomatosis. This is an acute necrotizing granulomatous disease of the upper respiratory tract involving arteries and veins and adjacent tissues (Fig. 15.18). It may be associated with focal or diffuse glomerulonephritis. The course is rapidly progressive. This condition responds to cyclophosphamide (see Chapter 21).

3 Takayasu's arteritis (non-specific aortoarteritis/pulseless disease/aortic arch syndrome). Takayasu's disease is a clinical syndrome of ocular disturbance and marked weakness of pulse in the upper extremities, related to fibrous thickening of the aortic arch with narrowing/obliteration of the origins of the great vessels. It is seen in young women with a female to male ratio of 9:1, most commonly in Japan. The average age of onset is 30 years. Aneurysms, haemorrhage and thrombosis are common. The disease is usually restricted to the aortic arch but the whole aorta is involved in 30% of cases and in 10% only in the ascending aorta.

Marked fibrosis is seen in all layers of the aortic wall, causing narrowing and occlusion of the vessels taking origin from the aorta. Histologically, there is infiltration of the media and adventitia by neutrophils and chronic inflammatory cells, particularly around the vasa vasorum. Occasionally, giant cell granulomas can be seen.

Occlusion of the aortic arch vessels results in loss of

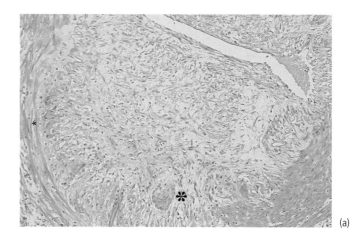

(a)

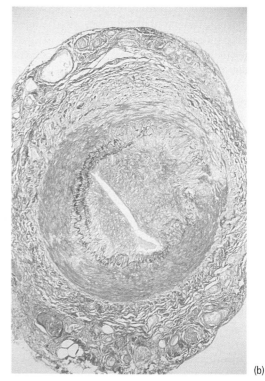

(b)

Fig. 15.17 (a) Giant cell arteritis in a temporal artery biopsy from an elderly woman with a history of headaches. Note the granulomatous inflammatory cell infiltrate with numerous giant cells (✳). (H&E.) (b) Giant cell arteritis. Note the granulomatous inflammatory cell infiltrate destroying elastic fibres and the intimal proliferation with occlusion. (EVG.)

radial pulses and ischaemic neurological lesions. There is commonly visual impairment. The course is variable.

4 Thromboangiitis obliterans (Buerger's disease). This is a segmental, thrombosing, obliterative, acute and chronic inflammation of arteries and veins (Fig. 15.19(a)), usually of the legs, leading to gangrene. It is almost exclusively seen in young **male cigarette smokers**. Although

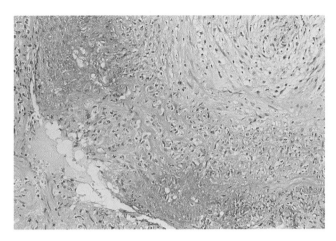

Fig. 15.18 Histology of acute necrotizing venulitis (left) seen in Wegener's granulomatosis in this lung biopsy. A granulomatous inflammation is seen (top right). (H&E.)

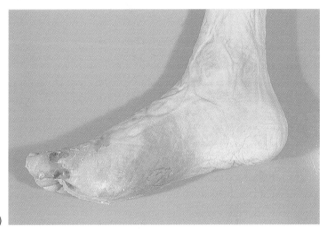

(a)

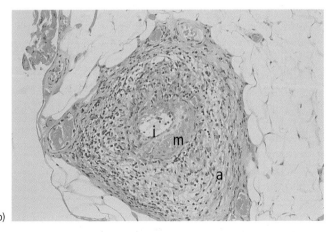

(b)

Fig. 15.19 Buerger's disease. (a) This young, male smoker presented with ischaemia and ulceration of the feet. (b) Histology of a small branch of the popliteal artery shows acute vasculitis with thrombotic occlusion of the vessel lumen. Note the inflammation extending out to the adventitial fat. (H&E.) i, intima; m, media; a, adventitial fat.

rare in the USA and Europe, it is a common cause of peripheral vascular disease in Israel, Japan and India.

In the acute phase, there is marked swelling and neutrophilic infiltration of the entire neurovascular bundle and thrombosis is common. Healing by organization and fibrosis produces thick cord-like vessels with occluded lumina.

Classically, there is progressive lower limb ischaemia with intermittent claudication and, eventually, pain at rest (Fig. 15.19(b)). Abstinence from smoking often results in remissions.

5 Rheumatoid arteritis/aortitis. This occurs in a small number of men with rheumatoid arthritis involving the spine (rheumatoid spondylitis). This is a true panarteritis with necrosis and fibrosis of the media, obliteration of vasa vasorum and intimal thickening.

6 Churg–Strauss syndrome (allergic granulomatosis and arteritis). This involves pulmonary and splenic vessels and is associated with bronchial asthma and eosinophilia. The vascular lesions resemble PAN histologically. This condition is discussed in more detail in Chapter 17.

7 Kawasaki's disease (mucocutaneous lymph node syndrome). Kawasaki's disease is an acute vasculitis of infancy and early childhood characterized by:

- fever;
- rash;
- lymphadenitis;
- conjunctival lesions;
- oral lesions.

An acute necrotizing vasculitis affects small and medium-sized arteries with a preference for the coronary arteries. The disease is self-limited and is thought to be of viral origin.

Degenerative diseases of arteries—arteriosclerosis

The term arteriosclerosis may be remembered as a collective term which is equivalent to what the lay person means by 'hardening of the arteries'. As the following account will reveal, there are many causes of 'hardening of the arteries' (arteriosclerosis) but the most prevalent and important is atherosclerosis (Table 15.15).

Definition of arteriosclerosis

Lobstein (1829)–'a generic term for all diseases of the arteries in which there is thickening and hardening of the vessel wall with reduction in diameter of the lumen'.

Atherosclerosis

Definitions. The term atheroma was introduced by Greek anatomists and popularized by von Haller (1735).

Table 15.15 Types and location of arteriosclerotic lesions.

Name	Predominant initial lesion	Arterial size
Atherosclerosis	Intima (inner media)	Large and medium
Mönckeberg's	Media	Large and medium
Diffuse intimal thickening (DIT)	Intima	Large and medium
Radiation vasculopathy	Intima	Large, medium and small
Arteriolosclerosis	Intima/media	Arterioles
Mucoid (cystic) medial necrosis	Media	Large
Endarteritis	Intima	Small
Polyarteritis	Intima/media/adventitia	Medium and small
Infectious arteritis	Adventitia/media	Large and medium
Giant cell arteritis	Media	Medium and small
Takayasu's arteritis	Intima and media	Large and medium

The World Health Organization (1958) gives the definition as 'a variable combination of changes in the intima of arteries consisting of focal accumulations of lipid, complex carbohydrates, blood and blood products, fibrous deposits and calcium deposits associated with medial changes'.

Atherosclerosis is a patchy, focal disease of the intima of large musculoelastic arteries including the aorta. It features cellular proliferation (smooth-muscle cells, macrophages, fibroblasts); lipid deposition; increase in ground substance and collagen and necrosis (i.e. the atheromatous plaque) (Fig. 15.20).

Epidemiology
- **Incidence.** Atherosclerosis and its complications are the leading cause of morbidity and mortality in the western world, accounting for > 50% of all deaths.
- **Prevalence.** This is a disease that increases in severity with age but there is 100% prevalence in adults. It has a variable pattern within individuals and a variable severity between individuals, probably due to the association of different predisposing or risk factors.
- **Sex.** Atherosclerosis has been found to be more extensive and more severe in men than in women. This difference disappears in women after the menopause and this is why oestrogen is thought to offer some degree of protection from atherosclerosis.
- **Heredity.** Heredity influences the severity of atherosclerosis by directly affecting arterial wall structure and function and indirectly via risk factors. There is thought to be a **polygenic inheritence**.

- **Risk factors.** These include:
  (**a**) smoking;
  (**b**) hypertension;
  (**c**) high-fat diets;
  (**d**) diabetes (hyperglycaemia);
  (**e**) obesity;
  (**f**) hyperlipidaemia (increased LDL).

Epidemiological studies (such as the Framingham study) have shown that certain habits, diseases and lifestyles are more significant than others and offer different degrees of risk.

It must be realized that advanced atherosclerosis and its clinical complications are uniquely human conditions. It is not possible to follow the progression of atherosclerosis within an individual and thus epidemiology has to rely on the assessment of clinical consequences of atherosclerosis, such as myocardial infarction, as they apply to populations. These risk factors may be important in the development of these clinical complications; they do not necessarily reflect what is going on at the level of the intimal lesion in a single individual.

Types of lesions
- **Fatty streaks.** These are yellow, flat lesions arising between the intima and internal elastic lamina, consisting of macrophages containing cholesterol and cholesterol esters derived from plasma (Fig. 15.21).
- **Fibrous plaques.** These are grey-white, elevated lesions consisting of subendothelial proliferations of smooth-muscle cells, collagen, elastin and variable amounts of extracellular lipid. They appear in the second and third decades at bifurcation points in arteries and aorta (Fig. 15.22(a)).
- **Complicated/advanced plaques.** These are pale yellow-grey/white, raised, of varying size involving the intima and inner media and giving rise to local complications (Fig. 15.22(b)).

Patterns of lesion distribution. The abdominal aorta is more severely affected than the thoracic aorta. Atheromatous plaques are rare in pulmonary arteries (unless pulmonary hypertension exists).

Sites most commonly affected include:
- coronary arteries;
- terminal abdominal aorta and its branches;
- innominate, carotid and subclavian arteries and their branches;
- visceral branches of the abdominal aorta including the renal arteries.

Pathogenesis. Multiple theories suggest multiple factors. Multiple theories of atherogenesis have been proposed (Table 15.16). Perhaps the earliest and best known the-

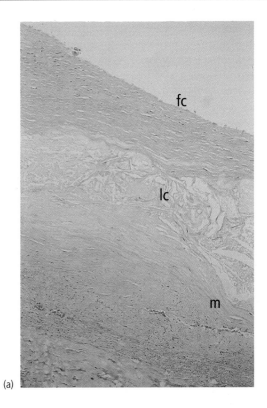

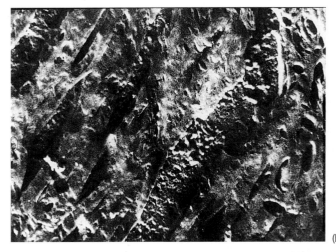

(a)

(b)

Fig. 15.20 Atherosclerosis. (a) Light microscopy of a coronary artery atherosclerotic plaque. Note the fibrous cap (fc), soluble lipid core (lc) with cholesterol clefts and macrophages (m) at the shoulder of the plaque. (H&E.) (b) Scanning electronmicrograph shows soluble lipid granules amid the cholesterol clefts and collagen fibres.

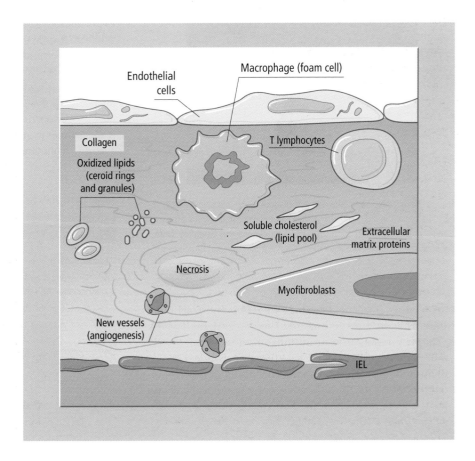

Fig. 15.20(c) Diagrammatic representation of the cellular and non-cellular components of atherosclerosis. IEL, internal elastic lamina.

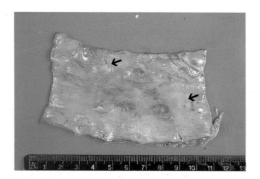

Fig. 15.21 Thoracic aorta from a road traffic accident victim aged 25. Note the numerous fatty streaks (arrowed) present in the intima. They are only slightly raised and yellow.

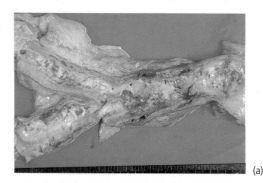

(a)

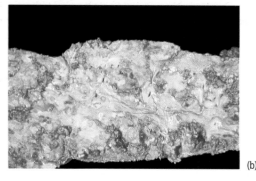

(b)

Fig. 15.22 (a) Fibro-fatty atheromatous plaques in the abdominal aorta from the patient in Fig. 15.21. (b) Advanced or complicated atheromatous plaques in the abdominal aorta from a 65-year-old business executive. Note the local complications of plaque ulceration, heamorrhage and thrombosis.

ories were those elaborated in 1844 by Carl von Rokitansky (the **thrombogenic** theory) and in 1835 by Rudolph Virchow (the **lipid imbibition** theory).

Virchow also believed that atheroma was a chronic inflammatory process involving the intima. It is now evident that platelets, fibrin, lipids and mononuclear cells do play a part in atherogenesis. The key question is, how?

Many theories of atherogenesis still abound and it is likely that multiple factors are involved and that these factors affect the status of the arterial wall and the composition and dynamics of the blood.

In the past decade, the cellular nature of atherosclerosis has been realized and more clearly understood. Much of this information has come from immunological and molecular biological studies on experimentally induced lesions in animal models. Increasingly, research is being undertaken on human material. We are only just beginning to understand how hypercholesterolaemia and hypertension might lead to the development of atherosclerosis.

It is now clear that the principal changes that take place in the artery wall during atherogenesis occur largely within the intima of medium and large arteries. The key factors include the entry of cells and non-cellular substances, including lipids (principally LDL), from the blood.

The role of the arterial wall in atherogenesis
1 Intimal injury and smooth-muscle cell proliferation. Injury to the intima causes smooth-muscle cell proliferation and the proliferation of myofibroblasts, cells with phenotypic characteristics of both smooth-muscle cells and fibroblasts, within the intima. This can be seen in experimental animal models and as part of an age-related phenomenon, known as **diffuse intimal thickening** (**DIT**) in humans. *In vitro* cell culture studies of smooth-muscle cells show that they are capable of synthesizing extracellular matrix components such as collagen, elastin and mucopolysaccharides. Smooth-muscle cells can metabolize lipoproteins and accumulate cholesterol esters.
2 Response to injury theory. Injury to the endothelium, arising from mechanical, chemical or immunological

Table 15.16 Theories of atherogenesis.

Theory	Main element
Haemodynamic	Endothelial cell injury
Encrustation	Thrombosis
Lipid imbibition (Virchow (1862))	Cholesterol–LDL–macrophage
Response to injury (Ross (1986))	Vessel wall and platelets
Neoplastic	Smooth-muscle cells
Viral	Endothelial/smooth-muscle cells
LDL uptake (Brown & Goldstein (1983))	Cholesterol–LDL–macrophages
Macrophage/oxidized lipid	Macrophage

LDL, Low-density lipoprotein.

damage, results in entry of plasma constituents such as lipoproteins and fibrinogen, together with cellular elements including platelets, monocytes and lymphocytes. **Platelet-derived growth factor (PDGF)** can induce smooth-muscle cell proliferation. The plaque then progresses with lipid infiltration and modification, monocytes, platelets and lymphocytes and further smooth-muscle cell proliferation and collagen production and degradation.

3 Monoclonal theory. Cells in the atheromatous plaque have been observed to be monotypic for the A or B isoenzyme of glucose-6-phosphate dehydrogenase (G6PD) in Negro females. This had been interpreted as evidence that atherosclerosis represents a neoplastic intimal lesion. In fact, there is a recognized tendency to monotypism in other benign, non-neoplastic proliferative lesions, like scar tissue.

4 Viral theory. Herpesvirus particles and viral DNA can be detected in early atherosclerotic lesions in humans. How this relates to atherogenesis is still unclear.

The role of lipids in atherogenesis

1 Dietary evidence. This remains a surprisingly controversial area. However, in studies of populations, dietary intake is probably important. Human populations consuming diets high in saturated fats and cholesterol have high mean serum cholesterol levels and have high mortality rates from coronary artery disease.

Recent studies have been performed on large numbers of hypercholesterolaemic individuals who have been treated with pharmacological agents that reduce plasma cholesterol levels. These trials have shown that decreasing cholesterol levels over time leads to a decreased incidence of the clinical sequelae of atherosclerosis.

2 Hyperlipidaemia. Patients with genetically determined hyperlipoproteinaemia (Table 15.8) and marked hypercholesterolaemia due to nephrotic syndrome, diabetes mellitus and untreated myxoedema have severe atherosclerosis. However, there remains an imperfect correlation between the severity of atherosclerosis and the cholesterol levels *per se* within an individual. The state of circulating lipids, rather than the level, may be of importance.

3 Low-density lipoprotein. LDL is the main carrier of plasma cholesterol to the tissues of the body. Studies on patients with familial hypercholesterolaemia (Brown and Goldstein) have shown that hepatocytes, fibroblasts and smooth-muscle cells contain **high-affinity receptors** for plasma LDL which are down-regulated when LDL is plentiful. Patients with familial hypercholesterolaemia have **defective LDL receptors**.

LDL can be modified by malonation and oxidation, principally by macrophages or exogenous agents. Macrophages, endothelial cells and smooth-muscle cells also contain **non-saturable scavenger receptors** or modified LDL receptors which are not down-regulated and which preferentially take up modified LDL.

High levels of circulating **HDL** appear to be protective even with raised cholesterol.

4 Oxidized lipids. Ceroid is the name given to the insoluble yellowish pigment present in mammalian tissues, especially in vitamin E deficiency. It is regularly seen in association with human atherosclerotic plaques and can be regarded as the hallmark of the advanced lesion. It is insoluble in lipid solvents and is therefore recognizable in routinely processed tissue sections by lipid stains such as oil red O (Fig. 15.23). It is thought to consist of polymerized products of oxidized lipoproteins, predominantly LDL, within macrophages.

Oxidized lipids are toxic and immunogenic, they can be chemoattractant for leukocytes and induce cell proliferation. Their effects could account for progression and some of the complications of atherosclerosis.

5 Experimental/animal models. Lesions resembling atherosclerosis can be induced in experimental animals by a combination of high-lipid diets and intimal injury.

*The role of macrophages in atherogenesis (the **macrophage hypothesis**; Table 15.17).* Recently, immunohistochemistry using monoclonal antibodies to human macrophages has shown that lipid-laden foam cells in early and advanced atherosclerotic plaques are monocyte-derived macrophages rather than smooth-muscle cells (Fig. 15.24(a)).

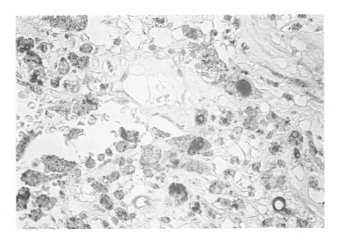

Fig. 15.23 Histology of an advanced atherosclerotic plaque stained with oil-red O in a routine paraffin section. Note the abundant insoluble lipid in granule and ring forms (stained red).

Table 15.17 Potential roles of macrophages in the pathogenesis of atherosclerosis.

Transport of LDL into the intima from blood-borne monocytes
Secretion of monokines which are chemoattractment for monocytes and smooth-muscle cells to the intima
Secretion of growth factors for smooth-muscle cells
Secretion of factors which induce phenotypic modulation of smooth-muscle cells from a contractile to a secretory state
Secretion of angiogenic factors that stimulate new vessel formation at the base of the plaque
The secretion of neutral proteases such as collagenases and elastases which contribute to the formation of the necrotic 'gruel'-like content of the advanced plaque and may be involved in aneurysm formation.
Degraded collagen is highly thrombogenic and is also a common site for dystrophic calcification
The production of toxic oxygen radicals which contribute to the above and which further oxidize free LDL, enhancing its uptake by macrophages
Macrophages secrete lipoprotein lipase, which leads to the uptake and degradation of lipoproteins by macrophages
Lipid-laden intimal macrophages may re-emerge into the blood. Although there is no evidence that this occurs in humans, it could be the mechanism for the regression of early lesions
Oxidation of lipid within macrophages leads to the production of ceroid
LDL which is oxidized by macrophages is antigenic, thought to be due to modification of lysine residues in the apolipoprotein B molecule
Macrophages are capable of acting as antigen-presenting cells and secrete monokines which recruit lymphocytes to the lesion

LDL, Low-density lipoprotein.

Table 15.18 Local complications of atherosclerosis.

Narrowing of lumen (stenosis) → ischaemia (Fig. 15.25(a))
Thrombosis (± thromboembolism) → ischaemia (Fig. 15.25(b))
Calcification (sclerosis)
Haemorrhage into the plaque (± sudden stenosis)
Ulceration and fissuring (± atheroembolism)
Chronic inflammation (chronic periaortitis)
Aneurysm (± thrombosis; ± rupture)
lead to the *clinical horizon* of atherosclerosis
Ischaemic heart disease
Peripheral vascular disease
Myocardial infarction
Acute heart failure
Congestive cardiac failure
Transient ischaemic attacks
Cerebrovascular accident
Acute renal failure
Sudden death

Until recently, research into atherosclerosis was centred upon the response to injury hypothesis. It is now apparent that foam cells which are present in fatty streaks and at the edges of most advanced plaques are macrophages and that macrophages are found in the necrotic base of the advanced atherosclerotic plaque. Smooth-muscle cells are present in diffuse intimal thickening and are increased in number in larger lesions.

The macrophage hypothesis can be seen as a unifying concept which may shed some light on the mechanisms of atherogenesis but may also permit some understanding of how atherosclerosis causes human disease (Fig. 15.24(b), Table 15.18).

Diagnosis of atherosclerosis. It is still true to say that the best way to assess the severity and extent of atherosclerosis in any individual is by examining the vascular system at autopsy. This is of no practical benefit to living patients!

At present, angiography and angioscopy may be used to evaluate localized occlusive lesions in coronary arteries in particular. More commonly, the severity of atherosclerosis is extrapolated from clinical effects, for example by electrocardiography (ECG) findings or by screening those with risk factors, for example by serum lipid measurements.

Treatment of atherosclerosis. **Surgical treatment** for localized disease includes local excision of the intimal plaque together with a portion of media (atherectomy or endarterectomy) or by coronary artery bypass grafting (CABG).

Balloon and laser angioplasty may remove or crush the plaque. In patients with end-stage ischaemic heart disease due to coronary artery atherosclerosis, **heart transplantation** may be the only treatment. In fact, the two most common reasons for referral for heart transplantation are **cardiomyopathy** and **ischaemic heart disease**.

Medical treatment is usually directed at the prevention of the development or propagation of thrombosis associated with the plaque (streptokinase and urokinase), or by the use of lipid-lowering drugs (clofibrate, cholestyramine, gemfibrozil). Trials are under way to assess the use of antioxidants such as probucol and vitamin E to prevent oxidation of LDL and atherogenesis. The future also holds the prospect of gene therapy to control smooth-muscle cell proliferation and macrophage migration into the intima.

Atherosclerosis is a disease that begins in childhood and, logically, control of this disease lies with the reduction of risk factors from childhood onwards.

Mönckeberg's sclerosis

This is an age-related and relatively common arteriosclerosis. It features medial calcification. Stenosis and atheroma may occur but the lumen remains patent. Sites affected are usually lower limbs, head, neck and pelvis (especially uterine arteries). It leads to 'pipestem' rigidity (Fig. 15.26).

The aetiology is uncertain, but it may reflect a more marked version of age-related degeneration with dystrophic calcification.

Cystic (mucoid) medial necrosis

This is a term introduced by Erdheim (1929) and is also known as **cystic medial degeneration**. It is a disorder of large arteries, especially the aorta, with focal degeneration of elastic tissue and muscle in media, and presence of mucoid material in media (Fig. 15.27). It is more frequent after the age of 40 years and has a male:female incidence of 2:1. It is an extremely important condition as it predisposes to dissecting aneurysm.

The aetiology is unknown but various hypotheses have been proposed:

- inherited abnormality of **fibrillin gene** (i.e. a *forme fruste* of Marfan's);
- ischaemia, which occurs earliest in the central media;
- hypertension, which is present in > 50% of cases;

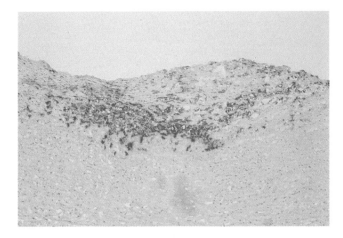

Fig. 15.24(a) Immunohistochemistry of an early atheromatous plaque shows positivity (red) for macrophage marker CD68. Note that the majority of cells are macrophages.

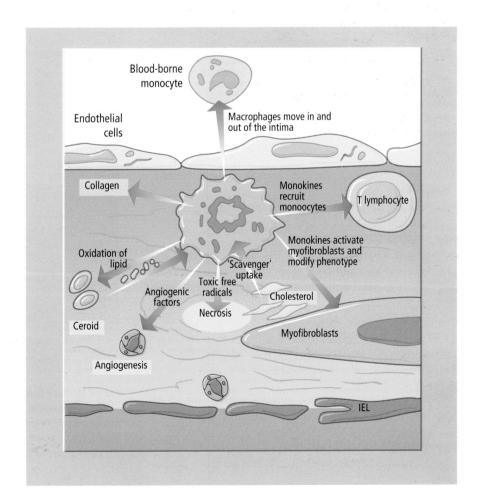

Fig. 15.24(b) The macrophage hypothesis: a central role of the macrophage in atherogenesis and in the progression of atherosclerosis.

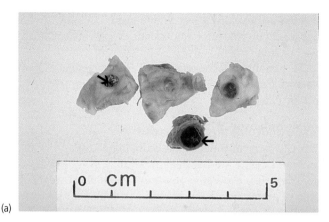

(a)

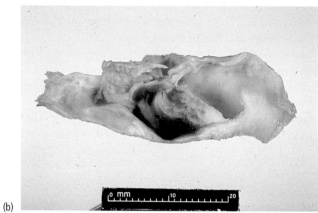

(b)

Fig. 15.25 (a) Coronary artery atherosclerosis and occlusive thrombosis (arrowed) from a patient with an acute myocardial infarction. (b) Carotid artery atherosclerosis and occlusive thrombosis from a patient with a cerebral infarct ('stroke').

- other associations, including bicuspid aortic stenosis, hypothroidism and pregnancy;
- certain amounts occur with normal advancing age.

Age-related vascular disease

Age-related changes occur in the aorta, arteries and arterioles and are commonly seen over the age of 70 years but there is marked individual variation. The commonest changes include:
- DIT (Fig. 15.28);
- fibrosis of the media;
- fragmentation of the elastic laminae (**elastopathy**);
- accumulation of mucopolysaccharide (mucoid or myxoid change).

These changes can cause arteriosclerosis, arteriolosclerosis, aortic or arterial ectasia or aneurysm formation.

Hypertensive vascular disease

Hypertension has the following effects on the vascular system:

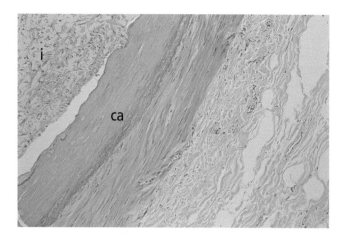

Fig. 15.26 Histology of Mönkeberg's medial calcification (ca) shows the intimal fibrous proliferation that stenoses the vessel lumen. i, intima.

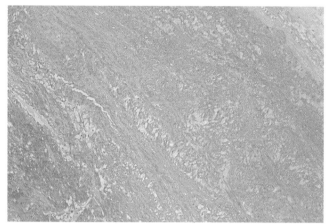

(a)

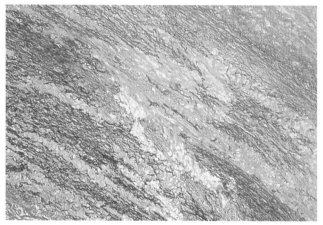

(b)

Fig. 15.27 Cystic medial necrosis in a patient with Marfan's syndrome. (a) Mucoid medial change with deposition of mucopolysaccharide in the media. (AB/PAS.) (b) Cystic medial necrosis in a patient with Marfan's syndrome. Note the severe fragmentation of the black elastin fibres or 'elastopathy'. (EVG.)

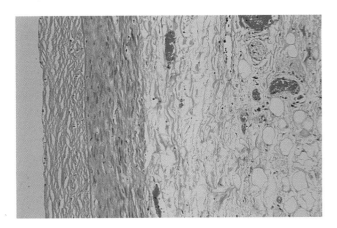

Fig. 15.28 Histology of diffuse intimal thickening (left) in an aorta from a patient aged 85. This is a 'normal' appearance for this patient's age. (H&E.)

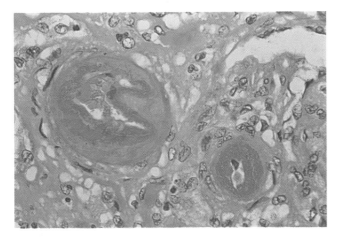

Fig. 15.29 Arteriole. Hypertensive hyaline vascular disease (hypertensive arteriolosclerosis) gives a homogenous, glassy, red thickening, resulting in stenosis. (H&E.)

- essential or benign hypertension is associated with hyaline arteriolosclerosis, thought to be due to insudation of plasma proteins (Fig. 15.29);
- malignant hypertension is associated with fibrinoid necrosis, which is a combination of fibrin deposition and necrosis of the vessel wall;
- concentric proliferation of smooth-muscle cells in small arteries and arterioles (hyperplastic arteriosclerosis/arteriolosclerosis);
- hypertension accelerates atherosclerosis;

These changes result in renal failure, cardiac failure and intracerebral haemorrhage.

Diabetic vascular disease

Patients with juvenile-onset, insulin-dependent diabetes may develop the following forms of vascular disease:
- accelerated atherosclerosis;
- hypertensive vascular disease;

- capillary microangiopathy with basement membrane thickening and intimal fibrosis ('onion-skin' lesions; Fig. 15.30). These lesions cause damage to the retina, nerves and kidneys.

The most serious complications include blindness, neuropathies, renal failure and gangrene.

Radiation vascular disease

Vascular endothelium is highly susceptible to radiation damage. With increasing use of radiotherapy in treatment of malignant disease, vascular complications are seen more commonly.

Radiation causes intimal thickening of arteries and arterioles and dilatation and occlusion of capillaries and venules (Fig. 15.31). The effects of local irradiation are those of locally induced ischaemia. Thus radiotherapy for

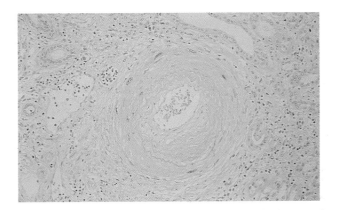

Fig. 15.30 Arteriole. Diabetic vascular disease with 'onion skinning' appearance ('diabetic arteriolosclerosis'). (H&E.)

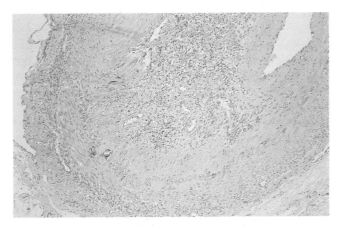

Fig. 15.31 Radiation vasculopathy in a mesenteric artery branch. This patient had radiotherapy for Hodgkin's disease and presented 2 years later with ischaemic colitis. Note the irregular fibrotic thickening of the vessel wall with stenosis. (H&E.)

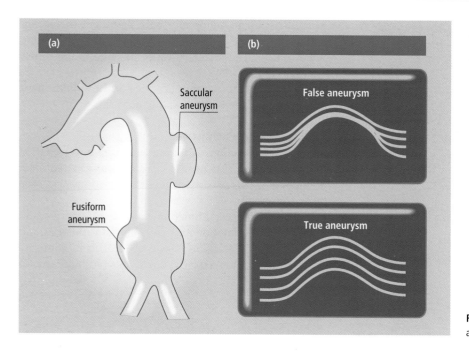

Fig. 15.32(a) and (b) Diagram of gross forms of aneurysms.

breast carcinoma may result in pulmonary or myocardial fibrosis; radiotherapy for cervical carcinoma may result in small-bowel or large-bowel ischaemia and stricture.

Vascular aneurysms

Aneurysms are more commonly seen in high-pressure systems such as the systemic arterial system and the aorta. They are rare in the pulmonary, portal and venous systems. They may occur in the wall of a vessel which has some congenital or acquired structural abnormality.

The most dramatic consequence of a vascular aneurysm is rupture. Common sites for aneurysm rupture are the aorta and cerebrovascular circulation. As the following account will reveal, as causes of sudden death in the young and elderly population, aneurysmal disease is very important.

Definition
An aneurysm is an **abnormal, localized dilatation of an artery or vein**. It results from damage to the vascular wall, particularly the media. Dilatation results from the distending forces of blood pressure on a weakened wall.

Gross forms (Fig. 15.32)
Fusiform. There is circumferential involvement of the vessel; elongated, spindle-shaped. It is usually seen in the aorta and common iliac arteries, most often due to atherosclerosis.

Saccular. These aneurysms are more circumscribed; there is sac formation which communicates with the vessel by a relatively narrow neck. It is commonly seen in syphilis in the thoracic aorta.

'True' versus 'false'. In a **true aneurysm**, the wall is altered (thinned) as in atherosclerotic, dissecting, syphilitic and congenital aneurysms. In a **false aneurysm**, the vascular wall has been breached and the wall of the aneurysm consists of periarterial tissue. Traumatic, mycotic and arteriovenous aneurysms are of this type.

Complications
- Thrombosis and its sequelae.
- External rupture.
- Erosion of neighbouring structures.

Specific forms
Atherosclerotic aneurysm (Fig. 15.33). This is the commonest form of aortic aneurysm and it occurs in association with atherosclerosis. The common sites are the abdominal aorta and common iliac arteries.

These aneurysms are 10 times more common in males than females. There is increasing incidence with age and they are rare before the age of 55 years. Deaths due to **abdominal aortic aneurysm (AAA)** rupture peak at 65–75 years and account for up to 1.7% of all deaths in men. The estimated prevalence of AAA in all men aged 65–75 years is 2.7% and the incidence is increasing.

Aneurysms <6 cm diameter have a 20% chance of rup-

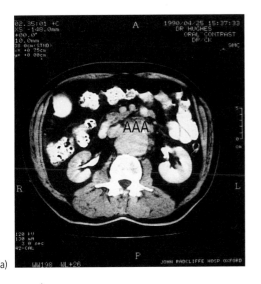

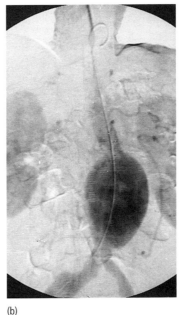

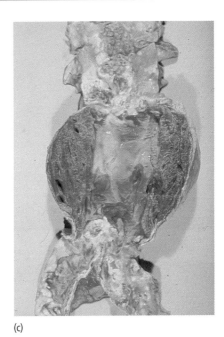

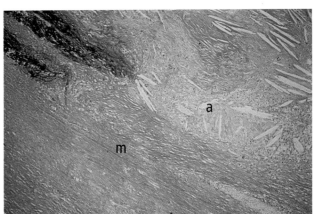

Fig. 15.33 (a) Computed tomographic (CT) scan of a 6.5 cm abdominal aortic aneurysm (AAA). (b) Angiography shows the common location for this disease, above the iliac bifurcation and below the renal artery origins. (c) The post mortem appearance of a ruptured AAA. The aorta is opened longitudinally. Note the abundant thrombus in the aneurysm wall. This patient had ischaemic feet prior to death. (d) Histology of the aneurysm wall shows intimal atheroma (a) eroding through the media (m). (EVG.)

ture within 1 year; > 6 cm diameter have a 50% chance of rupture within 1 year. Patients with AAAs of more than 6.0 cm maximum external diameter are advised to have elective repair. Operative mortality in Oxford is now of the order of 1.4%.

Syphilitic aneurysm (Fig. 15.34). Now a **rare** complication of tertiary syphilis, these aneurysms occur usually in the thoracic aorta, particularly in the ascending portion of the arch. They may lead to aortic incompetence. The saccular type may erode bone locally.

The suggested reason for apparent confinement to the aortic arch is that lymphatic drainage is in close relationship to pulmonary lymphatics – the lung may contain many spirochaetes in the secondary stage.

Dissecting aneurysm (Fig. 15.35). This is a common condition with an incidence of 1:10 000 hospital admissions and 1:400 autopsies. The cause is most often cystic medial necrosis in association with hypertension, aortic stenosis and Marfan's syndrome.

Histopathology shows haemorrhage into the media, commonly of the ascending aorta, with splitting into two layers. Haemorrhage may track upwards to give a double-barrelled aorta. Initial haemorrhage may be from the lumen or from within the wall due to rupture of vasa vasorum. The effects are:
• rupture with rapid death (occurs in 90%);
• occlusion of arteries – especially renals and mesenteric, leading to infarction of their territories;
• re-entry further down with formation of chronic

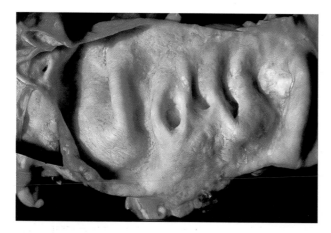

Fig. 15.34 Syphilitic aortitis. Note the rugose appearance of the intima. This patient presented with a pulsatile thoracic mass.

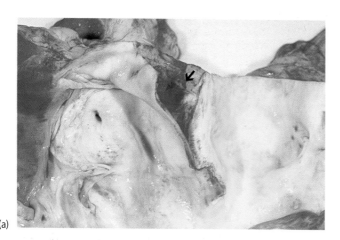

(a)

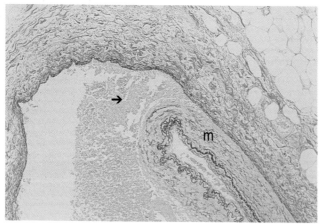

(b)

Fig. 15.35 Aortic dissection. (a) The origin of the dissection is in the proximal ascending aorta (arrowed). The patient died from cardiac tamponade. (b) Histology shows blood tracking (arrowed) between the media (m). (EVG.)

aneurysm or double-barrelled aorta. Usually, these aneurysms eventually rupture;

- haemorrhage from dissection may occur into the pericardium, mediastinum or pleural cavity.

Mycotic aneurysm. These may be caused by micro-organisms (all types, not just fungal) invading from within, often via an infected embolus during a pyaemic infection. They are seen most often as a complication of **acute bacterial endocarditis** (ABE; **not** subacute bacterial endocarditis). Most frequent sites are cerebral vessels, but mesenteric, splenic and renal arteries are not uncommonly affected. The aneurysms may rupture when quite small and rarely grow >1 cm.

Congenital (berry) aneurysm. These are saccular aneurysms seen at bifurcations of small arteries. Most commonly, they are found in the circle of Willis and major branches of base of brain. They are multiple in 12–15% of cases. The commonest sites are: (30%) middle cerebral artery at its first or second point of branching in the Sylvian fissure; (25%) junction of the anterior cerebral and anterior communicating arteries; (20%) terminal portion of the internal carotid and posterior communicating arteries (Fig. 15.11).

The cause is probably a congenital deficiency of medial muscle, exaggerated by hypertension which increases the chances of rupture with resultant haemorrhage at base of brain (subarachnoid haemorrhage), severe neurological symptoms and often death.

Traumatic aneurysm. These aneurysms are caused by direct injury to the vessel wall, usually forming false aneurysms (Fig. 15.36). Two anatomical sites are particu-

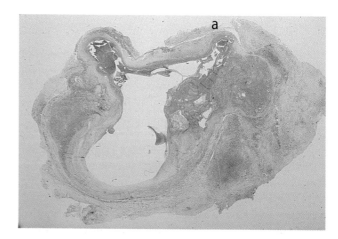

Fig. 15.36 Histology of a traumatic (false) aneurysm (a) of the aorta in a child who suffered a steering wheel injury in a road traffic accident. The aneurysm wall consists of only a portion of the true aortic wall. (H&E.)

larly susceptible; the junction of the arch and descending aorta and the proximal ascending aorta. They may be iatrogenic, due to cannulae inserted during cardiopulmonary bypass procedures or percutaneous insertion of arterial or aortic devices. This often results in dissection.

Arteriovenous aneurysm (or fistula). These are artificial communications between an artery and a vein. As such, the vein becomes the 'wall' of the aneurysm.

Causes include trauma, congenital anomaly (arteriovenous malformation (AVM) hereditary haemorrhagic telangiectasia, hemihypertrophy, Sturge–Weber syndrome), and rupture of an arterial aneurysm into a vein (rare). They result in the formation of an arteriovenous shunt with resultant haemodynamic consequences. There may be increased venous return with heart failure if the shunt is sufficiently large.

Aneurysms in vasculitis. These are most often seen in PAN, giant cell arteritis, rheumatoid arthritis, systemic lupus erythematosus (SLE), Wegener's, Churg–Strauss, ankylosing spondylitis and Takayasu's arteritis, but may occur in any case of vasculitis.

Microaneurysms
- Diabetic microangiopathy affects small arterioles, capillaries and venules with basement membrane thickening and endothelial cell loss.
- Hypertensive microangiopathies (Charcot–Bouchard aneurysm) are usually < 2 mm and occur in branches of cerebral arteries in 50% of hypertensives.

DISEASES OF VEINS

Normal venous anatomy

Veins consist of an intima, media and adventitia. They differ functionally from arteries in that they operate at low pressure and their structure reflects this. The media contains little elastin and the medial muscle is arranged in irregular bundles (Fig. 15.37).

Venous thrombosis

Thrombophlebitis

This is thrombosis secondary to acute inflammation of veins. It is commonly associated with infected wounds and ulcers. The affected vein shows all the features of acute inflammation, namely swelling, redness, tenderness, pain and warmth. This type of thrombus tends to be firmly attached to the vessel wall and fragments rarely become detached.

Rarely, thrombophlebitis occurs in multiple superficial leg veins (**thrombophlebitis migrans**) in patients with visceral cancers, most commonly pancreatic and gastric cancer (**Trousseau's sign**).

Phlebothrombosis

This is venous thrombosis in the absence of venous inflammation. It is seen most commonly in the deep veins (deep venous thrombosis; DVT). Less commonly, veins of the pelvis and prostatic venous plexuses are involved.

DVT is common and clinically important. Thrombus is easily detached and this leads to thrombo-embolus. Detached thrombus travels in the venous circulation to the lungs–a pulmonary thrombo-embolus.

Causes of **phlebothrombosis** *(deep venous thrombosis).* These have been described as Virchow's triad and include:
- endothelial injury;
- sluggish blood flow, commonly due to prolonged immobilization or to cardiac failure;
- increased tendency to coagulation (postoperatively, postpartum, associated with oral contraception).

Venous varicosities (varicose veins)

Abnormally dilated and tortuous veins occur at several sites–in the legs, rectum (**haemorrhoids**), oesophagus (**varices** in portal hypertension) or spermatic cord (**varicocoele**). They are associated with increased pressure in the affected vessels, obstruction to adequate venous drainage or increased blood flow in the affected vessels.

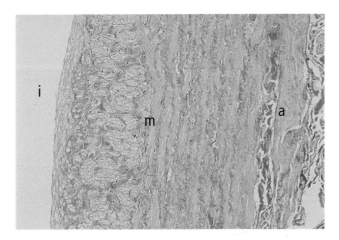

Fig. 15.37 Normal vein structure. The media contains bundles of muscle fibres without organized elastin. i, intima; m, media; a, adventitia.

Aetiology

In the legs, varicose veins involve the superficial saphenous system and have two main causes:

- obstruction to the deep veins of the leg causes the superficial varicosities to act as collateral venous drainage to the leg;
- incompetence of the valves of the saphenous veins and in the perforating veins that normally prevent flow of blood from the deep to the superficial veins. This is the commonest cause and is probably degenerative in nature.

Clinical features. Varicose veins are visible in a distribution that depends upon which valves are competent. They are associated with obesity and pregnancy and there is often a familial predisposition.

Effects.

- Swollen legs.
- Aching legs.
- Stasis dermatitis.
- Venous skin ulceration (Fig. 15.38).
- Thrombophlebitis.

Cardiac disease

Introduction

The discussion of the topic of myocardial disease will include normal cardiac anatomy, evaluation of cardiac function, clinical manifestations of cardiac disease and the commoner congenital diseases. The acquired cardiac diseases will be classified according to the 'pathological sieve'. It must be noted that cardiac disease may be primary and of known cause, primary and of unknown cause (strictly, cardiomyopathy) and that the heart may be involved secondarily in many systemic disease processes (Chapter 7; e.g. alcohol, haemochromatosis). Some diseases that are generally thought to have systemic effects may be isolated to the myocardium, for example amyloid heart disease and sarcoid heart disease.

Normal cardiac anatomy

Layers of the heart

The heart is composed of:

1 the **endocardium**, which lines the internal surface of the cardiac chambers and valves (Fig. 15.39(a));
2 the **myocardium**, containing cardiac myocytes which

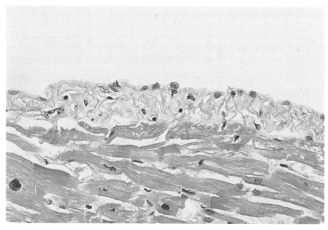

(a)

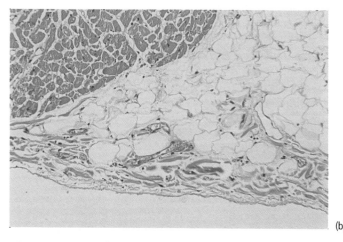

(b)

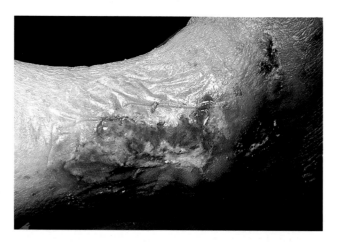

Fig. 15.38 Venous ulceration in the leg in a patient with longstanding varicose veins.

Fig. 15.39 Structure of the heart. (a) The normal endocardium. (b) The normal myocardium and pericardium. (H&E.)

normally possess regular cell nuclei and measure no more than 15 μm in diameter (Fig. 15.39(b));

3 the **pericardium**, composed of an inner visceral layer and an outer parietal layer completing the pericardial sac (Fig. 15.39(b));

4 the **specialized conducting system**, consisting of the sinoatrial (SA) node and atrioventricular (AV) node, the bundle of His and the Purkinje fibres (Fig. 15.40).

Walls of the heart

The muscular interatrial and interventricular septa divide the heart longitudinally into a right and left side.

Chambers of the heart

Each side of the heart is further divided into an atrium and ventricle by the atrioventricular valves. The muscular atrial walls have a thickness not exceeding 2mm.

The right ventricular wall has a thickness of less than 5mm; the left ventricle is no more than 15mm in thickness.

Valves of the heart

The cardiac valves enable the heart to function as a pump. The valves are thin, translucent fibrous membranes that the attached circumferentially to the valve ring. Blood flow through the normal open valve is non-turbulent and, when a valve closes, the free edges come firmly into apposition, thus completely closing the orifice.

Cardiac blood supply

The distribution of the coronary arteries is shown in Fig. 15.41.

Methods of evaluating cardiac structure and function

Examination of the patient

The most important aspects of the physical examination include:

- arterial pulse (bounding pulse of aortic valve incompetence; low-volume pulse of aortic valve stenosis);
- jugular venous pulse (increased in right heart failure and volume overload);
- cardiac apex beat (the apical 'heave' of left ventricular hypertrophy);
- auscultation of the heart (see below for valvular auscultation; a third heart sound may be due to rapid ventricular filling in diastole as in heart failure and mitral incompetence; a fourth heart sound in pulmonary or systemic hypertension and a friction rub in pericarditis).

Electrocardiography

The electrocardiogram (ECG) is a graphic display of electrical activity of the heart (Fig. 15.42; Tables 15.19 and 15.20).

Imaging

The most useful imaging modalities include the following.

Echocardiography. Pathologists who examine the heart at post mortem are accustomed to open the heart according to the pattern of blood flow. Indeed, most pathology reports will describe abnormalities from right atrium to right ventricle and from left atrium to left ventricle.

Table 15.19 The normal electrocardiogram tracing can be divided as follows.

The P wave due to atrial depolarization
The PR interval, which is a rough measurement of the conduction time through the atrioventricular node
The QRS complex due to ventricular depolarization
The T wave due to ventricular repolarization

Table 15.20 The electrocardiogram provides information for assessment of the following.

Cardiac hypertrophy
Arrhythmia
Myocardial ischaemia and infarction
Pericardial disease
Electrolyte disturbances (K^+, Mg^{2+}, Ca^{2+}) and drug effects (digitalis)

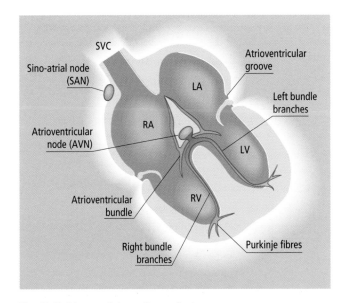

Fig. 15.40 Diagram of the cardiac conducting system.

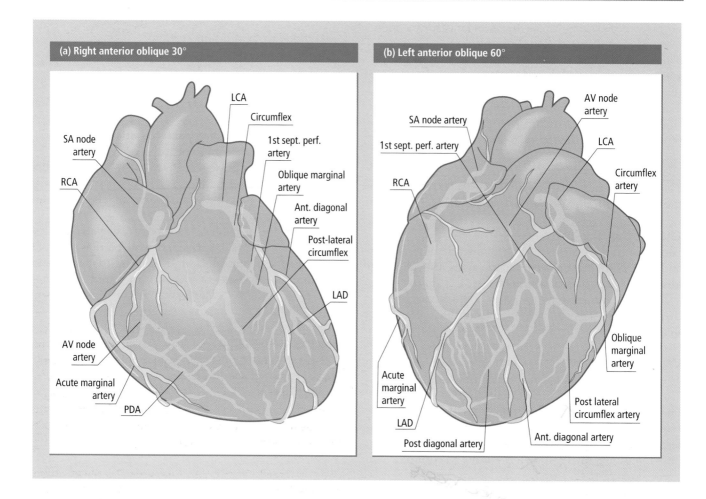

(a) Right anterior oblique 30°

LCA

Circumflex

1st sept. perf. artery

Oblique marginal artery

Ant. diagonal artery

Post-lateral circumflex

LAD

SA node artery

RCA

AV node artery

Acute marginal artery

PDA

(b) Left anterior oblique 60°

AV node artery

SA node artery

LCA

1st sept. perf. artery

Circumflex artery

RCA

Oblique marginal artery

Acute marginal artery

Post lateral circumflex artery

LAD

Post diagonal artery

Ant. diagonal artery

Fig. 15.41 (*Above*) Diagram of the coronary artery distribution. (a) Right anterior oblique 60°. (b) Left anterior oblique 60°. SA node art, artery to sino-atrial node; RCA, right coronary artery; AV node art, artery to the atrioventricular node; AcM, acute marginal; PDA, posterior descending artery; LCA, left coronary artery; circ, circumflex; ObM, obtuse marginal; Ant diag, anterior diagonal; Post lat circ, posterior lateral circumflex; LAD, left anterior descending.

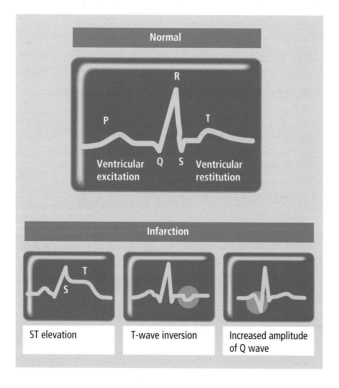

Normal

R

P

T

Ventricular excitation

Q   S

Ventricular restitution

Infarction

T

S

ST elevation

T-wave inversion

Increased amplitude of Q wave

Fig. 15.42 The echocardiograph (ECG).

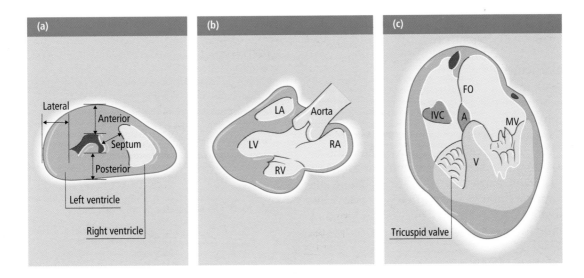

Fig. 15.43 Echocardiographic views of the heart. (a) Short axis view. (b) Long axis view. (c) Apical four chamber view. MV, mitral valve; A, atrial septum; IVC, inferior vena cava; V, ventricular septum. FO, foramen ovale.

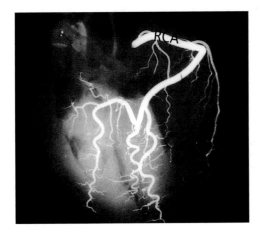

Fig. 15.44 Post mortem coronary artery angiography shows no evidence of stenosis. RCA, right coronary artery.

It is often more useful to open the heart in the echocardiographic planes which are understood by clinicians and which also allow for a good appreciation of normal and abnormal cardiac morphology (Fig. 15.43).

Chest radiograph. X-ray examination of the chest and lung fields and coronary artery angiography is part of the routine clinical work-up of patients presenting with heart failure.

Magnetic resonance imaging (MRI). This technique is of value in monitoring myocarditis and ischaemic heart disease.

Cardiac catheterization. This investigation requires insertion of a catheter through a vein to the right heart or artery to the left heart. This enables evaluation of pressures and oxygen saturation in the cardiac chambers. Injection of radiopaque dye (**angiography**) permits visualization of the heart and cardiac chambers. This technique may be used to visualize coronary artery stenosis *in vivo* or at post mortem (Fig. 15.44).

Endomyocardial biopsy (EMB). Cardiac catheterization permits biopsy of the endomyocardium. This is commonly done from the right ventricle (Table 15.21).

Table 15.21 Main indications for endomyocardial biopsy.

Evaluation of rejection after transplantation
Detection of myocarditis
Assessment of drug cardiotoxicity
Evaluation of cardiomyopathy, by exclusion of primary or secondary cardiac disease

Manifestations of cardiac disease

Pain

Ischaemic pain. Pain is due to stimulation of nerve endings by lactic acid produced during anaerobic glycolysis. This pain is usually retrosternal but may radiate into the neck or arms.

Angina pectoris is ischaemic pain which is brought on by exercise and relieved by rest.

Pericardial pain. Inflammation of the parietal pericardium will produce a sharp lower retrosternal pain that varies with posture and with respiration.

Cardiac enlargement

This may result from:
- dilatation of the ventricles;
- hypertrophy of the walls.

It is assessed at autopsy by measuring the ventricular wall thickness (right ventricle ≤3mm; left ventricle ≤15mm), weighing the heart (upper limit for an adult male heart is 380g; range 260–380g), or weighing the ventricular muscle (right ventriular free wall below the tricuspid valve ring; left ventricular free wall and septum below the mitral valve ring).

Abnormal cardiac rhythm

Arrhythmia (Tables 15.22 and 15.23) may reflect the following:
- altered activity of the SA node;
- the development of 'new' or ectopic foci that drive the heart at an accelerated or irregular rate;
- conduction defects.

Cardiac failure

The features of cardiac failure will be described below.

Congenital heart disease

There is no identiafible cause in most cases of congenital heart disease. However, many cases result from the actions of unidentified teratogens in the first trimester of pregnancy when fetal cardiac development occurs. Most congenital cardiac abnormalities are not inherited.

Table 15.22 Aetiology of cardiac arrhythmias.

Ischaemia
Myocarditis
Inflammatory diseases such as systemic lupus erythematosus, rheumatic fever, sarcoidosis
Drugs (digitalis, quinine, catecholamines, β-blockers)
Electrolyte abnormalities (K⁺)
Endocrine diseases (thyrotoxicosis)
Congenital abnormalities of the conducting system

Table 15.23 Effects of cardiac arrhythmias.

Reduced cardiac output
Ischaemia
Acute heart failure
Sudden death

Figure 15.45 illustrates the normal child's heart.

Aetiology

In a few patients, a specific cause can be identified.

Rubella. If there is transplacental infection of the fetus in the first trimester of pregnancy with the rubella virus, the following abnormalities may occur:
- patent ductus arteriosus;
- pulmonary stenosis.

Drugs. The most important drugs are thalidomide and alcohol. The latter is associated with **fetal alcohol syndrome**.

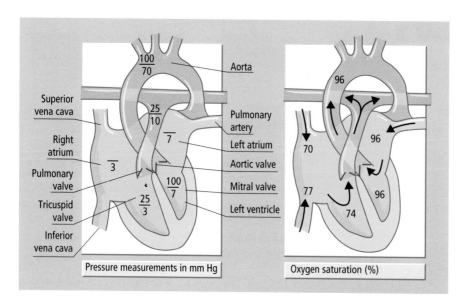

Fig. 15.45 Diagram of the normal child's heart.

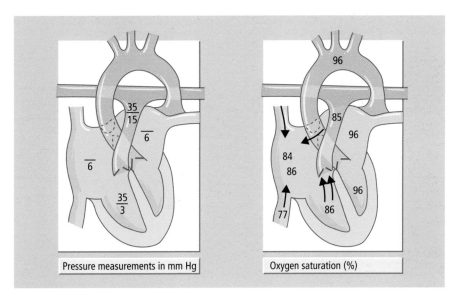

Pressure measurements in mm Hg

Oxygen saturation (%)

Fig. 15.46(a) Diagram of atrial septal defect (ASD).

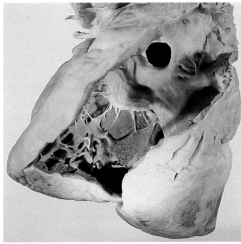

Fig. 15.46(b) ASD discovered incidentally at post mortem.

Chromosomal abnormalities. The following are the most important chromosome abnormalities associated with congenital heart disease:

• Turner's syndrome (45,XO); 20% will have cardiac abnormalities. The most common is coarctation of the aorta;
• Down syndrome (trisomy 21); 20% will have cardiac defects which include defects of the AV valves or the septa;
• trisomy 18; this is associated with a right ventricular origin of the aorta.

Classification

Congenital heart defects can involve the right side or left side of the heart, at the atrial, ventricular or aorto-pulmonary levels.

The common defects are classified according to:

• which side of the heart is involved;
• whether there is a communication or shunt between the two sides;
• in those defects where there is a shunt, the presence or absence of cyanosis.

Cyanosis is the bluish discoloration of the skin and mucous membranes caused by increased amounts of reduced haemoglobin in the arterial blood. In congenital cyanotic heart disease, cyanosis is caused by right-to-left shunts which allow unoxygenated venous blood to bypass the lungs and enter the systemic circulation (central cyanosis). The classification and frequency of congenital heart disease are shown in Table 15.24.

Table 15.24 Classification of congenital heart disease.

With shunt (80%)	
Acyanotic	
ASD	15%
VSD	25%
PDA	15%
Cyanotic	
Tetralogy of Fallot	10%
Transposition of great vessels	10%
Eisenmenger's syndrome	Rare
Without shunt (20%)	
Right-sided	
Pulmonary stenosis	10%
Ebstein's anomaly	Rare
Left-sided	
Coarctation of the aorta	10%
Aortic stenosis	Rare

ADS, Atrial septal defect; VSD, ventricular septal defect; PDA, patent ductus arteriosus.

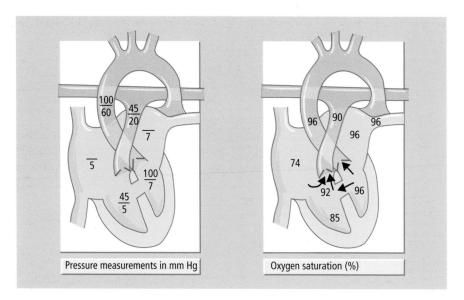

Pressure measurements in mm Hg

Oxygen saturation (%)

Fig. 15.47(a) Diagram of ventricular septal defect (VSD).

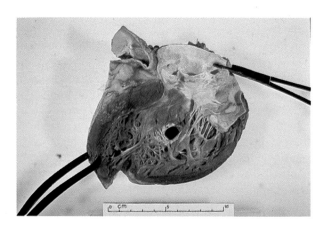

Fig. 15.47(b) Ventricular septal defect (VSD).

Atrial septal defect (ASD)

1 Ostium secundum ASD (Fig. 15.46). This is the commonest type of ASD and it is a defect in the development of the septum secundum in the interatrial septum.

It produces mild disease or may be asymptomatic, as often the defect is large enough (>2 cm) to cause near equalization of left and right atrial pressure with flow of blood from left to right through the ASD. Pulmonary blood flow is increased; the right ventricle becomes dilated and hypertrophied in response to the volume overload. This is usually well-tolerated and right ventricular failure is uncommon.

The main complications of ASD are:
- pulmonary hypertension;
- right heart failure;
- paradoxical embolism to the systemic circulation;

- infective endocarditis.

2 Ostium primum ASD. Ostium primum defects are rare, constituting about 5% of all cases of ASD. They are found as large defects in the lower portion of the interatrial septum. Because of their location, they often involve the mitral valve. Ostim primum defect is more common in Down's syndrome. Ostium primum ASD produces severe disease in childhood.

Ventricular septal defect (VSD; Fig. 15.47). VSD is the commonest congenital cardiac abnormality in children. Most defects occur in the membranous part of the interventricular septum just below the orifices of the aortic and pulmonary valves.

VSD may be classified according to size:

1 Small VSD (*maladie de Roger*). Small VSDs of <5 mm are common. They produce a low-volume shunt from the left to the right ventricle during systole. With a small defect, right ventricular pressure is only slightly increased but a loud systolic murmur is heard. Patients with small VSDs have few symptoms and the defect assumes less importance as the child grows and may eventually close spontaneously.

2 Large VSD. A large VSD will produce symptoms during early childhood. Initially, a large volume of blood is shunted from the left to the right ventricle during systole, producing volume overload, dilatation and hypertrophy of both ventricles. There is a pansystolic murmur. There is pulmonary hypertension. Thickening of the right ventricular wall and raised pulmonary pressure narrow the small pulmonary arteries, resulting in cyanosis (Eisenmenger's syndrome). Shunt reversal in VSD occurs some time after birth (**tardive cyanosis**) and may be associated with decrease or disappearance of the murmur.

The main complications of a large VSD are:
- pulmonary hypertension;
- right heart failure;
- cyanosis;
- paradoxical embolism to the systemic circulation;
- infective endocarditis.

Patent ductus arteriosus (PDA; Fig. 15.48). In fetal life, the ductus arteriosus is a normal structure that connects the pulmonary artery to the aorta. In fetal life, this permits right ventricular output to bypass the inactive fetal lungs. At birth when the lungs expand, pulmonary vascular resistance falls and flow across the ductus decreases. The ductus usually closes by muscle spasm. Permanent occlusion by fibrous tissue is usually complete by 8 weeks. In premature infants, anatomical closure may be delayed for several months. Promotion of closure may be induced by use of indomethacin.

1 Small PDA. A small PDA may lead to a small left-to-right shunt which is continuous through the cardiac cycle. This causes the typical '**machinery murmur**'. A small PDA will cause only mild elevation of pulmonary artery pressure and minimal symptoms. Infective endocarditis is a complication, even with a small PDA.

2 Large PDA. With a large PDA, the high aortic pressure is transmitted to the pulmonary artery, causing marked pulmonary hypertension and ultimately resulting in shunt reversal.

Tetralogy of Fallot. Tetralogy of Fallot is the commonest cyanotic congenital heart abnormality (Fig. 15.49(a)). It is characterized by:
- a large VSD;
- stenosis of the pulmonary outflow tract;
- dextroposition of the aorta which overrides the right ventricle;
- hypertrophy of the right ventricle.

Pulmonary stenosis raises the right ventricular pressure so that the shunt across the VSD is right-to-left. This results in mixing of venous and systemic arterial blood, causing severe cyanosis from birth. The prognosis is poor without surgery (Fig. 15.49(b)).

MYOCARDIAL DISEASE

Myocardial disease may be classified in the following way:
1 primary;
2 secondary;
3 idiopathic (cardiomyopathy);
4 myocarditis (features in primary, secondary and idiopathic myocardial disease).

Primary myocardial disease (excluding coronary artery disease, valvular heart disease, pulmonary and systemic hypertension) can be classified according to the 'pathological sieve' described in Chapter 1 (Table 15.25).

Primary myocardial disease (of known cause)

Definition
Primary myocardial disease excludes congenital heart

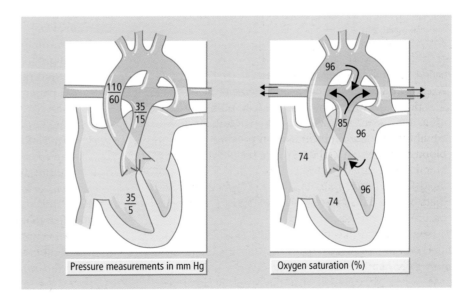

Fig. 15.48 Diagram of patent ductus arteriosus (PDA).

Pressure measurements in mm Hg

Oxygen saturation (%)

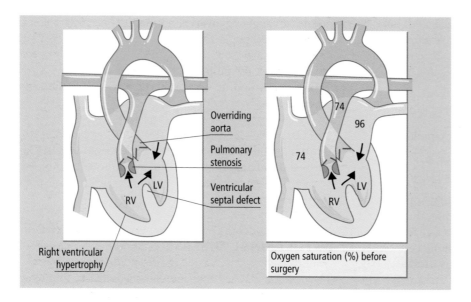

Fig. 15.49(a) Diagram of the components of tetralogy of Fallot.

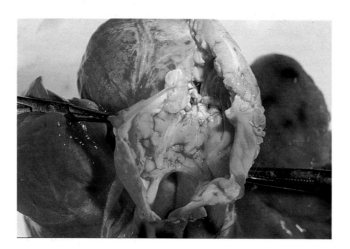

Fig. 15.49(b) Surgical repair of tetralogy of Fallot. Note the patch to enlarge the pulmonary outflow tract and to close the VSD. Note also the right ventricular hypertrophy.

disease (CHD), ischaemic heart disease (IHD), hypertensive heart disease, valvular heart disease or heart disease secondary to pulmonary disease (cor pulmonale). Primary myocardial disease may be of unknown cause (cardiomyopathy) or of known cause. Some of the more common diseases affecting the heart will be described.

Myocardial infections

The heart may be the site for a variety of infections. These infections are associated with myocarditis. Some of the most important infections will be given.

Bacterial

The myocardium may be infected with a variety of pyogenic bacteria, most commonly **staphylococci** and **streptococci**.

Myocardial disease in **diphtheria** is the result of exotoxin. The bacillus does not enter the blood stream but multiplies in the respiratory tract. Diphtheria toxin inhibits protein synthesis leading to myocyte degeneration.

The myocardium may be the site of *Mycobacterium tuberculosis* infection, although this is more commonly seen in the pericardium.

Protozoan

American **trypanosomiasis** (Chagas disease) is endemic in South America where it is a common cause of myocarditis. Acutely, the parasites cause necrosis of the myocytes; chronic disease is associated with the formation of parasite pseudocysts in the myocytes and a lymphocytic myocarditis. *Toxoplasma gondii* pseudocysts are seen in the myocytes in immunocompromised patients (see Chapter 8).

Parasitic

Trichinella spiralis infect the heart via the blood stream. The larvae cause necrosis and an eosinophilic inflammatory cell infiltrate.

Viral

Viruses are the most common cause of myocarditis in developed countries. **Coxsackie B** virus is the most common, but others include mumps, influenza, echo, polio, measles and influenza viruses. A variety of **rickettsial**

Table 15.25 Classification of myocardial disease.

CONGENITAL

ACQUIRED
*Infectious**
Bacterial (*Streptococcus* in rheumatic fever)
Protozoan (*Leishmania*, trypanosomes, malaria, *Toxoplasma*)
Parasitic (trichinosis, taeniasis)
Viral (Coxsackie B, echovirus 8, mumps, EBV, influenza, HIV)
Fungal

Neoplastic
Benign (atrial myxoma, rhabdomyoma)
Malignant
    Primary (angiosarcoma, rhabdomyosarcoma)
    Secondary (metastases)*

Vascular
Vasculitis

Inflammatory
Dressler's syndrome
Sarcoidosis*
Collagen vascular Rheumatoid*
    SLE*
    Sclerodema*
Hypersensitivity reactions

Traumatic
Surgery, radiation

*Endocrine**
Thyrotoxicosis, myxoedema, diabetes, mellitus, carcinoid,
phaeochromocytoma, acromegaly

Depositional
Amyloid,* haemochromatosis,* calcification, brown atrophy, fatty
degeneration

*Metabolic**
Potassium, magnesium, protein, vitamin B_6, uraemia, storage diseases

Nutritional

*Drugs/toxins**
Alcohol, cobalt, mercury, anthracyclines, busulphan, isoprenaline,
chloroquine, colchicine, adriamycin, vincristine

*Neuromuscular**
Duchenne muscular dystrophy, Friedreich's ataxia

EBV, Epstein–Barr virus; HIV, human immunodeficiency virus; SLE, systemic
lupus erythematosus.
* Myocardial diseases which develop in association with systemic disease and
may be secondary myocardial diseases.

diseases infect the heart, such as Q-fever, typhus and
Rocky mountain spotted fever. These infections give rise
to a lymphocytic myocarditis (see below).

Fungal

A variety of fungal infections infect the heart in the
immunocompromised patient and are increasingly seen
in association with the use of cardiac prostheses and in-
strumentation. The most important are *Nocardia*,
Aspergillus and *Mucor*.

Cardiac neoplasms

Primary tumours of the heart are rare.

Benign

Atrial myxoma (Fig. 15.50). Myxomas are the commonest
tumours of the heart. Up to 80% of cardiac myxomas arise
from the left atrium. They are commonly seen in adults.
They are pedunculated, well-circumscribed masses
measuring up to 5 cm and often have a recognizable stalk
attaching them to the atrial wall. They can be very friable
and are prone to fragment and embolize. Patients may
present with myoma emboli to the brain or limbs.

The histology is typical and consists of spindle cells
floating in a myxoid matrix (Figure 15.50(c)). This is
thought to be a true neoplasm arising from mesenchymal
cells of the subendocardium.

Clinical effects of atrial myxoma include:
- mitral stenosis or incompetence;
- cardiac murmur;
- fever;
- peripheral emboli.

Rhabdomyoma (Fig. 15.51). This tumour is composed of a
disorganized mass of cardiac muscle. It is very rare but
occurs in patients with tuberous sclerosis. It is probably a
hamartoma rather than a true neoplasm.

Mesothelioma. The commonest tumour of the pericardium
is mesothelioma. Histologically, the tumour consists of
bland spindle cells resembling fibrous tissue similar to
that described in the pleura (Chapter 17).

Malignant

The heart and pericardium are more commonly involved
by direct spread or metastasis of carcinoma from the lung
and breast, other carcinomas or by lymphomas from the
mediastinum or by metastatic malignant melanoma. In
patients with carcinomatosis, involvement of the heart
and pericardium (Fig. 15.52) can be found in up to 10% of
patients.

Primary malignant tumours of the heart include
angiosarcoma and rhabdomyosarcoma. These tumours
are very rare.

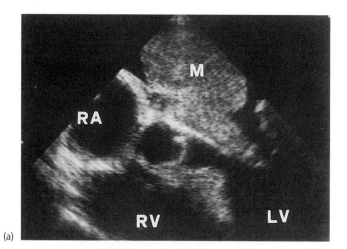

(a)

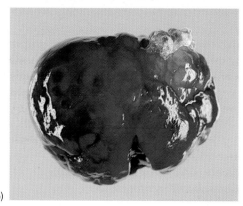

(b)

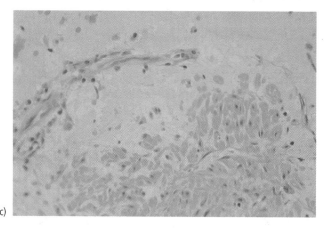

(c)

Fig. 15.50 (a) Echocardiogram (long axis view) of a left atrial myxoma. RA, right atrium; RV, right ventricle; LV, left ventricle; M, myxoma. (b) The surgically excised left atrial myxoma, note the stalk. (c) Histology of atrial myxoma including a stalk composed of atrial endocardium (bottom). (H&E.)

Ischaemic heart disease

Definition

'Cardiac disability, acute and chronic, arising from the

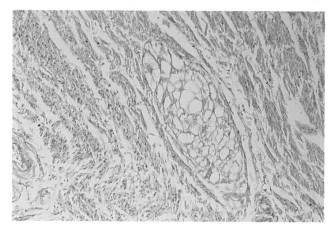

Fig. 15.51 Histology of a cardiac rhabdomyoma shows vacuolated primitive cells. (Trichome stain).

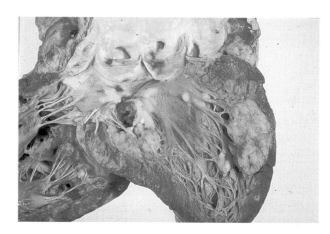

Fig. 15.52 Metastatic carcinoma involving the heart. This patient died from disseminated carcinoma of the breast.

reduction or arrest of blood supply to the myocardium in association with disease processes in the coronary arterial system' (World Health Organization, 1957).

IHD is a very important cause of death in the UK and USA: 40% of deaths are due to heart disease compared to 20% for malignancy.

Incidence

IHD has been falling gradually throughout the 1970s in the USA and Japan and more recently in western Europe.

Causes

Ninety per cent of the cases of IHD are due to **atherosclerosis** (Fig. 15.53).

Early atherosclerotic plaques and plaques with intact fibrous caps (they have a smooth outline on angiography and are referred to as **type I plaques**) do not tend to undergo thrombosis and by themselves rarely completely occlude the vessel lumen. In patients without coronary

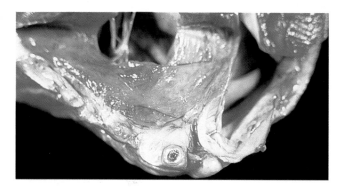

Fig. 15.53(a) Coronary artery atheroma and thrombosis seen in the lower field (brown).

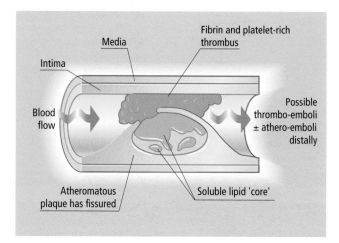

Fig. 15.53(b) Diagram showing the progression of coronary artery thrombosis.

thrombosis, it is a combination of increased demand by the myocardium (e.g. when a patient runs for a bus) and reduction in blood supply through a stenosed and poorly compliant vessel that causes lack of oxygenation of the heart muscle, and thus angina (ischaemic pain) or a myocardial infarction (heart attack).

Seventy-five per cent of cases of coronary thrombosis are initiated by **plaque rupture**; lipid-rich, eccentric plaques are more prone to rupture; patients with risk factors such as hypertension are also more prone to plaque rupture. These 'dangerous' lesions can be recognized angiographically by their ragged outline (**type II plaques**).

There are several consequences of coronary thrombosis which can be recognized histologically. If the patient survives and these thrombi do not lyse, then they heal. Occlusive thrombi tend to progress down the vessel distally. Angiographic studies have shown that, from the time a plaque fissures, active thrombosis occurs for a period of around 3 weeks, after which time the lesion either progresses to form a persistent occlusion with the risk of myocardial infarction or it organizes.

Therapeutic thrombolysis is more successful when there is little deep injury to the plaque. Lysis of the most recent thrombus, that which occludes the lumen, is known to occur first.

The remaining 10% of non-atheromatous causes of IHD include the following (Table 15.26).

Table 15.26 Non-atherosclerotic causes of ischaemic heart disease.

Stenosis of the coronary ostia
Arteritis
Embolism
Thrombotic disease
Neoplasms
Trauma
Aneurysms
Congenital anomalies

IHD may also result from reduced coronary artery perfusion. The commonest cause of this is shock, especially as a result of haemorrhage. Severe aortic valve stenosis or incompetence may also impair coronary blood flow. Severe anaemia may also produce symptoms of IHD.

As the preceding account of atherosclerosis has shown, atherosclerosis causes IHD by several local mechanisms. The most important ones include:
- luminal narrowing;
- thrombosis;
- haemorrhage into the plaque;
- plaque rupture;
- calcification (preventing vasodilatation).

Effects (Table 15.27)

Acute myocardial infarction (MI). Almost all infarcts occur in the **left ventricle**. The anterior descending branch of the left coronary artery is the most often affected (Fig. 15.53). The right coronary artery is involved in 25% of cases.

Macroscopically MI can be classified into three types:
- full-thickness;
- massive, not quite full-thickness;
- subendocardial.

1 Gross appearances of MI (Fig. 15.54). Very little is seen in the first 12 hours, then there is a paler, drier myocardium at the site of the infarct (15–24 hours); on days 4 to 8 increasing yellow appearance as neutrophils enter; on days 8–10 there is a purple periphery (granulation

Table 15.27 Effects of ischaemic heart disease.

Acute myocardial infarction
Angina pectoris
Sudden death
Chronic cardiac failure

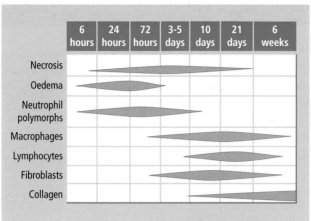

	6 hours	24 hours	72 hours	3-5 days	10 days	21 days	6 weeks
Necrosis							
Oedema							
Neutrophil polymorphs							
Macrophages							
Lymphocytes							
Fibroblasts							
Collagen							

(a)

Fig. 15.54 (a) Dating a myocardial infarct (MI). (b) The macroscopic features of an acute MI in the lateral wall of the left ventricle. (c) The microscopic features of an actue MI. (d) The macroscopic featues of an organizing MI. (e) The microscopic features of an organizing MI. (f) The macroscopic features of a healed MI, note the white fibrosis. (g) The microscopic features of a healed MI. (H&E.)

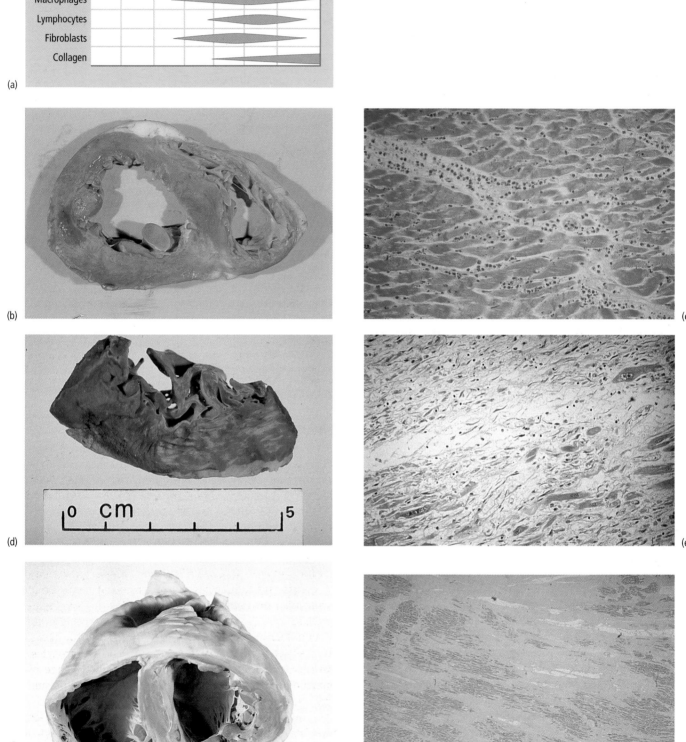

(b)

(c)

(d)

(e)

(f)

(g)

tissue) and thinning of ventricular wall and by 2–3 months a white scar forms.

2 Microscopic appearances of MI (Fig. 15.54). There is very little to see histologically immediately after an infarct. By 6–24 hours there is loss of muscle striations, eosinophilia of fibres, karyolysis, karyorrhexis and pyknosis, connective tissue necrosis and neutrophil infiltrate; at 2–4 days increasing numbers of neutrophils are seen; at 4–5 days there is phagocytosis by macrophages, granulation tissue formation occurs; by the second week, eosinophils, macrophages, fibroblasts and new collagen are found; by the third week more granulation tissue and collagen is laid down and by week 4–6 there is scar tissue and decreased vascularity (Table 15.28).

Angina pectoris.
- **Definition.** 'A clinical syndrome caused by inadequate oxygenation of the heart, characteristically precipitated by exertion or relieved by rest'.
- **Causes.** The main cause by far is **atherosclerosis**. Others include syphilitic aortitis; aortic stenosis; severe anaemia; hypertrophic cardiomyopathy; thyrotoxicosis; and coronary artery spasm.

Cardiac sudden death.
- **Causes.** Most commonly this is due to IHD where the mode of death is probably **arrhythmia**. Examination of the heart may reveal no macroscopic myocardial abnormality but the coronary arteries may show an acute thrombosis. Histology of the myopcardium may show contraction band ischaemic change (Fig. 15.59). However, there are also non-IHD causes (Table 15.29).

Chronic cardiac failure. When two- or three-vessel disease is present without acute occlusion, then long-standing ischaemia may cause a diffuse myocardial fibrosis with decreased muscular efficiency and consequently gradual

Table 15.28 Complications of myocardial infarction.

Death – 25% in the first 24 hours
Arrhythmias
Cardiogenic shock
External cardiac rupture (Fig. 15.55)
Rupture of the interventricular septum
Mitral incompetence, usually due to papillary muscle rupture (Fig. 15.56)
Mural thrombosis
Ventricular aneurysm (Fig. 15.57)
Pericarditis (Fig. 15.58)
Dressler's syndrome
Deep venous thrombosis
Cardiac neurosis
Angina/further infarction

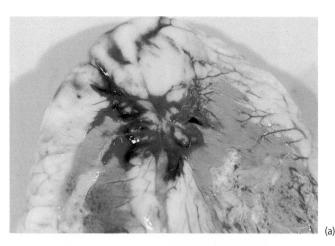

(a)

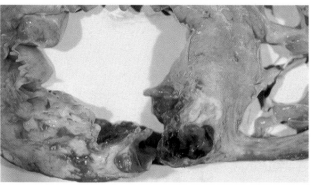

(b)

Fig. 15.55 Acute rupture of the left ventricle. (a) Shows the surface of the ruptured apex of the heart. (b) Note the yellow–red appearance at the site of rupture of the ventricle.

failure of both left and right ventricles. Back-pressure effects of right ventricular failure may be seen in the liver as a 'nutmeg' pattern and clinically as dependent oedema. The lungs will show the effects of chronic oedema and haemorrhage from congested alveolar capillaries in the form of 'heart failure cells' (haemosiderin-laden macrophages; Fig. 15.60).

Biochemical markers of myocardial ischaemia and infarction

Cardiac enzymes (Fig. 15.61). The changes in activity of certain plasma enzymes reflect recent myocardial ischaemia or infarction, although most are non-cardiospecific (Table 15.30).

1 Aspartate transaminase (AST). This is found in heart, liver, skeletal muscle, pancreas, kidney and erythrocytes. An increase in plasma activity results from leakage of enzyme from cells as a result of disruption of plasma membranes of damaged tissue.

In **myocardial** disease, plasma activity increases after MI and also in myocarditis. After an MI, AST begins to rise 6–12 hours postinfarct, reaches a peak by 24–36

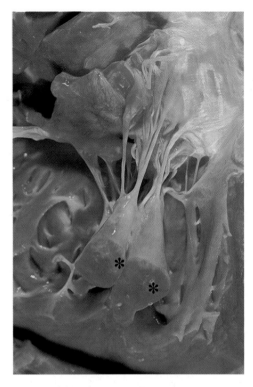

Fig. 15.56 Acute rupture of the infarcted papillary muscles (✱) results in acute mitral valve incompetence and death.

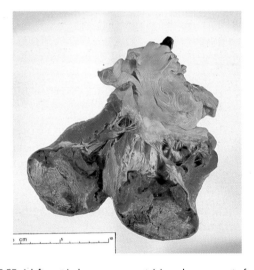

Fig. 15.57 A left ventricular aneurysm containing a large amount of thrombus.

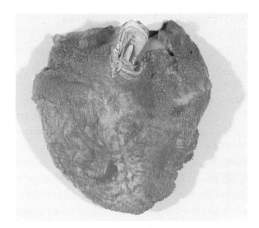

Fig. 15.58 Acute 'fibrinous' ('bread and butter') pericarditis 2 weeks following a myocardial infarction.

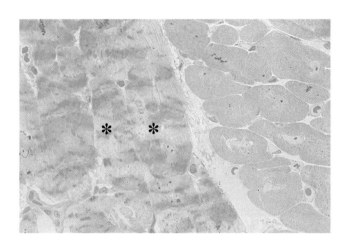

Fig. 15.59 Cardiac biopsy. This patient died from an acute arrythmia. The only visible change is contraction band necrosis (✱).

hours and then returns to normal after 3–5 days (if no complications).

Peak levels of AST reach 2–10 times the upper reference limit. The peak may reflect extent of infarct but not necessarily the prognosis. Plasma AST is also raised in liver disease (including that secondary to congestive cardiac failure post-MI; Table 15.31).

2 **Lactate dehydrogenase (LDH).** LDH is a widespread cytosolic enzyme that is found in greatest concentrations in heart, skeletal muscle, liver, kidney and erythrocytes. An increase in plasma activity results from leakage of enzyme from cells as a result of disruption of plasma membranes of damaged tissue.

In **myocardial** disease, plasma activities are raised after MI and in myocarditis (Table 15.32). Post-MI, LDH begins to rise 12–24 hours postinfarct and reaches a peak after 48–72 hours, returning to normal after 8–10 days (if no complications). The peak ranges from 2 to 10 times the upper reference limits.

3 **Creatine kinase (CK).** The major sources are muscle and brain. None is found in liver. Two subunits exist, designated M and B.
  • MM – skeletal and cardiac muscle;
  • MB – cardiac muscle (15–45% of total CK); skeletal muscle (trace only);

Table 15.29 Causes of sudden death.

Cardiac
Ischaemic heart disease
Myocarditis
Hypertrophic cardiomyopathy
Mitral valve prolapse
Conduction abnormalities (congenital, inflammatory, degenerative, neoplastic)
Arrhythmogenic right ventricular dysplasia
Dilated cardiomyopathy
Tetralogy of Fallot and other congenital heart diseases
Anomalous coronary artery origin

Vascular
Ruptured abdominal aortic aneurysm
   Atherosclerotic
   Dissecting

Neurological
Epilepsy
Cerebral haemorrhage

Pulmonary
Pulmonary embolus
Asthma

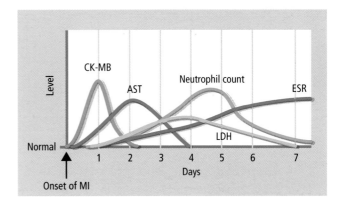

Fig. 15.61 Diagram of cardiac enzyme changes post myocardial infarction.

Table 15.30 Cardiac enzymes.

Non-cardiospecific	
Aspartate transaminase	AST
Lactate dehydrogenase	LDH
Creatine kinase	CK
Cardiospecific	
Creatine kinase-MB	CK-MB (or CK-2)
(Lactate dehydrogenase isoenzyme 1	LDH-1)
(α-Hydroxybutyrate dehydrogenase	HBDH)

Table 15.31 Non-cardiac causes of raised aspartate transaminase (AST).

Plasma AST is raised in the following *skeletal muscle* diseases:
• trauma
• muscular dystrophies
• dermatomyositis
• rhabdomyolysis

and in the following *miscellaneous* diseases:
• haemolysis
• renal infarction
• acute pancreatitis
• postsurgery and intramuscular injections
• hypothyroidism

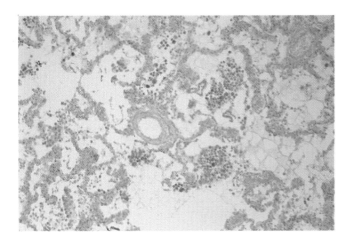

Fig. 15.60 Lung histology. Note the oedema and brown haemosiderin-containing macrophages ('heart failure cells').

• BB – brain.

Total CK (TCK) should be routinely available whilst. CK-MB (CK-2) is only of value in special circumstances. In myocardial disease, plasma levels rise following MI and in myocarditis (Table 15.33). Post-MI, TCK begins to rise 3–6 hours postinfarct and reaches a peak after 18–24 hours. It returns to normal by the third day (if there are no complications). The peak can be 2–10 times the upper reference limit.

4 CK-MB. Normal plasma activity is <6% of TCK and the half-life is 12 hours. Post-MI activity can reach 12–15% of TCK. The peak level correlates well with extent of myocardial damage.

CK-MB is most useful in distinguishing between skeletal and cardiac muscle damage when there is reasonable cause for both to be present, e.g. postintramuscular injections (morphine), postsurgery or mild muscle trauma (Tables 15.34–15.36). However, there is no point in measuring CK-MB activity if TCK activity is low/normal or very high (i.e. >5000 IU/l).

Table 15.32 Non-cardiac causes of raised lactate dehydrogenase (LDH).

Plasma LDH also raised in:
- liver disease
- skeletal muscle diseases
- haemolysis *in vitro* and *in vivo*
- leukaemia
- pernicious anaemia
- myeloproliferative disorders
- malignancy (all types)
- renal infarction
- pulmonary embolus
- congestive cardiac failure
- hypothyroidism

LDH-1 can be separated electrophoretically from total LDH to give cardiospecificity. This is seldom done in practice.

Table 15.33 Non-cardiac causes of raised creatine kinase (CK).

CK is raised in other diseases:
Skeletal muscle disorders
　Muscular dystrophies (high early in disease)
　Rhabdomyolysis
　Dermatomyositis
Hypothyroidism
CVA (CK-BB isoenzyme from brain)
Hyperthermia
Hypothermia
Intramuscular injections (very variable effect)

CVA, Cerebrovascular accident.

Table 15.34 Indications and uses of cardiac enzymes.

To assist in or confirm diagnosis of myocardial infarction – particularly useful if:
　Conflicting or absent clinical signs, e.g. in elderly
　Equivocal or absent ECG changes but clinical suspicion
　Conduction defects, e.g. bundle branch block
　In general practice (especially if no ECG available)
　Retrospective diagnosis
Monitoring progress and response to therapy
Assist in the prognosis if site of infarct is known

ECG, Electrocardiogram.

Myocarditis

Definition

The diagnosis of myocarditis can only be made if there is **myocyte necrosis** or **degeneration** or both, associated with an **inflammatory infiltrate** adjacent to the degenerating or necrotic myocytes (Dallas Criteria, (Aretz 1987); Table 15.37).

Table 15.35 Problems in the use of cardiac enzymes.

Need to have clear understanding of the time course of expected enzyme changes
Need to take samples at appropriate intervals with respect to the onset of symptoms
Sequential samples give the most useful information, especially in the case of creatine kinase
Need to be aware of the lack of cardiospecificity and therefore interference in interpretation
Cardiac enzymes are usually of *no value* in deciding whether antifibrinolytic agents are to be used
Different labs will offer different cardiac enzyme profiles

Table 15.36 Other biochemical markers of myocardial infarction.

- Myoglobin
- C-reactive protein (CRP)
- Serum amyloid A (SAA) protein

All have similar time responses to CK-MB following an uncomplicated infarct
All are relatively non-cardiospecific
Myoglobin and SAA protein are not easily measured quantitatively

Potential new marker – troponin T
Advantages
　Highly cardiospecific
　High sensitivity
　Early and sustained rise post-myocardial infarct
　Prognostic value
Disadvantages
　May be too sensitive (e.g. rises in unstable angina)
　No quick/easy/cheap assay available

CK-MB, Creatine kinase-MB.

Table 15.37 Causes of various forms of myocarditis.

Lymphocytic (Fig. 15.62)
Idiopathic, viral, hypersensitivity, polymyositis, sarcoidosis
Lyme disease, lymphoma, Kawasaki disease, drug toxicity

Neutrophilic
Idiopathic, infection, infarction, drug toxicity

Eosinophilic
Idiopathic, hypereosinophilic syndrome, restrictive cardiomyopathy, asthma, parasitic infestations, drug hypersensitivity

Giant cell (granulomatous; Figs 15.63 and 15.64)
Idiopathic, sarcoidosis, infection, rheumatoid, rheumatic, drug hypersensitivity

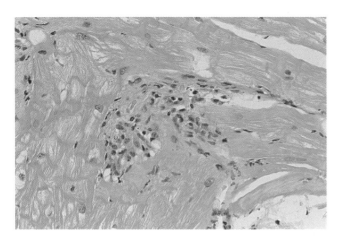

Fig. 15.62 Cardiac biopsy. Lymphocytic myocarditis. (H&E.)

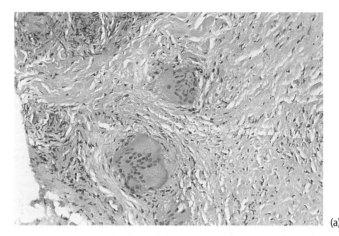

(a)

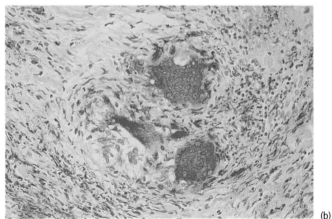

(b)

Fig. 15.63 Cardiac biopsy. (a) Idiopathic giant cell myocarditis. (H&E.) (b) Immunohistochemistry using a macrophage marker, CD68, shows that the giant cells are not of myocyte origin but of macrophage origin (red).

Vasculitis and the heart

Vasculitis can affect the coronary arteries and the smaller intramyocardial arteries, giving rise to IHD. The most important vasculitides affecting the heart include polyarteritus nodosa (PAN) and acute hypersensitivity vasculitis.

Inflammatory cardiac disease

Dressler's syndrome

This is thought to be an autoimmune inflammatory process directed against myocyte antigens. It occurs post MI, resulting in pain and fever.

Sarcoidosis

Sarcoidosis may produce extensive cardiac involvement as part of systemic sarcoidosis or as a disease process isolated to the heart. The cardiac conducting system may be involved, giving rise to arrhythmia as a presenting complaint. The lesions contain the typical non-caseating, well-circumscribed granulomas (Fig. 15.64).

Collagen vascular disease

Collagen vascular diseases have the following features in common:
- carditis;
- arthritis;
- vasculitis.
  They include:
- rheumatic fever;
- rheumatoid arthritis;
- SLE;

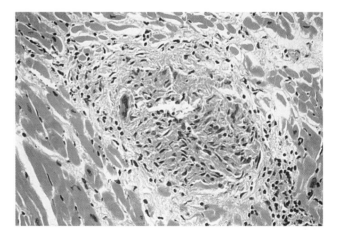

Fig. 15.64 Cardiac biopsy. Sarcoid granuloma.

- systemic sclerosis (scleroderma).
  The cardiac features include myocyte necrosis, lymphocytic infiltrates and fibrosis. Rheumatic fever also features Aschoff bodies.

Radiation and the heart

The myocardium is relatively resistant to ionizing radiation but endothelial cells are very sensitive. Small-vessel stenosis results in ischaemia to the myocardium which leads to cardiac fibrosis.

Endocrine disease and the heart

In patients with **acromegaly**, the heart undergoes massive hypertrophy with ultimate cardiac failure. In **thyrotoxicosis**, patients present with arrhythmia, particularly atrial fibrillation. The increase in metabolic rate may lead to high-output cardiac failure.

In **myxoedema**, there is bradycardia, ventricular dilatation and pericardial effusion.

Degenerative/depositional disease and the heart

Fatty change

The accumulation of fat in myocytes is associated with nutritional deficiency, ischaemia, carbon monoxide poisoning, septicaemia and alcohol intoxication. In childhood, the association of an acute encephalopathy and fatty degeneration of the viscera, including the heart, is seen in Reye's syndrome.

Storage diseases

The heart can be involved in type II (Pompe's) glycogen storage disease (Fig. 15.65), oxalosis, Fabry's disease, Whipple's disease (intestinal lipodystrophy), calcinosis and 'foamy transformation of infancy'.

Amyloid (Fig. 15.66)

Amyloid deposits may be seen in the heart in secondary systemic amyloidosis (AL), senile cardiac amyloid (AS) or as familial variants (AF, AA). Patients present with heart failure and a restrictive cardiac picture.

Haemochromatosis (Fig. 15.67)

Cardiac haemochromatosis may present with heart failure and a dilated cardiac picture. The iron is deposited in myocytes in a characteristic polar perinuclear distribution with deposits being more concentrated subepicardially than subpericardially.

Calcification

Cardiac calcification may be metastatic (as in hyperparathyroidism) or dystrophic (postinflammatory or degenerative). If deposits affect the vessel walls, they can inhibit

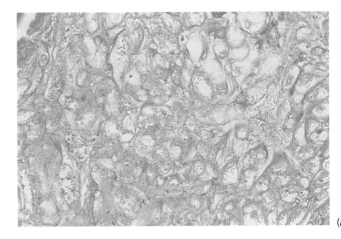

(a)

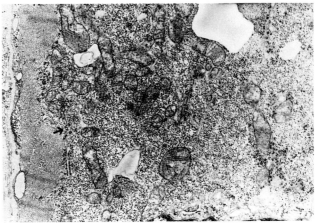

(b)

Fig. 15.65 Cardiac biopsy. Glycogen storage disease in a newborn baby girl. (a) Note the PAS-positive granules. (b) Transmission electronmicroscopy. Note the glycogen particles in membrane-bound structures. (×10 500).

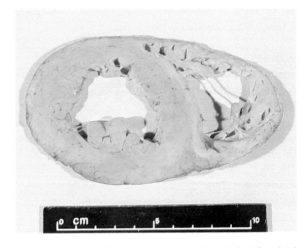

Fig. 15.66 Cardiac amyloid. A transverse section through the left and right ventricles shows the waxy pallor of the myocardium. This patient presented with a restrictive cardiac function.

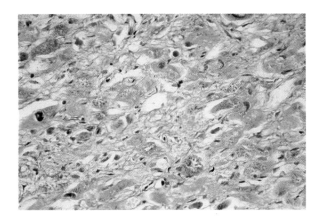

Fig. 15.67 Cardiac biopsy. Haemochromatosis. Note the brown colour in this H&E section.

vasodilatation and thus lead to ischaemia. If deposits occur in the conducting tissue, they may give rise to arrhythmia.

Drugs and toxins and the heart

Many drugs injure the heart. The more common ones include those shown in Table 15.38.

Table 15.38 Drugs and the heart.

Alcohol
Tricyclic antidepressants
Phenytoin
Cyclophosphamide
Adriamycin (doxorubicin)
Hydralazine
Procainamide

Cardiomyopathies (primary cardiac disease of unknown cause)

Definition

'Primary myocardial diseases of undetermined cause' (World Health Organization, 1980). Three main cardiomyopathies are recognized:
- **dilated (congestive)**;
- **hypertrophic**;
- **restrictive**.

But under this strict definition, one may also add:
- peripartum cardiomyopathy;
- arrhythmogenic right ventricular dysplasia;
- giant cell myocarditis;

- histiocytoid cardiomyopathy;
- keshan cardiomyopathy.

The student should be aware that the term cardiomyopathy is used clinically to refer to any myocardial diseases, so do not be surprised to hear the terms ischaemic cardiomyopathy or alcoholic cardiomyopathy.

Dilated cardiomyopathy (Fig. 15.68)

Characterized by dilatation and impaired contractile function of the left ventricle (LV) and/or right ventricle (RV), this disease presents at any age. The incidence is 6/100 000 and the prevalence is 38/100 000. Dilated cardiomyopathy may be familial in a certain percentage of cases.

Macroscopically there is an **enlarged**, heavy heart, often with **dilatation** of all four chambers. Unless the history is short, there is compensatory myocardial wall thickening. Epicardial coronary arteries are normal. LV and RV mural thrombi are often seen.

Histology shows non-specific **myocyte hypertrophy** with **interstitial fibrosis**. There may be a chronic inflam-

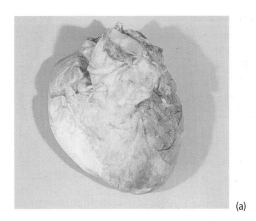

(a)

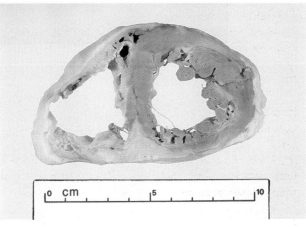

(b)

Fig. 15.68 Dilated cardiomyopathy. (a) Note the dilated, globular heart. (b) This section through the left and right ventricles demonstrates the dilatation and the myocardial fibrosis.

matory cell infiltrate. Dilated cardiomyopathy presents with heart failure, pulmonary or systemic thromboemboli or arrhythmias.

The aetiology is unknown but familial forms occur and there is an association with viral myocarditis which may be the precursor lesion. Raised antibodies to Coxsackie B and to cardiac autoantigens have been described in patients with dilated cardiomyopathy. An association with excessive alcohol intake has also been proposed.

In order to make a diagnosis of dilated cardiomyopathy, other causes of cardiac dilatation and failure should be excluded (Table 15.39).

Table 15.39 Differential diagnoses of dilated cardiomyopathy.

| Haemochromatosis |
| Ischaemic heart disease |
| Myocarditis |
| Alcoholic heart disease |

Hypertrophic cardiomyopathy (Fig. 15.69)

This disease is characterized by a hypertrophied and non-dilated LV or RV in the absence of cardiac or systemic disease. Stroke volume is reduced, but systolic ejection fraction is normal.

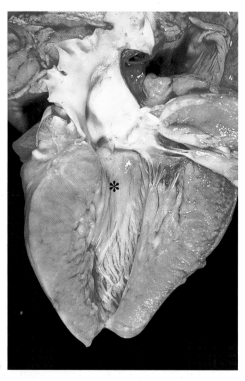

(a)

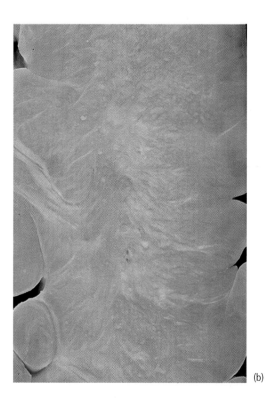

(b)

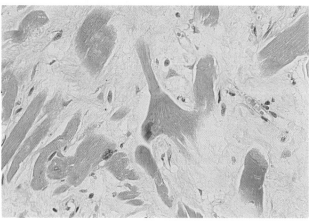

(c)

Fig. 15.69 (a) Hypertrophic cardiomyopathy. This long axis view demostrates the asymmetric hypertrophy of the interventricular septum and the sub-aortic valve fibrous ridge (✶). (b) This short axis section shows the grossly thickened septum with the whirls of fibrosis. (c) Histology shows the enlarged myocytes with bizarre nuclei, interstitial fibrosis and myocyte 'disarray'. (H&E.)

Familial, **autosomal dominant** forms exist (with incomplete penetrance) that involve abnormalities in genes encoding **β heavy chain myosin** (chromosome 14), **troponin T** (chromosome 1) and **α-tropomyosin** (chromosome 15).

Hypertrophic cardiomyopathy does not manifest itself until late adolescence but has an incidence in this age group of approximately 3/100 000 (incidence in the 40–50-year group of 5/1000). Grossly, the enlarged heart shows symmetric or asymmetric thickening of the septum. In the latter there may be obstruction to LV outflow and **subaortic endocardial thickening** due to abrasion from the anterior mitral valve leaflet on the thickened septum. Thrombi in cardiac chambers are not common. Myocyte hypertrophy, fibrosis and **myocyte disarray** are seen histologically and intramyocardial vessels show fibromuscular thickening.

Sudden death occurs due to arrhythmias. Systemic hypertension and prolonged physical activity ('athletic heart syndrome') are important causes to exclude. In order to make a diagnosis of hypertrophic cardiomyopathy, other causes of cardiac hypertrophy should be excluded (Table 15.40).

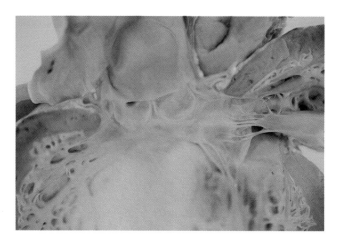

Fig. 15.70 Restrictive cardiomyopathy. Note the fibrosis of the endocardium involving the valves.

Table 15.40 Differential diagnoses of hypertrophic cardiomyopathy.

Amyloidosis
Hypertensive heart disease
'Athletic heart syndrome'
Obesity
Age-related angulation of the ventricular septum
Aortic stenosis
Glycogen storage disease

Restrictive cardiomyopathy (Fig. 15.70)

Characterized by loss of ventricular distensibility due to endocardial fibrosis, restrictive cardiomyopathy has the following two forms.

1 Restrictive cardiomyopathy associated with peripheral eosinophilia. This includes the hypereosinophilic syndrome, eosinophilic myocarditis and endomyocardial fibrosis. Associated diseases will include asthma, chronic parasitic infestation and Hodgkin's lymphoma. Restrictive features are due to thrombosis and fibrosis of the ventricular inflow tracts. Mural thrombus lines the ventricles and may obliterate much of the ventricular cavities with atrial dilatation. In the active form, fresh mural thrombus is seen, which contains many eosinophils. In the inactive form of the disease, there is dense endocardial fibrosis.

2 Non-eosinophilic restrictive cardiomyopathy. Myocardial fibrosis alone results in decreased ventricular compliance. The atria are dilated but mural thrombus is not a feature. There is patchy or diffuse myocardial fibrosis. Death is due to heart failure and arrhythmias.

In order to make a diagnosis of restrictive cardiomyopathy, other causes of restrictive function should be excluded (Table 15.41).

Postpartum cardiomyopathy

This presents as dilated cardiomyopathy in women within 3 months of childbirth. Approximately 40% will die. The aetiology is unknown.

Arrhythmogenic right ventricular dysplasia

This is an idiopathic, autosomal dominant condition characterized by replacement of myocytes of the RV (and LV) by fat and fibrous tissue. Patients present with ventricular arrhythmias or sudden death.

Giant cell myocarditis

This is a rare condition of young men presenting with syncope or sudden death and characterized by cardiac enlargement. It is sometimes referred to clinically as **Fiedler's myocarditis**. Histology of the myocardium features chronic inflammatory cells and numerous giant cells. To be classified as a cardiomyopathy, one must

Table 15.41 Differential diagnoses of restrictive cardiomyopathy.

Amyloid
Constrictive pericarditis
Haemochromatosis
Pseudoxanthoma elasticum
Hypertrophic cardiomyopathy

exclude all known causes of giant cell granuloma formation in the heart (Fig. 15.63).

Histiocytoid cardiomyopathy

This rare disease occurs in female children and is rapidly fatal in the first 2 years of life. It is characterized by severe ventricular and supraventricular arrhythmias. Both LV and RV are grossly hypertrophied and dilated. Histology features pale staining myocytes which resemble Purkinje cells.

Keshan cardiomyopathy

An endemic form of dilated cardiomyopathy seen in China, this disease is characterized by ventricular hypertrophy and dilatation with myocyte necrosis. It is possibly related to nutritional deficiencies.

Systemic arterial hypertension

Definitions

Essential or **benign hypertension** represents 80–95% of cases. It is defined as blood pressure >160/95 mmHg and is considered to represent an exaggeration of the tendency of the blood pressure to rise with age. No primary cause is found.

Secondary hypertension represents 5% of cases and here, an underlying cause is found.

Malignant hypertension occurs when the diastolic pressure >120 mmHg. The age range is 25–55 years.

Mean arterial pressure
= cardiac output × peripheral resistance

The general level of the systemic arterial blood pressure is maintained by three mechanisms:
- catecholamine production;
- renin–angiotensin system;
- aldosterone production.

This is regulated by the baroreceptor mechanism and the autonomic nervous system (Table 15.42).

Causes of essential hypertension

Even after thorough investigation, a specific cause for a raised arterial pressure is found only in about 5% of cases. A small proportion of hypertensives develop a sudden rise in blood pressure from benign to accelerated or malignant hypertension. The majority with malignant hypertension die within 6–12 months if untreated. About 2–3% are referred to hospital; the rest are managed in general practice.

Family history and genetic background are involved (Table 15.43). The best correlation is between siblings (better than between parents and children).

Table 15.42 What is hypertension?

There is no such thing as normal blood pressure
Variability in individual blood pressure can be due to: • Method of measurement   • Age   • Sex   • Personal variation
There is a common arbitrary upper limit for normal blood pressure, which is 140/90 mmHg
One needs to measure blood pressure on at least three occasions
If only one reading is taken, a third of the UK population will have diastolic pressure >90 mmHg
If six readings are taken, the frequency of hypertension in the population falls
General advice seems to be to take three readings over 3–4 weeks unless clinical signs of hypertension are evident
Should diastolic or systolic blood pressure reflect hypertension? Traditionally it is the diastolic, but the source studies suggest that systolic is a better predictor

Table 15.43 The following factors may also be involved in systemic hypertension.

High salt (NaCl) intake: Strong connection between average salt intake of different populations and incidence of high BP and cardiovascular complications. Many complicating factors, including other dietary factors, exist and there is no evidence from within-population studies. There is possibly a genetically determined defect in cell membrane transport which raises BP, or a combination of genetic defect and increased salt intake increasing intracellular sodium	
Extreme dietary salt restriction to <10 mmol/day will reduce arterial BP	
High dietary K^+	
High dietary Mg^{2+}	
High dietary Ca^{2+}	
There is good evidence that excessive alcohol intake raises BP	
Vegan diets	
Age	
Males	Show a steady rise in BP with age
Female	BP rises after menopause
Temperature	BP rises in winter
Coffee	
Smoking	Malignant hypertension more common in smokers than non-smokers
Sympathetic nervous system	Related to secretion of catecholamines
Physical fitness	BP is lowered acutely by exercise

BP, Blood pressure.

Causes of secondary hypertension

If a cause can be found and treated, this will spare the patient a lifetime of hypertension clinics and antihypertensive drugs (Tables 15.44–15.48).

Table 15.44 Causes of secondary hypertension.

RENAL
Parenchymal ischaemia
Heart failure
Aortic/renal artery atherosclerosis

Chronic renal failure
Chronic pyelonephritis
Acute or chronic glomerulonephritis
Diabetic nephropathy
Polyarteritis nodosa
SLE
Polycystic disease
Amyloidosis
Tumours
Hydronephrosis

CARDIOVASCULAR
Coarctation of aorta – hypertension in upper half of body

Renal artery stenosis
Fibromuscular dysplasia
Dissecting aneurysm
Pressure from tumours/ligatures

High cardiac output states

HORMONAL
Oral contraceptives

Cushing's syndrome
Primary
   Cortical adenoma/hyperplasia
   Adrenal carcinoma

Secondary
   Basophil adenoma of the pituitary
   Corticosteroid therapy
   ACTH therapy
   Oat cell carcinoma of the bronchus
   Islet cell tumour of the pancreas
   Medullary carcinoma of the thyroid

Primary aldosteronism (Conn's)
Cortical adenoma/hyperplasia
Adrenogenital syndrome due to deficiency of 11-β-hydroxylase

Phaeochromocytoma – a tumour of chromaffin cells in the adrenal medulla (90%) or in the sympathetic ganglia which secretes large quantities of adrenaline/noradrenaline (excess catecholamines due to treatment with indirect sympathomimetics (amphetamine, tyramine) in combination with monoamine oxidase inhibitors)

Acromegaly due to acidophil adenoma of the pituitary

Renin-producing tumours of the kidney

NEUROLOGICAL
Raised intracranial pressure
Trauma
Tumour
Abscess
Haemorrhage

Hypothalamus and brainstem lesions

Anxiety

TOXAEMIA OF PREGNANCY

SLE, Systemic lupus erythematosus; ACTH, adrenocorticotrophic hormone.

Biochemical investigation of secondary hypertension

Renal vascular disease (renal artery stenosis). It is important to investigate the renin–angiotensin system in renal vascular disease or renal artery stenosis, in particular the peripheral blood plasma renin activity. However, only about 50% of patients with surgically treatable lesions have a raised renin.

Measurement of **renal vein renin** is more sensitive but many false-negatives and positives occur. Look for ratio of greater than 1.6:1 between stenosed and intact sides; alternatively, measuring fractional renin secretion from each kidney can be helpful (i.e. (RV – IVC)/IVC). *n* value = 0.24).

In renal artery stenosis, value may be increased on the affected side with suppression to zero on the normal side.

Renin-secreting tumours. Benign haemangiopericytomas in the kidney may contain cells similar to those of juxtaglomerular apparatus; they produce renin and also angiotensin II and aldosterone, causing hypokalaemic alkalosis and hypertension. In this case, hypertension is usually very severe, affecting young people. This is very rare but there is a good response to surgery.

Hypersecretion of renin may also be seen in acute glomerulosclerosis, renal carcinoma or Wilms tumour. Extrarenal tumours of the lung, pancreas and liver may also produce renin.

Pulmonary vascular disease and the heart

Normal pulmonary vasculature (Fig. 15.71)

The normal pulmonary arterial tree is adapted to func-

Table 15.45 Effects of essential hypertension.

Blood vessels	
Arterioles	Hyalinization
Small/medium- sized arteries	Medial hypertrophy Intimal proliferation Microaneurysms
Large arteries	Increase in atheroclerosis
Heart	
Myocardium	Left ventricular hypertrophy Focal myocardial fibrosis
Coronary arteries	Increase in atherosclerosis
Kidneys	
Macroscopically (hypertensive nephrosclerosis)	Small and granular with thinned cortex
Vessels	Intimal fibrosis and reduplication of internal elastic lamina Medial hypertrophy and hyalinization
Glomeruli	Increase in mesangium with hyalinization and thickening of basement membrane Tubules—atrophy and casts Interstitium—fibrosis and chronic inflammation
Brain	
Arteries	Medial hypertrophy Elongation and spiralling of vessels Increased atherosclerosis Micro (Charcot–Bouchard) aneurysms Berry aneurysms Small and large haemorrhages—lentiform nucleus, cerebellar white matter, pons and midbrain
Retina	
Vessels	Constriction of arterioles Medial hypertrophy Linear and flare haemorrhages Lipid exudates Retinal ischaemia/infarction

Table 15.46 Effects of malignant hypertension.

Blood vessels	
	Fibrinoid necrosis Aneurysm formation Rupture
Kidneys	
Macroscopically	Enlarged and pale with petechial haemorrhages
Vessels	Fibrinoid necrosis Endarteritis obliterans
Glomeruli	Fibrinoid necrosis with epithelial crescent formation
Tubules	Hyaline droplet degeneration
Interstitium	Oedema and haemorrhage
Brain (hypertensive encephalopathy)	
Arteries	Fibrinoid necrosis Haemorrhage

Table 15.47 Criteria for investigation of hypertension.

Age
Sex
Family history
Mild increase in blood pressure
Response to simple treatment
Recent sudden change in blood pressure

- pulmonary capillaries;
- pulmonary venules and veins.

The pulmonary trunk. In the adult this differs from the aorta in that the media consists of short irregularly arranged elastic laminae (Fig. 15.72) interspersed with smooth-muscle fibres and connective tissue. The elastic fibres are widely spaced and irregular in shape.

In the fetus and neonate the pulmonary trunk resembles the aorta in that the configuration of the elastic tissue is similar with numerous concentrically arranged thick elastic laminae. In the normal subject this media involutes to the adult form by about the age of 9 months but if pulmonary hypertension is present from birth, such involution does not take place.

Conducting or elastic pulmonary arteries. These extend from the hilum of the lung to vessels of approximately 1 mm external diameter. They accompany the airways. Their distinguishing feature lies in the media where there is plentiful elastic tissue arranged in parallel concentric elastic laminae.

Muscular pulmonary arteries. These range from between 1 mm and 100 μm in external diameter and have a very

tional requirements of a low-pressure system. The pulmonary arteries represent a great contrast to the systemic vessels as they provide a **low-resistance system** for transmission of total cardiac output. Gravity, rather than constriction of muscular vessels, appears to play the most important role in directing blood flow to different portions of the pulmonary vascular bed. The structure of the pulmonary arteries reflects this difference.

The pulmonary vascular system consist of:
- conducting/elastic pulmonary arteries;
- muscular pulmonary arteries;
- pulmonary arterioles;

Table 15.48 Biochemical investigation of hypertension.

First-line	To help exclude
Urine	
Protein ⎤ test	
Blood ⎬ strips	Glomerulonephritides and diabetes
Sugar ⎦ initially	
(+ microscopy, culture)	
Blood	
Urea	Chronic renal failure
Creatinine	
Uric acid	CRF and gout
Fasting glucose	Diabetes
Electrolytes	Renal and endocrine causes
Calcium	Hyperparathyroidism
gGT	Alcoholism
Fasting lipids (Hb and ESR)	Evaluation of risk
Other investigations	
CXR	
ECG, particularly for LVH	
Echocardiography	
More detailed biochemical investigations if:	
Abnormal plasma: urea, creatinine, potassium, calcium	
Proteinuria, haematuria or glycosuria	
(+ clinical features suggesting primary cause, e.g. Cushing's, phaeochromocytoma)	
Hypertension under 30 years' age	
Malignant hypertension	
Uncontrolled hypertension	

CRF, Chronic renal failure; gGT, γ-glutamyltransferase; Hb, haemoglobin; ESR, erythrocyte sedimentation rate; CXR, chest X-ray; ECG, electrocardiogram; LVH, left ventricular hypertrophy.

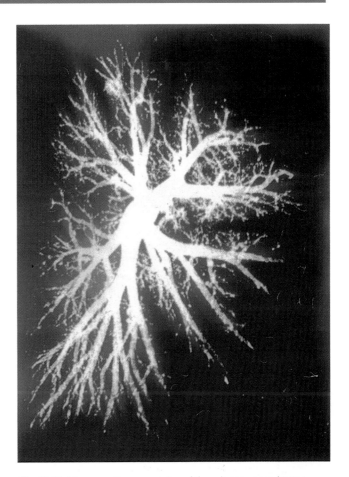

Fig. 15.71 Diagrammatic representation of the pulmonary vascular tree.

Fig. 15.72 The pulmonary trunk in an adult. The media contains short irregularly spaced elastic fibres. (EVG.)

thin media defined by distinct internal and external elastic laminae. The total thickness of the muscular media in normal subjects never exceeds 10% of the total vessel diameter and is often much less.

Pulmonary arterioles. These are vessels of less than 100 μm external diameter. They have exceedingly thin walls composed of endothelium and a single elastic lamina with no true media but an occasional spirally wound single smooth-muscle cell.

Pulmonary venules. These resemble pulmonary arterioles in structure but are situated, together with lymphatics, in the interlobular septa and only join the airways and arteries at the apex of the lobule.

Pulmonary hypertension

Definition. Pulmonary pressure >30/15mmHg (Tables 15.49 and 15.50).

Table 15.49 Causes of pulmonary hypertension.

PRIMARY OR IDIOPATHIC (rapidly fatal, found mainly in young women)

SECONDARY

Increased pulmonary venous pressure
Chronic left ventricular failure
Mitral stenosis (the picture of the lungs in pulmonary hypertension due to mitral stenosis is classical, with atheroma in the pulmonary trunk and elastic pulmonary arteries, medial hypertrophy, arterialization of veins, dilatation of lymphatics in oedematous interlobular septa, focal haemosiderosis and interstitial fibrosis and 'pulmonary ossification')
More rarely:
  Left atrial myxoma
  Pulmonary veno-occlusive disease (children <15 years? associated with alkaloids in tea)
  Compression of veins by a mediastinal neoplasm

Increased pulmonary vascular resistance
Obstruction to pulmonary arteries/arterioles
  Recurrent thromboemboli
  In situ thrombosis
  Tumour emboli
  Ova of *Schistosoma mansoni*
Destruction of pulmonary vasculature
  Severe pulmonary fibrosis, e.g. tuberculosis, silicosis
  Bronchiectasis
  Chronic bronchitis and emphysema
Destruction associated with alveolar–capillary diffusion block
  Pneumoconioses
  Sarcoidosis
  Scleroderma and SLE
  Fibrosing alveolitis
Vasoconstriction due to hypoxia
  Pulmonary oedema
  Chronic bronchitis and emphysema
  Primary pulmonary hypertension
  High altitude

Increased pulmonary blood flow
Resulting from left-to-right shunts
Pre-tricuspid shunts
  Atrial septal defect
  Anomalous pulmonary venous drainage into the right atrium or SVC
Post-tricuspid shunts
  Persistent ductus arteriosus
  Ventricular septal defect

Disorders affecting movement of the chest wall
Kyphoscoliosis, thoracoplasty, pleural fibrosis, poliomyelitis, obesity

SLE, Systemic lupus erythematosus; SVC, superior vena cava.

Table 15.50 Alternative classification of pulmonary hypertension. These may be roughly divided into cardiac causes and those secondary to pulmonary diseases with consequent hypoxia. A simple classification is as follows.

Cardiac causes

Congenital defects
pre-tricuspid shunts, e.g. ASD, anomalous pulmonary venous drainage
post-tricuspid shunts, e.g. VSD, patent ductus arteriosus

Acquired disease
e.g. mitral stenosis, atrial myxoma, pulmonary veno-occlusive disease, left ventricular failure

Primary pulmonary hypertension—cause unknown

Cor pulmonale
Diseases of airways and lung parenchyma, e.g. chronic bronchitis, emphysema, pulmonary fibrosis, pulmonary granulomas

Diseases affecting respiratory movement, e.g. kyphoscoliosis, obesity

Pulmonary embolism (recurrent thromboembolism) or thrombosis, e.g. sickle-cell anaemia

ASD, Atrial septal defect; VSD, ventricular septal defect.

Effects of pulmonary hypertension. If present since birth, the pulmonary trunk retains its fetal configuration. If hypertension develops after 9 months of age the following effects occur.

1 Mainly on the vasculature of the lung (Table 15.51; Fig. 15.73).

- **Pulmonary arterial changes in pulmonary hypertension:** These differ from case to case depending on the underlying cause. In some instances, for instance in chronic pulmonary emphysema, the lesions are minor, consisting only of a little hypertrophy of the media in muscular vessels, whereas in others they are dramatic with fibrinoid necrosis. In congenital heart disease and in primary pulmonary hypertension the following changes may occur.
- **Elastic pulmonary arteries:** These exhibit atheroma

Table 15.51 The effects of pulmonary hypertension of the pulmonary vasculature.

Elastic (pulmonary/conducting) arteries
Medial hypertrophy
Mucoid degeneration
Atherosclerosis

Muscular (bronchial) arteries
Medial hypertrophy
Intimal proliferation (± fibrinoid necrosis)
Fibroelastosis
Localized dilatations with rupture and haemosiderosis

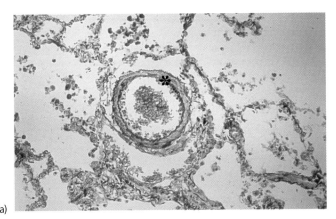

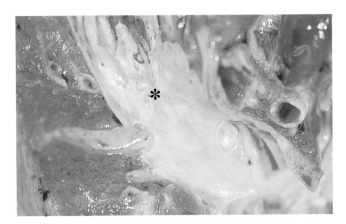

Fig. 15.74 Atheroma (✳) in conducting pulmonary arteries in pulmonary hypertension.

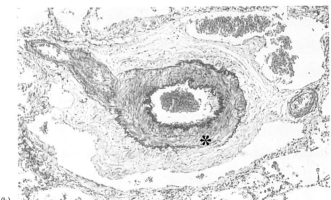

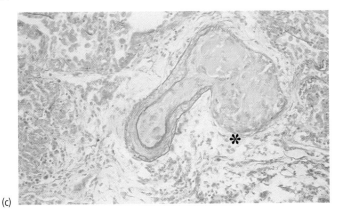

Fig. 15.73 The pulmonary vasculature in pulmonary hypertension. (a) A normal postnatal pulmonary artery. (EVG.) (b) In pulmonary hypertension, the changes mimic those seen in the fetal artery, with thickening of the media (✳). (c) Severe pulmonary hypertension leads to intimal thickening and 'blowout' aneurysms (✳).

and an increase in ground substance in the media (Fig. 15.74).

- **Muscular pulmonary arteries:** They may show: (i) medial hypertrophy; (ii) cellular intimal proliferation; (iii) fibrinoid necrosis; and (iv) dilatation lesions which affect smaller vessels and are composed of a variety of aneurysmal dilatations in their walls, re-

ferred to as **plexiform lesions**, which represent 'healing' areas of fibrinoid necrosis.

- **Arterioles** develop a thick muscular media: in addition there is intimal fibrosis and in severe cases fibrinoid necrosis.

Fibrinoid necrosis or necrotizing arteritis is the term used to describe the appearances of the vessel wall when it adopts the tinctorial staining reaction of fibrin. It is associated with rapid onset of extremely high levels of blood pressure.

In pulmonary hypertension associated with acquired heart disease similar changes may be seen but dilatation lesions are not found.

2 The heart: Right ventricular failure and hypertrophy occur. This is called **cor pulmonale** if the cause is a primary lung disease. The weights of the individual left ventricle and septum (LV and S) and right ventricle (RV) are used to assess right ventricular hypertrophy at post mortem (Fulton technique). The ratio of RV : LV + S is in the range of 2.5–3.5.

Cor pulmonale

Definition. 'Hypertrophy of the right ventricle resulting from diseases affecting the function and/or the structure of the lung – except when these alterations are the result of diseases that primarily affect the left side of the heart or are the result of congenital heart disease' (World Health Organization, 1961; Fig. 15.75; Table 15.52).

Heart failure

Definition

Heart failure is a clinical syndrome caused by an abnormality of the heart and recognized by a characteristic pattern of haemodynamic, renal, neural and hormonal

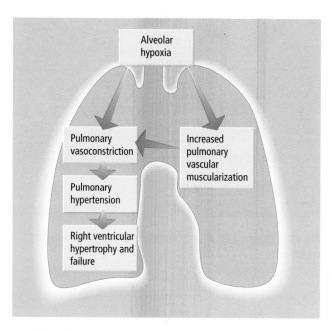

Fig. 15.75 The pathogenesis of cor pulmonale.

Table 15.52 Causes of cor pulmonale.

Hypoxic pulmonary vascular diseases
Chronic bronchitis (± emphysema)
Emphysema (± bronchitis or asthma)
Bronchial asthma
Pulmonary fibrosis (due to tuberculosis, pneumoconiosis, etc.)
Pulmonary granulomas and infiltrations (sarcoidosis, malignant infiltration, etc.)
Pulmonary resection
High-altitude hypoxia

Diseases primarily affecting the pulmonary vasculature
Arterial, e.g. primary pulmonary hypertension
Thrombotic disorders, e.g. sickle-cell anaemia
Pulmonary embolism

Diseases affecting movement of the chest wall
Kyphoscoliosis, etc.

responses. It is the inability to pump sufficient blood to meet metabolic demands (Table 15.53).

Practical terminology

It has been common for clinicians and pathologists to refer to right and left, forward and backward and congestive heart failure and cardiogenic shock.

For practical purposes, some clinicians use the terms:
- circulatory collapse;
- acute heart failure;
- chronic heart failure (Table 15.54).

Table 15.53 The response to heart failure. The body compensates for an abnormality of cardiac function in five ways.

Hypertrophy, dilatation and fibrosis in response to chronic pressure or volume overload
Increased cardiac output (Starling mechanism)
Vasoconstriction secondary to activation of the sympathetic and renin–angiotensin systems
Constriction of arterioles with redistribution of blood flow
Desensitization of vessels and myocardium

Table 15.54 Grading of heart failure according to the inability to exercise.

Grade I	No limitation of physical activity
Grade II	Slight limitation of physical activity
Grade III	Marked limitation of physical activity
Grade IV	Inability to carry out any physical activity without discomfort

Acute heart failure

This is a clinical syndrome resulting from sudden deterioration in left ventricular function. The clinical picture is characterized by:
- marked shortness of breath;
- cyanosis;
- pulmonary oedema;
- peripheral vasoconstriction.

An acute cause is usually present, such as an arrhythmia, MI or an abrupt deterioration in chronic heart failure.

Chronic heart failure

This is a syndrome dominated by the retention of sodium and water. Clinical features include:
- peripheral oedema;
- raised venous pressure;
- hepatomegaly;
- pulmonary oedema;
- an enlarged heart;
- a third heart sound.

In treated chronic heart failure, there may be few abnormal physical signs (Tables 15.55 and 15.56).

Circulatory collapse

This is characterized by:
- low blood pressure;
- poor urine output;
- peripheral vasoconstriction.

If the central venous pressure (CVP) is raised, the cause is likely to be pump failure. This is sometimes termed **cardiogenic shock**. Most conditions which affect the heart and lungs can precipitate circulatory collapse. A high CVP can be caused by RV infarction.

Table 15.55 Causes of left ventricular failure.

Systemic hypertension
Myocardial ischaemia
Rheumatic heart disease
   Mitral incompetence
   Aortic stenosis/incompetence
Calcific aorti stenosis
Cardiomyopathy/myocarditis
Coarctation of the aorta
High-output states
   Anaemia
   Thyrotoxicosis
   Beri-beri
   Pregnancy
   Pyrexia
   Paget's disease
Constrictive pericarditis

Table 15.56 Effects of left ventricular failure.

Lung
Pulmonary oedema
Chronic venous congestion
Pulmonary infarction
Pleural effusions

Systemic hypoperfusion
Infarcts
   Kidney
   Brain ('watershed areas')
   Intestine (ischaemic colitis)
Liver
   Fatty change
   Centrilobular necrosis
Kidney
   Decreased GFR with Na$^+$ and water retention
   Hydropic vacuolation of tubular epithelium

GFR, Glomerular filtration rate.

Circulatory collapse due to pump failure associated with a low CVP is commonly due to a LV infarction. Low arterial or venous tone following drug overdose or septicaemia is also a cause of circulatory collapse characterized by low CVP and vasodilatation. when venous tone is high, a low CVP indicates low circulatory volume due to;
- haemorrhage;
- gastrointestinal fluid loss;
- excess diuresis;
- diabetic ketoacidosis;
- Addisonian crisis (Tables 15.57–15.59).

Table 15.57 Causes of right ventricular failure.

Secondary to left ventricular failure
Pulmonary hypertension
Congenital heart disease
   Atrial septal defect
   Pulmonary stenosis
   Tricuspid anomalies
Myocarditis
Myocardial ischaemia

Table 15.58 Effects of right ventricular failure.

Liver
Hepatomegaly
'Nutmeg' appearance due to:
   Centrilobular congestion
   Peripheral fatty change
   Centrilobular necrosis/fibrosis
Ascites due to portal congestion

Spleen
Splenomegaly
Haemosiderin
Fibrosis of sinusoidal walls

Kidneys
Congestion
Fatty change due to hypoxia

Brain
Congestion and hypoxia

Limbs
Dependent oedema

Table 15.59 Diagnosis of heart failure.

There are six investigations that are essential for the diagnosis of heart failure:
Chest radiography
Electrocardiography
Echocardiography (the most useful diagnostic aid)
Full blood count
Measurement of plasma electrolytes
Measurement of plasma urea

Other tests which may be useful:
Thyroid function tests
Nuclear techniques to assess ejection fraction and cardiac function
Cardiac catheterization – performed when there is major diagnostic doubt or if a condition amenable to surgery is suspected
Exercise testing is helpful in assessing the severity of heart failure and determining the prognosis

VALVULAR HEART DISEASE

Definition

Valvular heart disease is cardiac dysfunction produced by structural and/or functional abnormalities of single or multiple cardiac valves. It can be classified according to the 'pathological sieve' described in Chapter 1 (Tables 15.60 and 15.61).

Congenital valve defects

The commonest congenital valvular disease is congenital bicuspid aortic valve. It is seen in 1–2% of the population. It is the inevitable fate of this defect to undergo dystrophic calcification in patients over the age of 60 years. This congenital valve disease is associated with aortic dissection.

Infective endocarditis

Introduction. The incidence of infective endocarditis has decreased dramatically in the western world with the availability of antibiotic therapy. Virulent organisms and defects in host defense mechanisms are associated with certain types of infection.

It has been customary to classify infective bacterial endocarditis as acute (ABE) or subacute (SBE) but there is considerable overlap and **infective endocarditis** is the preferred term. In general infections from staphylococci, *Streptococcus pyogenes*, *Neisseria* and *Pseudomonas* will produce a more acute clinical picture (Fig. 15.76).

Infective endocarditis will lead to valve destruction and valvular incompetence. Embolic phenomena are common and patients will present with septic emboli in

Table 15.60 Clinical features of acute and chronic valvular disease.

Features of acute valvular disease	Features of chronic valvular disease
Tachycardia	Gradual onset of reduced exercise tolerance
Fever	Heart murmurs
Heart murmurs	Inevitable cardiac failure secondary to stenosis or regurgitation
Embolic phenomena	
Splenic pain	Atrial dilatation and ball-valve thrombi
Renal infarcts	Arrhythmias
Cerebral infarcts	Increased susceptibility to endocarditis
Cardiac failure if valvular swelling and distortion cause sufficient haemodynamic disturbance	

Table 15.61 Causes of valvular heart disease.

Congenital
Acquired
Infective
Endocarditis
Syphilis
Inflammatory
Rheumatic
Rheumatoid
Ankylosing spondylitis
Systemic lupus erythematosus
Neoplastic
Carcinoid
Metastases
Traumatic
Balloon-tip catheters
Aortic dissection
Metabolic
Mucopolysaccharidoses
Marfan's
Degenerative
Calcific
Fibrotic
Lipidosis/atherosclerosis
Floppy' valve
Papillary muscle dysfunction

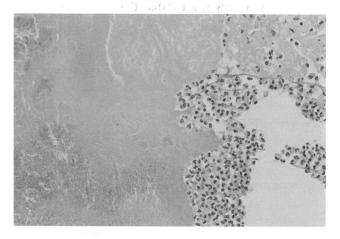

Fig. 15.76 The histology of an acute valvular vegetation in infective endocarditis. (H&E.)

the skin, spleen, kidney and brain. Infective endocarditis is associated with coronary artery emboli.

Microbiology

1 Endocarditis on natural valves. The dextran-positive species are able to adhere to the endocardial surface more effectively. There is an association between *Streptococcus bovis* endocarditis and carcinoma of the colon. Gram-

Table 15.62 Main organisms in endocarditis on natural valves.

Viridans streptococci	50%
Faecal streptococci	10%
Staphylococcus aureus	25%
Staphylococcus epidermidis	25%
Miscellaneous	
Gram-negative bacteria	4%
Fungi and yeast	4%
Coxiella burnetii	2%
Chlamydia psittaci	2%

No organisms are isolated in up to 11%

These figures refer to endocarditis on natural valves, in patients who are not drug addicts

The majority of viridans streptococci that cause endocarditis are dextran-positive species:
- *Streptococcus mitis*
- *Streptococcus mutans*
- *Streptococcus sanguis*
- *Streptococcus bovis I*

Table 15.63 Microbiology of prosthetic valve endocarditis.

Staphylococcus aureus	50%
Staphylococcus epidermidis	50%
Gram-negative bracteria	
Candida spp.	
Diphtheroids	

Differential diagnosis
Other causes of persistent or recurrent postoperative fever
    Chest infection, sternal wound infection, urinary tract infection
    Postperfusion syndrome
    Post pericardotomy syndrome

Mortality >40%

Table 15.64 Infective endocarditis in drug addicts.

Staphylococcus aureus	60% followed by
Staphylococcus epidermidis	
Faecal streptococci (enterococci)	
Group A streptococci	
Yeasts	
Aspergillus	
Diphtheroids	
Clostridium spp.	
Bacillus spp.	
Gram-negative bacilli, e.g. *Pseudomonas* spp., *Serratia* spp.	

Table 15.65 Diagnosis of infective endocarditis.

Blood culture is the single most important investigation

Take at least three samples of blood for culture over a 24-hour period (1–2 hours in critically ill)

The correct aseptic procedure and a no-touch technique are essential

Bacteraemia is persistent, so timing is unimportant

One blood culture 89%
Two blood cultures 95%   } of culture-positive cases
Three blood cultures 99%

Prolonged incubation of cultures may be necessary for some organisms

Special culture techniques required for cell-wall-deficient organisms, nutritionally variant streptococci, anaerobes, etc.

Interpretation of blood cultures—see below

negative endocarditis is very uncommon on natural valves, except in drug addicts (Table 15.62).

2 Prosthetic valve endocarditis

- **Acute-onset:** Eradication is difficult and there is a high mortality. The incidence is 2% and the aortic valve is more commonly affected than the mitral valve. Early onset of endocarditis is defined as occurring within 60 days of surgery.

Organisms gain access during perioperative period via the following routes; (i) contaminated cardiopulmonary bypass equipment; (ii) wound infection; and (iii) intravascular lines.

- **Late-onset:** This is endocarditis occurring more than 2 months after surgery. Clinically and microbiologically, this disease is similar to endocarditis on natural valves (Table 15.63). Mortality is 20%.

3 Infective endocarditis in drug addicts. This is a growing problem in intravenous drug abusers. The organisms arise from contaminated heroin and adulterants (starch, lactose). The endocarditis is more often on the **tricuspid valve** and the microbiology is very varied (Tables 15.64 and 16.65).

Interpretation of blood cultures. Isolation of any organism from at least two different sets of blood cultures is usually significant. Contaminants, e.g. *Staphylococcus epidermidis* or *Corynebacterium* spp. (skin diphtheroids) usually only grow in one or two bottles. Antimicrobial susceptibility testing and typing of isolates can help in distinguishing contaminants from pathogens (Tables 15.66–15.68). It may be necessary to take several more sets of cultures to validate the isolation of *S. epidermidis* or similar common contaminants.

Chemoprophylaxis of infective endocarditis. Indications for antibiotic prophylaxis include dental work, including extractions, scaling, root fillings, tonsillectomy and other surgery to the upper respiratory tract. Also included are genitourinary surgery—cystoscopy, prostatectomy, in-

Table 15.66 Antimicrobial treatment.

Determine antimicrobial susceptibilities of infecting organism as follows:
Minimum inhibitory concentration (MIC)
  Make doubling dilutions of antimicrobial in broth
  Controls
  Inoculate each tube with patient's organism
  Incubate 18 hours at 37°C
  Inspect visually
  MIC = highest dilution with no visible growth

Minimum bacterial concentrations (MBC)
  Highest dilution giving a 99.99% kill
  Bactericidal therapy is essential

Test combinations of antimicrobials for evidence of synergistic activity, e.g. penicillin and gentamicin

After treatment has started, check capacity of patient's serum to kill the infecting organism
Collect samples of clotted blood just before and 1 hour after dose of antimicrobials. Make doubling dilutions of patient's serum in serum broth and inoculate each tube with the patient's infecting organism:
  Incubate 18 hours at 37°C
  Inspect visually
  Bacteriostatic level = highest dilution with no visible growth

Subculture each tube on to blood agar
  Incubate 18 hours at 37°C
  Bactericidal level = highest dilution which kills 99.99% of organisms
  Bactericidal levels should be > one-quarter pre-dose (trough) > one-eighth post-dose (peak)

Choice of antimicrobial therapy:
  Close liaison between clinician and microbiologist is essential
  All dosages given are for adult patients
  Blind therapy—natural valves
  Benzylpenicillin and gentamicin
  If *Staphylococcus* is suspected, add flucloxacillin

Table 15.67 Antimicrobial treatment of infective endocarditis.

Viridans streptococci
Benzylpenicillin and gentamicin
If *Staphylococcus* is suspected, add flucloxacillin
If organism proves to be exquisitely sensitive to penicillin, stop gentamicin or give low dose of gentamicin, e.g. 40 mg b.d. for 2 weeks. Stop gentamicin after 2 weeks in most cases. Continue benzylpenicillin for 2–3 weeks then give oral penicillin or amoxycillin for a further 3–4 weeks.
Check bactericidal levels during parenteral and oral therapy

Faecal streptococci
In vitro studies necessary to determine optimal therapy—often ampicillin and gentamicin

Staphylococcus aureus ⎱ flucloxacillin, benzylpenicillin,
Staphylococcus epidermidis ⎰ gentamicin

Stop benzylpenicillin if penicillin-resistant strain
Stop flucloxacillin if penicillin-sensitive strain

In penicillin-hypersensitive patients, use Vancomycin and gentamicin or cephalosporin and gentamicin

Table 15.68 Treatment of prosthetic valve endocarditis.

Often require surgery
May need several months of treatment
Pyrexia during treatment
Temperature may remain elevated for 3–14 days after initiation of therapy

If temperature worsens or persists, consider:
  Drug reaction
  Superinfection
  Line-associated infection
  Lack of effective therapy—mixed infection

strumental obstetric delivery. Gastrointestinal surgery in high-risk groups (e.g. those with prosthetic valves) should also be covered by antibiotics.

Review of infective endocarditis cases in Oxford has shown that 14% of cases had undergone dental treatment within 3 months of start of illness; in a further 7% of cases, poor dental hygiene was incriminated. Edentulous patients with ill-fitting dentures are still at risk.

Other blood tests show no set pattern in infective endocarditis. A normochromic normocytic anaemia is seen in 50%; white cell count is variable, being low, normal or raised; the ESR is variable—20 >100 mm/hour; immunoglobulins are raised and rheumatoid factor is positive in 50%.

Serology is of value for Q-fever (*Coxiella burnetii*) phase I and II antibodies, *Candida*, *Chlamydia psittaci*, *Aspergillus* and *Brucella*.

If the patient has recently been or is still receiving antibodies, stop them and collect several sets of blood cultures over 10 days.

Other tests for infective endocarditis include ECG and echocardiography.

Non-bacterial thrombotic endocarditis

Sometimes called marantic thrombi, these are platelet-rich accumulations on valve cusps that are not associated with infectious organisms or inflammatory infiltrates. They are associated with wasting diseases, particularly carcinomatosis, thrombotic disorders, particularly SLE and high anticardiolipin antibody titres. When small and localized, they are of no pathological significance. However, when occurring as part of a thrombotic disorder they may lead to embolic phenomena.

Inflammatory valve disease

Rheumatic valve disease

- **Definition.** Inflammatory, non-suppurative systemic disease affecting predominantly the heart and joints, which has a tendency to relapse.
- **Incidence.** This disease has almost disappeared in developed countries but it is still a major problem in the Third World. It affects all races and has an equal sex distribution. Peak age range is 5–15 years.
- **Predisposing factors.**
  1 climate, particularly months of high humidity and wet areas with fluctuating temperatures;
  2 living conditions, particularly overcrowding and poor nutrition;
  3 hereditary tendencies do exist with human leucocyte antigen associations;
  4 infection with Lancefield group, A, β-haemolytic streptococci is known to be the cause.
- **Clinical details.** See Jones's criteria (revised by the American Heart Association) for guidance in the diagnosis of rheumatic fever (Tables 15.69 and 15.70).
- **Associated and complicating factors.** These include polyarthritis, subcutaneous nodules, chorea, heart failure, pulmonary hypertension, infective endocarditis (Fig. 15.77), atrial fibrillation, atrial thrombosis, embolism and chordal rupture.
- **Causes of death in rheumatic fever.** Death occurs most commonly in children who die from congestive cardiac failure with active carditis. In adults, the commonest cause of death is congestive cardiac failure and pulmonary hypertension. Twenty-five per cent develop infective endocarditis and 20% die from aortic incompetence. Death may also occur due to conduction defects and cerebral emboli (Table 15.71).

Rheumatoid arthritis. This is a generalized disease of unknown aetiology in which rheumatoid factor (antibodies to γ-globulin) is demonstrated in the serum.

This disease presents as a sacroiliac joint disease, mainly in young men. Cardiac manifestations are common associations with this condition (Table 15.72).

- **Cardiac lesions.** Aortic incompetence occurs secondary to dilatation of the aortic ring. The aortic valve cusps are thickened, fibrotic and contracted. The aortic media shows fibrosis and necrosis but no granulomas or inflammatory infiltrates are seen.

Systemic lupus erythematosus (SLE). This is a multisystem

Table 15.69 Jones' criteria for diagnosis of rheumatic fever

MAJOR MANIFESTATIONS
Carditis—almost always associated with a significant murmur/ cardiomegaly/CCF
Pericarditis—with or without a friction rub
Chorea
Erythema marginatum
Subcutaneous nodules

MINOR MANIFESTATIONS
Clinical
Previous rheumatic fever or rheumatic heart disease
Arthralgia
Fever

Laboratory
Acute-phase reactions (ESR, C-reactive protein, leukocytosis)
ECG—prolonged PR interval
The presence of two major criteria or of one major and two minor indicates a high probability of rheumatic fever

Supporting evidence for streptococcal infection
Increased titre of streptococcal antibodies (A50 anti-Streptolysin O)
Other antibodies—anti-DNAase, antistreptokinase, antihyaluronidase
Positive throat culture for group A streptococci
Recent scarlet fever

Differential diagnosis
Rheumatoid arthritis, systemic lupus erythematosus, bacterial endocarditis, serum sickness, penicillin sensitivity, gonococcal arthritis, sickle-cell anaemia, viral pericarditis or myocarditis, leukaemia, tuberculosis, septicaemia (e.g. meningococcal), undulant fever (brucellosis)

CCF, congestive cardiac failure; ESR, erythrocyte sedimentation rate; ECG, electrocardiogram.

disease in which antinuclear antibodies are seen in serum (Table 15.73).

The causes of stenosis and incompetence in the cardiac valves will now be summarized (Tables 15.74–15.77).

Valve surgery

Common surgical procedures

Stenotic valve lesions are more frequent (85%) than purely incompetent lesions. The most frequently excised stenotic valve is the aortic valve (50%), followed by the mitral valve (48%) and tricuspid valve (2%). The most frequently excised purely incompetent valve is the aortic (48%), followed by the mitral valve (45%). Univalvular replacement is three times more common than multiple valve replacements.

Table 15.70 Pathology of rheumatic fever.

Acute rheumatic fever is a pancarditis
The following lesions may be seen in the heart:
Pericardium—fibrinous pericarditis
Myocardium—dark red foci of necrosis ± hypertrophy
The pathognomonic histological lesion is the *Aschoff nodule* (Fig. 15.77)

Stages

Exudative	Basophilic ground substance, foci of fibrinoid necrosis with a few lymphocytes and plasma cells
Granulomatous	Central, amorphous eosinophilic material surrounded by *Aschoff cells* (large mononuclear or multinucleate cells with ragged edges), *Anitschkow* cells (owl-eyed nuclei), lymphocytes and plasma cells (Fig. 15.77)
Healing	Aschoff cells disappear, fibroblasts appear with scar formation
	Localization usually around blood vessels in the connective tissue between myocardial fibres

Endocardium
Valve cusps
  Most commonly the mitral valve
  Slight swelling, opaqueness, tiny vegetations ± fibrous thickening
Posterior surface of left atrium
  McCallum's patch (jet lesion)—accumulation of inflammatory cells and mucoid material, Aschoff nodules, fibrinoid necrosis. Vegetations composed of fibrin

Chronic rheumatic heart disease

Pericardium	Fibrous thickening, dense adhesions
Myocardium	Fibrosis, often perivascular
Endocardium	McCallum's patch and valve lesions

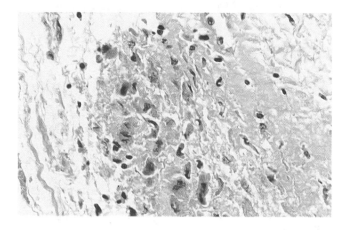

Fig. 15.77 Cardiac histology. The Aschoff nodule, a form of granuloma which is considered to be pathognomonic of rheumatic fever. (H&E.)

Table 15.71 Clinical consequences of rheumatic fever.

Aortic stenosis
Left-sided myocardial hypertrophy until heart failure supervenes and then bilateral ventricular hypertrophy

Aortic incompetence alone
Left ventricular hypertrophy and dilatation—mitral incompetence—left atrial dilatation—heart failure

Mitral incompetence alone
Dilatation and hypertrophy of all four chambers

Mitral stenosis
Dilatation of left atrium—right ventricular hypertrophy and dilatation—right atrial dilatation—tricuspid incompetence—heart failure and pulmonary hypertension

Table 15.72 Cardiac lesions of rheumatoid arthritis.

Pericarditis	Chronic fibrous type
Myocarditis	Non-specific—lymphocytes and plasma cells
	Specific granulomas—identical to subcutaneous nodules in rheumatoid arthritis
	Fibrinoid necrosis contains γ-globulin, palisading histiocytes, fibroblasts, multinucleate giant cells with an outer zone of fibrosis and chronic inflammatory cell infiltrate
Endocarditis	Granulomas involving the mitral and aortic valves
Coronary arteritis	

Table 15.73 Cardiac lesions in systemic lupus erythematosus (SLE).

Pericarditis	Gelatinous fibrous tissue
Myocarditis	Interstitial connective tissue, perivascular fibrinoid changes, infiltration of mainly fibroblasts, nuclei are pyknotic
Endocarditis (Libman–Sacks)	Small, flat, granular, firmly adherent vegetations composed of fibrin
	Mitral valve most commonly affected, in contrast to other types of vegetative endocarditis, the right side of the heart, in particular the tricuspid valve is most often involved.
	Histology—fibrinoid degeneration; fibrin and platelet vegetations may become infected.
Coronary arteritis	

Table 15.74 Aortic valve disease (Fig. 15.78).

Aortic stenosis
Congenital bicuspid valves
Rheumatic fusion of two or three commissures
Degenerative, nodular calcific deposits

Aortic incompetence
Infective endocarditis (active or healed)
Systemic hypertension (chronic, severe)
Discrete subaortic stenosis
Rheumatic (with or without commissural fusion)
Aortic tear or laceration
Degenerative, calcific
Rheumatoid arthritis
Prolapse from a VSD
Aortic wall disease
 Marfan's
 Syphilis
 Ankylosing spondylitis
 Dissection
 Cystic medial necrosis
 Aortic root dilatation

VSD, Ventricular septal defect.

Table 15.75 Pulmonary valve disease (Fig. 15.79).

Pulmonary stenosis
Congenitally bicuspid
Rheumatic disease
Carcinoid heart disease

Pulmonary incompetence
Pulmonary systolic hypertension
Infective endocarditis
Rheumatic

Complications of valve surgery

The outcome of valve surgery depends on the state of the myocardium and the degree of pulmonary vascular damage (Table 15.78).

PERICARDIAL DISEASE

Clinical syndromes of pericardial disease

Acute pericarditis (Fig. 15.83)

This is common among children and young adults. It is often viral in aetiology. Pericarditis is common in the first

Table 15.76 Mitral valve disease (Fig. 15.80).

Mitral stenosis
Congenital
Rheumatic
Infective endocarditis
Calcification
Drug-induced (methysergide)

Mitral incompetence
Leaflets
 Rheumatic
 Calcification
 Hypertrophic cardiomyopathy
Annulus
 Floppy mitral valve
 Rheumatic
 Infective endocarditis
Chordal rupture
 Infective endocarditis
 Floppy mitral valve
Papillary muscles
 Ischaemic heart disease

Floppy mitral valve (Fig. 15.80(f) and (g))
This condition is also known as floppy valve, billowing posterior leaflet syndrome, click-murmur syndrome, mitral valve prolapse, Barlow's syndrome, myxomatous degeneration

It is defined as increased annular circumference (>11.5 cm) associated with myxomatous change in the spongiosa layer of the valve ± chordal rupture

It is seen in Marfan's, Ehlers–Danlos, osteogenesis imperfecta, pseudoxanthoma elasticum

Table 15.77 Tricuspid valve disease (Fig. 15.81).

Tricuspid stenosis
Congenital
Carcinoid
Rheumatic (rarely isolated to tricuspid)

Tricuspid incompetence
Infective endocarditis (active or healed)
Floppy (tricuspid valve prolapse ± chordal rupture)
Papillary muscle dysfunction (ischaemia or trauma)
Right ventricular dilatation (pulmonary hypertension or cardiomyopathy)
Carcinoid
Rheumatic

week of a transmural MI. Recurrent of late pericarditis may occur from 2 weeks to 3 months after an MI and may be associated with an autoimmune phenomenon– Dressler's syndrome.

Normal aortic valve

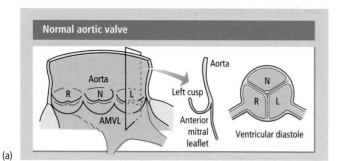

(a)

Degenerative

(b)

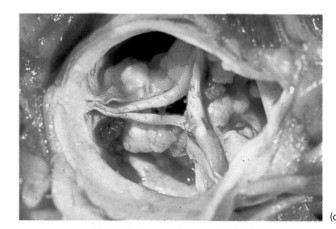

(c)

Infective endocarditis ((active or healed) tricuspid)

(d)

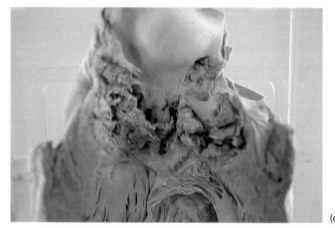

(e)

Rheumatic (with or without commissural fusion)

(f)

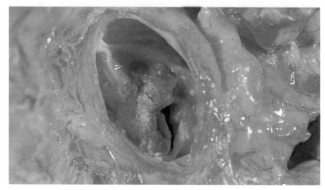

(g)

Fig. 15.78 (a) Diagram of normal aortic valve. (b) Diagram of aortic valve calcification. (c) Aortic valve calcification. (d) Diagram of aortic valve endocarditis. (e) Aortic valve endocarditis. (f) Diagram of aortic valve rheumatic stenosis. (g) Aortic valve rheumatic stenosis.

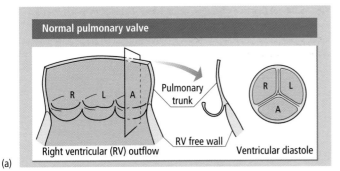

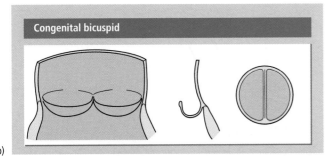

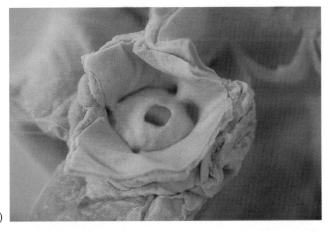

Fig. 15.79 (a) Diagram of normal pulmonary valve. (b) Diagram of congenital pulmonary valve stenosis. (c) Congenital pulmonary valve stenosis.

Table 15.78 Causes of valve failure in mechanical or biological prostheses.

Thrombotic obstruction
Prosthetic endocarditis
Paraprosthetic leak (Fig. 15.82)
Myocardial failure
Haemorrhage due to anticoagulation
Thromboembolism

Pericardial effusion

Effusions may accompany all forms of acute pericarditis. A small effusion occurs in most patients with severe congestive cardiac failure.

Table 15.79 Causes of pericarditis.

Infectious
Viral (Coxsackie B, echovirus 8, mumps, influenza, EBV)
Bacterial (streptococci, pneumococci), tuberculous, syphilis, fungal

Neoplasm
Benign (mesothelioma, pericardial cyst)
Malignant
   Primary (mesothelioma)
   Secondary—metastases

Vascular
Postmyocardial infarction, haemopericardium due to trauma or leakage from an aneurysm

Inflammatory
Acute rheumatic fever
Sarcoidosis
Collagen vascular disease—rheumatoid, SLE, scleroderma

Trauma
Radiation, postpericardiotomy

Endocrine
Myxoedema

Depositional
Amyloidosis

Metabolic
Uraemia

Drugs/toxins
Hydralazine, methysergide, isoniazid, procainamide

EBV, Epstein–Barr virus; SLE, systemic lupus erythematosus.

Pericardial effusion with tamponade

Pericardial effusion increases intrapericardial pressure and, in excess, impairs venous return with a subsequent fall in forward cardiac output. This is aggravated in inspiration. The rate of pericardial fluid accumulation is critical.

Chronic constrictive pericarditis

This may follow pericarditis due to most causes (particularly infection but also haemopericardium, radiation, uraemia, rheumatoid arthritis; Table 15.79). Cardiac filling is limited by the thickened, fibrosed or calcified pericardium. The clinical appearance is constrictive pericarditis includes right-sided heart failure, severe ascites, neck view congestion, hepatomegaly and splenomegaly.

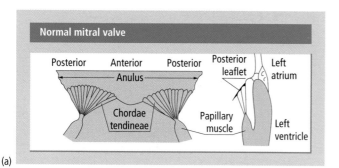

(a)

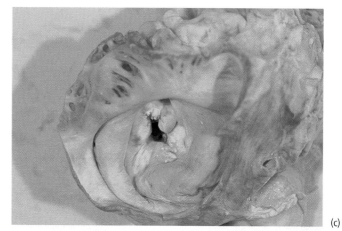

Fig. 15.80 (a) Diagram of normal mitral valve. (b) Diagram of rheumatic mitral valve stenosis. (c) Rheumatic mitral valve stenosis. (d) Diagram of mitral valve endocarditis. (e) Mitral valve endocarditis. (f) Diagram of floppy mitral valve. (g) Floppy mitral valve.

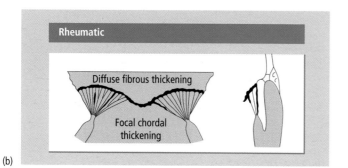

(b)

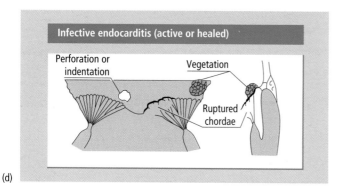

(d)

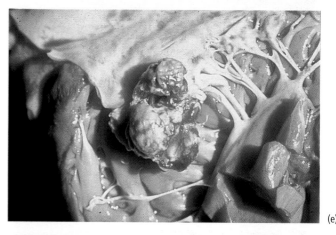

(e)

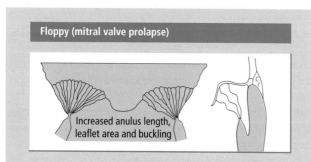

(f)

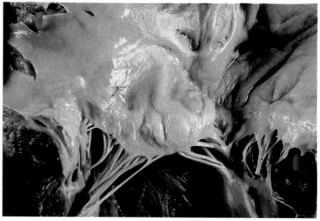

(g)

(c)

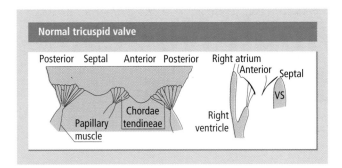

Fig. 15.81 Diagram of normal tricuspid valve.

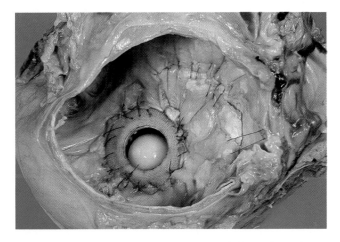

Fig. 15.82 Mitral valve replacement in a patient with chronic rheumatic valvular disease. The prosthetic valve has developed a leak because the entire valve ring and left atrium is fibrotic and calcified and stitches have not secured the prosthetic valve.

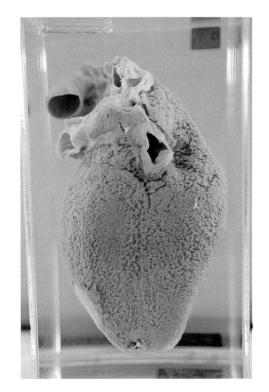

Fig. 15.83 Acute pericarditis in a patient with uraemia.

REFERENCES

Aretz H.T. (1987) Myocarditis: a histopathological definition and classification. *American Journal of Cardiovascular Pathology*; **1**:1.

Brown M.S. & Goldstein J.L. (1983) Lipoprotein metabolism in the macrophage; implications for cholesterol deposition in atherosclerosis. *Annual Review of Biochemistry*; **52**:223–261.

Lobstein J.G. (1829) *Traite d'Anatomie Pathologique*. Levrault, Paris.

Ross R. (1986) The pathogenesis of atherosclerosis – an update. *New England Journal of Medicine*; **314**:488–500.

Virchow R. (1862) Gesammelte Abhandlunger z. Wizentschaftlichen Medicin, In: *Phlogose und Thrombose in Gefassystem*. Max Hirsch, Berlin.

Von Haller A. (1735) *Opuscula Pathologica*. Bousquet, Lausanne.

World Health Organization (1958) Report of a study group: classification of atherosclerotic lesions. *World Health Organization Technical Report Series, 143*.

FURTHER READING

Becker A.E. & Andersion R.H. (1983) *Cardiac Pathology*. Churchill Livingstone, Edinburgh.

Knight B. (1983) *The Coroner's Autopsy*. Churchill Livingstone, Edinburgh.

Mitchinson M.J. (1996) *Essentials of Pathology* (Chapter 14). Blackwell Science, Oxford.

Stehbens W.E. & Lie J.T. (1995) *Vascular Pathology*. Chapman & Hall, London.

C H A P T E R   16

Diseases of Lymph Nodes, Spleen and Thymus

C O N T E N T S

Lymph nodes

THE NORMAL LYMPH NODE

Many organs are involved in the activity of the immune system and they can be divided, somewhat arbitrarily, into **primary** and **secondary lymphoid tissues** depending on their functions. Thus, the bone marrow and thymus, which are concerned with lymphocyte development, are referred to as the primary lymphoid tissues. Lymph nodes, the spleen, tonsils and mucosa-associated lymphoid tissue (MALT) belong to the secondary lymphoid tissues which are involved with lymphocyte function, both humoral and cell-mediated.

The normal lymph node is usually less than 1 cm in maximum diameter and has an oval or bean-shaped appearance (Fig. 16.1). The node parenchyma is divided into three main regions:
1 the **cortex**;
2 the **paracortex**;
3 the **medulla**.

The **cortex** contains primary and secondary follicles (Fig. 16.2). Primary follicles consist of collections of resting B lymphocytes that have not yet been stimulated by antigen, whilst the secondary follicles have in addition a central area of proliferating lymphocytes known as a germinal centre. The cortex contains predominantly B lymphocytes.

In contrast, the **paracortex** (the area between the follicles and the medulla) consists mainly of T lymphocytes and has a rich vascular supply.

The **medulla**, situated at the hilum of the node, drains the converging sinuses and is rich in macrophages and mature B lymphocytes, i.e. plasma cells.

It is not possible to tell if a lymphocyte is of B or T lineage using histological criteria alone. The ability to distinguish them in tissue sections has been made possible by the rapid and extensive developments which have taken place in immunocytochemistry, in particular, the use of monoclonal antibodies. This is illustrated in Fig. 16.3 where monoclonal antibodies have been used to reveal the topographical distribution of a lymph node's cellular constituents. A knowledge of these constituents within a normal node allows some insight into the types

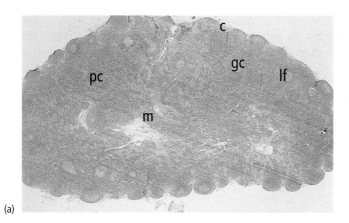

(a)

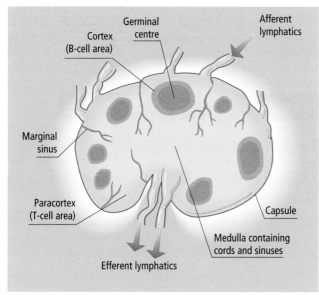

(b)

Fig. 16.1 (a) The normal lymph node. Low power histology. pc, paracortex; c, cortex; gc, germinal centre; lf, lymphoid follicle; m, medulla. (b) The normal lymph node.

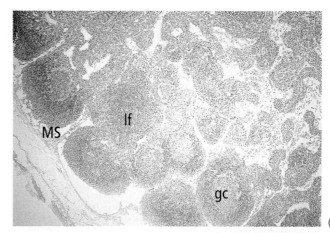

(a)

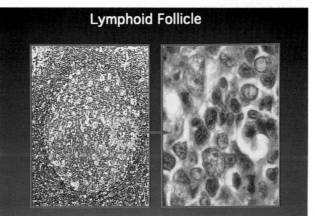

(b)

Fig. 16.2 The normal lymph node. (a) The cortex showing the marginal sunuses (MS), lymphoid follicles (lf) and germinal centres (gc). (b) The cells of the germinal centres.

of malignancy, i.e. lymphoma, which can arise within it (Fig. 16.4). Table 16.1 and Fig. 16.5 illustrate these cells in a schematic way.

LYMPHADENOPATHY

Lymphadenopathy implies **lymph node enlargement** which can be detected either clinically by palpation, or by other means, such as computed tomographic scans of less accessible sites such as the retroperitoneum or liver hilum (Fig. 16.6). A normal lymph node and an enlarged reactive node differ mainly in the degree to which they are being antigenically stimulated. During periods of markedly increased antigenic stimulation, e.g. infections, the lymph node reacts by increasing the number of lymphoid

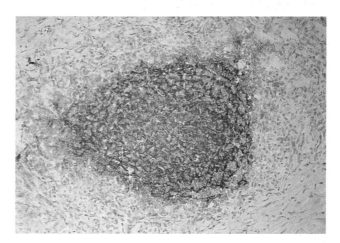

Fig. 16.3 Immunohistochemistry with antibodies to the cells of the lymph node constituents helps to define the normal and abnormal components. Here is a normal lymph node germinal centre stained with antibodies to CD20 (red) defining the B-cell populations.

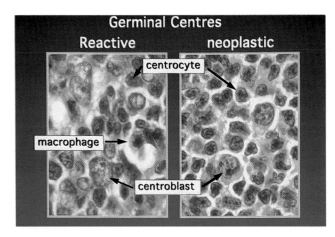

Fig. 16.4 The cells of the reactive and neoplastic germinal centres; centrocytes and centroblasts.

cells with a corresponding increase in the node's size. This is termed **reactive hyperplasia**. Although this is the commonest cause of lymphadenopathy, there are other conditions which can result in lymph node enlargement (Table 16.2). The primary malignancies of the lymph nodes (lymphomas) are dealt with later.

For the sake of clarity and simplicity, reactive hyperplasia can be divided into three separate histological patterns which are represented schematically in Fig. 16.7(b). It is important to realize that only rarely does a lymph node demonstrate exclusively one of these three patterns, there being almost invariably a mixture, with one pattern predominating. In addition, whilst certain infections may produce a typical histological picture it is rarely so characteristic as to be pathognomonic. Thus in diagnosing reactive hyperplasia the histopathologist can

Table 16.1 Lymphoid cell types.

Name	Characteristics	Figure
Small lymphocyte	Resting lymphoid stem cells Resting mature T cells bearing antigen receptors Resting mature B cells bearing antigen receptors (immunoglobulin) Cytotoxic, sensitized, killer or effector T cells Helper and suppressor T cells Natural killer cells	16.5(a)
Lymphoblast	Actively dividing stem cell	16.5(b)
Immunoblast (transformed lymphocyte)	Dividing, antigenically stimulated T cell Dividing, antigenically stimulated B cell	16.5(c)
Follicular centre cell	Intermediate B cell found during antigen-stimulated proliferation in lymphoid follicles	16.5(d)
Plasma cell	Immunoglobulin-secreting B cell	16.5(e)

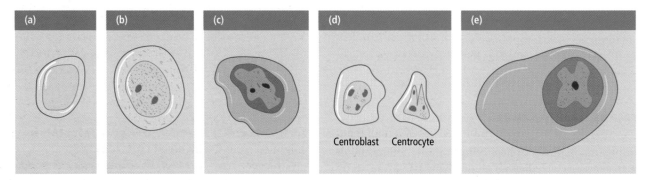

Fig. 16.5 (a) Small lymphocyte. (b) Lymphoblast. (c) Immunoblast. (d) Follicle centre cells – centroblast and centrocyte. (e) Plasma cell.

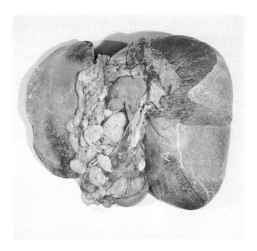

Fig. 16.6 The liver showing massive hilar lymphadenopathy.

Table 16.2 General causes of lymphadenopathy.

Benign
Follicular hyperplasia
Sinus histiocytosis
Paracortical expansion

Malignant
Primary, i.e. lymphoma
Secondary, i.e. metastases

often only give a differential diagnosis and suggest a list of possible aetiologies.

Follicular hyperplasia

This pattern is the most common type seen in reactive lymph nodes. A variety of conditions will produce enlargement of the secondary follicles and conversion of primary follicles into secondary ones (Fig. 16.7(a)). For example, rheumatoid arthritis may produce considerable follicular hyperplasia, as can measles infection. In the latter condition the germinal centres may contain characteristic multinucleated cells called Warthin–Finkeldey cells (Fig. 16.8). Follicular hyperplasia is also frequently seen in lymph nodes which drain the site of a malignant tumour. It is not uncommon to encounter lymphadenopathy during childhood and adolescence, displaying follicular hyperplasia, but for which no cause is ever established.

Sinus hyperplasia

In this pattern, the sinuses which drain the lymph fluid as

it passes through the nodal parenchyma become dilated and prominent. They are often filled with numerous macrophages, and the condition is then called **sinus histiocytosis**. This pattern, like that of follicular hyperplasia, is also seen in nodes draining a tumour. Whipple's disease, a cause of malabsorption in middle-aged males, may involve the lymph nodes and produce collections of macrophages, within dilated sinuses, containing periodic acid–Schiff (PAS)-positive material (Fig. 16.9). The lymphangiogram procedure may result in accumulation of the injected radiopaque material within the sinuses where it may elicit a foreign body multinucleated giant cell response (Fig. 16.10).

Paracortical expansion

Viruses such as Epstein–Barr (Fig. 16.11) and vaccinia often produce a picture which involves predominantly the paracortex (because T lymphocytes, which are mainly situated in the paracortex, play the major role in combating viral infections). Granulomatous disorders, e.g. tuberculosis (TB) and sarcoid, also involve this region of the node.

TB classically produces large confluent granulomas with areas of central coagulative necrosis; the necrosis appears macroscopically similar to soft cheese and is therefore known as caseous necrosis (Fig. 16.12). Sarcoidosis, a disease of unknown aetiology, produces smaller non-confluent granulomas without necrosis. Both conditions have multinucleated giant cells. Distinguishing between these two conditions and indeed the many other causes of granulomatous reactions is often not possible using histology alone. A Ziehl–Neelsen stain performed on a tissue section of an involved node may demonstrate acid-fast bacilli; however, the definitive diagnosis depends on microbiological investigations. Thus any suspected case of TB should always have part of the biopsy sent fresh to the bacteriology laboratory.

Certain skin conditions, e.g. eczema, may produce a reactive hyperplasia of the lymph nodes draining the affected site. This is known as dermatopathic lymphadenopathy, the paracortical expansion being due to the accumulation of Langerhans cells which have migrated from the involved epidermis.

Gaucher's and Niemann–Pick's disease are rare lipid storage disorders which cause paracortical expansion by the accumulation of either glucocerebroside or sphingomyelin within the macrophages.

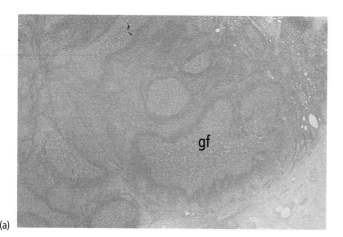

(a)

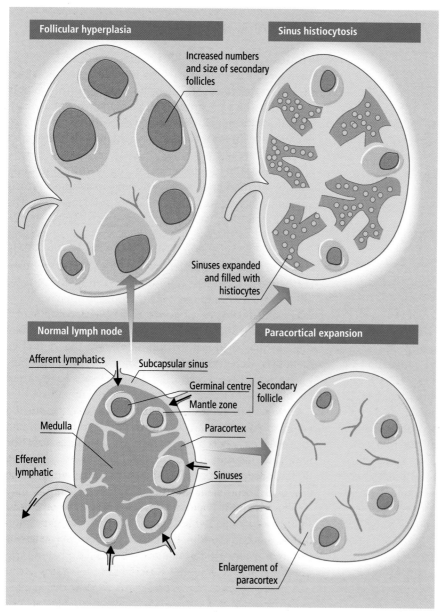

(b)

Fig. 16.7 Reactive hyperplasia. (a) Giant follicular hyperplasia. gf, giant follicle. (H&E.) (b) In lymph nodes.

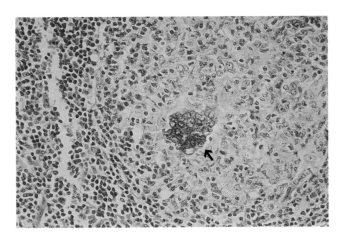

Fig. 16.8 Warthin–Finkeldy giant cells (arrowed) seen in measles. (H&E.)

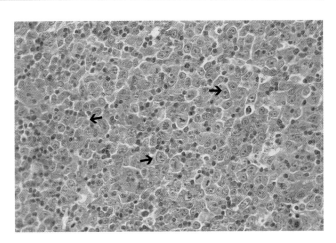

Fig. 16.11 Infectious mononucleosis is associated with expansion of the T-cell areas with atypical T lymphocytes (arrowed).

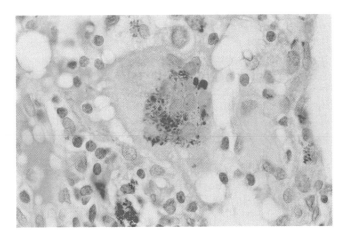

Fig. 16.9 Foamy multinucleate giant cells contain PAS-positive inclusions in Whipple's disease.

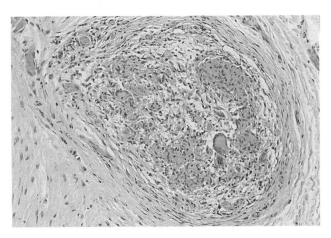

Fig. 16.12 Giant cell epithelioid granulomas seen in tuberculosis. (H&E.)

Mixed pattern

Infection by the protozoan *Toxoplasma gondii* produces a striking granulomatous picture in lymph nodes. Small collections (congeries) of epithelioid macrophages may be found located within the paracortex and at the periphery of secondary follicles (Fig. 16.13), follicular hyperplasia is usually prominent and the subcapsular sinuses may be filled with cells which were originally believed to be immature histocytes but have been shown, immuno-histochemically, to be B lymphocytes. Toxoplasmosis produces effects on all three zones of the lymph node and illustrates how overlap between the different patterns can occur. A reflection of reactive hyperplasia is the tingible body macrophage which contains remnants of cell material (Fig. 16.14).

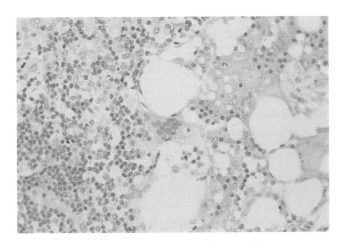

Fig. 16.10 Lipogranulomas seen post lymphangiogram. (H&E.)

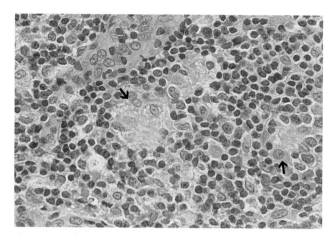

Fig. 16.13 'Congeries' of pale-staining macrophages (arrowed) seen in infectious toxoplasmosis. (H&E.)

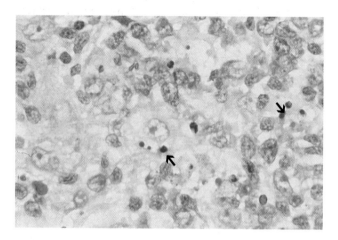

Fig. 16.14 Tingible body macrophages (arrowed) contain phagocytosed cell debris and are a common feature of reactive lymphadenopathy. (H&E.)

THE LYMPHOMAS

Lymphoma is a neoplastic proliferation in tissues of lymphocytes and their precursors. It is one of the less common malignancies, accounting for only 5% of malignant disease in adults, though its general responsiveness to current therapy makes it an important disease to recognize clinically. Two main groups are described—Hodgkin's and non-Hodgkin's lymphoma.

The diagnosis of lymphoma rests on surgical biopsy, although aspiration cytology is becoming increasingly important, particularly as a means of identifying reactive lymph nodes (and thus preventing an unnecessary operation). To give some idea of the numbers involved, over 10 years (1982–1992) 1740 lymph node biopsies were registered in the Oxford Lymphoma Clinic (Table 16.3).

It can be seen that non-Hodgkin's lymphoma (NHL) accounts for more than three-quarters of the diagnoses of lymphoma.

It should be borne in mind that about a quarter of all lymphomas present in an extranodal site, such as the gut or skin. In the Oxford series 446 (31% of all lymphomas) cases were located extranodally, of which only four were Hodgkin's disease. Because of its relative rarity, a lymphoma may be overlooked on a general medical unit as a treatable cause of a pyrexia of unknown origin (PUO), ill-defined malaise or unexplained weight loss. Conversely, lymphoma is not an uncommon incidental finding at an autopsy on an elderly patient dying of something else.

Hodgkin's disease

Hodgkin's disease is defined as a lymphoma characterized by the presence of large abnormal cells in a background of reactive-appearing lymphocytes, macrophages, granulocytes and fibroblasts.

At least a proportion of the abnormal cells must be **Reed–Sternberg cells** which are a characteristic binucleate cell with large eosinophilic nucleoli giving a so-called owl's eye appearance (Fig. 16.15). Dr Thomas Hodgkin, of Guy's Hospital, London, described the first cases in 1832.

Hodgkin's disease is about twice as common in males than females, and shows two peaks of incidence—one in young adults, the other in the elderly.

Histogenesis

The nature of the neoplastic mononuclear and multinuclear cells in Hodgkin's disease remains unclear, though it is now generally agreed that the cell is lymphoid in origin. Hodgkin mononuclear cells and Reed–Sternberg cells have a characteristic immunophenotype by expressing the antigens **CD15** and **CD30**.

Table 16.3 Lymph node biopsies in Oxford, 1982–1992.

Diagnosis	No. of cases	%
Non-Hodgkin's lymphoma	1105	63
Hodgkin's disease	319	18
Reactive	274	16
Non-lymphoid or undiagnosable	42	3
Total	1740	

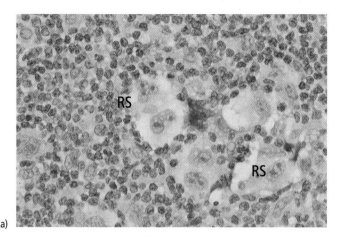

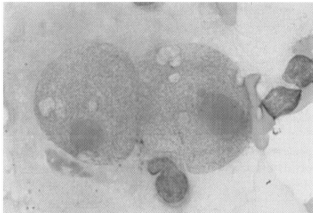

Fig. 16.15 Nodular sclerosing Hodgkin's disease (a) Lymph node biopsy showing a group of Reed–Sternberg cells (RS) with a background of lymphocytes, eosinophils and plasma cells and bands of fibrosis (not shown). (H&E.) (b) Lymph node imprint cytology showing a binucleate Reed–Sternberg cell. (H&E.)

Aetiology

The aetiology of Hodgkin's disease remains unknown. It is likely that no single event is responsible for the malignant transformation underlying the disease, and a series of possibly unrelated steps seems probable. Several lines of evidence suggest that at least one of these steps may involve an infectious agent.

One possibility comes from the presence of significantly raised antibody titres to the Epstein–Barr virus (EBV) in some patients. More recently the development of specific gene probes and antibodies for EBV have shown a high involvement of EBV in Hodgkin's disease. Unfortunately, EBV is also found in a number of other malignancies, both lymphoid and non-lymphoid, which suggests that EBV infection cannot be specific and is presumably acting in a manner synergistic to other transforming agents.

Pathological features

Histological diagnosis. In Hodgkin's disease the lymph node biopsy shows replacement of nodal architecture, with a proliferation of Hodgkin's mononuclear cells and the diagnostic Reed–Sternberg binucleate or multinucleate cells in a characteristic histological setting. In contrast to most NHL, early Hodgkin's disease may affect just part of a node, starting usually in the perifollicular areas.

In contrast to NHL, only **four subtypes** of Hodgkin's disease are generally recognized and have remained accepted by pathologists and clinicians alike since their inception at the Rye Conference in 1966. Virtually all studies have demonstrated distinct differences in survival between the different categories (Fig. 16.16).

1 Lymphocyte-predominant. The infiltrate consists mainly of small lymphocytes with a variable admixture of histiocytes but very few granulocytes or plasma cells. Reed–Sternberg cells are infrequent and are known as **L&H** (lymphocytic and histiocytic) cells to distinguish them from the classical Reed–Sternberg cells of other subtypes. Approximately **10–15%** of cases are lymphocyte-predominant at presentation.

There is now a growing consensus on clinical, histological and immunological grounds that this category of Hodgkin's disease is a distinct clinicopathological entity. The excellent prognosis and prompt response to

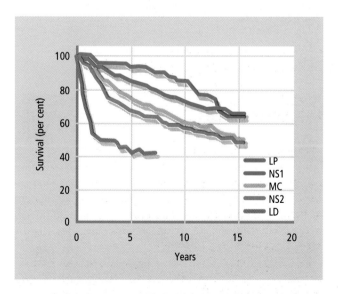

Fig. 16.16 Actuarial survival of patients with Hodgkin's disease. The data are subdivided according to a modified Rye histological classification with subdivision of nodular sclerosis (NS) into grades 1 and 2. (Data from the British National Lymphoma Investigation.) LP, lymphocyte predominant; MC, mixed cellularity; LD, lymphocyte depleted.

treatment have even raised the question whether it should be considered a malignant disease at all.

2 Nodular sclerosing. This subtype is characterized by nodules separated by bands of collagenous connective tissue, a thickened capsule and **lacunar cells** (large atypical cells which have broken away from their attachment to other cells, giving an impression of being an island in a lake; Fig. 16.17). Reed–Sternberg cells are usually easily found and there are variable proportions of lymphocytes, histiocytes, granulocytes (including eosinophils) and plasma cells within the tumour nodules. Approximately **20–50%** of patients present with this type of disease and the proportion of younger patients, often female and with mediastinal disease, is high.

Recently, the British National Lymphoma Investigation (BNLI) group has identified a subtype of nodular sclerosing Hodgkin's disease (accounting for about 20% of these cases) in which the histological picture shows areas of lymphocyte depletion or confluent groups of pleomorphic Reed–Sternberg and Hodgkin's cells. This is called **type II** nodular sclerosing Hodgkin's disease and has a more aggressive natural history than all other types of nodular sclerosis, which are known as **type I**.

3 Mixed cellularity. The architecture of the lymph node is diffusely effaced by a mixed infiltrate with conspicuous granulocytes, especially eosinophils, plasma cells, lymphocytes and histiocytes, and plentiful Reed–Sternberg cells. This type accounts for **20–40%** of cases at presentation.

4 Lymphocyte-depleted. This is characterized by large numbers of atypical mononuclear cells, often pleo-

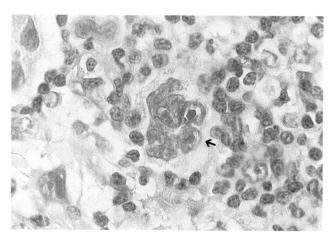

Fig. 16.18 Lymphocyte-depleted Hodgkin's disease. An atypical Hodgkin's cell (arrowed) with a multilobated or 'popcorn' shaped nucleus. (H&E.)

morphic with bizarre mitoses (Fig. 16.18) and many Reed–Sternberg cells, but a paucity of other cells. Often there is accompanying diffuse fibrosis. This form is rare at presentation, accounting for no more than **1–2%** of all cases of Hodgkin's disease.

Non-Hodgkin's lymphoma

The NHLs comprise a group of malignant disorders which by definition include all lymphomas which lack the characteristic histopathological features of Hodgkin's disease—in other words, Reed–Sternberg cells in the appropriate setting are absent and destruction of the normal architecture need not be present.

There is now clear evidence that most, if not all, of these disorders have a **clonal origin** from a single mutant cell. In most cases the malignant cells show characteristics of **B-cell** differentiation, with most of the remainder being of **T-cell** origin. A rather loose definition of lymphoid tissue enables cells of the monocyte macrophage lineage to be included: these cells are frequently described as histiocytes by pathologists, although in the context of lymphomas this term has not always been so precisely used (see below).

Of 729 NHLs immunophenotyped in Oxford from 1982 to 1992, 629 were of **B-cell** origin (**88%**) and 99 were **T cell** (**14%**). Only 1 case was unequivocally histiocytic.

Considerable effort has been made in recent years to characterize these disorders, particularly with respect to their aetiology, cellular and molecular biology, natural history and response to treatment.

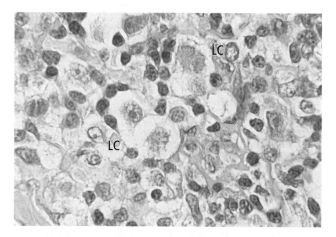

Fig. 16.17 Hodgkin's disease. 'Lacunar cells' (LC) surrounded by their own personal space. (H&E.)

Classification and pathology

Both the clinical and histopathological features of NHL are diverse, and this has led to a plethora of classifications. All of these schemes for classifying NHL suffer from the drawback that they are presented as if based on original scientific data, when in reality they are no more than hypotheses.

The hypothesis behind each lymphoma classification is twofold:
- first, that the scheme identifies distinct disease entities (with the implication that they differ in terms of aetiology and response to therapy);
- second, that the classification can be used reproducibly in practice, both by the expert haematopathologist and by the routine histopathologist.

In recent years our understanding of lymphoid differentiation has increased markedly, helped by immunological techniques which can pinpoint surface antigens on individual cells within suitable histological sections. More recent classifications of NHL have attempted to use this knowledge to relate the nature of the malignant cell to its normal counterpart. Several such schemes have evolved which vary mostly in their interpretation of the cytology and morphology of routine histopathological sections. All have **prognostic significance** because all

make a similar distinction between groups of tumours with a **good prognosis** (**low grade**) and a **bad prognosis** (**high grade**).

Unfortunately it is not easy to make direct translations between the various classifications, which makes comparisons of therapeutic trials difficult to interpret. The 1981 National Cancer Institute (NCI)-sponsored Working Formulation was an attempt to provide a translation between the six most commonly used classifications of NHL. This scheme was not meant to supplant any of those in use already, but is a common language through which, for example, comparison of results of clinical trials may be made (Fig. 16.19).

It should be noted that, in spite of all the efforts put into the classification of NHL, in all series up to 10% of cases cannot be accurately classified with the material or techniques available.

The classification most widely used in European centres is that devised by Lennert's group in Kiel (the Kiel classification; Fig. 16.20). This scheme was updated in 1988 (Table 16.4) to incorporate information gained from cell-marker studies and when combined with a cytological/haematological approach enables a considerable consensus to be reached by non-specialist histopathologists working with routine biopsies. It has **good prognostic correlations** and, like other classifications, separates NHL into those with a relatively good prognosis (low-grade) and others with high-grade or poor prognostic features. The rapid introduction of immunocytochemistry into histology now allows a more refined distinction of different tumour types. With this and other information from molecular and cytogenetic studies a new classification was proposed by the International Lymphoma Study Group

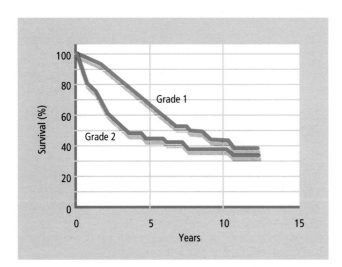

Fig. 16.19 Actuarial survival of patients with non-Hodgkin's lymphoma. The graph is divided into low-grade (1) and high-grade (2) forms of the disease. Patients with high-grade lymphoma have an initial high death rate but the survival curve forms a plateau at 5 years, indicating that a significant proportion of patients are cured of their disease. Low-grade lymphomas, although having an indolent initial course, show a continuing death rate after 5 years and appear to be incurable with current therapies. By 10 years, the survival rates of low and high grade lymphomas are similar. (Data from the British National Lymphoma Investigation.)

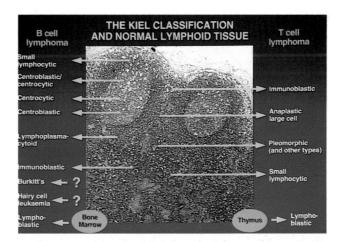

Fig. 16.20 The Kiel classification of non-Hodgkin's lymphoma (NHL).

Table 16.4 Updated Kiel classification of non-Hodgkin's lymphoma. (From *Lancet* 1988, **i**: 292–293.)

Low-grade B	Low-grade T
Lymphocytic–chronic lymphocytic and prolymphocytic leukaemia; hairy cell leukaemia	Lymphocytic–chronic lymphocytic and prolymphocytic leukaemia
Lymphoplasmacytic/cytoid (LP immunocytoma)	Small cerebriform cell–mycosis fungoides, Sézary's syndrome
Plasmacytic	Lymphoepithelioid (Lennert's lymphoma)
Centroblastic/centrocytic	Angioimmunoblastic (AILD, LgX)
Follicular ± diffuse	
Diffuse	T zone
Centrocytic	
	Pleomorphic, small cell (HTLV-1±)
High-grade B	**High-grade T**
Centroblastic	Pleomorphic, medium and large cell (HTLV-1±)
Immunoblastic	
Large cell anaplastic (Ki-1+)	Immunoblastic (HTLV-1±)
Burkitt lymphoma	Large cell anaplastic (Ki-1+)
Lymphoblastic	Lymphoblastic
Rare types	**Rare types**

AILD, angioimmunoblastic lymphoproliferative disease; LgX, lymphogranuloma X; HTLV, human T-lymphotropic virus.

in 1994, termed the revised European–American lymphoma (REAL) classification. Table 16.5 shows a current working classification based on the Kiel classification of 1988 which with minor modifications approximates closely to what many haematopathologists are using today.

The important points to note are that the grading system is morphological. Low-grade tumours have well-differentiated cytological or morphological features. They are composed predominantly of small cells recognizable as lymphocytes or germinal centre cells (Fig. 16.21). High-grade tumours are poorly differentiated, being composed of large, often obviously abnormal cells or smaller blastic cells resembling those seen in childhood acute leukaemia.

Primary extranodal lymphomas

Although NHL is generally discussed as a lymph node disease it should be realized that around 30% of cases at presentation involve structures other than lymph nodes either by direct invasion or by secondary spread, more remotely. Extranodal spread occurs rarely in Hodgkin's disease.

Table 16.5 A revised European–American lymphoma classification (REAL).

Morphology	% NHL	Immunotype
B-CELL LYMPHOMAS		
Low-grade (B)		
Lymphocyte: small lymphocytes	11	Surface Ig, CD5+, CD23+
Immunocytoma: lymphoplasmacytic	12	Cytoplasmic Ig, CD5+, CD23+
Follicular: centroblastic/centrocytic	21	Surface Ig, *bcl*-2+, CD5–, CD10+
Mantle cell: centrocytic	6	Surface Ig, CD5+, CD23–
High-grade (B)		
Large cell: centroblasts and immunoblasts	20	Surface Ig, CD10– (80%)
Burkitt's: cohesive lymphoblast-like	3	Surface Ig, CD10+
Lymphoblastic: lymphoblasts	1	Cytoplasmic Ig, CD10+
Anaplastic large cell: large pleomorphic blast cells with prominent nucleoli	<1	CD30+
T-CELL LYMPHOMAS		
Low-grade (T)		
Lymphocytic: small lymphocytes	1	pan T, CD4 or 8+
Cutaneous: small cerebriform cells	1	pan T, CD4+
Polymorphous: small pleomorphic cells with variable backgrounds	7	pan T, CD4+
High-grade (T)		
Polymorphous: medium and large pleomorphic cells, including immunoblasts	5	pan T, but may show Ag loss, CD4 or 8+, variable HTLV-1+
Lymphoblastic: lymphoblasts	3	pan T, CD7+, may be CD4 or 8+
Anaplastic large cell: large pleomorphic blast cells with prominent nucleoli	2	CD30+

NHL, Non-Hodgkin's lymphoma; Ig, Immunoglobulin; Ag, antigen; HTLV-1, human T-lymphotropic virus-1.

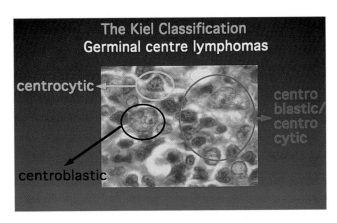

Fig. 16.21 Germinal centre lymphomas according to the Kiel classification.

Lymphomas of mucosa-associated lymphoid tissue

Primary extranodal presentations (without evidence of disease elsewhere) are less common and are almost exclusively confined to the non-Hodgkin's group. A wide variety of tissues may be involved. These most commonly involve the **MALT** of gut, thyroid, lung and salivary gland (the so-called MALTomas), the eye and the skin.

Maltomas may be low- or high-grade and are most common in the stomach. Low-grade tumours are composed of characteristic small centrocyte-like cells with a marked propensity for invading epithelial glands but remain localized to the organ site, be it stomach or thyroid, for many years. It is assumed that high-grade maltomas arise as a transformation of these low-grade tumours. Strikingly, even these high-grade lesions may remain localized for relatively long periods. This results in the important feature that fully resected maltomas have a much better prognosis than their nodal counterparts. Recent studies of **gastric maltoma** have demonstrated an important association with *Helicobacter* infection. It has been shown that treatment of this infection can result in remission of the lymphoma, though whether this will be permanent is currently awaiting long-term follow-up studies.

The histiocytoses

As noted above, true histiocytic lymphomas do occur but are uncommon. Many so-called histiocytic lymphomas, such as histiocytic medullary reticulosis, have been shown by immunohistochemistry to be T-cell lymphomas.

The histiocytoses represent reactive and neoplastic histiocytic disorders and are more common in children and young adults.

Histiocytosis X (Langerhans cell histiocytosis; LCH)

The term histiocytosis X is used to denote three related diseases that all feature Langerhans cell infiltrates (CDIa, S100 positive with Birbeck granules on electron-microscopy; see Chapter 26).

1 Eosinophilic granuloma is a relatively benign disease that involves bone, particularly the skull and ribs of children and young adults. Long bones may be involved. X-ray shows a well-demarcated lytic lesion. Histology demonstrates a diffuse infiltrate composed of histiocytes, giant cells and eosinophils.

2 Hand–Schueller–Christian disease is morphologically similar to eosinophilic granuloma but it is a multifocal disease and has a poor prognosis. It commonly involves the base of the skull to produce proptosis, lytic bone lesions in skull and diabetes insipidus due to destruction of the posterior pituitary.

3 Letterer–Siwe disease is an aggressive, disseminated disease that involves bone and lymphoid tissue in young children. Lymphadenopathy and skin lesions are due to infiltration by large pale neoplastic histiocytes.

LYMPH NODE METASTASES

An enlarged lymph node is commonly the method of clinical presentation of a carcinoma or malignant melanoma. The primary tumour may be occult and lymph node enlargement represents the first clinical feature.

For the histopathologist who examines the lymph node biopsy, the diagnosis of metastatic malignancy is easy if the tumour is well-differentiated (Fig. 16.22). When it is

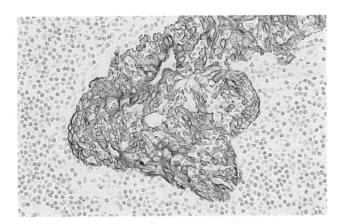

Fig. 16.22 Metastatic squamous carcinoma of the bronchus in a mediastinal lymph node. Immunohistochemistry shows the tumour deposits clearly as they stain positively with antibodies to cytokeratin (brown).

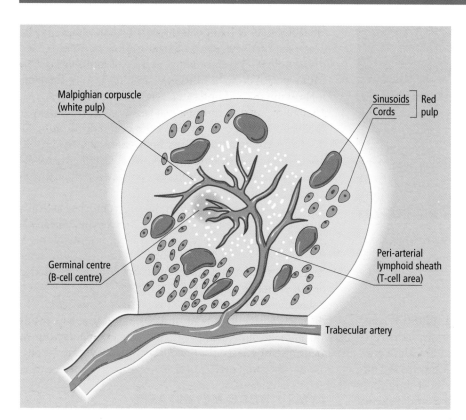

Fig. 16.23 The normal spleen – red pulp and white pulp.

poorly differentiated, the distinction between large cell anaplastic lymphoma, poorly differentiated carcinoma and amelanotic malignant melanoma may be very difficult to make on morphology alone. A panel of immunomarkers will be employed to determine the histogenesis of the tumour cell in such a case and would include a leukocyte marker (for lymphoid cells), cytokeratin (for epithelial cells), endocrine cell marker (chromogranin), melanoma marker (S100) and mesenchymal cell marker (vimentin) prior to use of more specific markers (e.g. for T and B cells, prostate-specific antigen, etc.).

The spleen

Normal structure

The spleen in located in the upper abdomen underneath the left ribcage. The normal splenic weight is between 120 and 140 g. The spleen comprises;

- **white pulp**, composed of the lymphoid follicles (Malpighian corpuscles), which contain B-cell (germinal centres) and T-cell (periarteriolar lymphoid sheath) zones;
- **red pulp**, composed of the sinusoids, lined by

endothelium and separated by the splenic cords (Fig. 16.23).

The main function of the spleen is as a **blood filter**. This function is performed by phagocytic cells or macrophages (littoral cells) that lie in the cords and sinusoids. These macrophages remove senescent erythrocytes from the blood and have Fc receptors that permit them to recognize antibody-complexed particles in the blood and phagocytose them. In patients with autoimmune haemolytic anaemias and thrombocytopenia, the spleen represents a major site of cell destruction.

In otherwise normal adults, splenectomy results in minimal immunodeficiency (Fig. 16.24). In young children, splenectomy is followed by an increased susceptibility to infection with encapsulated organisms such as *Streptococcus pneumoniae* and *Salmonella* spp.

Causes of splenomegaly

When splenic enlargement occurs, the spleen can be palpated under the left costal margin. Splenomegaly represents the commonest manifestation of splenic disease and can itself have clinical consequences (Fig. 16.25). The causes of splenomegaly are similar to the causes of

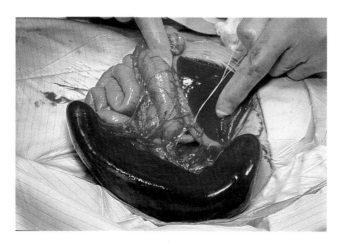

Fig. 16.24 A splenectomy being performed for splenomegaly in a 3-year-old child.

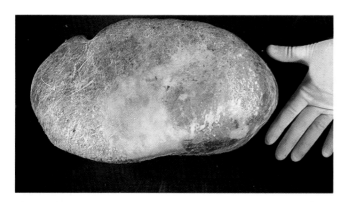

Fig. 16.25 Massive splenomegaly in a patient with myelofibrosis. This 5 kg spleen was received by the histopathologist as a routine surgical pathology specimen in the cut-up room.

lymphadenopathy (Table 16.6); however, additional features are included that relate to the role of the spleen as a blood filter for the blood and as a potential haematopoietic organ.

In acute and chronic infections, splenomegaly results from proliferation of immunologically reactive lymphocytes. Malpighian corpuscles are generally much enlarged and may show reactive B-cell proliferative centres. In most infections, a combined T- and B-cell response is seen. Histiocytic responses may predominate in certain diseases such as brucellosis and *Leishmania*.

Sarcoidosis produces numerous discrete granulomatous lesions resembling those seen in lymph nodes. Disseminated tuberculosis may produce a similar appearance. Storage diseases also show abundant histiocytes; splenomegaly being marked in Gaucher's disease, and Niemann–Pick disease.

In portal hypertension, initially, there is an expanded red pulp consisting of dilated sinuses filled with red

blood cells; in chronic portal hypertension, there may be fibrosis, haemorrhage and haemosiderin deposition.

The spleen is involved in a variety of leukaemias. The white pulp becomes infiltrated in chronic lymphocytic leukaemia; the red pulp is involved in hairy cell leukaemia, myelocytic and monocytic leukaemias. Extramedullary haemopoiesis is a common feature of leukaemias.

NHLs may involve the splenic white pulp. Hodgkin's disease produces multifocal disease in the spleen, initially within the white pulp but later forming large, diffuse confluent nodules.

A small, shrunken spleen may be seen in sickle-cell anaemia, in which the spleen fibroses and shrivels (autosplenectomy).

Hypersplenism

Splenic enlargement from any cause may rarely result in anaemia, leukopenia and thrombocytopenia due to increased **sequestration** and **destruction** of red cells, white cells and platelets in the spleen. Splenectomy is curative.

Table 16.6 Causes of splenomegaly.

Splenic cysts and hamartomas
Infections Infectious mononucleosis, typhoid fever, malaria, brucellosis, infective endocarditis, malaria, leishmaniasis
Lymphomas Non-Hodgkins's lymphomas, Hodgkin's disease
Leukaemias Chronic lymphocytic leukaemia, hairy cell leukaemia, monocytoid leukaemias, chronic myelocytic leukaemia, histocytosis X
Autoimmune disease Rheumatoid arthritis, systemic lupus erythematosus, idiopathic thrombocytopenic purpura
Sarcoidosis
Amyloidosis
Storage diseases Gaucher's disease; Niemann–Pick disease
Portal hypertension Cirrhosis, portal vein thrombosis
Haematological disorders Haemolytic anaemias (thalassaemia, autoimmune), extramedullary erythropoiesis, myelofibrosis, polycythaemia rubra vera

The thymus

The thymus is in the anterior superior mediastinum. It is most functionally active before birth, where it plays a vital role in the development and differentiation of T lymphocytes. This function is largely complete at birth, and thymectomy, even in the neonatal period, produces little immunological impairment.

The thymus undergoes gradual involution after childhood and in adults the thymus is replaced by fat in which are scattered occasional lymphoid nodules and Hassall's corpuscles (Fig. 16.26).

Abnormalities in thymic structure are associated with congenital immunodeficiency disease and have been described in Chapter 10.

Thymic hyperplasia

There is no thymic response that mirrors the normal hyperplasia of lymphoid tissue that occurs in the lymph nodes, spleen, or MALT in response to immune stimulation such as occurs in infection. However, the term thymic hyperplasia persists in current usage and denotes the presence of reactive follicles of B-cell proliferation seen in the thymic medulla. This phenomenon is rarely seen in normal individuals, but is the key feature of myasthenia gravis and, to a lesser extent, some other autoimmune diseases (Fig. 16.27).

Myasthenia gravis

Approximately 80% of patients with myasthenia gravis show germinal or reactive centres within the thymic medulla and another 10% of patients with myasthenia gravis have thymomas (see below).

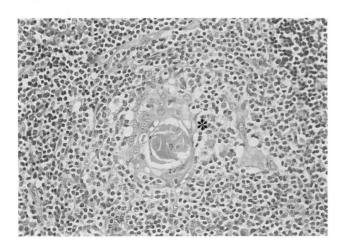

Fig. 16.26 The normal thymus. A Hassall's corpuscle (✳). (H&E.)

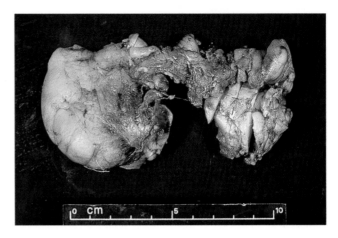

Fig. 16.27 Thymic hyperplasia in a patient with myasthenia gravis.

A variety of abnormal immunological findings have been described in myasthenia gravis, including:
- lymphocytic infiltrates in muscle;
- depressed mitogen responses for T cells;
- anti-DNA antibodies;
- antithymocyte antibodies, and, most importantly;
- **antibodies** to motor end-plate **acetylcholine receptors**.

Thymectomy leads to a gradual improvement in symptoms in many patients, possibly due to removal of a cross-reacting antigen or of a T-helper cell population within the thymus that promotes production of the antireceptor antibody.

Thymic neoplasms

Primary neoplasms of the thymus may result from any of its cell components, including lymphocytes, epithelial cells, fibroblasts, endothelial cells and neuroendocrine cells. Thymomas have some particular interesting features.

Thymic lymphomas

NHLs of T-cell type may involve the thymus and occasionally appear ro originate in the thymus. B-cell lymphomas are less common but may extend into the organ from involved mediastinal lymph nodes. Nodular sclerosing Hodgkin's disease typically involves the mediastinum and thymus.

Acute lymphoblastic leukaemia of T-cell type particularly involves the thymus. This disease presents as a mediastinal mass, and characteristically is a disease of young men and terminates in acute lymphoblastic leukaemia. The neoplastic T lymphoblasts show immuno-

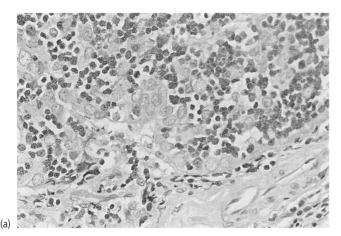

(a)

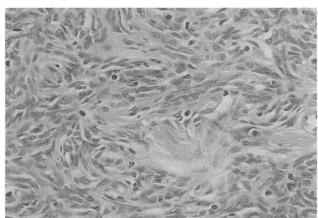

(b)

Fig. 16.28 Thymoma (a) Classical appearance in which the epithelial cells may be over-run by lymphocytes. (H&E.) (b) The epithelial variant of malignant thymoma. (H&E.)

Table 16.7 Classification of thymoma.

Traditional classification	Histogenetic classification
Non-invasive thymoma (benign)	Medullary thymoma Mixed thymoma
Invasive (malignant) thymoma	Cortical thymoma Well-differentiated thymic carcinoma
Thymic carcinoma	Epidermoid carcinoma Endocrine carcinoma Undifferentiated carcinoma

Table 16.8 Thymoma disease associations.

Myasthenia gravis: 10% of myasthenia patients have thymoma
Other (non-thymic) tumours
Other autoimmune diseases
Pure red cell aplasia: 50% of aplastic patients have thymoma
Neutropenia with or without thrombocytopenia
Hypogammaglobulinaemia
Polymyositis
Myocarditis
Systemic lupus erythematosus
Immunoglobulin A deficiency and multiple neoplasms

logical features in common with thymic lymphocytes and have a suppressor phenotype (CD8).

Thymoma

A thymoma is a neoplasm derived from thymic epithelial cells, which will often contain large numbers of non-neoplastic T lymphocytes. The lymphocytes may be so numerous and the epithelial cells so inconspicuous that the distinction from lymphoma is difficult (Fig. 16.28).

Thymomas may present due to local effects of compression (e.g. with stridor) or infiltration of adjacent structures, or they may produce a range of paraneoplastic syndromes (Tables 16.7 and 16.8).

Thymomas are rare tumours, but several histological subtypes have been described.

- **Well-differentiated thymomas** resemble normal thymus and are usually encapsulated and benign. In other cases, the epithelial cells are larger and more numerous.
- **Poorly differentiated thymomas** feature epithelial cells with a spindle appearance (spindle cell thymoma; Fig. 16.28(b)). Capsular invasion occurs in some tumours and may be followed by local invasion in a minority of cases. Distant metastases are rare.

Thymic seminoma and teratoma

Seminoma and seminoma with other germ cell neoplastic elements may occur in the thymus as primary extragonadal neoplasms. They resemble the corresponding tumours of ovary or testis. It is important to distinguish these seminomas from epithelial thymomas, as seminomas are radiosensitive.

C H A P T E R　17

Diseases of the Ear and Respiratory Tract

C O N T E N T S

continued

The ear

INTRODUCTION

The ear may be divided into these regions (Fig. 17.1):
- the **inner ear**, consisting of the semicircular canals and the cochlea;
- the **middle ear**, which is separated from the external auditory meatus by the tympanic membrane and which communicates with the pharynx via the eustachian tube and with the mastoid air sinuses;
- the **external ear**, which includes the external auditory meatus, pinna and auricle.

The skin of the pinna is prone to the range of infections and tumours described in Chapter 26. The following account will consider the conditions that are specific to the ear.

INFECTIONS

Otitis externa

The normal flora of the ear canal is similar to that found in the skin.
- *Staphylococcus aureus* and *Streptococcus pyogenes* are the main pathogens;

    Pseudomonas aeruginosa may colonize the canal and is

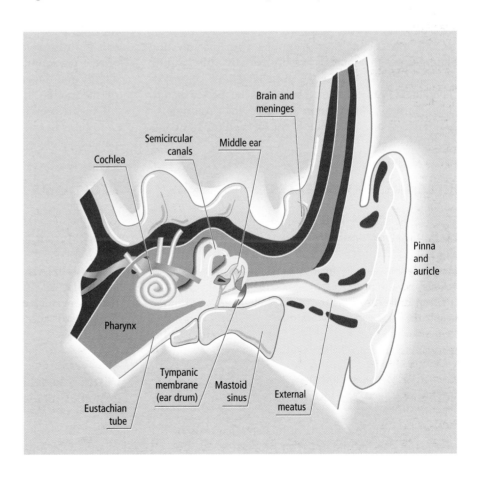

Fig. 17.1 The structure of the ear.

rarely pathogenic but is the infectious agent of **malignant otitis externa,** a severe necrotizing infection of all tissues which occurs especially in diabetics.

Aspergillus may be pathogenic. Management is by aural toilet and by use of drying agents (alcohol/acetic acid) and topical antimicrobials (combined with steroids).

Otitis media

Otitis media is very common in childhood with a peak incidence between 6 and 24 months. Recurrent attacks are an important cause of impaired hearing. The majority of infections are bacterial and common pathogens include *Streptococcus pneumoniae,* non-capsulated *Haemophilus influenzae, S. pyogenes* and *Moraxella catarrhalis.*

The cause of otitis media is a blocked eustachian tube, usually due to enlarged adenoid glands; this interferes with ventilation and drainage, leading to an accumulation of fluid (**glue ear**) which may become secondarily infected.

Clinical findings include ear pain, discharge, a redness of the tympanic membrane and, in the infant, irritability, fever and vomitting. Complications include recurrent attacks, chronic otitis media, deafness, mastoiditis and brain abscess.

Otitis media may be self-limiting with the infection undergoing spontaneous resolution by discharging via the tympanic membrane. Amoxycillin or co-amoxiclavulanate is advised for treatment of suspected pathogens. Surgical intervention involves the insertion of **grommets** to drain the middle ear through the tympanic membrane.

INFLAMMATORY DISEASES

Inflammatory dermatoses

Herpes zoster involving the facial nerve may result in vesicles on the outer ear.

Chondrodermatitis nodularis helicis is a common lesion that occurs due to trauma. It involves ulceration and inflammation of the skin with degeneration of the underlying cartilage of the helix.

Otosclerosis

This disease process results in bilateral **sclerosis of the ossicles** of the middle ear with progessive deafness. It

occurs during the third and fourth decades. The disease is of unknown cause but it has a familial tendency (autosomal dominant). It results in a progessive increase in density, loss of vascularity and fusion of the middle ear ossicles.

Acute labyrinthitis

Acute labyrinthitis commonly has a **viral** cause and may occur rarely as part of a systemic mumps or measles infection. Patients present with sudden hearing loss and vertigo. The disease is usually self-limiting.

Bacterial labyrinthitis is rarer and occurs due to extension of a suppurative otitis media. It may result in permanent deafness due to destruction of the middle ear ossicles.

Ménière's disease

This disease results in hydrops of the labyrinth due to an imbalance between secretion and absorption of endolymphatic fluid. This results in increased endolymphatic pressure in the cochlear duct, leading to degeneration of the cochlear hair cells, the end-organ of hearing.

It is a disease of middle age, is usually unilateral and affects predominantly men. The cause is unknown but allergy and degenerative vascular disease have been implicated in its aetiology.

Patients present with tinnitus, vertigo and a sensation of fullness in the ear. There is no effective treatment and patients often require surgery.

NEOPLASMS

The external ear

The external ear is a common site for neoplasms such as basal cell carcinoma, squamous cell carcinoma and malignant melanoma (see Chapter 26). Osteoma (see Chapter 20) and adenoma of the ceruminous glands are rare.

Extra-adrenal paraganglioma (glomus jugulare tumour)

Below the floor of the middle ear lies the jugular vein glomus which gives rise to a particular paraganglioma, the glomus jugulare tumour. This tumour may erode into the middle ear and produce deafness. These tumours may be locally aggressive but they do not metastasize.

Upper respiratory tract

INTRODUCTION

The respiratory system has two components. The upper respiratory tract (URT) comprises the oropharynx, nasopharynx, tonsils, epiglottis, larynx and trachea (Fig. 17.2). The lower respiratory tract comprises the bronchi and lungs.

The pathology of the mouth and salivary glands is discussed in Chapter 18.

INFECTIONS

Introduction

The upper respiratory tract is colonized with bacteria, including the potential pathogens *Streptococcus pneumoniae* and *Haemophilus influenzae*. The lower respiratory tract, beyond the terminal bronchioles, is normally sterile.

Viral infections make up the bulk of respiratory tract infections, although it is often difficult to distinguish between a bacterial and viral aetiology and antibiotics are often over-prescribed.

The common viruses and bacteria can infect several different sites of the respiratory tract and cause a variety of clinical conditions. The four main bacterial pathogens are:

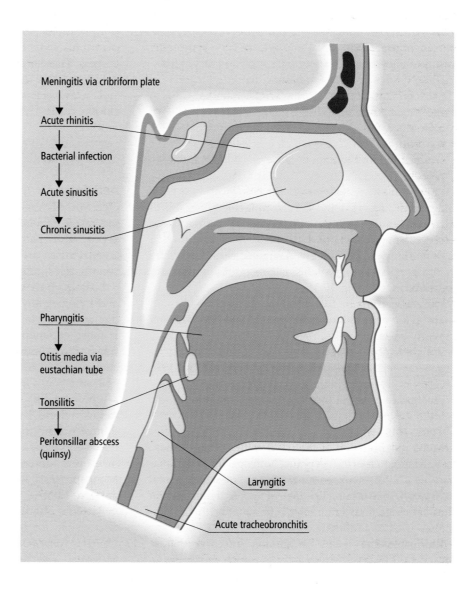

Meningitis via cribriform plate

Acute rhinitis

Bacterial infection

Acute sinusitis

Chronic sinusitis

Pharyngitis

Otitis media via eustachian tube

Tonsilitis

Peritonsillar abscess (quinsy)

Laryngitis

Acute tracheobronchitis

Fig. 17.2 Diseases of the upper respiratory tract.

- *S. pneumoniae*—in the UK, 97% of strains are sensitive to penicillin but resistance worldwide is increasing;
- *H. influenzae* b—non-capsulated strains cause the majority of less severe diseases; capsulated type b cause life-threatening diseases—85% sensitive to ampicillin;
- *S. pyogenes* (Lancefield group A streptococcus); 100% sensitive to penicillin;
- *Moraxella (Branhamella) catarrhalis*—15% are sensitive to ampicillin.

Rhinitis

Acute rhinitis

Acute infectious rhinitis (coryza) is almost always the result of a viral infection and is one of the commonest infections of humans.

A large range of viruses cause the **common cold syndrome**; in order of importance these are rhinovirus, coronavirus, parainfluenza and influenza viruses, respiratory syncytial virus (RSV) and adenovirus. Symptoms include rhinorrhoea, pharyngitis, cough and laryngitis.

These viruses have in common:

- predominant infection during winter months;
- short incubation period, 2–3 days;
- high attack rate;
- short duration of illness which is self-limiting;
- reinfections are common because of multiple antigenic types.

Rhinoviruses are responsible for 30% of all infections and consist of over 100 different antigenic types. Influenza viruses undergo periodic antigenic change, large changes being associated with pandemics resulting in high morbidity and mortality. Antigenic variation occurs in the surface viral proteins haemagglutinin (H) and neuramidase (N) (Fig. 17.3).

Variation occurs by two different mechanisms:

- **antigenic drift**; minor changes in H and N occur on a yearly basis;
- **antigenic shift**; major changes in H and N occur by genetic reassortment. Pandemics occurred in 1918 (H1N1), 1957 (H2N2), 1968 (H3N2) and 1977 (re-emergence of H1N1 in a susceptible population).

Chronic rhinitis

Chronic inflammation of the nasal cavity occurs in leprosy, leishmaniasis and syphilis. Non-specific inflammation also occurs with cocaine sniffing, in which septal perforation may occur. Histology of the nasal mucosa will show a foreign body granuloma inflammation due to substances used to adulterate cocaine.

Rhinoscleroma is an uncommon infection that is caused by *Klebsiella rhinoscleromatis*, which multiplies in macrophages in the nasal mucosa. **Rhinosporidiosis** caused by the fungus *Rhinosporidium seeberi*, occurs in India but is rare elsewhere. It typically forms large nasal polyps. Rhinosporidium cannot be grown in culture.

Sinusitis

The maxillary, ethmoid and frontal sinuses are normally sterile. However in chronic disease the sinuses become colonized with respiratory flora with infections representing acute exacerbations. The majority of infections are secondary bacterial invaders following a viral illness. *H. influenzae* and *S. pneumoniae* are the organisms found most commonly.

Sinusitis can cause local tenderness, postnasal discharge and headache, sometimes accompanied by fever and cervical lymph node enlargement. Extension of the inflammation to adjacent structures may lead to serious complications such as osteomyelitis, orbital cellulitis, cavernous sinus thrombophlebitis, meningitis and brain abscess. These are rare complications.

Management of sinusitis involves use of amoxycillin and co-amoxiclavulanate with drainage in complicated or chronic disease.

Pharyngitis

Aetiology

Over 90% of cases of pharyngitis (including tonsillitis) are the result of viral infections—influenza, parainfluenza, myxo- and paramyxoviruses, adenovirus, RSV and enteroviruses are the usual causes. Viral infections are usually self-limited.

Epstein–Barr virus (EBV; infectious mononucleosis) and cytomegalovirus produce pharyngitis as part of a distinctive systemic illness. Infectious mononucleosis is more common in children and young adults and is transmitted commonly by kissing. Patients present with acute onset of fever, sore throat, lymphadenopathy and splenomegaly. EBV infects B cells which possess a receptor for EBV on the cell membrane. Infected B cells induce a florid T-cell immune response with the production of transformed mononuclear cells in the lymphoid tissue and peripheral blood. Diagnosis is by detection of heterophil antibodies to EBV (Paul–Bunnell or the Monospot test), EBV membrane antigen (MA) or nuclear antigen (EBNA).

Bacterial infection, most commonly with *S. pyogenes*, is responsible for less than 10% of cases of pharyngitis. *Neisseria gonorrhoeae*, *Mycoplasma pneumoniae* and *Corynebacterium diphtheriae* are rare causes. Non-group A

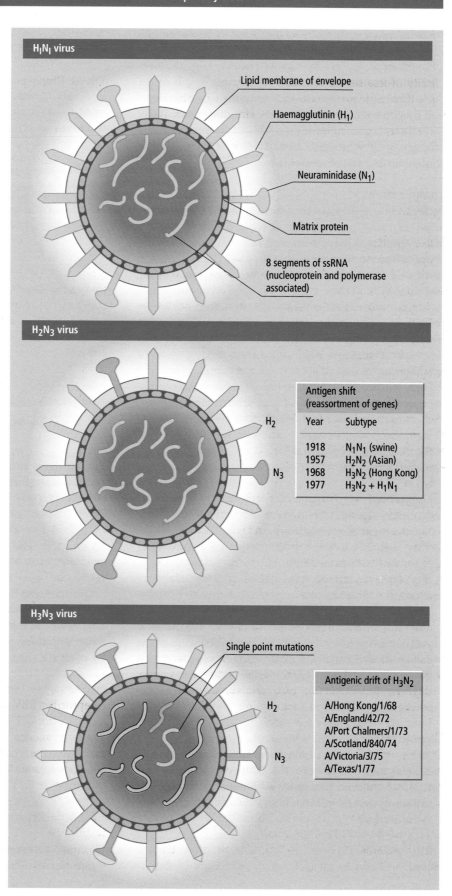

Fig. 17.3 The influenza viruses. Antigenic variation occurs in the surface viral proteins haemagglutinin (H) and neuraminidase (N).

β-haemolytic streptococci, group C and G, are occasionally associated with pharyngitis.

Clinical presentation

Clinically, **acute pharyngitis** and **tonsillitis** are characterized by hyperaemia of the mucosa with sore throat. Fever is commonly present. Certain strains of streptococci may produce an erythrogenic toxin, giving a characteristic erythematous rash of **scarlet fever**.

Complications

Bacterial infections may lead to suppuration around the tonsil to cause **peritonsillar abscess (quinsy)**. Quinsy may present as a mass, pain on swallowing and inability to open the mouth (trismus) due to spasm of the masseter. Abscesses may also occur in the retropharyngeal space and rarely involve the vertebral bone. Tonsils subject to recurring inflammation may be advantageously removed; otherwise, the enlarged tonsils and adenoids simply represent reactive hyperplasia of the lymphoid tissue of Waldeyer's ring, part of the body's defence mechanism.

Early treatment of streptococcal infections is important because it decreases the risk of suppurative complications and **acute rheumatic fever**, which occur as complications of streptococcal pharyngitis. There is no evidence that early treatment reduces the risk of poststreptococcal glomerulonephritis.

Management

Culture of a throat swab is essential for diagnosis.

Management of acute pharyngitis is as follows:

- Take a throat swab with the option of commencing treatment with penicillin V.
- If no bacterial pathogen is isolated, stop treatment.
- If group A streptococcus is isolated, complete a 10-day course.

The differential diagnosis of exudative tonsillitis is glandular fever (EBV). Penicillin V is used because of the possible idiosyncratic skin rash which is produced as a result of the interaction of amoxycillin and EBV infection.

Therapeutic failures of *S. pyogenes* pharyngitis are common because:

- antibiotic courses are too short;
- reinfection may occur with another strain;
- there is a possible role of β-lactamase-producing organisms;
- < 20% of children may be asymptomatic carriers of this organism and be falsely diagnosed as having a bacterial infection.

Epiglottitis and croup

The incidence of epiglottitis has declined due to an effective vaccination programme. It has to be distiguished from the commoner viral infection, croup, which represents as an acute laryngotracheobronchitis (Table 17.1).

Table 17.1 A comparison of croup and epiglottitis.

	Croup	Epiglottitis
Condition	Inflammation of subglottic area	Cellulitis of epiglottis (cherry-red epiglottis)
Agent	Viral, parainfluenza	*Haemophilus influenzae* type b (Hib)
Seasonal variation	Winter	None
Age range	3 months to 3 years	2–4 years
Preceding URTI	Yes	No
Barking cough	Yes	No
Drooling	Slight	Yes
Toxic	Mildly	Yes (100% bacteraemic)
Treatment	Supportive	Intravenous cefotaxime or chloramphenicol

URTI, Upper respiratory tract infection.

Epiglottitis is caused by *H. influenzae* type b and can be rapidly fatal. Inspection of the epiglottis may precipitate complete airway obstruction and throat swabs are rarely taken. The site of maximal involvement is the epiglottis, though in severe cases the entire larynx and trachea may be affected. The acute inflammation and its attendant swelling result in narrowing of the air passages, causing respiratory obstruction.

Croup (acute laryngotracheobronchitis) is acute respiratory difficulty with cyanosis in a child. The subglottic area is inflamed and narrowed, resulting in the characteristic inspiratory sounds of croup. It is commonly caused by parainfluenza virus.

Laryngitis

Acute laryngitis frequently accompanies viral and bacterial infections of the URT, causing pain and hoarseness. It is usually self-limited.

Diphtheria

Diphtheria is a systemic disease caused by the toxin of the Gram-positive bacillus *Corynebacterium diphtheriae*. It has become rare in developed countries because of effective immunization in childhood (the D in DPT vaccine represents diphtheria toxoid). However, imported cases do occur, especially where immunization programmes have been disrupted.

Diphtheria is transmitted by droplet infection. Nasal, facial, cutaneous and laryngeal forms of diphtheria are recognized depending on the site of maximum involvement. Laryngeal diphtheria is the most common form as well as the most dangerous. The bacterium infects the mucosa, causing acute inflammation with exudation and necrosis. A characteristic adherent grey membrane at the back of the throat is seen. Respiratory obstruction is a common cause of death in diphtheria and may require emergency tracheotomy. The toxin has systemic effects on the heart and nervous system.

The laboratory should be alerted to the possible diagnosis as culture of this organism is often not routine. Management includes treatment with diphtheria antitoxin, penicillin or erythromycin and contact tracing. Revaccination is recommended for some parts of the world.

Fungal infections

Aspergillus causes an acute nasal inflammation in immunocompromised patients. Extensive tissue necrosis occurs due to invasion of blood vessels with thrombosis, frequently spreading to the adjacent orbit and the cranial cavity. *Aspergillus* in culture features thin, dichotomously branching, septate hyphae.

Mucormycosis is a infection caused by fungi of the class Phycomycetes, most commonly *Mucor* species. Patients with diabetic ketoacidotic coma and patients being treated for cancer with immunosuppressive anticancer drugs are those usually affected. Irregularly branching non-septate hyphae can be identified by microscopy and culture.

INFLAMMATORY DISEASES

Allergic rhinitis

Type I hypersensitivity (atopy) is a common cause of acute rhinitis (hayfever). Susceptible patients are affected by a variety of allergens, most commonly pollens and dust.

Allergic polyps

Repeated episodes of acute rhinitis result in the development of nasal polyps. These common nasal 'tumours' occur mainly in young adults and are usually multiple.

Similar polyps may occur in the sinuses. Microscopically, they are composed of oedematous stroma in which are found numerous neutrophils, eosinophils, lymphocytes and plasma cells. Eosinophils are more numerous in allergic than inflammatory polyps. Nasal polyps may cause nasal obstruction and frequently need to be removed surgically.

Wegener's granulomatosis

Wegener's granulomatosis is a rare disease which in its fully expressed form involves the upper and lower respiratory tract (see below) and the renal glomeruli (Chapter 21). Nasal lesions occur in up to 60% of patients and are characterized clinically by destructive granulation tissue masses in the nasopharynx. Biopsies of the nasal lesions may show necrotizing granulomas and a severe vasculitis (see Chapter 15).

Lethal midline granuloma

This is a clinical term applied to a group of diseases characterized by a severe acute destructive ulcerative lesion of the middle of the face, including the nasal cavity. The cause may be bacterial or fungal infection, Wegener's granulomatosis or malignancy, particularly malignant lymphoma.

NEOPLASMS OF THE UPPER RESPIRATORY TRACT

Nasopharynx

Nasal neoplasms are uncommon but are variable in their nature and presentation (Table 17.2). They may present as polyps in the nasal cavity. Benign and malignant tumours may ulcerate and bleed, producing **epistaxis**. Malignant neoplasms tend to metastasize via lymphatics to the cervical lymph nodes.

Polyps
Any neoplasm of the nasal cavity may present as a polyp. The most common benign neoplasm is a squamous papilloma known as **inverted papilloma** which is locally infiltrative and has a tendency to recur. **Juvenile angiofibroma** is a benign, highly vascular lesion in the nose of young men which tends to bleed profusely.

Lymphoma
Waldeyer's ring of lymphoid tissue in the oropharynx is a

Table 17.2 Neoplasms of the nasopharynx.

Neoplasm	Location	Behaviour	Microscopic appearance	Age at presentation
Juvenile angiofibroma	Roof of nasal cavity	Benign	Large blood vessels and fibrous tissue	Mainly in young adult males
Squamous papilloma	Nasal cavity, septum, sinuses	Benign	Papillary squamous epithelium	Adults
Inverted papilloma	Nasal cavity, lateral wall	Benign but may recur	Papillary epithelial growth; infiltrative	Adults
Malignant lymphoma	Nasal cavity, sinuses	Malignant	Monoclonal lymphoid proliferation	All ages
Embryonal rhabdomyosarcoma (sarcoma botryoides)	Nasal cavity	Malignant	Primitive small cells; striated muscle, differentiation	Children
Olfactory neuroblastoma (aesthesioneuroblastoma)	Nasal cavity	Malignant	Primitive small cells; rosettes and neurofibrils	Children, adults
Squamous carcinoma	Nasal cavity sinuses, nasopharynx, hypopharynx	Malignant	Infiltrative proliferation of atypical squamous epithelium	Adults

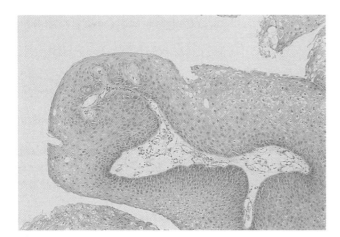

Fig. 17.4 Larynx. Histology of a benign squamous papilloma. (H&E.)

common site for occurrence of extranodal malignant lymphoma. Most are of B-cell origin and they tend to be high-grade.

Nasopharyngeal carcinoma

Squamous carcinoma of the nasopharynx has a striking geographic distribution, being very common in the **Far East** and East Africa. It has been linked to **EBV** infection. EBV viral genome has been identified in the tumour cells but the mechanism of EBV carcinogenesis is unknown. Nasopharyngeal carcinoma (NPC) may occur at all ages but is particularly common in younger patients. The incidence of the disease is also increased in smokers.

NPC metastasizes to cervical lymph nodes and may locally infiltrate the skull base, involving cranial nerves at the base of the brain.

Adenocarcinoma of the nasopharynx is a rare tumour that was first described in furniture makers in High Wycombe, UK. It is associated with the inhalation of hardwood dust.

Larynx

The larynx is a specialized structure that is responsible for converting expired air into specific sounds during speech. It is encased in cartilage and lined by a stratified squamous epithelium that changes to respiratory columnar epithelium inferior to the true vocal cords.

Benign neoplasms

The larynx is a common site for formation of **benign squamous papillomas** (Fig. 17.4). Laryngeal nodule, sometimes called singer's nodule, follows prolonged trauma and is found on the true vocal cord. These are not true neoplasms but consist of fibromyxoid tissue covered by epithelium. Although benign, these lesions may recur. Treatment is by surgical excision.

Squamous carcinoma

Laryngeal squamous carcinoma (Fig. 17.5) is a tumour of predominantly men in their middle age. This malignancy is seen more commonly in **smokers**.

As is common to many squamous carcinomas, laryngeal squamous carcinomas are often preceded by foci of intraepithelial neoplasia or severe dysplasia. These areas can be visualized as white patches or plaques.

Squamous carcinomas are classified anatomically as follows:
- **glottic**; arising in the vocal cords;
- **supraglottic**; arising in the epiglottis and aryepiglottic folds;
- **subglottic**; arising below the vocal cords.

Patients with these tumours may present with hoarseness or laryngeal obstruction. Laryngeal carcinoma may be well-differentiated (verrucous squamous carcinoma). Treatment is by surgical excision and radiotherapy.

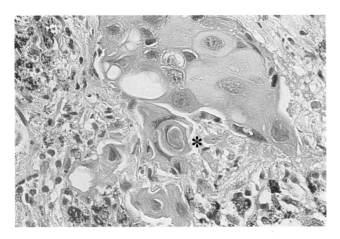

Fig. 17.5 Larynx. Histology of a squamous carcinoma. Note the keratin formation (✱).

Lower respiratory tract

ANATOMY AND DEFENCE OF THE LUNG

The anatomy of the lung represents a compromise between conflicting requirements of economy as regards tissue volume and efficiency of function, i.e. extensive alveolar surface area for gas exchange, combined with aerodynamic and other defence mechanisms.

The structure is adapted to gas transport in airways, gas mixing in acini and gas transfer across the alveolar–capillary membrane (Fig. 17.6).

The lung can be divided into three anatomical zones on the basis of these three functions.

- **Conducting zone.** Airways and elastic arteries.

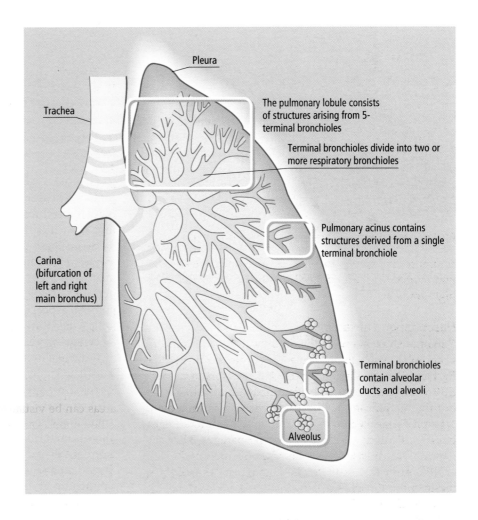

Pleura

Trachea

The pulmonary lobule consists of structures arising from 5-terminal bronchioles

Terminal bronchioles divide into two or more respiratory bronchioles

Pulmonary acinus contains structures derived from a single terminal bronchiole

Carina (bifurcation of left and right main bronchus)

Terminal bronchioles contain alveolar ducts and alveoli

Alveolus

Fig. 17.6 Structure of the lower respiratory tract.

- **Transition zone.** Terminal bronchioles and muscular pulmonary arteries.
- **Exchange zone.** Acini and alveolar capillary complex.

Conducting zone

- **Bronchi** (Figs 17.7 and 17.8) are defined as 'airways with cartilage in their walls'. They are lined by a pseudostratified columnar ciliated epithelium lying on a basement membrane deep to which there are seromucinous glands, smooth muscle and a variable quantity of connective tissue. Bronchi and bronchioles (see below) divide dichotomously with the total cross-sectional area of the daughter airways being greater than that of the parent airway. This results in a dramatic decrease in air flow in the more distal parts of the lung.
- **Cells of the bronchial mucosa** (Fig 17.9). Lying on the

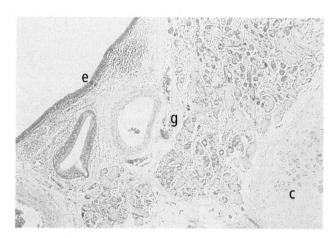

Fig. 17.7 Wall of bronchus containing cartilage (c) and seromucinous glands (g). e, epithelium. (H&E.)

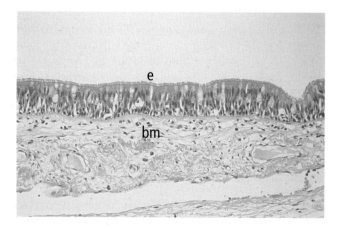

Fig. 17.8 Bronchial mucosa consisting of pseudostratified columnar ciliated epithelium (e) lying on a thin basement membrane (bm). (H&E.)

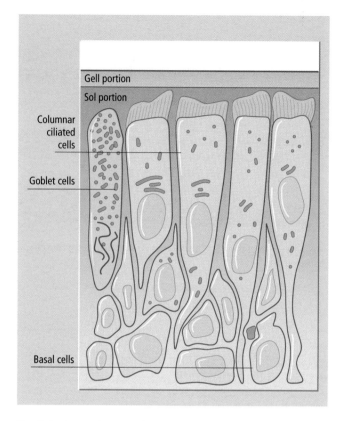

Fig. 17.9 Diagram showing cells in bronchial mucosa.

bronchial basement membrane is a layer of small cells with hyperchromatic nuclei and a high nuclear/cytoplasmic ratio; these are the basal or reserve cells. Interspersed between these there are occasional clear cells, known as Feyter cells, which contain in their cytoplasm dense core neurosecretory granules and which send thin cytoplasmic extensions towards the luminal surface. On the luminal aspect of the basal cells is a layer of intermediate cells which differentiate into either columnar ciliated cells or mucus-secreting goblet cells.

Bronchial mucosa has remarkable regenerative powers and if it is shed either as a result of trauma, mucosal oedema or infections, e.g. in influenza, the basal cells proliferate and differentiate firstly into a simple stratified squamous type epithelium (Fig. 17.10) which, providing there is no further insult to the mucosa, differentiates into normal ciliated epithelium in 3–4 weeks. During the period when the bronchus is lined by simple non-ciliated epithelium it is especially vulnerable to inhaled particles as a consequence of absence of the ciliary defence mechanism.

- **Bronchioles** (Fig. 17.11) differ from bronchi in that they do not have cartilage in their walls; seromucinous glands are less prominent and indeed absent in more distal

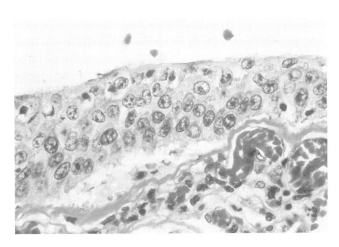

Fig. 17.10 Squamous metaplasia in regenerating bronchial mucosa. (H&E.)

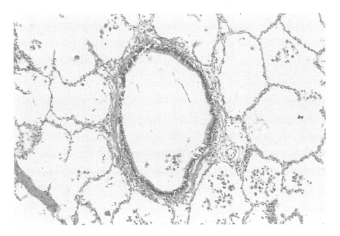

Fig. 17.11 Bronchiole with an absence of cartilage and seromucinous glands in its wall. (H&E.)

branches, and their walls are much thinner. Yet the proportion of the wall occupied by muscle is greater than in bronchi. Their mucosa is only one or two cells thick in the distal branches and contains occasional small pyramidal-shaped cells, interspersed between columnar ciliated cells, known as Clara cells. Their precise function is not understood but they probably secrete a surfactant-like substance.
• **Terminal bronchioles** supply the acinus which is the primary respiratory unit of the lung. They divide into two first-order respiratory bronchioles.

Pulmonary defence in the conducting zone

The structure of these airways assists in the defence of the lung. Most agents which are pathogenic to the lungs are inhaled. The disease produced depends upon the type of particle inhaled and the tissue reaction evoked to deal with it. Thus a relatively small number of bacterial organisms are needed to produce pneumonia in susceptible subjects whereas industrial diseases may only be found when the relevant dust particles have been inhaled over a number of years.

Aerodynamic defence. The branching tubular form of the airways results in larger inhaled particles becoming impacted on bronchial mucosa, particularly at points of bronchial bifurcation. The larger the particle, the greater the chance of inertial impaction taking place. Smaller particles, and in particular those of less than 5 μm diameter, escape this form of arrest and pass on to the level of the acinus. Those that are lodged on the bronchial mucosal surface are moved proximally on the mucociliary escalator (see below).

Shape, density, solubility and surface structure are also important in deciding the fate of inhaled particles. Asbestos fibres, for instance, which may be up to 300 μm in length but only 0.1 μm in diameter, reach alveoli because their long axis may lie parallel to the air stream. Solubility and surface area are important where toxic absorption of pharmacologically active agents is involved. Most pathogenic organisms are inhaled as droplet nuclei. When someone sneezes or coughs vigorously he or she may expel up to 10^6 droplets into the atmosphere. These can be up to 100 μm in diameter but evaporation takes place and the residue is known as a droplet nucleus. These nuclei vary from 0.5 to 5.0 μm diameter and some contain organisms. Particles of this size tend to lodge at the alveolar level.

Cough reflex. Cough and bronchoconstriction are direct mechanisms that have an immediate effect on inhaled particles. Constriction of bronchial smooth muscle occurs as a result of vagal reflex stimulation initiated by direct irritation of mucosal surfaces. Cough reflexes operate in larger airways, probably only down to the fifth generation.

Mucociliary transport mechanism. Cilia are found from the level of the larynx to the level of the terminal bronchiole, though they are far more numerous in proximal than distal airways. Cilia have a complex microstructure (Fig. 17.12) which, however, results in efficient and effective function so that normally they beat metachronously and this is often likened to the appearance seen when a gust of wind blows across a field of corn. Cilia beat in a fluid medium which has a sol component adjacent to the cell surface and a gel component lying on top of this and secreted by goblet cells in the bronchial mucosa.

Particles may lodge in the mucous or gel layer and are rapidly moved proximally by cilia which only touch this layer at the peak of their forward stroke. Many factors have an adverse effect on ciliary action:

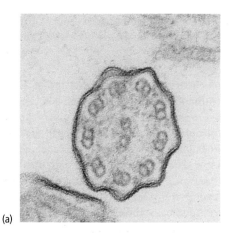

(a)

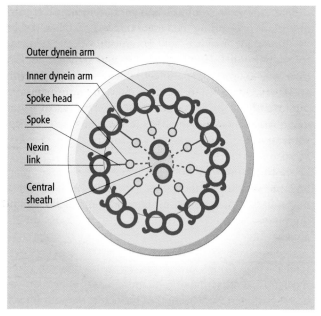

Outer dynein arm

Inner dynein arm

Spoke head

Spoke

Nexin link

Central sheath

(b)

Fig. 17.12 Cross-section of a cilium. (a) Electronmicrograph. (b) Diagram.

- abnormal structure, e.g. absence of dynein arms;
- purulent exudate;
- excess oxygen, e.g. in artificial and positive-pressure ventilation;
- excess carbon dioxide;
- air pollutants, e.g. smog, oxides of nitrogen and sulphur;
- cigarette smoke;
- anaesthetics, including intravenous anaesthetics.

Lysozyme. This antibacterial substance, which splits mucopeptide in bacterial walls, is secreted by the serous cells in bronchial seromucinous glands. If these serous cells are diminished in number, as occurs in chronic bronchitis, one of the major defences against bacterial infection is removed.

Immunoglobulin A (IgA). This immunoglobulin is secreted by plasma cells in bronchial-associated lymphoid tissue. To be effective it has to be formed into a dimer and a cysteine-rich polypeptide, known as the J piece, added in the cells of the bronchial glands. IgA inhibits adherence of micro-organisms to the surface of respiratory cells. Damage to mucosal glands prevents dimerization and this is an important factor in impairing bronchial defence mechanisms.

Transition zone

This is composed of structures at the level of the terminal and first-order respiratory bronchiole. It is in this region that conducting or elastic pulmonary arteries are replaced by muscular pulmonary arteries and it is here also that lymphatics originate. In these airways, as a consequence of the enormous increase in cross-sectional area, mass movement of gas gives way to diffusion which becomes the mode of gas mixing within the acini.

Exchange zone

This consists of the acini. An acinus is defined as 'that unit of lung supplied by the terminal bronchiole' and is made up of respiratory bronchioles, alveolar ducts and alveoli (Figs 17.13 and 17.14) together with the alveolar capillary network. It is in this region that exchange of gases between air spaces and blood takes place. (In some texts, the term secondary lobule is used to describe the unit which is outlined by connective tissue and lymphatics on the pleural surface of the lung. This unit contains from three to five acini. It is preferable to use the term acinus, as this

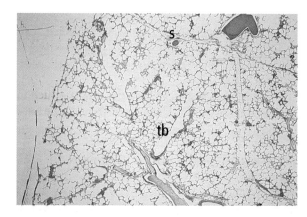

Fig. 17.13 A secondary lobule of lung outlined by connective tissue septa (s) and containing several acini, each of which is supplied by a terminal bronchiole (tb). (EVG.)

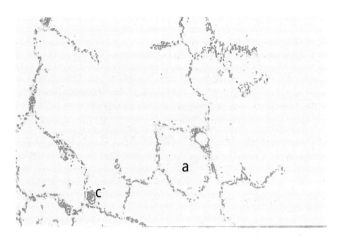

Fig. 17.14 A group of normal alveoli (a) showing their thin walls containing numerous capillaries (c). (H&E.)

is the functional respiratory unit.) Communication between adjacent alveoli is through the pores of Kohn. Within the alveolus there are three important cell types.

Type I pneumocytes

These cells have very attenuated cytoplasm, cover the greater portion of the alveolar surface and form an essential part of the barrier to gas exchange. Because of their large surface to volume ratio they are very susceptible to damage from noxious substances passing through the cell membrane.

Type II pneumocytes (Fig. 17.15)

These cells are cuboidal in shape and, although more numerous than type I pneumocytes, occupy only a very small part of the alveolar surface. They have two main functions:

1 secretion of surfactant which is contained in lamellated

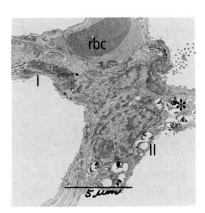

Fig. 17.15 Electronmicrograph of the junction between four alveoli. In the bottom right hand corner there is a type II pneumocyte containing lamellated bodies in its cytoplasm (∗). A red blood cell (rbc) in a capillary is at the top of the field and the remaining alveoli are lined by the attenuated cytoplasm of type I pneumocytes.

osmophilic intracytoplasmic bodies;

2 they act as progenitors of type I pneumocytes when the latter undergo necrosis, thus covering the denuded alveolar basement membrane.

Alveolar macrophages

These cells are derived primarily from the bone marrow, though some are formed from secondary division in the pulmonary interstitial tissues. They are the main defence against pathogenic particles and organisms at the alveolar level. Following ingestion of particles they may migrate to the level of the respiratory bronchioles where lymphatic commence. Some macrophages are resident in alveoli but further cells may migrate there as part of the inflammatory response. They have numerous membrane receptors, e.g. for the Fc component of IgG and C3b. Macrophages are activated in infections, probably by interaction with T lymphocytes, and when activated they phagocytose organisms. Phagosomes fuse with lysosomes and by enzymatic action and production of, among other substances, hydrogen peroxide, attack organisms. Many factors are known to depress macrophage effectiveness:

- irradiation;
- immunosuppressive drugs;
- cytotoxic drugs;
- metabolic acidosis, e.g. in diabetes mellitus and uraemia;
- ethanol;
- hypoxia;
- cold;
- cigarette smoke;
- virus infection.

CLINICAL MANIFESTATIONS OF RESPIRATORY DISEASE

Dyspnoea

This is the term used to indicate difficulty in breathing. Any alterations of the normal, subconscious state of respiration such as a sensation of obstruction or pain associated with breathing may be considered to represent dyspnoea. Dyspnoea may result from a variety of causes (Table 17.3).

Cyanosis

Cyanosis is a bluish discoloration of the skin and mucous membranes caused by the presence of increased amounts

Table 17.3 Some causes of dyspnoea.

Large airway obstruction	May cause respiratory difficulty with a coarse noise (stridor) on inhalation
Small airway obstruction	Produces an expiratory wheeze (as in asthma) which is worse on expiration
Painful lesions of chest or pleura	Produce limited expansion
Fluid in the parenchyma or alveoli	Produces decreased compliance and vital capacity
Collapse and consolidation	Reduces the vital capacity
Diffuse pulmonary fibrosis	Decreases compliance and diffusion
Hypoxaemia and hypercapnia	Stimulates the respiratory centre, increasing the ventilatory rate
Fluid or air in the pleural cavity	Reduces expansion of the lung
Pulmonary embolism and infarction	Perfusion defects and destruction of lung

*Anxiety and exercise produce temporary 'dyspnoea' in normal individuals.

of reduced haemoglobin in the blood (> 5g/dl). Two mechanisms may lead to cyanosis.

1 Central cyanosis is caused by a mixture of deoxygenated venous blood with oxygenated arterial blood in the heart and lungs. Central cyanosis occurs in:

(a) congenital cyanotic heart disease where there is a right-to-left shunt, e.g. Fallot's tetralogy (see Chapter 15);

(b) pulmonary arteriovenous fistula;

(c) extensive right-to-left shunting of blood in the lungs caused by lack of ventilation of adequately perfused alveoli.

Central cyanosis features blue discoloration of mucous membrane such as the tongue in addition to the skin.

2 Peripheral cyanosis usually results from slowing of blood flow, usually in the skin of the extremities, most commonly from cold and states of extreme cutaneous vasoconstriction such as shock.

In peripheral cyanosis, mucous membranes are normal in colour.

Chest pain

Most pulmonary diseases do not cause pain as the lung parenchyma is not sensitive to pain. The parietal pleura is sensitive to pain and so diseases that cause inflammation of the parietal pleura, such as lobar pneumonia and pulmonary infarction, cause chest pain.

Pleural pain is usually related to ventilatory chest movement and is often associated with a pleural friction rub that may be heard on auscultation.

Cough

Cough results from:
- stimulation of the cough reflex by the entry of foreign material into the larynx;
- the accumulation of secretions in the lower respiratory tract.

Cough may be dry, or non-productive, as occurs typically in intersitial lung diseases, or production of sputum in processes involving the air passages and alveoli.

Sputum production

Examination of sputum, usually performed by a microbiologist or a cytopathologist, is useful, in certain cases, in evaluating patients with suspected lung disease. A purulent appearance or foul odour suggests bacterial infection; the presence of blood may indicate infarction, infection or malignancy; Charcot–Leyden crystals (crystalline material produced by eosinophil degranulation) and Curschmann's spirals (inspissated bronchiolar casts) may suggest asthma (see below); acid-fast bacilli, *Pneumocystis* and fungi may be identified using special stains.

Respiratory failure

Respiratory failure may result from a failure in pulmonary diffusion, perfusion or ventilation. Measurement of arterial blood Po_2, Pco_2 and pH may help to determine the cause of respiratory failure, and will monitor its severity and progress (Table 17.4). Mechanisms of respiratory acidosis and alkalosis are discussed in Chapter 13.

Pulmonary oedema

Pulmonary oedema has many pulmonary and cardiac causes (Table 17.5).

Diffuse alveolar damage

This is the condition variously known as the **acute respiratory distress syndrome** or **hyaline membrane disease**. It occurs at all ages and is associated with a variety of

Table 17.4 Arterial blood gases in respiratory failure.

	P_{O_2}	P_{CO_2}	pH	Physiology
Ventilation failure	↓	↑	↓	Non-ventilated lung is effectively right-to-left shunt, allowing venous-type blood (low P_{O_2}, high P_{CO_2}) to pass directly to the left heart
Perfusion failure	↓	Normal	Normal	Effective dead space is increased; hyperventilation of remaining lung may correct P_{CO_2} level
Diffusion failure	↓	↓	↑	Diffusion failure affects only exchange of oxygen, not CO_2: resulting hypoxaemia may cause compensatory hyperventilation, causing hypocapnia

Table 17.5 Causes of pulmonary oedema.

Increased capillary permeability due to capillary wall damage
    Pneumonia
    Inhaled toxins, e.g. mustard gas, chlorine
    Circulating toxins, e.g. septicaemia, histamine
    Disseminated intravascular coagulation
    Renal failure
    'Shock lung' (posttrauma)
    Radiation pneumonitis

Increased capillary hydrostatic pressure (> in lower zones)
    Left ventricular failure, e.g. myocardial infarction or hypertension
    Increase in left atrial pressure, e.g. mitral stenosis
    Pulmonary venous obstruction
    Fluid overload (especially intravenously administered)

Decreased plasma oncotic pressure e.g. hypoalbuminaemia

Lymphatic obstruction

Unknown mechanism
    Raised intracranial pressure ('neurogenic oedema')
    High altitude
    Heroin overdose
    Pulmonary embolism
    Eclampsia

clinical situations, all with severe damage to the integrity of the alveolar–capillary barrier. The prognosis is usually grave. The most important causes are:
- shock, e.g. trauma, burns, anaphylaxis, fat embolism;
- severe infections, e.g. influenza, Gram-negative septicaemia;

- drowning;
- toxic gases, e.g. O_2, O_3, SO_2, NO_2;
- radiation;
- drugs, e.g. cytotoxic drugs, heroin;
- paraquat.

As a result of the action of these toxic agents or as a consequence of severe under-perfusion, there is damage to alveolar capillary endothelium and to type I pneumocytes with consequent exudation of protein-laden fluid into alveolar spaces. This fluid, together with cell debris derived from necrotic pneumocytes, constitutes the **hyaline membranes** which are one of the cardinal morphological features of the condition (Fig. 17.16).

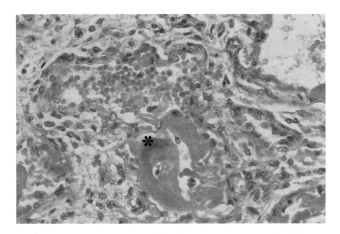

Fig. 17.16 Shock lung showing severe collapse and a hyaline membrane (✳). (H&E.)

This **exudative phase** is rapidly followed by a **proliferative phase** in which Type II pneumocytes divide to cover the denuded alveolar basement membrane. This is followed, if the patient survives long enough, by interstitial infiltration with lymphocytes and plasma cells and fibroblastic proliferation.

Some patients may survive and have a return to normal pulmonary function but in others there is extensive residual fibrosis. It shoud be noted that treatment of these patients is difficult as they require artificial respiration with high concentrations of oxygen which itself is toxic to the alveolar lining.

PULMONARY INFECTIONS (Fig. 17.17)

Acute bronchial infection

Acute bronchitis
Acute bronchitis is usually part of a generalized viral infection (e.g. common cold syndrome) and treatment is

supportive. Important non-viral causes are *Mycoplasma* and *Bordetella pertussis*. Chronic bronchitis is a clinical diagnosis and both viruses and bacteria play an important role in the progession of the disease by causing acute exacerbations (see below).

Whooping cough

B. pertussis is a Gram-negative coccobacillus (Fig. 17.18). The infection is endemic with epidemics occurring every 3–5 years. It is very contagious, occurring in childhood, between ages 1 and 5 years, and is commoner in females.

Whooping cough is not a single toxin-mediated disease. Apart from the pertussis toxin, which is responsible for systemic effects, other locally acting virulence factors are surface bacterial components (filamentous haemagglutinin) and other toxins (adenylate cyclase and necrotic toxins).

Whooping cough has the following phases:
- a **catarrhal** phase, with URT symptoms lasting 1 week;
- a **paroxysmal** phase–characteristic cough paroxysms lasting the second week;
- a **convalescent** phase, lasting a further week.
Recovery of the organism via a pernasal swab is more common in weeks 1 and 2.
Complications include;
- **bacterial infections**, e.g. aspiration pneumonia;
- physical consequences of paroxsymal coughing, e.g. subconjunctival haemorrhages;
- **central nervous system abnormalities**, e.g. encephalitis.
Prevention is by whole-cell vaccine, as part of DPT.

Concerns about vaccine reactions such as encephalitis have been unfounded. Erythromycin reduces the severity and duration of whooping cough.

Bronchiolitis

An acute viral illness occurring within the first 2 years of life, **RSV** causes the majority of infections. The peak incidence of infection is between 2 and 10 months of age. Outbreaks of RSV occur each year, from January to March (other viruses have their own seasonal peaks in the winter months). Immunity to RSV is incomplete and reinfections in older children and adults as URT infections (URTIs) are common. Adults may act as reservoirs for infection.

Necrosis and proliferation of bronchiolar epithelium and ultimately sloughing of cells occur. Young infants are very vulnerable to obstruction because of a relatively small lumen. Recovery of the respiratory epithelium is slow.

Bronchiolitis starts as a URTI, often with fever and otitis media. It progresses to involve the lower tract, producing cough, dyspnoea, tachypnoea and retractions of the chest wall. The classic signs of bronchiolitis are wheezing and hyperaeration of the lung.

Pneumonia may accompany the bronchiolitis. Infants with severe disease may be at increased risk of developing chronic obstructive disease in later life. Diagnosis is usually made on the characteristic clinical and epidemiology findings. A nasopharyngeal aspirate may be used for rapid detection by an immunofluorescence technique.

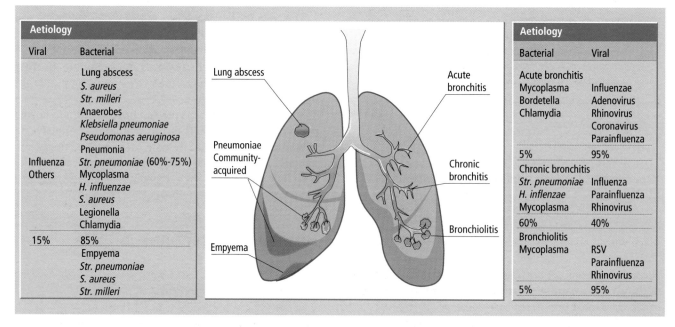

Fig. 17.17 Infections of the lower respiratory tract.

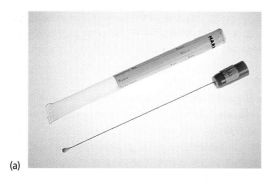

(a)

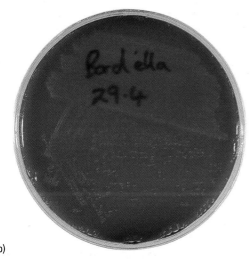

(b)

Fig. 17.18 (a) Isolation of *Bordetella pertussis* is done using a swab passed along the floor of the nose until the posterior wall of the nasopharynx is reached. (b) Ideally, the swab should be plated at the bedside on to Bordet–Gengou agar (cough plate) as shown here.

Management is mainly supportive, although **ribavirin** (a broad-spectrum antiviral) may be used in hospitalized patients. Attempts at producing an effective vaccine have been unsuccessful and may even have predisposed the recipient to more severe disease.

Pneumonia

Introduction

Pneumonia is the term applied to acute inflammation of the lung caused by micro-organisms.

Alveolitis is sometimes used to describe this condition but it is a term best reserved for allergic reactions taking place within alveoli, as in extrinsic allergic alveolitis.

Pneumonitis is a term often used to describe inflammation due to physical agents. However, all three words are unfortunately often used in an interchangeable fashion.

The term **'compromised host'** is used to describe patients whose defence mechanisms have been impaired by disease, e.g. in leukaemia, malabsorption, megaloblastic

anaemia, etc., or by therapy, e.g. with cytotoxic drugs, steroids, radiotherapy, etc. Certain organisms have a predilection for patients with specific forms of immune impairment:

- **neutropenia** and **phagocytic** defects tend to be associated with infections by Gram-negative bacilli or fungi;
- **humoral defects** are often associated with infections due to *Streptococcus pneumoniae* or *Haemophilus influenzae*;
- those with **defective cellular immunity** tend to be infected by fungi, mycobacteria, *Toxoplasma, Pneumocystis carinii* or viruses.

It is useful in trying to identify the aetiology of pneumonia, and hence empiric treatment, to divide pneumonias into the following categories:

- community-acquired;
- hospital-acquired;
- atypical;
- aspiration;
- recurrent and chronic pneumonias.

Acute, community-acquired pneumonia

Classically pneumonia is divided into two varieties according to the gross and microscopic characteristics (Fig. 17.19), **lobar pneumonia** and **bronchopneumonia** (Fig. 17.20). The distinction between the two morphological forms is to some extent arbitrary and imprecise from a microbiological perspective.

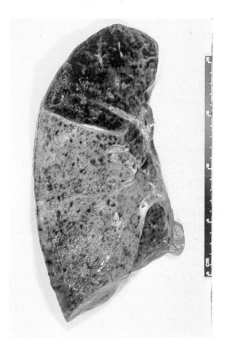

Fig. 17.19 Lower lobar pneumonia in the stage of red hepatization. There is a very clear demarcation between consolidated lower lobe and the upper lobe which is not affected.

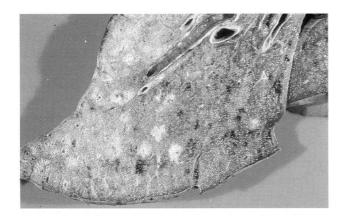

Fig. 17.20 Lower lobar bronchopneumonia. Rounded discrete areas of pneumonic consolidation can be seen surrounded by normal lung in this formalin fixed specimen.

The precise type of pneumonia depends upon a balance between rapid formation of infected fluid and localization of infection by leucocytes.

S. pneumoniae is the commonest cause of community-acquired pneumonia, although of late its incidence is declining (Fig. 17.21). *Mycoplasma pneumoniae* in epidemic years accounts for 10–20% of cases of pneumonia. *Staphylococcus aureus* is important as a secondary invader in influenza epidemic years.

Lobar pneumonia. Before the advent of antibiotics pneumococcal lobar pneumonia was a frequent cause of death in young adults. It remains an important cause of morbidity and mortality both among patients in the community and hospital patients.

Risk factors include:
- extremes of age;
- pre-existing lung disease;
- following surgery involving intubation;
- alcoholism;
- diabetes mellitus;
- congestive cardiac failure;
- in congenital and acquired immune deficiency syndromes.

Pneumococcal pneumonia typically occurs in the elderly and in the case of bacteraemic pneumonias may have a mortality rate of 60%. Peaks occur from winter to early spring.

Clinically pneumococcal lobar pneumonia is a disease of rapid onset with a severe rigor followed by pleuritic pain, high pyrexia, cough and tenacious 'rusty' sputum. Clinical and radiological examination reveals consolidation of one or more lobes. In the untreated patient either death ensues or there is resolution by crisis when the patient undergoes a dramatic improvement as a consequence of a good immune response to the infection. Infec-

tion occurs by inhalation of infected droplets which lodge in peripheral alveoli and, in those who lack specific antibody, this excites outpouring of oedema fluid. This infected fluid spreads rapidly throughout the lobe via the pores of Kohn.

Four classical stages are described:
- **hyperaemia**–the alveoli are filled with oedema fluid and numerous pneumococci;
- **red hepatization**–(Fig. 17.22) the affected lobe has a dry, rough and red cut surface and there is a fibrinous pleurisy. Histologically alveoli are filled with red cells enmeshed in a fibrinous exudate. Neutrophils are present but not numerous;
- **grey hepatization**–the lung remains consolidated but the cut surface is wet and grey. The alveoli are filled with neutrophils and fibrin is inconspicuous as it has been digested by fibrinolysins released from leucocytes;
- **resolution**–which is often incomplete, is characterized by alveoli filled with macrophages removing intra-alveolar cellular debris resulting from disintegration of polymorphs and bacteria.

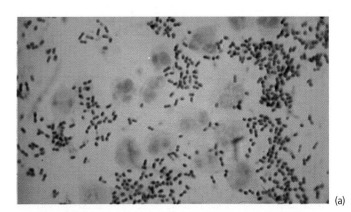

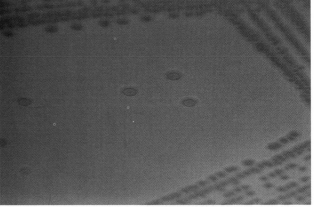

(a)

(b)

Fig. 17.21 *Streptococcus pneumoniae.* (a) Isolation in sputum using Gram stain shows pus cells and the presence of diplococci. (b) Grown on blood agarie shows alpha haemolysis and typical draughtsman colonies.

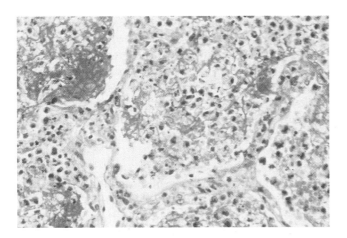

Fig. 17.22 Lobar pneumonia in the stage of red hepatization. Alveoli are filled with a mixture of fibrin and neutrophils. (H&E.)

Complications include non-resolution with resultant fibrosis, abscess formation, pleural effusion, empyema and systemic effects such as endocarditis, meningitis and arthritis. Pneumococcal and influenza vaccines are available for those at risk.

Sputum microscopy and culture have low sensitivity and specificity as the organisms colonizing the respiratory tract are the same potential pathogens. Blood culture should always be taken. A pathogen is not found in 40% of cases. In the latter, antigen testing may be necessary.

Empiric treatment of pneumonia depends on whether it is **community-acquired** (likely to be pneumococcal) or **hospital-acquired** (due to Gram-negative bacteria). Empiric treatment of pneumonia in the community includes oral amoxycillin or co-amoxiclavulanate. In patients requiring hospitalization, intravenous benzylpenicillin is advised. In patients with severe pneumonias empiric treatment with intravenous cefuroxime and erythromycin (the latter for atypical pathogens such as *Mycoplasma* and *Legionella*) is recommended.

Bronchopneumonia. Bronchopneumonias are usually secondary pneumonias occurring in patients with predisposing conditions such as:
• prematurity;
• old age;
• malignancy;
• immune suppression;
• viral infection;
• malnutrition;
• aspiration (due to absent cough reflex) with bronchial damage due to gastric acid.

The pneumonic consolidation is **patchy** and usually originates from a **bronchiolitis**. Areas of consolidation may become confluent and lead to abscess formation.

Bronchopneumonia does not undergo resolution. Healing is by organization and fibrosis.

Pneumococci are present in 80% of cases together with mixed bacterial flora including pharyngeal commensals.

Other community-acquired bacterial pneumonias
• *Haemophilus influenzae.* Infection with this organism may affect infants and adults, often as a secondary invader following a viral infection. It can give rise to a lobar pneumonia, particularly if type b organisms are involved. Alternatively there may be a miliary bronchopneumonia, a condition found sometimes in middle-aged or elderly cigarette smokers. Severe inflammation accompanied by necrosis is often present within bronchiolar walls.
• *Staphylococcus aureus.* Pulmonary infection with this organism may produce a variety of morphological forms:
  1 haemorrhagic bronchopneumonia, often occurring in severely debilitated subjects and rapidly fatal;
  2 purulent bronchopneumonia;
  3 lobar pneumonia;
  4 multiple abscesses in septicaemia.
Complications include abscess formation, fibrosis and empyema. When the disease occurs in infants it may resolve following treatment to leave cysts in the lung, known as pneumatocoeles, which can give rise to respiratory distress but which frequently resolve spontaneously.

Viral pneumonias. Virus infection in the lung involves an attack on the epithelial cells and results in necrosis of either bronchial epithelial cells, or alveolar lining cells, or both.
• **Influenza.** The virus attacks the columnar ciliated respiratory epithelial cells in airways where it can be identified using an immunofluorescent antibody technique. The resultant necrosis of respiratory mucosa leaves the lung in an undefended state and susceptible to secondary infection, especially by staphylococci, streptococci and *Haemophilus influenzae*. In severe cases alveolar epithelium undergoes necrosis and there is hyaline membrane formation characteristic of the diffuse alveolar damage syndrome (see above). In fatal cases there is extensive haemorrhage in the airways and the lung parenchyma is oedematous and haemorrhagic. Histology may reveal, in addition to secondary bronchopneumonic changes, interstitial inflammation.
• **Measles.** Although unusual in Europe and the USA, measles pneumonia is common among malnourished children is Africa where it gives rise to a high mortality. Grossly the appearance of the lungs is non-specific. They are heavy and oedematous. Histologically there is a striking giant cell pneumonia (Fig. 17.23). Both airways and

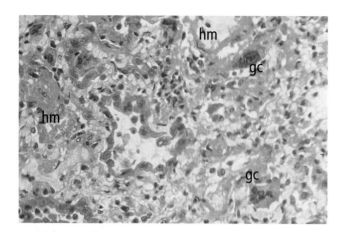

Fig. 17.23 Histology of measles pneumonia. Giant cells (gc) and hyaline membranes (hm) are present. (H&E.)

interstitial tissues are involved with infiltration by lymphocytes, plasma cells and multinucleate giant cells and there is also hyaline membrane formation.

• **Cytomegalovirus.** Since the introduction of immunosuppressive and cytotoxic drugs this disease has become prominent in adults receiving them. It often coexists with infection by *Pneumocystis carinii*. The condition gives rise to a panlobular interstitial pneumonia. Alveolar walls are thickened and infiltrated with lymphocytes and plasma cells and in severe instances there is oedema and hyaline membrane formation. Cytomegalic inclusions (Fig. 17.24) can be seen in macrophages, endothelial and alveolar epithelial cells. Affected cells are large and the inclusions are intranuclear, pinkish in colour in haematoxylin and eosin preparations and are usually surrounded by a halo separating them from the nuclear chromatin.

• *Other viral infection.* **Herpes simples** and **varicella** can both cause interstitial pneumonia in susceptible subjects.

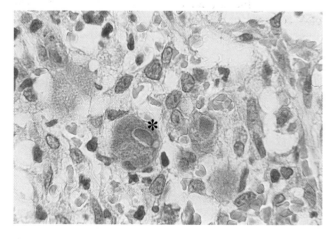

Fig. 17.24 Cytomegalic inclusion viral pneumonia. A large inclusion (✻) can be seen in the nucleus of a detached type I pneumocyte. (H&E.)

Adenovirus infection of the upper respiratory passages is common but rarely serious in adults. Yet in infancy, infection with types 7 and 21 may prove fatal due to severe necrotizing bronchiolitis and bronchopneumonia. In those that survive there is a high incidence of bronchiolar obliteration and bronchiectasis. **RSV** accounts for many infections in infants and young children and gives rise to acute bronchiolitis and interstitial pneumonia.

Hospital-acquired pneumonia

This accounts for 10–20% of all hospital-acquired infections. This pneumonia has a high mortality and risk factors include:
• severe underlying disease;
• intubation;
• surgery;
• previous antibiotic treatment.

Prolonged hospitalization, stress and antibiotics cause a loss of fibronectin, a non-specific receptor for the resident Gram-positive flora, from the respiratory tract. As a consequence, the respiratory tract becomes colonized with enteric bacilli. Only in a few cases does this result in infection.

Gram-negative bacilli predominate, e.g. *Klebsiella pneumoniae*, *Enterobacter* spp. and *Pseudomonas* spp. These are all opportunistic infections (see Chapter 10).

• *K. pneumoniae.* Infection with this organism, formerly known as **Friedländer's pneumonia**, has clinical features somewhat similar to pneumococcal lobar pneumonia. It particularly affects elderly male alcoholics but may occur in any debilitated state. Pathologically there is consolidation of one or more lobes, the cut surface of which reveals a foul-smelling mucoid exudate. In those that survive empyema is a frequent complication, as are abscess formation and cavitation.

• *P. aeruginosa.* Pulmonary infection typically complicates severe burns but may sometimes follow surgery or occur in ventilated patients. Two forms are described – bacteraemic pneumonia, in which confluent small abscesses are found and the condition is occasionally accompanied by a pulmonary arteritis, and an inhalation pneumonia with extensive necrosis.

Diagnosis of hospital-acquired pneumonias can be difficult. Suggestive features are:
• a fever;
• elevated white cell count;
• increase in oxygen requirements in intubated patients;
• chest X-ray changes.

Sputum culture is unhelpful and a bronchoalveolar lavage is often required. Empiric treatment is governed by a knowledge of local sensitivity patterns but often includes third-generation cephalosporins, aminoglycosides and antibiotics with pseudomonal activity.

Atypical pneumonias

The agents causing atypical pneumonias are so named because the clinical illness follows an atypical cause. The illness begins with a mild respiratory tract infection followed by shortness of breath and cough but little or no sputum production. Other features may include a predominance of constitutional symptoms, for example, legionnaire's disease features abdominal pain, vomiting, diarrhoea and confusion with diffuse, pulmonary involvement.

Mycoplasma pneumoniae. The commonest pathogen causing an atypical pneumonia is *Mycoplasma pneumoniae*. This accounts for 1–10% of all community-acquired pneumonias. It occurs in epidemics every 4–5 years. It has a peak incidence in children and young adults, producing a mild disease in the majority of cases.

Legionnaire's disease. Legionnaire's disease is caused by a small Gram-negative coccobacillus, *Legionella pneumophilia*. This was first identified in 1976 and affects especially alcoholics, the elderly and immune-suppressed patients. A non-pulmonary form exists, Pontiac fever. Although infection is air-borne, the organism may reside in water tanks in hospitals and hotels, with infection occurring via contaminated aerosols. The condition carries a high mortality.

Post-mortem examination reveals both lungs to be very heavy due to extensive consolidation (Fig. 17.25),

haemorrhage and oedema. A fibrinopurulent pleurisy with an effusion is often present. Abscesses with extensive necrosis of lung tissue and cavity formation may occur. Hyaline membranes, intra-alveolar neutrophils and a pulmonary vasculitis are other features. The organism is difficult to identify but can be seen in the intra-alveolar exudate using silver stains or an immunofluorescent antibody method.

Fungal infections. These are found not only in immunocompromised patients but also as secondary infections in those with pre-existing lung disease such as bronchiectasis.

• *Pneumocystis carinii.* Infection with this organism is frequent in immunosuppressed patients and those with acquired immune deficiency syndrome (AIDS; see Chapter 10). Taxonomic classification of *Pneumocystis* has been a subject of controversy as it has some characteristics associated with protozoa but it is now classified as a fungus.

The organism appears in two forms:
(a) a cyst 5–10 μm diameter containing up to eight intracytoplasmic bodies known as merozoites;
(b) a sickle-shaped form representing a collapsed cyst from which the merozoites have been discharged. The latter undergo binary fission, enlarge and eventually form the cysts, so completing the life cycle.

The disease presents as a diffuse or focal pneumonia involving the lower lobes. Histologically there is an interstitial inflammation but the most typical feature is the foamy intra-alveolar exudate in which organisms can be easily found in methenamine silver preparations. If treatment is to be effective rapid diagnosis is of the utmost importance and for this examination of sputum, or even better bronchiolar–alveolar washing, must be undertaken when the organisms can be readily detected in smears using silver stains (Fig. 17.26). Treatment is with high-dose co-trimoxazole, although in AIDS patients, toxicity problems may arise.

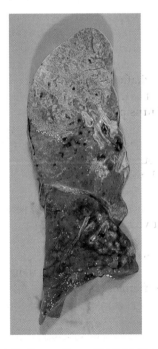

Fig. 17.25 Legionnaire's disease with consolidation of the upper lobe and abscess formation in the lower lobe.

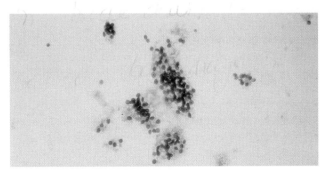

Fig. 17.26 *Pneumocystis carinii* stained black by the methenamine silver method in bronchiolo–alveolar lavage fluid.

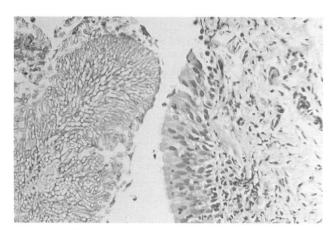

Fig. 17.27 Hyphae of aspergillus in the lumen of a bronchus (left). (H&E.)

- *Aspergillus fumigatus* is probably the most commonly encountered organism and can give rise to a necrotizing bronchopneumonia (Fig. 17.27), a granulomatous reaction, multiple abscesses or, if it has invaded blood vessels, pulmonary infarction. Allergy to the fungus can also give rise to an asthmatic reaction.

Other species pathogenic to lung include cryptococci, *Candida*, phycomycetes, *Coccidioides immitis*, *Blastomyces*, actinomycetes and, especially in the USA, *Histoplasma*.

Other agents causing atypical pneumonias are:
- *Chlamydia psittaci* (psittacosis), transmitted via birds, especially parrots.
- *Chlamydia pneumoniae* (TWAR), transmitted via person-to-person spread.
- *Coxiella burneti* (Q-fever), transmitted via sheep, goats and cattle.

Diagnosis and management of atypical pneumonias. Culture of these infectious agents may be difficult and is not routinely done. Detection of Legionella antigen in urine is performed. Otherwise, serology is the mainstay of diagnosis, via measurement of either IgM or IgG titres.

These atypical agents may be intracellular parasites and require an antibiotic that achieves acceptable intracellular levels. Erythromycin is used for empiric treatment.

Recurrent pneumonias

These infections usually occur as a result of a diminished host response and the defect may be congenital or acquired:
- cystic fibrosis—*Staphylococcus aureus*; *Pseudomonas aeroginosa* and *P. cepacia*;
- bronchial obstruction (e.g. bronchial carcinoma)—respiratory pathogens;
- immunosuppressed host (e.g. immunosuppressive therapy or AIDS) opportunistic infections; Gram-negative bacilli; *Mycobacterium*; fungi; *Aspergillus*; *Candida*;

Pneumocystis carinii; protozoa; *Toxoplasma gondii*; viruses; herpes zoster; cytomegalovirus.

Chronic pneumonias

Tuberculosis is the most common cause of chronic pneumonia in both immune-competent and immune-compromised individuals. In the immune-compromised, other agents such as atypical mycobacteria, *Mycobacterium avium-intracellulare* (MAI), complex, *Histoplasma* and other dimorphic fungi are also important.

Tuberculosis (Fig. 17.28). Tuberculosis is still a major cause of death worldwide and was of epidemic proportions in the UK in the 19th century. Both incidence and mortality have fallen dramatically in the west due to public health measures and improved treatment but because of this the disease is in danger of being overlooked in differential diagnosis. Yet it is one of the infections to which the immunocompromised patient is particularly susceptible. Reactivation of latent infection is also liable to occur in the elderly who then act as a potential source of infection to those with whom they come in contact.

Primary infection with *M. tuberculosis* usually takes place by inhalation of bacilli into the lung, though the infection may sometimes primarily occur in the ileum, if the organism is ingested, or in the tonsil.

Inhaled bacilli lodge in the subpleural region, often in the upper or middle zones, and set up the **Ghon focus**, an inflammatory lesion approximately 1cm diameter in which bacilli are contained but not killed. The organisms track along lymphatics to hilar lymph nodes where they are detained and initiate a caseating epithelioid granulomatous reaction. This combination of the Ghon focus and the enlarged hilar lymph nodes is known as the **primary tuberculous complex**:
- this complex may heal completely with calcification of the nodes and Ghon focus and this is indeed the usual outcome;
- the lymph nodes may erode into a bronchus; infected material may be inhaled into the lung, giving rise to bronchopneumonia;
- the lymph nodes may erode into a pulmonary vein resulting in bacillaemia when the effect will depend upon the numbers of bacilli entering the blood stream. A small number may lodge at a single site, e.g. bone, kidney or brain, whereas if there is a heavy bacillaemia **miliary tuberculosis** occurs (Fig. 17.29). **Tuberculous meningitis** arises when organisms lodge in the subependymal region and subsequently seed into the cerebrospinal fluid.

Reinfection, sometimes referred to as postprimary, secondary or adult tuberculosis, takes place when a subject who has had a primary infection inhales further ba-

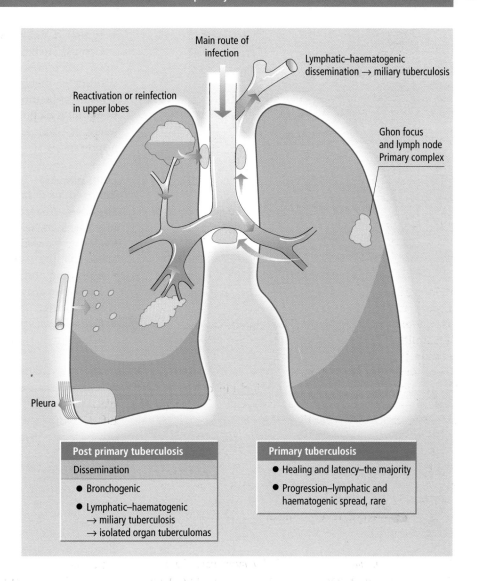

Fig. 17.28 Pulmonary tuberculosis.

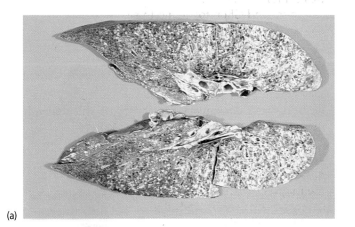

(a)

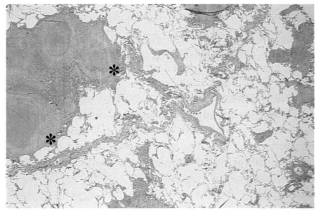

(b)

Fig. 17.29 Miliary tuberculosis in the lung. (a) There are numerous small, white caseating granulomas. (b) Miliary tuberculosis in the lung. Histology shows caseating granulomas (✳). (H&E.)

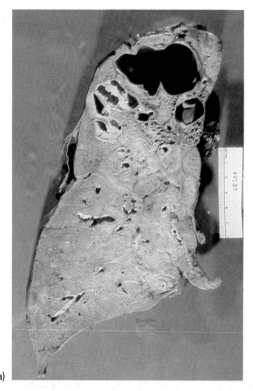

(a)

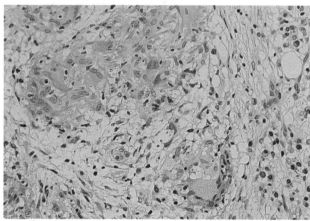

(b)

Fig. 17.30 Tuberculous cavities in the upper lobe in a patient with reinfection. (b) Histology shows caseating, giant cell, epithelioid granulomas. (H&E.)

cilli. This results in caseating granulomatous lesions, often situated in the upper zones (Fig. 17.30(a)), which frequently necrose and form cavities (Fig. 17.30(b)). Unlike the primary infection the lymph nodes are not involved.

Management of tuberculosis is with triple or quadruple chemotherapy (Fig. 17.31):
- isoniazid;
- rifampicin;
- pyrazinamide;
- ethambutol, which is included if resistance is suspected for the first 2 months, followed by;

- isoniazid and rifampicin for a further 4 months.

Complicated disease may require longer therapy. In open tuberculosis cases (cavitating lesions, where the sputum is Ziehl–Neelsen-positive), respiratory precautions must be undertaken for the first 2 weeks of therapy to reduce infection risk. Tracing of contacts and follow up (chest X-rays, sputum, Heaf testing) is also of great importance.

Lung abscess

Endogenous flora are responsible for the majority of lung abscesses. Anaerobic or microaerophilic streptococci are important causes and often present in mixed culture. Underlying conditions predisposing to abscess formation are as follows:
- aspiration and periodontal disease: infection with oral anaerobes are common;
- necrotizing pneumonias (*Staphylococcus aureus*, *Klebsiella pneumoniae*, *Pseudomonas aeruginosa*);

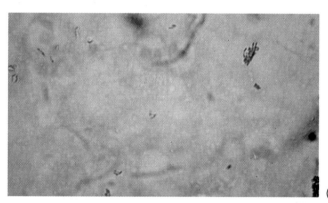

(a)

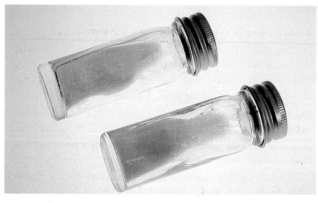

(b)

Fig. 17.31 (a) Sputum smear from a patient with open tuberculosis showing numerous acid and alcohol-fast bacilli, stained with Ziehl–Neelsen (courtesy M. Crow). (b) *Mycobacterium tuberculosis* produces colonies with a buff-coloured, breadcrumb-like appearance when grown on Löwenstein–Jensen medium. In contrast, opportunistic mycobacteria may produce yellow- or orange-pigmented colonies.

- obstructive or necrotizing lung pathology;
  a bronchiectasis;
  b bronchial carcinoma;
- septic emboli from right-sided endocarditis;
- bacteraemia; where abscesses may be multiple (*S. aureus, Streptococcus milleri* and *Nocardia*; Fig. 17.32).

The onset is insidious with weight loss, fevers and foul-smelling sputum. Complications include empyemas and, rarely, brain abscesses.

Management includes prolonged antimicrobial therapy (2–4 months) depending on the organisms isolated from sputum or drainage of the abscess. Metronidazole is often included for its anaerobic cover and good penetration into tissues.

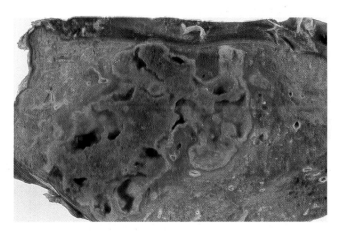

Fig. 17.32 Lung abscess due to *Nocardia* infection.

ASTHMA

This has been defined clinically as a condition in which there is widespread narrowing of bronchial airways which changes in severity over short periods of time either spontaneously or as a result of treatment and is not due to cardiovascular disease. Two broad categories are recognized.

1 Atopic or extrinsic asthma usually starts in childhood and is initiated by a variety of air-borne allergens such as house dust mites, grass pollens and animal danders. It is mediated by an IgE type I hypersensitivity reaction and is associated with positive wheal-and-flare skin tests to appropriate allergens. Peripheral blood eosinophilia is common.

2 Non-atopic or intrinsic asthma occurs mainly in adults, is often associated with respiratory infections and does not exhibit any evidence of a hypersensitivity reaction. (**Allergic bronchopulmonary aspergillosis** is a form of asthma due to inhalation of fungal spores causing both an immediate type I reaction and also an immune complex-induced type III reaction.)

Pathology

The **gross appearances** in the lung in patients dying with asthma are typified by extreme over-distension in the absence of destructive emphysema. There is widespread occlusion of airways by viscid tenacious mucoid exudate, focal areas of collapse, most marked along the anterior borders of the upper lobes, and sometimes small areas of bronchiectasis.

Histologically the exudate in the lumen (Fig. 17.33) can be seen to contain desquamated columnar ciliated respiratory epithelial cells, eosinophils, albumen and mucus. The bronchial mucous membrane itself is oedematous and shows separation and shedding of epithelial cells. In many areas only basal cells are present and there is often evidence of regeneration of mucosa with formation of non-ciliated simple squamous epithelium. The submucosa shows all the evidence of an allergic reaction with oedema, vasodilatation and infiltration with eosinophils. Mast cells may be prominent in both mucosa and submucosa, as may eosinophil major basic protein. There is hypertrophy of bronchial smooth muscle.

Relation of pathology to clinical findings

The airways obstruction is a consequence of the exudate in the bronchial lumen and contraction of bronchial smooth muscle. The main defect in the asthmatic bronchus is failure to clear the exudate due to its rapid formation and loss of ciliary activity in the mucous membrane. Those cilia that remain may be ineffective as they suffer from malfunction when beating in fluid with a high plasma protein content.

The exudate in the bronchial lumen is formed from mucus derived from the mucous glands and from a protein-laden fluid present in the submucosa, derived as a result of increased permeability, which passes across the delicate respiratory mucosa into the bronchial lumen – a process which itself plays a major role in mucosal shedding and loss of ciliary activity.

Pathogenesis of atopic asthma

This is not fully understood but it is considered that patients are sensitized to an allergen the antibodies to which are the IgE attached to mast cells. In an asthmatic

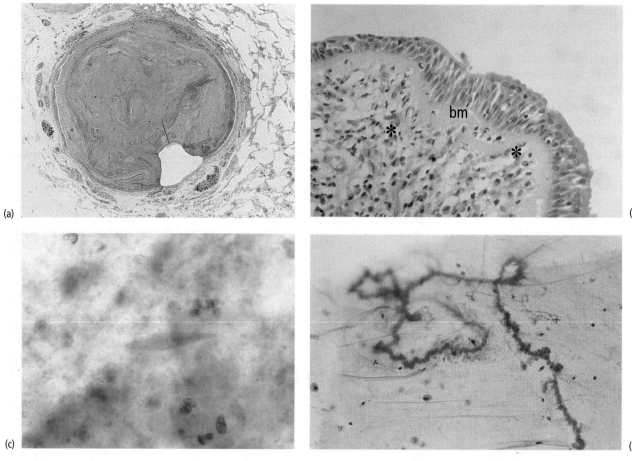

Fig. 17.33 Asthma. (a) Low power view of a bronchus plugged with mucus in a patient who died in status asthmaticus. (b) Asthmatic bronchus. The mucosa has a variable appearance with some squamous metaplasia (✱). There is thickening of the basement membrane (bm) and submucosal eosinophil infiltration. (H&E.) (c) Sputum cytology. The Charcot–Leyden crystal (orange) represents eosinophil degranulation material. (d) Sputum cytology. Curschmann's spiral represents coughed up inspissated mucus casts from a small bronchiole.

attack the inhaled antigen binds to the Ig, causing the mast cells to release a cascade of mediators including histamine. These account for the mucosal oedema seen in acute asthma.

CHRONIC OBSTRUCTIVE AIRWAYS DISEASE

Chronic obstructive airways disease (COAD) features chronic obstruction to air flow and is associated with two pathological conditions–chronic bronchitis and emphysema.

COAD is a common disease, second only to ischaemic heart disease, in the western world. The FEV_1 (forced expiratory volume): FVC (forced vital capacity) ratio is normally over 75%. In COAD this ratio is decreased and the degree of reduction correlates with disease severity and with survival (Fig. 17.34).

Chronic bronchitis

The clinical condition of chronic bronchitis refers to subjects with chronic or excessive mucus secretion in the bronchial tree. This is associated with **air flow obstruction** which is largely **irreversible** (cf. asthma, where it is largely reversible).

Pathologically one of the main features of the condition is an increase in the volume of the mucous glands in the bronchial wall (Fig. 17.35). There is a variety of methods that have been employed to measure the volume of bronchial glands but they all demonstrate a continuous distribution, comparable to that seen in population studies of blood pressure, with no obvious cut-off point between normal and disease values.

Histological findings
The mucosa shows either goblet cell transformation or,

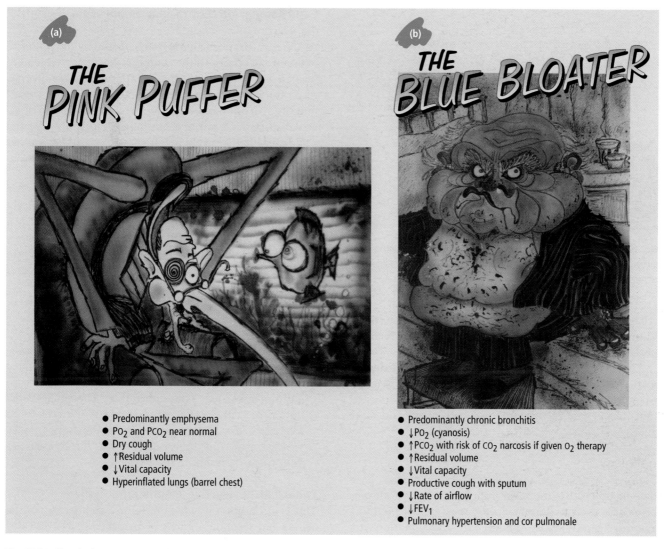

Fig. 17.34 Chronic obstructive airways disease (COAD). (a) Chronic bronchitis. (b) Emphysema.

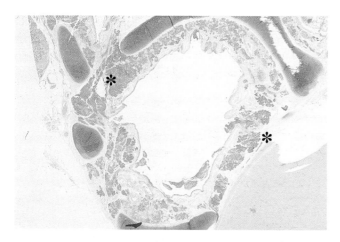

Fig. 17.35 Cross-section of a segmental bronchus showing considerable enlargement of the mucous glands (✱). (H&E.)

more commonly, **squamous metaplasia** (Fig. 17.36). The latter is a regenerative phenomenon following desquamation of the mucosa which occurs in bronchial infection.

Smooth muscle in the bronchial wall is not constantly increased. Mucous glands are enlarged due to both hypertrophy and hyperplasia of the mucus-secreting cells at the expense of the serous cells with consequent reduction in secretion of lysozyme and also deficiency of IgA secretion. As a result of excess mucus production and infection in the upper airways, mucus is inhaled into smaller airways where the cough reflex does not operate. This gives rise to focal areas of alveolar collapse. Secondary infection, often with *Haemophilus influenzae*, frequently occurs due to stasis distal to the bronchiolar obstruction and impaired local resistance due to de-

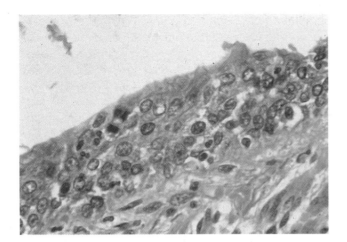

Fig. 17.36 Histology of the bronchial epithelium showing squamous metaplasia—the replacement of one differentiated cell type (glandular) by another differentiated cell type (squamous). (H&E.)

creased lysozyme and IgA. This secondary infection may ultimately give rise to focal areas of fibrosis in the lung parenchyma.

Air flow obstruction observed clinically is due to increased resistance in smaller airways consequent upon peribronchiolar fibrosis and inflammatory and mucoid exudate in the lumen of both small and large airways.

Aetiology

Both epidemiological and experimental studies have demonstrated that the most important cause of chronic bronchitis is air pollution and the most potent polluting agent is cigarette smoke, though industrial pollution with oxides of sulphur and nitrogen and urban smog formation are also significant factors.

Emphysema

Pulmonary emphysema is defined as an abnormal, permanent increase in size in the respiratory portion of the lung (i.e. distal to the terminal bronchiole) known as the acinus, accompanied by destructive changes. Thus simple overdistension without destruction as occurs in asthma is not strictly emphysema.

Diagnosis

Diagnosis can only be satisfactorily made at necropsy from examination of lungs fixed in the distended state. If this procedure is carried out it readily becomes apparent that there are several different morphological forms of the disease, though these often occur in mixed forms.

Centrilobular or centriacinar emphysema
(Fig. 17.37)

As the name implies, this is characterized by the presence of abnormal spaces in the centre of the acinus which are formed as a result of destruction of first- or second-order respiratory bronchioles. Thus terminal bronchioles lead into the spaces; third-order respiratory bronchioles or alveolar ducts lead out of them to peripheral alveolar tissue. Typically the emphysematous spaces are surrounded by normal alveolar tissue. Upper lobes are usually more severely affected than lower lobes.

Aetiology. Essentially this is a disorder affecting elderly cigarette-smoking males. In all probability it occurs as a result of enzymatic digestion of alveolar walls in respiratory bronchioles. The principal enzymes involved are proteases, mainly elastases, derived from neutrophils and macrophages.

Both these cell types tend to accumulate in the walls of respiratory bronchioles in smokers. Cigarette smoke is known to:
- cause cytoplasmic disturbance with release of proteolytic enzymes from polymorphs and macrophages;
- interfere with the antiproteolytic action of serum antiproteases such as α_1-antitrypsin. The zonal distribution of centrilobular emphysema is thought to be related to the poorer perfusion in the upper zones which results in less exposure of these areas to antiprotease present in the blood.

Panacinar destructive emphysema

This is a condition in which the entire architecture of the acinus and secondary lobule is disturbed (Figs 17.38 and 17.39) with no obvious localization of the disease process. Alveoli, alveolar ducts and respiratory bronchioles are

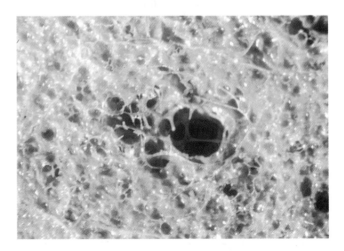

Fig. 17.37 Lung. Typical centrilobular emphysematous space.

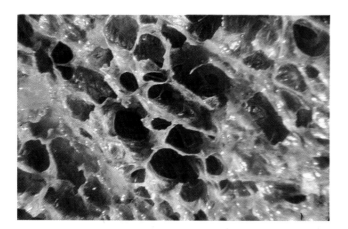

Fig. 17.38 Close up view of lung with panacinar emphysema.

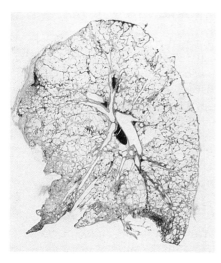

Fig. 17.39 Panacinar destructive emphysema as seen in a whole lung paper mounted section; all acini are replaced by abnormal air spaces.

replaced by a series of abnormal, large, irregular air spaces. Lower lobes are often more extensively affected than upper lobes. The aetiology of this form is thought to be related to a protease–antiprotease imbalance at the level of the alveolar wall. This may be due to a primary deficiency of antiprotease, as in familial α_1-antitrypsin deficiency (see below) or due to an increase in protease activity due to release of enzymes by neutrophils in alveoli. The latter may occur if noxious gases, for instance SO_2, are absorbed in the upper airways and excreted in peripheral alveoli where they excite a neutrophil response and subsequent release of proteases. Occasionally severe lung infections may result in destruction of alveolar walls with formation of emphysematous spaces, but this is unusual. One explanation for this apparent anomaly is that pneumococci, for instance, contain a powerful elastase inhibitor.

Familial emphysema and α_1-antitrypsin deficiency

This is a rare condition inherited as an **autosomal recessive**. Females are as frequently affected as males. The disease presents in the third and fourth decades, that is, much earlier than in the common form of the disease in cigarette smokers, and is of the panacinar variety affecting the lower lobes. Chronic bronchitis is seldom prominent, in contrast to centrilobular emphysema. The homozygotes are affected and have a very low level of antiprotease in their serum. Heterozygotes have only half the normal level of protease inhibitor but their lungs appear to be unaffected. The condition is much more complicated than first thought and there are at least 30 different alleles recognized. It is important because its discovery led to the idea that protease–antiprotease imbalance at the alveolar level was the main factor in the development of emphysema.

Other forms of emphysema

Abnormal air spaces are found around areas of scarring, often termed paracicatricial emphysema, and in zones of dust deposition—so-called focal emphysema. Rarer forms of the disease include congenital lobar emphysema and unilateral emphysema (MacLeod's syndrome), whose aetiology and pathogenesis are obscure.

Airways obstruction in emphysema

Emphysema is one of the causes of chronic obstructive lung disease. The reasons for the obstruction are multiple but one of the most important is the diminution in the number of airways of less than 2 mm diameter and the presence of peribronchiolar fibrosis and exudate in the bronchiolar lumens.

Complications

Patients with emphysema, particularly of the centrilobular variety, are liable to develop carbon dioxide retention and hypoxia. Secondary infection with development of pneumonia is common and this increases the hypoxia which in turn raises the pulmonary artery pressure and often precipitates cor pulmonale.

Bullous disease of the lung

In this condition large air-filled cysts or bullae are found in the subpleural regions, usually along the anterior margins of upper lobes or on the diaphragmatic surface of lower lobes. They are a striking finding at post-mortem examination but the underlying parenchyma may be normal or may be the seat of one of the other forms of emphysema. Bullae are in communication with the rest of the lung parenchyma and, when punctured in the living patient, rapidly refill with air. They may cause respiratory distress due to compression of underlying lung tissue as they act as a space-occupying lesion.

BRONCHIECTASIS

Bronchiectasis is the name given to the condition in which there is widespread and usually permanent dilatation of bronchi. It most often presents clinically when there is secondary infection.

Aetiology and pathogenesis

The condition is most commonly initiated by bronchial obstruction following inhalation of a foreign body in children, mucous plugs in asthma, tumours, especially bronchial carcinomas or carcinoids, or compression of a bronchus from without by enlarged reactive, tuberculous or tumorous lymph nodes.

The bronchus to the right middle lobe or that to the lingula is particularly susceptible to pressure from without due to their long, relatively unsupported course. As a consequence of the obstruction there is collapse of distal lung tissue, retention and secondary infection of retained secretions and weakening of the wall of the affected bronchus. This, with the changes following collapse (i.e. compensatory expansion of surrounding lung tissue together with chest wall, mediastinal and diaphragmatic shift towards the collapsed portion of lung) which result in increased negative pressure being transmitted across collapsed lung parenchyma to the bronchial wall, give rise to dilatation of the bronchial lumen.

Pathology

Grossly the affected airways (Fig. 17.40) exhibit varying morphological appearances described as fusiform, cylindrical or saccular but these carry no aetiological significance and are purely descriptive terms.

Histologically there is pus in the bronchial lumen with infiltration of the bronchial wall by neutrophils and lymphocytes. Mucosal ulceration may take place resulting in haemoptysis from the dilated submucosal veins. There is one form, known as follicular bronchiectasis, in which lymphoid follicles are prominent in the walls of the bronchiectatic sacs and in lung parenchyma, and this is said to be associated with adenovirus infection.

In all forms of the disease persistent infection results in focal areas of parenchymal fibrosis.

Complications include pneumonia, metastatic abscess

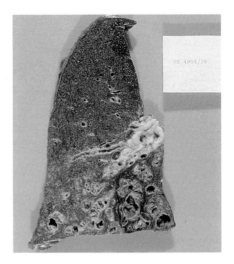

Fig. 17.40 Severe lower lobe bronchiectasis.

formation and, in cases which are of long standing, amyloid disease. In severe widespread disease extensive anastomoses are formed in the bronchial wall between the bronchial and pulmonary arterial circulations with resultant strain on the right side of the heart.

PULMONARY FIBROSIS

Pulmonary fibrosis may be **focal,** taking the form of an area of scarring as a sequel to an infection, e.g. tuberculosis, or **diffuse.** In the latter instance the disease may be idiopathic or caused by inhaled noxious agents often in an industrial environment, as in the pneumoconioses.

Fibrosing alveolitis (synonym: usual interstitial pneumonia; idiopathic diffuse pulmonary fibrosis)

Clinically these patients present with increasing dyspnoea which may or may not be accompanied by fever. There is little or no sputum and physical examination reveals a few rales over both lungs, which is in contrast to the chest radiograph where there is extensive patchy shadowing over both lungs with accentuation at the bases.

Pathology

Gross appearances. At necropsy both lungs are small, firm and have a typical nodular pleural surface described as bosselation (Fig. 17.41). The cut surface reveals numerous small cyst-like spaces surrounded by fine areas of fibrosis—an appearance sometimes described as honey-

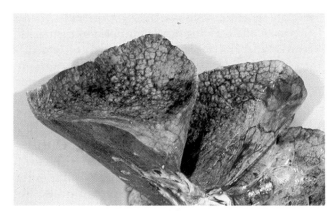

Fig. 17.41 Pleural surface of lung, which is the seat of severe interstitial fibrosis, showing bosselation.

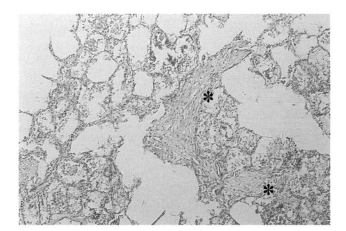

Fig. 17.42 Bronchiolitis obliterans with fibrous tissue (✱) growing in lumen of respiratory bronchiole. (Trichome stain.)

comb lung. Terminal infection may mask the cyst spaces which are then filled with purulent exudate and oedema fluid.

Histological findings. These are characterized by some diversity but two features are consistently present, fibrous thickening of the walls of the air spaces and metaplastic changes in the cells lining the air spaces. In cases of some standing smooth-muscle proliferation may be pronounced, so much so that in early literature some cases were referred to as 'muscular cirrhosis of the lung'. Many air spaces are lined by cuboidal type II pneumocytes and there may be frank squamous metaplasia. A focal lymphoplasmacytic infiltrate of varying intensity is present and in areas of dense fibrosis foci of calcification or ossification may be found. In some patients granulation tissue and fibrosis in the lumen of respiratory bronchioles are striking features and are known as bronchiolitis obliterans (Fig. 17.42). It is important to

identify this change as there is some evidence that cases showing it may respond to treatment with steroids.

Pathogenesis

Diffuse pulmonary fibrosis represents the end-result of diffuse alveolar damage which may occur following an acute incident (e.g. paraquat poisoning) or as a slowly developing process as in many industrial lung diseases but the majority of cases are of unknown aetiology. It represents a response to inflammation and many of the potentiating factors, which include release of proteolytic enzymes and generation of oxygen radicals, are derived from granulocytes. Studies of bronchioloalveolar lavage fluid and immunocytochemical investigations indicate that autoimmunity has an important but as yet undefined role in initiating the disease. The varied morphological appearances are probably a result of tissue being examined at different stages of the disease (Table 17.6).

Occupational lung disease

Pulmonary disease which develops as a result of conditions at work is an important cause of morbidity and mortality in certain industries, notably mining, but also in any occupation where workers are exposed to dust or toxic fumes.

Pneumoconiosis is the term used to describe lung changes brought about by inhaled dust. Although in general the extent and severity of lung lesions reflect the dose and length of exposure, individual susceptibility and the fibrogenic properties of the dust are important. Small quantities of silica and asbestos may produce extensive fibrosis, whereas a considerable quantity of coal dust can be inhaled with only mild fibrosis.

Silicosis

This is caused by inhalation of silicon dioxide which is the main constituent of quartz and thus those working in

Table 17.6 Conditions associated with diffuse pulmonary fibrosis. These are legion in number and a few general categories are listed in the table.

Idiopathic
Rheumatoid disease, scleroderma, dermatomyositis, Sjögren's syndrome
Oxygen toxicity, nitrous oxide fumes
Drugs, e.g. amiodorone
Industrial lung disease, the pneumoconioses
End-stage granulomatous disease, e.g. sarcoid, allergic alveolitis
Viral pneumonias
Histiocytosis X
Radiation fibrosis

mining of any variety necessitating drilling through rock containing quartz are liable to develop silicosis. In addition, workers in occupations such as sandblasting, stone masonry, pottery and ceramic manufacture, quarrying and metal grinding may develop the disease.

Pathology. There are three main forms described:

1 Simple silicosis. This is the commonest form and is found in most workers exposed to the dust. It takes the form of nodules 2–4 mm in diameter composed of concentrically arranged collagen fibres with some surrounding lymphocytic and macrophage infiltration. Calcification may be present and hilar lymph nodes can be involved. Unless very extensive, it is unlikely to result in clinical symptoms. **Progressive massive fibrosis** is the term applied when the nodules exceed 1 cm in diameter and are often much larger. Situated in upper zones of the lungs they often undergo cavitation and are frequently complicated by tuberculous infection which may indeed play a major role in the pathogenesis of the cavitation. Such patients experience increasing respiratory difficulty.

2 Acute silicosis. This is seldom encountered in modern times and is due to sudden heavy exposure to the dust, as in sandblasting. In the acute stage the histological appearances are those of alveolar proteinosis with intra-alveolar filling with finely granular, intensely positive periodic–acid Schiff material but intact alveolar walls and an absence of inflammatory cell infiltration.

3 Coal workers' pneumoconiosis. Coal miners may develop silicosis due to boring through rock in order to reach the coal but coal dust in itself may produce distinctive lung lesions.

(a) *Simple coal workers' pneumoconiosis* (Fig. 17.43). Working in the absence of silica, as occurs in those loading the holds of cargo ships with coal, results in coal dust particles being inhaled into the lungs. These particles are then phagocytosed by macrophages which migrate in and around respiratory bronchioles. These air spaces dilate, giving rise to an appearance similar to centrilobular emphysema but without any accompanying inflammation. This condition, sometimes called focal emphysema is associated with a fine mottling on the chest radiograph but little in the way of functional disability.

(b) *Progressive massive fibrosis (PMF;* Fig. 17.44). This condition is similar to the disorder of the same name occurring in silicosis. Its precise aetiology is unknown but it is probably due to the presence of silica in the rock being worked by the coal miners. It is also frequently associated with tuberculosis.

(c) *Caplan's syndrome.* In these patients rheumatoid arthritis is associated with progressive massive fibrosis of the lung. It is also found in patients with silicosis and asbestosis.

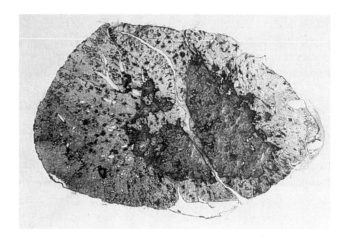

Fig. 17.44 Whole lung section from the lung of a coal miner showing progressive massive fibrosis.

Pathogenesis. The precise mechanism whereby the disease develops is not fully understood but it is certain that macrophages ingest silicon particles and stimulate them to produce cytokines which in turn promote fibroblast growth. Unfortunately, the silicon particles kill macrophages and are thus released back into the tissues, where they are once again ingested by macrophages and the whole cycle is repeated, leading to extensive and continual production of fibrous tissue.

Asbestos-associated lung disease

Asbestos-related lung disease, in contrast to silicosis and coal workers' pneumoconiosis, can occur following exposure to relatively small quantities of dust.

Asbestosis. Pathologically the primary lesion is one of in-

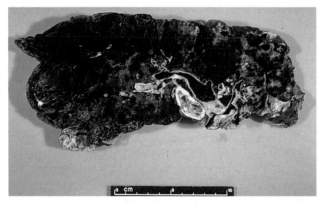

Fig. 17.43 Simple coal workers' pneumoconiosis with extensive dust deposition (black) and emphysema.

terstitial fibrosis in which typical asbestos (i.e. ferruginous) bodies (Fig. 17.45) can be detected. These bodies consist of an asbestos fibre, usually 10–20 μm in length and 0.1 μm diameter, covered with a beaded layer of ferritin and protein. The asbestos fibres are attacked by macrophages but the latter cannot engulf them as they are too large and they become coated with mucopolysaccharide, protein and ferritin.

The macrophages release a fibroblast-stimulating factor that promotes fibrogenesis that is the hallmark of the disease. Grossly the lower zones are more severely affected and there is disorganization of pulmonary architecture with development of fibrocystic disease or 'honeycomb' lung.

Mesothelioma. There is a strong relationship between exposure to the crocidolite form of asbestos and development of this malignant tumour (see below).

Carcinoma of the lung. There is an increased incidence of carcinoma of the lung among asbestos workers when compared with the general population. This increase is much more marked in those workers who smoke.

Extrinsic allergic alveolitis

This disease was originally known as farmer's lung as it was first described in agricultural workers handling mouldy hay. It was found to be due to inhalation of thermophilic actinomycetes, *Micropolyspora faeni*. Since this first description, numerous other foreign proteins have been found to induce the disease, giving rise to a variety of disorders, e.g. bird fancier's lung, bagassosis, wood pulp worker's lung, etc.

Clinically the disease has an acute and chronic phase.

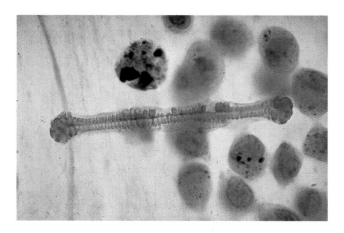

Fig. 17.45 Intra-alveolar ferruginous (asbestos) body.

The acute form is an influenza-like illness which occurs shortly after exposure to the allergen and is characterized by acute respiratory distress. In the chronic phase there is steadily increasing dyspnoea and in severe cases this may lead on to **cor pulmonale** (see Chapter 15).

Pathologically, in the acute phase there is extensive interstitial lymphoplasmacytic infiltration. Poorly formed granulomas are found in respiratory bronchioles and alveoli. In the chronic phase there is fibrosing alveolitis with eventual total architectural disorganization and formation of irregular cystic spaces, giving rise to the appearance known as **honeycomb lung**.

PULMONARY NEOPLASMS

Benign neoplasms

Benign tumours of the lung are relatively uncommon, whereas carcinoma of the lung is the major cause of cancer death in men and is appearing with an increasing frequency in women. Although the term cancer of the lung is commonly used, the vast majority of tumours are carcinomas arising in bronchi.

Carcinoma of the bronchus

Epidemiological studies have clearly demonstrated that the main aetiological factor in this disease is cigarette smoking. The latent period between onset of smoking and development of tumours is approximately 20 years and in the UK, where cigarette smoking became popular during the First World War, the incidence of lung cancer started to rise dramatically in the late 1930s and 1940s in men, whereas in women, who developed the habit somewhat later, the increase in the number of cases was delayed. Less frequent are occupational factors, notably exposure to uranium and asbestos.

Gross appearances
The majority of tumours arise centrally and careful dissection will usually reveal the bronchus of origin, though sometimes the condition is so advanced that this may not be possible. Ulceration of bronchial mucosa (Fig. 17.46) may give rise to the common symptom of haemoptysis. Occlusion of the lumen of the airway causes collapse of distal lung, retention of secretions, bronchiectasis and frequent secondary infection (Fig. 17.47). A common presentation is as an unresolved pneumonia. The mediastinal shift, due to the collapse, together with the rigidity imposed on the bronchial tree by the tumour,

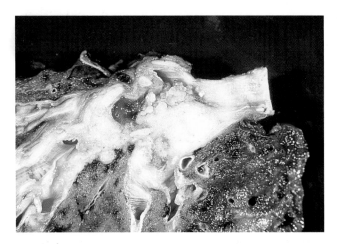

Fig. 17.46 Carcinoma of main bronchus ulcerating the mucosa and invading surrounding tissues.

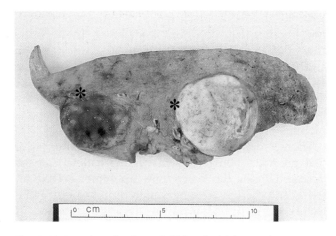

Fig. 17.48 Lung. Secondary 'canon ball' deposits (✳) from a primary carcinoma of the kidney.

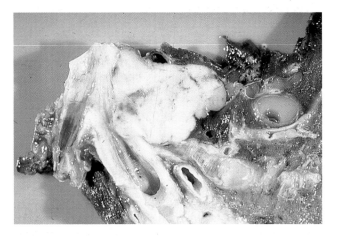

Fig. 17.47 Lung. Occlusion of a bronchus with tumour may produce collapse, consolidation and bronchiectasis distal to the tumour.

Although the 'pure' histological types listed below are those commonly encountered, mixed varieties may be found.

Squamous or epidermoid carcinoma (Fig. 17.49). This is the commonest tumour. It is characterized by pleomorphic but rather angulated cells with hyperchromatic nuclei, scanty cytoplasm and fairly frequent mitoses. The diagnostic feature is the finding of intercellular bridges or, in the better differentiated cases, individual cell keratinization or keratin pearls. If the site of origin of the tumour can be found, changes of carcinoma-*in-situ* can often be detected in adjacent mucosa.

probably accounts for the dyspnoea experienced by many of these patients. Peripheral tumours are less common and initially give rise to few symptoms, though later they may undergo necrosis and cavitate. It is essential in all cases of peripheral tumours to exclude the possibility that they represent secondary deposits from an extrapulmonary primary neoplasm (Fig. 17.48).

Histological types

Although the bronchus is lined by pseudostratified mucus-secreting epithelium, only approximately 25% of lung cancers are adenocarcinomas. This is perhaps not surprising considering the constitution of the epithelium and its capacity for regeneration following injury and the frequency with which metaplastic change is encountered.

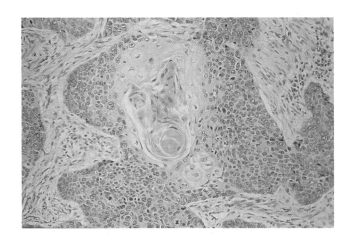

Fig. 17.49 Squamous carcinoma arising in a bronchus. Histology shows the characteristic squamous cell morphology with areas of keratin production and necrosis. (H&E.)

Adenocarcinomas (Fig. 17.50). These are of variable differentiation. In well-differentiated tumours there is evidence of glandular formation and secretion of mucus in haematoxylin and eosin preparations but in those that are less well-differentiated histochemical stains for mucus or electronmicroscopy may be needed to establish the diagnosis. These tumours are often peripheral and in such cases it is important to establish that the lesion is primary in the lung and not a secondary deposit.

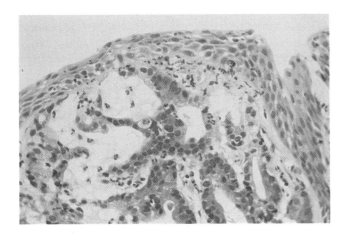

Fig. 17.50 Adenocarcinoma arising in a bronchus. There is squamous metaplasia of overlying bronchial mucosa. (H&E.)

Small cell carcinoma (Fig. 17.51). Originally known as oat cell carcinoma, this is the most malignant of lung cancers and carries a grave prognosis. It is composed of sheets or ribbons of small, somewhat oval, closely packed cells with very scanty cytoplasm and densely staining nuclei. There tends to be parallel orientation of the long axis of the cells. No obvious differentiation can be seen. Electronmicroscopy reveals that some of the cells contain electron-dense core granules of the neuroendocrine type in their cytoplasm, which is taken to indicate a relationship to the Kultchitsky cells found in the basal layer in normal bronchial mucosa.

Large cell undifferentiated carcinoma. As its name implies, this is a tumour in which on light microscopy no clear differentiation can be discerned. However, most such tumours when subjected to histochemical or ultrastructural investigation, show evidence of a squamous or glandular origin.

Bronchioloalveolar carcinoma

This is a peripheral carcinoma which arises in alveolar or bronchiolar epithelium. The tumour may thus resemble type I or II pneumocytes or mucus-secreting bronchiolar cells. They are described in the World Health Organization classification of lung neoplasms as a special form of adenocarcinoma and characteristically they grow on the walls of pre-existing alveoli (Fig. 17.52), a process known as lepidic growth. These tumours may present as a 'coin' lesion, as consolidation of a lobe or sometimes as multiple lesions scattered through the lung fields. Males and females are equally affected and there is not thought to be any relationship to smoking. Distinction from a solitary metastatic adenocarcinoma may be difficult, particularly

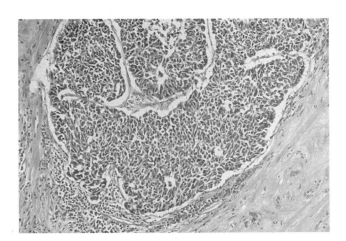

Fig. 17.51 Small or oat cell bronchial carcinoma composed of uniform darkly staining, closely packed cells with high nuclear cyoplasmic ratio. (H&E.)

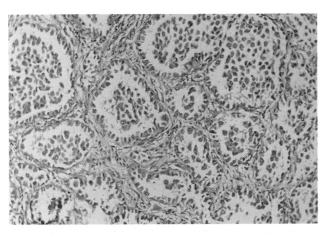

Fig. 17.52 Bronchiolo-alveolar carcinoma with tumour cells growing along alveolar walls. (H&E.)

as tumours from the alimentary canal, e.g. stomach and pancreas, may exhibit lepidic growth in secondary pulmonary deposits.

Carcinoid tumour

These tumours usually involve bronchi near the hilum, though occasionally they are situated peripherally, when they may be multiple. They can ulcerate the overlying bronchial mucosa giving rise to haemoptysis but more commonly either partially or entirely obstruct the bronchial lumen and present with pulmonary collapse, secondary infections or unresolved pneumonia (Fig. 17.53(a)).

Histologically, they show evidence of their origin from the Kultchitsky cells of the bronchial mucosa. The tumours are composed of small aggregates, sheets or inter-lacing trabeculae of cells that are uniform in appearance (Fig. 17.53(b)). They have small darkly staining nuclei and rather scanty pale pink cytoplasm. Superficially resembling carcinoids found in the alimentary canal, they differ in their staining reactions to silver. Being foregut derivatives, they are **argentaffin** or Fontana-negative but are **argyrophilic**, that is **Grimelius-positive**, whereas carcinoids of the ileum are both argentaffin and argyrophil-positive. There is a vascular fibrous stroma surrounding groups of tumour cells. Electronmicroscopy reveals typical intracytoplasmic dense core granules characteristic of a neuroendocrine tumour.

These tumours are always locally invasive and sometimes metastasize to lymph nodes and via the blood stream to distant organs and bone.

Other tumours

Other rarer lung tumours which are locally invasive include:
- cylindroma or adenocystic carcinoma;
- mucoepidermoid tumours;
- Pleomorphic adenomas.

Spread of malignant lung tumours

Carcinoma of the bronchus frequently metastasizes early in its natural history and indeed a solitary metastasis may be the presenting feature. It readily invades the surrounding pulmonary tissue and the mediastinum and pleural involvement occurs in peripheral tumours. Invasion of hilar and mediastinal lymph nodes is seen early and spread to cervical nodes is common. Blood spread takes place to liver and brain. Carcinoma of the bronchus is one of the tumours which has a tendency to produce bone metastases and the disease may present with a pathological fracture.

Pathological diagnosis

This is established by exfoliative cytology of sputum or from bronchial biopsy material.

Systemic effects

Lung cancer is a condition in which there is a high incidence of paramalignant disorders unrelated to the physical effects of the primary tumour. These include weight loss, finger clubbing, normocytic anaemia

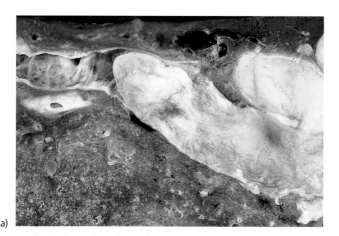

(a)

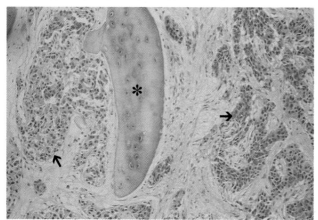

(b)

Fig. 17.53 Bronchial carcinoid (a) obstructing lower lobe bronchus and giving rise to collapse and secondary infection. (b) Histology with groups of cells (arrowed) with uniform appearance. Bone (✱) is present in the stroma, a feature associated with some of these tumours. (H&E.)

(leukoerythroblastic anaemia if there are bone secondaries), neuromyopathies (these are possibly autoimmune in origin) and the following endocrine disorders:
• ectopic adrenocorticotrophic hormone production;
• hypercalcitoninaemia;
• inappropriate antidiuretic hormone production;
• hyperthyroidism;
• carcinoid syndrome;
• gynaecomastia;
• hypercalcaemic syndrome;
• growth hormone production;
• hypocalcaemia.

PULMONARY EMBOLISM

Definition

Pulmonary embolism is defined as the transportation of undissolved material in the blood stream and its impaction in the pulmonary arteries. Embolism may be due to fat, trophoblast, tumours, brain, air, cotton wool or bone marrow, but is most often due to thrombus.

Pulmonary thromboembolism (Fig. 17.54)

This is an extremely common condition, occurring not only in hospital patients but also in patients at home. Pulmonary embolism arises as a result of detachment of thrombi present in leg or pelvic veins (Table 17.7). Massive pulmonary embolism is a cause of sudden death but non-fatal pulmonary embolism is probably very much more common than is realized (Fig. 17.55(a)). If the lungs are distended with fixative at post-mortem examination and carefully sliced, over 50% of hospital patients will be found to have had some small emboli (Fig. 17.55(b)).

Table 17.7 Pulmonary thromboembolism.

Site
Deep veins of the calf muscles
Pelvic veins
Prostatic venous plexus
Right ventricle

Risk factors
Virchow's triad
Surgery
Carcinoma
Coagulation disorders

Incidence
The cause of over 20 000 deaths per year in the UK
52% of necropsies
1–2/100 000 pregnancies

Classification
Acute, massive, resulting in sudden death or severe shock
Silent
Recurrent, giving rise to cor pulmonale
Resulting in pulmonary infarction

Pulmonary infarction

Pulmonary infarction (Fig. 17.56) is unusual unless there is also pulmonary venous congestion as, for instance, in mitral stenosis. When present the infarcted lung is solid, dull red, raised and sharply demarcated from surrounding lung. There is a fibrinous pleurisy over the infarcted zone and a small pleural effusion is a frequent finding. Histologically there may be true necrosis of alveolar walls or, more commonly, alveolar walls appear viable but the air spaces are filled with blood. In the first instance the infarct undergoes necrosis, organization and ultimate fibrosis. In the second type of lesion there may be complete resolution with removal of blood by alveolar macrophages and restoration of normal aeration (Table 17.8).

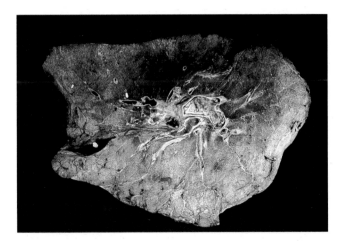

Fig. 17.54 Lung from a patient who died suddenly from a massive pulmonary embolus. Note the large mass of thrombus lodged in the pulmonary artery.

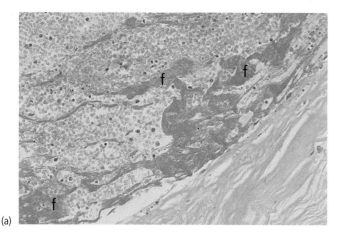

(a)

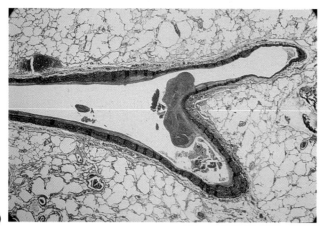

(b)

Fig. 17.55· (a) Acute pulmonary thrombo-embolus lodged in a pulmonary artery showing pink fibrin (f) containing enmeshed platelets, red cells and white cells. (H&E.) (b) A small, organizing pulmonary thrombo-embolus lodged at the bifurcation of a conducting pulmonary artery. (EVG.)

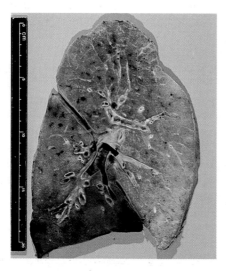

Fig. 17.56 Pulmonary embolus and infarction. This patient had longstanding congestive cardiac failure before suffering a large pulmonary thrombo-embolus. Note the wedge-shaped, red pulmonary infarction in the lower lobe.

Table 17.8 Variants of pulmonary infarction.

Complete infarct
True necrosis which organizes and undergoes fibrosis (often associated with infection)

Incomplete infarct
Alveolar walls are viable and filled with blood which resolves completely

VASCULITIC AND GRANULOMATOUS PULMONARY DISEASE

These are rare diseases.

Wegener's granulomatosis

This is a disorder which may on occasion be limited to the lung but more usually consists of glomerulonephritis, systemic vasculitis and necrotizing granulomas in the upper and lower respiratory tract. In the lung the lesions are characterized by an irregular outline, described as serpiginous or geographical, and are surrounded by a granulomatous cellular reaction, often with numerous Langhans-type giant cells. This inflammatory reaction involves branches of the pulmonary arterial tree with disruption of vessel walls. The aetiology is unknown but many of these patients have a circulating **antineutrophil cytoplasmic antibody (ANCA)**.

Lymphomatoid granulomatosis

This is a disease which may involve organs other than the lung but which may present with pulmonary manifestations. There are often multiple nodules scattered through the lungs and histologically these are described as angiocentric and angioinvasive. The cellular infiltrate is made up of lymphocytes, plasma cells and some neutrophils but also typically contains bizarre immunoblasts and atypical cells of the lymphoid series. The majority of these cases eventually reveal themselves as one or other form of lymphoma.

Churg–Strauss syndrome

Some asthmatic patients have nodules throughout the lung parenchyma which histologically are necrotic granulomas containing a heavy concentration of eosinophils.

These granulomas are accompanied by a pulmonary vasculitis. There is in addition a systemic vasculitis and a profound peripheral blood eosinophilia. The condition is probably related to systemic polyarteritis nodosa and responds to treatment with systemic steroids.

Sarcoidosis

This disease affects most frequently the lung and lymph nodes. The lesions consist of multiple, discrete, well-defined non-caseating epithelioid granulomas with a variable number of Langhans-type giant cells. There is hilar lymph node involvement. In the lung the granulomas are situated in walls of blood vessels, where there is accompanying destruction of elastic tissue, and in interlobular septa and walls of small airways. The condition, which is of unknown aetiology, may result in extensive interstitial fibrosis with resulting restrictive lung disease. Bronchioloalveolar lavage fluid contains a greatly increased lymphocyte count which is a feature that may be used in diagnosis.

DISEASES OF THE PLEURA

Pleural effusion

Fluid may accumulate in the pleural cavity as a result of exudation or transudation (Table 17.9).

Table 17.9 Types of pleural effusion.

Transudate (<2 g protein/100 ml fluid)	Heart failure, nephrotic syndrome, hepatic failure
Exudate (>2 g protein/100 ml fluid)	Pneumonia, malignancy, tuberculosis, pulmonary infarction, collagen vascular disease, subphrenic abscess, Meig's syndrome

Transudates occur in conditions where there is increased capillary pressure, as in left ventricular failure, or decreased plasma osmotic pressure secondary to hypoproteinaemia, as in liver cirrhosis or the nephrotic syndrome. The fluid when aspirated has a low protein content, less than 3 g/dl and few white cells.

Exudates are found in inflammatory or neoplastic disorders where there is increased capillary permeability with the result that the fluid has a high protein and cell content. The high protein may cause the fluid to clot and

examination of the cell content often provides diagnostic features, particularly in malignant disease. Other important causes of effusions of this type include tuberculosis, any form of pneumonia, rheumatoid disease, systemic lupus erythematosus and pulmonary infarcts (Table 17.10). Chylous effusions are encountered when there is obstruction of the thoracic duct usually by tumour in mediastinal lymph nodes. Haemothorax is most commonly due to trauma but is also found in malignancy and in pulmonary infarcts.

Table 17.10 Causes of pleural effusion.

Increased systemic venous pressure (causing obstruction to lymphatics resulting in transudate through the parietal pleura) e.g. heart failure
Obstruction to lymphatics e.g. malignancy, infection
Damage to capillary walls in the parietal pleura e.g. infection, inflammation, infarction, collagen vascular disease (SLE)
Unknown mechanism Hepatic failure, nephrotic syndrome, Meig's syndrome (associated with ovarian fibroma)

SLE, Systemic lupus erythematosus.

Empyema

The most important cause is local extension secondary to pneumonia. Mechanisms of infection and pathogens involved are shown in Table 17.11. In chronic disease it is important to consider tuberculosis.

Clinical presentation is non-specific. Radiological changes and persisting fever following treatment of pneumonia with appropriate antimicrobials are highly

Table 17.11 Organisms isolated from empyemal fluid.

Mechanism	Common pathogens isolated
Secondary to pneumonia	Streptococcus pneumoniae
Aspiration	Anaerobes, Streptococcus milleri, oral flora: often polymicrobial
Secondary to mediastinal and subdiaphragmatic disease	Anaerobes, Gram-negative bacilli: often polymicrobial
Posttraumatic	Staphylococcus aureus

suggestive of empyema. Complications include broncho-pleural fistula.

Diagnosis is by Gram stain (Ziehl–Neelsen for mycobacteria) and culture of pleural aspirate. Pleural biopsy is especially important for the diagnosis of tuberculosis. Pneumococcal antigen testing may be useful if therapy has already been initiated.

Drainage of fluid is the most important therapeutic option with decortication in chronic disease. Antibiotics are selected on the basis of the organism or presumed flora.

Pneumothorax

This condition may complicate many forms of lung disease, notably asthma, bullous disease, chronic bronchitis, emphysema, tuberculosis and pulmonary infarction. Most commonly, however, spontaneous pneumothorax occurs in young otherwise fit individuals without any obvious serious underlying parenchymal disease. In these subjects the pleura is punctuated by one or more small thin-walled cysts which are in all probability congenital defects. In cases where there have been one or more episodes of spontaneous pneumothorax histology reveals an exuberant proliferative pleuritis with abundant eosinophils, termed reactive eosinophilic pleuritis. The reason for this response is not known.

Pleural plaques (Fig. 17.57)

These are a common finding at post-mortem examination. They consist of hard shiny white masses most often found on the diaphragmatic pleura and on the parietal pleura of the lower chest wall. Histologically they consist of interlacing bundles of rather acellular collagen. They are considered to occur as a result of exposure to low levels of asbestos.

Pleural tumours

Benign pleural mesothelioma

This is a rare tumour arising usually from the visceral pleura and often attached to it by a thin vascular pedicle. It is usually single and may achieve a considerable size. Histologically it is composed of interlacing bundles of fibroblasts and collagen with few, if any, mitoses. Sometimes these tumours are associated with hypoglycaemia and electronmicroscopy reveals dense core granules in the cytoplasm of some of the tumour cells.

Malignant mesothelioma

This relatively common neoplasm is strongly associated with exposure to crocidolite, the blue form of asbestos. There is a latent interval of 10–40 years between exposure and clinical presentation with the tumour. At post-mortem examination there is a striking appearance, as often the entire lung is encased in tumour (Fig. 17.58). The condition may be unilateral or bilateral.

The histological appearances are variable due to the ability of mesothelium to differentiate into both spindle cell and epithelial-like forms. The main appearances encountered are:
- a tubulopapillary epithelial form;
- a fibromatous form;
- an undifferentiated form (Fig. 17.59).

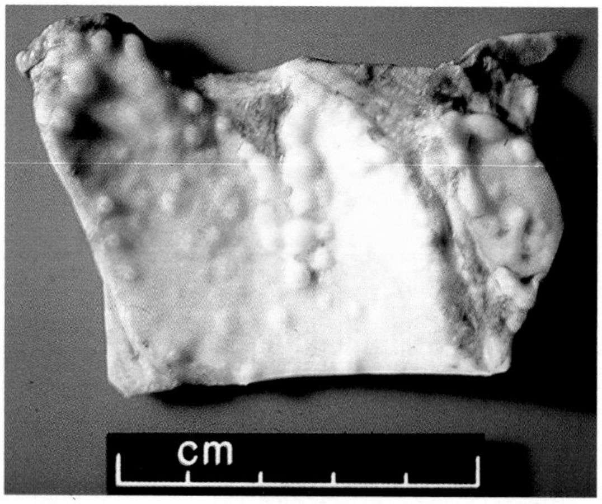

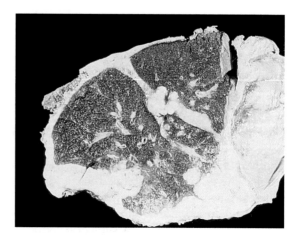

Fig. 17.57 Pleural plaque removed from the parietal pleura in a patient with a history of asbestos exposure from working in a brake-lining factory.

Fig. 17.58 Lung. Pleural mesothelioma with the entire lung encased by tumour.

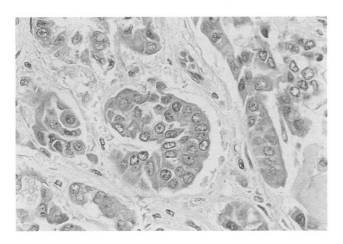

Fig. 17.59 Undifferentiated form of malignant mesothelioma. Histology shows large, atypical cells with prominent nucleoli. There is no keratin or mucin-production. (H&E.)

Diagnosis during life is established from examination of pleural fluid if this can be aspirated or from pleural biopsy material, but this is not always easy to differentiate from a truly epithelial neoplasm. Immunohistochemistry and the use of electronmicroscopy may help determine the diagnosis (see Chapter 1). The distinction is important as the disease, if acquired through an occupation, is one that may give rise to claims for compensation.

REFERENCE

The World Health Organization (1982) The World Health Organization histological typing of lung tumours. *American Journal of Clinical Pathology*; **77**: 123–136.

FURTHER READING

Dunnill M.S. (1982) *Pulmonary Pathology*. Churchill Livingstone.
Wenig B.M. (1993) *Atlas of Head and Neck Pathology*. WB Saunders, Philadelphia.
Woods G.L. & Gutierrez Y. (1993) *Diagnostic Pathology of Infectious Diseases*. Lea & Febiger, Philadelphia.

CHAPTER 18

Diseases of the Gastrointestinal Tract

CONTENTS

INTRODUCTION

In this chapter, diseases of each of the components of the gastrointestinal tract will be discussed, from mouth to anus. The approach taken will be according to the pathological sieve.

THE SALIVARY GLANDS

Normal anatomy

Major salivary glands
The parotid, submandibular and sublingual glands secrete in response to parasympathetic activity. The parotid

gland consists of superficial and deep lobes separated by the facial nerve and a few small lymph nodes.

Minor salivary glands
Minor salivary glands are scattered throughout the oral cavity and they secrete continuously.

Normal histology

Secretory acini are supported by myoepithelial cells and drain into a system of ducts. The parotid gland consists largely of serous glands and produces thin secretions which are low in protein. The sublingual gland consists of mucous glands which produce thicker secretions with a higher protein content and the submandibular gland consists of a mixture of both.

Function

Saliva contains mucins, enzymes (e.g. amylase and lysozyme), antibodies and inorganic ions. It has a role in digestion and in protection of the oral cavity.

Infection

Ascending bacterial infection may be seen in patients with a dry mouth, as a result of radiotherapy to the head and neck or as a consequence of autoimmune disease (Sjögren's syndrome – see below).

Causative organisms include *Streptococcus viridans*, *Staphylococcus aureus* and *Streptococcus pyogenes*.

Inflammatory diseases

Sialolithiasis – salivary calculi
Calculi are commonest in the submandibular gland because secretions here are richer in calcium salts. Stones may have a foreign body or bacterial nidus. They block ducts, leading to swelling of the distal salivary tissue. The gland becomes inflamed, with associated fibrosis and destruction of acini. Secondary bacterial infection may occur.

Histology. Dilated ducts undergo squamous metaplasia, chronic inflammation, fibrosis and acinar atrophy.

Sjögren's syndrome
This is an autoimmune disease with lymphocytic infiltration of exocrine glands, including the lacrimal and salivary glands (see Chapter 9). It may be primary (with dry eyes and dry mouth alone) or secondary (associated with other autoimmune disorders, particularly rheumatoid arthritis). There is an increased risk of lymphoma.

Histology. Infiltration of the gland by lymphoid cells forming germinal centres is seen. Islands of proliferated myoepithelial cells are present with atrophy of acini.

Irradiation sialadenitis
This occurs following irradiation to the head and neck and leads to destruction of acini with fibrosis.

Salivary gland tumours

The most recent World Health Organization classification (Seifert *et al.*, 1990) divides salivary gland tumours into:
- adenomas;
- carcinomas;
- non-epithelial tumours;
- malignant lymphomas;
- secondary tumours;
- unclassified tumours;
- tumour-like conditions.

Examples of the most commonly encountered tumour types are shown in Table 18.1.

Benign tumours
Pleomorphic adenoma (Fig. 18.1). These comprise 65–80% of tumours in the major salivary glands. The majority

Table 18.1 Salivary gland neoplams.

	Incidence (%)	Behaviour
Adenomas		
Pleomorphic adenoma (mixed parotid tumour)	60	Benign but can recur
Adenolymphoma (Warthin's tumour)	10	Benign
Monomorphic adenomas (various subtypes)	3	Benign
Carcinomas		
Mucoepidermoid tumour	5	Variable degree of malignancy
Acinic cell carcinoma	3	Low-grade malignancy
Adenoid cystic carcinoma	5	Malignant and invasive
Carcinoma in a mixed tumour	3	Variable degree of malignancy
Undifferentiated carcinoma	3	Highly malignant
Others include adenocarcinomas, lymphomas and squamous carcinomas		

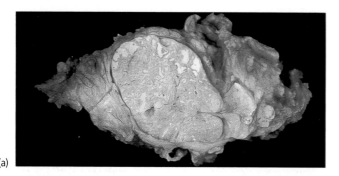

(a)

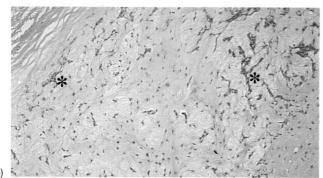

(b)

Fig. 18.1 Pleomorphic adenoma arising in the parotid gland. (a) Note how well circumscribed the tumour is. (b) Histology shows a mixture of epithelial elements (✳) in a chondromyxoid stroma. (H&E.)

arise in the **parotid** (superficial lobe 75%, deep lobe 25%).

They can occur at any age, but are commonest in the fifth and sixth decades and are more common in women than men.

Histologically, they consist of a mixture of epithelial, mucoid, myxoid and chondroid tissues in variable proportions. Generally they are well-circumscribed but have tongue-like projections which may be left behind after surgery. Wide excision and long-term follow-up are essential.

In 5–10% of cases there is **malignant transformation** of the epithelial component.

Adenolymphoma (Warthin's tumour; Fig. 18.2). These comprise 10% of all salivary gland tumours. They occur almost exclusively in the **parotid gland** and are bilateral in 10–15% of cases.

They are commonest in the sixth and seventh decades and in men (M/F = 2:1). Histology shows a multicystic mass of lymphoid tissue with cysts and papillae lined by a double layer of large eptithelial cells with granular pink cytoplasm.

These tumours are cured by excision.

Malignant tumours

Mucoepidermoid carcinoma. This is **rare**, representing 5% of all salivary gland tumours in adults. It is the commonest malignant salivary gland tumour in children.

The majority present in the **parotid** gland but they may also occur in the minor salivary glands. Histologically, they consist of a mixture of mucinous, squamous, intermediate and clear cells. They may be high-grade (5-year survival 56%) or low-grade (5-year survival 98%). These tumours can recur locally and have the potential for metastasis to regional lymph nodes and/or distant sites.

Acinic cell tumour. These tumours are **rare**. The majority occur in the **parotid**. They have solid, microcystic, papillary or follicular patterns. It is important to carry out wide local excision. Five-year survival is 89% and 20-year survival 56%. Acinic cell tumours metastasize particularly to the regional lymph nodes.

Adenoid cystic carcinoma. This is the commonest malignant tumour in the **minor salivary glands**. They can occur at any age but are commonest in the elderly.

Histologically they have a cribriform pattern with a mixture of tubular and solid areas. Invasion of perineural lymphatics is common.

Prognosis depend on the pattern of growth (solid pattern is worst), completeness of excision, size, anatomical site, degree of atypia and presence or absence of lymph node metastases. Five-year survival is 70% but 20-year survival is only 15%.

Lymphoma. Lymphoma may arise within intraparotid lymph nodes or from within the gland itself (see Sjögren's syndrome, above).

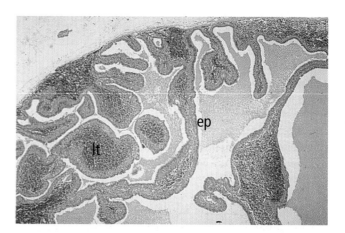

Fig. 18.2 Adenolymphoma of the salivary gland. Histology shows island of lymphoid tissue (lt) associated with epithelium (ep) featuring pink, granular cells. (H&E.)

THE MOUTH AND OROPHARYNX

Normal anatomy

The mouth and oropharynx are lined by stratified squamous epithelium, although with varying patterns of keratinization according to the site; for example, the hard palate is lined by keratinized epithelium and the soft palate by non-keratinized epithelium. The epithelium overlies vascular connective tissues.

Food is held in the mouth as it is chewed before being swallowed and passed on to the oesophagus.

Infectious diseases of the oropharynx

A variety of infectious diseases may be recognized in the oropharynx, the majority being of viral origin (Table 18.2).

Inflammatory diseases of the oropharynx

The oral mucosa may be affected by lichen planus, pemphigoid, pemphigus, erythema mutiforme and other mucocutaneous inflammatory diseases (Table 18.3).

Trauma to the oral tissues may result in a localized overgrowth of fibrous connective tissue forming an **epulis** or **fibroepithelial polyp**.

Aphthous ulcers may be single or mutiple. They heal spontaneously and are of unknown aetiology, although they are more common in patients with inflammatory bowel disease, particularly Crohn's disease.

Neoplasms of the oropharynx

Benign

Squamous papilloma is the most common benign tumour. These may be found on the tongue, lips or palate.

Malignant

Squamous cell carcinoma (Fig. 18.3). Oral squamous carcinoma represents 2% of cancers in the UK but there is wide variation in incidence worldwide. This tumour is commonest in the elderly and in men. It is often painless and is detected late.

The commonest site of presentation varies. In the west it is the floor of the mouth and the ventrolateral aspect of the tongue. In other parts of the world the lip or buccal mucosa may be predominantly affected.

Table 18.2 Infections of the oral cavity.

Disease	Causes
Infections	
Herpes simplex	Herpes simplex
Herpangina	Coxsackie virus A
Candidiasis	*Candida albicans*
Aphthous stomatitis	Unknown
Foot and mouth disease	Virus
Vincent's angina (gingivitis)	Vincent's spirochaete and fusiform bacilli
Tuberculosis	*Myobacterium tuberculosis*
Actinomycosis	*Actinomyces israelii*
Syphilis	*Treponema pallidum*
Measles	Measles virus
Koplik's spots (papules) on cheeks	
Diphtheria	*Clostridium diphtheriae*
Adherent membrane of fibrin and exudate on pharynx	
Leishmaniasis (espundia)	*Leishmania*

Table 18.3 Oral manifestations of systemic disease.

Skin disease	
Bullous pemphigoid	
Pemphigus vulgaris	
Erythema multiforme (Stevens–Johnson syndrome)	
Lichen planus	
Systemic disease	
Iron deficiency (Plummer–Vinson syndrome)	Atrophic glossitis
Telangiectasia (Osler–Weber–Rendu)	Telangiectases of mucosa and lips
Behçet's syndrome	Ulcers of mouth, conjuctiva, genitals
Metal poisoning (lead, silver, arsenic, gold, mercury)	Pigmented lesions of oral mucosa
Phenytoin	Hypertrophied gums
Scurvy (vitamin C deficiency)	Bleeding from gums
Vitamin B complex deficiency	Glossitis, angular cheilitis
Addison's disease	Pigmentation of oral mucosa
Haemochromatosis	Pigmentation of oral mucosa
Peutz–Jeghers syndrome	Pigmentation of oral mucosa

- **Aetiology.** Tobacco and alcohol are the most important factors. Others factors include ultraviolet light and iron-deficiency anaemia.
- **Macroscopic appearance.** This is most commonly as an ulcer with rolled edges and an indurated base.

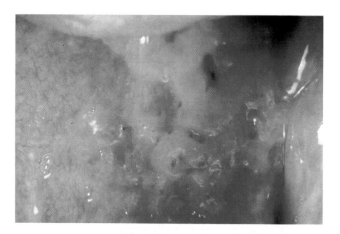

Fig. 18.3 Oral squamous cell carcinoma is a common malignancy but it may present late due to lack of pain associated with its growth. This illustrates the appearance of as lightly raised, white plaque in an early oral squamous cell carcinoma.

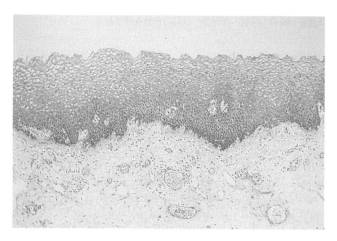

Fig. 18.4 Histology of the normal oesophagus which is lined by stratified squamous epithelium.

- **Histology.** The majority are well or moderately differentiated keratinizing squamous carcinomas.
- **Spread.** Initially local spread is seen. Involvement of cervical lymph nodes occurs relatively late in the disease's history.
- **Premalignant lesions.** Leukoplakia is a clinical term to denote a raised white area of hyperkeratosis. It is not indicative of malignancy but of an increased risk of malignancy, particularly if associated with red patches –erythroplakia. Other risk factors include site, a lesion on the tongue is more worrying than one on the hard palate, and smoking.

A biopsy of a worrying lesion might show hyperplasia, hyperkeratosis and dysplasia of keratinocytes (i.e. disordered architecture with nuclear and cytoplasmic changes similar to those seen in malignancy but without evidence of invasion through the basement membrane).

THE OESOPHAGUS

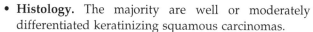

Normal anatomy

The oesophagus is a muscular tube extending from the pharynx to the cardia of the stomach, with sphincters at its upper and lower ends.

The lower sphincter is physiological rather than anatomical. The oesophagus is lined by non-keratinizing stratified squamous epithelium overlying muscularis mucosae, submucosa (loose vascular connective tissue and mucous glands) and muscularis propria (inner circular and outer longitudinal layers; Fig. 18.4).

Congenital stenosis of the oesophagus occurs. Congenital oesophageal atresia is associated with tracheo-oesophageal fistula in 80–90% of cases.

Motility disorders

Primary motility disorder–achalasia

Achalasia represents failure of relaxation of the lower oesophageal sphincter with absence of peristalsis in the oesophageal smooth muscle. The condition leads to a delay in emptying.

Symptoms include dysphagia (i.e. difficulty in swallowing), retrosternal fullness and pain with regurgitation.

Epidemiology. The incidence is 1:100000 of the population with an equal male to female ratio. It is commonest between the ages of 35–45 years.

Aetiology. This is unknown but it may be familial in some cases.

Pathology. Macroscopic features include oesophageal dilatation with thickening of the wall. The oesophagus may develop secondary changes such as diverticula or mucosal ulceration.

Histology shows **loss** or absence of **ganglion cells** in the myenteric plexus. Changes secondary to denervation and stasis occur, particularly hypertrophy of oesophageal smooth muscle and varying degrees of mucosal inflammation.

Other findings include degenerative changes in

extrinsic innervation; parasympathetic nerves, vagal trunk and decrease in vasoactive intestinal polypeptide fibres.

Complications include aspiration pneumonia, haemorrhage and carcinoma.

Secondary motility disorders

There are many acquired causes of dysmotility:
- Chagas disease (*Trypanosoma cruzi*);
- connective tissue diseases;
- muscular dystrophy;
- amyloid and diabetic neuropathy;
- idiopathic muscular dystrophy.

Mechanical disorders

Oesophageal rings and webs

These are uncommon.

Webs occur above the aortic arch. **Postcricoid webs** occurring in women and associated with iron-deficiency anaemia are known as **Plummer–Vinson** or **Paterson–Brown–Kelly syndrome** and are associated with an increased risk of squamous carcinoma in the oropharynx and oesophagus.

Rings occur below the aortic arch: 15% are associated with hiatus hernia.

Oesophageal diverticula

Diverticula may be congenital or acquired and occur in the upper, mid or lower oesophagus. Causes of acquired oesophageal diverticula include motility disorders, foreign-body penetration of the wall, hiatus hernias and strictures.

Hiatus hernia

Hiatus hernia involves the presence of part of the stomach above the diaphragmatic orifice. There are two main types:
1 **Sliding hiatus hernia.** These comprise 90% of hiatus hernias.

Aetiology is multifactorial. Factors such as age-related replacement of elastic fibres by collagen, congenital shortening and postinflammatory fibrous scarring, in conjunction with increased intra-abdominal pressure, result in a portion of the stomach sliding into the thorax. This is accentuated during swallowing.

Complications include reflux oesophagitis. Less frequently, minor haemorrhage may occur.
2 **Paraoesophageal 'rolling' hiatus hernia.** These comprise 5–10% of hiatus herniae. There is a female to male ratio of 4:1.

Aetiology involves increased intra-abdominal pressure

from whatever cause. Complications include haemorrhage, ischaemia, strangulation and infarction.

Inflammation–oesophagitis

Acute oesophagitis

Causes include bacterial infection, viral infection (e.g. herpes simplex, cytomegalovirus), fungal infection (e.g. *Candida*).

Acute oesophagitis may be corrosive, chemical or drug-induced (e.g. tetracyclin, clindamycin). Radiation oesophagitis is seen more commonly associated with radiotherapy of thoracic malignancy.

Chronic oesophagitis

Reflux oesophagitis is common and occurs at any age. It results in transient or persistent loss of tone of the lower oesophageal sphincter.

Common associated conditions are sliding hiatus hernia, pyloric stenosis and pregnancy. Less common associations are diabetic autonomic neuropathy and scleroderma.

At endoscopy, the mucosa is red, oedematous and may be ulcerated.

Histology. Histology of reflux oesophagitis is typical and includes basal hyperplasia, inflammation, ulceration, fibrosis and glandular metaplasia.

Complications. These include fibrous stricture, peptic ulceration and glandular metaplasia (Barrett's oesophagus).

Barrett's oesophagus (columnar cell-lined lower oesophagus)

This condition is found in 10% of patients with symptomatic reflux oesophagitis. The mucosa may resemble gastric or intestinal epithelium. There is an increased risk of malignancy in the latter (by 30–40 times).

Other rare causes of oesophagitis include tuberculosis, mucocutaneous diseases such as pemphigus, graft-versus-host disease, sarcoid, Crohn's disease, syphilis and Chagas disease.

Oesophageal neoplasms

Benign neoplasms

Leiomyoma. These benign tumours are commoner in men than women and may be single or multiple. They are usually an incidental finding.

An intramural site is most common and these tumours are usually less than 3 cm in size.

Other benign tumours are rare but are of numerous types, including lipoma, haemangioma and squamous papilloma.

Malignant neoplasms

Oesophageal carcinoma. This malignanacy has an incidence in the UK and USA of 5–10/100000 and represents 2–5% of all deaths from malignant disease. It is commonest in patients over 50 years of age and is more common in men (M:F = 1.5–3:1 except for Plummer–Vinson syndrome).

There is a wide geographical variation with a high incidence in North China, Iran and Russia. There may be a widely differing incidence in areas separated by only a few hundred miles.

Predisposing factors include:
- oesophageal strictures and achalasia;
- Plummer–Vinson syndrome (affects women more than men);
- Barrett's oesophagus, in which there is an 8–10% risk of developing **adenocarcinoma**;
- alcohol;
- smoking (risk increased 40 times if >40 years of smoking and >80g of alcohol a day);
- coeliac disease;
- tylosis–this is an extremely rare autosomal dominant condition in which there is hyperkeratosis of the palms and soles and a high risk of developing squamous carcinoma of the oesophagus.

Dietary factors are thought to be involved, including fungal contamination of food; food with a high nitrite content; deficiencies of vitamins and trace metals.

- **Site.** Approximately 50% occur in the middle third of the oesophagus; these are usually squamous carcinomas. Thirty per cent occur in the lower third; these may be squamous or adenocarcinomas. Twenty per cent occur in the upper third; these are squamous carcinomas.
- **Presentation.** Progressive dysphagia (difficulty in swallowing, initially just solids but later also liquids); decreased weight and decreased appetite.
- **Diagnosis** involves radiology; endoscopy, particiularly the combination of cytology and biopsy, gives 95% diagnostic accuracy.
- **Macroscopic appearances.** Oesophageal carcinoma presents as a flat, ulcerated or warty mass which may result in the formation of a stricture.
- **Histology.** Ninty per cent are squamous carcinomas; 10% adenocarcinoma (if carcinomas of the cardia with upward spread are excluded).
- **Spread** may be directly to bronchi, lungs, pleura, aorta and superior/posterior mediastinum or to regional lymph nodes (50% of patients who come to surgery have positive nodes at the time of operation)–paratracheal, parabronchial, paraoesophageal, posterior mediastinal, coeliac, upper deep cervical. Vascular metastases occur to the liver, lungs and adrenals.
- **Prognosis.** Resection is only possible in up to 50%. The others are treated by radiotherapy. The 5-year survival is only 5–10% with 70% dead within 1 year.

Other malignant oesophageal tumours are rare but include adenoid cystic carcinoma, malignant melanoma, small cell carcinoma, leiomyosarcoma and metastases from malignant tumours at other sites.

Vascular diseases of the oesophagus

Oesophageal varices

Varices are seen as a complication of portal hypertension with formation of portosystemic venous shunts (see Chapter 19).

The commonest cause is cirrhosis. There is a 40% risk of mortality at each episode of bleeding.

Oesophageal lacerations

These are uncommon and usually occur as result of prolonged vomiting (e.g. in alcoholics).

THE STOMACH

Normal anatomy and histology

The stomach is situated in the upper-left-hand part of the abdomen and is important for the mixing and digestion of food. It can be divided into three distinct regions:
- the **cardia**–situated immediately below the gastro-oesophageal junction and lined by mucus-secreting glandular epithelium;
- the **fundus** and **body**, lined by mucosa within which there are tight coiled tubular glands with parietal cells (acid and intrinsic factor) in their upper part and chief cells (pepsinogen) in their lower as well as mucus and endocrine cells;
- the **gastric antrum**–situated between the incisura on the lesser curve to the pylorus and lined by glands with mucus cells and endocrine cells, the latter secreting gastrin and other hormones (Fig. 18.5).

The mucosa overlies muscularis mucosae, submucosa and muscularis propria with inner circular and outer longitudinal layers. Congenital abnormalities of the stomach include diaphragmatic hernias (see above) and pyloric stenosis.

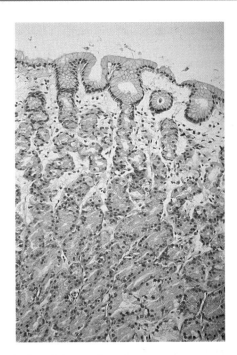

Fig. 18.5 Histology of the normal gastric mucosa.

Congenital pyloric stenosis

Pyloric stenosis is one of the commonest congenital disorders to affect the gastrointestinal tract (Fig. 18.6). This condition occurs in approximately 1 in 500 live births and is four times more common in males than females, with a tendency to affect the first-born infant. Although there is a familial tendency, no clear pattern of inheritance has been established.

As Fig. 18.6 shows, the condition is associated with concentric hypertrophy of the muscle at the pyloric

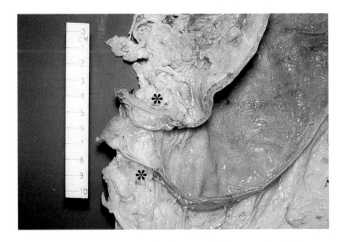

Fig. 18.6 Hypertrophic congenital pyloric stenosis from a newborn baby. ✳, marks the region of the pylorus. Note the thickened wall.

sphincter. Symptoms of gastric outlet obstruction are seen within a week or two after birth and include **projectile vomiting** with visible gastric peristalsis. Treatment is highly successful and consists of myotomy or splitting of the hypertrophied muscle to the level of the mucosa.

Inflammation–gastritis

Acute gastritis

Acute gastritis may be idiopathic or associated with duodenal ulcer, hiatus hernia, uraemia, cirrhosis, acute alcoholism, shock, drugs (e.g. aspirin, non-steroidal anti-inflammatory drugs–NSAIDs–ferrous sulphate). Acute gastritis is potentiated by smoking.

Inflammation may involve the mucosa only (haemorrhagic, erosive) or the full thickness of the wall (phlegmonous).

Histology. Histology of acute gastritis features oedema, haemorrhage, acute inflammation and variable necrosis.

Aetiology. Breakdown of the balance between aggressive (i.e. peptic secretions) and defensive (i.e. surface mucus–bicarbonate layer, tissue prostaglandins) factors are involved in the aetiology of acute gastritis. For example, aspirin inhibits prostaglandin synthesis, and mucosal hypoxia may damage the mucosal barrier, allowing back-diffusion of hydrogen ions.

Chronic gastritis

Chronic gastritis is a non-specific histopathological sequela to diffuse, long-standing and multifactorial injury.

There is little correlation between the endoscopic and histological appearances.

Classification of chronic gastritis. Classification **histologically** is on the basis of the type of gastric mucosa affected, distribution of inflammation and presence or absence of atrophy into:
• superficial chronic gastritis;
• chronic atrophic gastritis;
• gastric atrophy.

The presence of neutrophils denotes activity. Presence or absence of *Helicobacter pylori* may give another clue as to the aetiology.

Gastritis can be divided on a **clinicopathological** basis into the following:
• **Type A (autoimmune):** Involves the body and features circulating antibodies to parietal cells and to **intrinsic factor**. Hypo-/achlorhydria is a feature with raised gastric pH. Hypergastrinaemia occurs with loss of pa-

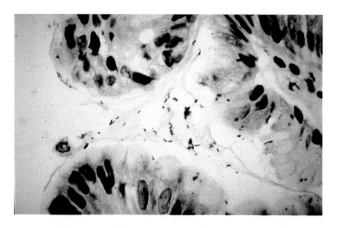

Fig. 18.7 *Helicobacter pylori* adheres to the gastric epithelium. Note the curved shaped of the bacteria, shown here using a silver stain (black).

rietal cells, gastric atrophy and intestinal metaplasia. Ten per cent develop overt **pernicious anaemia**; 2% develop hyperplasia of antral G cells. Type A gastritis is often associated with other organ-specific auto-immune disorders and with an increased risk of gastric cancer.
- **Type B (bacterial):** This is not associated with auto-antibodies but is associated with *H. pylori* in over 90% of cases (Fig. 18.7).
  H. pylori is a Gram-negative spiral bacterium that lives on the surface epithelium beneath the protective mucous layer. It is thought to produce cellular damage with a consequent acute inflammatory response. There are two subtypes;
  (a) **Hypersecretory** (associated with duodenal ulcer). Intestinal metaplasia is not conspicuous and there is no association with carcinoma.
  (b) **Environmental**. Associated with metaplasia. This is seen in areas with a high incidence of gastric carcinoma.
- **Type C (chemical):** Associated with enterogastric reflux, NSAIDs and alcohol. Type C gastritis is characterized by normal numbers of inflammatory cells together with foveolar hyperplasia, increased vascularity and increased smooth-muscle fibres.
- **Other types of gastritis** include hypertrophic (Ménétrier's), varioliform, eosinophilic, bacterial, fungal, viral, sarcoid, tuberculosis, portal hypertensive gastropathy, uraemia and irradiation gastritis.

Peptic ulceration (including duodenal ulcer)

Peptic ulcers occur in areas exposed to peptic secretions:
- lowest end of the oesophagus;
- the lesser curve of the stomach;
- the antral and prepyloric regions;
- the anterior and posterior walls of first part of duodenum;
- in the area around the anastomosis following gastroenterostomy;
- in the second, third and fourth parts of the duodenum and upper jejunum in Zollinger–Ellison syndrome;
- in or adjacent to a Meckel's diverticulum.

Peptic erosions
Erosions involve less than the full thickness of the mucosa and may be multiple. Site depends on cause but they are most common in the body. The aetiology of gastric erosions is similar to acute gastritis and, in particular, stress appears to be involved.

Acute ulcers
Ulcers involve the full thickness of the mucosa and are common in the body. The aetiology is as above.

Chronic peptic ulcers (Fig. 18.8)
Chronic peptic ulcers are usually single and are rare in the body. They are usually less than 2 cm in size and are round or oval with typical 'punched-out' edges. A grey base contains blood clot and acute inflammatory exudate. There may be submucosal, muscular and serosal fibrosis with adherence to underlying structures. The surrounding mucosa may appear atrophic.

Duodenal ulcer. Anterior duodenal ulcers are more common than posterior ulcers. Two per cent occur distal to the first part of the duodenum. Chronic antral gastritis is invariable and is associated with *H. pylori* in 90–100% of cases.

Complications of chronic peptic ulcer. Complications are common and include:
- perforation;
- haemorrhage;
- fibrosis and stenosis;
- involvement of adjacent organs, e.g. pancreas, large bowel;
- risk of developing carcinoma in a chronic peptic ulcer is probably <1%.

Prevalence and incidence. There is marked fluctuation in the incidence from time to time and from place to place. The male/female ratio is 2–3:1 with duodenal ulceration being more common than gastric ulceration in both sexes. The decrease in incidence over the last 25 years is thought to be due to changes in birth cohort risk.

Aetiology. Two distinct groups are duodenal and prepyloric ulcer and gastric ulcer (Table 18.4).

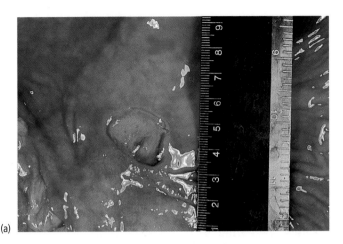

(a)

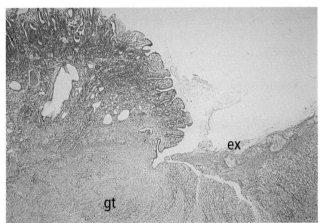

(b)

Fig. 18.8 (a) A chronic gastric ulcer. Macroscopic appearance. Note the punched-out margin. (b) The histological appearance of a benign chronic gastric ulcer reveals inflammatory exudate (ex) in the surface of the ulcer with granulation tissue (gt) in the ulcer base. (H&E.)

Neoplasms of the stomach

Benign polyps

Benign polyps may be hamartomatous, inflammatory or neoplastic.

Cystic fundic polyps are common multiple, small, transparent, sessile polyps seen in middle-aged women and increased in frequency in patients with familial adenomatous polyposis. They are harmless. **Peutz–Jeghers polyps** and **juvenile polyps** are found in the stomach. **Heterotopic pancreas** may also present as a benign gastric polyp. **Inflammatory polyps** are not truly neoplastic. Hyperplastic polyps are common at this site.

Benign tumours

Adenomas of the stomach are rare but they have malignant potential and there is a high risk of coexistent carci-

noma. **Leiomyoma** usually measures less than 4 cm and is submucosal with central ulceration of overlying mucosa (Fig. 18.9). Leiomyoma may present with haemorrhage. Behaviour may be unpredictable and distinction of benign from malignant tumour may be difficult. **Lipoma** of the submucosa may be found.

Malignant tumours

Carcinoma is the most common malignant neoplasm (90–95%), followed by lymphoma (4%), gastric carcinoid (< 3%) and leiomyosarcoma (2%).

Carcinoma

- **Epidemiology.** Incidence in the UK and USA is 20/100 000, where it is the third most fatal carcinoma, causing 10% of deaths from malignancy. It has been decreasing in incidence in recent years.

  Gastric carcinoma is commoner in men than women (1 : 1 in the young to >2 : 1 in the elderly) with an increas-

Table 18.4 Aetiology of duodenal and prepyloric ulcer.

Duodenal ulceration
Hyperacidity
Increase in meal stimulated acid secretion of 50%
Increase in parietal cell mass correlates with acid output
Increased speed of gastic emptying
Genetic factors
Association with blood group O and non-secretors
Risk increased 2–3 times in relatives
50% of patients have elevated serum pepsinogen I; 50% do not
Multiple endocrine neoplasia type 1 (MEN1)
Stress is probably involved to some extent but direct evidence is lacking
Gastric ulceration
Normal or hypoacidity
Gastritis is more extensive and severe than in duodenal ulcer
The mechanism is unknown
Theories include:
Reflux of duodenal contents leading to a chronic inflammatory reaction and an increase in susceptibility to action by acid or pepsin
Removal of surface mucin by bile acids resulting in the breakdown of the gastric mucus barrier causing back-diffusion of hydrogen ions
But normal controls show same degree of bile reflux as gastric ulcer patients
Factors common to both types
Smoking: adverse affect on healing
Drugs particularly aspirin and NSAIDs
Role of *Helicobacter pylorii* is unclear

NSAIDs, Non-steroidal anti-inflammatory drugs.

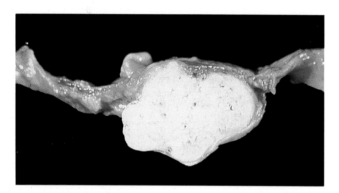

Fig. 18.9 The macroscopic appearance of a benign gastric leiomyoma. Note how it pushes up the mucosa.

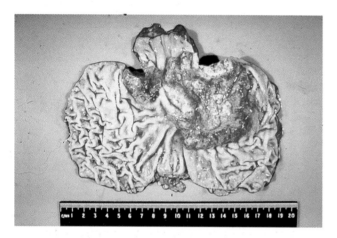

Fig. 18.10 The macroscopic appearance of a fungating gastric carcinoma originating at the base of the oesophagus.

ing incidence with age. There is wide geographical variation, with a high incidence in Japan and Scandinavia and a relatively low incidence in the USA and UK.

- **Aetiology and pathogenesis.** Gastric carcinoma is multifactorial with many predisposing factors:
  (a) chronic gastritis;
  (b) pernicious anaemia;
  (c) previous partial gastrectomy;
  (d) adenomatous polyps;
  (e) dietary factors.
  High-risk populations seem to have high intakes of salt and complex carbohydrate and low intakes of animal fat, protein, leafy greens, vegetables and fruit.
- **Site.** 50–60% occur in the pylorus and antrum; 25% in the cardia; 40% on the lesser curve and 12% on the greater curve.
- **Symptoms.** Weight loss, abdominal pain, anorexia,

vomiting, altered bowel habit, dyspepsia, anaemic symptoms and haematemesis.
- **Diagnosis.** Barium meal and endoscopy with cytology and biopsy.
- **Macroscopic appearances.** Polypoid, ulcerated or diffusely infiltrating (linitis plastica or leather bottle stomach; Figs 18.10 and 18.11(a)).
- **Histology.** This is an adenocarcinoma (Fig. 18.11(b)). Several different classifications exist. The simplest is **Lauren's classification** which divides gastric adenocarcinoma into two types:
  (a) **intestinal** (with glandular differentiation); and
  (b) **diffuse** (tumour cells single or in small clumps. Often 'signet-ring' cells.
- **Spread.** Direct spread to the pancreas and transverse colon may occur. Lymphatic metastases occur to lymph nodes on the lesser curve, greater curve, porta hepatis, coeliac axis and supraclavicular fossa (70% have positive nodes at surgery, 90% at autopsy). Haematogenous metastases to the liver, lung, skin

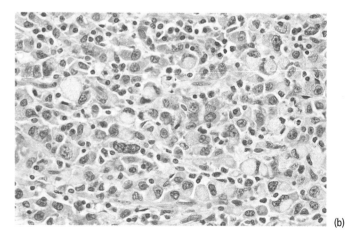

(a)

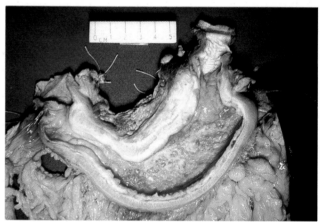

(b)

Fig. 18.11 Infiltrating gastric adenocarcinoma. (a) Macroscopic appearance or 'linitis plastica' ('leather-bottle stomach'). (b) Histological appearance. Note the mucin-containing 'signet-ring' adenocarcinoma cells. (H&E.)

and ovaries may occur (10% have liver metastases at surgery).
- **Prognosis.** This is poor with a 5-year survival of only 20–30%.

Early gastric cancer. This is a carcinoma which is limited to the mucosa or mucosa and submucosa, irrespective of whether or not metastasis to lymph nodes has occurred. It can be subclassified on the basis of the endoscopic and macroscopic appearances. This malignancy evolves slowly and may take up to 8 years to become invasive. Early gastric cancer forms 35% of cases of gastric cancer in Japan where there is a screening programme aimed at detecting early gastric cancers. It forms 10% of cases elsewhere. The 5-year survival is 80–90%.

Primary gastric lymphoma (Fig. 18.12). The gut is a common site of **secondary involvement** in disseminated lymphoma. Therefore for **diagnosis** of a **primary lesion** there should be:
- no palpable lymphadenopathy at presentation;
- no enlargement of mediastinal lymph nodes on chest X-ray;
- normal white cell count (total and differential);
- at laparotomy the bowel lesion predominates, with any obviously involved nodes being related to the affected organ;
- the liver and spleen appear free from tumour at laparotomy.

   Gastric (and other gastrointestinal) lymphomas are probably increasing in incidence because of acquired and therapeutic immunosuppression.
- **Macroscopic appearances.** Gastric lymphomas occur in the body or antrum and only rarely in the cardia.

Table 18.5 Histological classification of primary gastrointestinal lymphomas.

Low-grade
B-cell
   Small cell (lymphoma of mucosa-associated lymphoid tissue; MALT)
   Mediterranean lymphoma (immunoproliferative small intestinal disease)
   Malignant lymphomatous polyposis (centrocytic)
   Others (rare) e.g. follicular, plasmacytoma
T-cell
   Small cell pleomorphic (± enteropathy)

High-grade
B-cell
   Large cell
   Burkitt-type (immunoblastic)
   Others (rare), e.g. pure centroblastic, pure immunoblastic
T-cell
   Medium/large cell pleomorphic (± enteropathy ± tissue eosinophilia)
   Others (rare), e.g. immunoblastic, large cell anaplastic

True histiocytic lymphoma

Unclassified

They may be single, multiple or diffuse, nodular or polypoid and are often ulcerated (Table 18.5).
- **Treatment.** Surgery or radiotherapy if there is lymph node involvement.
- **Prognosis.** Stage is the most important variable. Low-grade lymphomas confined to the mucosa and submucosa have a good prognosis; prognosis is poor if the tumour is more advanced.

Carcinoid tumours. Carcinoid tumours of the stomach tend to be aggressive (see below).

THE SMALL INTESTINE

Normal anatomy

The small intestine consists of the **duodenum**, **jejunum** and **ileum**. The main functions of the small intestine are **digestion** and **absorption**.

   The small intestine is composed of **glandular** mucosa, with **villi** (functional compartment) and **crypts** (proliferative compartment) overlying **muscularis mucosae**, **submucosa** (includes Brunner's glands in the duodenum) and **muscularis propria** (Fig. 18.13).

   Covering the villi there are **absorptive cells**, **goblet cells** and occasional **neuroendocrine cells**. Lining the

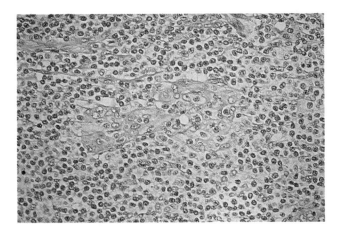

Fig. 18.12 The histological appearance of a gastric lymphoma of MALT-type. Note the lymphocytic infiltration and destruction of the glands. This is a 'lympho-epithelial lesion'. (H&E.)

crypts are **goblet cells**, **neuroendocrine cells**, undifferentiated **stem cells** and, at the base of the crypts, **Paneth cells**.

Congenital abnormalities

Congenital abnormalities of the small intestine include malpositions, omphalocoele, aplasia, agenesis, atresia, stenosis, duplications, diverticula, cysts, heterotopias, hamartomas and aganglionosis. The commonest is Meckel's diverticulum.

Meckel's diverticulum

Meckel's diverticulum represents persistence of the proximal part of the **vitellointestinal duct** and is seen in 1–4% of the population, equally in males and females.

The diverticulum is seen on the antimesenteric border of the small bowel, 90 cm from the ileocaecal valve in adults and may contain heterotopic tissue (e.g. gastric or large intestinal epithelium, pancreas). Complications include:

- peptic ulceration;
- perforation and haemorrhage;
- volvulus;
- obstruction;
- intussusception;
- perforation by a foreign body.

Meckel's diverticulum may be the site of tumours, but these are rare.

Malabsorption syndromes

Maldigestion may occur if there are defects in gastric,

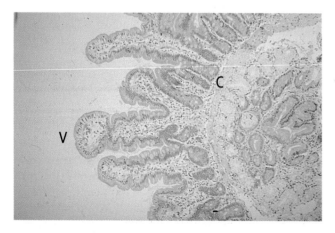

Fig. 18.13 The histology of the small intestine. Note the normal villous (V) to crypt (C) ratio. (H&E.)

pancreatic or hepatobiliary function (Table 18.6). Malabsorption falls into three main categories:

- inborn abnormalities, e.g. disaccharidase deficiency, glucose-6-phosphatase deficiency, a-β-lipoproteinaemia;
- acquired damage to surface enterocytes, crypts or both (see below);
- local organic disease or previous surgery, e.g. diverticula, stagnant loops, short circuits of bowel which decrease the surface area available for absorption and/or disturb the normal small intestinal ecology.

Clincial features of malabsorption

Steatorrhoea and anaemia are the commonest presenting features (Table 18.7).

Investigations

Naked-eye examination of stools, estimation of faecal fats, routine haematology, barium meal and follow-through, small-bowel enema, ultrasound, measurement of small intestinal transit times and carbohydrate absorption by hydrogen breath tests, tests for calcium and bile absorption may be necessary. Ultimately, biopsy and histology may provide the diagnosis.

Malabsorption due to damage to enterocytes

Coeliac syndromes (coeliac disease and idiopathic steatorrhoea). The incidence of coeliac syndromes in the UK is in the region of 1:1500–2000.

Ninety-eight per cent respond to a gluten-free diet—**coeliac disease**. Two per cent do not respond to a gluten-free diet—**idiopathic steatorrhoea**.

Coeliac disease. Coeliac disease usually presents in children. The following are required for diagnosis:

- abnormal villous pattern on biopsy;
- clinical and mucosal improvement on withdrawal of gluten from the diet (usually within 3–6 months);
- if there is still clinical doubt—symptomatic and mucosal relapse following the reintroduction of gluten into the diet.

Histology. This shows villous atrophy with some degree of crowding and overlapping of surface enterocytes; crypt hyperplasia; increased numbers of intraepithelial lymphocytes and increased numbers of chronic inflammatory cells in the lamina propria (Fig. 18.14).

Aetiology and pathogenesis

- **Gluten.** The probable toxic component is gliadin but the exact mechanism is still unknown (see below).
- **Genetic factors.** Human leucocyte antigen (HLA) associations (in northern Europe the disease is associated with HLA B8, DR3 and DQ2).

Table 18.6 Mechanisms and causes of malabsorption syndrome.

Inadequate digestion
Postgastrectomy
Deficiency of pancreatic lipase
Chronic pancreatitis
Cystic fibrosis
Pancreatic resection
Zollinger–Ellison syndrome (high acid inhibits lipase)

Deficient bile salt concentration
Obstructive jaundice
Bacterial overgrowth (leading to bile salt deconjugation)
Stasis in blind loops or diverticula
Fistulas
Hypomotility states (diabetes, scleroderma, visceral myopathy)
Interrupted enterohepatic circulation of bile salts
Terminal ileal resection
Crohn's disease
Precipitation of bile salts
Neomycin and cholestyramine

Primary mucosal abnormalities
Coeliac disease
Tropical sprue
Whipple's disease
Amyloidosis
Radiation enteritis

Inadequate small intestine absorption
Intestinal resection
Crohn's
Mesenteric vascular disease with infarction
Jejunoileal bypass

Lymphatic obstruction
Intestinal lymphangiectasia
Malignant lymphoma

Possible ways in which mucosal damage could be sustained
- **Direct effect** of a breakdown product of **gluten**–no evidence.
- A **defect** in **enzyme synthesis** within enterocytes leading to incomplete breakdown of gluten and the presence of gliadin fractions toxic to enterocytes.
- **Immunologically mediated.**
  (a) **Humoral.** Coeliac disease may be associated with a selective deficiency of immunoglobulin A (IgA). Serum antibodies to gluten and gliadin fractions are found in the majority of coeliac patients.
  (b) **Cellular.** Antibody-dependent and cell-mediated cytotoxicity.
  (c) **Adenoviruses.** There is a region of homology between α-gliadin and the early region E1β protein of

human adenovirus 12. Cross-reacting antibodies occur and it is possible that loss of tolerance to gluten could occur following adenovirus infection in susceptible individuals.

Complications and associated conditions
- splenic atrophy;
- dermatitis herpetiformis–60–80% of these patients also have coeliac disease;
- perforating ulceration;
- small intestinal lymphoma;
- carcinoma of the small intestine and even oesophagus.

Malabsorption due to infections

Tropical sprue. Tropical sprue has similar clinical features to coeliac disease and is acquired by visitors to the Caribbean, South America, West Africa, South-east Asia and the Philippines. This disease is caused by enteric pathogens, mostly coliforms, which produce enterotoxins acting directly on enterocytes and crypt cells. Tropical sprue responds to treatment with antibiotics.

Table 18.7 Systemic effects of malabsorption.

Dietary factor	Clinical effect
Total calories	Weight loss, general weakness
Protein	Muscle wasting (increased gluconeogenesis), osteoporosis, oedema, ascites
Decreased pituitary hormones	Amenorrhoea
Calcium	Hypocalcaemia, tetany, paraesthesias, secondary hyperparathyroidism, osteomalacia, osteitis fibrosa cystica
Magnesium	Hypomagnesaemia, tetany
Iron	Hypochromic microcytic anaemia, glossitis, koilonychia
Folic acid	Macrocytic megaloblastic anaemia, peripheral neuropathy
Vitamin B_{12}	Macrocytic megaloblastic anaemia, peripheral neuropathy, subacute combined degeneration of the spinal cord
Vitamin B complex	Macrocytic megaloblastic anaemia
Vitamin K	Hypoprothrombinaemia, haemorrhagic diathesis
Vitamin D	Hypocalcaemia, osteomalacia
Vitamin A	Night blindness, xerophthalmia

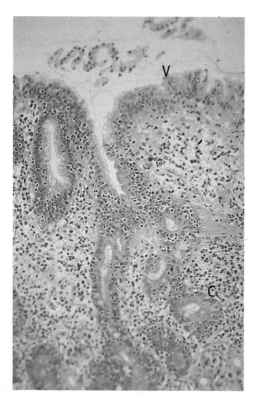

Fig. 18.14 Histology of a biopsy from a patient with coeliac disease shows atrophy of the villi (V), crypt (C) hyperplasia and abundant chronic inflammatory cells including plasma cells.

Giardiasis. Chronic infestation may result in malabsorption (Fig. 18.15).

Whipple's disease. This is an extremely rare systemic disorder with fever, anaemia, skin pigmentation, peripheral lymphadenopathy and arthralgia.

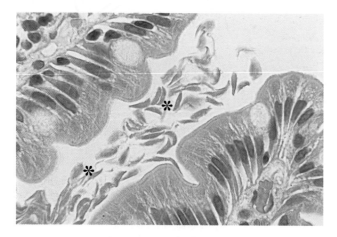

Fig. 18.15 A duodenal biopsy from a patient with abdominal pain and weight loss shows numerous giardia lamblia (✱) between the villi. (H&E.)

Involvement of the small intestine results in malabsorption with weight loss and diarrhoea. Biopsy of the small intestine reveals numerous granular macrophages filling the lamina propria. Electronmicroscopy shows that these are filled with rod-shaped micro-organisms, the exact nature of which is as yet unknown. Patients respond to treatment with tetracyclines.

Immune deficiency syndromes. Malabsorption may be associated with defects in either the cellular or humoral arms of the immune system. Patients with acquired immune deficiency syndrome (AIDS) may present with malabsorption secondary to small-bowel infections (see below).

Malabsorption related to drugs and chemicals
Broad-spectrum antibiotics such as chloramphenicol are most commonly involved.

Biochemical aspects of enteral and parenteral nutrition

Patients in need of nutritional support should be fed enterally whenever possible as this provides the most natural, cheap and simple means and avoids the well-recognized metabolic complications of intravenous feeding.

Enteral feeding is provided either by **oral supplementation** to increase intake, particularly of energy and protein-rich foods to prevent or correct protein-energy malnutrition. If this supplementation process is not possible or adequate, a liquid formula diet may be given directly into the stomach via a tube placed in the stomach or small intestine. These are available with a variety of different calorie contents, are usually isotonic and lactose-free and recently have included fibre. These latter three features have helped to reduce the incidence of diarrhoea which is the main complication of this process. The other **complications** include infections, nausea, vomiting, dehydration and constipation if inadequate water is supplemented.

Parenteral feeding must be considered in patients in whom malnutrition is accompanied by intestinal failure, fistulae in the small intestine or pancreas or in severe catabolic states when the energy requirements can only be met by this process (Table 18.8).

The feed provided parenterally is usually complete of all main nutrients and hence is termed **total parenteral nutrition (TPN)**. TPN has been shown to be effective in the primary management of short-bowel syndrome, enterocutaneous fistulae, end-stage liver failure, renal failure with acute tubular necrosis (ATN) and for burns, as well as effective support for radiation- and chemotherapy-induced enteritis and in some perioperative situ-

Table 18.8 Indications for nutritional support.

Severe under-/malnutrition
Patients in significant negative nitrogen balance
Cachexia
Post-GI resection for malignancy
Postsurgical
Severe gastrointestinal disease
Severe sepsis
Trauma
Burns
Adjunct to radio- or chemotherapy

GI, Gastrointestinal.

Table 18.9 Metabolic complications of total parenteral nutrition (TPN).

Glucose metabolism
Hyperglycaemia
Hypoglycaemia
Hyperglycaemic, hyperosmolar non-ketotic coma
Fluid and acid–base balance
Dehydration
Overhydration
Acidosis
Alkalosis
Electrolytes
Hypernatraemia
Hyponatraemia
Hypocalcaemia
Hypercalcaemia
Hypomagnesaemia
Hypophosphataemia
Liver and biliary tract
Cholestasis
Hepatocellular fatty infiltration
Lipids
Hypertriglyceridaemia
Fatty acid deficiencies
Vitamin deficiencies
Trace element deficiencies

ations. The feeds usually contain glucose and fatty acid emulsions as energy sources, amino acids as protein sources, fluid, electrolytes, vitamins and trace elements. The composition of each of these can be adjusted depending on assessed requirements and the type of condition initiating the requirement. As these solutions are hypertonic they have to be administered into a central vein in order to reduce the risk of severe damage to the vascular endothelium and of inducing thrombosis.

Because of the wide range of serious metabolic complications of parenteral feeding (Table 18.9), together with the need to monitor response to the therapy, regular biochemical measurements should be performed.

Parameters that should be monitored regularly (most should be done daily), in order to predict and prevent complications, include:

- plasma electrolytes;
- calcium;
- magnesium;
- phosphate;
- glucose;
- bicarbonate;
- urea;
- creatinine;
- liver enzymes and bilirubin;
- routine haematological investigations.

Plasma trace elements should be monitored less frequently but are essential in long-term therapy. **Nitrogen balance** may also be monitored as well as plasma proteins to assess response, although interpretation may be difficult. **Hepatic complications** involve both cholestasis and hepatocellular fatty infiltration and damage occurs during TPN, but these processes are reversible and are not considered to be of significance to alter TPN management.

Inflammatory disorders of the small intestine

There are many inflammatory conditions of the small intestine (Table 18.10, page 414).

Neoplasms of the small intestine

Benign neoplasms

These are rare and take the form of adenomas or papillomas, smooth-muscle tumour, fibroma, lipoma or Peutz–Jeghers polyps. Most are found incidentally at autopsy but they may present clinically with intussusception, obstruction, bleeding or volvulus.

Malignant neoplasms

These are rare. In decreasing order of frequency they include carcinoid tumours, lymphomas, adenocarcinoma and leiomyosarcoma.

Carcinoid tumours (Fig. 18.16). Carcinoid tumours arise from endocrine cells or their precursors in the foregut,

Table 18.10 Inflammatory disorders of the small intestine.

Solitary ulcer of the small intestine
  Congenital, vascular, inflammatory, neoplastic, drugs (e.g. potassium salts, NSAIDs), associated with malabsorption

Gold-induced enterocolitis

Duodenitis
  Either associated with peptic ulcer disease or with specific causes such as Crohn's disease

Chronic ulcerative (non-granulomatous) jejunoileitis
  Unknown aetiology

Benign lymphoid hyperplasia

Irradiation damage

Behçet's syndrome

NSAIDs, Non-steroidal anti-inflammatory drugs.

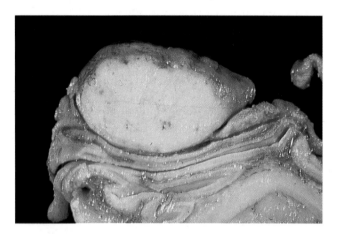

Fig. 18.16 The macroscopic appearance of a small bowel carcinoid tumour. Note how well circumscribed it is and its yellow-grey colour.

midgut or hindgut. Some 60–80% occur in the midgut (appendix and terminal ileum) and 10–20% in the hindgut (rectum).

The behaviour of carcinoid tumours correlates with:
• the site of origin (those arising in the appendix and rectum are usually benign, whilst those in the stomach and ileum are frequently malignant);
• size (66% of those larger than 2 cm have metastasized at the time of diagnosis whereas only 5% of those less than 1 cm have metastasized).

Carcinoid tumours contain a variety of secretory granules depending on the individual tumour, e.g. 5-hydroxytryptamine, gastrin, somatostatin, insulin, calcitonin, adrenocorticotrophic hormone, etc. (see Chapter 14).

Morphologically, they may present as round, plaque-like tumours causing submucosal elevation or as a polypoid projection into the lumen. They may be bright yellow in colour. In the appendix they frequently affect the tip.

Histology of carcinoid tumours is varied with trabecular, insular, mucinous and mixed forms. Carcinoid tumours are subdivided into **argentaffin** and **argyrophil** groups depending on their ability to reduce silver with or without the addition of an external reducing agent.

They are often an incidental discovery, particularly in the appendix, but may present with obstruction, bleeding or functional syndromes (carcinoid, Zollinger–Ellison, Cushing's syndrome), particularly if there are hepatic metastases. If malignant, carcinoid tumours are slowly but relentlessly progressive.

Lymphoma (Fig. 18.17). Predisposing factors include coeliac disease, Crohn's disease and selective IgA deficiency.

Adenocarcinoma. These are rare tumours and small-bowel adenocarcinomas represent only 3–6% of all gastrointestinal tumours and less than 1% of malignant tumours of the small bowel. This is possibly because of the rapid transit time of fluid and relatively sterile bowel contents.

Adenocarcinomas are commonest in the duodenum (periampullary). The prognosis for periampullary tumours is good but most of the other small-bowel carcinomas have spread widely at the time of diagnosis and have only a 20% 5-year survival.

Predisposing factors include Crohn's disease, coeliac disease and familial adenomatous polyposis.

Ischaemic bowel disease

Apart from the first part of the duodenum, the entire

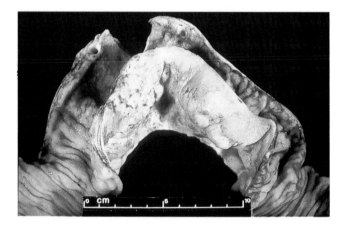

Fig. 18.17 The macroscopic appearance of small bowel lymphoma. These tumours may infiltrate extensively along the bowel wall.

small intestine receives its blood supply from the **superior mesenteric artery**. The distribution of ischaemic change depends on the level of any vascular lesion. Changes may be acute or chronic and may affect the full thickness of the bowel wall or just part of it.

Pathogenesis

Pathogenesis depends on whether the underlying vascular disease is occlusive or non-occlusive.

Occlusive vascular disease. Arterial occlusion may be due to atheroma, thrombus or embolus; arteritis is a rarer cause. Venous occlusion (5–10%) may be due to external pressure or to conditions predisposing to intravascular thromboses, e.g. appendicitis, pelvic inflammation.

Non-occlusive vascular disease (low-flow states). Non-occlusive vascular causes of small-bowel ischaemia include hypotension due to left ventricular failure, aortic insufficiency and shock.

Small-vessel disease associated with vasculitis, irradiation or disseminated intravascular coagulation may be associated with small-bowel ischaemia.

Small-bowel obstruction

Intestinal obstruction might be the result of a lesion within the lumen, within the wall or outside the wall. Common causes are fibrous adhesions, twisting (torsion) of the bowel and tumours.

Pseudo-obstruction may be secondary to paralytic ileus (due to peritoneal irritation or metabolic disturbances) or to disorders of smooth muscle or nerves.

THE APPENDIX

Normal anatomy

The appendix is a vestigial organ in humans with its base in the caecum and its tip at variable positions behind the caecum and colon or overhanging the pelvic brim. The appendix is lined by mucosa consisting of simple tubular glands rich in goblet and endocrine cells. The lamina propria contains abundant lymphoid tissue. The appendix may be the site for a wide range of disease processes (Table 18.11).

Inflammatory disorders (Fig. 18.18)

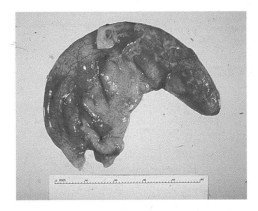

Fig. 18.18 The macroscopic appearance of acute appendicitis. Note the yellow inflammatory exudate on the surface.

Acute appendicitis

This is the commonest acute abdominal emergency in children and young adults in the developed world. The peak age at presentation is in the teens and 20s but appendicitis may occur at any age.

Aetiology and pathogenesis. It is likely that **obstruction of the lumen** leads to distension and accumulation of secretions with ischaemic damage to the mucosa and invasion of the appendix wall by enteric pathogens.

Possible causes of obstruction include mucosal inflammation, hyperplasia of lymphoid tissue within the wall, formation of a **faecolith** (calcified faeces) within the lumen or torsion.

Table 18.11 Disorders of the appendix.

Congenital diseases
Mucocoele

Infections
Tuberculosis, yersiniosis, actinomycosis, schistosomiasis, *Enterobius vermicularis* (pinworms), lymphoid hyperplasia (viral lymphadenitis)

Inflammatory diseases
Crohn's disease, polyarteritis nodosa, sarcoidosis, neoplasms
Benign
   Endometriosis (in women), lipoma, fibroma, adenoma, carcinoid

Malignant
   Primary – adenocarcinoma, carcinoid
   Secondary – colonic adenocarcinoma, gynaecological malignancy

Vascular diseases
Angiodysplasia, ischaemia

Pathology. In the early stages, the appendix may just appear to be congested, but in established disease it becomes haemorrhagic and soft with purulent exudate on the serosal surface. In severe cases perforation may be present.

Histology shows ulceration and transmural infiltration by polymorphs. If perforation is present there may be venous thrombosis and ischaemic necrosis.

Complications. These include perforation, peritonitis, abscess formation (local, subphrenic, pelvic), adhesions, fistulae and hepatic abscess (via infected thrombosed veins in the mesoappendix).

Mucocoele

A mucocoele is distension of the appendix lumen secondary to accumulation of mucin. Postinflammatory fibrosis and faecolith are causes of simple mucocoele. Other causes are mucinous cystadenoma and cystadenocarcinoma.

The mucocoele may rupture and give rise to deposits of mucin throughout the peritoneal cavity – **pseudomyxoma peritonei**. Pseudomyxoma peritonei regresses following appendicectomy unless the cause is a carcinoma.

THE LARGE INTESTINE

Normal anatomy

The large intestine extends from the ileocaecal valve to the anus. It is approximately 150 cm long and can be divided anatomically into six regions:
- the caecum;
- the ascending colon (from the caecum to the hepatic flexure);
- the transverse colon (hepatic to splenic flexure);
- the descending colon (splenic flexure to left iliac fossa);
- the sigmoid colon;
- the rectum.

The main functions of the large intestine are absorption of water and electrolytes and the storage of faeces. The mucosa is lined by straight tubular glands with absorptive, goblet, endocrine and stem cells (Fig. 18.19).

Congenital abnormalities

Hirschsprung's disease

Hirschsprung's disease is a congenital absence of ganglion cells from the distal rectum and colon. It can, in very rare instances, affect the length of the bowel.

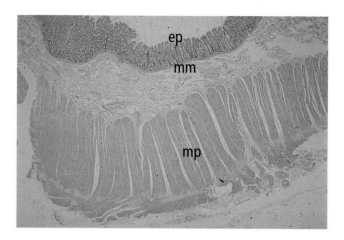

Fig. 18.19 The histology of the large intestine. ep, epithelium; mm, muscularis mucosa; mp, muscularis propria. (H&E.)

Clinical presentation is usually in the neonatal period or in early infancy and is related to delayed passage of meconium or constipation with signs of bowel obstruction. Occasionally, presentation may not occur until childhood or even adulthood when, retrospectively, chronic constipation may be recognized as having been present since birth. Rarely, Hirschsprung's disease can present as a life-threatening enterocolitis.

The incidence is approximately 1 in 4000–5000 births with a male/female ratio of about 4 : 1. A familial element is present in nearly 10% of cases and an association with trisomy 21 (Down syndrome), congenital heart disease and Ondine's curse (central hypoventilation) indicates cytogenetic factors are significant in a proportion. The majority of cases are sporadic.

Conventionally, Hirschsprung's disease is attributed to a failure of normal migration of neural crest cells destined to become bowel ganglion cells, during the embryonic period. However, there is some evidence that there may be an abnormality of the bowel into which the cells migrate that inhibits or prevents normal maturation. The distal rectum or rectosigmoid is always affected but up to 25% of cases will exhibit longer segments of aganglionosis.

Confirmatory diagnosis is by an inability to demonstrate ganglion cells within a rectal biopsy serially sectioned and examined by light microscopy. An additional valuable feature is that, within the aganglionic segment, there is proliferation of parasympathetic nerve fibres in both the myenteric and submucosal plexus. Further, proliferation of thickened nerve fibres within the muscularis mucosa and mucosa itself can be revealed by specific staining for acetylcholinesterase using a histochemical technique on frozen sections (Fig. 18.20).

Following diagnosis, therapy usually involves resec-

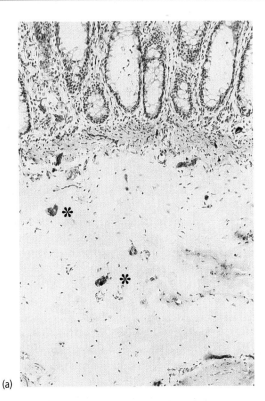

(a)

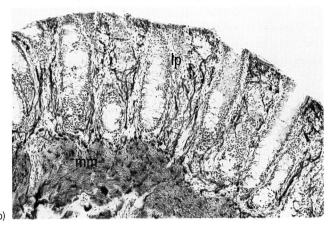

(b)

Fig. 18.20 Segment of colon from a child with Hirschsprung's disease. (a) Normal acetyl-cholinesterase staining, of a ganglionic segment (✱). (b) Acetyl-cholinesterase staining of the distal, aganglionic segment. The comparative increase and thickening of nerves is clearly present within the muscularis mucosa (mm) and extending into the lamina propria (lp).

ting the aganglionic segment and pulling normal ganglionated bowel down to the internal sphincter.

Gastrointestinal infections (Table 18.12)

The normal flora

Anaerobes predominate in the normal flora of the

Table 18.12 Laboratory diagnosis of gastrointestinal infections.

Microscopic stool examination	Neutrophils absent: toxigenic bacteria, viruses, protozoa Neutrophils present: invasive bacterial infections (*Shigella*, *Salmonella*, *Yersinia*, *Campylobacter*, pathogenic *Escherichia coli*)
Stool examination for organisms	Gram stain for *Staphylococcus aureus*, *Vibrio cholerae* Electronmicroscopy for viruses Wet prep for *Entamoeba*, *Giardia*, helminth ova Acid-fast stain for mycobacteria, *Cyptosporidium*, *Isospora*
Stool culture	*Shigella*, *Salmonella*, *Yersinia*, and *Campylobacter* (selective media) Vibrios can be cultured on thiosulphate-citrate-bile salt agar)
Blood culture	Typhoid fever (positive blood culture in 90% of cases)
Serological tests	*Salmonella* H, O, Vi antibodies in diagnosis of typhoid fever Antibodies against *Entamoeba histolytica*
Demonstration of enterotoxin	*Clostridium difficile* cytotoxin in stool and blood; heat-labile enterotoxin of *Vibrio cholerae* and *Escherichia coli*

gastrointestinal tract from the mouth to the large intestine. Faeces consist of 25% of bacteria by weight (= 10^{12} organisms/g). More than 99% are anaerobes, including *Bacteroides* spp., *Clostridium* spp., *Escherichia coli*, other coliforms and enterococci.

Bacterial infections

Cholera

The infectious agent is *Vibrio cholerae*. Cholera is a disease of humans with no animal reservoirs. There are two biotypes—classic and El Tor.

For centuries, cholera has been endemic in the common delta of Ganges and Brahmaputra rivers. There have been well-documented cholera pandemics throughout world history:
- 1814   First pandemic—Iran and Russia;
- 1852–62   Third pandemic—Crimea, Europe, London;
- 1863–75   Fourth pandemic—Middle East, Europe, Edinburgh;
- 1961   El Tor pandemic—China, Africa, Europe.

Pathogenesis. The organisms colonize the small bowel to release a potent enterotoxin (choleragen). The toxin binds to the GMI-ganglioside recepter on cell membrane via binding (B) units. The active portion (A2) of the A subunit enters the cell and activates adenyl cyclase. Adenyl cyclase activity results in accumulation of cyclic adenosine monophosphate (AMP)–active secretion of Na^+, Cl^-, K^+, HCO_3^- and H_2O into the intestinal lumen.

The incubation period is 24 hours. Symptoms include profuse, watery diarrhoea (**ricewater stool**) and vomiting with ultimate dehydration and collapse.

Diagnosis is made by microscopy and culture. Treatment is by fluid replacement and tetracycline (for adults).

Bacillary dysentery

There is no animal host for *Shigella* spp. and the ID_{50} is up to 200 organisms. The following subtypes are responsible for causing bacillary dysentery:

- *Shigella sonnei* > 90% UK cases;
- *S. flexneri*;
- *S. boydii*;
- *S. dysenteriae*.

Pathogenesis. The bacterium invades superficial colonic mucosa causing acute inflammation. The incubation period is 2 days and symptoms include diarrhoea, malaise, fever, vomiting, blood and mucus. Outbreaks are seen in nurseries (50% cases <10 years old), mental and geriatric institutions.

Diagnosis is made by stool culture. The infection is usually self-limiting and no treatment is necessary.

Campylobacter

Campylobacter jejuni is the commonest cause of gastroenteritis. The organism is a zoonosis found in sheep, cattle and fowl. Sources of infection include contaminated food, poultry, meat, water, unpasteurized milk and transmission may occur via kittens and puppies. The ID_{50} is 10^5 organisms.

Pathogenesis. Campylobacter colonizes the jejunum, ileum and colon with local invasion of the epithelium. *Campylobacter* produces a cholera-like toxin and one or more cytotoxins.

The incubation period is 1–7 days (average 3 days). Symptoms include a prodromal fever, headache, myalgia for 1–2 days, proceeding to diarrhoea with blood and mucus and vomiting.

Complications. Complications are uncommon and include transient bacteraemia. Systemic campylobacteraemia is of no consequence in a healthy individual but may produce complications in those with immune deficiency or a predisposing abnormality, such as damaged heart valves. In 1% of cases, there may be a reactive arthritis, and very

rarely a peripheral polyneuropathy (Guillain–Barré syndrome).

Diagnosis. Diagnosis is made by culture-selective media at 42°C.

Treatment. Campylobacter infection is usually self-limiting but may last 1–2 weeks. If severe, erythromycin is the treatment of choice. Chronic carriage is unknown in healthy people.

Salmonella

Infection with *Salmonella typhi*, and *S. paratyphi* results in enteric fever. *Salmonella* exists as a zoonosis with infection resulting from meat, meat products, dairy products, poultry, eggs (*S. enteritidis*), pets (terrapins, *S. java*) and human carriers. The ID_{50} is 10^5 organisms.

Pathogenesis. The exact mechanism of diarrhoea is unknown but is presumed to be via activation of cyclic AMP. The incubation period is 12–36 hours. Symptoms include vomiting, diarrhoea and abdominal cramps and these symptoms may lasts 2–5 days.

Complications. Complications of salmonellosis include bacteraemia (*S. dublin, S. virchow*), neonatal meningitis and osteomyelitis (in sickle-cell anaemia and human immunodeficiency virus–HIV).

Diagnosis. Diagnosis is made by culture.

Treatment. In the majority of cases infection is benign and self-limiting. Antibiotics are usually unnecessary. The organism is readily killed by heat (60°C for 15 minutes).

Escherichia coli

Certain strains (or serotypes) of *E. coli* can produce diarrhoea:

- **enterotoxigenic** *E. coli* (ETEC) produces enterotoxins;
- **enteroinvasive** *E. coli* (EIEC) produces a dysentery-like illness;
- **enteropathogenic** *E. coli* (EPEC) produces diarrhoea by an unknown mechanism;
- **enterohaemorrhagic** *E. coli* (EHEC) produces haemorrhagic colitis, and haemolytic–uraemic syndrome produces one or more verotoxins (cytotoxic to Vero green monkey kidney).

Tuberculosis

Tuberculosis usually affects the terminal ileum and caecum but may rarely affect the colon. It is important in the differential diagnosis of Crohn's disease, particularly amongst high-risk groups.

Yersinia enterocolitica

This may cause a colitis which is either self-limiting or easily treated with antibiotics. Infection may be associated with systemic symptoms such as erythema nodosum, arthritis and pericarditis.

Pseudomembranous colitis

Pseudomembranous colitis was first described as a complication of gastrointestinal surgery but has increased markedly in incidence following the introduction of broad-spectrum antibiotics. Some 97% of cases are caused by *Clostridium difficile* and its associated toxins.

Pathology. Raised creamy yellow patches separated by congested but otherwise normal mucosa are seen (Fig. 18.21). In severe disease a diffuse necrotic membrane may be seen which is indistinguishable from that seen in ischaemic enterocolitis.

Histology shows crypts distended with mucin, fibrin, degenerate epithelial cells and neutrophil polymorphs which 'erupt' on to the mucosal surface. The mucosa between these lesions is characteristically normal or only mildly inflamed, although in severe cases there is necrosis through its full thickness. Treatment is with metronidazole.

Antibiotic-associated colitis. Clostridium difficile and its toxin are found in 38% of cases. The mucosa shows mild changes similar to those seen in infectious colitis.

Antibiotic-associated diarrhoea. C. difficile and its toxin is seen in 6% of cases. The mucosa is normal.

Protozoal infections

Amoebiasis (Fig. 18.22)

Amoebiasis is caused by *Entamoeba histolytica*. Infection is prevalent worldwide but spread is by the faecal–oral route and is associated with poor hygiene. Infection is commoner in underdeveloped countries.

Infection can be seen in patients who have not travelled abroad. Diagnosis is based on the presence of cysts in the stools, serology and the presence of erythrophagocytic amoebae on biopsy (only pathogenic strains ingest red blood cells).

Schistosomiasis (Fig. 18.23)

Schistosoma mansoni (Africa and central South America) and *S. japonicum* (Far East) are the species responsible for most colonic disease, although infection can occur with *S. haematobium*.

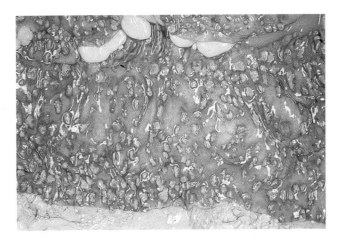

Fig. 18.21 Large bowel specimen from a case of pseudomembranous colitis. Note the focal areas of purulent exudate and mucus.

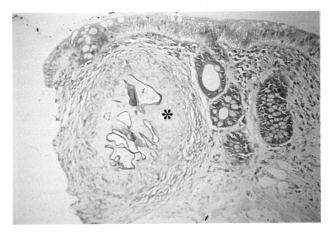

Fig. 18.22 Intestinal amoebiasis from a patient who presented with colitic symptoms. Note the pale-staining amoebae (✻) that have phagocytosed red cells. (H&E.)

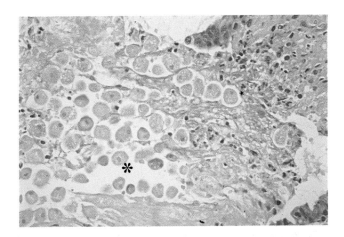

Fig. 18.23 Intestinal schistosomiasis has produced granulomtous inflammation and fibrosis within the bowel wall. Ziehl–Neelsen stain highlights the remnants of ova (✻) within the bowel wall.

Humans may be infected by the larval stage of the fluke (the cercaria) as they wade or bathe in contaminated water (see Chapter 8). The larvae penetrate the skin and pass in the blood stream to the liver where they mature into adults. The adults mate and then migrate to other tissues to lay their eggs – the exact site depends on the species. In the intestine the eggs pass through the mucosa into the faeces. If the faeces are deposited in fresh water the eggs hatch, releasing larvae (miracidia) which infect the intermediate host – the snail. The cycle is complete when the free-swimming cercaria leave the snail and infect humans.

Pathological changes are due to the presence of eggs within the bowel wall which elicit a granulomatous inflammatory response.

Cryptosporidium

Cryptosporidium parvum is a protozoan and zoonosis that was first recognized in 1976 as a cause of diarrhoea in patients with AIDS. It is now known commonly to cause diarrhoea in children aged 1–5 years.

Sources of infection include animals, person-to-person contact, water, unpasteurized milk and family outbreaks. The ID_{50} is 10–100 oocysts and the incubation period is 1 week.

Symptoms include profuse watery diarrhoea, fever and abdominal cramps. Infection is self-limiting and no specific treatment is available.

Diagnosis. A modified Ziehl–Neelsen stain will demonstrate the organism in faeces. Auramine fluorescence is sometimes used. The oocysts are highly resistant to disinfectants including bleach but are killed by 5–10 minutes at 55°C or a few seconds at 100°C.

Giardiasis

Giardia lamblia is a flagellate, pear-shaped protozoan, found worldwide in contaminated food or water.

Pathogenesis. Following an incubation period of 1–3 days, trophozoites in the duodenum adhere to the villi. Symptoms occur in 20% and include abdominal discomfort, flatulence and diarrhoea. If untreated, infection lasts for 4–6 weeks and may lead to steatorrhoea and malabsorption.

Diagnosis. Diagnosis is made on microscopy of faeces, duodenal aspirate or duodenal biopsy. Prevention requires adequate chlorination and filtration of water supplies.

AIDS and gastrointestinal infection

Infection of the gastrointestinal tract is a common compli-

cation of AIDS. Patients may present with diarrhoea and/or malabsorption. Possible pathogens include:

- *Cryptosporidium;*
- cytomegalovirus;
- *Mycobacterium avium-intracellulare;*
- *Entamoeba histolytica;*
- *Giardia lamblia;*
- *Campylobacter* spp.;
- *Mycobacterium avium-intracellulare* (MIA) (see Chapter 10).

'Gay bowel' syndrome

This term refers to a group of infective conditions which can affect homosexual or bisexual patients and are spread by the anorectal route:

- *Campylobacter* spp.;
- *Clostridium difficile;*
- *Entamoeba histolytica;*
- *Enterobius vermicularis;*
- *Giardia lamblia;*
- *Chlamydia trachomatis;*
- herpes simplex;
- HIV;
- *Neisseria gonorrhoeae;*
- *Treponema pallidum.*

Food poisoning

Food poisoning is defined as an acute attack of abdominal pain and diarrhoea, with or without vomiting, lasting 1–2 days (sometimes up to 1 week). The onset may be sudden (1–2 hours) or delayed (up to 40 hours) after eating contaminated food (Table 18.13).

One important problem is the distinction between infective colitis and idiopathic inflammatory bowel disease, i.e. ulcerative colitis and Crohn's disease. The organisms that might cause confusion are those that invade the mucosa, i.e. *Salmonella* spp., *Shigella* spp. and *Campylobacter* spp. Stool culture should establish the correct diagnosis but occasionally biopsy is necessary. The char-

Table 18.13 Causes of food poisoning.

Bacterial (*Escherichia coli*, *Salmonella*, *Campylobacter*, *Shigella*)
Viral food poisoning, e.g. hepatitis A shellfish
Poisonous food intrinsically poisonous, e.g. deadly nightshade
Parasites in meat, e.g. *Taenia*, *Trichinella*
Chemicals, e.g. insecticides
Food allergies in individuals, e.g. to strawberries, peanuts
Poisonous fish, e.g. scombrotoxin histamine intoxication 1–3 hours after eating scombroid fish – mackerel and tuna
Red kidney beans (*Phaseolus vulgaris*) 2–4 hours after ingestion due to lectins that impair intestinal absorption – avoided by boiling beans
Chinese restaurant syndrome due to excessive monosodium glutamate

acteristic histological features are only seen in the early stages of infection (Table 18.14).

Inflammatory bowel disease

Ulcerative colitis

Ulcerative colitis is a chronic disease characterized by exacerbations and remissions in which the rectum alone or the rectum and the contiguous large intestine become diffusely inflamed and may ulcerate. The patient suffers from diarrhoea with blood, mucus and pus.

Aetiology. The aetiology is unknown. Approximately 25% of family members have either ulcerative colitis or Crohn's disease. Smokers have a decreased risk of developing ulcerative colitis (but an increased risk of developing Crohn's disease).

Possible causes are infective, immunological (but many immunological phenomena that are observed in ulcer-

ative colitis, e.g. presence of autoantibodies that cross-react with gut-associated bacteria may be secondary to the disease rather than causative) and psychosomatic (no convincing evidence). The true aetiology is likely to be multifactorial with an abnormal immune response to an environmental agent in genetically susceptible individuals.

Epidemiology. Both sexes are equally affected. The peak incidence is in the third decade with a second peak in the eighth decade. Ulcerative colitis has a global distribution but it is commonest in the west with a prevalence in north-west Europe of $5-8/10^5$ population.

Macroscopic appearances (Fig. 18.24(a)). The mucosa of the rectum and a variable amount of proximal large bowel are inflamed with a granular or ulcerated appearence. The diseased areas are continuous, there are no fissures or spontaneous fistulae and the serosa (except in fulminating acute colitis) is normal. Inflammatory polyps are com-

Table 18.14 Gastrointestinal infections.

Organism	Source	Illness
Toxigenic bacterial infections		
Vibrio cholerae	Contaminated water	Diarrhoea
Escherichia coli (toxigenic)	Food, water	Traveller's diarrhoea
Staphylococcus aureus	Toxin in food	Food poisoning
Clostridium perfringens	Reheated food	Food poisoning
Bacillus cereus	Reheated rice	Food poisoning
Vibrio parahaemolyticus	Shellfish	Diarrhoea and dysentery
Clostridium botulinum	Neurotoxin in food	Botulism
Invasive viral infections		
Rotaviruses and advenoviruses	Person to person	Infantile diarrhoea
Parvoviruses	Person to person	Gastroenteritis
Cytomegalovirus	Person to person	Enterocolitis (in immunocompromised patients)
Invasive bacterial infections		
Salmonella spp.	Food, milk, water	Food poisoning
Salmonella typhi	Food or water	Typhoid
Shigella spp.	Food or water	Dysentery
Campylobacter spp.	Animals, infected persons	Childhood diarrhoea
Mycobacterium tuberculosis	Infected person or milk	Chronic infection
Atypical mycobacteria	Infected person or soil	Chronic diarrhea (mainly in immunocompromised patients)
Protozoal infections		
Entamobea histolytica	Faecal contamination (cysts)	Amoebic colitis
Non-invasive infections		
Giardia lamblia	Contaminated water	Giardiasis
Cryptosporidium, Isospora	Contaminated food, water	Diarrhoea (mainly in immunocompromised patients)

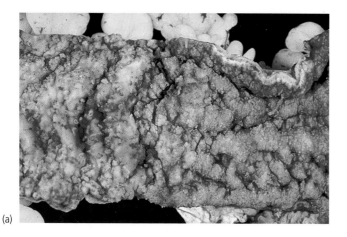

(a)

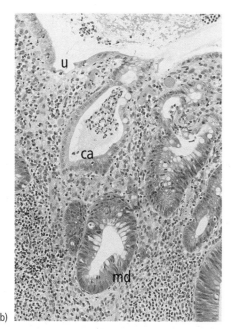

(b)

Fig. 18.24 Active ulcerative colitis. (a) The rectum shows diffuse superficial ulceration. (b) Histology shows ulceration (u), crypt abscess (ca) formation, mucus-depletion (md) and acute-on-chronic inflammation. (H&E.)

mon but fibrous strictures are rare. The involved mucosa is often very haemorrhagic. The terminal ileum is involved in 10% (backwash ileitis) and the anus in < 25%. Malignant change is well-recognized. Although continuous, the disease may vary in severity at different sites, giving a false impression of segmental involvement and causing confusion with Crohn's disease.

Histology (Fig. 18.24(b)). The inflammation is confined to the mucosa and submucosa with destruction and distortion of the normal regular glandular architecture. Mucin secretion is impaired. Neutrophil polymorphs invade glands to form crypt abscess. Sarcoid-type granulomas are not seen and fissures are only present in acute fulmi-

nating disease. Vascularity rather than oedema is prominent and the submucosa is normal or even reduced in width. Paneth cell metaplasia is common and precancerous epithelial changes (dysplasia) may be seen in longstanding disease. Anal lesions show non-specific chronic inflammatory changes (Table 18.15).

Crohn's disease

Definition. Granulomatous inflammation affecting any part of the gastrointestinal tract, frequently in discontinuity and with a tendency to form fistulae.

Aetiology. The aetiology is unknown. Theories are as for ulcerative colitis. There is an increased incidence in smokers. Other possible causes include vasculitis, dietary factors (increased incidence in those with a high sugar intake) and infection with atypical mycobacteria or cell-wall-deficient bacteria.

Epidemiology. The peak age is the third decade with smaller peaks in the sixth and eighth decades. There is worldwide incidence but the disease is commoner in the west, with a prevalence in the UK of $26–56/10^5$ population.

Distribution. Seventy per cent of patients present with small-bowel disease. Eventually 30–35% will have small-bowel disease alone, 30–40% will have disease affecting both small and large bowel and in 25–35% of cases the large bowel alone will be involved.

Table 18.15 Complications of ulcerative colitis.

Haemorrhage
Malnutrition
Electrolyte disturbance
Perforation (rare – a complication of toxic megacolon)
Toxic megacolon, stricture formation (rare)
Fistula formation (rare)
Malignancy
   Carcinoma – the risk of developing carcinoma for patients with total
     colitis for over 20 years is 5–10%
   Lymphoma – there is a small but definite risk of developing a
     gastrointestinal lymphoma
Liver disease
   Primary sclerosing cholangitis
   Non-specific reactive hepatitis
   Fatty change
   Pericholangitis

Miscellaneous complications include pyoderma gangrenosum, polyarthritis, ankylosing spondylitis, iridocyclitis and carcinoma of the bile ducts (rare).

Macroscopic appearances (Fig. 18.25(a)). Characteristically the disease is discontinuous, with skip lesions being seen on X-ray. Oedematous but otherwise normal mucosa lies between discrete ulcers, giving a cobblestone appearence. Fissures, fistulae (enterocutaneous or intestinal), strictures, serositis and adhesions are common. Anal lesions are seen in over 75% of cases. Malignant change (carcinoma and lymphoma) is increasingly recognized but still very rare and less common than in ulcerative colitis.

Histology (Fig. 18.25(b)). Characteristically, inflammation is patchy but involves the full thickness of the bowel wall (i.e. it is transmural). Fissure-type ulceration is common but glandular destruction, mucin depletion and crypt abscess formation are less severe than in ulcerative colitis. Focal lymphoid hyperplasia is seen in the mucosa, submucosa, serosa and pericolic tissues. Neuronal

Table 18.16 Complications of Crohn's disease.

> Haemorrhage
> Malabsorption
> Intestinal obstruction
> Stricture formation (common)
> Fistula formation (10%)
> Perforation
> Malignancy (the risk is less than for ulcerative colitis)
> Liver disease
>   Primary sclerosing cholangitis (rare)
>   Gallstones
>   Fatty change
>   Chronic active hepatitis
>   Cirrhosis

Miscellaneous complications include—aphthous ulceration, pyoderma gangrenosum, erythema nodosum, acute arthropathy, conjunctivitis, uveitis, sacroiliitis, ankylosing spondylitis and amyloid.

hyperplasia may be seen in the submucosal and myenteric plexuses. Paneth cell metaplasia is rare but pyloric metaplasia is often seen. Sarcoid-type granulomas are seen in the bowel and/or lymph nodes in 60% of cases. They may also be seen in the anal lesions (Table 18.16).

Table 18.17 compares and contrasts the features of ulcerative colitis and Crohn's disease.

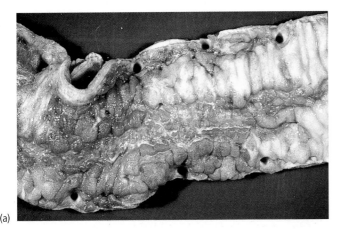

(a)

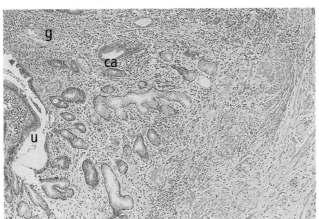

(b)

Fig. 18.25 Active Crohn's disease. (a) The colon shows patchy, deep ulceration with a cobblestone appearance of the mucosa. (b) Histology shows deep ulceration (u), crypt abscess (ca) formation, acute-on-chronic inflammation and granulomas (g). (H&E.)

Table 18.17 A comparison of ulcerative colitis and Crohn's disease.

Clinical features	Ulcerative colitis	Crohn's colitis
Mucosal ulceration	Continuous	Skip lesions
Mucosal appearance	Diffusely involved	Aphthous linear with cobblestoning
Ileal disease	10% mild inflammation	50% have combined ileal and colonic involvement
Perianal involvement	Rare	Common
Strictures	Not seen	Common
Fissures	Not seen	Common
Perforation	Rare	Rare
Haemorrhage	Common	Rare
Depth of inflammation	Mucosal (submucosal)	Transmural
Thickening of wall	Not seen	Common
Crypt abscesses	Common	Common
Pseudopolyps	Common	Common
Granulomas	Not seen	Common
Dysplasia	Common	Rare
Carcinoma	10%	Rare

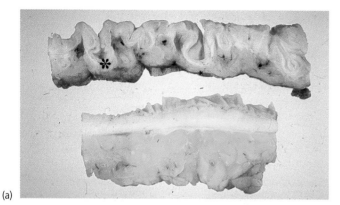

(a)

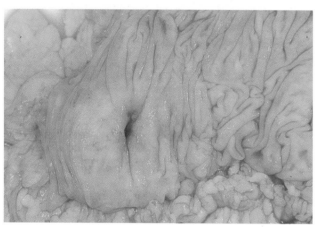

(b)

Fig. 18.26 (a) A comparison between normal large bowel (bottom) and bowel involved with diverticular diseases (top). Note the diverticula and the thickened, fibrotic wall (✷). (b) Large bowel diverticulum viewed from above showing some recent bleeding.

Diverticular disease (Fig. 18.26)

Diverticular occur throughout the gastrointestinal tract but are commonest in the sigmoid colon. They consist of outpouchings of mucosa through the muscularis propria at the points where blood vessels pass into or out of the bowel wall.

Epidemiology

Diverticular disease increases in incidence with increasing age and occurs in populations with a low-fibre diet (e.g. the UK).

Pathogenesis

A low-fibre diet leads to disordered sigmoid motility and the generation of high luminal pressures which may cause the mucosa to be pushed through the bowel wall at points of weakness. However the exact mechanism is unknown.

Pathology

The bowel wall is thickened due to hypertrophy of the muscularis propria and outpouchings of the mucosa can be seen extending through the muscle into pericolic tissues. Elsewhere the mucosa lies in prominent folds.

Complications

These include inflammation (diverticulitis), haemorrhage, perforation, peritonitis, abscess formation, fistulae and intestinal obstruction.

Tumours of the large intestine

Benign, non-neoplastic polyps

Hyperplastic polyps represent more than 90% of the polyps removed at autopsy and 15–29% of the polyps removed surgically. These polyps are commonest in the rectosigmoid, are often multiple, less than 5 cm, have a sawtooth profile on histology and show no malignant potential.

Hamartomatous polyps include juvenile polyps and Peutz–Jeghers polyps (see below). **Inflammatory polyps** are seen in conditions such as ulcerative colitis. **Lymphoid polyps** are also seen in the colon.

Benign, neoplastic polyps

Adenomas. These polyps are usually asymptomatic but may present with bleeding or altered bowel habit. Large villous adenomas may present with mucoid diarrhoea and electrolyte depletion. They may be single or multiple. Microscopically they may be composed predominantly of tubular glands (Fig. 18.27), of frond-like villi (Fig. 18.28)

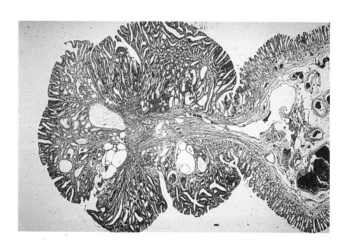

Fig. 18.27 A low power histological view of a benign, tubular adenoma of the colon. (H&E.)

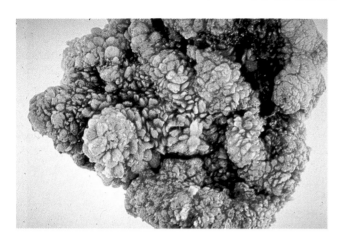

Fig. 18.28 The macroscopic appearance of villous adenoma.

Table 18.18 Evidence for the adenoma–carcinoma sequence.

Adenomas are commoner in surgical resection specimens for carcinoma than in controls

Metachronous carcinoma (i.e. two separate primary tumour presenting on two different occasions) is twice as common in patients with multiple adenomas

Adenomas are present in 75% of resections for synchronous carcinoma (i.e. two separate primary tumours presenting at the same time)

Focal carcinoma may be observed in adenomas

Adenomas occur at an earlier age than carcinomas

Adenomas are larger and more numerous in populations at high risk for colorectal carcinoma

An increase in dysplasia within adenomas is accompanied by an increase in DNA aneuploidy

Removing adenomas decreases the risk of carcinoma developing in that segment of the bowel

The steps involved in the transformation probably involve the activation of an oncogene followed by the loss of several tumour suppressor genes

or of a mixture of the two (tubulovillous). All show some degree of dysplasia. The risk of malignant change is increased if the adenoma is large (>2 cm) and/or villous (Table 18.18).

The polyposis syndromes (Table 18.19)

Peutz–Jeghers syndrome. Peutz–Jeghers syndrome is an autosomal dominant condition. Patients present with pigmented spots in the mouth, fingers and toes, and perianal region. Multiple polyps (50–100) are found in the gastrointestinal tract, especially the **small bowel**. These polyps represent hamartomas and their malignant potential is in the region of 5%.

Juvenile polyposis. This is an autosomal dominant condition in which several hundred polyps are present throughout the bowel, particularly the **large intestine**. These are hamartomatous polyps with a malignant potential in the region of 10%.

Familial adenomatous polyposis. This is an autosomal dominant condition in which hundreds of polyps (maybe thousands) are seen throughout the bowel (Fig. 18.29), particularly in the **colorectum** and periampullary regions. The polyps are **adenomas** (although hamartomas lacking in malignant potential occur in the stomach). The malignant potential of the adenomas is 100%.

Malignant tumours
Carcinoma
• **Epidemiology.** These are common malignancies, representing 19 000 deaths per year in the UK. There is marked geographical variation with a high incidence in the west and a relatively low incidence in countries such as India and Japan. Japanese immigrants to the USA acquire the risk of their new country.

Colonic carcinoma is generally a disease of affluence. It tends to be right-sided in low-incidence areas and left-sided in high-incidence areas, but the pattern is changing with a shift towards right-sided tumours in the west—

Table 18.19 Familial polyposis syndromes.

Syndrome	Polyp	Locations	Cancer risk
Polyposis coli	Adenoma	Colon	100%
Gardner's syndrome	Adenoma	Colon	100%
Turcot's syndrome	Adenoma	Colon	100%
Peutz–Jeghers syndrome	Hamartoma	Jejunum	Slight increase
Juvenile polyposis	Hamartoma	Colon	Slight increase

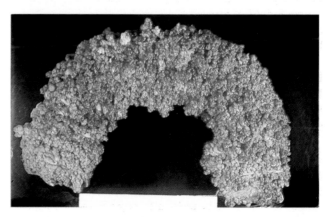

Fig. 18.29 The colon in familial adenomatous polyposis (FAP). There are hundreds of polyps.

perhaps because of the use of flexible sigmoidoscopy and removal of adenomas. The peak incidence is in the seventh decade.

Rectal tumours are twice as common in men but the sex incidence is equal for tumours elsewhere in the large bowel.

- **Predisposing dietary factors.** Low content of unabsorbable vegetable fibre; high intake of refined carbohydrate and high fat content are factors that possibly act through faecal stasis (prolonged exposure to carcinogens).
- **Other predisposing factors** include:
  (a) adenomas;
  (b) polyposis syndromes;
  (c) ulcerative colitis;
  (d) crohn's disease.
- **Site.** 30% occur in the rectum; 30% in the sigmoid and 30% in the proximal colon.
- **Macroscopic appearance.** The tumours may be annular (Fig. 18.30), polypoid or fungating.
- **Histology.** Adenocarcinoma (Fig. 18.31).
- **Spread.** Direct spread to adjacent structures and to local lymph nodes occurs. Haematogenous spread is to the liver, lungs or skeleton.

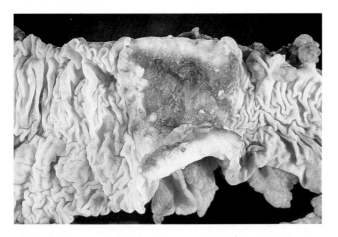

Fig. 18.30 A circumferential adenocarcinoma of the colon.

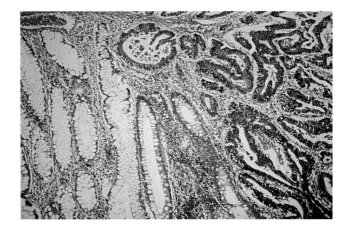

Fig. 18.31 Histology of a well-differentiated colonic adenocarcinoma shows well-formed glands. (H&E.)

- **Staging: Dukes' classification** (Fig. 18.32):
  (a) stage A, tumour confined by the muscularis propria, 15% of operated case, 80% 5-year survival (Fig. 18.33);
  (b) stage B, tumour through the muscularis propia, no lymph node involvement, 35% of operated cases, 60% 5-year survival;
  (c) stage C, lymph node metastases present, 50% of operated cases, 30% 5-year survival (60% if 1 lymph node involved, 35% if 2–5 nodes, 20% if > 6 nodes).

There are many modifications of the Dukes' system (Fig. 18.32) some of which can cause confusion but the above is still the most commonly used staging system for colorectal cancer.

- **Others.** The Jass classification also assesses the character of the tumour margin (infiltrating or pushing) and the degree of peritumoral lymphocytic infiltrate.
- **Diagnosis.** Faecal occult bloods, rectal examination, sigmoidoscopy, barium enema, ultrasound and computed tomographic scan all have their place. Carcinoembryonic antigen is not specific for large-bowel carcinoma but assessment of plasma levels may be used in order to detect recurrence.

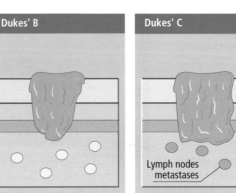

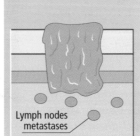

Dukes' A	Dukes' B	Dukes' C

Epithelium

Muscularis mucosa

Mucosa   Tumour

Submucosa

Muscularis propria

Lymph nodes

Lymph nodes metastases

Fig. 18.32 Diagram of Dukes' staging of colonic carcinoma.

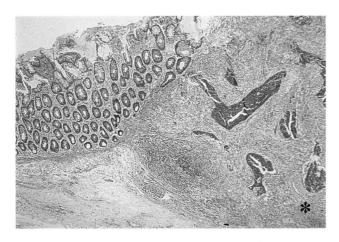

Fig. 18.33 Histology of a Dukes' stage A carcinoma (✳) that has not reached the muscularis propria. (H&E.)

- **Other malignant tumours.** Undifferentiated carcinoma, carcinoid, stromal tumours and lymphomas.

THE ANUS

Normal anatomy

The anus extends from the rectum to the perineal skin. It is 2–3 cm long and has internal and external sphincters, the normal function of which is required for faecal continence.

The upper part of the anal canal is lined by large-bowel-type mucosa and the lower part is lined by stratified squamous epithelium. Between the two there is a variable length of transitional mucosa composed of a mixture of columnar and squamous cells.

Inflammatory disease

The commonest lesions are fistulae, fissures and abscesses. These may occur in isolation or in association with Crohn's disease.

Pilonidal sinus is particulary common in young, hairy men. It is thought to be due to penetration of the skin of the natal cleft by hair shafts. Secondary infection may lead to abscess formation.

Infections

Syphilis, tuberculosis, lymphogranuloma inguinale and herpes simplex may all affect the anal and perianal region.

Haemorrhoids

Haemorrhoids result from dilatation of the internal haemorrhoidal venous plexus. Complications include haemorrhage, thrombosis, strangulation, prolapse and infection.

Tumours of the anus

Benign and precancerous tumours
These include:
- viral warts (condyloma acuminata);
- giant condyloma (clinically progressive);
- verrucous carcinoma (a low-grade squamous carcinoma);
- Bowen's disease (squamous carcinoma-*in-situ*);
- benign sweat gland tumours;
- extramammary Paget's disease.

Malignant tumours
Carcinoma. One in 50 colorectal carcinomas arise from the anus (Fig. 18.34). There is an increasing incidence amongst male homosexuals with or without AIDS. Carcinomas of the anal margin are more common in men (male/female ratio of 4:1) whereas carcinomas of the anal canal are commoner in women (male/female ratio of 2:3). The peak incidence is in the sixth and seventh decades.

- **Histology.** These are usually squamous carcinomas, either small-cell, non-keratinizing (basaloid, cloacogenic, transitional) or large-cell keratinizing squamous carcinoma.

  Other, rare anal tumours include mucoepidermoid carcinoma, malignant melanoma, basal cell carcinoma

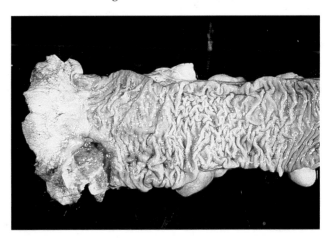

Fig. 18.34 A squamous carcinoma is seen here arising from the anus (left).

and endocrine tumours. It is important to remember the possibility of spread of tumour from the female genital tract.

- **Spread**. Spread may be direct to the rectum, perineum and perianal tissue with a tendency to spread upwards in the submucosal plane. Downward spread is limited by the tethering of the dentate line by the underlying sphincter.

  Lymphatic spread is to inguinal, superior haemorrhoidal and pelvic wall nodes. Haematogenous spread is usually a late event.

- **Treatment and prognosis.** Treatment is surgical. Radiotherapy and chemotherapy are increasingly popular but, for the commoner types, prognosis is related to the surgical stage rather than to the histological type. The 5-year survival is 50%.

REFERENCE

Seifert G., Brocheriou C., Cardesa A. & Eveson J.W. (1990) WHO international histological classification of tumours: tentative histological classification of salivary gland tumours. *Pathological Research Practise*; **186**: 555–581.

FURTHER READING

Mitros F.A. (1988) *Atlas of Gastrointestinal Pathology*. Lippincott, Philadelphia.

Morson B. (ed.) (1990) *Morson and Dawson's Gastrointestinal Pathology*. (3rd edn.) Blackwell Scientific Publications, Oxford.

Royal College of Surgeons of Edinburgh. (1983) *Color Atlas of Demonstrations in Surgical Pathology*. Williams & Wilkins, Baltimore.

Diseases of the Liver, Biliary Tract and Exocrine Pancreas

C O N T E N T S

continued

Liver

INTRODUCTION

In this chapter, diseases of the **liver** and **biliary tract** will be discussed together with diseases of the **exocrine pancreas**. Diseases of the endocrine pancreas (pancreatic islets) will be discussed in Chapter 14.

The first section of this chapter deals with the biochemistry and hepatic manifestations of jaundice but the detailed pathology of the biliary tract will be covered in the second section.

The classifications of liver disease are all, to a greater or lesser extent, based on pathological groupings. However, the pathology of liver disease can be approached in a number of ways:

- the **area** of the liver affected – parenchyma or portal tract;
- the **cells** or structure mainly affected – hepatocyte, bile duct, blood vessel, sinusoid, Kupffer cell;
- the **morphological abnormality** on liver biopsy – fatty change, hepatitis, fibrosis, cirrhosis, cholestasis, bile duct abnormalities, tumour;
- the **clinical presentation** – jaundice, abdominal pain, non-specific symptoms, chronic liver disease, liver failure;
- **specific disease** – alcoholic hepatitis, primary biliary cirrhosis, etc.;
- **primary** or **secondary** (i.e. reactive) **changes**;
- **biochemical parameters** – cholestatic, hepatitic or mixed pattern;
- **aetiological agent** causing the liver damage – virus, toxin, drug, etc.

None of these can be used exclusively, and any patient or patient's liver biopsy should be categorized with reference to all of these classification methods, the synthesis of all these different descriptions being the pathology in a particular case.

Like most branches of systemic pathology, it is impossible to consider a sample of liver tissue without reference to the **clinical history** of the patient, **clinical impression** of the disease process, **biochemical tests** and other investigations. There are only a limited number of types of histological abnormality that can occur in the liver, and the combinations or pattern of these abnormalities are also limited. Identical appearances can be seen in different conditions (e.g. alcoholic hepatitis and acute diabetic-related changes), thus clinical data may be all-important.

ANATOMY AND PHYSIOLOGY

The average **liver weight** in adult females is **1400 g**, and in males **1800 g**. It is normally non-palpable, but the lower border may be felt beneath the right costal margin on deep inspiration. It has two lobes anatomically, with the right being six times the size of the left. This anatomical division does not correspond exactly with the functional division into right and left lobes as related to blood supply and biliary drainage.

The liver has a **dual blood supply**, with up to 40% being delivered by the **hepatic artery** (a branch of the coeliac artery), the rest by the **hepatic portal vein** (which supplies it with venous blood from the intestine and spleen; Fig. 19.1).

Bile drains eventually into the **left** and **right hepatic ducts** which emerge from their respective liver lobes and unite to form the **common hepatic duct**. This is joined by the **cystic duct** (which allows passage of bile to and from the gallbladder), at which point it becomes the **common bile duct**. This runs out into the second part of the duodenum at the **ampulla of Vater** (or duodenal papilla). The **pancreatic duct** may join the common hepatic duct at the ampulla, proximal to it, or may drain separately into the duodenum (Fig. 19.2).

The liver has many functions relating to metabolism, with roles both in **synthesis** and **breakdown**. It synthesizes proteins and enzymes, forms and secretes bile, is involved in the intermediary metabolism of protein, and breaks down drugs, toxins and endogenously produced waste products.

At a microscopic level, the liver is essentially a solid mass of parenchyma composed of **hepatocytes** and cells lining **sinusoids**, pierced by **portal tracts** and tributaries

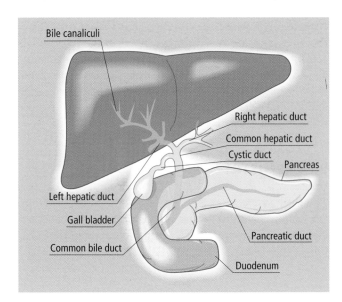

Fig. 19.1 The architecture of the liver.

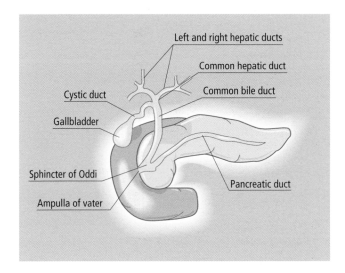

Fig. 19.2 The biliary tract.

of the **hepatic veins**. These latter structures do not directly interconnect, and tend to run in planes perpendicular to each other. The portal tracts usually contain one branch each of the **hepatic artery** and **hepatic portal vein**, and one **interlobular bile duct**, thus representing the point of access of blood to the parenchyma, and the point to which the bile produced by the hepatocytes drains. If a section is cut through the liver in virtually any plane, the same pattern will be produced.

This pattern is dominated by the relatively regular arrangement of the **portal tracts** and central veins, the distance between these structures being approximately 0.5 mm. The framework of the liver is classically considered as a series of **lobules**, with a tributary of the

hepatic vein at the centre (**central vein**), and **portal tracts** at alternate apices of a hexagon (Fig. 19.3). Thus the blood flows from the edges of the hexagon towards the centre, and the bile drains in the opposite direction to the portal tracts.

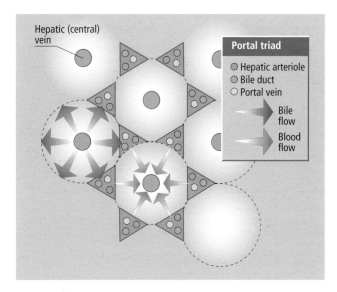

Fig. 19.3 The architecture of the liver lobule. Branches of the portal vein and hepatic artery deliver blood to the sinusoids. This drains into the central vein. Bile drains in the opposite direction, to the portal tracts.

Another way of looking at the structure of the liver is by dividing it into **acini**. Acini represent areas of the liver defined by blood supply, and do not correspond to the classical lobules. **Acinar zone 1** represents the best oxygenated hepatocytes (which are around the borders of the classical lobules), **acinar zone 3** the worst (the hepatocytes in the areas joining portal tracts to central veins; Fig. 19.4). This acinar concept is useful when explaining patterns of damage in the liver such as bridging necrosis and fibrosis between portal tracts and central veins, as the hepatocytes originally occupying these areas would have been the most hypoxic and hence the most vulnerable to damage (Table 19.1).

The **hepatocytes** represent approximately 80% of the cell population of the liver, are responsible for most of its metabolic functions, and are arranged in liver cell plates which are one cell thick, being bordered on both sides by **vascular sinusoids**, and forming **bile canaliculi** within the junctions between adjacent hepatocytes. Most of the cells are diploid, but a proportion are polyploid, and this proportion increases with age. This results in the nuclear pleomorphism and binucleation seen with ageing. They usually contain large amounts of glycogen, and occasionally fine lipid vacuoles. Ultrastructurally there are large numbers of mitochondria and endoplasmic reticulum,

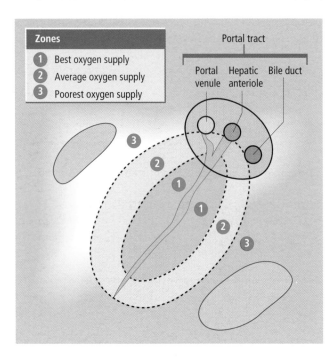

Fig. 19.4 The acinar zones of the liver.

Table 19.1 Regional changes and liver disease.

Three zones	
Zone 1	Closest to the portal tract
Zone 3	Closest to the hepatic vein
	More susceptible to anoxia and injury
Enzymic localization relates to differences in oxygenation of the three zones	
Zone 1	Alkaline phosphatase, aminotransferases
Zone 3	Glutamate dehydrogenase
	3-Hydroxybutyrate dehydrogenase
Viral hepatitis features hepatocyte necrosis in zone 3 more commonly	
Ethanol affects zone 3	
Piecemeal necrosis is zone 1	
Bridging necrosis which occurs between central veins and central vein to portal tract in viral hepatitis is zone 3	

reflecting the cells' metabolic activity, but there are no organelles peculiar to the liver. Hepatocytes may contain **lipofuscin**, which is a degenerative pigment. The amount of this pigment tends to increase with age, but is very variable between individual subjects. Other pigments and substances can be seen in various disease states, which will be discussed later.

The sinusoids are lined by **endothelial cells** and

Kupffer cells. Kupffer cells represent 15% of the cells of the liver, and are macrophages fixed in the liver which can phagocytose and endocytose, effectively performing a sieving function for the circulation. **Ito cells** are found in the **space of Disse** (between the hepatocytes and endothelial cells), and store fat and vitamins, and are also thought to synthesize collagen.

BIOCHEMISTRY

The liver synthesizes carbohydrates, lipids and proteins (including albumin), forms bile, detoxifies drugs and carcinogens, and excretes many other compounds into the bile (Table 19.2).

Table 19.2 Major functions of the liver.

Carbohydrate metabolism
Synthesis and storage of glycogen
Glycogenolysis
Gluconeogenesis
Protein metabolism
Synthesis and degradation of proteins (except immunoglobulins)
Amino acid metabolism
Urea formation
Lipid metabolism
Synthesis of cholesterol, lipoproteins and phospholipids
Fatty acid metabolism
Bile salt synthesis
Excretion and detoxification
Bilirubin and bile acid excretion
Drug detoxification and excretion
Steroid hormone inactivation and excretion
Storage of iron and vitamins
(A, D, E, B$_{12}$)

Biochemistry of jaundice

Composition of bile

Bile is composed mainly of bile acids, cholesterol and phospholipids.

Bile acids (cholic and deoxycholic acids) are made by hepatocytes from cholesterol, conjugated with amino acids (glycine or taurine), and secreted in the bile. There is a very efficient recycling of these bile acids as they

Table 19.3 Steps in bilirubin transport.

Bilirubin formation and transport in plasma
80% bilirubin from red cells (lymphoreticular system)
20% from red cell precursors (bone marrow)
    Myoglobin
    Cytochromes
    Peroxidases
Bilirubin is lipid-soluble
Bound to albumin in plasma
Not filtered at the glomerulus

Transport across the hepatocyte
Hepatic uptake of bilirubin
Binding of bilirubin (glutathione *S*-transferase)
Conjugation of bilirubin with glucuronic acid catalysed by bilirubin-UDP-
    glucuronyltransferase
Secretion of bilirubin glucuronides into bile

Further metabolism of bilirubin in the gut
Bilirubin glucuronides not reabsorbed
Deconjugated and converted into urobilinogen by bacterial action
Excretion into faeces → urobilin
Urobilinogen reabsorption → enterohepatic circulation
Excretion in the urine

Measurements of plasma bilirubin
Two forms of bilirubin in plasma:
    Unconjugated, lipid-soluble, bound to albumin, indirect
    Conjugated, water-soluble, direct
Total bilirubin 2–17 µmol/l
Unconjugated 85% of total
Third form
    Conjugated bilirubin irreversibly bound to albumin

UDP, Uridyl diphosphate

Jaundice

Jaundice is apparent when the plasma bilirubin concentration is > 50 µmol/l (Table 19.6). The causes for this can be conveniently split into three groups:
- **prehepatic**–haemolytic anaemia, excessive ineffective erythropoiesis;
- **hepatocellular**–hepatitis, cirrhosis, congenital disorders (e.g. Gilbert's syndrome), drugs, other primary liver diseases;
- **posthepatic**–mechanical obstruction of biliary tree.

Neonatal (physiological) jaundice (Table 19.7)
Mild jaundice in the first few days of life is common and is a result of immaturity of the liver enzyme system. Up

Table 19.4 Causes of hyperbilirubinaemia.

Prehepatic
Haemolysis
Ineffective erythropoiesis
Bleeding into tissues
Sepsis

Hepatocellular
Hepatic uptake
Gilbert's syndrome
Hepatitis
Cirrhosis
Conjugation
    Premature infants
    Hepatitis
    Cirrhosis
    Gilbert's syndrome
    Crigler–Najjar
    Competitive inhibition of the enzyme
Secretion
    Rotor syndrome
    Dubin–Johnson
    Hepatitis
    Cirrhosis

Cholestatic
Intrahepatic
    Hepatitis
    Cirrhosis
    Intrahepatic carcinoma
    Drugs (phenothiazines)
    Primary biliary cirrhosis
    Biliary atresia
    Infiltrations
Posthepatic
    Cholelithiasis
    Carcinoma of the pancreas, biliary tree
    Cholangitis
    Stricture of bile duct

are reabsorbed in the terminal ileum, removed from the portal blood by the liver, and re-excreted in the bile.

Bilirubin is derived from haemoglobin, myoglobin, cytochromes and peroxidase (Table 19.3). Most of the bilirubin in the plasma is **unconjugated** and bound to albumin, with only a small amount **conjugated**. Eighty per cent is derived from broken-down **red blood cells** (which have reached the end of their life span), the rest from **ineffective erythropoiesis** in the marrow and other haem proteins. It is bound mainly to albumin in the blood (which makes it soluble but non-filtrable by the kidney), taken up by hepatocytes (by an unknown mechanism), conjugated with glucuronic acid (making it water-soluble), and secreted into the bile. It is converted in the colon by bacterial action to **urobilinogen** which is mainly lost in the faeces, with only a small proportion reabsorbed. This is then either re-excreted by the liver, or excreted in the urine (Tables 19.4 and 19.5).

Table 19.5 Investigation of the jaundiced patient.

Haemolytic jaundice
Unconjugated hyperbilirubinaemia
↑ Urine urobilinogen
↑ LDH
↑ Reticulocytes
↓ Haemoglobin
Evidence of haemolysis on blood film
↓ Plasma haptoglobin
Normal ALT, AST

Hepatocellular jaundice
ALT, AST   6–100× increase
ALP   < 2× increase

Cholestatic jaundice
ALT, AST   Slight ↑
ALP   2–10× ↑
Conjugated hyperbilirubinaemia
Bilirubinuria
Urobilinogen may or may not be present in urine

Acute hepatitis
Preicteric
    ↑ ALT, AST
    Bilirubin slightly ↑
    Urobilinogen, bilirubin present in urine
    Normal ALP
Clinical jaundice
    ALT, AST 6–100× ↑
    Bilirubin > 50 μmol/l
    Urobilinogen disappears from urine
    ALP: slightly ↑
    Pale stools
    ↑ BSP retention

ALT, Alanine aminotransferase; AST, aspartate aminotransferase; ALP, alkaline phosphatase; LDH, lactate dehydrogenase; BSP, bromsulphthalein.

Table 19.6 Causes of prolonged or late-presenting jaundice.

Breast-feeding
Perinatal infection
Rhesus/ABO isoimmunization
Total parenteral nutrition
Biliary atresia
α_1-Antitrypsin deficiency
Hypothyroidism
Alagille's syndrome
    Intrahepatic biliary disease
    Characteristic facies
    Pulmonary artery hypoplasia
Galactosaemia
Tyrosinaemia type I
Zellweger's syndrome
Glucose-6-phosphate dehydrogenase deficiency
Crigler–Najjar types I and II
Cystic fibrosis

Table 19.7 Physiological jaundice.

Mechanism of physiological jaundice
Normal postnatal haemolysis
Immaturity of the conjugating enzyme
Exaggerated enterohepatic circulation of bilirubin
Risk of kernicterus if plasma bilirubin exceeds 500 μmol/l

Pathological factors aggravating physiological jaundice
Prematurity
Dehydration
Haemolysis
Polycythaemia
Infections
Hypoxia
Hypoglycaemia
Hypothyroidism
Inadequate calories
Meconium retention
Intestinal obstruction
Breast-feeding
Cephalohaematoma
Use of oxytocins during delivery

Management
Phototherapy
Exchange transfusion
Phenobarbitone

to 50% of babies develop physiological jaundice after 48 hours of age. Total bilirubin may be up to 200 μmol/l (mainly unconjugated). This falls to normal by day 7–10. It is more severe in more extreme degrees of prematurity and can reach dangerous levels (**kernicterus**; Chapter 25).

In addition, there is a group of familial disorders known as the hereditary hyperbilirubinaemias.

Hereditary hyperbilirubinaemia (Table 19.8)
They are **rare conditions** that present with **jaundice** but otherwise normal liver function tests, and do not show any specific histological appearances on biopsy except for pigment in Dubin–Johnson syndrome. They may be split into unconjugated and conjugated types, depending on the site of the defect.

Unconjugated hyperbilirubinaemias
• **Crigler–Najjar syndrome, type 1.** This is due to **absent glucoronyltransferase activity**. It is autosomal recessive and fatal in neonates due to progressive kernicterus (jaundice).

Table 19.8 Congenital hyperbilirubinaemias: inherited defects in the mechanism of bilirubin transport.

Gilbert's syndrome
Asymptomatic unconjugated hyperbilirubinaemia
Autosomal dominant
2–3% of the population
Bilirubin < 50 μmol/l
Bile acids are normal
Increases on fasting and with intercurrent illness
Abnormality of hepatic uptake of bilirubin and mild deficiency of
    bilirubin-UDP-glucuronyltransferase

Crigler–Najjar syndrome
Type I
    Autosomal recessive
    Absence of conjugating enzyme
    Severe unconjugated hyperbilirubinaemia
    Kernicterus leads to early death
Type II
    Autosomal dominant
    Partial defect of conjugating enzyme
    Severe unconjugated hyperbilirubinaemia
    Responds to phenobarbitone, phototherapy
    Survival to adulthood occurs

Dubin–Johnson syndrome
Autosomal recessive
Decreased hepatic excretion
Mild conjugated hyperbilirubinaemia
Bilirubinuria
Increased coproporphyrin I/III ratio in urine
Normal lifespan

Rotor syndrome
Autosomal recessive
Defect: unknown
No hepatic pigmentation

UDP–Uridyl diphosphate

- **Crigler–Najjar syndrome, type 2.** This is due to variably **decreased glucoronyltransferase activity**. It is autosomal dominant with variable penetrance. A few patients may survive to adolescence.
- **Gilbert's syndrome.** This is the **most common** of these disorders (1–2% prevalence), usually recognized between age 10 and 30 years. It is probably **autosomal dominant**. There appear to be multiple variable defects in bilirubin metabolism. Patients may become jaundiced on occasion, but have a normal life expectancy. Liver biopsy is normal.

Conjugated hyperbilirubinaemias
- **Dubin–Johnson syndrome.** This is due to impaired biliary secretion and is **autosomal recessive**. Liver biopsy is characterized by pigment within hepatocytes, the nature of which is obscure.

- **Rotor syndrome.** This is due to impaired uptake and storage of organic anions and is an **autosomal recessive** disease.

Liver function tests

Table 19.10 gives a summary of liver function tests and their most important findings.

Albumin
Albumin is produced in large amounts by the liver (10–20 g of albumin is synthesized daily) and its plasma concentration falls in chronic hepatic failure from any cause. There are many reasons why measurement of this protein in plasma may give misleading information on hepatic function. Albumin has a long half-life in plasma (20 days) and so even an abrupt reduction in its rate of synthesis will not be manifest immediately.

Caution is needed when extrapolating plasma albumin levels to hepatic protein synthetic rates. There can be a fall in plasma albumin of up to 15% following 30 minutes of recumbency (e.g. from 40 to 34 g/l).

In most individuals, protein depletion is associated with an increased plasma volume. Loss of albumin following haemorrhage is short-lived and the plasma concentration will subsequently tend to rise. There is a significant loss of albumin following burns and this will be sustained until significant skin recovery is achieved.

The mechanism of low albumin in liver disease is not straightforward as there is often a variable rate of hepatic protein production. The main effect on serum levels is via fluid retention and only late in cirrhosis is there a demonstrable fall in hepatic protein synthesis.

Assessment of **plasma protein abnormalities** is also useful in considering liver function and liver disease.
- **Albumin** is synthesized by the hepatocytes, and falls in chronic liver disease.
- **Coagulation factors** (fibrinogen, factors II, V, VII, IX, X, antithrombin III) are also synthesized by hepatocytes.
- **Prothrombin time** may be prolonged in liver disease, either due to cholestasis resulting in failed absorption of vitamin K (fat-soluble vitamins II, VII, IX, X), or due to change to or decreased numbers of hepatocytes.

Other plasma proteins made in the liver can also be measured specifically.

Measurement of **plasma immunoglobulins** is important in some liver diseases.
- In **cirrhosis, immunoglobulin A (IgA)** may be two to three times the normal level, with rises in IgG and IgM.
- In **primary biliary cirrhosis (PBC)**, IgM is greatly raised, with smaller rises in IgG and IgA, and **antimito-**

Table 19.9 Summary of laboratory findings in jaundice.

Type of jaundice	Blood						Urine		Stool colour
	Haematocrit	Conjugated bilirubin	Unconjugated bilirubin	Alkaline phosphatase	ALT and AST	Cholesterol	Bilirubin	Urobilinogen	
Haemolytic	↓	N	↑↑	N	N	N	0	↑	N
Hepatocellular									
Gilbert's syndrome	N	N	↑	N	N	N	0	N or ↓	N
Abnormal conjugation	N	N	↑	N	N	N	0	N or ↓	N
Hepatocyte damage	N	↑	↑	↑	↑↑	N	↑	↑	N
Obstructive									
Defective excretion	N	↑	N	N	N	N	↑	N	N
Intrahepatic cholestasis	N	↑	N	↑	N	N or ↑	↑	↓	Pale
Extrahepatic biliary obstruction	N	↑	N	↑↑	N or ↑	↑	↑	↑	Pale

ALT, Alanine transaminase; AST, aspartate transaminase.

Table 19.10 A summary of liver function tests.

Test	Significance
Serum bilirubin (conjugated)	↑ in hepatocellular failure or biliary obstruction
Serum bilirubin (unconjugated)	↑ in haemolysis or defective bilirubin uptake
Urine bilirubin	↑ in biliary obstruction
Urine urobilinogen	↓ in biliary obstruction
	↑ in haemolysis and hepatocellular failure
Dye excretion tests (BSP)	↓ in hepatocellular damage and biliary obstruction
Serum alkaline phosphatase	↑ in biliary obstruction and liver masses
Serum transaminase (AAT and ALT)	↑↑↑ in liver cell necrosis and ↑ in obstruction
Serum albumin (albumin:globulin levels)	↓ in hepatocellular failure
	↑ globin levels in chronic liver disease
Serum ammonia (NH_3)	↑ in hepatocellular failure
Serum cholesterol	↓ in hepatitis and cirrhosis
	↑ in biliary obstruction
Plasma glucose	↓ in acute liver failure
Prothrombin time	↑ in biliary obstruction and liver damage. This test reflects ↓ synthesis of prothrombin and coagulation factors V, VII and X
Serum iron	↑ in haemochromatosis
Serum free copper	↑ in Wilson's disease (lesser ↑ in primary biliary cirrhosis)
Serum caeruloplasmin	↓ in Wilson's disease
Serum A1AT	↓ in A1AT deficiency
Serum AFP	↑ in haemochromatosis

BSP, Bromsulphthalein; AST, aspartate transaminase; ALT, alanine aminotransferase; ALAT, α_1-antitrypsin; AFP, α-fetoprotein.

chondrial antibodies are found in 95–99% of cases.
• In **chronic active hepatitis (CAH)**, IgG is raised (with **antismooth-muscle antibodies**, and occasionally antinuclear or mitochondrial antibodies).
A clinical biochemistry request for **liver function tests** will usually initiate measurement of certain plasma enzymes, even though they are not a direct measure of liver function. However, changes in their levels are good indicators of liver disease, and are of two main types.

Alanine transaminase (ALT) and aspartate transaminase (AST)

The cytoplasmic enzyme **ALT** and the cytoplasmic and mitochondrial enzyme **AST** are released from the hepatocytes when damaged by virus, toxin or other insult.

AST is also found in significant quantities in the heart and smooth muscle (liver:heart:smooth muscle = 7:8:5), ALT to a lesser extent (liver:heart:smooth muscle = 30:4:3), thus both enzymes may be raised by damage to organs other than the liver. However, ALT is more liver-specific. The rise in ALT is usually more marked than AST in early hepatocellular damage, but AST is more markedly increased with chronic damage.

Alkaline phosphatase and γ-glutamyltransferase

The two main membrane-associated enzymes measured are **alkaline phosphatase** and γ-glutamyltransferase **(GGT)**.

Alkaline phosphatase is found in clinically significant quantities in the liver, bone, placenta and intestine, and thus may be released in bone diseases such as Paget's disease, or from the placenta in pregnancy. The tissue source of the alkaline phosphatase may be determined by various techniques, as different isoenzymes are produced by different tissues.

GGT is found in the kidney, liver, biliary tract and pancreas. The largest concentration is found in the kidney, but is not released into the plasma, and is therefore not of clinical relevance. Small amounts of alkaline phosphatase and GGT may be released secondary to hepatocellular damage, but the most marked increases are seen in cholestatic conditions. Alkaline phosphatase is the one most commonly measured, but is less specific and sensitive than GGT.

Thus liver enzyme test abnormalities can be divided into:
- those indicating **hepatocellular damage** as seen in hepatitis (raised AST and ALT);
- those indicating **cholestasis** (raised alkaline phosphatase and GGT).

However most cases of liver disease are not purely hepatitic or cholestatic, and thus the proportionate rise in the enzyme levels needs to be considered.

Other tests

Dynamic tests of liver function have been developed and used in some circumstances, although they have generally been shown to be of limited value outside a research environment. They include tests of hepatic metabolic capacity such as galactose elimination capacity, bromsulphthalein (BSP) excretion test and measurements of the maximum rate of elimination of indocyanine green, tests of microsomal function such as caffeine clearance and tests of hepatic perfusion such as galactose clearance.

MORPHOLOGICAL CHANGES AND PATHOPHYSIOLOGY

There are a relatively limited number of morphological changes that can be seen in liver tissue. These changes are, on the whole, not specific to one pathology/aetiology, but it is more the combination of the changes taken in conjunction with the clinical setting. These will be dealt with more fully in subsequent sections.

Fatty change

This may be either **macrovesicular** or **microvesicular** depending on the size of the fat vacuoles (Fig. 19.5). The most common type is macrovesicular, where there is one large vacuole filling and distending the cell, displacing the nucleus to the periphery of the cell. Fatty change may occur due to abnormality at any point in the sequence between fatty acid entry into the liver and lipoprotein exit from the liver. Common causes include alcoholic liver disease, diabetes, obesity, other gastrointestinal disease and hypoxia.

Hepatocyte swelling

Swelling of hepatocytes is usually seen as **ballooning degeneration** in alcoholic liver disease (Fig. 19.6) and viral hepatitis.

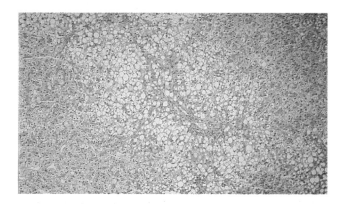

Fig. 19.5 Liver biopsy. Micro and macrovesicular fatty change seen in acute alcoholic hepatitis. (H&E.)

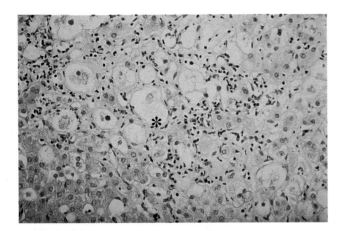

Fig. 19.6 Liver biopsy. 'Balloon cell' (✻) degeneration seen in acute alcoholic hepatitis. (H&E.)

Intracellular deposits

Lipofuscin

This is a golden brown pigment seen in hepatocytes on haematoxylin and eosin (H&E) staining and is a so-called 'wear-and-tear' pigment which increases with increasing age. It represents the indigestible remnants of autophagic vacuoles, and as such does not cause damage to the hepatocyte.

Iron, copper, copper-binding protein, and α_1-antitrypsin

These may be seen within hepatocytes. Iron is identified with Perl's Prussian blue (PPB) stain (Fig. 19.7). Copper may be identified by rubeanic acid or orcein (copper and copper-binding protein; Fig. 19.8) and α_1-antitrypsin (A1AT) by diastase–periodic acid–Schiff (PAS) (Fig. 19.9).

Mallory bodies

These are derived from the intermediate filament framework of the cells, and are seen as rather amorphous eosinophilic deposits within the hepatocytes (Fig. 19.10), particularly around the nucleus. They are thought of by many as being a specific indicator of alcoholic liver disease, but are not, being seen in primary biliary cirrhosis, diabetes, Wilson's disease, intestinal bypass surgery and some drug reactions. They tend to be concentrated in the perivenular area and in areas of alcoholic hepatitis, or around the periphery of the nodules in cirrhosis. They tend to disappear within 6–8 weeks of abstension.

Megamitochondria

These are mitochondria which are swollen enough to become visible by light microscopy (2–10 μm), being seen as

round, oval or spindle-shaped bright red inclusions in the hepatocytes on H&E staining. They are also not specific for alcohol, but when seen in large numbers they are very highly suggestive of acute alcoholic damage.

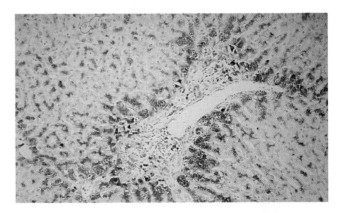

Fig. 19.7 Liver biopsy. Perl's Prussian Blue. (PPB.) Staining for iron in haemochromatosis.

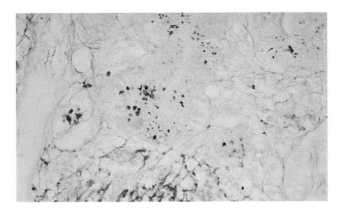

Fig. 19.8 Liver biopsy. Orcein staining black for copper binding protein in primary sclerosing cholangitis. (PSC.)

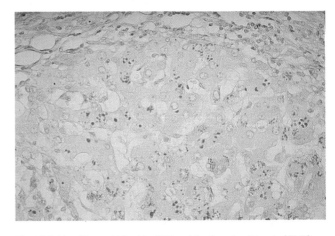

Fig. 19.9 Liver biopsy. Alcian blue/PAS staining in α-1-antitrypsin (A1AT) deficiency shows purple PAS-positive granules in hepatocytes.

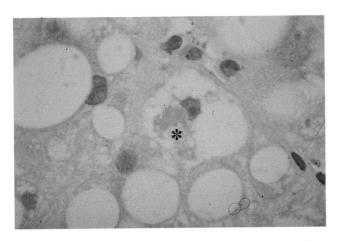

Fig. 19.10 Liver biopsy. Mallory body (✻) in alcoholic liver disease. (H&E.)

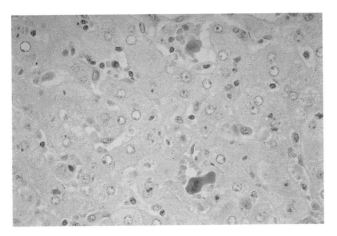

Fig. 19.11 Liver biopsy. Intra-canalicular bile (brown) in large duct obstruction. (H&E.)

Bile (cholestasis)

Although bile is synthesized by hepatocytes, it is not usually visible in the cells. It can be seen as bile plugs within canaliculi (Fig. 19.11), or droplets within hepatocytes or Kupffer cells. Bile may accumulate in many different diseases, the main ones being obstruction of bile ducts or hepatitis due to drugs or virus. Accumulation of bile within hepatocytes is associated with **feathery degeneration**, which is thought to be due mainly to the retained bile acids. The hepatocytes appear swollen with pale staining strands of cytoplasm. They may also form **rosettes** (gland-like formations) if the cholestasis is long-term.

Necrosis

This may take the form of scattered **single-cell necrosis**, which might take on the appearance of **acidophil cells** or **Councilman bodies** (Fig. 19.12). These latter are cells undergoing **apoptosis** (programmed cell death), which 'drop out' of the liver framework. **Focal necrosis**, when a few adjacent cells undergo necrosis and drop out of the normal lobular network, is typical of viral hepatitis, and will usually be associated with focal collections of inflammatory cells. Necrosis may be **zonal**, i.e. a consistent area within the lobule or acinus, which may be seen with a number of different aetiologies. These constant patterns depend on zonal differences in enzyme distribution, cell metabolism and blood supply. **Confluent necrosis** involves substantial areas of the liver, and is most often due to viral or drug-induced hepatitis. It may take the form of bridging necrosis, where the necrotic areas run between adjacent vascular structures. This is usually seen in severe viral hepatitis and is a poor prognostic sign. **Piecemeal necrosis** is the degeneration of hepatocytes at the junction between the portal tracts and hepatic lobules associated with a chronic inflammatory cell infiltrate which characteristically extends out from the portal tracts into the adjacent liver cell areas and surrounds the hepatocytes (Fig. 19.13). **Panacinar necrosis** involves all areas within the lobule. **Submassive** and **massive necrosis** are macroscopic descriptions (at laparotomy or post mortem) to describe large areas of necrosis affecting a large proportion of the liver.

Collapse

This results from loss of hepatocytes with resulting collapse of the reticulin framework, resulting in apparent convergence of the vascular structures within the liver (Fig. 19.14).

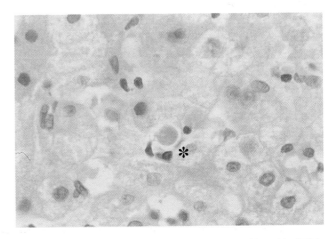

Fig. 19.12 Liver biopsy. Councilman body (✻) in acute viral hepatitis. (H&E.)

Fibrosis

Fibrous tissue may be produced by various sinusoidal lining cells (especially Ito cells) and fibroblasts, and both Kupffer cells and hepatocytes have some role if not in the direct synthesis of fibrous tissue. It is most commonly laid down in the **portal tracts** (Fig. 19.15), but may also be increased around **central veins** (outflow obstruction, alcohol), form around hepatocytes in a **pericellular pattern** (alcohol), or may be laid down in areas of collapse. Thus it may be both a repair mechanism and a response to direct stimulation by a number of agents. Cirrhosis will be discussed later (see page 457).

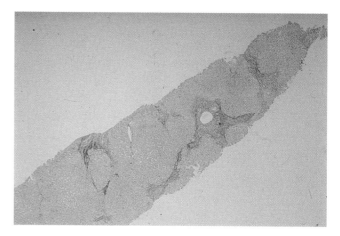

Fig. 19.15 Liver biopsy. Portal tract fibrosis stains dark red with EVG.

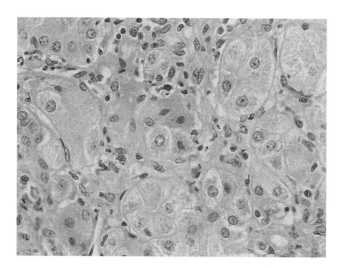

Fig. 19.13 Liver biopsy. Piecemeal necrosis (centre) in autoimmune chronic active hepatitis. (H&E.)

Architectural changes

This usually refers to disturbance of the relationships between the **portal tracts** and **central veins**, resulting from loss of hepatocytes and collapse with subsequent regeneration of surviving hepatocytes.

Portal tract changes

A number of changes may occur in the portal tracts. Increased numbers of inflammatory cells (mainly chronic) may be seen in many conditions, but this is a very nonspecific finding. **Neutrophils** may be seen as a minor component of such infiltrates, but if excessive this raises the possibility of **large duct obstruction** (see Fig. 19.14). This may be also seen in a few drug reactions, in particular that to dextropropoxyphene. So-called **bile duct proliferation** may also be seen in large duct obstruction and other primary chronic biliary diseases, due to increased tortuosity of ducts and hence apparent proliferation, but also probably due to true proliferation and **ductular transformation of hepatocytes** at the edges of tracts. Fibrosis and subsequent expansion of the tracts is a sign of more chronic damage to the portal areas.

METABOLIC DISORDERS

The most important metabolic disorders affecting the liver include primary and secondary haemochromatosis, Wilson's disease and A1AT deficiency. These disorders have been covered in detail in Chapter 7 but the liver manifestations are discussed here.

There are numerous other metabolic disorders affect-

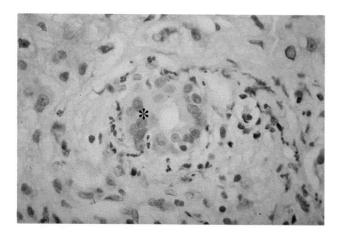

Fig. 19.14 Liver biopsy. Neutrophil poymorphs (✳) in portal tracts in large duct obstruction. (H&E.)

ing the liver, including glycogen storage diseases, porphyrias, lipid storage disorders and amino acid disorders. Reference should be made to more specialized texts for the rarer metabolic disorders.

Haemochromatosis

Haemochromatosis is defined as 'iron overload associated with tissue damage'. It is a result of progressive accumulation of iron with an increase in the body stores. This accumulation occurs in many organs throughout the body and causes damage at a number of sites.

Nomenclature is rather confused, as a number of different terms are used to describe the same conditions. There are essentially two main diseases, **primary** and **secondary** haemochromatosis. In the past, the term **haemochromatosis** has been used to describe the genetic form of the disease, and **haemosiderosis** to describe acquired forms of iron overload.

Liver pathology

Primary haemochromatosis. When small amounts of iron are seen in the liver, for example due to haemolysis, it is usually in the **Kupffer cells**.

In primary haemochromatosis, however, it is seen mainly as haemosiderin within hepatocytes (which stains blue with techniques utilizing the Prussian Blue reaction; see Fig. 19.7), although there will be some in Kupffer cells too. It initially accumulates in periportal hepatocytes, but eventually spreads to involve all areas of the liver. It is graded on a scale of 0–4 (normal liver contains no stainable iron).

The granules also appear larger with increased levels of deposition. Eventually deposition will be seen within macrophages and bile duct epithelium in the portal tracts, the latter being rare in non-genetic forms of iron overload. There is an increase in **fibrosis** in the **portal tracts**, which progresses to the formation of fibrous septa and ultimately regeneration, nodule formation and **cirrhosis**.

Hepatocellular carcinoma will often develop if the patient becomes cirrhotic before therapy is initiated.

Secondary haemochromatosis. Other primary liver diseases may show **secondary iron overload**. This is the case with **alcoholic liver disease**, where iron is commonly seen in the liver. This does not usually cause confusion with primary haemochromatosis; however, in those cases where liver iron is very high, the patients probably do actually have genetic haemochromatosis too. It is interesting that 25–40% of patients with the genetic form of the disease

have excessive alcohol intakes, a finding that is as yet unexplained.

Investigations
- Raised serum iron concentration together with decreased serum transferrin, increased transferrin saturation and markedly raised serum ferritin is the characteristic pattern.
- Quantitation of iron stores is best done as a chemical measure of iron on liver derived from a biopsy sample.
- Both computed tomography (CT), and, more promisingly, nuclear magnetic resonance, are being used to attempt to assess body iron stores in a non-invasive manner.

Wilson's disease (hepatolenticular degeneration)

The incidence of this disease is 1:30000. **Copper deposition** occurs in the liver, brain, and kidney. **Kayser–Fleischer rings** are copper deposits in the corneas. The liver is unable to excrete copper into bile and incorporate it into caeruloplasmin. This results in a decreased plasma caeruloplasmin and a decreased plasma copper.

Measurement of raised urinary copper output is the most significant among the non-invasive tests but liver copper is also raised.

Liver pathology
Initially there may be **fatty change** and glycogenic vacuolation of hepatocyte nuclei with some mild portal fibrosis. **Chronic hepatitis** may then develop, with histological features like other forms of CAH but with **copper** and **copper-binding protein** evident in periportal hepatocytes (see Fig. 19.8). **Cirrhosis** may ultimately develop, which may be active and show fatty change, hepatocyte ballooning, cholestasis and **Mallory body formation**.

α₁-Antitrypsin deficiency

Liver pathology
A1AT is produced by hepatocytes, and is an **acute-phase reactant** and **protease inhibitor**, most importantly of an **elastase** from neutrophils which degrades most structural proteins.

A1AT globules are seen in the periportal hepatocytes as eosinophilic globules which stain with PAS–diastase (see Fig. 19.9) and can be more specifically labelled by immunocytochemistry. There may be portal fibrosis, CAH or cirrhosis.

CLINICAL PRESENTATION OF LIVER DISEASE

As a complex organ receiving a large blood supply and performing numerous functions including many synthetic and degradative metabolic processes, diseases of the liver may present in many different ways:
- presymptomatic;
- acute (non-recurrent disease);
- chronic due to:
  (a) hepatocellular failure; or
  (b) portal hypertension;
- biliary obstruction.

With the increasing incidence of **health screening**, which often includes the measuring of liver enzymes, more liver disease is being picked up in a **presymptomatic** or **asymptomatic** phase.

There are also a number of diseases with an **acute** presentation (e.g. hepatitis A) which do not have any long-term sequelae.

The more significant presentations are those of **chronic liver disease**. This is somewhat of a misnomer in that the word chronic is often taken to indicate a slow and progressive course. Although this may well be the case, in others the presentation may be acute with the sudden appearance of ascites or jaundice, representing a stage where the increasing damage to the liver can no longer be coped with and the liver enters a phase of decompensation with dramatic effect. Chronic liver disease may also consist of a series of crises or illnesses with a relatively healthy existence between attacks. The features seen in chronic liver disease may be divided into two main categories from a pathophysiological view – those relating to **hepatocellular failure** (Fig. 19.16) and those to **portal hypertension** (Fig. 19.17). Invariably there is a degree of overlap between these two groupings.

The fourth category is that of **biliary obstruction**, which may either occur as a **mechanical effect** on the biliary ducts outside the liver, or may be a result of **stagnation of bile** within the liver due to factors affecting the biliary canaliculi and intrahepatic ducts. This category of diseases will be discussed in the second section of this chapter.

Hepatocellular failure

Hepatocellular failure can occur in a number of situations including severe acute diseases and advanced chronic

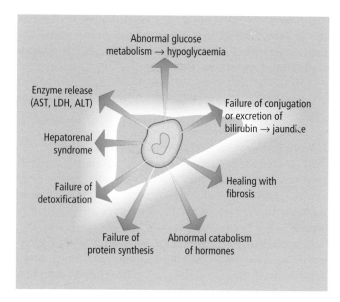

Fig. 19.16 Pathophysiological effects of liver cell failure.

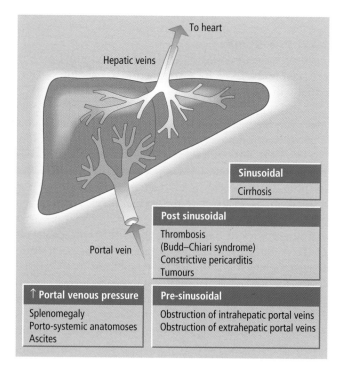

Fig. 19.17 Pathophysiological effects of portal hypertension.

conditions. It may occur as a result of a drug-induced hepatitis, and may complicate viral hepatitis at any stage, or may occur in the later stages of chronic diseases such as primary biliary cirrhosis (see Fig. 19.16).

Hepatocellular failure is a **clinical syndrome** rather than a single condition. It is definable from a histopathological view, as it may be precipitated by a number of different agents with a different pattern of histo-pathological changes. In a situation such as paracetamol overdose where there may be extensive necrosis and loss of hepatocytes in centrilobular areas, it might be antici-pated from the histological features alone. In other cases, such as a relatively chronic cirrhosis, it may occur sud-denly as the liver finally decompensates, but without any dramatic change in histological features.

The various changes which may occur in hepatocellular failure may be considered from a systemic point of view (Fig. 19.18).

General

There may be **weakness**, fatigue and **anorexia**, a low-grade constant fever (**pyrexia of unknown origin**) and **fetor hepaticus** (breath with a rather sweetish faecal smell).

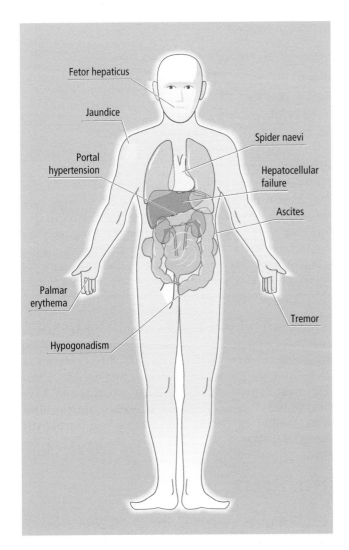

Fig. 19.18 The clinical features of hepatocellular failure.

Skin changes

Jaundice occurs as hepatocytes are unable to metabolize the normal load of bilirubin produced. There may also be haemolysis which increases the bilirubin load.

Spider naevi are small vessels radiating out from a central arteriole and these occur in the vascular territory of the superior vena cava. They are usually seen in cirrhotics (i.e. chronic disease) but may occur transiently in acute viral hepatitis.

Palmar erythema occurs with bright red palms and warm hands. It may affect the soles of the feet too.

Leuconychia or white nails may occur.

Mechanisms. The spider naevi and palmar erythema are thought to be vasoactive and due to oestrogen excess secondary to failure of hepatic inactivation of oestrogens.

Endocrine changes

Males tend towards feminization, females towards masculinization with gonadal atrophy. Males show de-creased libido, impotence, sterility, testicular atrophy and may develop gynaecomastia. Females show decreased libido, infertility, erratic or decreased menstruation, breast and uterine atrophy.

Cardiovascular/pulmonary changes

There is cyanosis and finger clubbing with hyperkinetic circulation (increased cardiac output, rate, and blood vol-ume). **Hepatopulmonary syndrome** may develop with pulmonary vasodilation, arteriovenous shunting and ventilation/perfusion imbalance.

Renal changes

Hepatorenal syndrome is renal failure secondary to chronic liver disease with decreased glomerular filtration rate and progressive oliguria. There is no morphological change on renal biopsy and the mechanism of patho-genesis is unknown.

Coagulation defects

Coagulation defects occur due to decreased coagulation factors produced by the liver. Thrombocytopenia occurs due to hypersplenism. Disseminated intravascular coagu-lation is a particular feature in acute hepatic necrosis. Increased blood loss in the gut is due to raised portal venous pressure.

Ascites/oedema

Ascites is detectable clinically when the **peritoneal fluid volume** exceeds 500 ml. This is usually serous fluid with < 3 mg/dl of protein. An abundance of neutrophils present suggests secondary infection.

A number of factors are involved in the formation of

ascites, including a reduction in colloid osmotic pressure of plasma ($\downarrow$ albumin production lowers osmotic pressure); raised portal venous pressure ($\uparrow$ with portal hypertension); renal retention of sodium and water and increased hepatic lymph formation.

Neurological changes (hepatic encephalopathy)

These are usually seen in cirrhosis or viral hepatitis. The features include progressive confusion, apathy, disorientation, flapping tremor, drowsiness and coma. There appears to be an increased sensitivity of the brain due to **abnormal cerebral metabolism**. Both hepatocellular damage and portal–systemic shunting are important in hepatic encephalopathy. Most hypotheses relate to some disturbance of nitrogen metabolism and passage of some toxic substance from the gut to the brain, but it is likely that it is a multifactorial process.

Portal hypertension

Anatomy

The **portal venous system** consists of the veins carrying blood from the alimentary canal, spleen, pancreas and gallbladder to the liver. The **portal venous pressure** is normally 7 mmHg (i.e. venous pressure). When the flow of blood in the portal system is obstructed, a collateral system expands to carry the portal blood into the veins of the systemic venous system.

These points of contact between the **portal (p)** and **systemic (s)** venous systems are in five areas:
1 left and short gastric veins (**p**) $\Rightarrow$ intercostal, diaphragmo-oesophageal and azygous minor veins (**s**) leads to varices in lower oesophagus and upper stomach;
2 superior haemorrhoidal vein (**p**) $\Rightarrow$ middle and inferior haemorrhoidal vein (**s**) leads to varicosities in lower rectum/anus (haemorrhoids);
3 in the falciform ligament between the left branch of the portal vein (**p**) $\Rightarrow$ superficial veins of the anterior abdominal wall via the paraumbilical veins (**s**) leads to varicosities in the anterior abdominal wall radiating out from the umbilicus (**caput medusae**);
4 points of contact between abdominal organs and the posterior abdominal wall (e.g. liver $\Rightarrow$ diaphragm, veins in the lienorenal ligament, omentum, lumbar veins, veins in laparotomy scars) result in **internal varicosities**;
5 splenic vein (**p**) $\Rightarrow$ left renal vein (**s**).

Causes

Classically, they are divided into prehepatic, intrahepatic and posthepatic causes (Table 19.11; see also Fig. 19.17, p. 442).

Table 19.11 Causes of portal hypertension.

Prehepatic
Portal vein thrombosis
Portal vein invasion (tumour)
Portal vein compression (tumour, nodes)
Splenomegaly (increased blood flow from spleen)
Splenic vein thrombosis/invasion/compression

Intrahepatic
Cirrhosis
Fibrosis, e.g. schistosomiasis, congenital hepatic fibrosis
Diffuse fibrosing granulomatous reaction, e.g. sarcoidosis
Massive fatty change
Focal nodular hyperplasia
Acute alcoholic hepatitis
Alcoholic central sclerosing hyaline necrosis
Veno-occlusive disease
Drugs (cytotoxics, vinyl chloride, arsenic, copper, vitamin A excess)
Tumour (primary or metastatic)
Idiopathic portal hypertension

Posthepatic
Hepatic vein thrombosis/tumour invasion/compression
Inferior vena cava thrombosis/tumour invasion/compression
Budd–Chiari syndrome
Right heart failure
Constrictive pericarditis

Effects

Haemorrhage from oesophagogastric **varices** is the commonest presentation but haemorrhage may also occur from other varicosities, e.g. rectal haemorrhoids. **Splenomegaly** may occur. **Ascites** may be acute and transient if there is, for instance, a sudden thrombosis precipitating the portal hypertension, lasting until the collaterals open up adequately. Ascites may be chronic if the patient also has depressed hepatocellular function for other reasons.

There may be **visible portosystemic shunts** such as prominent periumbilical veins or haemorrhoids. Blood bypassing the liver may result in raised blood levels of toxins from the gut which may aggravate the effects that coincident depressed hepatocellular function may have on the central nervous system and other systems. This may result in adults presenting with **hepatic encephalopathy**.

LIVER BIOPSY

Liver biopsy is a powerful tool in the diagnosis and categorization of liver disease. As well as a necessary step in **primary diagnosis**, it is also used in a number of situations for **monitoring** the progression of disease. In alcoholic liver disease it is useful for bringing home to patients that they are continuing to damage themselves by persisting in drinking (and may give evidence of recent abuse despite it being denied). It may be necessary when considering if **drug therapy** is appropriate (e.g. immunosuppressive drugs for autoimmune CAH, interferon therapy in viral hepatitis). It is also used for monitoring **response in drug trials**, and is also essential as a regular procedure when using some hepatotoxic drugs (such as methotrexate for psoriasis).

Rather than being part of a planned admission specifically for a diagnostic biopsy, it may also be used **peroperatively** during the course of an intra-abdominal operation when an unexpected abnormality in the liver is aparent. A **frozen-section diagnosis** may be required if malignancy is suspected.

A sample of liver can be obtained either as a percutaneous needle biopsy or a needle or wedge biopsy at laparotomy. If the liver is small, or a focal lesion is suspected, biopsy under ultrasound or CT guidance is usually recommended. Biopsy as an open procedure (at laparotomy or laparoscopy) may also give higher success rates for focal lesions.

Needle biopsy is usually performed with a Menghini needle (1.4 mm diameter) by aspiration, or a cutting biopsy may be performed with a Tru-cut needle. The usual approach is via an intercostal space on the right side, although focal lesions in the right lobe of the liver require an approach through the epigastrium with imaging assistance. The technique is obviously operator-dependent, but failure may also be due to other reasons such as a cirrhotic liver being too hard to pierce, or other anatomical variations.

Mortality of the procedure in most series is approximately **0.01%**, usually as a result of haemorrhage in those with severe liver disease.

One must also be aware of the shortcomings of deriving an impression of the state of the liver from examination of one tiny fraction of the whole (a needle biopsy represents approximately 2×10^{-5} of the whole liver). Some liver diseases are diffuse, affecting the whole liver in the same manner throughout, whereas others may be very focal.

ALCOHOLIC LIVER DISEASE

Clinical features

For the diagnosis of alcoholic liver disease to be made, it is most important for the doctor to have a high index of suspicion. This is because the presenting symptoms may be vague and non-specific, such as **anorexia** and **weight loss**, and **denial** of alcohol abuse is also very common even upon direct challenging.

The symptoms and signs depend on the stage of disease, and may range from biochemical abnormalities in asymptomatic patients picked up on routine screening, to patients with florid signs of **portal hypertension** and **hepatocellular failure**. And even in cirrhotic patients, signs of decompensation of liver function may not be present.

Patients tend to be divided into three main groups— patients with early disease (fatty liver); alcoholic hepatitis; and cirrhosis.

Early disease (fatty liver)
These patients will often be asymptomatic, but may have symptoms such as nausea/vomiting. Examination might reveal hepatomegaly, the liver appearing smooth and firm.

Alcoholic hepatitis
Symptoms may vary dramatically from anorexia/weight loss to features of severe decompensated liver disease. There may be tender hepatomegaly, sometimes with an audible bruit. Ascites and gastrointestinal bleeding may occur despite the absence of cirrhosis. Biochemistry may only show a relatively mild increase in AST, and haematology may reveal a **polymorph leukocytosis** (which depends on the severity of the hepatitis).

Cirrhosis
Signs of portal hypertension and hepatocellular failure may be evident.

Investigations

Biochemistry
Any of the liver blood tests may be abnormal, with raised AST and GGT being most likely in early disease. **Raised GGT** is a commonly used **screening test** for alcohol abuse, as it is an enzyme which is induced by alcohol, as well as being released secondary to hepatocellular damage and cholestasis. Blood alcohol levels may be taken in clinic.

Haematology
Macrocytosis ($> 95 \mu m$) is a useful screening test. The effect of alcohol on red cells is due mainly to a direct e[ffect] of alcohol on the bone marrow, but malnutriti[on] chronic alcoholics may contribute (folate and vi[tamin] deficiency).

Risk factors

Drinking patterns

Alcohol **dose** is the most important factor with the following regarded as danger levels–> 60–80 g/day (male), >20 g/day (female). **Duration** of intake is important with 50% of those consuming high levels of alcohol for over 21 years developing cirrhosis. Continuous drinking is felt to be more damaging than 'binge' drinking.

Sex

Females are more susceptible to liver damage and more likely to relapse. Women develop higher blood levels on standard alcohol doses than males and are more likely to develop progressive disease.

Genetics

There is some evidence that drinking behaviour is partially inherited. Different rates of elimination may be related to genetic polymorphism of liver enzymes. Some human leucocyte antigen (HLA) associations are associated with the development of alcoholic hepatitis, but this varies between countries (B8 in UK). However, social and behavioural patterns are probably most important.

Aetiology and pathogenesis

A healthy person can metabolize up to 180 g of alcohol per day, but enzyme induction in alcoholics may allow more to be metabolized. Alcohol is oxidized to acetaldehyde which is very reactive and toxic, damaging membranes and causing cell necrosis. This oxidation alters the redox potential of the hepatocyte, which inhibits protein synthesis and increases lipid peroxidation. This oxidation and consequent consumption of oxygen tends to damage particularly those cells in **acinar zone 3** (as these are the least well-oxygenated and hence most susceptible to damage). These cells also contain the highest levels of enzymes metabolizing alcohol.

Thus alcohol produces toxic metabolites, it depresses enzymes which remove fat and results in increased synthesis of fatty acids, and may directly stimulate ˜˜˜˜˜ well as causing cell necrosis which in turn

occurs in the centrilobular ˜˜d throughout all areas. It ˜˜˜ but may occasionally be

microvesicular. It is the earliest and most common indicator of alcoholic damage, but is non-specific, being seen in many other conditions. It disappears after 2–4 weeks of abstinence from alcohol. Rupture of fat-laden hepatocytes may produce an inflammatory reaction of lymphocytes and macrophages (**lipogranulomas**). Other indicators of acute alcoholic damage are **Mallory body** formation (see Fig. 19.10) and increased numbers of **megamitochondria**.

Alcoholic hepatitis tends to occur in the **centrilobular area**, but may become very widespread. It consists of swollen degenerating hepatocytes surrounded by inflammatory cells (neutrophils and lymphocytes; Fig. 19.6), and showing **pericellular fibrosis** on special staining. The hepatocytes may well contain Mallory bodies, but they are not essential for the diagnosis. The picture is very characteristic, but may occasionally be seen in **diabetes**, which should always be excluded if alcohol is denied.

Fibrosis may thus be seen in alcoholic hepatitis, but may occur in the absence of inflammation. It may occur in a rather non-specific fashion in portal tracts, but more specifically as a thickening around the central veins and as pericellular extensions in this area.

Ultimately, the patient may become **cirrhotic** (Figs 19.19 and 19.20). This does not always occur, although the presence of alcoholic hepatitis or central/pericellular fibrosis are indicators of more likely progression. A biopsy may show cirrhosis without any of the indicators of acute alcoholic damage, especially if the patient has cut down on the drinking.

Treatment and prognosis

The most important treatment is to persuade the patient to **abstain** from alcohol. Withdrawal from alcohol may

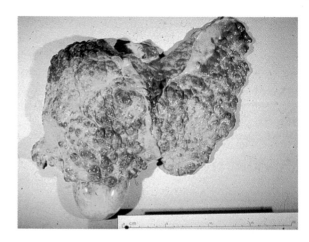

Fig. 19.19 Liver. Micro- and macronodular cirrhosis. Note the yellow colour due to fatty deposition.

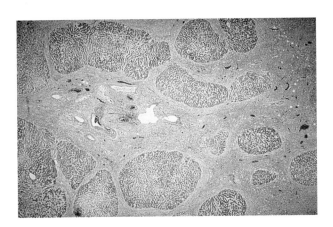

Fig. 19.20 Liver biopsy. Alcoholic cirrhosis. Trichome stain shows broad bands of collagen (blue).

be helped by the use of **chlormethiazole** or **chlordiazepoxide**. Dietary supplementation with protein and vitamins may be necessary. Most therapy will be directed towards the complications of chronic liver disease, namely portal hypertension, encephalopathy and ascites. Transplantation is not normally performed on alcoholic cirrhotics, due mainly to psychological factors and frequent continued abuse.

Up to 50% of patients with alcoholic hepatitis will develop **cirrhosis** after 10 years of continued drinking. If an alcoholic cirrhotic can abstain from alcohol, the prognosis is much better than for other types of cirrhosis, with up to 60% 5-year survival. Women tend to do worse than men. Some 5–15% of alcoholic cirrhotics will develop **hepatocellular carcinoma** (Fig. 19.21). Cirrhotics ultimately die secondary to variceal bleeding, infection, hepatic coma or hepatorenal syndrome.

INFECTIONS OF THE LIVER (Table 19.12)

Bacterial infections

Non-suppurative infections

Bacterial infections of the liver usually result from bacteraemia associated with systemic infection. Miliary tuberculosis may be diagnosed on liver biopsy by the finding of caseous granulomas (Fig. 19.22). Typhoid fever, leptospirosis and brucellosis may all produce focal necrosis and inflammation of the liver.

Liver abscess

Epidemiology. This is relatively uncommon despite the frequency of infectious sources including cholecystitis, appendicitis, diverticulitis and any source resulting in peritonitis. They are often polymicrobial in nature and may be singular or multiple. Characteristically infections via the portal vein feature as a single abscess in the right lobe of the liver and biliary disease as multiple abscesses.

Organisms involved include anaerobes including *Streptococcus milleri* which account for the majority of infections either as a pure or mixed culture, coliforms mixed with the above and, less commonly, pyogenic organisms, e.g. *Staphylococcus aureus* and *Streptococcus pyogenes*. Other organisms such as *Candida* spp. in neutropenic leukaemic patients, are opportunistic.

Management. Ultrasound and CT techniques have revolutionized the management of these infections. Drainage of abscesses by these techniques is most important, following by long courses of appropiate antibiotics. Metronidazole is often added because of the propensity

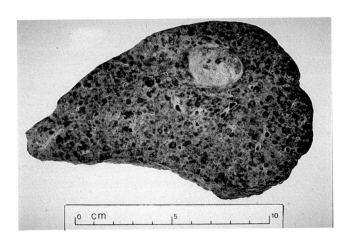

Fig. 19.21 Liver. Co-existence of macronodular cirrhosis and hepatocellular carcinoma (top).

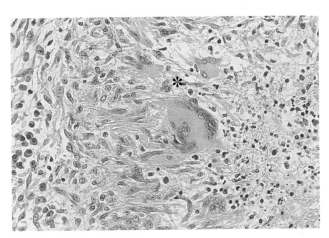

Fig. 19.22 Liver biopsy. Caseous granuloma (✳) in miliary tuberculosis. Note the necrosis (right). (H&E.)

Table 19.12 Infections of the liver.

Disease	Organism	Features
Abscess	Various	Secondary to portal pyelophlebitis (with abdominal sepsis) or septic emboli
Ascending cholangitis	Escherichia coli, etc.	Cholangitis, abscesses. Large duct obstruction predisposes (especially calculus)
Granulomatous hepatitis	Mycobacterium Brucella Histoplasma	Tuberculosis, atypical mycobacteria, tuberculoid leprosy
Leptospirosis	Leptospira	A spirochaete causing fever with jaundice Cholestasis, inflammation and necrosis on liver biopsy
Syphilis	Treponema pallidum	Congenital syphilis results in diffuse inflammation and pericellular fibrosis. Acquired syphilis causes hepatitis; granulomas in secondary disease ultimately heal with fibrosis
Amoebic abscess	Entamoeba	E. histolytica may cause hepatic abscesses (spread from gut via portal vein)
Leishmaniasis (visceral)	Leishmania	L. donovani accumulate in Kupffer cells ± granulomas and fibrosis
Malaria	Plasmodium	P. falciparum infection results in haemozoin pigment accumulation in Kupffer cells and portal macrophages
Schistosomiasis	Schistosoma	S. mansoni infests hepatic portal vein. Ova deposited in liver cause granulomas and 'pipestem fibrosis'. May cause portal hypertension
Fascioliasis	Fasciola	F. hepatica (common liver fluke) from sheep (via water cress). Liver fluke infests the bile ducts and causes obstruction and inflammation
Opisthorchiasis	Opisthorcis	O. sinensis (Chinese liver fluke) from raw fish. Duct infestation causing obstruction and cholangiocarcinoma
Hydatid cysts	Echinococcus	E. granulosus (primary host carnivores, especially dogs). Ovum ingestion results in cysts in many organs, including liver
Ascariasis	Ascaris	A. lumbricoides migrates through the liver and causes inflammation, necrosis and granulomas

of anaerobic infections. Repeated imaging of the liver allows assessment to determine the duration of antibiotics.

Viral hepatitis

Inflammation of the liver (hepatitis) can be caused by many agents, including viruses. Five well-characterized hepatotropic viruses are associated with primary hepatitis (hepatitis A–E; Table 19.13). Structurally they are quite distinct but cannot be differentiated on clinical grounds. They typically cause necrosis and inflammation of the liver.

Other much rarer causes include viruses which secondarily invade the liver as part of a systemic infection such as Epstein–Barr virus (EBV), cytomegalovirus (CMV), herpes simplex virus (HSV), adenovirus, coxsackie and enteroviruses; yellow fever virus and other zoonoses which are geographically restricted and other viruses which have yet to be fully characterized, e.g. hepatitis F. **Viral hepatitis** is usually taken to mean the hepatotropic viruses (Fig. 19.23).

Hepatitis A (Table 19.14)

This is so-called **infectious hepatitis** (a bit of a misnomer in that all types of viral hepatitis are, by definition,

infective). It is a relatively benign, self-limited infection, more common in younger age groups (<15 years) and lower socioeconomic groups, causing up to 25% of acute viral hepatitis in the developing world. It occurs both endemically and in epidemic forms–75% of cases are acquired by ingestion of **contaminated food** or **water**, 25% from close personal contact and **faecal/oral** contamination.

The hepatitis is usually mild, especially in children in whom it may be subclinical. It is more serious–often a distinct febrile illness–in adults. Only a small proportion (0.1%) have a fulminant/fatal course.

The virus replicates and is released from hepatocytes without directly damaging the cells, the damage being caused by an immune response to the infected cells. The hepatitis never becomes chronic, and does not predispose to hepatocellular carcinoma.

Hepatitis B (Tables 19.15 and 19.16)

Hepatitis B (HBV) infection is **more serious**, with often a more severe acute attack than hepatitis A (HAV). Fulminant hepatitis with massive liver necrosis and death may occur. **Chronic hepatitis** may also occur, in both those who suffer an initial acute illness, and also those in whom the initial infection is asymptomatic.

Ten per cent of adult infections become chronic, whereas virtually all neonatal infections do. Up to 10% of

Table 19.13 Viral hepatitis.

Hepatitis virus	A	B	C	D*	E
Family	Picorna	Heptadna	Flavi/Pesti	Viroid	Calici
Nucleic acid	ssRNA	dsDNA	ssRNA	ssRNA	ssRNA
Transmission	Faecal–oral	Parenteral Sexual Congenital	Parenteral	Parenteral with HBV	Faecal–oral
Incubation period (months)	c. 1	1–6	1–6	As for HBV	1–2
Incidence in UK	++	+/–	+/–	+/–	–
Chronicity	No	c. 10%	c. 50%	Yes with HBV	No
Fulminant liver failure	< 1:1000	1:100	Minimal	Greater risk than HBV	High risk in pregnancy
Subclinical	Usually in childhood	30–50% are anicteric	75% are anicteric	?	?
Vaccine	Introduced 1992	Introduced 1982	None	None but HBV vaccine protects	None

* Hepatitis D only occurs in association with hepatitis B virus (HBV).

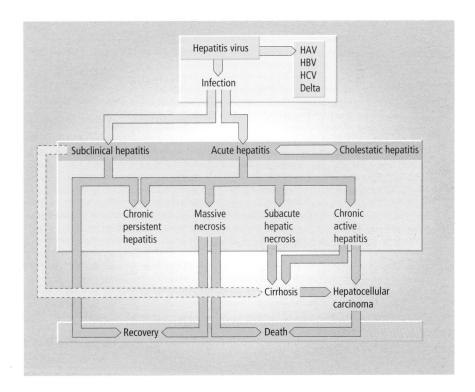

Fig. 19.23 Clinical syndromes associated with viral hepatitis.

Table 19.14 Hepatitis A virus (HAV).

Not as severe or as long-lasting as hepatitis B

No chronic or carrier state

Outbreaks can be epidemic in nature via contamination of water and foods, especially shellfish

HAV is endemic in developing countries and poses a particular hazard for travellers, for whom vaccination is recommended

Table 19.15 Hepatitis B virus (HBV).

Propensity to cause chronic infections

Associated with hepatocellular carcinoma

High incidence in South East Asia where infection at an early age is associated with chronic disease and its sequelae

Increased incidence in homosexuals, intravenous drug abusers and haemophiliacs

Health care workers are at increased risk of acquiring HBV and vaccination of this group is recommended. Strict hospital infection control measures are in place to prevent transmission of this virus

Table 19.16 Serodiagnosis and significance of markers for hepatitis B.

Infection	Test	Comments
Acute	Anti-HBc IgM+	Mainstay of diagnosis
	HBsAg+	c. 20% clear HBsAg at presentation
	HBeAg+	c. 80% clear HBeAg at presentation. HBeAg correlates with active infection and a highly infectious state
Past infection or immunization	Anti-HBc IgG+	
Past infection	Anti-HBs IgG+	
Immune, past or chronic infection	HBsAg+	
Chronic carriage	Anti-HBc IgG+	
	HBeAg+/–	Highly infectious
	Anti-HBe IgG+/–	Low infectious risk

HBc IgM, Hepatitis B core immunoglobulin M; HBsAg, hepatitis B surface antigen; HBeAg, hepatitis B e antigen.

acute infections in adults will also lead to the patient becoming an **asymptomatic carrier**, i.e. have hepatitis B surface antigen (HBsAg) in the blood, but remain asymptomatic. These patients may have anything from minor abnormalities to active cirrhosis on biopsy, but the majority (95%) will have only very minor changes.

Three distinct antigens can be detected–HBsAg (blood and liver), which is the **surface coat** of the virus; hepatitis B core antigen (HBcAg; liver) which is associated with the **central core** of the virus; hepatitis B e antigen (HBeAg; blood) which is an envelope breakdown product of the HBcAg (Fig. 19.24).

Presence of HBeAg in the **blood** or HBcAg in the **liver** indicates **active viral replication** and hence **infectivity**.

HBV DNA can also be detected in the **serum**, which is a more sensitive measure of replication.

As with HAV, the virus is not itself cytotoxic, the injury to the hepatocytes being secondary to an immune response mediated by cytotoxic T cells.

HBV may lead to **chronic hepatitis** and **cirrhosis** (macronodular), but also may predispose to **hepatocellular carcinoma (HCC)**, with a 200× increased risk of HCC in male HBV carriers. This increased susceptibility is not just because of HBV leading to cirrhosis (which is in itself a predisposition to HCC). It is most important in those with HBV infection established from an early age. HBV DNA integrates into the host genome at multiple sites, which probably initiates cell transformation due to the inserted sequences' effects on adjacent cellular oncogenes. Separate secondary events are probably also necessary to produce tumour formation.

Hepatitis D (Table 19.17)

δ Virus is an **incomplete RNA virus** requiring a **protein coat** (HBsAg) derived from HBV (Fig. 19.25). Thus it can only occur as an infection in the presence of HBV, being initiated either as an acute coinfection or **superinfection** on top of hepatitis B.

Table 19.17 Hepatitis D virus (HDV or δ agent).

Defective virus requiring HBV to replicate
Results in more severe disease than HBV infection alone
Infection is uncommon in the UK
Infection is common in parts of Europe, South America and Africa
Infection is either by coinfection or superimposed on HBV

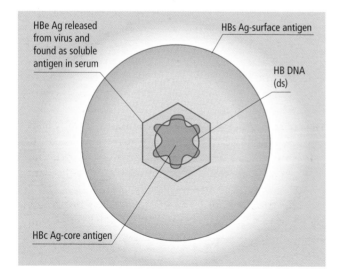

HBe Ag released from virus and found as soluble antigen in serum

HBs Ag-surface antigen

HB DNA (ds)

HBc Ag-core antigen

Fig. 19.24 The hepatitis B virus.

HBV, Hepatitis B virus.

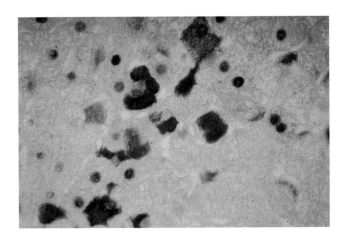

Fig. 19.25 Liver biopsy. Double immunohistochemistry shows HBs (blue) and HBc (brown).

It is endemic in southern Europe, Africa, the Middle East and South America, with 50% of HBsAg carriers in southern Italy also having hepatitis D virus (HDV). In the western world it is mainly spread **parenterally**, predominantly by intravenous drug abuse. It invariably causes liver damage, and is thought to have a direct cytopathic effect on hepatocytes. Those with acute HDV coinfection are more likely to present with severe or fulminant hepatitis than those with acute HBV alone, and those who develop chronic disease are more likely to progress ultimately to cirrhosis.

The non-A, non-B viruses

This designation was given to a putative third type of acute viral hepatitis, thought to include at least three different viruses–a **blood transfusion-transmitted** virus; a **coagulation factor-transmitted** virus and an **epidemic water-borne** virus. Two of these have recently been characterized.

Hepatitis C virus (HCV; Table 19.18). HCV accounts for 95% of hepatitis cases in blood transfusion recipients, and 50% of cases of sporadic non-A, non-B (NANB) hepatitis. It is a single-stranded RNA virus. It can be detected by tests for anti-HCV antibodies in the serum, although early tests gave a high false-positive rate.

At present there are no tests for HCV antigens in the serum, although they can be detected by immunoperoxidase with specific antibodies in liver sec-

Table 19.18 Hepatitis C virus.

The cause of the majority of transfusion-related hepatitides before the routine screening of blood products
Sexual transmission of the virus is rare
Strongly associated with chronic disease

tions. Polymerase chain reaction (PCR) for HCV RNA can be done on both liver and serum.

Prevalence of HCV is approximately 1% (0.7% western Europe, 1.4% USA). Only 60% of these have had any possibility of parenteral or sexual transmission of the virus, the mode of spread to the other 40% being obscure. HCV is much **less infectious** than **HBV**. Well over half of patients infected with HCV will develop **chronic hepatitis**, and at least 20% of these will progress to **cirrhosis**. HCV also predisposes to **HCC**, being considered four times as important as HBV in the genesis of the tumour in Japan.

Hepatitis E virus (HEV; Table 19.19*).* Hepatitis E is another distinct virus, again being composed of single-stranded RNA. It is transmitted by the *faecal–oral* route, usually by sewage-contaminated water in developing countries, and occurs both in **sporadic** and **epidemic** forms. Especially worrying is the high mortality (20–39%) in pregnant women. It is not thought to lead to chronic disease.

Table 19.19 Hepatitis E virus.

Responsible for large outbreaks of water-borne infections in developing countries
Generally mild infection
Has a high mortality in pregnant women

There are also one or more viruses yet to be characterized to account for the 5% of transfusion-associated hepatitis cases and the 50% of sporadic cases which are HCV-negative.

Clinical features of viral hepatitis

Acute viral hepatitis. Acute viral hepatitis can vary very widely from mild malaise to jaundice to fulminant disease with hepatic coma and death.

A, B and C tend to have similar disease courses, with B and C generally more severe. Mild cases will be characterized by non-specific features and a rise in serum transaminase levels. Others have more obvious symptoms with nausea/anorexia and abdominal pain, which lessens when jaundice appears. The jaundice usually lasts 1–4 weeks. Tender hepatomegaly is also a usual feature. Up to 15% of cases of acute hepatitis may relapse, but usually in a milder form. Rarely it may lead a fulminant course over a period of aproximately 10 days.

Patients tend to feel generally 'run-down' for a few weeks to months (the posthepatitis syndrome), but recover (both clinically and biochemically) within 6 months.

Chronic viral hepatitis. Chronic viral hepatitis may occur with hepatitis B, D and C, and is defined as 'chronic inflammation of the liver continuing without improvement for at least 6 months'. As well as being classified as to the virus involved, the chronic hepatitis is also separated morphologically into chronic persistent, chronic active, chronic lobular or chronic septal hepatitis (see later).

Investigations (Table 19.20)

Biochemically the changes are predominantly those of hepatocellular damage, with **bilirubin AST** and **GGT** showing modest rises (Fig. 19.26). Serum autoantibodies are usually not present, but there may be **smooth-muscle**

Table 19.20 Serodiagnosis and significance of markers for viral hepatitis.

Hepatitis antigen	Acute infection	Immune/past infection or immunization		Chronic infection
		IgM	IgG	IgG
A	HAV in faeces	Anti-HAV	Anti-HAV	
C	HCV in serum			Anti-HCV
D	HDV in serum	Anti-HDV	Anti-HDV	
E		Anti-HEV	Anti-HEV	

IgM, Immunoglobulin M; HAV, hepatitis A virus; HCV, hepatitis C virus; HDV, hepatitis D virus; HEV, hepatitis E virus.

antibody in chronic HBV. A viral screen would be performed to look for hepatitis A, B and possibly C (depending on local availability of the test), and also CMV/EBV.

Macroscopic pathology

The liver may be swollen and red with a tense capsule; there may be focal areas of collapse visible beneath the capsule; if cholestasis is severe, the liver may appear bright yellow; if fulminant, the liver would appear shrunken and wrinkled.

Microscopic pathology

The features may be similar for all the viruses. The liver is infiltrated by **chronic inflammatory cells** which may be seen in the lobules and portal tracts. There is parenchymal damage with swelling of hepatocytes and acidophilic change in others (forming acidophil cells or **Councilman bodies** (see Fig. 19.12).

Cell necrosis and drop-out are most marked around the central veins. Loss of hepatocytes, swelling, regeneration and inflammatory cell infiltration result in lobular disarray. Cholestasis would usually be seen, with bile both within hepatocytes and canaliculi. Changes in the hepatocytes (feathery degeneration) may be seen secondary to this. **Fatty change** may be a feature of **hepatitis C**. The inflammatory involvement of the portal tracts may spill over into the surrounding liver tissue (not to be

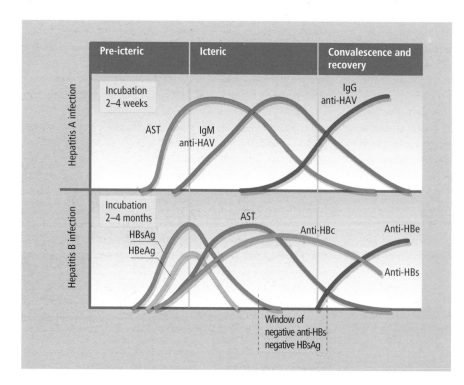

Fig. 19.26 Hepatitis A and B. Serum antigen and antibody levels.

confused with the piecemeal necrosis of CAH). Damage to bile ducts may be seen in hepatitis C, which may mimic large duct obstruction, and the infiltrate in the tracts may be focal with lymphoid follicle formation.

Bridging necrosis may be seen (between portal tracts and central veins), which is a sign of poorer prognosis and increased risk of progression to chronic liver disease. Necrosis may be even more widespread, e.g. panacinar, massive.

This pattern of acute viral hepatitis may be mimicked by drugs, such that without a known aetiological agent a biopsy may be diagnosed as 'viral/drug hepatitis', hopefully initiating the appropriate further investigations.

Diagnosis

The diagnosis of hepatitis B is complicated by the carrier state and the serodiagnosis and significance of markers are shown in Table 19.16.

Parasitic infections

These organisms are discussed in more detail in Chapter 8.

Hepatic amoebiasis/amoebic cysts

Entamoeba histolytica infection of the liver complicates 3–9% of amoebic dysentaries. The liver contains large abscesses filled with reddish brown pus (likened to **anchovy paste**). Trophozoites of *Entamoeba histolytica* may be found in the abscess wall.

Hydatid cyst

In the UK, especially in sheep-farming areas of Wales, *Echinococcus granulosus* causes hydatid disease with solitary or multiple cysts in the liver (Fig. 19.27). Histology of the cysts shows a thick wall lined by germinal epithelium of the larva. Numerous scolices or **brood capsules** are present which are highly immunogenic. The diagnosis may be made by radiology as the cyst walls commonly calcify.

Hepatic schistosomiasis

Schistosomiasis of the liver complicates intestinal schistosomiasis. *Schistosoma mansoni*, which causes intestinal infection in the Middle East, and *S. japonicum*, which causes intestinal infection in the Far East, are involved. Hepatic schistosomiasis causes **pipestem fibrosis** of the portal tracts with **portal hypertension** and **ascites**.

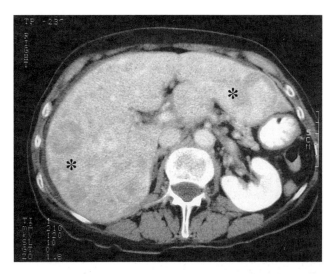

Fig. 19.27 Liver CT scan. Cysts (✳) in hydatid disease.

NON-INFECTIOUS CAUSES OF HEPATITIS

Drug hepatotoxicity

Virtually any clinical or pathological presentation of liver disease may be caused by drugs (Fig. 19.28). 'Drugs' include prescription medications, medicines bought over the counter, recreational drugs (mainly illegal substances) and herbal remedies.

Thus a **clinical history** of a patient presenting with liver disease (or in fact with any disease) should always include a thorough enquiry into what drugs are taken. This should not simply be a throw-away line such as 'do you take any drugs?', to which most people's answer would be 'no' (thinking you were asking if they were heroin addicts), but should be a detailed investigation

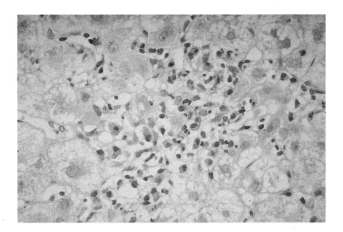

Fig. 19.28 Liver biopsy. Acute hepatitis associated with Voltarol. Note the eosinophil infiltrate. (H&E.)

into the various categories of medication listed above, with specific reference to when they were taken in relation to the onset of jaundice or other symptoms/signs.

Herbal remedies in particular are being used more and more, and as there are no controls as to what goes into these, and usually little indication on the packaging, increasingly they are being recognized as a cause of liver disease. Most people would not volunteer information about their taking of herbal remedies, as they do not consider them to be drugs. Another problem with drug histories is that many junior doctors seem to assume that they know which drugs are hepatotoxic ('if it's a common drug it can't be hepatotoxic') and thus do not record them if they think they are irrelevant.

Importance of drug reactions

Two per cent of jaundice in a hospital inpatient setting is due to drug reactions, and in certain groups, e.g. geriatric inpatients, this may be up to 20%.

Drug reactions may go **unrecognized**, thus prolonging the hepatic injury; they may initiate **chronic disease** with CAH, despite the drug being stopped; they may cause **cirrhosis**; and they may lead to the formation of **liver tumours**.

Classification of drug reactions

The reaction may be assessed on the general character of the injury caused:

- **cytotoxic**;
- **cholestatic**;
- **mixed cytotoxic/cholestatic**.

Perhaps rather more useful, from a morphological viewpoint, the injury can be described with reference to more specific pathological changes (Table 19.21):

- fatty change;
- hepatitis;
- fibrosis/cirrhosis;
- necrosis;
- cholestasis;
- granulomas;
- vascular changes;
- neoplastic change.

They can be classified on the basis of **presumed mechanism**:

- **intrinsic** or **predictable**: these reactions are **dose-related**–the injury may be as a result of **direct** action on the cells or by **indirect** means;
- **idiosyncratic**: these are not dose-related, and are due to either a hypersensitivity reaction in a patient or an individual's metabolic aberration.

And finally they can be classified as:

- **iatrogenic**;
- **toxicological** (overdose).

Table 19.21 Some examples of drug hepatotoxicity.

Fatty change	Alcohol, methotrexate (macrovesicular); sodium valproate, tetracycline (microvesicular)
Hepatitis	Halothane, methyldopa
Fibrosis/cirrhosis	Methotrexate, vitamin A
Necrosis	Paracetamol, halothane
Cholestasis	Chlorpromazine, oral contraceptives
Granulomas	Phenylbutazone, allopurinol, carbamazepine
Vascular changes	
Sinusoidal dilatation/peliosis hepatis	Oral contraceptives
Veno-occlusive disease	Herbal teas, azathioprine
Hepatic vein thrombosis	Oral contraceptives
Neoplastic change	
(Hepatocellular adenoma/carcinoma)	Anabolic steroids and oral contraceptives
(Angiosarcoma)	Thorotrast, vinyl chloride

In certain cases, there may be an interaction between metabolic abnormalities or infection and drugs. An example is **Reye's syndrome**, or 'encephalopathy and fatty degeneration of the viscera'. A disease seen almost exclusively in children, it is usually preceded by a viral infection such as influenza B. **Aspirin** is thought to play a role and is now considered an inappropriate drug to give to young children (Table 19.22).

Liver biopsy shows severe microvesicular fatty change and in this respect the disease resembles urea cycle defects and acute fatty liver of pregnancy, conditions which may also be precipitated by or exacerbated by drugs.

Table 19.22 Features of Reye's syndrome.

Children aged 6–11 years
Prodromal viral illness (varicella or influenza B)
Protracted vomiting
Neurological changes (lethargy, confusion, stupor, coma)
Hepatomegaly
Mitochondrial dysfunction in the hepatocyte
↑ ALT, AST from liver + muscle
↑ Ammonia
Hyperaminoacidaemia
↑ Fatty acids
↑ Urate
↓ Prothrombin unresponsive to vitamin K
Hypoglycaemia
Liver biopsy characteristic yellow to white colour

ALT, Alanine aminotransferase; AST, aspartate aminotransferase.

Impaired perfusion due to vascular disorders

The **blood supply** of the liver is 1.5 l/minute which comes from the **hepatic artery** (25%) and the **hepatic portal vein** (75%), with the former having a higher oxygen saturation (95%) than the latter (85%). Infarcts of the liver are rare due to this dual blood supply. The blood drains via the **hepatic vein** into the **inferior vena cava**.

The **perfusion** of the liver may be affected by generalized vascular disease, disease processes having a local effect on vessels, and pathology primarily affecting the liver.

The supply from the **hepatic artery** may be affected by thrombosis, hypotension or anaemia. The hepatic portal vein may be obstructed by intrahepatic causes (cirrhosis, primary or secondary tumours invading vessels) or extrahepatic causes (thrombus, compression by tumour at the porta hepatis, pylephlebitis due to peritoneal sepsis). Drainage via the hepatic vein may be affected by thrombosis, tumour, and high back-pressure due to right-sided heart failure.

Hepatic congestion

The classic appearance of the liver in patients with chronic passive venous congestion due to right-sided heart failure is a **'nutmeg liver'** (Fig. 19.29), appearing as dark congested centrilobular areas surrounded by paler areas at the periphery of the lobules. Microscopically there is central congestion, atrophy and necrosis of hepatocytes in severe cases (**central haemorrhagic necrosis**), with the more peripheral hepatocytes suffering less severe hypoxia and undergoing fatty change.

In severe chronic cases the atrophic and necrotic hepatocytes are replaced by fibrous tissue around the

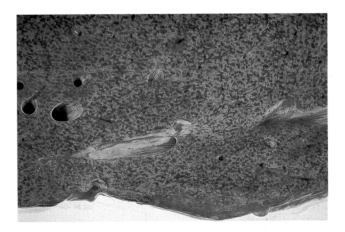

Fig. 19.29 'Nutmeg liver'. This patient had chronic congestive cardiac failure. Chronic passive venous congestion results in areas of fat (yellow) and congestion (dark red/brown).

central veins. In extreme cases, e.g. with tricuspid insufficiency, the fibrosis may be so severe as to produce fibrous bridging between adjacent central veins (**cardiac cirrhosis**).

Budd–Chiari syndrome

This term was first used to describe a clinical syndrome of abdominal pain, hepatomegaly and ascites secondary to hepatic vein thrombosis, but is now more loosely used to describe the result of occlusion of medium or large hepatic veins or the inferior vena cava by thrombus, tumour or fibrous tissue.

Thirty per cent of cases occur with no known predisposing factor (**idiopathic**). The rest are due to a variety of causes such as polycythaemia rubra vera, pregnancy, the postpartum state and oral contraceptive use.

Macroscopically the liver appears **swollen** and has a red/purple discoloration. **Microscopically** there is severe centrilobular **sinusoidal dilatation** and **congestion** with extensive **necrosis** of **hepatocytes** (much more severe changes than those seen in cardiac failure). It may be treated in the acute situation by the surgical formation of portosystemic venous shunts to allow reverse flow through the portal vein.

Veno-occlusive disease

In this condition, the small tributaries of the hepatic vein (**terminal hepatic venules**) become obstructed by fibrous tissue, and may even become obliterated. Superadded thrombosis may occur, and may be associated with central congestion and necrosis.

Causes include the ingestion of pyrrolizidine alkaloids in 'bush tea', irradiation, immunosuppressive drugs (azathioprine) and cytotoxic drugs.

Autoimmune hepatitis

Autoimmune CAH (**lupoid hepatitis**) is associated with a variety of non-specific autoantibodies (antinuclear, anti-smooth-muscle, antimitochondrial) and organ-specific autoantibodies (liver membrane and liver microsomal). This disease is seen in **young** and **perimenopausal women** who have other forms of autoimmune disease such as thyroiditis, arthritis, vasculitis and Sjögren's syndrome.

Miscellaneous causes of hepatitis

These include malignant infiltration of the liver, hyperthermia, Wilson's disease, partial hepatectomy and liver transplantation.

CHRONIC HEPATITIS

Chronic hepatitis is defined as 'inflammation of the liver which has occurred without improvement for over 6 months' as evidenced by symptomatic, biochemical, serological or morphological features.

It may be classified by aetiology, but more usually is split into one of three groups which are based on liver biopsy appearances and then subclassified on the basis of clinical grouping or aetiology. These groups are chronic persistent, chronic active and chronic lobular hepatitis (Table 19.23). This subdivision into three main groups is currently evolving into a new classification, recognizing that chronic hepatitis is a spectrum of disease through which the diseases of individual patients may evolve. More descriptive groupings incorporating numerical scoring for inflammation and fibrosis and immunohistochemical findings are currently being used.

Chronic persistent hepatitis

Clinical features

It is seen in **males** more than females, often in the age group 30–50 years. The disease may be symptomatically remitting or relapsing, with generalized or, more specifically, abdominal symptoms with or without jaundice.

It tends to be a relatively mild disease with a generally benign course. There may be tender hepatomegaly, but signs of chronic liver disease are absent.

Biochemically the **AST** and possibly **bilirubin** may be **raised**, and serum IgG may be **slightly raised**.

Table 19.23 Chronic hepatitis: hepatic inflammation persisting without improvement for 6 months.

Chronic persistent hepatitis (CPH)
Better prognosis
Raised transaminases 2× in CPH
Chronic active hepatitis (CAH)
Causes
Autoimmune
Chronic infection with hepatitis B virus
Alcohol
Drugs
CAH → cirrhosis
Raised transaminases 2–10× in CAH
Alkaline phosphatase is normal
Albumin, prothrombin time, globulins may be abnormal in CAH

Aetiology

This is usually viral, either **hepatitis B** or **C**.

Pathology

The liver biopsy will show portal tract expansion by a chronic inflammatory cell infiltrate which is the same in most of the portal areas. The borders of the portal tracts are well-defined, with no piecemeal necrosis. There may be a mild increase in portal fibrosis, possibly with formation of small fibrous spurs extending outwards. There may be a very minor lobular component to the inflammatory infiltrate. If due to hepatitis B, then HBsAg will usually be demonstrable.

Course

Only a small minority of patients will change to mild chronic CAH, and they do not tend to progress to cirrhosis. Thus specific therapy is not required.

Chronic active hepatitis

Clinical features

Women are more often affected than men (3:1), but if due to hepatitis B there is a majority of males. The most common age at presentation is 20–50 years. They may be asymptomatic, but may have severe symptoms with exhaustion and signs of chronic liver disease and portal hypertension (in the later stages).

Biochemically the AST, IgG and bilirubin will be increased. Autoantibodies may be present, depending on the aetiology of the CAH.

Aetiology

The three major types of CAH are hepatitis B, hepatitis C and autoimmune or lupoid. Rarer causes include drugs, Wilson's disease, A1AT deficiency and alcohol.

Chronic biliary disease may have many similar features, both clinically and pathologically, and there are some patients who seem to fall somewhere between the diagnoses of CAH and primary biliary cirrhosis.

Autoimmune CAH tends to occur in young women (F:M = 8:1), is associated with high titres of both organ-non-specific, antibodies (antinuclear and anti-smooth muscle) and organ-specific antibodies (liver-specific protein, liver membrane antigen, liver microsomes), and is strongly associated with HLA-B8, DR3. There is also concurrence of other autoimmune diseases.

Pathology

The essential feature for the diagnosis is the presence of **piecemeal necrosis** (Fig. 19.30), which may be classed as mild, moderate or severe. There is a chronic inflamma-

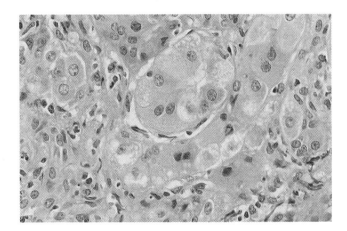

Fig. 19.30 Liver biopsy. 'Piecemeal necrosis' in chronic active hepatitis (CAH). Note the eosinophilic necrotic cells and inflammatory cells. (H&E.)

tory cell infiltrate in the portal tracts which is not contained by the limiting plate of the tracts, but extends into the adjacent hepatic parenchyma with lymphoid cells surrounding hepatocytes and evidence of cell necrosis. There may be ductular proliferation at the edges of the portal areas, but marked bile duct damage or abnormalities are not a feature of the disease. Rosette formations of hepatocytes may be seen surrounding the portal tracts. Fibrosis is also seen, and there may be both **bridging necrosis** and **bridging fibrosis** between the various vascular structures (portal–portal, portal–central or central–central).

Course

Lupoid CAH is treated with corticosteroids. It usually responds well in the first instance. The mean survival is 12 years after diagnosis. Ultimately, cirrhosis develops in virtually all cases. CAH due to hepatitis B may be treated with **antiviral therapy** if there is evidence of viral replication (**HBeAg-positive**). Clinical course varies widely, depending on such factors as degree of activity, response to therapy (and conversion to CPH), and superinfection with hepatitis D. Cirrhosis (with or without HCC) will develop if the disease continues to be active.

Chronic lobular hepatitis

Clinical features

This is a rare form of chronic hepatitis. It is seen in hepatitis B carriers and in hepatitis C. The course is intermittent with serum transaminases raised during periods of activity.

Pathology

It is diagnosed when there is **lobular inflammation** without evidence of significant portal inflammation (note that there can also be lobular inflammation in CAH). Foci of necrosis and even bridging necrosis may be seen.

CIRRHOSIS

Liver disease may resolve or become chronic. If it becomes chronic, the ultimate end-stage is cirrhosis (which may result in the development of HCC if the patient survives long enough).

Cirrhosis is a **diffuse** process occurring throughout the whole liver (Fig. 19.31). There is no such thing as a focal cirrhosis. It is also an **irreversible** process. It is seen as regenerative nodules of hepatocytes completely surrounded by bands of fibrous tissue (Fig. 19.32). As a consequence of the regenerative nature of the hepatic structure, the normal vascular relationships are lost. The parenchymal architecture is also abnormal, with the nor-

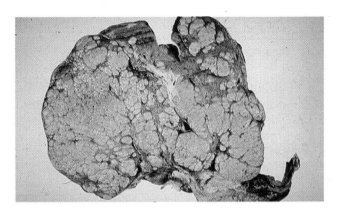

Fig. 19.31 Liver. Macronodular cirrhosis. Broad bands of fibrosis are seen macroscopically.

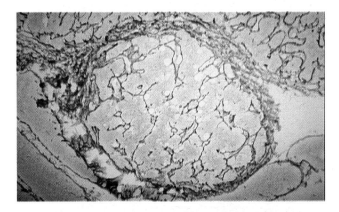

Fig. 19.32 Liver biopsy. Macronodular cirrhosis. Note the black bands of fibrosis shown in this reticulin (silver) stain encircling regenerating liver nodules.

mal one-cell-thick liver plates being replaced by more **disorganized liver plates**, two or three or more cells thick.

Classification

Cirrhosis may be classified in three main ways, all of which have their uses.

The classical/anatomical classification

This has an anatomical basis, namely the size of the nodules. If most are <3 mm, then this is a **micronodular cirrhosis**; if most are >3 mm, then this is a **macronodular cirrhosis**.

However, there is often a mixed micro-/macronodular picture, and in addition the nodules may be subdivided by fibrous septa. There is in fact very little clinical relevance to this purely morphological classification, except that an unexpected micronodular cirrhosis would most likely be due to alcohol, and HCCs are more likely to arise in a macronodular than a micronodular cirrhosis.

Aetiological classification (Table 19.24)

Table 19.24 Cirrhosis.

Causes
Alcoholism
Viral hepatitis B
Prolonged cholestasis
Wilson's
Cystic fibrosis
α_1-Antitrypsin deficiency
Galactosaemia
Haemochromatosis
Primary biliary cirrhosis
Autoimmune disease
Investigations
Mild or latent
↑ Plasma bile acids
↑ BSP retention
↑ GGT in heavy drinkers without cirrhosis
Severe
Jaundice
↑ ALT, AST, ALP, GGT
↓ Albumin
↑ Immunoglobulins
Prolonged prothrombin time
↑ Ammonia
↓ Urea
AST may be low because of exhaustion of hepatocytes

BSP, Bromsulphthalein; GGT, γ-glutamyl transferase; ALT, alanine transaminase; AST, aspartate transaminase; ALP, alkaline phosphatase.

The aetiological agent resulting in the cirrhosis may be suspected or known clinically, and may also be evident morphologically. However, in a proportion of cases the cause of the cirrhosis is not evident (**cryptogenic cirrhosis**). Broadly speaking, the cases can be broken down into the following groups:
- alcohol;
- drugs/toxins;
- virus;
- biliary obstruction;
- metabolic;
- autoimmune CAH;
- vascular;
- miscellaneous;
- cryptogenic (idiopathic).

In the western world the majority of cirrhoses are due to alcohol–the approximate proportions are 60% alcohol, 15% cryptogenic, 10% viral, 10% biliary, 5% other causes. In Africa and the Far East, the proportion of cases due to virus (mainly hepatitis B) is much higher.

Classification based on disease activity

Third, a cirrhosis may be described as being either **active** or **inactive**. This is assessed on the basis of inflammatory activity in the fibrous septa and hepatocyte nodules, and continuing evidence of hepatocyte necrosis.

The three major mechanisms involved in the **pathogenesis** of cirrhosis are:
1 cell injury and death;
2 fibrosis;
3 regeneration.

Cell death is usually continuous, thus a patient suffering an episode of massive necrosis due to virus or toxin may die or fully recover, but would not tend to become cirrhotic. The mechanism of the cell death is variable depending on the agent involved–immunological, metabolic disturbance or toxin.

All of these various factors may act through a final common pathway involving calcium flux into the hepatocytes. Fibrosis is stimulated directly by cell death and by lymphokines derived from inflammatory cells associated with areas of cell death. Types I and III collagen are produced by various cells. However the exact mechanism of this regulation of fibrogenesis is not fully understood. Regeneration is also stimulated by cell death–the human liver can restore three-quarters of its mass in 6 months, indicating its great regenerative potential, but the precise mechanism is again unclear.

LIVER TUMOURS

Liver tumours can be divided up into **benign** tumours,

malignant tumours, and lesions which are 'tumour-like' but are not true neoplasms.

Malignant tumours may be **primary** or **secondary**, with secondary tumours being far more common than primary in the western world. Of the primary tumours (both benign and malignant), most are derived from **hepatocytes**, with a minority being of **bile duct** origin. There are also some rare primary vascular tumours.

Benign tumours

Liver cell adenoma

Clinical. These arise mainly in **women** and are related to the use of **oral contraceptives**. They are also seen in **men** related to the use of **anabolic/androgenic steroids**. Rarely they may arise in children or young adults in the absence of drug use. The patients presents with either an abdominal mass or pain (related to haemorrhage into the tumour).

Pathology. They are usually well-defined solitary nodules composed of rather bland-appearing hepatocytes arranged in trabeculae. The reticulin pattern tends to be maintained. Vessels are prominent. A key feature in the differential from non-neoplastic liver or focal nodular hyperplasia is the absence of fibrous septa, portal tracts and bile ducts within the nodules. There are sometimes problems differentiating them from HCC.

Bile duct adenoma

These are usually small white subcapsular nodules which are usually submitted for histology when a laparotomy is being performed (e.g. for colonic carcinoma resection) and are mistaken for metastatic tumour. Histologically they are composed of numerous small bile ducts packed close together within a small amount of fibrous stroma. They are actually quite common if a liver is thoroughly examined.

Haemangioma

These are relatively common (prevalence 5% at autopsy) well-defined nodules composed of thin-walled vessels (cavernous or capillary, depending on the size of vessels) set within fibrous stroma. They are also often **subcapsular**, and again may be mistaken for metastatic tumour at laparotomy. They may become thrombosed, sclerosed or calcified. They rarely rupture.

Benign tumour-like lesions

Focal nodular hyperplasia

This may occur at any age, in either sex, and the aetiology is uncertain but may be related to an abnormal blood supply to part of the liver. They are well-defined nodules of 1–5cm diameter which often have a prominent central fibrous scar and are divided up by fibrous septa. Histologically they resemble cirrhosis, but are obviously not as they are only focal lesions (and are thus by definition **not cirrhotic**).

Nodular regenerative hyperplasia

In this condition the liver appears nodular, but the nodules are not associated with fibrosis around the edges (although the reticulin pattern may be rather compressed around the edges). They may show **reverse lobulation** with portal tracts apparently at their centre. It is associated with a number of conditions, including chronic venous congestion, rheumatic diseases and myeloproliferative disorders. It may be related to portal vein thrombosis. It may present with **portal hypertension**.

Malignant primary liver tumours

Hepatocellular carcinoma (also known as hepatoma)

Incidence. The world can be split up into areas of high, intermediate and low incidence. In parts of Africa and South-east Asia it is the commonest malignant tumour, with an incidence of up to 150/100000 population/year. In Japan, the Middle East and southern Europe there are 5–20 cases/100000/year. In the UK, northern Europe, the Americas, India and Australia the incidence is low (<5/100000/year), with the UK incidence being approximately 3/100000 per year, representing 0.5% of all cancers.

Age. In the high-incidence areas the patients are younger (20–50 years); in the low incidence areas they are older (50–70 years).

Sex. In high-incidence areas the M:F ratio is up to 8:1, but in the low-incidence areas it is 2–3:1. This is mainly related to higher carriage rate of hepatitis B in males.

Aetiology
- *Cirrhosis.* Usually macronodular or of mixed type. In the west, 5–15% of cirrhotics develop HCC.
- *Hepatitis B.* Worldwide this is the most important aeti-

ological factor, and its effective control would lead to a great reduction in mortality due to HCC (i.e. HBV vaccine is in effect an 'anticancer vaccine').

Others causes include **aflatoxins** (from *Aspergillus flavus* contamination of food); **chemicals** (many are carcinogenic in animal models, but none have been definitely implicated in human HCC); **genetic effects** (40% of patient with hereditary tyrosinaemia develop HCC); **alcohol** (because of increased hepatitis B in alcoholics).

Clinical presentation. Patients tend to present late. There may be a sudden deterioration in a known cirrhotic patient. There is usually pain, weight loss and hepatomegaly. Jaundice is present in <50%; a bruit is audible over the tumour in 25%. There may be haemorrhage into the tumour and rupture into the peritoneal cavity. **Paraneoplastic syndromes** may be seen (see Chapter 11), with various manifestations such as hypoglycaemia, hypercalcaemia, sexual changes and erythrocytosis.

Investigations. Serum α-fetoprotein (**AFP**) may be raised up to 500 ng/ml in hepatitis/hepatic metastasis/other tumours (normal up to 20 ng/ml), but levels above this are really only seen in HCC, hepatoblastoma or germ cell tumours (yolk sac elements in testis and ovary). Up to 95% of patients in high-incidence areas and 80% in low-incidence areas have levels >500 ng/ml. There are other less specific markers such as **carcinoembryonic antigen (CEA)** and **acidic isoferritin** which may be raised.

The tumours may be seen by various **imaging** modalities (ultrasound, isotope scans, CT scans, magnetic resonance imaging (MRI). **Hepatic angiography** is also useful in diagnosis, localization and assessment of operability, and for monitoring the effects of therapy.

Macroscopic appearances. The tumour may be a solitary mass, multiple nodules (implying multiple primaries or intrahepatic spread) or may diffusely infiltrate the liver. There is a tendency for the nodules to become necrotic centrally. The liver harbouring the tumour will usually be cirrhotic (Fig. 19.21; metastatic tumours may be seen in cirrhotic livers, but much more rarely). The right lobe is more commonly affected than the left. There may be infarction of the tumour, haemorrhage or rupture.

Microscopic appearances (Fig. 19.33). The main feature is that the tumour cells resemble normal hepatocytes, although they will usually show cytological and architectural features of malignancy. The tumour may show a number of different architectural patterns–trabecular,

pseudoglandular or solid. The cells may show only minor cytological differences from normal hepatocytes, or they may be pleomorphic and mitotically active. Clear cell and pleomorphic variants are seen. The tumour cells may contain fat, glycogen, Mallory bodies, globular hyaline bodies (AFP, fibrinogen, A1AT, albumin, ferritin). Reticulin stains will usually show almost complete loss of reticulin from the tumour (a useful diagnostic feature, if somewhat variable).

Immunocytochemistry is usually disappointing, as AFP is only rarely demonstrated (despite claims to the contrary in other texts) and other markers are non-specific.

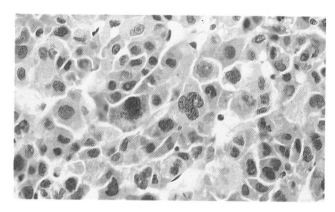

Fig. 19.33 Liver biopsy. Hepatocellular carcinoma. Note the large cells with large, irregular nuclei. (H&E.)

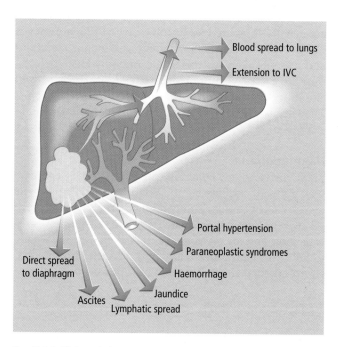

Fig. 19.34 Clinicopathology of hepatocellular carcinoma.

Course (Fig. 19.34). Some surgeons might resect the tumour if amenable to surgery. Results of transplantation are so appalling (with early recurrence) that most centres now do not transplant patients with HCC. Various cytotoxic drugs have been used, and attempts are also made to treat by hepatic artery embolization. HCC spreads into veins and there will be evidence of metastasis in 50% at post mortem (lungs, local nodes). Death is due to cachexia, gastrointestinal haemorrhage, hepatic failure and coma.

Fibrolamellar carcinoma

This is a relatively rare variant of HCC seen in adolescents and young adults. It is commoner in females than males. It is not associated with cirrhosis or hepatitis B, and the serum AFP is not raised.

It is usually large and solitary (Fig. 19.35), and most are in the **left lobe** of the liver. It is composed of groups of densely eosinophilic tumour cells separated by dense fibrous lamellae (Fig. 19.36). It has a better prognosis than

the normal type of HCC (survival 3–5 years), and is treated by resection or transplantation.

Hepatoblastoma

There are rare tumours occurring in **infancy** and **early childhood** in both sexes. There are two types–**epithelial** (embryonal and fetal cells) and **mixed** (epithelial and mesenchymal elements). Resection may be possible, and there is a 36% 5-year survival.

Angiosarcoma

This is a rare (0.2 cases/million per year), highly malignant tumour. It may be associated with chronic **arsenic** intoxication (occupational or therapeutic), **thorotrast, vinyl chloride** monomer or **copper**-containing sprays in vineyards. The tumours are often multicentric and very vascular, and are composed of elongated cells which surround hepatocytes and extend along sinusoids. They are derived from **endothelial** cells. They metastasize in 20% of cases.

Metastatic tumours

Metastases are the most common tumour in the liver in the western world. The liver is the most common site for blood-borne metastases in malignancy, being found in one-third of cases. The most common primary sites are the stomach, breast, lung and colon (Fig. 19.37). The clinical presentation may be related to the primary or the metastasis (or both). There may be malaise and weight loss, pain, hepatomegaly, but jaundice is only slight or absent.

Biochemistry may be abnormal with a **raised alkaline phosphatase**. The metastases may be visualized by ultrasound, CT or MRI. The diagnosis should be confirmed by guided biopsy. If metastases are suspected at laparotomy, they should be biopsied, as benign lesions (bile duct adenomas and haemangiomas) are often mistaken for metastases by surgeons. Attempts at therapy yield disap-

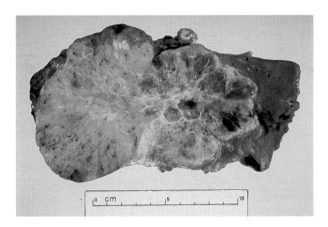

Fig. 19.35 Liver. Fibrolamellar carcinoma. Note how well circumscribed this tumour is.

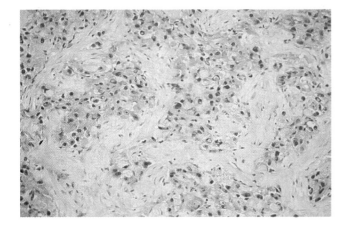

Fig. 19.36 Liver biopsy. Fibrolamellar carcinoma. Bands of fibrous tissue 'strangle' groups of atypical hepatocytes. (H&E.)

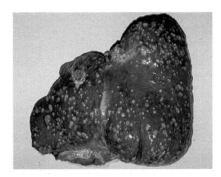

Fig. 19.37 Liver. Multiple nodules of metastatic colonic adenocarcinoma.

pointing results, but surgical resection may be feasible in some cases. The prognosis is poor, with death usually within a year.

LIVER TRANSPLANTATION

Liver transplantation was first performed successfully in man in 1963. The rate of transplantation worldwide is now approximately 1000/year, with a 1-year survival between 50 and 75% depending on the patient group.

With improving survival, patients with progressive chronic disease are being offered earlier transplantation, before reaching the end stages, as the results in healthier patients are better than in severe liver failure.

The largest group of patients transplanted are those with **cirrhosis**, in particular **primary biliary cirrhosis**. Patients with HCC used to make up a sizeable proportion of cases, but most centres do not transplant these patients now due to almost inevitable recurrence of the disease (although a few have been apparently cured in the past).

Pathology of rejection

Immunosuppression with **cyclosporin A** is utilized to counter graft rejection. Rejection may be **acute (reversible)** or **chronic (irreversible)**. It is a **T-cell-mediated** response directed against cells expressing major histocompatibility complex (MHC) class II antigens, namely the epithelium of the bile ducts and endothelium of vessels. Hepatocytes do not express class II antigens.

An episode of **acute rejection** occurs in up to 70% of

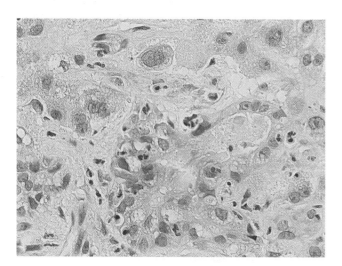

Fig. 19.38 Liver biopsy. Acute transplant rejection. The biliary tract epithelium is the immunological target. Note the damage to the epithelial cells and the inflammatory infiltrate. (H&E.)

patients within a month of transplantation (mostly 10–15 days). Biopsy shows portal inflammation and damage to bile ducts; endothelialitis (attachment of lymphocytes to the endothelium of vessels); and minor damage to centrilobular hepatocytes (Fig. 19.38). It responds to steroids.

Chronic rejection occurs in 5–20% of cases, usually presenting within the first year. It is characterized by **'vanishing bile duct syndrome'**, where there is inexorable loss of bile ducts with fibrous replacement. There is also an obliterative vasculopathy involving large and medium-sized arteries, and perivenular cholestasis with hepatocyte necrosis. Most cases are unresponsive to immunosuppression and progress to graft failure which requires retransplantation.

Biliary tract

ANATOMY OF THE BILIARY TRACT

Bile is excreted from **hepatocytes** into **canaliculi** between the hepatocytes within the liver cell plates. It then passes into interlobular/septal/intrahepatic ducts (with everincreasing size) which are situated within the portal areas, then into the right or left hepatic ducts which unite to form the common hepatic duct. After being joined by the cystic duct from the gallbladder, this becomes the **common bile duct**. It passes down to enter the second part of the duodenum on its posteromedial wall at the ampulla of Vater. In 70% of people the pancreatic duct joins it at the **ampulla**–in the remainder, the pancreatic duct **drains** separately into the duodenum (Fig. 19.2).

The **gallbladder** is a sac up to 10 cm long which lies in the gallbladder bed on the lower aspect of the liver, with its tip close to the liver's anterior border.

The biliary tree is lined throughout by **columnar epithelium**. There are **mucus glands** in the stroma underlying the epithelium of the neck of the gallbladder and the more distal portions of the extrahepatic biliary tree.

Bile has many constituents–water (97%), bilirubin, bile acids, cholesterol, phospholipids, various excreted metabolites, mucus. It is needed for absorption of fat, fatsoluble vitamins and calcium in the ileum (Table 19.1). It also acts as an excretory pathway for bilirubin, cholesterol and hormone and drug metabolites.

Bile is stored and concentrated by up to 90% in the gallbladder (which acts like a railway siding), and is expelled into the **common bile duct** and hence **duodenum** when fatty food enters the duodenum (mediated via **cholecystokinin** secreted from the duodenal and jejunal neuroendocrine cells and other hormones).

SYMPTOMS AND SIGNS OF BILIARY DISEASE

The clinical presentation of biliary disease is varied. There are some non-specific features, and others which are more specific to the liver and biliary tract:

- weight loss, pain, nausea, vomiting, fevers/rigors, cholesterol deposits;
- pruritus, jaundice, skin pigmentation;
- signs of portal hypertension and liver failure if cirrhosis ensues.

The presentation will depend on the type and site of lesion. Some forms of biliary disease have a very insidious onset and progression. Diseases such as primary biliary cirrhosis may be picked up in asymptomatic people on a routine health screen. Others, such as a gallstone lodged in the common bile duct, may be a very dramatic presentation with severe colicky pain and vomiting.

INVESTIGATION OF BILIARY DISEASE

Biochemistry

This has been covered in some depth in the preceding section of this chapter and is summarized in Table 19.9; however some of the main points will be emphasized again here.

Bile pigments

Serum bilirubin may be raised. Raised conjugated bilirubin is suggestive of a posthepatic or obstructive (i.e. biliary) lesion (although also seen in some of the familial hyperbilirubinaemias and in cholestatic forms of hepatocellular disease, e.g. cholestatic viral hepatitis). Raised unconjugated bilirubin suggests a prehepatic or hepatic lesion.

Urinary bilirubin is not detectable in normal people or those with unconjugated hyperbilirubinaemia. It is seen in cholestatic patients (and is responsible for the darkness of their urine).

Urobilinogen, normally present in urine, is absent from the urine in cholestatic patients. It is raised in those with hepatocellular disease (when the hepatocytes cannot re-excrete all the pigment reabsorbed from the small intestine).

Serum enzymes

Alkaline phosphatase is a hepatocyte membrane-associated enzyme released in cholestatic conditions. It also shows lesser rises with hepatocellular disease. It can be distinguished from bony forms of alkaline phosphatase by iso-enzyme fractionation.

GGT is also a membrane-associated enzyme, and concomitant rise confirms a liver origin for a raised alkaline phosphatase. However it is raised in both biliary and hepatocellular disease.

Transaminase AST and **ALT** are released when hepatocytes are damaged. There may be minor rises in biliary disease.

Bile acids

Serum bile acids may be raised, and may also be detected in the urine (not seen in normal subjects).

Lipids

Serum **cholesterol** may be raised (retained due to lack of its normal excretion in the bile). **Plasma triglycerides** are increased in both obstructive and hepatocellular disease. Abnormal **lipoproteins** may be found.

Plasma proteins

Albumin will only be decreased if the patient becomes cirrhotic. **Immunoglobulins** are not raised except if cirrhotic, or in primary biliary cirrhosis (raised IgM mainly).

Imaging

Plain radiology

A plain abdominal film may show **gallstones**, a **calcified gallbladder** or **gas** in the biliary system (due to fistula).

Ultrasound

This is the main **screening** procedure for assessment of the biliary tract. It may be used to look for **dilatation** of the **hepatic ducts** (as seen in large duct obstruction), **gallstones**, thickening of the gallbladder wall in **cholecystitis**.

CT scan

This may also be used to assess **bile duct dilatation**, but the only advantage over ultrasound is better visualization of the more distal portion of the common bile duct. It is not very useful for gallbladder disease.

Oral cholecystogram

This is good at detecting gallstones and lesions of the gallbladder wall. The common bile duct is also visualized.

Endoscopic retrograde cholangiopancreatography

This involves endoscopy with **cannulation** of the common bile duct or pancreatic duct and production of a cholangiogram or pancreatogram respectively (after injection of contrast). This is probably the investigation of choice in diseases of the bile ducts, as it visualizes the whole of the biliary tree, and may be used for therapy by sphincterotomy (for calculi) or stenting of the common bile duct (for strictures). In primary sclerosing cholangitis, it is the characteristic endoscopic retrograde cholangiopancreatography (ERCP) appearance which is diagnostic.

DISEASES OF THE BILE DUCTS

Developmental diseases

There are anatomical variations in the biliary tree in one-quarter of people if studied. However, not all of these lesions are of any pathological significance. There may be variations in number of bile ducts (duplication, accessory ducts); the common bile duct may be absent (agenesis); there may be defects in the bile duct walls resulting in biliary leakage in the neonatal period; bronchobiliary fistulas may rarely be present.

Extrahepatic biliary atresia

Epidemiology. The incidence of this disorder is 1 in 10 000 births, with females being more commonly affected than males.

Aetiology/pathogenesis. It may develop in the intrauterine or in the neonatal period and is thought to be probably due to an infective cause, possibly viral, *in utero.*

Clinical presentation. This is with unremitting jaundice (obstructive picture) in the first week after birth with severe pruritus. Xanthomas may develop.

Macroscopic/microscopic appearances. The site of the lesion is variable, as is the extent. The ducts may be completely absent, or replaced by connective tissue. On liver biopsy the appearance will depend on the timing. There will be cholestasis, periportal ductular proliferation, portal fibrosis, and eventually secondary biliary cirrhosis will develop if the condition is not treated. There may be some giant cell transformation of hepatocytes, but not as marked as in neonatal hepatitis (its main clinical differential diagnosis).

Course. The only treatment is surgery or transplantation. Surgery (**Kasai procedure**, hepatic portoenterostomy) must be performed before 4 months of age, and has a 33% 5-year survival. Transplantation gives an 80% 1-year survival.

Paucity of the intrahepatic bile ducts

This may be either syndromatic (Alagille's syndrome) or non-syndromatic.

Non-syndromatic. These patients usually present within a few days of birth, but may not present in some cases until the age of 6 years. They may be **idiopathic** or associated with a definable cause such as **A1AT deficiency**. They have persistent **jaundice** and severe pruritus. Early on, liver biopsy shows changes similar to neonatal hepatitis, and only later do the bile ducts disappear (suggesting a link with some infective agent). This is associated with portal fibrosis but only rather minor inflammation.

Patients are treated with **cholestyramine** (which binds bile acids in gut to reduce reabsorption), which produces symptomatic improvement. Biliary cirrhosis may occur, but this is relatively rare.

Alagille syndrome (arteriohepatic dysplasia)

This condition is **autosomal dominant**. The bile duct disappearance is associated with abnormal facies, skeletal and cardiac abnormalities and eye changes. There is also growth and sometimes **mental retardation**. Progression to cirrhosis is again rare, and patients tend to improve in adulthood.

Cystic and dysplastic lesions

These conditions are associated with abnormal development of the ductal plate (also called **ductal plate malformations**), and there are similarities between the different conditions and considerable cross-over pathologically.

Congenital hepatic fibrosis

This is an uncommon condition which is associated with polycystic renal disease (Chapter 21). A prehepatic form of **portal hypertension** may develop.

This disease is **autosomal recessive** or **sporadic**. Patients usually present in childhood, but may not present until adulthood. Histologically there are broad fibrous bands containing dilated abnormally shaped bile ducts. The liver may appear nodular, but is not cirrhotic, and there is good preservation of hepatocyte function (Fig. 19.39).

Caroli's disease

This is **non-familial** and has a male/female ratio of 3:1. Patients present as children or young adults with **cholangitis/septicaemia**. Pathologically there are dilatations of the intrahepatic ducts, with infection of the bile

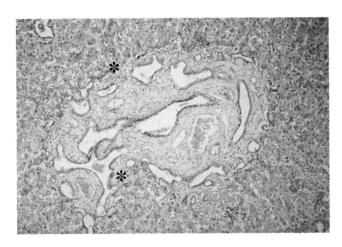

Fig. 19.39 Liver biopsy. Congenital hepatic fibrosis. Note the von Meyenburg complexes (✳).

and possible stone formation. It is often seen in association with congenital hepatic fibrosis. Cholangitis tends to be recurrent, and the prognosis is not very good.

Von Meyenburg complexes

These are microhamartomas consisting of fibrous nodules containing a cluster of abnormal bile ducts, and may be multiple (Fig. 19.40). They are usually **incidental** findings, and may be mistaken macroscopically for metastatic disease at laparotomy.

Polycystic liver disease

This may be **infantile** (autosomal recessive) or **adult** (autosomal dominant). In the infantile form, irregular biliary channels are seen but only rarely large cysts. Prognosis depends on the extent of the associated renal cystic disease.

In the adult form there are large cysts (see Fig. 19.40). There are associations with cystic disease in the kidneys, pancreas, spleen, ovaries and lungs. If patients present in life, they are usually in their 30s or 40s and have symptoms either relating to their enlarged liver or associated renal cystic disease. Haemorrhage may occur into a cyst (with pain), which may be treated by deroofing. Severe involvement may rarely necessitate transplantation.

Choledochal cysts

These are cysts of the common bile duct presenting in both children and adults (M/F = 1:4). Patients have pain and intermittent jaundice. Treatment is by excision.

Large bile duct obstruction

This condition consists of mechanical obstruction to

the large ducts (common bile duct or hepatic ducts) outside the liver or at the porta hepatis. A similar histological picture can be seen in obstruction of the larger intrahepatic ducts.

Aetiology. It may be due to obstruction within the lumen, within the wall or from outside.
- Within the lumen: gallstones (most common cause of obstruction).
- Within the wall: atresia, choledochal cysts; benign strictures (97% are post-biliary surgery, usually cholecystectomy); cholangiocarcinoma, ampullary adenocarcinoma.
- Outside duct: nodes at porta hepatis, carcinoma of head of pancreas.

Clinical features. There will usually be **jaundice**, which may be acute in onset (e.g. due to gallstone lodging in the common bile duct) or more insidious (benign and malignant duct strictures). If there is an acute obstruction, it will usually be accompanied by pain. Any case may be associated with fever and rigors (i.e. associated ascending cholangitis).

Macroscopic appearances of the liver. The liver will be **green** (bile-stained) and swollen. On sectioning, dilated intrahepatic ducts may be seen, which will contain bile and possible biliary sludge/small calculi. Secondary infection would result in pus and abscess formation. If more chronic, fibrous septa and nodularity may be seen.

Microscopic appearances on liver biopsy. **Cholestasis** will be seen as bile plugs within canaliculi and bile within hepatocytes in the centrilobular area. These hepatocytes might become swollen and undergo feathery degeneration. Larger areas of degeneration and necrosis that occur

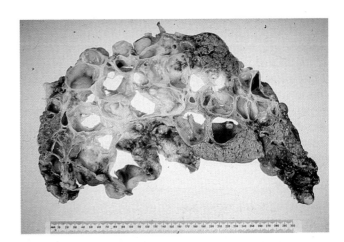

Fig. 19.40 Liver. Adult polycystic liver disease.

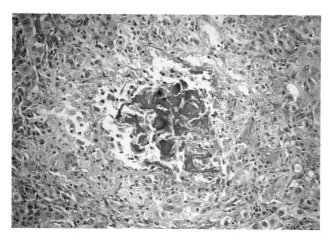

Fig. 19.41 Liver biopsy. 'Bile infarct' in cholestasis due to large duct obstruction. Note the brown-staining bile. (H&E.)

in some patients are called **bile infarcts** (Fig. 19.41). The portal tracts enlarge with oedema, show bile duct proliferation and an **inflammatory infiltrate** composed mainly of neutrophils is seen closely associated with the biliary epithelium, to such an extent that the inflammatory cells may infiltrate between the epithelial cells and be seen within the lumen.

If the obstruction is unrelieved, portal fibrosis occurs with **periductal sclerosis** indistinguishable from that seen in primary **sclerosing cholangitis**. The portal tracts become expanded, fibrous spurs form with bridging fibrosis and ultimately **secondary biliary cirrhosis** will ensue. This may have a characteristic jigsaw appearance, with irregular-shaped nodules fitted close together.

Course. Obstruction may be intermittent and, if due to calculus, the stone may be passed. Treatment will depend on the cause, but ERCP may allow a stone to be extracted, a sphincterotomy to be performed and a stent to be inserted. Laparotomy may be required to perform a resection and reconstitute the bile excretory pathway.

Secondary biliary cirrhosis

If unrelieved, secondary biliary cirrhosis will develop. The time course varies with the aetiology, possibly relating to the nature (i.e. constant or intermittent) or completeness of the obstruction. One study has shown the mean time for onset of cirrhosis to be 7.1 years for benign common duct stricture, 4.6 years for common bile duct calculi, 0.8 years for malignant obstructions.

Primary sclerosing cholangitis

PSC is a disease characterized by **inflammation** and

fibrosis resulting in irregular stricturing of both **intra-** and **extrahepatic** bile ducts which progresses ultimately to **biliary cirrhosis**.

Epidemiology

It is less common than PBC (see below). PSC presents mainly in patients from age 20 to 50 years, and is seen more commonly in males than females (M/F = 2–3:1). Some 50–70% of patients also have **ulcerative colitis** (UC), and some studies give even higher percentages. UC may develop in these patients either before or after the diagnosis of PSC is made. There is also some association with **Crohn's disease**, and a few other rare associations.

There is an association with HLA B8 DR3 (as in UC). Despite various observations as to genetic factors and immunological abnormalities, it is not classically an autoimmune disease, and the association with UC is not understood. It is assumed that there is some common factor in the two diseases, not that one causes the other.

Clinical presentation

Patients present with non-specific symptoms, **pruritus** and **intermittent jaundice**. Increased screening of patients with UC by biochemical methods is resulting in more diagnoses being made in patients with a **raised alkaline phosphatase** but no other symptoms or signs of liver disease.

Investigations

Biochemical investigations show **cholestatic changes** such as raised alkaline phosphatase (and GGT). However there is no rise in IgM, and antimitochondrial antibodies are not present. A low titre of antinuclear antibodies may be found in up to one-third of patients. A positive polymorph binding test is characteristic of PSC.

ERCP (together with **biopsy**) is probably the **main diagnostic test**. It shows irregular strictures and **beading** of both intra- and extrahepatic ducts, with either normal or dilated ducts between these areas. A 'pruned tree' appearance may be seen in later stages.

Liver biopsy appearances

Most of the histological changes are similar to those of secondary sclerosing cholangitis, so causes of the latter have to be excluded clinically before a confident diagnosis is made.

There is **portal fibrosis** with a characteristic 'onion skin' arrangement of fibres around bile ducts (**periductal sclerosis**; Fig. 19.42). Inflammation is usually less marked than in PBC, but focal chronic and mixed inflammatory infiltrates may be seen. **Disappearance of ducts** may be found, with small hyalinized scars representing the origi-

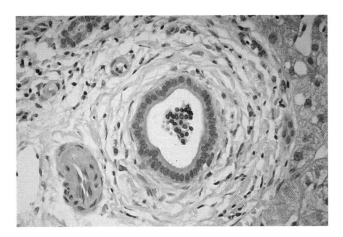

Fig. 19.42 Liver biopsy. Primary sclerosing cholangitis (PSC). Note the dilated bile ductule surrounded by fibrosis. (H&E.)

nal site. Copper-binding protein is usually found in the periportal hepatocytes (Fig. 19.8).

PSC progresses in a rather similar and focal manner as PBC. It may also be staged as for PBC:

- stage 1, portal lesion;
- stage 2, periportal hepatitis with piecemeal necrosis;
- stage 3, fibrous scarring and septum formation;
- stage 4, cirrhosis.

Dysplasia of bile ducts indicating development of cholangiocarcinoma should be sought on biopsy.

Course

PSC is a progressive disease, with the mean time from diagnosis to death being approximately 7 years, although some studies show rather better survivals. There is no specific treatment, although there are ongoing drug trials. Death is usually associated with **cholangitis**, consequences of **portal hypertension** or the development of cholangiocarcinoma. It is the third most common indication for transplantation, with good results (57% 5-year survival).

Primary biliary cirrhosis

PBC is a **progressive** disease, culminating ultimately in **cirrhosis**, characterized by inflammatory destruction of intrahepatic bile ducts.

Epidemiology

In the UK, the incidence of PBC is 5–10/million per year, with a prevalence of approximately 50/million population. It is seen from 30 to 70 years, with a peak in those between 40 and 60 years. There is a distinct **female** preponderance, with a F/M ratio of 10–15:1. Although seen in all races, there are more cases in the west than in Africa and India.

The **aetiology** is **unknown**, but it is assumed to be an **autoimmune** disease. Evidence for this includes **family clustering**, association with other autoimmune diseases and the observation of cytotoxic T-cell destruction of ducts. Environmental factors may also be involved (possibly a triggering infective agent), as suggested by geographical clustering. There is no apparent HLA association.

Clinical presentation

Patients usually present with intense **pruritus**, but **jaundice** is a feature of later stages of the disease. There may also be **increased skin pigmentation** and **hepatosplenomegaly**. Increasingly patients are being diagnosed at a presymptomatic stage due to increased biochemical screening.

Investigations

Biochemistry shows a **cholestatic picture** with a markedly raised alkaline phosphatase and associated raised GGT. Transaminases may be marginally raised. Bilirubin is not usually increased at presentation. Serum cholesterol may be raised, albumin is normal, serum globulins are marginally raised.

One of the most important diagnostic tests is finding **antimitochondrial antibodies (AMA)**. These are present in from 95 to 100% of patients with PBC, this figure depending on the antibody test used and the clinician's definition of the disease (i.e. some say that if AMA is not present then the patient does not have PBC). These antibodies may also be found in up to 30% of patients with autoimmune CAH. However there are nine different mitochondrial antigens identified, and anti-M2 and M8 are probably specific for PBC. Anti-M9 may be seen in early PBC.

Liver biopsy appearances

This is useful for diagnosis and also staging of the disease. It is a disease centred on the portal tracts, in particular on the **bile ducts**. The disease progresses through a number of different stages, ultimately resulting in **true cirrhosis**. This rate of progression is very variable between individual patients.

In **stage 1** disease (Fig. 19.43) there is focal chronic inflammation in the portal tracts, usually centred on the bile ducts. These may show focal damage, and in fact progressive damage and loss of bile ducts is a hallmark of the disease. **Granulomas** may also be seen.

In **stage 2** disease the inflammation extends into liver tissue surrounding the portal tracts and there is **piecemeal necrosis**.

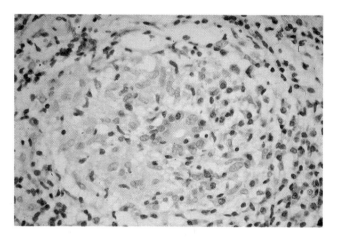

Fig. 19.43 Liver biopsy. Stage I primary biliary cirrhosis (PBC). Note the granulomas surrounding the central bile duct. (H&E.)

In **stage 3** disease there is fibrous scarring with formation of **fibrous septa** between adjacent portal tracts.

Stage 4 disease is the development of **cirrhosis**.

PBC is a rather focal disease, and even within a small-needle biopsy there may be variation in stage from one end of a biopsy to the other. Patients may have features of portal hypertension before cirrhosis is evident on biopsy. However, staging by biopsy is a useful procedure.

Course

Progression is very variable and hence difficult to predict in an individual patient. Some patients do not appear to progress for years. Patients diagnosed at a presymptomatic stage will usually survive at least 10 years, and may have a normal life expectancy. In those with symptomatic disease and jaundice mean survival is about 7 years.

Therapy includes treatment for relief of itching and steatorrhoea, and parenteral vitamin supplementation. Various drugs are being tried, including urodeoxycholic acid, but none have as yet been shown to affect progression. Patients with PBC are one of the main groups undergoing transplantation, and results are relatively good with 70% 1-year survival.

Cholangiocarcinoma

Cholangiocarcinoma may arise from the biliary epithelium anywhere in the biliary tree, i.e. from the common bile duct to the smallest intrahepatic ducts.

Epidemiology

It represents 7–10% of all **liver carcinomas** in the UK (20% in South-east Asia). It arises in patients in their 60s, and slightly more **males** than females are affected.

Aetiology

There are various associations. The most important in the west is with primary sclerosing cholangitis and UC. Developmental anomalies of the biliary tree may be complicated by cholangiocarcinoma. In South-east Asia the disease is associated with **liver fluke infestation** (*Clonorchis sinensis* and *Opisthorchis viverrini*). Various chemicals have also been implicated, including **thorotrast** and carcinogens in the rubber and car industries.

Clinical presentation

These patients usually present with **jaundice** and **pruritus**. There may be epigastric pain in 50%, and weight loss. There are three main clinical groupings depending on the site of the tumour:

- **Intrahepatic tumours** are the most common, are usually solitary, and affect the right lobe more than the left. Patients present with fever, malaise and pain, with jaundice in one-third.
- **Hilar tumours (Klatskin's tumour)** represent 30% of cholangiocarcinomas, and arise from the bifurcation of the main hepatic ducts. It may mimic primary biliary cirrhosis clinically. Patients present with **obstructive jaundice** and may develop secondary biliary cirrhosis.
- **Extrahepatic tumours** present with painless jaundice, pruritus and distension of the gallbladder.

Investigations

Biochemistry will show an **obstructive picture**. AFP is not raised. Imaging techniques may show dilated bile ducts but the tumour itself is often difficult to visualize. The best method of localization is endoscopic retrograde percutaneous cholangiography (ERPC).

Macroscopic appearances

The tumours are white in colour and appear tough and scirrhous.

Microscopic appearances

It is an **adenocarcinoma** composed of mucin-secreting glands lined by cuboidal or columnar epithelium set within a dense fibrous stroma (Fig. 19.44). This stroma is a characteristic feature, and helps to differentiate it from HCC (also HCC also does not secrete mucin). There may be evidence on biopsy of dysplasia of ducts which are not frankly malignant, which can be helpful in differentiating the tumour from metastatic adenocarcinoma.

Course

The tumour is **slow-growing** and metastasizes late, and the prognosis is possibly slightly better than HCC. Although most patients die within 6 months, some may survive up to 5 years. Surgical resection is possible

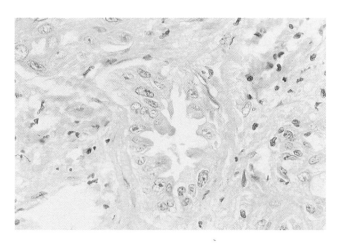

Fig. 19.44 Liver biopsy. Cholangiocarcinoma. The tumour cells are seen to form glands in this case. (H&E.)

in 20%, and bypass operations or stenting may be performed.

DISEASES OF THE GALLBLADDER

Developmental abnormalities

These include **duplication**, **agenesis**, **ectopia** (including intrahepatic gallbladders) and formation of septa. These are generally rare, but may be of significance due to predisposition to stone formation and to torsion (if there is a long mesenteric attachment) and may also be of significance at surgery.

Cholelithiasis (gallstones)

Prevalence
They are very common in the west, with a prevalence of between 10 and 20%. They are much less common in Third World countries, presumably due to dietary factors, with a 4% prevalence.

Age
They are more common with increasing age, with most patients presenting in their 50s or 60s, but teenagers may present with symptoms from gallstones.

Sex
They are more common in females, with a F:M ratio of 3:1.

Types of gallstone

Gallstones consist of **cholesterol**, **pigment** (calcium bilirubinate) and **calcium carbonate**. In the west, 10% are pure cholesterol, 10% are pigment, and 80% are mixed stones (50–70% cholesterol + pigment). In other areas (especially the Far East) there is a higher proportion of pigment stones. The different types may be seen together in the same gallbladder.

Cholesterol stones (Fig. 19.45) are usually solitary, cream/yellow in colour, have a rough surface, and may be up to 5 cm diameter. **Pigment stones** are smaller and multiple, being either black, sharp and brittle or brown and softer (Fig. 19.46). **Mixed stones** are of variable size from tiny pieces of grit to larger stones a couple of centimetres in diameter. They are yellow/brown in colour, often smooth and multifaceted, and usually multiple (sometimes thousands of stones in one gallbladder; Fig. 19.47). These stones may be so fine and so numerous as to form a 'sludge' within the gallbladder (Fig. 19.48).

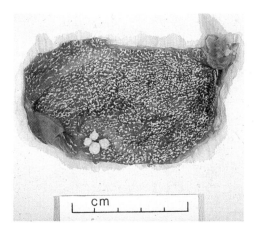

Fig. 19.45 Gallbladder. Cholesterol stones are yellow in colour. Note the cholesterolosis of the gallbladder mucosa ('strawberry gallbladder').

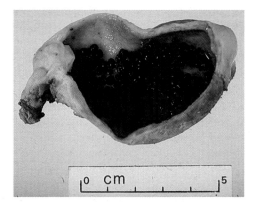

Fig. 19.46 Gallbladder. Pigment stones. These are small and dark in colour.

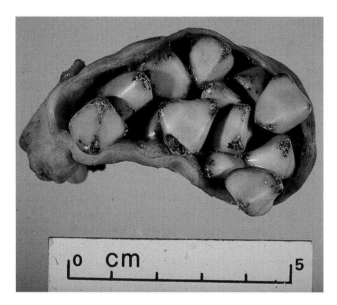

Fig. 19.47 Gallbladder. Mixed stones. Many of these are large and faceted.

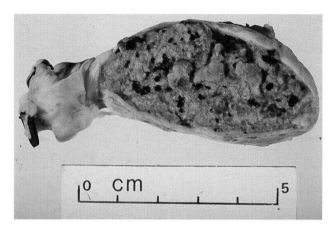

Fig. 19.48 Gallbladder. Biliary sludge.

Aetiology/pathogenesis

The three main factors resulting in gallstone formation are **abnormal bile composition**, **bile stasis** and **infection** (more common in stasis).

Once the bile has become saturated with the various components of the calculi, nucleation around a particle may occur (usually any old particle, but may be a small aggregate of cholesterol crystals), and the calculi then grow by continuing precipitation on to this core.

There are a number of specific risk factors for the formation of stones.

Cholesterol (and mixed) stones are more common in **women** (due to oestrogen effect), and there are also some racial influences (not only those tied in with diet). **Obesity** and high-calorie diets predispose to stone formation,

as does **ileal disease** (related to decreased reabsorption of bile acids leading to alteration of bile composition).

Pigment stones are more common in the **Far East**. There appear to be some racial factors (e.g. high incidence in Japan). They are seen in patients with haemolytic anaemias, haemolysis due to malarial infection, and in other parasitic infestations and infections. **Cirrhosis** also predisposes to the formation of pigment stones.

Clinical presentation

This depends on the associated syndrome:

'Silent' stones. These are commonly discovered in the course of another investigation. They have a low chance of becoming symptomatic, but there is controversy as to how to manage the patients, especially with such low morbidity/mortality procedures as laparoscopic cholecystectomy when weighed against the problems of emergency surgery in elderly patients.

Biliary colic. This is due to short-term obstruction of cystic or bile duct leading to severe right subcostal pain with vomiting.

Acute cholecystitis. If the stone continues to cause obstruction, a chemical cholecystitis ensues. If the pain persists, fever and toxaemia ensue.

Chronic cholecystitis. This is associated with recurrent bouts of pain.

Obstructive jaundice with or without ascending infection. Biliary colic with obstructive jaundice may be associated with rigor, high intermittent fever and severe toxaemia.

Sequelae of gallstones

See Table 19.25.

Table 19.25 Sequelae of gallstones.

Acute or chronic cholecystitis
Biliary obstruction
Ascending infection (cholangitis) ± hepatic abscesses
Mucocoele or empyema
Common hepatic/bile duct stricture, fistula formation, gallstone ileus
Acute pancreatitis (stone lodged at ampulla resulting in bile reflux along pancreatic duct)
Carcinoma of the gallbladder

Treatment of gallstones

See Table 19.26.

Table 19.26 Treatment of gallstones.

Cholecystectomy—usually laparoscopic now, but also at laparotomy
Medical dissolution—chenodeoxycholic acid, ursodeoxycholic acid (often long-term therapy)
Solvent dissolution—catheterize gallbladder and instil methyltenbutyl ether
Shock-wave therapy
Common duct stones may be removed by sphincterotomy, Dormia basket removal (± prior mechanical crushing)

Cholecystitis

Acute cholecystitis

Aetiology. A total of 96% of cases of acute cholecystitis are associated with **outflow** (cystic duct) **obstruction** by gallstones.

Presentation. Usually obese, middle-aged females are involved. Patients present with more **constant pain** than that seen in biliary colic and there is often associated **nausea**. On examination the patients are ill, with **fever**, shallow respirations and **abdominal tenderness**.

Investigations. Leucocytosis (10 000 white blood cells/mm³) is present. Ultrasound or CT may show gallstones and a thickened gallbladder wall.

Pathology. The gallbladder is enlarged with a congested/haemorrhagic wall which is usually markedly thickened. The gallbladder may contain pus and blood (and the offending gallstones), and the mucosal surface appears haemorrhagic. Histologically there is haemorrhage into the mucosa, neutrophil infiltration and ulceration.

Treatment. Fifty per cent of cases will resolve with conservative (medical) therapy, consisting of bedrest, intravenous fluids, pain relief (pethidine and Buscopan) and antibiotics. However early surgery has its advocates, due to the low mortality of the procedure (0.5% if in first 3 days from presentation) when compared with the problems encountered with later interventions.

Sequelae. These include empyema, cholangitis, necrosis and perforation and chronic cholecystitis.

Chronic cholecystitis

Aetiology. Virtually all cases are associated with **gallstones**. There may be previous attacks of acute cholecystitis, or more commonly it develops insidiously.

Presentation. Symptoms are often ill-defined, hence making diagnosis difficult. Epigastric discomfort, pain, nausea and abdominal distension are present.

Investigations. Gallstones will usually be demonstrated by imaging.

Pathology. The gallbladder will usually contain calculi. Otherwise there may be surprisingly little on macroscopic and microscopic examination. There may be **cholesterolosis ('strawberry gallbladder')** in association with the gallstones (yellow flecks on the mucosal surface which histologically consist of collections of foamy macrophages in the lamina propria). The gallbladder wall may be thickened. Histologically there may be chronic inflammation through all layers of the wall of variable degree, usually associated with at least some fibrosis. A number of other conditions or types of chronic cholecystitis may be seen (Table 19.27).

Treatment. Surgery is indicated if the patient is repeatedly symptomatic. Medical measures to attempt to remove stones may be tried.

Complications. These include choledocholithiasis (stones in common bile duct), pancreatitis, fistula and gallbladder carcinoma.

Carcinoma of the gallbladder

Epidemiology

Gallbladder carcinoma is the fourth commonest gastrointestinal cancer (large bowel > stomach > pancreas >

Table 19.27 Types of chronic cholecystitis.

	Histology
Cholegranulomatous reaction	Cholesterol clefts, multinucleate giant cells, pigment-containing macrophages
Ceroid granuloma	Ceroid-containing macrophages
Xanthogranulomatous cholecystitis	Numerous foamy macrophages
Follicular cholecystitis	Lymphoid follicles (± reactive centres) within the mucosa
Eosinophilic cholecystitis	A relatively pure infiltrate of eosinophils in the gallbladder wall
Porcelain gallbladder	Fibrosis with calcification

gallbladder). There are 2.5 cases/100 000 population per year with an average age at presentation of 65 years and a female:male ratio of 3:1. **Gallstones** and **chronic cholecystitis** frequently coexist/predispose.

Presentation

This is usually **late** and most are inoperable by time of presentation. Patients have **pain**, nausea, vomiting, weight loss and **jaundice**.

Macroscopic appearances

Most involve large portions of the gallbladder, and 90% have spread into the liver and surrounding tissues. The tumour may diffusely infiltrate the wall, or be polypoid (Fig. 19.49).

Microscopic appearances

Most (>80%) are **adenocarcinomas**, with a small percentage of squamous carcinomas and anaplastic carcinomas. They show malignant glands of variable differentiation,

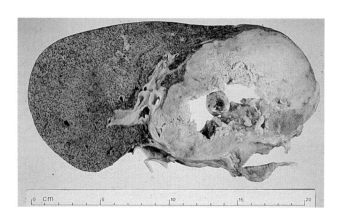

Fig. 19.49 Gallbladder. Gallbladder carcinoma (right) with invasion into the liver.

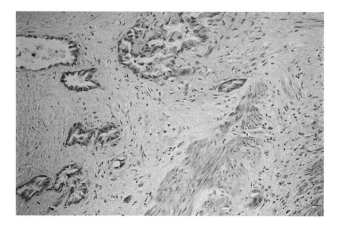

Fig. 19.50 Gallbladder histology. Gallbladder carcinoma is seen (left) invading muscle of the gallbladder wall (right).

and there is usually a markedly sclerotic background. They may show mucinous areas or papillary formations (Fig. 19.50).

Prognosis

The prognosis is **appalling** with only 4.5-month mean survival from diagnosis. There is a 5% 5-year survival, the survivors usually being patients with incidental tumours discovered at cholecystectomy.

The exocrine pancreas

INTRODUCTION

The pancreas develops from two outgrowths of the foregut, a ventral and dorsal bud, which fuse after rotation of the gut. Each bud includes **endocrine** and **exocrine** components, all developing from a single stem cell which first forms the ducts which in turn form outpushings that produce the acini and islets. Many developmental abnormalities of the pancreas (Table 19.28) can be explained from a knowledge of these processes and, inevitably, within all examples both exocrine and the endocrine components occur. All of these abnormalities are uncommon but some are now easily demonstrated with sophisticated invasive and non-invasive imaging techniques.

In this chapter, the **exocrine** components will be discussed. The **endocrine** pancreas and the pathology of diabetes mellitus are discussed in Chapter 14.

The pancreas, lying behind the stomach, liver and transverse colon, is inaccessible to direct clinical examination and can only be palpated if gross changes are

Table 19.28 Congenital abnormalities of the pancreas.

Agenesis and hypoplasia	Varying degrees; potentially life-threatening
Duct abnormalities	Many variations
Pancreas divisum	Failure of the two embryological buds to fuse; 25% incidence in idiopathic pancreatitis
Choledochal cyst	Associated with abnormal junction of pancreatic and common bile ducts
Annular pancreas	Encircling duodenum and intimately attached to the wall
Heterotopic pancreas	70% in upper gastrointestinal tract; 6% in Meckel's diverticulum
Cysts	Solitary and multiple with or without cysts in other organs, e.g. kidney, liver, lung and brain
Nesidioblastosis	Budding of islet cells into acinar cells with functional abnormalities

present and the patient is thin. Ancillary approaches include:

- direct **sampling** of the **pancreatic juices** with cannulation of the ampulla of Vater;
- **imaging** procedures which are aided by the extensive blood supply from the coeliac axis and superior mesenteric artery and their extensive intrapancreatic anastomoses;
- **fine-needle aspiration**.

Biopsy of the pancreas, involving a laparotomy, is **avoided** if possible because of the high incidence of subsequent fistula, haemorrhage and pancreatitis, but monitoring blood hormone levels provides an invaluable method of observing endocrine abnormalities.

CONGENITAL PANCREATIC DISEASE

The most important congenital process to affect the pancreas is **cystic fibrosis (CF)**.

Cystic fibrosis

Cystic fibrosis is an **autosomally recessively** inherited multisystem disease that affects approximately 1:2500 infants. It is due to a defect in the gene that codes for the CF transmembrane conductance regulator (CFTR), a cyclic adenosine monophosphate-regulated membrane protein whose main demonstrated function is to act as a chloride channel across epithelium.

It is recognized, that whilst normal chloride transport does seem important for normal secretion in some tissues, e.g. the pancreatic duct, in other sites there is evidence for an associated or additional defect in sodium reabsorption. Thus, in addition to defective chloride transport, airway epithelia may have increased capacity for sodium resorption leading to drying of the surface.

Genetics

The gene that codes for CFTR is present on **chromosome 7**, and a large number of different gene defects have been identified. The commonest in the UK is δF-508, present in some 75–80% of cases (δ = deletion; F = phenylalanine; 508 = position 508). Of note, whilst two abnormal genes need to be inherited–the abnormal genes do not have to be identical to produce CF. Further, it is possible that the different genetic defects may account for the wide clinical spectrum of CF encountered.

Clinicopathology of cystic fibrosis (Fig. 19.51)

Gastrointestinal tract. As noted above, CF is a **multisystem disorder** and presentation may depend on which organ or system is most affected but symptoms attributable to gastrointestinal dysfunction are the most common. In 10–15% of neonates, inspissated secretions in the small bowel cause a **meconium ileus** and present with delayed passage of meconium and signs of obstruction. **Volvulus** and **perforation** are additional potential complications at this stage. Later, **steatorrhoea** due to defective pancreatic enzyme and bicarbonate secretion is a feature in 80–90% of children. Other less common presentations include vomiting, appendicitis, intussusception, pancreatitis and rectal prolapse.

Histologically, the small bowel may show crypts distended by inspissated mucus. Similar features are seen in the appendix. The pancreas will show abnormalities in almost all cases, many of which are present before birth. Ducts and acini contain eosinophilic concretions and there is also morphometric evidence that there is an early increase in connective tissue relative to exocrine glands. Progressive fibrosis with relatively little chronic inflammation but increasing pancreatic insufficiently proceeds postnatally. Almost all changes can be attributed to duct obstruction from thickened secretions.

Respiratory system. Respiratory complications often dominate the clinical course and may be the major cause of serious morbidity and mortality in the CF patient and, ultimately, determine the outcome. The tenacious mucus predisposes to chest infection, particularly with *Pseudomonas aeruginosa,* or, following the repeated use of antibiotics, fungal infection such as **aspergillosis**. Recurrent infection may eventually lead to damage of bronchial walls and **bronchiectasis**.

Liver and biliary tract. The occurrence of liver disease in association with CF is extremely variable with only a relatively small proportion of patients presenting with early and severe disease. Whilst this may be more frequent in some CF haplotypes than others, no clear reason for this degree of variability is apparent.

The main site of damage appears to be in the **biliary epithelium** and, as elsewhere, is presumably due to the presence of abnormal chloride channels; it should be stressed, however, that to date there are little available data on the mechanism of bile epithelial damage in CF.

Pathologically, portal tracts are expanded with fibrous tissue and proliferating bile ducts are occluded by inspissated secretion. In general, hepatocytes appear relatively well-preserved. In some cases, evidence of damage to larger bile ducts is also present and this may be associated with **fibrosis** and stricture. **Portal hypertension** associated with splenomegaly, ascites and sometimes variceal haemorrhage are the eventual complications of this disease process.

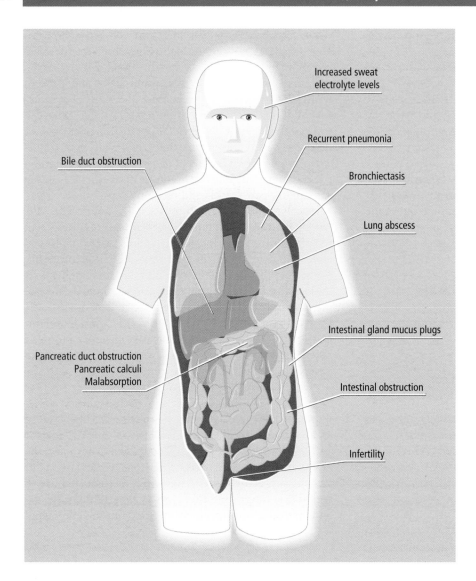

Fig. 19.51 Clinicopathology of cystic fibrosis.

Diagnosis of cystic fibrosis has relied for some years on increases in sweat concentrations of sodium and chloride and, providing adequate sweat is collected after stimulation with pilocarpine and iontophoresis, this is the most reliable diagnostic procedure and is easier and cheaper to perform than any battery of genetic tests which still will not reach the same efficiency. Measurement of serum or blood spot immunoreactive trypsin (IRT) in the first 6 weeks of life has recently been demonstrated to be a reliable diagnostic method at this stage of life when it is important to reach a diagnosis and when the sweat test may be difficult to perform accurately. These procedures can now be supported by DNA analysis for the most common gene defects although genetic analysis is currently unsuitable for screening as it has a lower sensitivity and higher cost than conventional tests.

NORMAL ASPECTS OF THE EXOCRINE PANCREAS

Structure

In the adult the pancreas weighs between 85 and 100 g with a smaller mass in women, and is divisible into head, neck, body and tail, all having a lobular arrangement to the parenchyma.

The greater part of each lobule is exocrine tissue; endocrine tissue forms about 1% of the total pancreatic mass. Acini and their ducts form the exocrine tissue and the ducts drain from the lobules in a herringbone pattern to the main duct. The **main duct** and common bile duct in 80% of pancreases form a common duct draining into the

ampulla of Vater but a wide range of anatomical variations occur. The lobules are separated by loose thin septa in which run the vascular channels feeding and draining the pancreas together with the lymphatics, the latter draining to lymph nodes both entrapped within the pancreas and lying around its borders.

The acini are not arranged in a regular pattern and popular comparisons to a bunch of grapes are hence inappropriate. They are characterized by the **zymogen granules** in the cytoplasm of their cells which are membrane-bound storage sites of inactive pancreatic enzymes. These enzymes are released into the lumen of the acini by exocytosis (emicytosis) and contribute substantially to the 6–20g of **digestive enzymes** the pancreas produces daily.

The duct system transports the enzymes to the lumen of the duodenum and also secretes **bicarbonate** and fluid to a total volume of 2.5 l/24 hours. The role of the nervous system in these processes is incompletely understood, although parasympathetic and sympathetic innervation is recognized and also an interplay between these systems and neuroregulatory peptides.

Hyperplasia and atrophy

The pancreas functionally has an immense **reserve capacity** since not until about 90% is lost does steatorrhoea become evident and about 75% before clinical diabetes develops. This functional reserve, however, is not due to regeneration or **hyperplasia**. Mitoses in the acini and islets are a very rare phenomenon, although commoner in the ducts, and following surgical resections do not become more evident. In keeping with this observation is the decrease in the number of islets that naturally occurs in the first 5 years of life and the absence of sustained hyperplasia or hypertrophy in association with exocrine or endocrine disorders.

In contrast atrophy, functionally and structurally, is seen with pancreatic disorders and as part of others, particularly kwashiorkor.

PANCREATITIS (Table 19.29)

Introduction

Inflammation of the pancreas is the basis of pancreatitis and in the majority of patients this is associated with alcohol (Table 19.29). Biliary calculi and duct obstruction from stenosis, congenital abnormalities and spasm are factors in others while rarer causes include drugs, viruses (mumps) and A1AT deficiency.

Table 19.29 Pancreatitis—aetiological factors and pathways of disease.

Alcohol	Obstruction
Biliary calculi	Increased intraduct pressure
Pancreatic calculi	Ductule disruption
Duct stenosis	Acinar cell injury
Congenital duct abnormalities	Enzyme activation
Pancreas divisum	Autodigestion
	Neutrophil polymorph activation
Sphincter spasm	
Bile reflux	
Duodenal juice reflux	
Drugs (steroids, azathioprine, etc.)	
Viruses (mumps, cytomegalovirus, etc.)	
Hypothermia	
α_1-Antitrypsin deficiency	

Bacterial infection plays no part in initiating the disorder and pancreatic changes in **mucoviscidosis** and **haemochromatosis** are part of these disorders and not examples of pancreatitis. The perceived pathway for the inflammation is **duct disruption**, following obstruction and raised intraluminal pressure, with the release of pancreatic enzymes and consequent autodigestion, a pattern of events individually supported experimentally but unproven clinically. A major difficulty is that, although there is clear-cut epidemiological evidence linking alcohol with pancreatitis, exactly how the effect is produced remains unclear.

Alcohol and pancreatitis

Pancreatitis is commoner in countries and urban areas associated with a high intake of **alcohol** and where many patients have consumed large amounts for 8–10 years. Experimentally, dogs unused to alcohol have an increase in exocrine secretions following exposure and the pancreatic juice includes a high protein content which is matched by hyaline casts within the ducts and potential duct obstruction. Stimulation to secretion, however, is not sustained and once the animal is used to alcohol the effect is lost and even reversed and amongst patients there are a significant number in whom no evidence of chronic alcohol abuse is evident.

The possibility exists that **alcohol** directly **harms the acinar cells** provoking enzyme release but even if this is so excess enzyme release *per se* will not necessarily produce pancreatitis since the enzymes are only activated when they reach the lumen of the duodenum.

Other factors that might come into play are reflux of bile and spasm of the sphincter of Oddi. Bile can alter the permeability of the pancreatic ducts by impairing the integrity of the mucosal barrier and so contribute to pancreatic enzymes entering the pancreatic tissues, but experimentally bile within the pancreatic ducts does not produce pancreatitis and clinically there is also no support for such an event. Reflux of duodenal juices could activate the pancreatic enzymes but this too has not been demonstrated. Spasm of the sphincter of Oddi with functional obstruction to the pancreatic ducts is produced transiently by alcohol and also by disorders such as pancreatic carcinomas which additionally may physically obstruct the pancreas duct system. When obstruction is sustained, pancreatitis can be produced by the oxidative stress induced, a phenomenon possibly involving neutrophil polymorphs and leading to a sequence of events similar to those thought to underlie the adult respiratory distress syndrome.

Obstruction and pancreatitis

Obstruction to the outflow of the pancreatic juices is clearly involved in some examples of pancreatitis such as those arising behind an area of **congenital stenosis**.

Biliary calculi also appear to be involved since there is a high incidence of these calculi in the stools of patients following acute pancreatitis and, further, removal of obstructing calculi relieves pancreatitis. Obstruction from such calculi can only arise if the common bile duct and the pancreatic duct share a common terminus and if the biliary calculus becomes lodged in this region. Clearly, pre-existing stenosis or inflammatory stenosis following previous calculi and spasm in the sphincter may predispose to such an event but in most patients the common pathway following fusion of the common bile duct and the pancreatic duct is probably too short to entrap and produce significant obstruction of the passage of biliary calculi. Also obstruction at this site would probably not lead to either a rise in the intraluminal pressure of the duct system or to reflux of bile into the pancreas. Pressure within the biliary duct system is lower than that in the pancreas and pancreatic juices are more likely to reflux into the biliary system than in the reverse direction. The effect of bile within the pancreas, as already outlined, also may not necessarily be harmful.

Obstruction sufficient to produce pancreatitis must involve the main pancreatic duct before any fusion with the common bile duct and in these circumstances the increase in intraluminal pressure contributes to rupture of smaller ductules and a potential pathway for pancreatic juices into the pancreatic parenchyma. An alternative and additional process is that the effect of the increase in pressure is to impair acinar secretions, provoking breakdown of the zymogen granules, activation of their enzymes and tissue destruction.

Classification

This is a matter of uncertainty and something that is still evolving. The difficulties are that pancreatitis is often extremely difficult to recognize clinically, lacking any precise serum markers, and therefore that biopsies have not been studied of the early phases or in fact even at later stages. Nevertheless, it is appreciated that an **acute state** (Fig. 19.52) and a **chronic state** exist and that some acute attacks arise within chronic pancreatitis and that acute attacks can recur.

The patient with an acute attack of pancreatitis may recover completely from the disorder or die and when death occurs local and systemic complications have intervened.

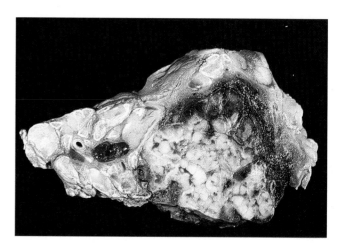

Fig. 19.52 Pancreas. Acute pancreatitis. A transverse section through the body of the pancreas taken at autopsy. The organ is pale and oedematous with large areas of established haemorrhage (black coloured zones) and foci of yellow necrotic tissue.

Chronic pancreatitis gives rise to persistent and progressive functional and structural insufficiency, often developing in a very insidious pattern, so making its clinical recognition difficult. In any pattern of disease there will be some exocrine and endocrine dysfunction but matching histopathological appearances with these clinical variants is inevitably partly conjecture and partly based on autopsy studies of the end-stage disorder (Fig. 19.53).

Histopathology

Acute pancreatitis

This produces appearances that will obviously vary at the stage at which the disorder is encountered, its dura-

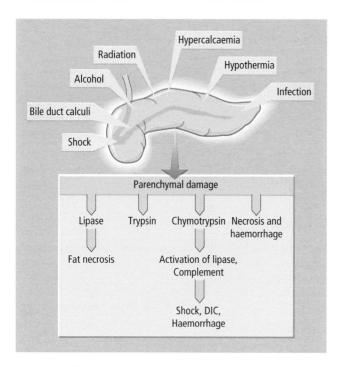

Fig. 19.53 Clinicopathology of acute pancreatitis.

tion and whether it is superimposed upon chronic pancreatitis.

When mild, oedema and inflammation, mainly confined to the interstitial tissues, is the principal change but in more severe examples haemorrhagic necrosis results, both in and around the pancreas. The necrosis may arise from acinar and/or ductular damage with consequent involvement of the vessels and connective tissue, including fat, associated with a marked infiltration of acute and chronic inflammatory cells (see Fig. 19.52). These changes may be focal or lobular but ultimately diffuse and produce swelling of the affected regions with bleeding and necrosis.

Biochemical diagnosis

Acute pancreatitis is usually accompanied by the release into the blood of a variety of enzymes including pancreatic **amylase** and **lipase**. A rise of plasma **amylase** is commonly detectable within 2–12 hours of the onset of acute pancreatitis reaching a peak of often greater than five times the upper limit of normal between 12 and 72 hours, usually returning to normal within 3 to 4 days. Although the magnitude of the rise in plasma amylase activity does not correlate well with the severity of the condition a greater rise will inevitably give a greater probability of acute pancreatitis. Up to 20% of proven cases of acute pancreatitis are normoamylasaemic. Sig-

nificant rises can occur in other abdominal emergencies including severe peptic ulceration, mesenteric infarction and acute biliary tract obstruction (see Table 19.30). Salivary amylase usually contributes little to plasma enzyme activity but may cause very high levels in acute parotitis or following parotid surgery. Recurrent bouts of acute pancreatitis may be reflected in fluctuating plasma levels of amylase activity. Renal excretion of amylase may be impaired in acute oliguric renal disease causing significant rises in plasma amylase activity and similar rises can occur when amylases form a polymer or a complex with immunoglobulin causing macroamylasaemia. This is probably the only situation when estimation of urinary amylase activity is useful although some claim a diagnostic value in this investigation, particularly in the amylase/creatinine clearance ratio. Measurement of amylase activity in ascitic, fistula or drain fluid may be of use in establishing pancreatic disease or the existence of it's complications although interpretation may be difficult.

Table 19.30 Causes of hypermylasaemia and hypermylasuria.

PANCREATIC DISEASE
Pancreatitis
  Acute
  Acute on chronic
  Complications
    Pseudocyst
    Ascites and pleural effusion
    Abscess
Pancreatic trauma
Pancreatic carcinoma

NON-PANCREATIC DISEASE
Renal insufficiency
Bronchogenic or ovarian Ca (usually S-type, up to 50 X ↑)
Salivary gland lesions, e.g. mumps (S-type)
Macroamylasaemia (predominantly S-type)
Biliary tract disease (± secondary pancreatic disease)
Intra-abdominal disease
  Perforated duodenal ulcer
  Intestinal obstruction
  Mesenteric infarction
  Peritonitis
  Acute appendicitis
  Ruptured ectopic pregnancy (S-type)
  Aortic aneurysm with dissection)
Cerebral trauma (uncertain mechanism)
Burns and traumatic shock
Post-operative (~20% of cases—pred S-type)
Diabetic ketoacidosis (very common, cause uncertain)
Acute alcoholism
Opiates
Renal transplantation

Plasma lipase activity rises within 4–8 hours of onset of acute pancreatitis reaching a peak at about 24 hours and remaining elevated for up to 14 days. Measurement of plasma lipase activity is carried out in some centres and the assay is now automatable but recent data suggests that it offers little advantage over amylase.

Diagnosis of **chronic pancreatitis** is more complicated and is often reached from predominantly clinical assessment and radiological evidence of pancreatic calcification. Plasma amylase and lipase activity are usually normal or subnormal except in acute on chronic attacks. Malabsorption will occur in severe cases leading to steatorrhoea and assessment by the semi-quantitation of faecal fat globules may help in the diagnosis. Faecal activity of pancreatic enzymes trypsin and chymotrypsin are now used widely and are relatively easy to perform. Various methods have been devised to assess pancreatic exocrine function either directly by measurement of trypsin, amylase or lipase activity in duodenal fluid following pancreatic stimulation with endogenously administered secretin/CCK-PZ or a meal (in the Lundh test) or indirectly by tests which rely on pancreatic enzyme activity in the duodenum to hydrolyse substrates, the products of which process are then measured over time in the urine. Such substrates include BT-PABA-[^{14}C]-PABA or fluorescein dilaurate. Although they have the advantage of being less invasive than tests requiring jejunal or duodenal fluid sampling, these tests are often considered impractical to perform and thus are rarely used although there has been a recent revival in interest in the fluorescein dilaurate test.

Chronic pancreatitis

This is characterized by progressive fibrosis and consequent loss of exocrine tissue, especially acinar. Ducts may initially survive but are dilated and may even become cystic and contain calculi. The islets, surprisingly, survive as isolated islands within the fibrosis and at any stage small numbers of inflammatory cells, most conspicuously chronic types, may be found (Fig. 19.54).

The regions involved are firm to palpation and shrunken, mimicking carcinoma, and rarely cysts may be recognized within the stroma. If there is main duct obstruction the entire duct system can be dilated, a condition which will resolve if the source of the obstruction is removed.

Complications

Local and systemic complications occur and in acute episodes of pancreatitis these are largely responsible for the high mortality (Table 19.31). The development of the local

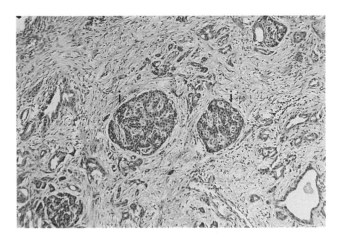

Fig. 19.54 Pancreas histology. Chronic pancreatitis. The islets (i) are the only recognizable structures. Much of the exocrine tissue has been destroyed and that remaining is degenerate and atrophic. Fibrous tissue has replaced the exocrine tissue and includes a diffuse mononuclear cell infiltrate. (H&E.)

Table 19.31 Systemic complications of pancreatitis.

Hypovolaemia	This is contributed to by capillary leakage, transudation and exudation of fluid locally and a decrease in intravascular osmotic pressure from low albumin levels
Hypoalbuminaemia	Protein loss and leakage from the pancreas are the basis
Hypotension	A release of myocardial-depressant factor impairs cardiac responses to fluid loss and also produces a low peripheral resistance
Pulmonary failure	This is analogous to the adult respiratory distress syndrome with lowered surfactant from circulating phospholipidases
Renal failure	A phenomenon involving sepsis, hypotension and circulating immune complexes
Hypocalcaemia	Combining the effects of low calcium levels from the albumin loss, loss of calcium into necrotic fat and lowered parathormone levels

complications can be explained but the systemic changes are less well-understood.

Local

Intrapancreatic abscess. This follows the necrosis seen in acute pancreatitis and colonization by Gram-negative organisms. These abscesses are found in over 50% of patients dying from acute pancreatitis and in these patients they have usually ruptured into the peritoneal cavity and may have eroded adjacent structures such as the transverse colon. They have a high association with the systemic complications.

Cysts and pseudocysts. These differ in that true cysts have an epithelial lining and pseudocysts do not. True cysts develop from dilated components of the duct system but if they become inflamed they may lose their lining, making them indistinguishable from pseudocysts. The origin of pseudocysts is inflammation associated with potentially expansile tissue and bacterial infection, usually precipitated by rupture of small ducts in acute pancreatitis and the coalescence of microcysts in chronic pancreatitis. More than 50% of alcohol-associated pancreatitis patients have pseudocysts and from these local haemorrhage, rupture and fistula formation may result.

Ascites. Ascites is found principally in those patients with alcohol-related disease and mainly men. It is distinguished by the **high amylase** content and related to a leaking pseudocyst.

Pleural effusions. These may occur following tracking of ascitic fluid through the retroperitoneal tissues into the pleural cavity or in response to inflammation beneath the diaphragm.

Diabetes mellitus. This supervenes in **acute** and **chronic pancreatitis**, although the condition should resolve eventually when associated with the acute disorder. Almost 40% of patients with alcohol-related pancreatitis can expect to develop diabetes mellitus, and slightly fewer when alcohol is not involved, with a time scale of 8 and 12 years respectively from the onset of the disorder.

Systemic

These (see Table 19.31) are all interrelated and will adversely affect the course of the pancreatitis as well as one another. Their appearance is hence ominous and related with a high morbidity and a high mortality.

EXOCRINE TUMOURS

Introduction

Exocrine and endocrine tumours occur, although both are uncommon (Fig. 19.55).

Exocrine tumours have shown an increasing incidence which is now levelling off and immunocytochemistry has helped to define the different patterns of endocrine tumours, although not distinguishing between the benign and malignant variants. There is evidence that genetic and environmental features contribute to all of these tumours but no single agent has been identified (Table 19.32).

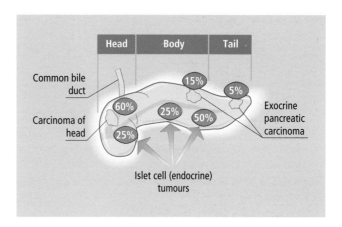

Fig. 19.55 Tumours of the pancreas. Islet cell (endocrine) tumours are commonly adenomas. Twenty per cent of exocrine carcinomas are diffuse.

Table 19.32 Factors involved in pancreatic tumours.

Smoking	Increased risk
Alcohol	May be involved if combined with a high-protein diet and high caffeine intake
Family history	Rarely
Diabetes mellitus	Possibly related but difficult to separate whether this precedes or follows
Pancreatitis	A definite complication of 30% of those with familial pancreatitis
Radiation	Involved with endocrine tumours only

Exocrine tumours of the pancreas

Over 90% of these arise from the **duct epithelium** and most are malignant (Table 19.33). The rare tumours with origin from the acinar cells are uniformly malignant. The life expectancy from diagnosis of the ductular adenocarcinomas is 2–3 months and the 5-year survival 2%. Underlying this abysmal prognosis is the finding at the time of diagnosis of metastatic tumour in lymph nodes in 90% of patients and in the liver in 80%, usually attributed to the insidious and non-specific presentation characterized by **weight loss** with sometimes **obstructive jaundice** and **pain** as later symptoms.

Carcinomas can occur in any part of the pancreas but 60–70% are found in the **head** and most of these alongside the intrapancreatic portion of the common bile duct (Fig. 19.56).

A group of particular interest are the **periampullary carcinomas** (Table 19.34) which are increasingly recognized following the greater sophistication of endoscopy

Table 19.33 Exocrine pancreatic tumours.

Benign
Duct adenoma
Intraduct papilloma
Serous cystadenoma
Solid/cystic tumour

Malignant
Duct adenocarcinoma
Mucinous
Adenosquamous
Giant cell
Acinar cell carcinoma

Potentially malignant
Mucinous cystadenoma
Pancreatic blastoma

Table 19.34 Tumours in the vicinity of the ampulla of Vater.

Ampulla of Vater and duodenal part of the common bile duct
Duodenum surrounding the ampulla of Vater (periampullary)
Mixed ampullary and periampullary
Head of the pancreas involving the ampulla of Vater

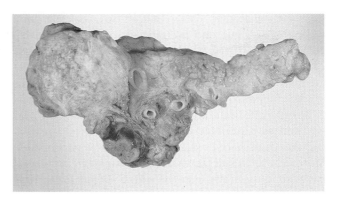

Fig. 19.56 Pancreas. Adenocarcinoma of the head of the pancreas. The pancreas has been sectioned longitudinally and includes a round yellowish tumour replacing the head of the gland.

procedures. All tumours vary in size according to the time of diagnosis but may reach 10 cm in diameter; small tumours in the region of the ampulla of Vater are notoriously difficult to distinguish from benign lesions. Histologically the tumour is an **adenocarcinoma** but variants are recognized which will influence the macroscopic appearances, especially the mucinous type. Most tumours are fairly well-defined, firm-to-hard, grey/white masses. Squamous metaplasia and several patterns of duct cell hyperplasia can precede the tumour but none is invariable or a predictive precursor and no antibodies specific to the tumour cells have been developed.

Spread is potentially to the main **lymph nodes** around and within the pancreas, via local infiltration to surrounding organs including the peritoneum, and haematogenously to distant sites. The pathways differ according to the site of the tumour within the pancreas but the timing of presentation will also influence the extent of the spread. Tumours in the head relative to those in the tail produce symptoms at an early stage and their spread at this time is usually local with only the **portal lymph nodes** affected while tumours in the tail of the pancreas where presentation is late may be widely disseminated by the time of diagnosis.

FURTHER READING

MacSween R.N.M., Anthony P.P. & Scheuer P.J. (1994) *Pathology of the Liver*, 3rd edn. Churchill Livingstone, Edinburgh.

Diseases of Bone and Joint

Bone

NORMAL STRUCTURE AND FUNCTION
(Fig. 20.1)

The main functions of the bony skeleton include:
• structural support;
• protection of internal organs;
• haematopoiesis;
• metabolic (reservoir of calcium).

Like other connective tissues, bone has both cellular and extracellular components. The extracellular component or osteoid is composed predominately of type I collagen together with smaller amounts of other proteins, phosphoproteins, lipids and growth factors. In order

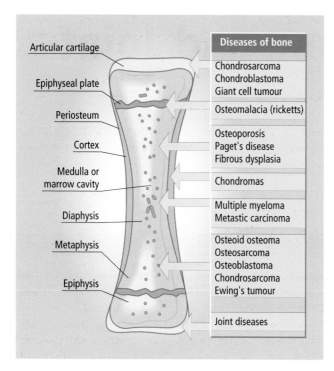

Diseases of bone
Chondrosarcoma Chondroblastoma Giant cell tumour
Osteomalacia (ricketts)
Osteoporosis Paget's disease Fibrous dysplasia
Chondromas
Multiple myeloma Metastic carcinoma
Osteoid osteoma Osteosarcoma Osteoblastoma Chondrosarcoma Ewing's tumour
Joint diseases

Labels: Articular cartilage, Epiphyseal plate, Periosteum, Cortex, Medulla or marrow cavity, Diaphysis, Metaphysis, Epiphysis

Fig. 20.1 The normal structure of the long bone.

to give the necessary rigid structure, this organic matrix is mineralized by deposition of calcium phosphate (hydroxyapatite). The organic and mineral content of bone may be assessed histologically in undercalcified sections using special histochemical stains (Fig. 20.2).

Flat bones, such as those of the skull, develop via **intramembranous ossification** from fibrous tissue. Long bones increase in length at the line of cartilage known as the **epiphyseal** or **growth plate** (Fig. 20.3). The **epiphysis** is the region between the growth plate and the joint; the **diaphysis** is the region between the growth plates and the

metaphysis is the region of bone adjacent to the growth plate on the diaphyseal side.

There are two main types of bone—lamellar bone and woven bone.

Lamellar bone

This is mature bone. The osteoid contains parallel sheets (lamellae) of collagen fibres. There are two types of lamellar bone—compact (e.g. the cortex of long bones) and cancellous (e.g. the medulla of long bones).

In compact bone the lamellae are arranged concentrically around haversian canals which contain blood and lymphatic vessels and nerves (Fig. 20.4). In cancellous bone there is a loose network of trabeculae which lack the organized structure of compact bone.

Woven bone

This is immature bone and is found in situations where there is rapid bone formation, e.g. in fracture callus. A haphazard arrangement of collagen fibres is found within the matrix (Fig. 20.5).

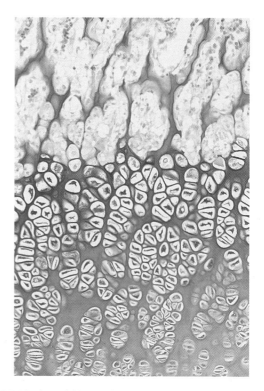

Fig. 20.3 Histology of the normal organized epiphyseal growth plate showing columns of cells in the proliferating zone (top) and the zone of mineralization of chondrocytes (bottom). (H&E.)

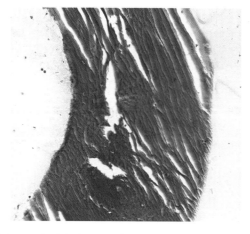

Fig. 20.2 An undecalcified section of normal bone stained with Picro–Mallory which stains mineralized bone blue and non-mineralized osteoid red.

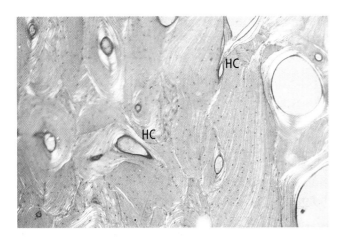

Fig. 20.4 Histology of mature lamellar bone (polarized) showing the Haversian canals (HC).

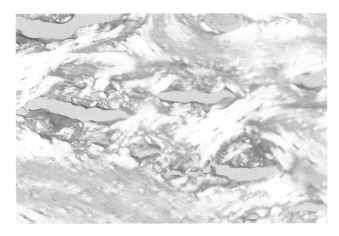

Fig. 20.5 Histology of woven bone (polarized) showing the haphazard arrangement of collagen.

Periosteum

This is a dense layer of connective tissue which surrounds bone and is capable of osteogenesis.

Cell types

There are three main cell types in bone.

Osteoblasts

These are mononuclear cells derived from bone marrow stromal cells (Fig. 20.6). They are found on the surfaces of bone trabeculae, the inner surface of the periosteum and the lining of the haversian canals. Osteoblasts synthesize bone matrix.

Osteocytes

These are osteoblasts that have become trapped within the bone trabeculae and have ceased to synthesize bone matrix.

Osteoclasts

Osteoclasts are often multinucleated and are derived from the mononuclear phagocyte system. Osteoclasts are responsible for bone resorption (see Fig. 20.6).

CONGENITAL DISEASES OF BONE

Achondroplasia is transmitted as an autosomal dominant trait and is characterized by failure of proliferation of cartilage cells in the epiphyseal plate of long bones. The result is shortening of limbs. Membranous ossification is not affected so the axial skeleton, skull and facial bones develop normally. Life expectancy is normal.

Osteogenesis imperfecta (brittle bone disease) has an autosomal pattern of inheritence with variable penetrance. The disease involves defective synthesis of collagen by fibroblasts and osteoid by osteoblasts, leading to bone fragility, hernias, blue sclera and thin skin. Survival into adulthood occurs.

Osteopetrosis (marble bone disease) is very rare with two forms, a mild autosomal dominant form associated with the overdevelopment of cortical bone and a lethal autosomal recessive form.

BONE BIOCHEMISTRY

Bone is constantly being remodelled and reformed in life by teams of bone cells that make up the **bone remodel-**

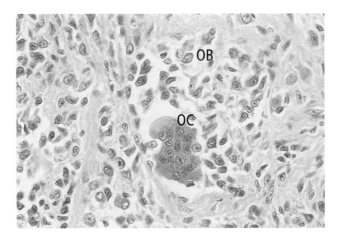

Fig. 20.6 Histology of osteoblast (OB) and osteoclast (OC) giant cells in an area of fracture callus.

ling unit (**BRU**). A specific series of events occurs, beginning with osteoclastic bone resorption followed by osteoblastic synthesis of the organic matrix. This passes through a 10–15-day period of maturation before mineralization of the matrix occurs. Bone remodelling is under the control of hormonal factors, some of which are described in Chapter 14.

Calcium biochemistry

Calcium is the most plentiful cation in the body. Some 98–99% is stored in bone and teeth, with bones forming a large reserve; 1–2% is found in plasma and other extracellular fluid.

Physiological functions of calcium

Intracellular function. Calcium is a prime inorganic messenger for regulation of cell functions in determining activity of enzymes (e.g. adenylate cyclase, phosphodiesterase) through reversible combination with **calmodulin**.

Calmodulin is a small protein (mol wt 16790) that is present in all nucleated cells. It is involved in regulation of:
- fertilization;
- mitosis;
- cell motility;
- ciliary action;

and many other complex functions. Each molecule of calmodulin contains four binding sites for Ca^{2+}.

Striated muscle. In striated muscle, Ca^{2+} activates contraction of the myosin fibril through combination of **troponin** (similar to calmodulin).

Plasma membrane. Secretions of several other endocrine glands are controlled by extracellular Ca^{2+} concentration at the cell surface, most notably;
- parathyroid glands;
- thyroid C cells;
- pancreatic β cells.

Calcium is also involved in cell-to-cell adhesion and possibly communication. It plays a vital role in blood coagulation and is a principal constituent of hydroxyapatite, found in bones and teeth.

Calcium requirements and sources

Calcium requirements depend on age, growth, pregnancy and lactation. Dairy products constitute 70% of dietary Ca^{2+} (in the west). Recommended daily dose is 800 mg/dl for adults and children >1 year of age, plus additional 400 mg/day in adolescence, pregnancy and lactation.

Plasma calcium (normal range: 2.12–2.62 mmol/l)

Forty per cent of plasma calcium is protein-bound and 60% is free (mostly ionized; 10% complex-bound to citrate).

Control of plasma calcium concentration is by:
- parathyroid hormone (PTH);
- calcitonin;
- 1,25-dihydroxycholecalciferol (DHCC).

It occurs in:
- bone;
- kidney;
- gut.

Dietary calcium

The average dietary intake is 25 mmol Ca^{2+}. Normally, 10 mmol (30–35%) is absorbed (mainly under the influence of DHCC); the rest is lost in the faeces. There is a urinary loss of 5 mmol, so the daily net absorption is 5 mmol.

Other factors affecting absorption are:
- gut pH;
- fat absorption;
- Ca/PO_4 ratio;
- phytates;
- oxalates.

Bone

Exchange of calcium between bone and the extracellular fluid is quantitatively much the largest and is regulated by PTH and DHCC via osteoclast activity.

Kidney

Daily 200 mmol of calcium is filtered by the glomeruli and 98% is reabsorbed under the influence of PTH and DHCC.

Phosphate biochemistry

The normal adult contains 20 mol (620 g) of phosphorus, entirely in the form of phosphate. This is equally distributed extracellularly and intracellularly. Intracellularly, phosphate is an integral component of phospholipids and phosphoproteins. A small but very important fraction exists intracellularly as inorganic phosphate, participating in high-energy transfer reactions. Eighty-five per cent of extracellular phosphate is inorganic as hydroxyapatite. In the plasma (serum) most phosphate is inorganic.

Physiological functions of phosphate

Phospholipid is a structural component of cell membranes. Phosphoprotein is found in high-energy nucleotides and nucleic acids.

Sources of phosphate include most foods, especially meat and milk. Phosphate has the same mg/day allowance as for calcium.

Parathyroid hormone

PTH is produced by parathyroid gland. The release of PTH is stimulated by **hypocalcaemia** and also by:

- hypomagnesaemia;
- prostaglandins;
- catecholamines;
- hydroxy vitamin D metabolites.

PTH is an 84 amino acid peptide released from the parathyroid gland with a biologically active NH_2-terminus. Amino terminus fragments from this peptide are generated by Kupffer cells in the liver. The role of parathyroid hormone is to maintain plasma calcium homeostasis and it achieves this by three separate mechanisms: enhancing bone resorption via a direct stimulatory effect on osteoclast activity, enhancing reabsorption of calcium by the glomerular filtrate and indirectly via it's stimulatory effect on renal 1-α hydroxylation of 25 OH vitamin D with subsequent enhancement of gastrointestinal calcium absorption. The effects on these three tissues are not simultaneous with the renal effect being most rapid followed by a biphasic bone response, the first occurring within three hours. The effect on gastrointestinal absorption of calcium occurs over days. Certain tumours, including hypernephromas and squamous cell carcinomas, can produce a peptide with identical biological activity and similar structural identity to PTH which is now known to be responsible for the humoral hyper-calcaemia of often non-metastatic malignancies. This peptide is termed PTH-related peptide (PTHrP) and is not detected by routine PTH assays.

Calcitonin

Calcitonin is produced by the C cells in the thyroid. Its main function is to increase osteoblast activity, thus reducing bone resorption (Table 20.1).

Vitamin D

Vitamin D should be considered as a hormone, its most significant role in calcium homeostasis being to enhance gastrointestinal calcium absorption but it also probably has some effects on enhancement of bone mineralization and on bone resorption (Fig. 20.7).

Table 20.1 New markers for bone disease.

BONE FORMATION
Osteoblasts produce:
- Type 1 collagen
- Alkaline phosphatase
- Osteocalcin
- Osteonectin
- Osteopontin
- Others
Osteocalcin is the most sensitive and reflects bone formation but is difficult to measure and affected by renal excretion

BONE RESORPTION
Collagen degradation products:
- Hydroxyproline (poor marker)
- Products of crosslink maturation (telopeptides)
- Pyridinoline
- Deoxypyridinoline
Pyridinoline is probably the best but poor assay at present

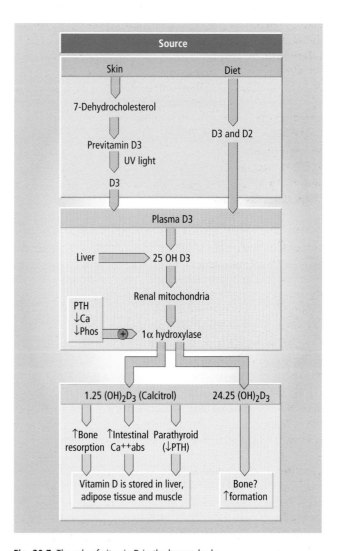

Fig. 20.7 The role of vitamin D in the human body.

Hypercalcaemia

See Tables 20.2 and 20.3.

Table 20.2 Clinical features of hypercalcaemia.

Gut
Abdominal pain
Nausea
Vomiting
Constipation
Weight loss
Anorexia
Polydipsia

Renal
Polyuria
Renal calculi
Renal failure

Depression
Tiredness, weakness
Sudden cardiac arrest
Corneal calcification

Table 20.3 Causes of hypercalcaemia.

Parathyroid disease
Primary or tertiary hyperparathyroidism

Bone disease
  Carcinoma
  Myeloma
  Leukaemias
  Paget's disease

Excess vitamin D intake

Excess calcium intake

Milk alkali syndrome

Familial (rare)

Drug-induced—thiazide diuretics

Others
  Sarcoid
  Thyrotoxicosis
  Adrenal insufficiency
  Phaeochromocytoma
  Haemodialysis
  Hypocalcaemia

Hypocalcaemia (Table 20.4)

Table 20.4 Clinical features of hypocalcaemia.

Tetany
Depression
Perioral paraesthesia
Carpopedal spasm
  Trousseau's sign
Neuromuscular excitability
  Chvostek's sign
With osteomalacia
  Bone pain
  Fractures, especially long bones, scapula
  Proximal myopathy
  (Rickets—deformities)

Causes

Causes of hypocalcaemia include hypoparathyroidism and pseudohypoparathyroidism, drugs (e.g. calcitonin, diuretics, phosphate, biphosphonates), metastatic carcinoma (particularly prostatic) and surgical hypoparathyroidism.

Primary hyperparathyroidism

Incidence

Primary hyperparathyroidism is seen in 42/100000 of the western population with an increased incidence after the age of 50 years. The female/male ratio is 3:1.

It is most commonly diagnosed on a routine biochemical screen. If symptoms are present, they will be those of hypercalcaemia (see above). The bone pathology is that of osteitis fibrosa cystica (see below; Table 20.5).

Table 20.5 Causes of primary hyperparathyroidism.

Single adenoma	83%
Multiple adenoma	4.3%
Carcinoma	1.7%
Hyperplasia	
Clear cell	7.6%
Chief cell	3.6% (associated with MEN type I or II)

MEN, Multiple endocrine neoplasia.

Secondary hyperparathyroidism

Secondary hyperparathyroidism is commonly due to a raised PTH secondary to hypocalcaemia and is seen in chronic renal failure and chronic intestinal malabsorption. Hyperplasia of all four parathyroid glands occurs.

Tertiary hyperparathyroidism

Tertiary hyperparathyroidism is commonly due to an autonomous adenoma of parathyroid as a complication of secondary hyperparathyroidism.

Hypoparathyroidism

There are many causes of hypoparathyroidism (Table 20.6).

Table 20.6 Causes of hypoparathyroidism.

Inadequate secretion of PTH Surgical—following thyroid, parathyroid and radical neck surgery Familial Sporadic DiGeorge syndrome
Suppression of PTH secretion from normal parathyroids Neonatal—from maternal hypercalcaemia Severe magnesium depletion
Defective end-organ response to PTH Pseudohypoparathyroidism types I and II (pseudopseudohypoparathyroidism)

PTH, Parathyroid hormone.

Alkaline phosphatase

Source

Alkaline phosphatase is present in most tissues. The richest sources are:
- osteoblasts in bone;
- bile canaliculi in the liver;
- small intestinal epithelium;
- the placenta;
- proximal tubules in kidney;
- breasts in lactation.

Function

The main function of alkaline phosphatase is in phosphate transport across cell membranes. The maximum activity is at pH 9.0–10.5. In normal adults alkaline phosphatase is mainly derived from liver and bone (Tables 20.7–20.9).

Table 20.7 Causes of a raised alkaline phosphatase.

Bone—only with increased osteoblast activity Paget's disease Rickets/osteomalacia Hyperparathyroidism Carcinoma with osteoblastic metastases
Liver—cholestasis causes increased enzyme production due to increased cell leakage
In carcinoma—a raised alkaline phosphatase is either due to osteoblastic bone metastases or to liver metastases causing cholestasis
Interpretation of a high alkaline phosphatase—look at other LFTs including GGT. If the GGT is raised, the most likely origin is the liver

LFT, Liver function test; GGT, γ-glutamyltransferase.

Table 20.8 Reference interval of alkaline phosphatase in childhood.

Birth	245–490 iu/l
2 weeks	310–740 iu/l
6 months	400–770 iu/l
4 years	380–620 iu/l
10–14 years	410–700 iu/l
Adult	30–300 iu/l

Table 20.9 Summary of calcium, phosphate and alkaline phosphatase biochemistry in different diseases.

	Calcium	Phosphate	Alkaline phosphatase
Osteoporosis	N	N	N
Osteomalacia	↓	↓	↑
Hyperparathyroidism	↑	↓	N or ↑
Hypoparathyroidism	↓	↓	N
Paget's disease	N	N	↑
Myeloma	↑	↑	N

N, Normal.

Treatment of hypercalcaemia

The aim of treatment is to reduce the high serum calcium levels and remove the underlying cause of hypercalcaemia. If severe, emergency treatment is required. Treatment is based on the understanding of the underlying cause and awareness of renal and hydration state. If asymptomatic or non-progressive, treat the underlying cause. If serum calcium is greater tha 3 mmol/l, intravenous rehydration with normal saline is advised.

Treatment of hypocalcaemia

Oral calcium supplements may be of help. In hypoparathyroidism, intravenous calcium gluconate may help in tetany. Vitamin D metabolites may be of value but response to their use must be monitored.

Magnesium

Magnesium (Mg) is the fourth most abundant cation in the body (2nd intracellular). Fifty to sixty per cent is found in bones (one third of which acts as an intracellular reservoir of Mg) and 1% in plasma and ECFs (normal plasma Mg is 0.75–0.95 mmol/l). Seventy to seventy five per cent is ionized, the rest is bound to plasma proteins, mainly albumin. The highest intracellular Mg is found in cells with high metabolic activity.

Physiological roles of Mg
The following are enzyme substrate and direct enzyme activation and membrane properties.
Cellular energy metabolism
- glycolysis;
- oxidative phosphorylation.

Cell replication
- nucleotide metabolism;
- protein biosynthesis.

Cell regulation
- adenylate cyclase;
- phosphoinositol turnover.

Mg metabolism
The kidney is the principal organ of Mg hemeostasis. Filtration and reabsorption occur in the kidney. Twenty to thirty per cent of reabsorption occurs in the proximal tubule (passive—related to blood flow), and 60% occurs in the thick ascending loop of Henlé (by ? active and NaCl-related transport systems). No hormones or factors are involved in the control of renal Mg handling. In the intestine, major sources of Mg are nuts, cereals, green, leafy vegetables and meats. Thirty to fifty per cent of Mg ingested is absorbed, maximum absorption occurs in the ileum and jejunum. There are possible Vitamin D effects of Mg absorption.

Mg deficiency
Mg deficiency is found in around 10% of hospital patients but may occur in over 50% of patients in intensive care. There is an increasing awareness of this condition (Tables 20.10, 20.11 and 20.12).

Table 20.10 Hypomagnesaemia—symptoms and signs.

| NEUROMUSCULAR |
| Mimic hypocalcaemia |
| Positive Chvostek and Trousseau seizures |
| Ataxia |
| Weakness |
| Tremor |
| Depression |
| Psychosis |
| |
| CARDIAC ARRYTHMIAS |
| Atrial tachycardia/fibrill |
| Ventric tachycardia/fibrill |
| Junctional arraythmia |
| Sensitivity to digitalis intox |
| Torsade de pointes |
| ECG changes |
| |
| HYPOCALCAEMIA |
| Impaired PTH secretion |
| Renal and skeletal resistance to PTH |
| Resistance to vitamin D |
| |
| HYPOKALAEMIA |
| Renal K wasting |
| Decreased intracellular K |

METABOLIC BONE DISEASE

Osteoporosis

Osteoporosis is a disease of **decreased bone mass** but with a normal ratio of mineral to organic matrix.

Osteoporosis results from an **imbalance** between **bone production** by osteoblasts and **bone resorption** by osteoclasts. This imbalance is a normal feature of ageing and osteoporosis is seen to some degree in all elderly patients. Accelerated bone loss occurs in women following the menopause. Clinically significant osteoporosis is therefore commoner in this group.

Other causes of generalized osteoporosis include:
- endocrine disease (e.g. Cushing's disease, thyrotoxicosis, hypopituitarism, hypogonadism, hyperparathyroidism, corticosteroid therapy);
- liver disease;
- chronic renal failure;
- immobility.

Table 20.11 Causes of hypomagnesaemia.

GASTROINTESTINAL DISORDERS
Malabsorption
Diarrhoea
Bowel resection
Fistulae

RENAL LOSS
Osmotic diuresis
   glucose
   mannitol
   urea
   hypercalcaemia
Alcohol
Drugs
   diuretics
   aminoglycosides
Metabolic acidosis
Renal diseases
   chronic pyelonephritis
   interstitial nephritis and GN
   ATN (diuretic phase)
   postobstructive nephropathy
   renal tubular acidosis
   post renal transplant

ENDOCRINE AND METABOLIC
Diabetes mellitus
Phosphate depletion
1° hyperparathyroidism
Hypoparathyroidism
1° aldosteronism

Table 20.12 Magnesium excess (hypermagnesaemia).

SYMPTOMS AND SIGNS
Mild (1.1–2.25 mmol/l)
• hypotension
• flushing
• somnolence
Moderate (< 4.0 mmol/l)
• nausea/vomiting
• ECG changes
• mental status changes
Severe (> 4.0 mmol/l)
• decreased respiration
• coma
• cardiac arrest

CAUSES
Excessive intake
• oral antacids
• rectal purgation
• parenteral treatment of low Mg
Renal failure
• chronic—usually with administration of Mg,
  GFR usually < 30 ml/min with antacids etc.
• acute—rhabdomyolysis
Familial hypocalciciuric hypercalcaemia
Lithium ingestion
Endocrine disorders
Others

Localized osteoporosis occurs following imobilization, for example, of a fracture or of painful joints in patients with rheumatoid arthritis. It also occurs in Paget's disease and in areas of infiltration of bone by tumour.

Complications

Deformity and vertebral compression are common, leading to loss of height. Bone pain and fractures occur, particularly of the wrist and hip. These are an important cause of morbidity and mortality in the elderly.

Rickets and osteomalacia

Both conditions feature deficient mineralization of the organic bone matrix; the amount of bone is normal.

Rickets occurs in children and affects both bone and growth cartilage. This leads to characteristic deformities:
• enlargement of epiphyses (swelling of the costochondral junctions is known as rachitic rosary);
• bossing (flattening) of the skull;
• bowing of long bones;
• short stature.

Osteomalacia occurs in adults. It is associated with bowing deformities of the long bones and incomplete pathological fractures (Looser's zones).

Aetiology

Causes include:
• vitamin D deficiency due to:
  (a) inadequate intake;
  (b) malabsorption (commonest cause in adults);
  (c) deficient synthesis (e.g. dark-skinned races living in the UK where there is little sunshine);
• renal disease;
• anticonvulsant therapy–drugs such as phenytoin induce liver enzymes which degrade vitamin D to inactive metabolites.

Histology

Examination of undercalcified sections shows incomplete mineralization of osteoid (Fig. 20.8).

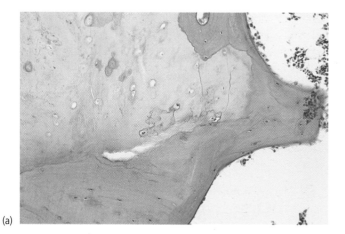

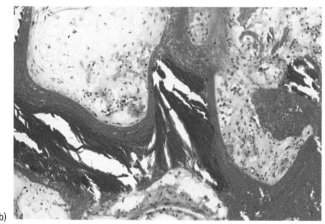

Fig. 20.8 Osteomalacia. (a) Histology shows the incomplete mineralization of bone. (b) Picro-Mallory stain on an undecalcified section of bone shows the areas of unmineralized bone.

Renal osteodystrophy

Patients with renal disease may suffer from any of the following.

1 **Osteomalacia:**
   (a) inadequate production of active vitamin D metabolites because of a decrease in the amount of functional renal tissue;
   (b) hyperphosphataemia may inhibit enzymes responsible for vitamin D metabolism;
   (c) the high levels of aluminium that used to be found in haemodialysis fluid were a possible cause of inhibition of calcification of osteoid;

2 **Hyperparathyroidism:**
   (a) impaired vitamin D metabolism in patients with renal failure results in a low serum calcium. This leads to stimulation of the parathyroid glands and secondary hyperparathyroidism;

3 **Osteoporosis and bone necrosis:**
   (a) may result from treatment with corticosteroids.
   Soft-tissue calcification is also seen in patients with renal failure.

Bone lesions in primary hyperparathyroidism (osteitis fibrosa cystica; brown tumours)

Primary hyperparathyroidism results from an adenoma (or rarely a carcinoma or diffuse hyperplasia) of the parathyroid glands. In primary hyperparathyroidism the serum calcium is raised so other causes of hypercalcaemia (e.g. metastatic bone disease, ectopic production of parathyroid hormone by malignant tumours, sarcoidosis, renal failure) should be excluded before making the diagnosis.

X-ray findings
Subperiosteal erosions are characteristically seen in the small bones of the hands.

Pathology
Generalized changes result from an increase in both osteoblastic and osteoclastic activity. Focal changes may also be seen. These consist of areas where the bone is totally removed and replaced by fibrous connective tissue containing numerous osteoclasts and showing evidence of haemorrhage with deposition of haemosiderin pigment. The latter gives a characteristic brown colour to these lesions, which are sometimes known as **brown tumours** (Fig. 20.9).

Histologically they may be confused with giant cell tumours of bone. It is therefore very important to check the serum calcium, phosphate and alkaline phosphatase

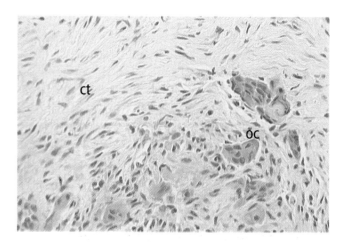

Fig. 20.9 Primary hyperparathyroidism, the brown tumour shows numerous osteoclasts (oc) and connective tissue (ct).

before diagnosing the latter. The radiological and pathological changes of hyperparathyroidism regress following treatment.

Paget's disease of bone (osteitis deformans)

This is a disease of unknown aetiology that affects mature bone and which is characterized by greatly increased osteoclastic and osteoblastic activity (Fig. 20.10).

Clinical presentation
Presentation is usually over 40 years of age. Any bone may be involved but the commonest sites for involvement are the lumbar spine, pelvis, skull, femur and tibia.

Epidemiology
There is a wide geographical variation in incidence. Paget's disease is commonest in northern Europe where between 2 and 3% of the population over 50 years show radiological evidence of the disease. The incidence in men is slightly higher than that in women. It is rare in certain parts of the world, including Asia.

Aetiology
The aetiology is unknown, but a genetic component is likely. Possible slow viral inclusions can be seen on electronmicroscopy, but there is no other evidence for a viral aetiology.

Clinical features
Paget's disease may affect part of one bone, a single bone or many bones. The disease may be asymptomatic. Exacerbations and remissions occur. Disease activity is best assessed by measuring serum alkaline phosphatase and hydroxyproline (and urinary hydroxyproline) which are both increased. Serum calcium and phosphate are usually normal.

Complications
Complications of Paget's disease include:
- fractures;
- degenerative arthritis;
- bone pain;
- neural compression (e.g. leading to deafness or spinal nerve deficits);
- spinal cord compression;
- high-output cardiac failure (because of greatly increased vascularity in affected bones);
- malignant change to a high-grade sarcoma.

Between 2 and 5% of patients develop osteosarcoma, chondrosarcoma or fibrosarcoma.

X-ray findings
- **Early.** Radiolucency without any thickening of the bone.
- **Late.** Combinations of increased density, lytic areas, honeycombed sections and striated appearances in thickened bone.

Pathology
The increase in osteoblastic and osteoclastic activity leads to bone trabeculae of irregular thickness with enlarged haversian canals. Overall the bone becomes thickened but because of its abnormal structure it is weak. Histology shows short bundles of collagenous matrix in a haphazard arrangement separated by cement lines (mosaic pattern; Fig. 20.10(b)). The marrow is replaced by highly vascular fibrous connective tissue.

(a)
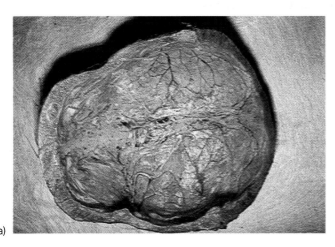

(b)
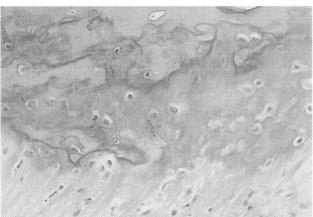

Fig. 20.10 Paget's disease of bone. (a) The skull plate is thickened. (b) Histology shows the haphazard arrangement of collagen and mineralization giving a 'mosaic' pattern. (H&E.)

BONE INFECTIONS

Acute osteomyelitis (Fig. 20.11)

Staphylococcus aureus is the most common cause of osteomyelitis in all age groups. Other organisms causing osteomyelitis relate to the age of the patient, route of infection and underlying clinical condition (Table 20.13). Primary osteomyelitis in the UK is relatively uncommon whereas osteomyelitis secondary to prosthetic joint infections is much commoner.

Clinical features

Acute osteomyelitis usually presents as a hot, painful bony lesion with fever. In the infant this may translate as restricted movement of a limb. Translucency on X-rays representing lytic areas does not become apparent until at least 10 days after the onset of the disease.

Diagnosis and management

Wherever possible the microbiology should be defined by obtaining a bone biopsy as the patient will be committed to long courses of parenteral antibiotics. The exception to this in the infant and child where *Staphylococcus aureus* is the commonest pathogen and specific empiric treatment is started. Shorter courses of antibiotics are also effective in this age group. In general, blood cultures are often positive. For *S. aureus*, flucloxacillin for at least 4 weeks is the recommended treatment. Clindamycin is used as an alterative in penicillin-allergic patients and it acheives good therapeutic levels in bone.

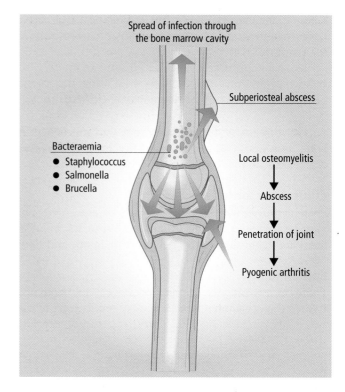

Fig. 20.11 Osteomyelitis of bone.

Chronic osteomyelitis

Chronic osteomyelitis may follow inadequately treated acute disease or follow an indolent infection (e.g. tuberculosis). Tuberculous osteomyelitis is rare in countries where there is good control of pulmonary and gastroin-

Table 20.13 Features of the major types of osteomyelitis.

	Haematogenous spread		Secondary to contagious foci
Age	Infants–children	Adults	Adults–elderly
Common site	Long bones with associated arthritis	Long bones, vertebrae	Long bones, skull and facial bones, feet
Underlying condition	Bacteraemia	Bacteraemia	Trauma, surgical procedures, soft-tissue infections, e.g. infected sinuses, teeth, chronic ulcers, diabetes and peripheral vascular disease
Organisms	*Staphylococcus aureus* (*Haemophilus influenzae* b) *Salmonella* spp.	*S. aureus* Enteric organisms Tuberculosis	*S. aureus* Mixed, often with enteric organisms (*Salmonella* spp.), tuberculosis and anaerobes

Special circumstances are:
- In children acute haematogenous osteomyelitis involves the growing end (metaphysis) of long bones. In the infant, extension to the adjacent joint occurs. *H. influenzae* type b as a cause of osteomyelitis is on the decline with the introduction of the vaccine
- In patients with sickle-cell disease and the immunocompromised there is an increased risk of *Salmonella* infections
- In diabetics and patients with peripheral vascular disease the feet are particularly prone to osteomyelitis. Anaerobic organisms, coliforms and *Pseudomonas* spp., often in mixed infections, are found

testinal tuberculosis but remains common in many developing countries. The vertebral column is a common site for infection (**Pott's disease** of the spine).

Necrotic bone, foreign bodies and sinus formation promote the setting-up of persistent infections. Biopsies of bone are essential as the microbiology of the sinus tract does not predict underlying pathology. Debridement is an important aspect of management and, in contrast to acute disease, the optimal duration of antibiotics has not been established.

THE HEALING FRACTURE

Fractures

Fractures may occur in normal or diseased bone. In normal bone a substantial force is usually required, although repeated episodes of minor injury (e.g. during intensive training for sport) may result in a stress fracture.

Fractures may occur in diseased bone either spontaneously or after minor injury. Common conditions that predispose to **pathological fractures** are:
- osteoporosis;
- metabolic bone disease;
- Paget's disease;
- malignancy.

Simple fractures do not communicate with the body surface.

Compound fractures communicate with the body surface via a wound at the site of the fracture.

Healing

For healing to occur the bone ends must be brought together and immobilized. Wide separation of the bone ends, movement, poor blood flow, interposition of soft tissue, infection, underlying bone pathology and systemic factors such as poor nutrition or steroid therapy may all impair fracture healing.

Sequence of events following a fracture
- Disruption of the soft tissues around and blood supply to the bone results in formation of a haematoma between the bone ends and beneath the adjacent periosteum.
- Neutrophil polymorphs (and later macrophages) infiltrate the area and remove necrotic tissue.
- Granulation tissue composed of fibroblasts and capillaries forms within the haematoma.
- The two bone ends become united by fracture callus.

Callus is composed of a mixture of fibroblasts, osteoblasts and woven bone with variable amounts of cartilage. It is produced by proliferation of periosteal and endosteal osteoprogenitor cells. External callus forms a cuff or splint around the bone ends. Internal callus lies within the medullary cavity. Formation of fracture callus is maximal by 2–3 weeks in an uncomplicated fracture.
- Active bone remodelling takes place over the next few months or even years until the bone attains its normal shape and strength.

BONE TUMOURS

Primary bone tumours are comparatively **rare** neoplasms. By far the commonest tumours to be found in bone are **metastases** from primary sites in:
- breast (Fig. 20.12);
- thyroid;
- bronchus;
- prostate;
- kidney.

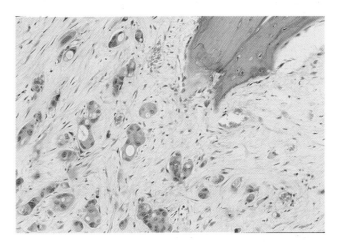

Fig. 20.12 Histology of metastatic breast carcinoma in bone. Note the malignant cells forming glandular structures. (H&E.)

Classification

Bone tumours may be classified according to the tissue of origin. Table 20.13 outlines this histogenic classification.

Diagnosis

The diagnosis of bone tumours depends on a combination of:

Table 20.14 Classification of bone tumours.

BONE-FORMING TUMOURS	*Low-grade malignancy*
Benign	Haemangiopericytoma
Osteoma	
Osteoid osteoma	*Malignant*
Osteoblastoma	Angiosarcoma
Malignant	CONNECTIVE TISSUE TUMOURS
Osteogenic sarcoma	*Benign*
	Non-ossifying fibroma
CARTILAGE-FORMING TUMOURS	Desmoplastic fibroma
Benign	Lipoma
Chondroma	
Osteochondroma	*Malignant*
Chondroblastoma	Fibrosarcoma
	Malignant fibrous histiocytoma
Malignant	Liposarcoma
Chondrosarcoma	Undifferentiated sarcoma
GIANT CELL TUMOUR	OTHER TUMOURS
	Neurofibroma
EWING'S SARCOMA	Neurilemmoma
	Chordoma
MARROW TUMOURS	Adamantinoma
Myeloma	
Lymphoma	METASTATIC TUMOURS
VASCULAR TUMOURS	
Benign	
Haemangioma	
Lymphangioma	
Glomus tumour	

- the clinical history – age, past medical history, family history, duration of symptoms, pain, swelling, tenderness;
- clinical examination – site, size, tenderness;
- X-ray findings – localization, extent, shape, borders, bone reaction, calcification;
- histopathology;
- laboratory investigations – serum PTH and alkaline phosphatase levels, white cell count, etc.

Bone-forming tumours

Benign

Osteoma. These lesions consist of well-differentiated mature, compact lamellar bone. They are found in the skull bones, especially around the orbit and the paranasal sinuses and are seen in association with Gardner's syndrome.

Osteoid osteoma and osteoblastoma (ossifying fibroma). Both

these lesions are composed of a mixture of bone and osteoid. They are distinguished from each other on clinical and radiological grounds. Osteoid osteoma is the more frequent tumour.

Osteoid osteoma (Fig. 20.13)
- **Site.** Shafts of long bones especially the tibia and femur.
- **Age.** Adolescent and young adult (10–30 years).
- **Sex.** Commoner in men (M/F 2:1).
- **Signs and symptoms**. Painful and tender, relieved by aspirin, does not appear to enlarge clinically.
- **X-ray.** Rounded zone of radiolucency; if cortical, often surrounded by massive bone sclerosis.
- **Histology.** Bone and osteoid are arranged in the form of trabeculae with no organized pattern of growth. Plump osteoblasts are present with occasional osteoclasts. There is highly vascular intertrabecular tissue with spindle cells and fibroblasts.
- **Treatment.** Excision.

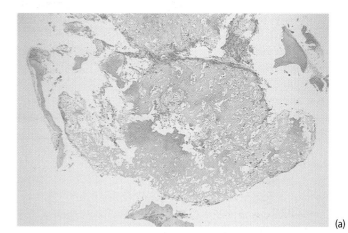

(a)

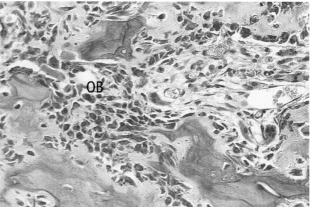

(b)

Fig. 20.13 Osteoid osteoma. (a) This small tumour measures less than 1 cm. (b) High power view shows numerous plump osteoblasts (OB) in fibrovascular tissue. (H&E.)

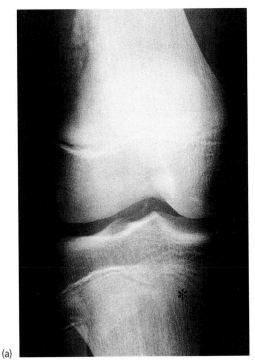

(a)

(b)

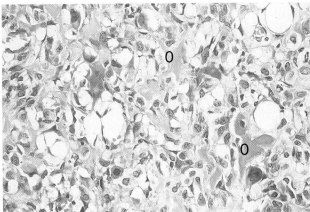

(c)

Fig. 20.14 Osteosarcoma. (a) The X-ray appearances show typical lifting of the periosteum (✳) in the region of the tibial metaphysis. (b) Metaphysis of the femur shows the typical sun-ray spicules (✳) (Codman's triangle) formed as the tumour lifts the periosteum. (c) Histology shows pleomorphic spindle cells amid areas of osteoid (O). (H&E.)

Osteoblastoma
- **Sites.** Short or flat bones (e.g. vertebrae/hands and feet).
- **Age.** Ten to thirty years.
- **Sex.** M = F.
- **X-ray.** Variable. Expansion with intact shell of reactive bone. Osteoblastoma is larger than osteoid osteoma (over 1 cm) and more commonly central.
- **Histology.** Similar to osteoid osteoma.
- **Treatment.** Excision, as for osteoid osteoma; 10% recur.

Malignant
Osteosarcoma (Fig. 20.14). This highly malignant tumour is characterized by the formation of bone and/or osteoid. It is the most common malignant primary tumour of bone (excluding myeloma).
- **Age.** It occurs before closure of the growth plate in the second decade (10–30 years). It occurs in older patients as a complication of Paget's disease.
- **Sex.** M/F = 2:1.
- **Site.** Metaphysis ± diaphysis of lower femur, upper tibia, upper humerus.
- **Predisposing factors.** Previous irradiation of bone and Paget's disease of bone.

- **Clinical features.** Pain, swelling and heat; often rapidly increasing in severity.
- **X-ray.** Osteoblastic, sclerosing in approximately 35%; osteolytic in 25% and mixed in the remaining 45%.
- **Pathology.** This tumour begins in the medulla of the metaphysis and spreads through the cortex (elevation of periosteum is seen on X-ray as **Codman's triangle**). The tumour is grey/white with areas of haemorrhage and necrosis.
- **Histology.** Highly variable. Malignant osteoblasts (pleomorphic with bizarre hyperchromatic nuclei and many mitoses) produce irregular disorganized spicules of osteoid and bone. Osteosarcomas may contain areas of haemorrhage and necrosis as well as foci of fibrosarcomatous or chondrosarcomatous differentiation.

Highly vascular variants (telangiectatic) are said to have a worse prognosis.

- **Spread.** Via the blood stream, particularly to the **lungs**.
- **Treatment.** Surgery and chemotherapy. Radiotherapy is rarely used.
- **Prognosis.** 5-year survival <60% if adequately treated.

Juxtacortical (paraosteal) osteosarcoma. This variant of osteosarcoma is characterized by its origin on the external surface of the bone and has a highly differentiated structure.

- **Age.** >30 years.
- **Site.** Metaphysis of the upper tibia, upper humerus and lower femur.
- **Prognosis.** Approximately 80% 5-year survival.

Cartilage-forming tumours

Benign

Chondroma (Fig. 20.15). Chondroma is characterized by the formation of mature cartilage. It may be single or multiple. In **Ollier's disease** multiple unilateral lesions are present, whereas in **Mafucci's disease** multiple chondromas are associated with soft-tissue haemangiomas.

- **Age.** Twenty to thirty years.
- **Sex.** M = F.
- **Clinical features.** Pain, swelling, deformity, pathological fracture.
- **Sites.** Commonest in the short bones of hands and feet, metaphysis to shaft.
- **X-ray.** Radiolucent, well-defined, may have spotty calcification.
- **Pathology.** The tumour is a lobulated cartilaginous swelling.

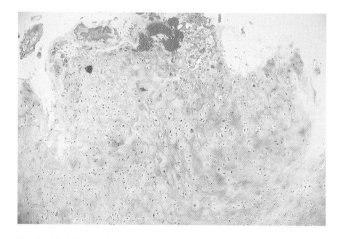

Fig. 20.15 A benign chondroma contains mature cartilage and chondrocytes.

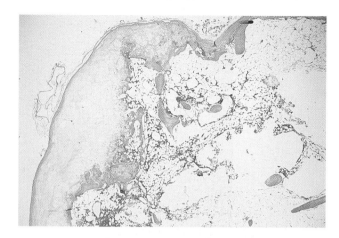

Fig. 20.16 Osteochondroma. Note the cartilage cap (left). (H&E.)

- **Histology.** Mature hyaline cartilage which is often paucicellular; calcification and ossification areas may be present.
- **Prognosis.** Malignant transformation (to chondrosarcoma) is unusual in solitary enchondromas but is seen in 30% of multiple lesions, especially of long bones.
- **Treatment.** Surgical excision.

Osteochondroma (enchondroma, exostosis; Fig. 20.16). Osteochondroma is a cartilage-capped projection on the surface of bone. This is the commonest primary bone tumour. The outer shell and the medulla are continuous with bone whilst the cap is cartilaginous (undergoing endochondral ossification at its lower border).

These tumours may be single or multiple (there is a form of autosomal dominant hereditary multiple exostosis).

- **Age.** First decade.
- **Sex.** M = F.
- **Clinical.** This tumour presents as a swelling and is rarely painful or tender.
- **Site.** Lower femur, upper tibia, upper humerus (only bones formed in cartilage).
- **X-ray.** Characteristic.
- **Pathology.** This tumour has a sessile or pedunculated, cartilage cap.
- **Histology.** Shows that the tumour is covered by periosteum then cartilage then bone.
- **Prognosis.** Malignant change is rare (<1%) in solitary tumours but commoner (20%) in multiple tumours.
- **Treatment.** Surgical excision.

Malignant

Chondrosarcoma (Fig. 20.17)
- **Age.** Thirty to sixty years; this tumour is rare under the age of 20 years.

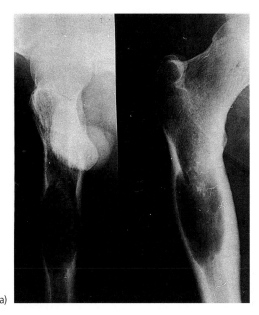

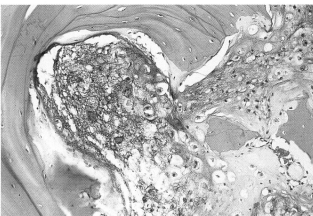

Fig. 20.17 Chondrosarcoma. (a) The X-ray shows a cloudy translucency of bone with bone expansion. (b) Pleomorphic cartilage cells showing multinucleation. (H&E.)

- **Sex.** Commoner in men (M/F 2:1).
- **Site.** Pelvis, ribs, shoulder girdle and humerus; 10% arise from pre-existing benign cartilaginous lesions.
- **Clinical.** Presentation is with pain and swelling.
- **X-ray.** There is a tumour shadow, bone expansion, cloudy translucency with spotty calcification.
- **Pathology.** This tumour may be central or peripheral. It is lobulated, slimy, mucoid, with foci of calcification giving it a gritty cut surface. Penetration of soft tissue, cortex, epiphysis and joint occurs with extension along the medulla.
- **Histology.** Cartilage cells with pleomorphism, occasional mitoses, double nuclei and multinucleated cells. Divided into three grades depending on the severity of these changes. This tumour may dedifferentiate into

undifferentiated spindle cells. Differentiation between benign and malignant is often difficult and one must take history, site, size and age of the patient into consideration.
- **Treatment.** Radical excision.
- **Prognosis.** Important factors are the site of the tumour, the size and the presence of multiple cartilage tumour syndrome. This tumour may recur if not adequately excised. It often has a prolonged course. Vascular spread is late and the direct involvement of local structures is the most likely cause of death.
- **Variants.** Clear cell chondrosarcoma (low-grade), mesenchymal chondrosarcoma (high-grade).

Giant cell tumour (Fig. 20.18)

Giant cell tumour is an osteolytic tumour composed of osteoclast-like giant cells and plump spindle/oval mononuclear cells.
- **Age.** 20–40 years. This tumour is very rare under 20 years. It occurs in bones that have stopped growing.
- **Sex.** Commoner in women.
- **Site.** Epiphyseal ends of long bones. This tumour is commonest in the lower femur, upper tibia and lower radius but any bone can be affected.
- **Clinical presentation.** Pain, swelling and pathological fracture.
- **X-ray.** Epiphyseal involvement with a translucent 'soap bubble' appearance. Cortical thinning is seen with no reactive bone formation.
- **Pathology.** This tumour has a thin shell of bone surrounding a red/grey tumour with haemorrhage and necrosis.
- **Histology.** Osteoclast-like giant cells and mononuclear

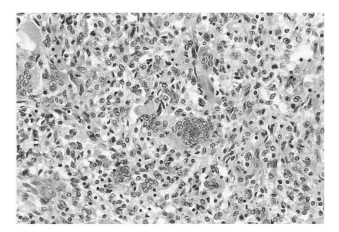

Fig. 20.18 Giant cell tumour of bone. Note the numerous osteoclast giant cells. (H&E.)

cells are present associated with haemorrhage and necrosis.

- **Differential diagnosis.** Includes cysts, hyperparathyroidism, chondroblastoma, non-ossifying fibroma and giant cell-rich osteogenic sarcoma (all of these lesions may contain numerous osteoclast-like giant cells).
- **Treatment.** Thorough surgical excision.
- **Prognosis.** These tumours frequently recur if incompletely removed. They are locally aggressive. Metastases are uncommon and occur in 15%. If treated with radiotherapy, they may recur as fibrosarcoma or osteosarcoma.

Ewing's sarcoma (Fig. 20.19)

This is a rare malignant bone tumour of uncertain

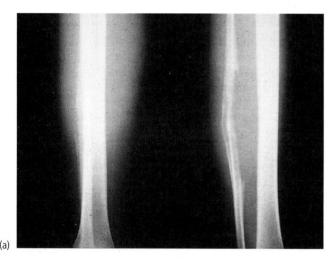

(a)

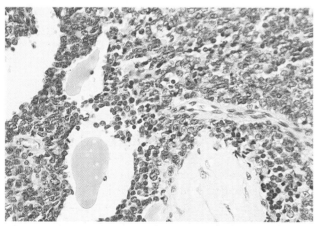

(b)

Fig. 20.19 Ewing's sarcoma of bone. (a) The X-ray shows a lytic lesion in the fibula (right). (b) The tumour consists of uniform, round cells with scanty cytoplasm. (H&E.)

histogenesis but which is likely to be part of the peripheral neuroectodermal tumour (PNET) group.

- **Age.** Five to fifteen years. This tumour is rare under 2 years and over 30 years.
- **Sex.** There is an equal incidence in males and females.
- **Site.** This tumour arises in the medullary cavity of the shaft and metaphysis of long bones such as femur, tibia, humerus, fibula and some flat bones.
- **Clinical presentation.** Pain, swelling, tenderness, fracture, raised temperature, raised white cell count and raised erythrocyte sedimentation rate (may present as possible osteomyelitis).
- **X-ray.** Lytic, moth-eaten, mottled appearance. There is medullary involvement, cortical destruction, elevation of the periosteum, and reactive bone formation in parallel layers gives rise to an 'onion-skin' appearance.
- **Pathology.** Ewing's sarcoma originates in the medulla and results in osteolysis, cortical destruction, elevation of the periosteum and reactive bone formation. The tumour is white, it may be firm or soft and may contain areas of haemorrhage and/or necrosis.
- **Histology.** Uniform round polyhedral cells. Pale nuclei are present with dispersed chromatin, indistinct, scanty cytoplasm and intracellular glycogen. There may be pseudorosette formation with sparse reticulin;
- **Differential diagnosis.** Secondary neuroblastoma, lymphoma, eosinophilic granuloma, osteosarcoma and secondary carcinoma (e.g. oat cell carcinoma).
- **Treatment.** Combination radiotherapy/chemotherapy/surgery.
- **Prognosis.** Very poor without treatment (metastases to lung, liver and bones occur early). There is a 5–8% 5-year survival; with treatment this is increased to 40–70%.

Tumours of bone marrow

Myeloma (Fig. 20.20)

When seen in bone, myeloma is usually disseminated (multiple myeloma) or rarely solitary (plasmacytoma). Myeloma is associated with the production of monoclonal immunoglobulin or immunoglobulin components.

- **Age.** Forty to seventy years.
- **Sex.** Commoner in men than women.
- **Site.** Sites of active haemopoesis, e.g. skull, spine, pelvis and ribs.
- **Clinical features.** Weakness, anaemia, raised erythrocyte sedimentation rate, predisposition to infections. Hypercalcaemia, pain, fractures, renal problems and amyloid.
- **X-ray.** Osteolytic lesions in the axial skeleton.

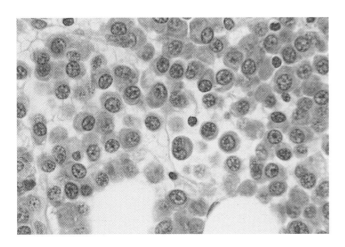

Fig. 20.20 Myeloma of bone. Note the atypical plasma cells. (H&E.)

- **Histology.** Plasma cells showing variable differentiation.
- **Treatment.** Chemotherapy.

Primary malignant lymphoma

Primary malignant lymphoma of bone is uncommon and occurs equally in both sexes. The majority of patients are over 30 years.

- **Clinical features.** Pain, swelling and involvement of long bones. Nodal disease should be excluded as lymphoma in bone is usually secondary to this.
- **X-ray.** Osteolytic lesions in the metaphysis and diaphysis of the bone give rise to a moth-eaten appearance.
- **Histology.** Rich reticulin network around each cell, generally B-cell in type.
- **Treatment.** Surgery/radiotherapy/chemotherapy.
- **Prognosis.** Thirty to sixty per cent 5-year survival, depending on the stage at presentation.

Connective tissue tumours

Malignant fibrous histiocytoma

This tumour presents in the adult and is found in the lower femur and lower tibia. It features cortical destruction, with minimal periosteal new bone formation. There are variable subtypes, the commonest being storiform or pleomorphic. Histology shows bundles and whorls of pleomorphic spindle cells. Treatment is by radical surgery.

Chordoma (Fig. 20.21)

Chordoma is a tumour which arises from notochordal remnants and which usually develops within or in close proximity to the axial skeleton.

All ages are affected, but the tumour is commonest in those over 40 years. It is commoner in men than women and is found in the **sacrococcygeal** and **spheno-occipital** region. It is slow-growing, recurrent after excision and presents with pressure symptoms on the spinal cord. X-ray findings show a **lytic** lesion with a soft-tissue shadow and patchy calcification.

Macroscopically, this is a lobulated, greyish, semi-translucent and gelatinous tumour. Histology shows clusters or cords of cells (some of which are vacuolated) lying in abundant mucoid stroma. Treatment is by surgery and/or radiotherapy. These tumours are generally fatal, with repeated local recurrence; distant metastases occur late.

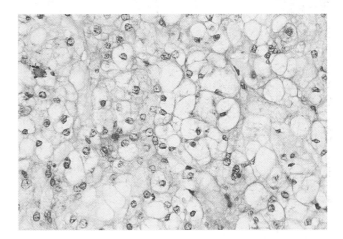

Fig. 20.21 Chordoma. Histology shows cords of vacuolated cells. (H&E.)

The joint

NORMAL JOINT STRUCTURE (Fig. 20.22)

Joints may be freely mobile (e.g. shoulder or knee), permit slight movement (e.g. intervertebral joints) or be fixed and rigid (e.g. skull sutures). They may be synovial (see below), cartilaginous (e.g. spinal joints) or fibrous (e.g. skull sutures).

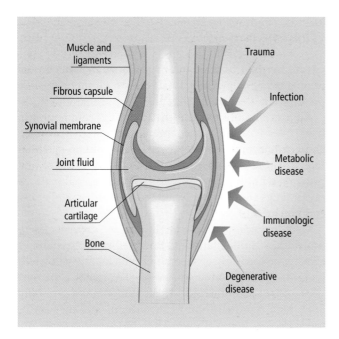

Fig. 20.22 Normal joint structure.

Synovial membrane

The synovial membrane is lined by two types of cell (distinguishable by electronmicroscopy). Type A are phagocytic. Type B are fibroblastic and secrete hyaluronic acid and the other proteins of synovial fluid.

Synovial fluid

Normal joints contain only a small amount of synovial fluid, the function of which is to lubricate the joint. Synovial fluid is a dialysate of plasma together with hyaluronic acid and proteoglycan secreted by the synovial lining cells.

INFECTIOUS ARTHRITIS

Septic arthritis

Staphylococcus aureus is the commonest cause of septic arthritis. Haematogenous spread of organisms to joints (Table 20.15) usually presents as a monoarticular suppurative arthrtis; trauma-related infection is a less common route of infection. The knee and hip joints are the most commonly affected, and patients with diabetes,

Table 20.15 Pathogens of infectious arthritis.

Type	Organism	Comments
Acute septic arthritis Usually monoarticular	*Staphylococcus aureus*	Commonest cause in all age groups
Culture positive	β-haemolytic streptococci	Usually group A, group B in neonates, culture positive
	Salmonella, Haemophilus influenzae b (Hib)	Occurs in children, vaccine available for Hib
	Neisseria gonorrhoeae	Occurs in adolescents, may also be of a a reactive type
Chronic septic arthritis	*Mycobacterium tuberculosis*	Occurs in weight-bearing joints
	Borrelia burgdorferi	Occurs in tertiary Lyme disease
	Candida spp.	Rare but commonest fungal cause in UK
Reactive arthritis (Culture negative) Often with rash	Hepatitis B	Occurs in the preicteric phase; polyarticular
	Mumps	Occurs mostly in men, culture negative
	Rubella	Occurs in young women often with rash
	Arboviruses, e.g. dengue virus	Often with rash
	Campylobacter, Yersinia Chlamydia	Often with rash Reiter's syndrome (urethritis, arthritis, uveitis) Associated with HLA B 27

HLA, Human leucocyte antigen.

rheumatoid and osteoarthritis are at an increased risk of infection.

Reactive arthritis or postinfectious arthritis is another catogory of disease. In these cases organisms are not isolated from the joint as the underlying process is immunological. Multiple joints are affected with a predeliction for the small joints of the hand.

Clinical features

Fever, joint swelling, pain and restricted movement of the affected joint are the presenting features.

Diagnosis and management

Appropriate antibiotic treatment relies on defining the microbiology by obtaining a joint aspirate. Blood cultures may also be useful. Open surgical drainage and irrigation are often required in suppurative arthritis.

Prosthetic joint infections

Hip and knee prostheses are common and about 1–5% will become infected. Infection may be:

- locally introduced at and around the time of operation, e.g. skin-type flora is common, such as coagulase-negative staphyloccoci;
- haematogenous spread, e.g. *Staphylococcus aureus*.

Infection occurs in the osseous tissue adjacent to the prosthesis and the organisms may survive on foreign material by forming a biolayer. X-ray changes may show loosening and areas of translucency but the changes are not specific. A joint aspirate may enable the diagnosis to be made, although sometimes a diagnosis is not made until operative samples are available. Treatment of these infections is difficult and requires removal of the prosthesis and long courses of intravenous antibiotics.

NON-INFECTIOUS ARTHRITIS

Osteoarthritis

Osteoarthritis is a non-inflammatory degenerative disease of large weight-bearing joints. It is a common, severe disease that affects up to 20% of elderly men and women in developed countries.

Previous damage to the joint is a predisposing factor. Secondary arthritis may develop in patients with pre-existing bone or joint disease such as rheumatoid arthritis or gout.

Pathology

Early features. These include fragmentaion and fibrillation of the articular cartilage. It is seen as part of normal wear and tear and does not necessarily progress to full-blown osteoarthritis.

Late. Erosion of cartilage occurs, leading to reactive proliferation and subsequent deformity of the subchondral bone plate. A vicious circle develops in which the resulting abnormal mechanics leads to further damage to residual articular cartilage. The subchondral bone plate may develop cysts. Bony outgrowths (**osteophytes**) at the margins of the articular surface are characteristic. In the distal interphalangeal joints they are recognized clinically as **Heberden's nodes**. The synovium may show reactive changes of focal hyperplasia and chronic inflammation.

Clinical features

Pain, stiffness, audible creaking, small effusions and joint crepitus are all common.

X-ray findings

There is loss of joint space with reactive proliferation of the subchondral bone plate and osteophyte formation.

Rheumatoid arthritis

The pathogenesis and extra-articular manifestations of rheumatoid disease have been described in Chapter 9.

Rheumatoid arthritis is a chronic, non-suppurative, progressive and often disabling disease. It predominantly affects the peripheral synovial joints in a symmetrical fashion.

Epidemiology

Rheumatoid arthritis is commoner in women and there is a female to male ratio of 3:1. All ages are affected but the disease is commonest between 35 and 50 years. In 75% of patients there is an association with human leucocyte antigen (HLA) DR4.

Circulating autoantibodies (usually immunoglobulin M (IgM) anti-IgG) are found in the majority of adult patients. High levels correlate with severe arthritis and multisystem disease. The underlying stimulus is unknown.

Clinical features

Rheumatoid arthritis affects the small joints of the fingers and toes, the knees, elbows, wrists and hips.

Synovial effusions may occur and these may contain neutrophil polymorphs and fibrin, even in the absence of infection. Progressive damage to the joint capsule and ligaments leads to joint instability and subluxation. Healing and fibrosis lead to characteristic fixed deformities.

Pathology

There is a chronic **inflammatory synovitis** with **villous hyperplasia** and an inflammatory cell infiltrate, including lymphocytes (with formation of lymphoid follicles) and plasma cells. Some fibrin and small numbers of neutrophil polymporphs may be seen. A layer of inflam-

Table 20.16 Causes of high serum uric acid.

Increased production with normal excretion, e.g. following chemotherapy for lymphoma and leukaemia

Decreased excretion with normal production, e.g. secondary to treatment with thiazide diuretics and in chronic renal failure

75% of cases of clinical gout have an idiopathic decrease in uric acid secretion

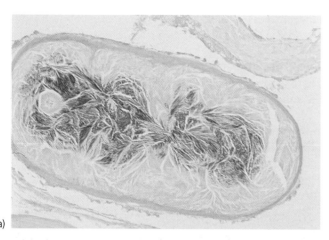

(a)

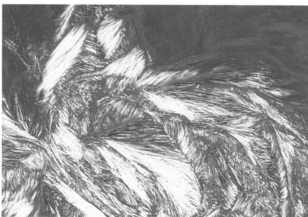

(b)

Fig. 20.23 A gouty tophus. (a) Note the surrounding fibrosis and the central dark staining crystalline material. (b) Polarized light microscopy shows that these crystals have the characteristic fine, feathery appearance of urate crystals.

matory granulation tissues—**pannus**—extends inwards from the synovial margin and erodes the articular cartilage. Adhesion to the synovium may lead to fibrous or **bony ankylosis**.

Pseudocysts form in adjacent weakened, osteoporotic bone. Secondary osteoarthritic changes may occur.

Similar histological changes may be seen in other chronic inflammatory joint diseases such as ankylosing spondylitis, Reiter's disease, psoriatic arthritis and enteropathic arthritis.

Classic rheumatoid nodules are only rarely found in the synovium.

Prognosis

This is variable:

- 10% of patients are severely disabled;
- 20% of patients have only slight symptoms and minor disability;
- 5–15% develop systemic amyloid.

Gout

In gout, crystals of monosodium urate are deposited in joints and other tissues, resulting in a painful acute inflammatory response.

Not all cases of hyperuricaemia develop gout. Local factors such as pH, low temperature and the presence of sulphated glycosaminoglycans are also important.

Clinical features

Over 90% of cases occur in men. The most commonly affected age group is 40–60 years. Ninety per cent of cases occur as an acute monoarthritis and 10% affect more than one joint.

Gout affects the toes (particularly the first metatarsophalyngeal joint), knees, ankles, elbows and fingers and may be confined to periarticular and extraskeletal soft tissues).

Pathology

Synovial fluid. In acute disease the synovial fluid contains neutrophil polymorphs. Urate crystals can be seen in suitably collected specimens.

Synovial biopsy. Fibrin, acute inflammation and urate crystals are seen.

Established lesions. These contain urate crystals surrounded by a chronic inflammatory cell infiltrate including macrophages and multinucleated giant cells with fibrosis (the 'gouty tophus'; Fig. 20.23).

Complications

Damage to cartilage and bone, calcification (to give a gouty tophus) and formation of fistulae from deep lesions to the skin occur. Renal failure is a recognized complication.

FURTHER READING

Unni K.K (ed.) (1988) *Bone Tumours.* Churchill Livingstone, New York.

Diseases of the Urinary Tract

C O N T E N T S

The kidney

RENAL BIOCHEMISTRY AND PHYSIOLOGY

The glomerulus

Approximately 150 litres of filtrate is produced per day by glomerular ultrafiltration. This filtrate is normally iso-osmolar with the plasma. Macromolecules are not filtered; the threshold size is equivalent to the albumin molecule (i.e. molecular weight of 65 000–70 000).

The proximal tubule

The proximal tubule is a site of active and passive reabsorption (Table 21.1).

The loop of Henlé (Fig. 21.1)

This is a site for **sodium chloride reabsorption**; up to 15% of filtered sodium is reabsorbed here. Production of hyperosmolar renal interstitium occurs as the osmolality increases towards the tip of the loop, using a counter-current multiplier mechanism. This mechanism is vital

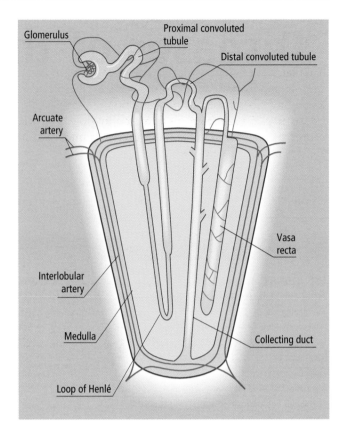

Fig. 21.1 The nephron.

for the production of **concentrated urine** in the collecting ducts.

Countercurrent multiplier mechanism

Tubular fluid passes through the descending limb of the loop of Henlé before the ascending limb.

In the **descending limb**, there is passive movement of sodium into the tubule and water moves out under the influence of the increasing sodium chloride concentration in the interstitium. Movement continues towards the tip of the loop (this increasing concentration having been produced by active pumping from the ascending limb).

Vasa recta, blood vessels which supply the medulla, are also loops and they follow the course of the loops of Henle. Their looped structure minimizes the 'washing-out' of sodium chloride from the interstitium which would otherwise occur.

The **ascending limb** is impermeable to water. Active pumping of chloride from the tubule into the interstitium (with sodium following passively) leads to trapping of sodium chloride in the medullary interstitium.

Table 21.1 The proximal tubule.

Active reabsorption of:	
Glucose	Normally all reabsorbed unless plasma glucose higher than threshold level which is usually about 10 mmol/l (180 mg/dl)
Sodium	Approximately 80% reabsorbed influenced by 'third factor' mechanisms
Potassium	Approximately 80% reabsorbed
Hydrogen ion	Results indirectly in the reabsorption of bicarbonate
Phosphate and calcium	Affected by parathyroid hormone
Amino acids	
Passive reabsorption of:	
Water	
Chloride	

Distal tubule

Tubular fluid entering the distal tubule is hypotonic to plasma because of the active pumping occurring in the ascending limb of the loop of Henle. Sodium reabsorption occurs in exchange for potassium and hydrogen ion and represents fine tuning of sodium excretion under the influence of aldosterone.

Collecting duct

Antidiuretic hormone (ADH) acts here. ADH increases the permeability of the collecting duct to water, so water passes out by osmotic action as the collecting duct passes through the area of increasing osmolality towards the tip of the renal papilla.

In the absence of ADH, the collecting duct is impermeable to water and the hypotonic fluid from the distal tubule passes out unaltered as urine (resulting in polyuria).

Assessment of renal function

Renal failure can be defined as a significant reduction in glomerular filtration rate (GFR).

Estimation of GFR is the most important and most frequently performed assessment of renal function.

Glomerular filtration rate

Estimates of GFR can be obtained from measurements of plasma urea, plasma creatinine and clearance measurements.

Plasma urea is the most widely used routine test. The disadvantages of using this test alone are that the urea production rate is affected by protein intake and by cellular catabolism. Urea clearance (and hence plasma urea) is affected by urine flow rate.

Creatinine production rate is proportional to skeletal muscle mass. If muscle mass is constant, serial measurements of creatinine provide a very good assessment of renal function.

Clearance measurements are shown in Table 21.2.

Creatinine clearance

This is an example of a steady-state clearance. Such tests depend on the plasma concentration of the compound being measured remaining constant during the test, and in the case of creatinine this is normally true because it is

Table 21.2 Calculation of glomerular filtration rate (GFR) from clearance measurements.

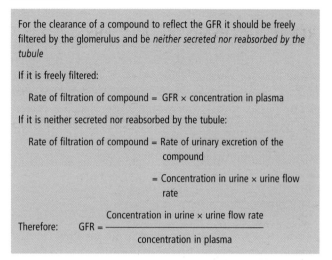

For the clearance of a compound to reflect the GFR it should be freely filtered by the glomerulus and be *neither secreted nor reabsorbed by the tubule*

If it is freely filtered:

Rate of filtration of compound = GFR × concentration in plasma

If it is neither secreted nor reabsorbed by the tubule:

Rate of filtration of compound = Rate of urinary excretion of the compound

= Concentration in urine × urine flow rate

Therefore: $$GFR = \frac{\text{Concentration in urine} \times \text{urine flow rate}}{\text{concentration in plasma}}$$

produced at a constant rate by muscle. A timed urine collection (normally 24 hours) and a simultaneous blood sample must be obtained.

Creatinine clearance is not ideal for GFR determinations because creatinine is secreted by the tubule to a small extent, thus it tends to overestimate the GFR, especially when low.

Chromium-51-labelled ethylenediaminetetraacetic acid (EDTA) clearance

This is normally performed as a single-shot technique in which a bolus of the compound is injected intravenously and the plasma decay curve is plotted by counting the radioactivity in serial blood samples. From this the GFR can be calculated mathematically (Table 21.2 and Fig. 21.2).

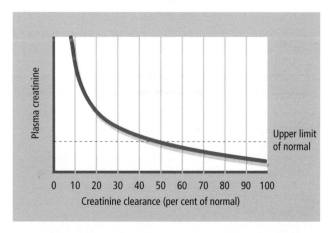

Fig. 21.2 Relationship between plasma creatinine and creatinine clearance.

Creatinine clearance versus plasma creatinine

It will be seen from Fig. 21.2 that plasma creatinine may be normal until creatinine clearance has dropped to 50% of normal (i.e. for a patient with low muscle mass whose plasma creatinine started at the low end of normal). Also, the curve is fairly flat until creatinine clearance has fallen below 50% of normal. Thus, it is in cases where the plasma creatinine is normal or slightly elevated that creatinine clearance is worthwhile. After that, it is preferable to monitor renal function by means of serial plasma creatinine measurements (this also overcomes the inaccuracies of 24-hour urine collections).

The glomerular filter

Leakiness of the glomerular filter is detected by:
- proteinuria – its presence and quality;
- haematuria;
- examination of the urinary deposit.

Selectivity of proteinuria

The greater the damage to the glomerular filter, the higher will be the molecular weight of proteins 'leaked' into the urine. This can be assessed by comparing the clearance of two proteins of different size, often transferrin and immunoglobulin G (IgG). The ratio of these clearances is expressed as a **selectivity index**.

Tubular function

Tests of tubular function are not performed very frequently but are of value in the following (Table 21.3).

Renal failure

Renal failure may be defined as a significant reduction in GFR, but other biochemical features are seen (Table 21.4).

Table 21.3 Tests of tubular function.

Acute renal failure
Renal tubular acidosis – urine pH/urinary acidification test
Nephrogenic diabetes insipidus – water deprivation/desmopressin tests
'Phosphaturic' rickets – phosphate clearance/creatinine clearance ratio
Fanconi syndrome } Simply showing the presence in urine of abnormal amounts of compounds normally reabsorbed by Aminoacidurias } the renal tubule
Also tubular proteins (e.g. albumin, β_2-microglobulin)

Table 21.4 Biochemical features of renal failure.

Elevated urea and creatinine levels

Disturbed sodium and water balance
Most commonly: sodium and water retention with, if anything, water retention being greater → dilutional hyponatraemia

Acidosis
When GFR < 20–30 ml/min
Caused by failure of excretion of the acid load normally excreted daily by the kidneys

Potassium disturbances
Most commonly: potassium retention → hyperkalaemia

Calcium and phosphate disturbances
Normally: phosphate retention
Normally: hypocalcaemia caused by:
      • acidosis reducing the level of protein-bound calcium in serum
      • high phosphate level within renal tubular cells inhibits production of 1,25-dihydroxycholecalciferol → poor calcium absorption from the gut
Hypocalcaemia → secondary hyperparathyroidism
In chronic renal failure, if these changes are not prevented, they lead to renal osteodystrophy

Middle molecule retention
Compounds with molecular weights of 1000–2000
Not routinely measured
Believed to be responsible for many of the symptoms of 'uraemia' (malaise, nausea, etc.)

Urate retention

Secondary hyperlipidaemia

GFR, Glomerular filtration rate.

Acute renal failure

There are many causes of acute renal failure (ARF) (Tables 21.5 and 21.6).

Acute-on-chronic renal failure

Acute deterioration of renal function in a patient with chronic renal failure may occur with dehydration or infection.

Features of acute renal failure. **Oliguria** or **anuria** is usually present in untreated ARF. The other features are as outlined already for renal failure in general. **Infection** is a common cause of death in ARF.

Prerenal ARF/acute tubular necrosis. Table 21.6 illustrates the differentiation of these two conditions. In either case,

Table 21.5 Causes of acute renal failure.

Prerenal
Poor renal perfusion because of hypovolaemia and/or reduced cardiac output
Recovers if renal perfusion is restored

Renal
Acute tubular necrosis
- Occurs if prerenal failure is not corrected fairly quickly
- A better name would be acute ischaemic renal failure
- See below for differentiation of this from prerenal failure
Glomerulonephritis
    Especially rapidly progressive (i.e. crescentic) glomerulonephritis (e.g. Goodpasture's syndrome)
Nephrotoxins and drug reactions
Disorders of the renal vasculature
    Large vessels
- Renal artery (embolism, thrombosis, etc.)
- Renal vein thrombosis
    Small vessels
- Disseminated intravascular coagulation
- Thrombotic microangiopathy (e.g. haemolytic–uraemic syndrome)
Renal tubule blockage, e.g. myeloma kidney (light chains)—amyloid protein

Postrenal
Urinary tract obstruction

Table 21.6 Differentiation of prerenal failure from acute tubular necrosis. In prerenal acute renal failure the kidney is responding to poor renal perfusion by retaining sodium and water; this leads to a low urine sodium and a concentrated urine with high osmolality.

As acute tubular necrosis develops, any glomerular filtrate produced passes out as urine with progressively less and less tubular modification, so the urine composition approaches that of plasma.

	Prerenal acute renal failure	Acute tubular necrosis
Urine osmolality	High	Falls to a level similar to plasma
Urine/plasma osmolality ratio	> 1.5	< 1.1
Fract excr sodium = [(U/V)Na/(U/V)Creat]	< 1.0	> 1.5
Urine sodium	< 10 mmol/l	> 20 mmol/l
Response to diuretics	Yes	No

Fract excr, Fraction excreted.

the patient should be rehydrated appropriately (if hypovolaemic) and given a diuretic (usually frusemide).

In prerenal ARF, if renal perfusion is restored, this will normally lead to immediate recovery of the renal failure.

In acute tubular necrosis, rehydration must be performed very carefully, because if it is overdone, the patient's kidneys will be unable to excrete the excess fluid/electrolytes and the circulation will be overloaded. Management should then be as described below for established ARF. Renal function will normally return within 3 weeks if predisposing causes have been removed and the patient can be kept alive.

Management of acute renal failure. Prerenal failure should be treated as described above. Postrenal obstruction should be excluded and relieved if found. Otherwise, the management of established ARF is as follows.

- **Fluids.** Maintain balance by giving a volume equivalent to the previous day's losses plus an allowance for insensible losses (insensible loss is normally about 500 ml/day). If the patient is fluid-overloaded, the volume given should, of course, be reduced until the overload is corrected.
- **Sodium.** Adjust sodium intake such that any overload or depletion is corrected, then give an allowance equivalent to the previous day's losses. This will normally involve a **low-sodium diet**.
- **Potassium.** A **low-potassium diet** and **treatment of hyperkalaemia** should be undertaken:
  (a) acutely by giving glucose and insulin (which causes potassium to enter cells) or calcium gluconate (calcium antagonizes the effect of hyperkalaemia on the heart);
  (b) giving calcium ion exchange resins orally or by enema (these remove potassium from the body and exchange it for calcium).
- **Protein.** A **low-protein diet** will reduce the production of nitrogenous waste products such as the 'middle molecules' which give rise to many of the symptoms of 'uraemia'. Since the advent of renal dialysis, very-low-protein diets (20 g/day) are no longer used because they increase the likelihood of infection.
- **Acidosis.** A low-protein diet will also reduce the production of acid and hence the severity of acidosis. Do not treat with sodium bicarbonate as this would lead to sodium overload.
- **Infection.** All possible precautions should be taken to prevent infection and any which do occur should be treated vigorously.
- **Drugs.** The dosage of drugs which are eliminated by the kidney should be adjusted.
- **Diuretic phase of acute tubular necrosis.** At the time of recovery from acute tubular necrosis, the GFR usually starts to increase before tubular function has returned to normal. This leads to large volumes of dilute urine being passed which may contain considerable amounts of sodium and potassium. Careful monitoring of losses may be required at this stage.

Renal dialysis may be required if conservative measures fail.

Chronic renal failure

In chronic renal failure (CRF), the range of homeostatic adjustment of urine composition becomes progressively curtailed.

Initially, this has little effect except that the kidney is unable to concentrate urine as much as normal at night. This leads to nocturia. Later, the kidney is unable to maintain homeostasis with the patient's existing dietary intake of fluid and electrolytes. In most cases, this is because the dietary load is too high for the failing kidney to be able to excrete it, the result being:

- sodium retention → hypertension and perhaps oedema;
- water retention → hyponatraemia;
- potassium retention → hyperkalaemia.

In rare cases, the maximum retaining ability of the kidney may be impaired more, and then the normal dietary load of sodium may be less than the ability of the failing kidney to retain it, resulting in a **sodium-losing nephropathy**.

The range over which the urine osmolality is adjustable becomes smaller and smaller until eventually the kidney is only able to produce urine with a similar osmolality to plasma (i.e. **isosthenuria** is present).

These features of CRF can be explained by the **reduced nephron hypothesis**. As nephrons are progressively destroyed the plasma level of urea and other waste compounds rises. Thus the concentration of these compounds in the glomerular filtrate of the still-functioning nephrons also rises and this leads to an osmotic diuretic effect in the tubules.

Anaemia is a feature of CRF, predominantly because of deficient erythropoietin production by the kidney (Fig. 21.3).

Assessment of the rate of deterioration of renal function. Referring to Fig. 21.2, it will be seen that GFR is inversely proportional to the plasma creatinine. GFR decreases linearly in CRF if there are no complicating factors.

Guidelines for management of chronic renal failure
1 Assess the rate of deterioration of renal function (see above); if it accelerates, look for correctable factors.
2 Control blood pressure carefully.
3 Control water and salt balance – patients are at risk of fluid overload or dehydration, especially after intercurrent infections and surgery.
4 As necessary, modify doses of those drugs which are eliminated by the kidney.

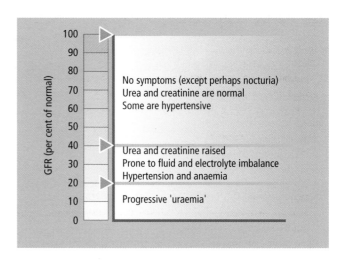

Fig. 21.3 Features of chronic renal failure related to glomerular filtration rate (GFR).

5 Control calcium and phosphate levels in an attempt to prevent renal osteodystrophy by giving:
  (a) phosphate binders;
  (b) calcium supplements;
  (c) vitamin D analogues (e.g. 1-α-OH cholecalciferol) which do not need to be hydroxylated by the kidney.
6 Reduce dietary protein when gastrointestinal symptoms develop.
7 Renal transplantation or chronic dialysis will eventually be required.

Nephrotic syndrome

This is defined as proteinuria which causes hypoalbuminaemia sufficient to cause oedema.

Normally proteinuria will need to exceed 0.05 g/kg body weight per day for the nephrotic syndrome to develop. Thus it will only occur with glomerular disease (Table 21.7).

Table 21.7 Some causes of glomerular damage which may be sufficient to produce nephrotic syndrome. It should be stressed that nephrotic syndrome is, as its name implies, simply a syndrome which results from heavy proteinuria of any cause, and it should *not* be considered a final diagnosis in its own right.

Minimal-change glomerulonephritis – this is a common cause of the nephrotic syndrome in children
Other idiopathic forms of glomerulonephritis
Connective tissue disorders
Infections (e.g. malaria, syphilis, hepatitis B)
Diabetes mellitus
Amyloidosis
Drugs (e.g. gold, penicillamine)

Table 21.8 Associated biochemical findings in the nephrotic syndrome.

Serum protein electrophoresis
Albumin will, of course, be reduced
α_2-Globulin is increased (α_2-macroglobulin has a high molecular weight, so it is not readily leaked into the urine)
γ-Globulin may be decreased if the proteinuria is non-selective

Secondary hyperlipidaemia

Investigation of nephrotic syndrome (Table 21.8)
- Adults: a renal biopsy will normally be required (see below).
- Children: if there is a highly selective proteinuria it is highly likely that minimal-change glomerulonephritis is the cause and a renal biopsy can be avoided.

INFECTION OF THE KIDNEY

Acute infection of the kidney

Acute renal infection is often divided into two main morphological types, acute pyelitis and acute pyelonephritis. However, from an aetiological or microbiological point of view it is more appropriate to consider upper urinary tract infection due to:
- **ascending infection** – the more common route, due to infection with *Escherichia coli*, *Proteus* spp., *Pseudomonas aeruginosa* and *Enterococcus faecalis*;
- **haematogenous spread** – associated with bacteraemia or septicaemia, due to infection with *Staphylococcus aureus* and *Mycobacterium tuberculosis*.

Acute pyelitis
This is common and may be protean in its manifestations but often presents as a **pyrexia of unknown origin**. It is usually an **ascending infection** from the bladder and is most often found in children and pregnant women. The main aetiological factors are the short female urethra and urinary obstruction by the gravid uterus. In men, urethral stricture and prostatic obstruction are the main predisposing causes.

Acute pyelonephritis
Urinary tract obstruction is a predisposing factor and is considered to be an important cause of the infection localizing in the kidney. The kidney is enlarged and oedematous due to intense inflammation. On the cut surface numerous small abscesses can be seen and there are wedgeshaped purulent areas streaking upwards from the medulla into the cortex with normal areas of intervening kidney. Histology reveals extensive interstitial neutrophil infiltration, marked tubular destruction and some abscess formation.

Pathogenesis of acute renal infection
The source of infection is most often the flora of the perineum, hence the predominance of faecal organisms but blood-borne infection is also possible. Stagnant urine and urinary obstruction together with vesicoureteric reflux are also necessary. Infection of the renal parenchyma via this route requires penetration of renal papillae by the organisms, a phenomenon particularly likely to take place in the concave compound papillae at the upper and lower poles of the kidney (Fig. 21.4).

Chronic pyelonephritis

In the past this condition has been diagnosed without adherence to rigid criteria and at one time it was fashionable to consider any shrunken scarred kidney as chronic pyelonephritis. It is in fact a chronic disease resulting from bacterial infection of the kidney. It is important to distinguish it from analgesic abuse, drug-induced interstitial nephritis or other disorders giving rise to interstitial infiltration by lymphocytes and plasma cells.

Clinically there may or may not be a history of recurrent attacks of an acute urinary infection. Often the disease is 'silent' until renal insufficiency occurs. Urinary obstruction is a common aetiological factor.

Pathology
The appearances depend on the presence or absence of

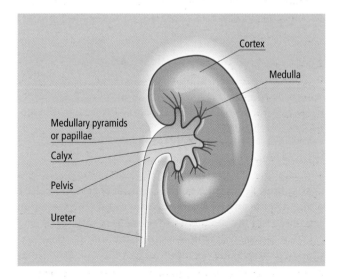

Fig. 21.4 The structure of the kidney.

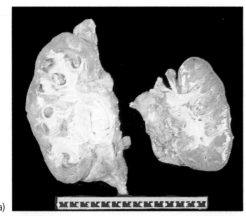

(a)

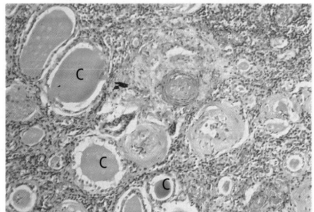

(b)

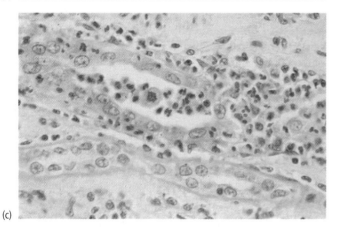

(c)

Fig. 21.5 The kidneys in chronic pyelonephritis. (a) They are unequal in size and the renal pelves are dilated and deformed. (b) Histology shows eosinophilic casts (C) in the tubules with interstitial inflammation and fibrosis. (c) H&E.

obstruction. Yet the outstanding feature is the focal nature of the disease and as a consequence of this there is often asymmetrical involvement of the kidneys (Fig. 21.5).

When associated with vesicoureteric reflux, the scarring first affects the compound papillae at the upper and lower poles but, if associated with obstruction, all papillae tend to be affected. Isolation of organisms

from renal parenchyma is unusual in chronic pyelonephritis but damage to the calyces and pelvis is always found. It is possible that reflux of urine alone can produce changes in renal parenchyma typical of chronic pyelonephritis in the absence of infection but this is a matter of controversy.

Histology of the kidney reveals further the focal nature of the disease with areas where kidney is normal alternating with abnormal areas. This makes use of renal biopsy in diagnosis of limited value. The main features in scarred areas are in the interstitium where there is fibrosis, intense lymphoplasmacytic infiltration and marked tubular atrophy. The atrophic tubules are lined by flattened epithelium and often filled with protein, giving rise to an appearance known as **thyroidization**. Occasional tubules may contain neutrophils. Periglomerular fibrosis is prominent. Examination of medullary pyramids and the pelves shows fibrosis and chronic inflammatory cell infiltration. Vascular changes are inconstant but intimal fibrosis in arcuate and interlobular arteries is often found and may be of a profound nature, no doubt contributing to the scarring process. Chronic pyelonephritis is one of the causes of secondary hypertension and, if present, this in itself may result in accentuation of vascular pathology.

GLOMERULAR DISEASE

Introduction

Diseases of the glomerulus (Fig. 21.6) may have a variety

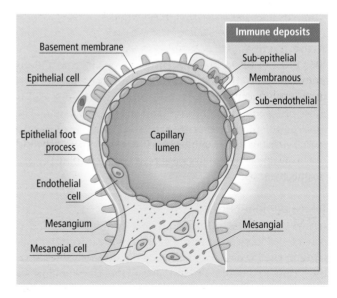

Fig. 21.6 The renal glomerulus.

of clinical manifestations. These can be broadly classified into five main categories, as follows.

Acute nephritic syndrome

These patients present with acute onset of haematuria which may be macroscopic or microscopic, proteinuria, hypertension and oedema. There is usually anuria or oliguria and both this and the oedema are associated with decreased glomerular filtration and sodium and water retention.

Rapidly progressive glomerulonephritis syndrome

There is either an acute or insidious onset of haematuria, proteinuria, anaemia and rapidly progressive renal failure, usually with oliguria or anuria. Unless effective dialysis treatment is instituted the condition is rapidly fatal.

The recurrent haematuria syndrome

These patients have intermittent acute attacks of painless haematuria, occasionally accompanied by proteinuria, often following an upper respiratory infection. This differs from the acute nephritic syndrome in that there is no hypertension or oedema.

Chronic nephritic syndrome

This is characterized by the insidious onset of renal failure which is progressive and often accompanied by haematuria, proteinuria and hypertension.

Nephrotic syndrome

This is one of the most frequent modes of presentation of renal disease and can occur in both primary glomerulonephritis or secondary to glomerular involvement in systemic disorders. There is massive proteinuria, hypoalbuminaemia, oedema and often hypercholesterolaemia.

It is important to understand that each of these clinical syndromes is not associated with a specific disease or group of diseases, thus the acute nephritic syndrome may be associated with not only acute postinfectious, glomerulonephritis but also with systemic lupus erythematosus and Henoch–Schönlein purpura. Similarly, almost any form of glomerulonephritis may give rise to the nephrotic syndrome. Needle biopsy of the kidney is necessary in many patients in order to obtain a true tissue diagnosis.

Histological classification of glomerular disease

It is all too easy to become obsessed with classification of glomerular histology on the basis of light microscopy but this does not always give an indication of aetiology and prognosis. The glomerulus, as with many other organs

and systems, has only a limited number of responses to pathological stimuli. Certain terms, however, require definition and these are listed below.

- **Diffuse** is a term used to describe a lesion which involves all glomeruli.
- **Focal** refers to lesions affecting some but not all glomeruli.
- **Segmental** is applied to a lesion which affects only part of the glomerulus and may or may not involve all glomeruli.
- **Global** is a term given to a process that involves the entire glomerulus.
- **Proliferative** is a term used to indicate an increased cell population within the glomerulus itself. In most cases this is based solely on a subjective impression with little in the way of firm quantitative data to support the concept. Proliferation implies multiplication of cells normally present in the glomerulus and in many instances this involves mesangial cells. Yet much of the increased cellularity may be due to infiltration of the capillary tufts by inflammatory cells, notably neutrophils and macrophages. Some pathologists attempt to distinguish between these two processes of proliferation and infiltration by using the term exudative to describe the condition where glomeruli are infiltrated by neutrophils.

Immunological classification of glomerular disease

As a result of experimental work on animals and also the study of fresh frozen renal biopsy material using immunofluorescent techniques two distinct forms of glomerular disease can be defined.

1 The first is **immune complex disease** which is characterized by granular deposition of immunoglobulins and complement within the glomerulus, usually on or in the capillary basement membrane. Using fluorescent conjugated antibodies to various immunoglobulins and complement components, these complexes can be demonstrated, using a fluorescent microscope, to be deposited in discrete granules in the glomerulus, giving rise to the so-called lumpy bumpy appearance. Under the electronmicroscope the complexes are seen as discrete electron-dense deposits. The actual mechanism whereby these immune complexes are deposited in the glomerulus is considered below.

2 The second form of disease is known as **antiglomerular basement membrane antibody disease** and is characterized by striking linear deposition of immunoglobulins and complement along the glomerular capillary basement membrane. As the name implies, it is due to a circulating antibody to glomerular capillary basement membrane. This is very uncommon and probably accounts for less than 5% of all cases.

These two forms of immunological disease do not always relate directly to light microscope appearances within the glomerulus. Furthermore, not all forms of glomerulonephritis can be grouped into one or other of these categories. Thus some types of glomerulonephritis are associated with a circulating **antineutrophil cytoplasmic antibody** (ANCA) and there are further varieties where there is as yet no detectable immunological abnormality.

Deposition of immune complexes

In early experimental work on acute glomerulonephritis associated with serum sickness it was noted that immune complex deposits, identified by immunofluorescent techniques and as electron-dense masses in electronmicrographs, were found in the subepithelial region of the glomerular capillary wall. It was postulated that antigen was deposited in that position and there combined with antibody. An alternative hypothesis considered that antigen–antibody complexes formed in the circulation were filtered through the glomerular capillary wall and were arrested at the subepithelial site; this was thought to take place either by direct filtration or following dissociation of the complexes with reaggregation after initial binding of antigen to subepithelial sites on the glomerular basement membrane. In some instances of glomerular disease there is evidence of an autoimmune process in which antibody aggregation with intrinsic glomerular antigen takes place.

Immune complexes may be detected at varying sites within the glomerulus (Fig. 21.6), notably in the subepithelial position and in the mesangium. The precise site depends on a number of factors, including the nature of the antigen and the number of its antibody binding sites, the molecular weight of the complexes, their charge and glomerular haemodynamics and permeability. The removal of complexes from the glomerulus is ill-understood. Mesangial cells resemble macrophages in many respects and it is considered by some authorities that they are responsible for removal of complexes but direct proof is lacking. The complement system is activated by immune complexes and this is important in causing glomerular damage but it is also known that complement depletion will inhibit removal of deposits, though the mechanism is once again ill-understood.

Secondary mediators of glomerular damage

Neutrophils. In many forms of glomerulonephritis neutrophils are prominent in the glomerular tuft (e.g. in antiglomerular basement membrane antibody disease and in acute proliferative glomerulonephritis; see below). This is due to activation of the complement cascade by immune complexes deposited within the glomerulus and generation of chemotactic substances from C3 and C5. Release of proteolytic enzymes from neutrophils is then thought to be of significance in causing damage to the capillary wall and resultant leakage of protein and red cells.

Monocytes. In many instances of glomerular disease neutrophils are not prominent even when there is hypercellularity of the glomerular tuft which is due instead to infiltration by monocytes. These cells can be identified by immunocytochemical techniques.

Glomerular recruitment of these cells could be due to one of several mechanisms:
- attraction by lymphokines released by activated T cells;
- Fc receptors on monocyte surfaces binding to IgG;
- binding to activated complement components;
- chemotaxis to activated C5a;
- binding to components in the glomerulus, e.g. laminin, fibronectin, attraction by fibrin.

Similarly, the mechanism whereby monocytes might potentiate glomerular damage could be by release of proteolytic enzymes.

Other mediators of glomerular injury

Undoubtedly, there are many other possible mechanisms whereby glomerular damage may occur but these are still under investigation. Among the more prominent of these are the following.

Free oxygen radicals. These are generated by the respiratory burst of infiltrating granulocytes and may cause damage by lipid peroxidation of cell membranes or by direct degradation of the glomerular basement membrane.

Prostanoids and eicosanoids. Arachidonic acid metabolites are generated during the process of immune complex deposition in the glomerulus and, although prostaglandin B_1 may protect against glomerular injury thromboxane A_2 is thought to disturb glomerular function.

Coagulation products. Evidence for involvement of the blood coagulation cascade in glomerular injury is largely of an indirect nature, though fibrin is readily demonstrated in some forms of proliferative glomerulonephritis and is known to be associated with crescent formation. Furthermore, in patients with nephritis there is elevation of serum and urinary levels of fibrinogen and fibrin-related antigens.

Diagnosis of glomerular disease

In any patient with glomerulonephritis the diagnosis should contain three elements:

1 the predominant clinical symptoms such as nephrotic syndrome, haematuria, etc.;

2 the histological appearances;

3 the immunopathological findings.

The diagnosis is usually made following a **renal biopsy** – an essential procedure in investigation of any patient with the nephrotic syndrome. It is important to submit tissue for **light microscopy**, **immunofluorescence** and **electronmicroscopy** as in some cases of renal disease the appearances in the glomeruli may be difficult to distinguish from normal on light microscopy alone, e.g. minimal change (see below).

Proteinuria

The **nephrotic syndrome** is a major presenting feature in many renal diseases. In some instances this is associated with inflammatory changes in the glomerulus and neutrophil infiltration. Enzymes released from these neutrophils damage the capillary basement membrane and result in increased permeability to protein. Yet in many forms of glomerular disease proteinuria occurs in the absence of neutrophils. Proteinuria could result from any or all of three causes, namely excessive leak of protein into the glomerular filtrate, lack of reabsorption of protein normally present in the filtrate or tubular excretion of protein. In fact in the vast majority of cases it is due to excessive leakage of protein via the glomerulus.

The glomerular capillary wall contains fixed negatively charged sites which are the most important factor in retaining negatively charged, i.e. anionic, protein molecules in the circulation. Glomerular filtration itself depends upon the structural and physical properties of the filter (Fig. 21.7), physical properties of the molecules undergoing filtration and flow dynamics within glomerular capillaries.

Physical properties of filtration molecules

- **Size** is of major importance as clearance studies demonstrate conclusively that with molecules of increasing radius filtration diminishes and clearance is reduced.
- **Molecular charge** is also of considerable significance and clearance studies using dextrans carrying varying charges have been employed to illustrate this. These show that for any given molecular radius fractional clearance of cationic dextrans is greater than that of neutral dextrans of the same radius and similarly that of neutral dextrans is greater than that of anionic dextrans of the same size.
- The **shape of filtration molecules** is important as molecules of the same radius and weight may show differing degrees of permeability due to their differing shape. Dextran molecules are particularly flexible and can uncoil to pass through the interstices of the

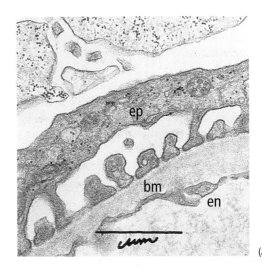

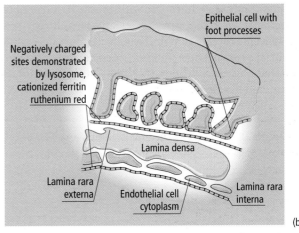

Fig. 21.7 The glomerular capillary wall. (a) Electronmicrograph showing the endothelium (en), basement membrane (bm) and epithelial foot (ep) processes. (b) Diagram showing the negatively charged sites.

glomerular basement membrane in a manner which a tightly bound rigid globular protein would be unable to achieve.

Appearances of the glomeruli in proteinuria

One of the characteristic appearances noted in the glomerulus in patients with proteinuria is **deformity** and **fusion** together with **flattening** of the **foot processes** of the epithelial cells when the glomerulus is viewed under the electronmicroscope. Indeed, in some forms of disease, notably minimal-change glomerulonephritis, this may be the only pathological finding.

Experimentally it has been shown that this alteration in epithelial cells of the glomerulus occurs prior to proteinuria. Because it results in a very considerable loss of epithelial cell surface area there is a corresponding reduction in the number of negatively charged sites which thus allows escape of protein into the urinary space.

Acute, postinfectious, diffuse, proliferative glomerulonephritis

This is one of the classical forms of **immune complex disease**. These patients present with the **acute nephritic syndrome**, which features:

- oedema, often in the loose connective tissues around the face and backs of hands;
- oliguria with urine of high specific gravity, or even anuria;
- albuminuria;
- haematuria, the urine often being described as smoky but it may be bright red in colour;
- hypertension.

In a typical case the disease follows 1–2 weeks after an upper respiratory infection with group A β-haemolytic streptococcus and occurs particularly in children. Today **poststreptococcal glomerulonephritis** is rare but this form of postinfectious nephritis has been described following a variety of other infections, including not only bacterial but also viral and parasitic diseases (Table 21.9).

Table 21.9 Diseases which may be associated with acute glomerulonephritis.

Bacterial causes
Group A β-haemolytic streptococcus
Streptococcus pneumoniae
Staphylococcus aureus
Neisseria meningitidis
Klebsiella pneumoniae
Treponema pallidum
Brucella melitensis
Leptospira spp.
Salmonella typhi
Mycoplasma pneumoniae
Viral diseases
Varicella
Mumps
Epstein–Barr virus
Hepatitis B
Cytomegalovirus
Coxsackievirus
Rickettsial diseases
Typhus
Rocky Mountain spotted fever
Parasitic diseases
Trichinosis
Falciparum malaria
Toxoplasmosis

Furthermore, advent of renal biopsy resulted in the realization that the acute nephritic syndrome could occur in other forms of nephritis and in glomerular lesions associated with systemic disease.

Pathology

Today death is unusual in the acute stage but, if it does occur within a week or so of the onset, the kidney is swollen with a smooth subcapsular surface punctuated by petechiae. On the cut surface the cortex may be rather pale but glomeruli can often be seen with the naked eye standing out as grey glistening dots.

Light microscopy reveals that all glomeruli are affected and show:

- increased cellularity (Fig. 21.8);
- neutrophil infiltration;
- focal fibrin deposition in the capillaries (Fig. 21.9);
- focal areas of necrosis in the capillary tuft.

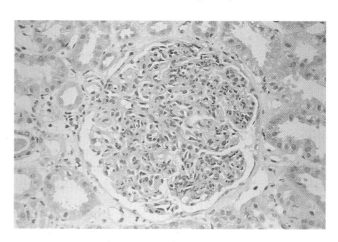

Fig. 21.8 The glomerulus in acute proliferative post-infectious glomerulonephritis. The glomerulus shows increased cellularity and many neutrophils are present. (H&E.)

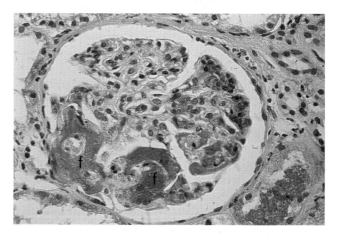

Fig. 21.9 Fibrin (f) deposition and capillary thrombosis in acute proliferative post-infectious glomerulonephritis. (Martius Scarlet blue (MSB).)

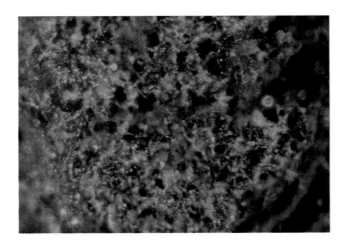

Fig. 21.10 Acute proliferative post-infectious glomerulonephritis. Immunofluorescent preparation using a fluorescein conjugated anti-C3 antibody shows granular deposition of C3 scattered throughout the mesangium and on the capillary basement membrane.

On **immunofluorescence microscopy** there is irregular granular distribution of the C3 component of complement on the epithelial aspect of the glomerular basement membrane and in the mesangium (Fig. 21.10), as well as IgG, though occasionally IgM may be seen. Bacterial antigen is seldom demonstrated but in a few cases it has been reported.

On **electronmicroscopy** scattered electron-dense deposits of variable size (Fig. 21.11) may be seen in the subepithelial position but also occasionally elsewhere. There is swelling of both endothelial and mesangial cell cytoplasm, and fibrin deposition. Neutrophils are often encountered and may be seen applied directly to glomerular basement membrane.

Correlation of clinical and pathological findings

The oliguria is mainly the result of obliteration of capillary lumens by swollen endothelial cells and the general increase in cellularity obliterating Bowman's space while haematuria comes from necrosis of the glomerular tuft. Oedema is probably mainly the result of water and salt retention but if protein loss is considerable it may form part of the nephrotic syndrome. The reason for hypertension is less clear as it has been reported to precede the onset of albuminuria. Ischaemia of the kidney may be responsible but hypervolaemia and sodium retention are also probably of considerable importance.

Progression

The ultimate prognosis in most patients with postinfectious glomerulonephritis has been thought to be good but there are no reliable modern statistics. Some patients proceed to a fulminant course and today many cases of acute proliferative glomerulonephritis are part of a systemic disease such as systemic lupus erythematosus where the outcome may be governed by factors other than the renal lesion.

Glomerulonephritis with crescents

It has long been recognized that widespread presence of epithelial crescents in the glomerulus indicated a poor prognosis. They are a feature of severe glomerulonephritis and are associated with fibrin in the urinary space beneath Bowman's capsule. Ultrastructural, immunocytochemical and cell culture techniques have demonstrated that crescents consist not only of epithelial cells but also of macrophages, which is not surprising as the latter ingest and process exuded fibrin.

Crescentic nephritis may be classified into three main groups:
1 severe **immune complex disease** of any type;
2 cases which on immunofluorescent investigation show an absence of immunoglobulins or complement deposition—so-called **pauci-immune glomerulonephritis**, of which the outstanding examples are **Wegener's granulomatosis** and **micropolyarteritis** (see below);
3 antiglomerular basement membrane (**anti-GBM**) glomerulonephritis.

Disorders in which crescents are commonly found are given in Table 21.10.

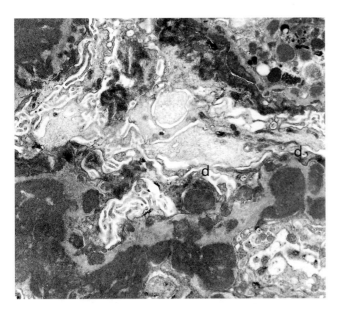

Fig. 21.11 Acute proliferative post-infectious glomerulonephritis. Electronmicrograph of the glomerulus shows electron dense subepithelial deposits (d). (×8700).

Table 21.10 Diseases associated with glomerular crescents.

> *Crescents are frequently seen in:*
> Antiglomerular basement antibody disease
> Postinfectious immune complex glomerulonephritis
> Henoch–Schönlein purpura
> Micropolyarteritis
>
> *Crescents are sometimes seen in:*
> Systemic lupus erythematosus
> Wegener's granulomatosis
> Membranoproliferative glomerulonephritis
> Membranous glomerulonephritis (very rare)
> Cryoglobulinaemia
> Malignant hypertension
> Haemolytic–uraemic syndrome

Antiglomerular basement membrane disease

This may occur at any age and both sexes are equally affected. The disease may follow an infection but this is by no means always so and most cases appear to arise without any predisposing cause. Clinical features are variable but patients present with a fairly acute onset of oliguric renal failure with haematuria. Renal biopsy is essential for diagnosis.

On **light microscopy** extensive numbers of epithelial crescents are seen (Fig. 21.12). In many cases up to 95% of glomeruli may be involved. Appearances depend on the stage in the disease at which the biopsy is taken but certainly in the early days fibrin can be readily demonstrated in the crescents. The initial lesion in the glomerular tuft may be segmental necrosis and this is accompanied by neutrophil infiltration and followed by diffuse infiltration of the whole glomerulus.

Immunofluorescence microscopy is essential for definitive diagnosis. There is striking linear fluorescence (Fig. 21.13) outlining glomerular capillaries when sections are treated with the appropriate fluorescent conjugated antibody. Most frequently IgG and C3 are detected but rarely IgM or IgA may be found.

On **electronmicroscopy** there is an absence of electron-dense deposits of the type seen in immune complex disease. There are no clear diagnostic changes. The lamina densa in the basement membrane is thought by some to show a uniformly increased density but this remains a subjective judgement. However, using immunohistochemical methods it has been demonstrated that the antibody is localized to the inner aspect of the basement membrane along the lamina rare interna. Electron-dense material with the periodicity of fibrin is readily identified in capillaries, in the urinary space and in crescents. Discontinuities in the basement membrane of Bowman's capsule are often described.

Goodpasture's syndrome

This is a well-recognized variant of anti-GBM antibody disease in which pulmonary symptoms, usually haemoptysis, accompany renal changes. Although it may occur at any age, it is most often encountered in young men. There is severe intra-alveolar haemorrhage but findings in the kidney are identical with those seen in anti-GBM antibody disease described above. Recently it has been shown that those patients with anti-GBM disease who have lung haemorrhage are almost invariably cigarette smokers. This may be related to release of proteolytic enzymes from neutrophils which are sequestrated in alveolar capillaries during cigarette smoking.

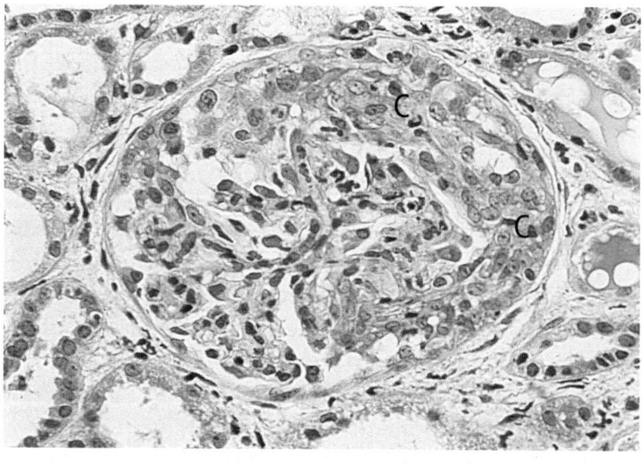

Fig. 21.12 Glomerulus shows a large epithelial crescent (C). (H&E.)

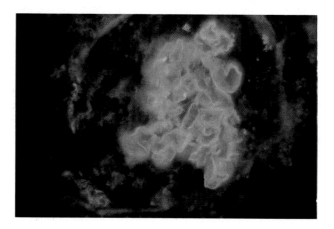

Fig. 21.13 Immunofluorescent preparation using a fluorescein conjugated anti-IgG antibody shows linear deposition of IgG along the length of the glomerular basement membrane.

On **immunofluorescent investigation** linear deposits of IgG and C3 are found on the alveolar basement membrane.

Pathogenesis. The pathogenesis of anti-GBM antibody disease is somewhat obscure but the antigens involved have been well-characterized and involve an epitope within the globular domain of type 4 collagen found in glomerular and alveolar basement membranes.

Several possible mechanisms have been suggested:

- The disease sometimes occurs following a **viral infection** and it is possible that there is a **cross-reaction** between **basement membrane** and antibodies to **viral antigens**.
- The disease has occasionally followed chronic exposure to **hydrocarbon solvents** and one theory that has been postulated is that these may alter the patient's tissues in some way to render them immunogenic.
- Environmental factors of a microbiological or chemical nature may **damage** pulmonary tissues to expose **basement membrane** antigens normally excluded from the circulation, allowing them to react with circulating anti-GBM antibodies.
- The antigenic stimulus may lie within the patients themselves. There is a high incidence of the phenotype human leucocyte antigen **(HLA) DR2** among these patients.

Membranous glomerulonephritis

The **nephrotic syndrome** may occur in many forms of renal disease but historically the best known of these is membranous glomerulonephritis. Experimentally a disease resembling this condition has been produced in rabbits by giving repeated small injections of foreign protein, usually bovine serum albumin. Investigation of the kidney in such animals reveals typical changes of chronic, as opposed to acute, immune complex disease very similar to the findings described below.

Clinically this disease presents with insidious onset of oedema, proteinuria, hypoproteinaemia and hypercholesterolaemia. It can occur at any age and both sexes are equally involved. Untreated, the majority of cases die in 5 years, either from intercurrent infection or from CRF, though initially renal function may be normal. Spontaneous remissions do sometimes occur.

Pathology

The gross appearance of the kidney in a patient dying with the fully developed nephrotic syndrome is very characteristic. It is large with a very yellow cortex due to the presence of lipid in proximal tubular epithelial cells.

Light microscopy. In established cases glomeruli appear larger than normal but show no increase in cellularity. Capillaries are patent and the capillary wall is thickened (Fig. 21.14). Methenamine silver preparations may reveal spikes on the epithelial aspect of the capillary wall due to basement membrane material being drawn up in between the deposits (Figs 21.15 and 21.16) but for definitive diagnosis immunofluorescent preparations are needed and show striking glomerular deposits of immunoglobulins, usually IgG, and complement components outlining the capillary loops (Fig. 21.17).

On **electronmicroscopy** these deposits are seen on the subepithelial aspect of the basement membrane (Fig. 21.18) accompanied by fusion of foot processes of epithelial cells. Basement membrane protrudes between

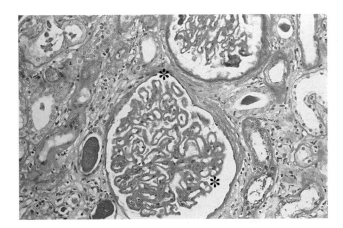

Fig. 21.14 Membranous glomerulonephritis. A periodic-acid–Schiff (PAS) preparation. The glomerulus is not unduly cellular and the capillaries are patent but their walls are thickened (✳).

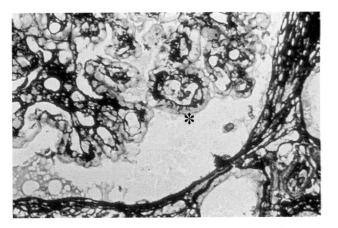

Fig. 21.15 Membranous glomerulonephritis. A methenamine silver preparation shows 'spikes' (✳) on the capillary basement membrane at a relatively early stage of the disease.

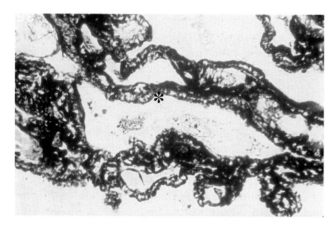

Fig. 21.16 Membranous glomerulonephritis. A methenamine silver preparation shows that the spikes have joined to form a chain (✳) on the capillary basement membrane at an advanced stage of the disease.

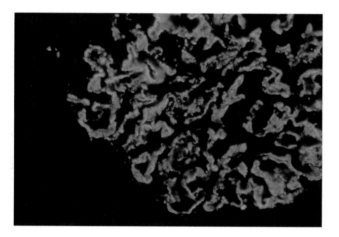

Fig. 21.17 Membranous glomerulonephritis. Immunofluorescent preparation showing granular deposition of IgG on the epithelial aspect of the capillary basement membrane.

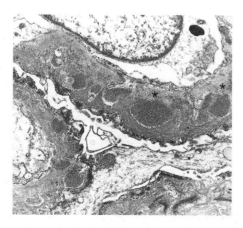

Fig. 21.18 Membranous glomerulonephritis. Electronmicrograph showing scattered electron-dense deposits (✳) on the epithelial aspect of the capillary basement membrane (×178 000).

the deposits and is the material that forms the spikes in silver preparations.

Staging

There is some evidence that an assessment of the stage of the disease is a guide to prognosis. Four stages are usually described, though some pathologists fuse stages 2 and 3 together.

- **Stage 1.** On electronmicroscopy there are a small number of subepithelial deposits. Spikes are difficult to identify in light microscope preparations at this stage.
- **Stage 2.** Light microscopy shows thickened glomerular capillary walls with well-formed spikes present in methenamine silver preparations. On electronmicroscopy there are numerous deposits covering the entire capillary loops.
- **Stage 3.** In methenamine silver preparations the spikes tend to join together to enclose deposits which then appear intramembranous on electronmicroscopy.
- **Stage 4.** This is characterized by deposits enclosed within basement membrane and difficult to distinguish from it. In occasional cases this may represent a repair stage.

In some series those patients who have undergone remission have been confined to stages 1 and 2. It should be borne in mind that these stages are those that occur with a single generation of deposits. In patients who do not recover there is continual formation of deposits due to constant exposure to antigen and no reparative phase is seen.

Proteinuria in membranous glomerulonephritis bears no relationship to the degree of basement membrane thickening. It is of the unselective variety, that is, high- as well as low-molecular-weight proteins appear in the urine. It is likely that proteinuria is due to a number of factors, foremost among which is occupation by immune complexes of negatively charged sites on the basement membrane and on the epithelial cell surface.

Membranoproliferative glomerulonephritis

This is a primary chronic progressive form of nephritis for which there are a variety of synonyms—mesangiocapillary, lobular, chronic latent and mixed membranous and proliferative glomerulonephritis.

Two types are described, with type 1 being much more frequently encountered, but both types have similar clinical presentations.

Type I

Clinical features. The primary form of the disease occurs mainly in children and young adults, often, but not always, following an upper respiratory infection. In certain forms of glomerulonephritis secondary to systemic disease identical morphology of the glomerulus may sometimes be present, e.g. in some types of systemic lupus erythematosus and in shunt nephritis (Table 21.11).

The disease usually presents insidiously with the nephrotic syndrome but differs from many other causes of this syndrome in that there is either microscopic or macroscopic haematuria and occasionally there may be a full-blown acute nephritic picture. It is thus essential to examine the urine in all cases of the nephrotic syndrome. Most patients have hypertension. The progress of the disease is variable and there are remissions and exacerbations, with the disease taking up to 10 years in 50–60% of cases before renal failure requiring dialysis or transplantation ensues.

A characteristic feature is a low level of serum C3 – found in 30–50% of cases at presentation and often being depressed at subsequent examinations in those where initial estimation was within normal limits.

Pathology. Renal biopsy is essential for diagnosis during life to distinguish this condition from other forms of nephrotic syndrome.

On **light microscopy** (Fig. 21.19) glomeruli are enlarged, cellular and often show striking lobulation. This is a consequence of an increase in mesangial cells with crowding of nuclei in the centre of the lobules. As the disease progresses mesangial matrix increases and patent capillaries are confined to the periphery of lobules. In some instances neutrophils may be prominent. The glomerular capillary walls are thickened and in methenamine silver preparations there often appears to be a reduplication of the peripheral basement membrane – so-called '**tram lining**' (Fig. 21.20). Epithelial crescents are unusual.

Immunofluorescent preparations reveal interrupted granular deposits on peripheral capillary walls (Fig. 21.21) and in the mesangium of C3 and immunoglobulins, usually IgG, occasionally IgM and rarely IgA. Occasionally only C3 is present.

Table 21.11 Systemic diseases associated with a nephritis resembling membranoproliferative glomerulonephritis on light microscopy.

Systemic lupus erythematosus
Malaria
Cryoglobulinaemia
Liver cirrhosis with α_1-antitrypsin deficiency
Atrioventricular shunt nephritis
Chronic allograft rejection

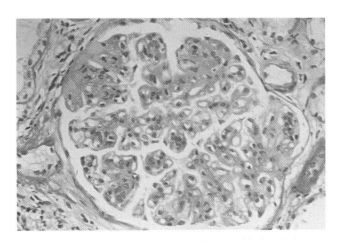

Fig. 21.19 Membranoproliferative glomerulonephritis. The glomerulus shows increased cellularity and lobularity. (H&E.)

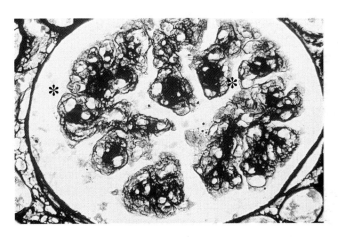

Fig. 21.20 Membranoproliferative glomerulonephritis. A methenamine silver preparation shows duplication (tram-lining) (✳) of the capillary basement membrane.

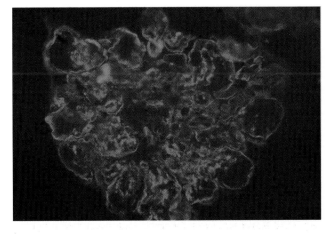

Fig. 21.21 Membranoproliferative glomerulonephritis. Immunofluorescent preparation showing C3 outlining the capillaries.

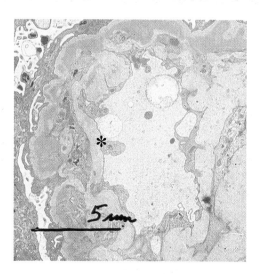

Fig. 21.22 Membranoproliferative glomerulonephritis type I. Electronmicrograph showing splitting (✳) of the capillary basement membrane. Electron-dense deposits can be seen in the capillary wall. (×180 000)

On **electronmicroscopy** electron-dense deposits are found most frequently in a subendothelial location (Fig. 21.22) but also are seen in the mesangium, in the intramembranous situation and even in the subepithelial position. In some capillaries there is intrusion of mesangial cell cytoplasm in between endothelium and basement membrane with the formation of a new basement membrane immediately beneath the endothelium. This gives rise to the tram track appearance seen on light microscopy and described above.

Type II

Very much less common than type I disease, this is probably an entirely separate entity but has been included under the general umbrella title of membranoproliferative glomerulonephritis because the clinical features and light microscopic appearances are similar in both forms of disease.

Clinical features. It presents more often as an overt acute nephritic picture, often with recurrent macroscopic haematuria. It tends to be a more aggressive disease, clinical remissions are less common and the nephritis tends to occur in a younger age group than type I. Hypertension is common.

Complement levels are more persistently depressed than in type I disease and very often a C3 nephritic factor is detected in the serum. Furthermore in some cases there is a strong association with partial lipodystrophy which may precede the nephritis by several years.

The reasons for considering this a disease entity separate from type I membranoproliferative glomerulonephritis are:

- the younger age at onset;
- more persistent depression of serum C3;
- C3 nephritic factor found in most patients;
- distinctive electronmicroscopic findings;
- association with lipodystrophy;
- the regular recurrence in renal transplants.

Pathology. **Light microscopy** shows similar appearances to those seen in type I disease but peripheral capillary walls appear thicker and are brightly eosinophilic.

On **immunofluorescent microscopy** there is smooth, often linear staining of peripheral capillary walls for C3 and this may also be seen in the basement membrane of Bowman's capsule and of the tubules. Immunoglobulins are not encountered as often but IgM is said to be predominant, followed by IgG. Early components of complement, C1q and C4, are only rarely found.

Electronmicroscopy discloses characteristic diagnostic lesions, namely thickening of the basement membrane due to the presence of electron-dense material in the lamina densa (Fig. 21.23). This material stains much more intensely than normal basement membrane or immune complex deposits and involves peripheral capillary loops and often also the basement membrane of Bowman's capsule and adjacent tubules. This material is not composed of immune complexes – there is an absence of staining for immunoglobulin in the deposits and the C3 staining seen on immunofluorescence only involves their outer margins and not the deposits themselves. The precise nature of the dense deposits is not known but they are composed

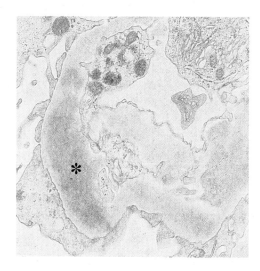

Fig. 21.23 Membranoproliferative glomerulonephritis type II (dense-deposit disease). Electronmicrograph shows a sausage-shaped deposit (✳) in the capillary wall. (×180 000).

of glycoproteins, do not contain immunoglobulin or complement and are not antigenic.

Pathogenesis. **Type I** disease is most often regarded as a form of **immune complex nephritis**. Evidence for this is provided by the presence of immunoglobulins and complement in the glomerulus, and the presence of C1q binding immune complexes in the serum. Furthermore there are several disorders known to be associated with circulating immune complexes which are deposited in the glomerulus giving rise to identical appearances in the kidney (see Table 21.11).

In **type II** disease immune complexes may be of importance but their role is, to say the least, obscure. It is likely that, as the disorder is often associated with partial lipodystrophy and recurs regularly in renal transplants, there is a fundamental systemic mechanism of **unknown aetiology** at work.

IgA nephropathy, recurrent haematuria syndrome (Berger's disease)

Clinically this usually presents in children and young adults and is often coincident with an **acute respiratory infection**, thus contrasting with acute postinfectious glomerulonephritis (see above) which occurs 1–2 weeks after an infection.

Haematuria, which may be very slight, tends to recur every time the patient has an upper respiratory infection and is accompanied by mild proteinuria. The majority of cases are said to carry a **good prognosis** but a few do progress to renal failure. It is of interest that in those patients who undergo **renal transplantation** the disease may **recur** in the allograft.

Renal biopsy is of considerable importance in investigation of this disease and is necessary to exclude other causes of recurrent haematuria of renal origin. The condition can only be satisfactorily diagnosed by a combination of light, immunofluorescence and electronmicroscopy.

Pathology

Light microscopy may show very few changes in some cases but typically there is localized crowding together of mesangial cell nuclei in a segment of the glomerular capillary tuft (Figs 21.24 and 21.25). The precise source of haematuria is difficult to determine as fibrinoid necrosis and capillary thrombosis are only very rarely encountered. In established cases segmental areas of hyalinization may be seen and there are occasional tuft adhesions between the glomerular capillaries and Bowman's capsule. The typical lesion is thus a focal segmental

glomerulonephritis. Tubulointerstitial tissues are normal apart from occasional red cells within tubular lumens. The presence of interstitial fibrosis and tubular atrophy are reliable signs of a poor prognosis but are rarely encountered.

Immunofluorescence microscopy (Fig. 21.26) reveals plentiful IgA in the mesangium, even in glomeruli that on light microscopy appear within normal limits. IgG is less often found and C1q and C4 are not present, pointing to the alternate pathway of complement activation.

Electronmicroscopy (Fig. 21.27) may require extensive sampling and careful searching to reveal typical well-defined electron-dense mesangial deposits. These are found at the base of capillary loops and only rarely extend into the subepithelial position. Generally the epithelial foot processes are normal.

Pathogenesis

The role of IgA, which is not normally complement fixing,

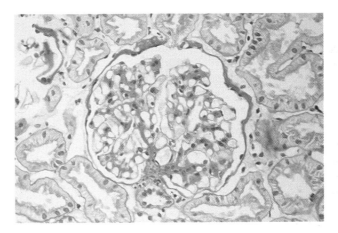

Fig. 21.24 IgA nephropathy. Focal increased cellularity and an increase in mesangium in the glomerulus. (PAS.)

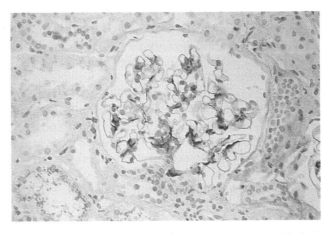

Fig. 21.25 IgA nephropathy. Immunohistochemistry using the APAAP technique shows IgA deposits (red) in the mesangium.

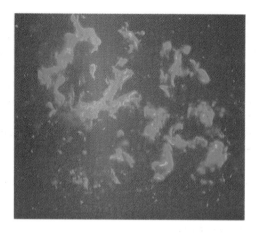

Fig. 21.26 IgA nephropathy. Immunofluorescent preparation shows IgA in the mesangium.

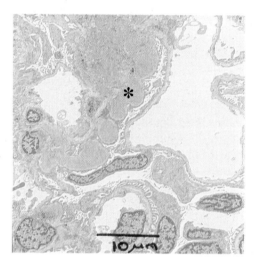

Fig. 21.27 IgA nephropathy. Electronmicrograph shows deposits (✳) in the mesangium.

in production of this disease is unclear. Both serum and nasal levels of IgA may be elevated. It has been suggested that following a respiratory infection of possibly viral origin products of the organism become sequestered in the mesangium. Further infections give rise to an IgA response and the antibody then reacts with antigen present in the mesangium, giving rise to the changes in the glomerulus. Unfortunately, this goes no way to explaining recurrence of the disease in transplants.

Relationship to Henoch–Schönlein purpura

There are certain striking similarities between IgA nephropathy and Henoch–Schönlein purpura (see below) in that both conditions are characterized by a segmental glomerulonephritis with IgA deposition.

This forms the basis of the suggestion that the two conditions may represent different forms of a single disease process – IgA nephropathy being a monosymptomatic form of Henoch–Schönlein purpura. In both diseases renal findings are usually found to be identical and it is only the presence of a rash, abdominal pain and the rather more severe proteinuria that distinguishes Henoch–Schönlein purpura.

Minimal change

This is the **commonest cause** of the **nephrotic syndrome** and accounts for 30% of all cases. In children under 5 years the proportion is much higher. There is a preponderance of males to females of the order of 2:1.

Clinically, it presents with the insidious onset of oedema and investigation reveals hypoalbuminaemia accompanied by heavy proteinuria, often of a selective variety, i.e. consisting of predominantly low-molecular-weight proteins. Blood pressure and renal function are within normal limits. The disease often appears to follow an infection but no sound aetiological connection between infection and the disease has been established.

Although haematuria is absent in the majority of cases, in up to 10% blood may be detected on microscopy. When the disease occurs in those over 15 years, the proteinuria may be unselective and there may be slight depression of renal function, making it difficult to distinguish between this and other causes of the nephrotic syndrome on clinical grounds alone. Renal biopsy is thus essential for diagnosis. Patients with minimal change usually respond dramatically to exhibition of steroids and the prognosis is good. Before the advent of antibiotics, death from intercurrent infections, often of a somewhat bizarre nature, such as pneumococcal peritonitis, was frequent. Now it is very rare.

Pathology

At post mortem the kidneys are enlarged and have a bright yellow cortex due to lipid in the proximal tubular epithelium. Because of this, the condition is often referred to in older textbooks as 'lipoid nephrosis'.

Light microscopy shows glomeruli which appear within normal limits (Fig. 21.28) in the majority of cases. Occasionally there may be prominence of mesangial stalks but if areas of segmental sclerosis are found, this immediately raises the possibility of the condition known as focal segmental glomerulosclerosis (see below). There is no tubular atrophy or interstitial fibrosis but suitably prepared frozen sections reveal lipid in the proximal tubules in untreated cases.

On **immunofluorescence microscopy** there is complete

Pathogenesis

The **aetiology** of this disease is unknown. There are numerous theories but one which finds favour with some authorities is that it is related to a disorder of cell-mediated immunity and in particular of T-cell function. Evidence for this is circumstantial and not conclusive but is suggested by the following.

- **Remissions** of the condition occurring following **measles** infection. The measles virus is known to have an effect on cell-mediated immunity.
- **Susceptibilities of patients to infection.** Although antibodies to, for instance, pneumococcal antigens, are produced by B cells, these need the help of T cells for antibody synthesis.
- **Remissions induced by steroids** and cyclophosphamide which are known to affect T-cell function.
- **Hodgkin's disease** may sometimes give rise to the nephrotic syndrome and this is thought, almost certainly wrongly, to be a T-cell disorder. Renal biopsy in such cases reveals appearances identical to those of minimal change.

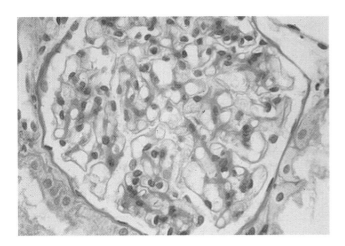

Fig. 21.28 Minimal change. The glomerulus appears normal on light microscopy.

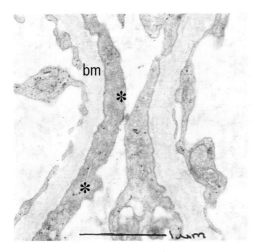

Fig. 21.29 Minimal change. Electronmicrograph shows fusion (✱) of epithelial foot processes on the glomerular capillary basement membrane (bm).

Focal segmental glomerulosclerosis

Some patients, both children and adults, present with clinical features suggesting the diagnosis of minimal-change disease but fail to respond to treatment. Renal biopsy in these patients may show identical changes to those seen in minimal change if the pathologist is not fortunate enough to sample affected glomeruli. More often the tissue will contain one or more glomeruli which show segmental sclerosis without localized hypercellularity (Fig. 21.30).

absence of any deposition of immunoglobulins or complement components.

Electromicroscopy fails to reveal any electron-dense deposits in the glomerulus and the only abnormality is fusion of epithelial foot processes (Fig. 21.29). This loss of extensive epithelial surface area reduces the negative charge on the glomerular capillary wall and thus probably plays a major role in allowing protein to leak through the glomerular filter.

In summary, the diagnosis depends upon:

- normal glomeruli being found on light microscopy;
- negative immunofluorescent staining;
- fusion of epithelial foot processes on electronmicroscopy;
- selective proteinuria;
- a good response to steroids.

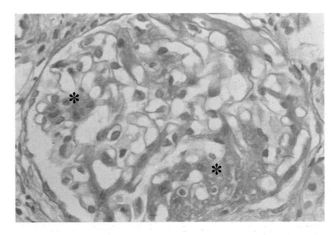

Fig. 21.30 Focal segmental glomerulosclerosis (✱) in the renal glomerulus. (H&E.)

Occasionally foam cells may be identified in the mesangium. Affected glomeruli are often in the juxtamedullary region. Care must be exercised in interpretation of these findings as occasional sclerosed glomeruli may be seen in otherwise normal subjects. Over several years this sclerotic process extends throughout the cortex with focal segmental sclerosis becoming global followed by tubulointerstitial fibrosis and subsequent renal failure.

It should be noted that focal segmental sclerosis may be found in association with many other conditions and in adults these should be excluded before the idiopathic form is diagnosed. Such conditions include:

- heroin addiction;
- acquired immune deficiency syndrome (AIDS);
- sickle-cell disease;
- healed segmental glomerulosclerosis as in, for instance, systemic lupus erythematosus.

Immunofluorescent studies have produced variable findings. In some series negative staining has been described, whereas in others IgM and C3 have been detected in sclerotic areas within the glomerulus.

On **electronmicroscopy** there is widespread loss of epithelial foot processes, though occasionally normal capillaries may be seen. In sclerotic regions there is an increase in mesangial matrix. In some cases scanty electron deposits have been reported in the mesangium in the sclerosed areas but there are no consistent findings. Another feature seen in many instances is lipid in mesangial cell cytoplasm, also observed on light microscopy, but whose significance is not understood.

Pathogenesis

The aetiology of this disease is not known. It is important to establish the diagnosis as the prognosis is not good and ultimately renal failure occurs, though this may take some years. Features which should alert the pathologist to the diagnosis in a patient who apparently has minimal change are moderate to severe tubular atrophy, interstitial fibrosis, frequent sclerotic glomeruli, segmental deposits of immunoglobulins or C3, diffuse enlargement of mesangial regions and failure to respond to steroid treatment.

Glomerular involvement in systemic disease

Glomerulonephritis in one of its many morphological forms described above may occur as part of a variety of systemic diseases. Frequently this renal involvement may be not only the presenting feature, as in some cases of the nephrotic syndrome, but in addition the severity of the renal changes may provide the key to prognosis. A short résumé of the renal features in a variety of systemic diseases is given below but for detailed description of the diseases themselves reference should be made to the relevant chapters.

Henoch–Schönlein purpura

These patients are usually **children** or **young adults** and the typical features of the disease are:

- purpura;
- abdominal pain;
- joint pains;
- nephritis with haematuria.

In the skin, joints and mesentery a vasculitis is found. Not all patients have evidence of renal involvement but when present the patient has haematuria.

Renal lesions vary from a mild segmental proliferative glomerulonephritis with focal hypercellularity to a disorder with diffuse glomerulonephritis accompanied by crescents. The latter is of grave prognostic significance if found in more than 45% of glomeruli.

Immunofluorescent preparations reveal diffuse granular deposition of IgA and often some IgG together with variable quantities of C3 and fibrinogen.

On **electronmicroscopy** there is mesangial hypercellularity and electron-dense deposits in the mesangium, sometimes extending to the subendothelial regions of the capillaries.

The invariable deposition of IgA is one of the reasons for considering that Henoch–Schönlein purpura represents an especially serious form of IgA nephropathy. As with the latter disorder, the precise pathogenesis of Henoch–Schönlein purpura has not been elucidated, though some immunological mechanism must be involved. Indeed, increased levels of circulating IgA-containing complexes have been detected in the serum. It is possible that the IgA response is a reaction to antigens presented to respiratory or gastrointestinal mucosa; indeed, the disease is often associated with an upper respiratory infection or food allergy.

Systemic lupus erythematosus

A classical form of **immune complex disease**, this is a multiple-system disorder in which every tissue of the body may be involved. It has long been recognized that renal disease in this condition is of serious prognostic significance. Yet histological appearances in the glomerulus vary greatly, as all forms of nephritis may be found.

Because of this the **World Health Organization** attempted to classify lupus nephritis and their **classification** is now in general use. It is of value because it incorporates immunofluorescent and ultrastructural features as well as light microscopy and gives some indication of prognosis.

- **Class I–normal glomeruli** on electronmicroscopy with no immunoglobulins or complement found on immunofluorescence and normal electronmicroscopy.
- **Class II–mesangial involvement.** There is mesangial prominence and hypercellularity. Immune complexes are detected on immunofluorescence and on electronmicroscopy deposits are seen in mesangial regions.
- **Class III–segmental and focal proliferative glomerulonephritis.** On light microscopy there is segmental increase in cellularity and in severe cases necrosis with exudation of fibrinoid. In later stages sclerosis is found. Immunofluorescence reveals extensive granular deposition of immune complexes and on electronmicroscopy there are subendothelial as well as mesangial deposits. Clinically these patients have a more aggressive course than classes I and II.
- **Class IV–diffuse proliferative glomerulonephritis.** This is a full-blown lupus nephritis and is probably the most common form of disease seen. All glomeruli are involved and exhibit diffuse hypercellularity and focal fibrinoid necrosis. Occasional capillary loops are thickened and exhibit bright eosinophilic staining–the so-called **'wire loop lesion'**. Crescents may be found in varying numbers. Immunoglobulins and complement components are detected arranged in a coarsely granular pattern in the mesangium and on peripheral capillary loops. On electronmicroscopy there are prominent subendothelial deposits. There is endothelial cytoplasmic swelling and some neutrophil infiltration. The **prognosis** in these patients is **poor** without treatment.
- **Class V–membranous glomerulonephritis.** The appearances here may be identical with those described in idiopathic membranous glomerulonephritis, i.e. capillary basement membrane thickening with spikes seen on silver preparations, granular deposits of IgG and C3 and extensive subepithelial electron-dense deposits on electronmicroscopy. In lupus this condition may coexist with lesions of class II, III and IV. Clinically there is nephrotic-range proteinuria and this tends to be resistant to treatment.

Other renal lesions. Tubulointerstitial changes with fibrosis and tubular atrophy may be extensive and carry a poor prognosis. Acute vasculitis involving the larger intrarenal arteries is unusual.

Bacterial endocarditis

One of the important clues to diagnosis of bacterial endocarditis is detection of **haematuria**, often of the microscopic variety, in a patient with known congenital or acquired valvular disease of the heart. In recent years with declining incidence of acute rheumatism the pattern of the disease has altered somewhat and the increased prevalence of right-sided acute endocarditis as a complication of drug addiction has tended to favour an acute form of the disease. A wide variety of organisms has been implicated.

Pathology. Involvement of the kidney has classically been referred to as **focal, embolic nephritis**, indicating erroneously that the disorder was due to microemboli from diseased valves lodging in glomerular capillaries. These were thought to cause small petechial haemorrhages visible to the naked eye on the subcapsular aspect of the kidney–an appearance referred to as **'flea-bitten' kidney**. In fact, when such embolism occurs, larger vessels are occluded and this results in small infarcts of the cortical parenchyma.

In practice, on renal biopsy, there is in most cases evidence of immune complex disease with a focal segmental proliferative glomerulonephritis in which, on immunofluorescence microscopy, IgG and C3 can be detected. Ultrastructural study shows electron-dense deposits in varying sites within the glomerulus.

Occasionally an acute diffuse glomerulonephritis may be present, often when the organism involved is *Staphylococcus aureus*. In other cases, notably those of congenital heart disease with shunts, the morphological appearances are identical with membranoproliferative glomerulonephritis.

Shunt nephritis

A condition analogous to nephritis in bacterial endocarditis complicating congenital heart disease has been described in patients with hydrocephalus treated by shunts from the cerebral ventricles to the left atrium of the heart. Such shunts are liable, as are ventricular septal defects and patent ductus arteriosus, to infection by organisms such as *Staph. aureus*.

The renal lesion in these cases is identical to that found in membranoproliferative glomerulonephritis. There is increased lobularity in the glomerulus, thickening of peripheral capillary loops and increased mesangial cellularity. Peripheral deposition of granular deposits of C3 and, less frequently, IgG or IgM is seen on immunofluorescence and electronmicroscopy reveals deposits in the subepithelial zones of the glomerular capillaries. In addition, splitting of the capillary basement membrane with interdeposition of mesangial cell cytoplasm is present. The condition has all the hallmarks of an immune-complex nephritis resulting from steady, slow release of antigen into the circulation.

Systemic sclerosis

Renal changes are not often found until late in the course of this disease and are not invariable. The lesions mainly affect arterial vessels and three classical features are cortical microinfarcts, concentric intimal thickening of interlobular arteries and fibrinoid necrosis of afferent glomerular arterioles. These changes are identical to those seen in malignant hypertension but are said to be found in the absence of this in scleroderma.

Glomerular lesions have been described with focal segmental areas of cellular proliferation and epithelial crescent formation but these are rare and often unsubstantiated. Focal capillary thrombosis and fibrinoid change are well-recognized and are secondary to the vascular changes.

RENAL INTERSTITIAL DISEASE

Interstitial nephritis

This term has been used by pathologists for nearly 100 years to describe disease in which there is severe tubulointerstitial change in the absence of glomerular lesions.

Before the advent of antibiotics it is claimed that such a condition was often present in those dying from acute infectious fevers. Indeed, reactive tubulointerstitial inflammation is found in patients with glomerulonephritis and renal infections. Today the commonest cause of primary interstitial nephritis associated with renal failure is a drug-induced lesion.

Clinical features

As indicated above, the frequent mode of presentation is renal failure with no previous history of kidney disease. Apart from signs of uraemia, there is often accompanying fever, a rash and arthralgia. Eosinophilia may be present. There is usually oliguria with the urine containing small quantities of protein, red cells and granular casts.

Pathology

The gross appearance of the kidney in those coming to necropsy may be unremarkable or may show diffuse cortical or medullary scarring with normal pyramids and calyces. The latter point serving to distinguish the condition from pyelonephritis and renal papillary necrosis described below.

Histology of renal biopsy provides the diagnosis. Glomeruli are essentially normal. There is an intense focal interstitial infiltrate composed of lymphocytes and plasma cells but also often including some eosinophils and occasional neutrophils (Fig. 21.31). Both cortex and medulla are involved. Cortical involvement of tubules is striking with erosion by the inflammatory infiltrate and

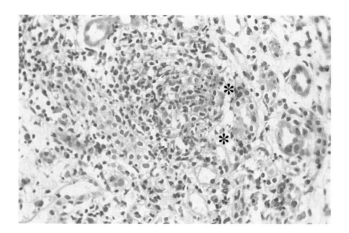

Fig. 21.31 Interstitial nephritis. There is a striking interstitial inflammatory infiltrate (✱) which includes many eosinophils. (H&E.)

focal necrosis of epithelium. In lesions of some standing, tubular atrophy is prominent with dilatation and cast formation. Small granulomas are sometimes found.

Immunofluorescent studies reveal an absence of immunoglobulins and complement in glomeruli but in some instances the third component of complement may be found on the tubular basement membrane accompanied by varying amounts of IgG.

Aetiology

As already mentioned, many of these cases are drug-induced and a wide variety of drugs have been reported as responsible for the condition. Yet non-steroidal anti-inflammatory drugs, diuretics and antibiotics, particularly of the β-lactam type, are most often incriminated. Recovery may be dramatic when administration of the offending drug is stopped and steroids are given.

The pathogenesis of renal failure is not fully understood, though back-filtration through necrotic tubular epithelium has been proposed.

Analgesic nephropathy

A special form of drug-induced renal disease is **renal papillary necrosis** which accompanies **abuse of analgesics**.

Phenacetin is the drug most commonly implicated but it has usually been used in combination with aspirin and codeine. Large quantities consumed over several years are required to produce the disease and there may be a history of long-standing painful disorders such as rheumatoid arthritis. Psychiatrically disturbed middle-aged women are the most frequently affected but it can occur in adults of either sex.

Because of severe **involvement of the medulla** urinary concentration is impaired with patients experiencing **polyuria**, **nocturia** and **polydipsia**. The urine tends to be of low specific gravity and pale. The onset is often insidious with symptoms of an indefinite nature. Dramatic improvement may follow if patients cease to take the drugs. Intravenous pyelography reveals the necrotic papillae.

Pathology

The classic lesion is necrosis of one or more of the **renal papillae** (Fig. 21.32). Renal parenchyma proximal to involved papillae shows extensive interstitial lymphoplasmacytic infiltration with interstitial fibrosis and tubular atrophy. The necrotic papilla is sharply demarcated from viable kidney but, unless secondary infection has supervened, there is no inflammatory reaction at the line of demarcation as may be seen in other forms of papillary necrosis (Fig. 21.33). The diagnosis may be made on renal

Table 21.12 Causes of renal papillary necrosis.

Analgesic abuse is not the only cause of this condition, though it is the commonest in adults. Renal papillary necrosis may be found in:
Analgesic abuse (phenacetin)
Severe acute pyelonephritis, often when this coexists with diabetes mellitus
Following severe hypotensive shock, particularly in the neonatal period
Sickle-cell disease

biopsy if the papilla is sampled but must be suspected in the presence of a suitable clinical setting and severe tubulointerstitial disease (Table 21.12).

Acute tubular necrosis

ARF usually presents as **anuria** or **oliguria**, though sometimes there may be a decrease in renal function leading to nitrogen retention with a urine output in the normal range or even with **polyuria** (e.g. in disorders of the renal medulla).

ARF is usually classified as:
- prerenal, e.g. due to hypovolaemia;
- intrarenal;
- postrenal, e.g. due to bilateral ureteric calculi or bladder lesions.

Intrarenal causes include obliteration of arterial blood supply due to intrarenal arterial thromboses or severe intimal fibrosis, glomerular capillary occlusion as in acute glomerulonephritis or the group of disorders known as **tubular necrosis**.

Traditionally **acute tubular necrosis** is divided into two varieties:
- following acute hypotension and hypovolaemia;
- toxic tubular necrosis due to tubular poisons.

In practice there is overlap between these two forms and histological changes are similar though more pronounced in toxic damage. The common causes are listed in Table 21.13.

Clinical features

Minor forms of the condition are seen following hypotensive periods during and after major surgical operations. Clinically, most significant cases occur following severe trauma, burns and Gram-negative septicaemia.

Classically four stages are described:
- the **first phase** lasting 1–10 hours from the initial insult until the onset of oliguria;

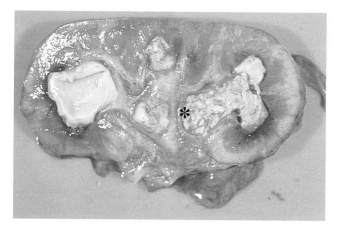

Fig. 21.32 Renal papillary necrosis (✱) in analgaesic nephropathy.

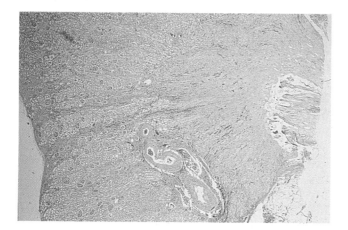

Fig. 21.33 Analgaesic nephropathy. There is renal papillary necrosis without an inflammatory infiltrate. (Trichome stain.)

Table 21.13 Conditions associated with acute tubular necrosis.

Extensive trauma
Burns
Crush injury

Postoperative shock
Pancreatitis
Peritonitis
Obstetric shock
Abortion

Intravascular haemolysis, e.g. blackwater fever, incompatible blood
   transfusion
Rhabdomyolysis

Renal poisons, e.g. mercury compounds, carbon tetrachloride, ethylene
   glycol, antibiotics, etc.

- 'anuric' phase lasting from 1 to 2 days to over 28 days depending on the severity of the lesion;
- a **diuretic phase** lasting 2–14 days when the urine resembles glomerular filtrate;
- a **recovery phase** with urine concentration returning with improved tubular function.

Pathology

Two or 3 days after the initial injury, the kidney is swollen due to oedema and there is cortical pallor. Histology based on necropsy material is notoriously difficult to interpret due to post-mortem autolysis, particularly affecting proximal tubules. Biopsy studies have indicated subtle changes.

The glomeruli are essentially within normal limits. The main changes are seen in tubules. It is often difficult to distinguish distal from proximal tubules as there is extensive loss of the brush border of the latter. Many tubules are

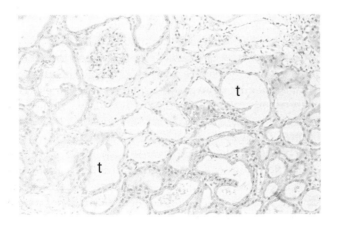

Fig. 21.34 Acute tubular necrosis. There is dilatation of the tubules (t) which are lined by flattened epithelium. (H&E.)

dilated and often lined by rather nondescript cuboidal-type epithelium (Fig. 21.34). In early cases proximal tubular epithelial cytoplasm is swollen, possibly in some cases due to treatment with intravenous hypertonic saline.

Ultrastructural examination reveals dissolution of mitochondria followed by complete necrosis of isolated cells; extensive epithelial necrosis is rare. Intratubular casts are found in both cortex and medulla but are seldom extensive enough to account for the oliguria. There is often evidence of epithelial regeneration in tubules and mitoses may be seen. Interstitial oedema is quite prominent but there is little or no accompanying lymphocytic infiltration (cf. interstitial nephritis). Occasional areas of tubular rupture, referred to as tubulorrhexis, have been reported in some cases.

An interesting and largely unexplained finding is the presence of collections of mononuclear cells in the vasa recta. Many of these are thought to be haemopoietic cells.

Pathogenesis

The cause of renal failure in this condition is much debated. The possibility of back-leak through tubular epithelium has been favoured by some authorities and evidence for this is provided by radiology. If an intravenous injection of contrast medium is given, a dense nephrogram is found which persists for several hours, whereas in normal kidneys it is cleared in 30 minutes. For a nephrogram to be formed, glomerular filtration must occur. In acute tubular necrosis it is thought that persistence of the nephrogram is due to back-leak from the tubules with the presence of contrast material in the interstitium. Some back-leak does take place but it is unlikely that this is the entire explanation for the oliguria. Other workers have demonstrated decreased cortical arterial blood flow and in some cases diminished GFR. Finally, it has been suggested that tubular obstruction due to casts formed from cellular debris might be of importance. It is likely that the pathogenesis of the oliguria is multifactorial but at the present time no convincing and unifying hypothesis exists.

RENAL INVOLVEMENT IN SYSTEMIC DISEASE

Myeloma

Myeloma is an important cause of renal failure and indeed this may be the first manifestation of the disease and is also a frequent cause of death.

Aside from the '**myeloma kidney**' described below, the kidney may be involved in several ways:

- a plasma cell tumour;
- tubular changes resulting in the Fanconi syndrome;
- secondary chronic pyelonephritis;
- amyloid disease.

The urine in myeloma

Abnormal constituents are found in the urine in most patients with myeloma whether or not they have renal symptoms. Albuminuria is frequent. Yet the typical finding is of monomers or dimers of immunoglobulin light chains known as Bence Jones protein. This is readily detected by heating urine when the protein precipitates at 55°C and redissolves at 65–70°C.

Myeloma kidney (light chain cast nephropathy)

The gross appearance of the kidney in myeloma is usually unremarkable. The diagnosis is usually made on renal biopsy material when histology (Fig. 21.35) reveals the classical tubular lesions. These consist of

- tubular casts;
- a giant cell reaction to the casts;
- tubular atrophy, and sometimes
- focal calcification.

The casts have a characteristic appearance described variously as fractured or laminated. Proximal, distal and collecting tubules may be involved. The number of casts is variable but on occasion they may be extensive. There is a reaction in adjacent tubular epithelium with formation of giant cells. Casts are composed of a variety of constituents, including albumin and fibrinogen as well as light chains.

There is some interstitial fibrosis but often surprisingly sparse plasma cell infiltration. Glomeruli are normal, contrasting with the severe tubulointerstial lesions.

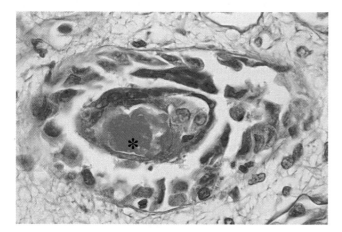

Fig. 21.35 Myeloma kidney. Note the typical 'fractured casts' (✱) and the syncytial reaction of the tubular epithelium. (H&E.)

Pathogenesis of renal failure

As with acute tubular necrosis, the precise cause of renal failure is not known but is probably multifactorial. A major contribution is thought to be toxicity of light chains on tubular epithelium. Casts to which light chains contribute may also be important.

Diabetes mellitus

The kidney may be involved in diabetes mellitus in several ways.

- In the untreated diabetic, rarely seen today, there is a striking increase in glycogen in renal tubular epithelial cells and this is responsible for the terracotta colour of the gross kidney in such cases.
- Diabetic kidneys in general show more advanced arteriosclerosis than kidneys of those of the same age without diabetes.
- There is an increased incidence of both acute and chronic pyelonephritis, sometimes accompanied by acute papillary necrosis.
- Diabetic glomerulosclerosis.

Diabetic glomerulosclerosis

This is sometimes referred to as the **Kimmelsteil–Wilson kidney** or alternatively as **diabetic nephropathy** but this latter term is best avoided as it can be taken to indicate any renal disease in a diabetic.

Clinically, albuminuria is the first sign of this condition. As the disease progresses the nephrotic syndrome may develop and finally renal failure, usually accompanied by hypertension, supervenes.

Pathology

Grossly the kidneys are unremarkable apart from subcapsular scarring due to arteriosclerotic changes.

Histology of biopsy material (Fig. 21.36) reveals the following typical glomerular appearances.

- the **nodular lesion**, which is a spherical hyaline mass, containing a few elongated nuclei, most often situated near the periphery of the glomerular tuft and usually surrounded by patent capillaries. This is often called nodular intercapillary glomerulosclerosis and is the most characteristic of the glomerular lesions.
- the **diffuse lesion** or diffuse intercapillary glomerulosclerosis affects, as the name implies, the entire glomerulus. There is thickening of mesangial lobular stalks and this is followed by increased thickness of the capillary basement membrane. It differs from the appearance seen in membranous glomerulopathy in that the thickening is more uniform and there is an

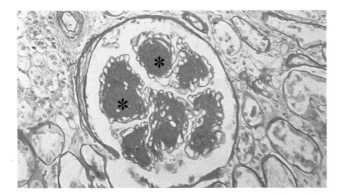

Fig. 21.36 The Kimmelstiel–Wilson lesion (✻) in diabetic glomerular nephropathy. This shows the nodular lesion.

absence of bristles or spikes in methenamine silver preparations.
- the **capsular drop** lesion is a homogeneous, waxy, eosinophilic mass of variable size situated between the basement membrane and overlying epithelium of Bowman's capsule. It is not specific for the disease.
- the **'fibrin' cap** lesion is an exudative change which is not specific of diabetes. It is an eosinophilic lipo-hyaline structure found on the top of a capillary loop and is situated between endothelium and basement membrane.

The pathogenesis of these diabetic lesions is not understood. In spite of many attempts to implicate an immunological mechanism, none has been substantiated. Immunoglobulins and complement when found in glomeruli are considered to be the result of non-specific trapping rather than deposition of immune complexes.

Amyloid

Renal involvement with amyloid is one of the important causes of proteinuria and the **nephrotic syndrome**. The diagnosis of amyloid depends upon:
- affinity for Congo red and its dichroism when viewed with polarized light;
- a characteristic fibrillar pattern on electronmicroscopy;
- its X-ray diffraction pattern.

The kidney is involved in both primary, amyloid light chain (AL), and secondary amyloid of the AA type associated with chronic inflammatory diseases but it may also be found on occasion in other forms, e.g. amyloid associated with myelomatosis of the AL type (see Chapter 7).

Pathology

In early stages of the disease the kidney is large. This is an important point when considering the differential diagnosis of the nephrotic syndrome as in many other causes the kidney is of normal size. The cut surface has a strikingly yellow appearance to the cortex.

Histology

The diagnosis is based on renal biopsy. On occasion amyloid infiltration may be relatively inconspicuous, making it imperative to stain every renal biopsy with Congo red so as not to overlook the diagnosis. A similar argument may be applied for routinely subjecting all biopsies to electronmicroscopy.

Although all parts of the kidney may be involved, it is the glomerular infiltrate that usually predominates. The mesangium is affected first, often at the hilum of the glomerulus, with mesangial cell nuclei being displaced by amorphous eosinophilic material. Later, capillary walls are infiltrated and eventually the glomerulus may be obliterated. Before this stage is reached, amyloid can be easily seen in tubular basement membranes and in blood vessels. Distinction between AA or AL amyloid can be made on immunofluorescence microscopy using specific monoclonal antibodies. On electronmicroscopy amyloid is seen as randomly arranged non-branching fibrils 8–10 nm in width and varying considerably in length.

Polyarteritis nodosa

Two forms of polyarteritis are recognized.

The first or **classical** form affects larger muscular arteries in many organs and is characterized by an inflammatory cell infiltrate involving all layers, including the adventitia. It often involves arterial vessels at their bifurcations, causing small aneurysms to form – hence the term nodosa. Many different organs including kidney may be affected.

In the second form, known as **micropolyarteritis**, it is smaller vessels and especially glomerular capillaries that are involved and there is a focal necrotizing glomerulitis with fibrinoid change and crescent formation. Immunofluorescent studies often do not reveal any deposition of immune complexes or complement, this being a form of so-called pauci-immune glomerulonephritis in which a circulating anti-neutrophil cytoplasmic antibody (ANCA) is often found.

Wegener's granulomatosis

This is a special form of vasculitis in which there is:
- necrotizing granulomatous inflammation and vasculitis of the upper and lower respiratory tract;

- necrotizing glomerulonephritis with crescents;
- disseminated small-vessel vasculitis.

Thus, apart from the upper respiratory lesions, the condition is identical to micropolyarteritis, described above. These patients also fail to exhibit any consistent deposition of immunoglobulins and complement in the glomeruli and also have a circulating ANCA in their serum. Thus it seems likely that micropolyarteritis and Wegener's granulomatosis represent two ends of a spectrum of disease (see Chapter 15).

The kidney in pregnancy

The urine during normal pregnancy contains an increased quantity of protein; this reverts to normal after delivery. In **pre-eclamptic toxaemia**, or the specific hypertensive disease of pregnancy, proteinuria is greatly increased. This condition is commoner during the first pregnancy and usually presents in the third trimester. Arterial pressure is raised and may reach considerable levels. In severe cases eclampsia with convulsions occurs – nowadays mercifully very rare.

Pathology

It is difficult to obtain renal biopsies during pregnancy and only a few studies have been performed in pre-eclampsia. There is generalized glomerular enlargement with narrowing of capillary lumens due to endothelial swelling and an increase in mesangium. Fibrin is not present in the capillaries unless full-blown eclampsia supervenes and there is no neutrophil polymorphonuclear leucocytic infiltration. Oedema of the wall of small arteries and arterioles is often present.

Electronmicroscopy has demonstrated, in addition to endothelial and mesangial cytoplasmic swelling, an amorphous subendothelial deposit which immunofluorescence microscopy has revealed to contain fibrin and IgM.

The aetiology of this condition is not understood but there are two hypotheses:
- that it is related to a **disorder of blood coagulation** with a slow low-grade intravascular coagulation as the primary process;
- that it is a **consequence of placental ischaemia**, possibly brought about by intravascular coagulation in the uterine vascular bed.

Renal cortical necrosis

A rare cause of acute renal failure, this condition accompanies a catastrophic hypotensive episode of **severe shock** associated with hypovolaemia or endotoxaemia.

It is by no means solely allied to pregnancy, though many descriptions of its pathology have been related to obstetric disasters. It is a recognized complication of acute pancreatitis and may sometimes be found in fatal cases of shock due to multiple fractures, haemorrhage and burns. In the neonate it can complicate dehydration following gastroenteritis and in adults has been described in cholera. Since all these conditions have also been associated with acute tubular necrosis, it is likely that the two conditions are opposite ends of a single spectrum.

Pathology

The lesions found have been graded into focal, minor and gross. In the fully developed or gross lesion at between 5 and 15 days the kidneys appear normal in shape but are enlarged. The cut surface presents a remarkable appearance as, apart from a very thin rim of subcapsular cortex, which obtains its blood supply from capsular vessels, the entire cortex is necrotic and yellow in colour, contrasting with the sharply demarcated red medulla. Histology confirms that there is total infarction of the cortex.

The pathogenesis of this condition, which is always related to severe shock, is thought to be due to spasm of intrarenal arteries followed by thrombosis.

Haemolytic–uraemic syndrome

This syndrome is characterized by a haemolytic anaemia, thrombocytopenia and renal failure. This syndrome is associated with **excessive platelet activation**.

The condition is rare but is found in the following situations:
- as part of the symptom complex of postpartum renal failure occurring up to 10 weeks after delivery;
- in cases of renal allograft rejection;
- severe hypertension;
- malignant disease;
- systemic lupus erythematosus;
- in infants as oliguria or anuria accompanied by diarrhoea, hypertension, neurological manifestations, a bleeding diathesis and anaemia, where it is associated with *Escherichia coli* 0157 infection in summer months. The organism and its verocytotoxin may be isolated from the stool.

The renal changes are similar in adult and childhood forms of haemolytic–uraemic syndrome. On renal biopsy the main early changes are in glomeruli where capillaries are occluded by fibrin thrombi and there is segmental necrosis of the glomerular tufts. After a few days mesangial and endothelial cell proliferation occurs and there is crescent formation. In post-mortem material from an early case thrombosis and necrosis are found in larger intrarenal vessels but in later cases there is concentric mucoid intimal fibrosis and smooth-muscle proliferation.

The kidney and tropical disease

In western countries the commonest cause of the **nephrotic syndrome** in childhood is minimal change (see above). Yet in children worldwide it is most often associated with *Plasmodium malariae* infection. The nephritis in these children is of the immune-complex variety. On light microscopy there is thickening of peripheral capillary walls and an increase in mesangium associated with mesangial cell proliferation. On ultrastructural study there are electron-dense deposits, usually but not always situated in the subendothelial position. Immunoglobulins, most often IgM, and C3 can be demonstrated on the glomerular capillary basement membrane distributed in a granular fashion consistent with an immune-complex nephritis.

Malaria is not the sole cause of the nephrotic syndrome in the tropics as similar forms of nephritis have been described in Senegal where infection with *P. malariae* is low but no convincing aetiological agent has been demonstrated in these cases. Similarly nephritis of the immune-complex type has been described in leprosy and, in Brazil, in association with *Schistosoma mansoni*.

Sickle-cell disease may involve the kidney in a variety of ways:

• segmental glomerular fibrosis and necrosis associated with blockage of glomerular capillaries by sickle-cell aggregation;
• acute tubular necrosis following sickle-cell crisis;
• medullary scarring;
• papillary necrosis—both of the latter associated with ischaemia.

Haematuria is a frequent occurrence in this disease.

Renal osteodystrophy

Osteitis fibrosis (± osteomalacia) 2° to 2° hyperparathyroidism affects up to 50% of patients with chronic renal failure and involves a high rate of bone turnover. Calcitonin levels remain (N) until creatinine clearance is < 40 ml/min, then a linear decline to undetectable levels at 5 ml/min. 2° hyperparathyroidism develops early in renal disease. Plasma phosphate shows a positive correlation with intact PTH levels so to maintain plasma Ca there is increased phosphate loss from bone and ↑ bone tumour and osteitis fibrosa.

The aim of vitamin D (1αOHD or 1,25(OH)2D) replacement, in large doses, is fourfold.

1 To replace vitamin D.
2 ↑ Ca absorption from the gut.
3 To suppress PTH release (direct and indirect).
4 To suppress bone turnover (measured by alkaline phosphatase activity).

Parathyroidectomy is an option if this therapy is unsuccessful.

RENAL TUMOURS

Benign renal tumours

Benign tumours of the kidney are **rare** and of little importance (Table 21.14).

Angiomyolipoma may occur either in isolation or as part of the syndrome of **tuberous sclerosis**.

Simple **fibromas** may be found in the medulla. Tubular **adenomas** are more frequent in kidneys that are the seat of chronic disease but are difficult or impossible to distinguish from renal tubular adenocarcinoma on histological grounds alone.

Wilms tumour and renal adenocarcinoma are the two most important malignant tumours.

Wilms tumour or nephroblastoma

This is one of the most frequently encountered malignant tumours in young children. It is notable for being found with equal frequency throughout the world and is said to affect 1 in 200000 children. The vast majority occur before the age of 5 years. Cytogenetic studies have shown that the tumour is associated with deletion of a portion of the short arm of chromosome 11 (see Chapter 11).

Clinically it may present as an abdominal mass associated with microscopic haematuria. Half the patients have hypertension. There is an association with certain congenital abnormalities, notably aniridia and hemihypertrophy.

Pathology

Usually only one kidney is involved but bilateral cases do occur. Tumours are large, sharply demarcated round masses which may almost completely replace the renal parenchymal tissue and attain weights of up to 600 g (Fig. 21.37). The cut surface is greyish white in colour and punctuated by areas of haemorrhage and necrosis. Invasion of the renal vein is a common feature.

On histological examination (Fig. 21.38) three elements are present:

Table 21.14 Renal neoplasms.

	Frequency	Appearance	Histology	Clinical features	Additional features
Benign					
Renal cortical adenoma	Common	<3.0 cm; firm circumscribed yellowish nodule in the renal cortex	Cytologically clear cells usually an incidental	Asymptomatic; differentiation from a finding	When found during life, small renal adenocarcinoma depends upon behaviour
Renal oncocytoma	Rare	May be large. Brown in colour	Uniform large cells with small, regular nuclei and granular cytoplasm	Slowly growing	Difficult to differentiate from oncocytic renal adenocarcinoma
Angiomyolipoma	Uncommon	May be large, solitary or multiple	Mature fat, vessels and smooth muscle	Mass. Presents with haematuria	Associated with tuberous sclerosis
Juxtaglomerular apparatus tumour	Very rare	Small, solid mass in cortex	Small, round cells arranged in nests and sheets	Hypertension due to increased renin secretion by tumour	Rare cause of secondary hypertension in a young patient
Congenital mesoblastic nephroma	Rare	May be large; circumscribed, firm, pale mass; whorled surface	Benign fibroblastic spindle cell proliferation	Mass during neonatal period	Occurs in first 3 months of life
Malignant					
Renal adenocarcinoma	Common	Usually large	Clear cells of varying cytological appearance	Mass or haematuria	1–2% of all cancers in adults
Transitional cell carcinoma	Common	Papillary mass in renal pelvis	Papillary urothelial neoplasms of varying grades	Haematuria or mass	Multiple tumours may be present
Primary sarcomas	Very rare	Large masses; usually in capsule and fat	Depends on type of sarcoma	Mass	
Nephroblastoma (Wilms tumour)	Common in children	Large; firm, solid mass	Primitive small spindle cells	Abdominal mass	25–30% of cancers in children under 10 years

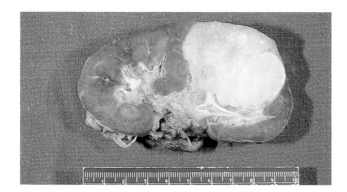

Fig. 21.37 Wilms tumour of the kidney seen here in a child.

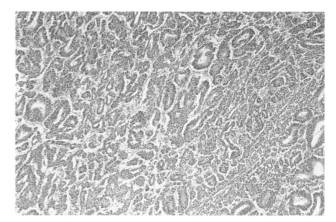

Fig. 21.38 Wilms tumour. Histology shows small cells (of the blastoma) arranged in trabeculae. (H&E.)

- metanephric blastema, similar to normal embryonic tissue;
- primitive epithelial elements;
- immature stroma.

The tumour cells in general show much nuclear variability and a high nuclear cytoplasmic ratio. A considerable diversity of appearance is encountered, including skeletal muscle, neural tissue, bone and a variety of epithelia. Primitive renal differentiation with proglomeruli and primitive tubules is often present.

The prognosis is poor, though improving with modern therapy. It is said to be more favourable if well-differentiated elements such as striated muscle are present.

Adenocarcinoma (clear cell carcinoma, hypernephroma, Grawitz tumour)

This is the commonest malignant tumour of the kidney with a peak incidence between 50 and 60 years. Males are more often affected than females and there is an association with cigarette smoking. Clinically it usually presents with haematuria, loin pain and abdominal mass but systemic effects such as hypertension and pyrexia are common.

Pathology

The tumour involves renal cortex at first and is typically spherical with a false capsule formed by compression of adjacent normal tissue (Fig. 21.39). The cut surface has a variegated appearance. It is often predominantly bright yellow in colour due to lipid in the tumour cell cytoplasm and there are prominent areas of haemorrhage and necrosis. It invades the renal pelvis and renal vein.

There is considerable histological diversity. The commonest type of lesion consists of solid sheets together

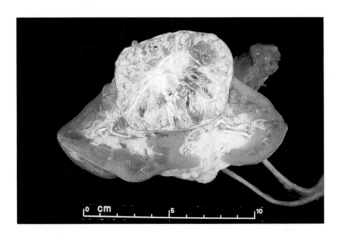

Fig. 21.39 Renal adenocarcinoma arising in the renal cortex. Note the striking yellow colour.

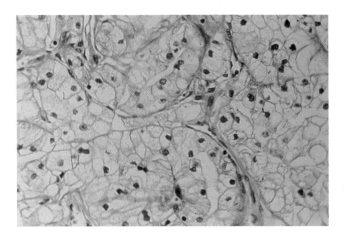

Fig. 21.40 Renal adenocarcinoma. Histology of a well-differentiated tumour. Note the large clear cells that are produced by removal of fat during routine processing of the tissue.

with alveolar or tubular collections of clear cells (Fig. 21.40). However, papillary and spindle cell patterns are also frequently encountered. Sometimes tumour cells have plentiful pink granular cytoplasm, known as oncocytic change, associated with giant mitochondria. The cell of origin is thought to be in the proximal convoluted tubule.

The tumour spreads by direct invasion, by lymphatics and especially via the blood stream. Pulmonary, bone and brain metastases are frequent.

The prognosis depends upon the stage of the disease. Four stages are described:
1 tumour confined to the kidney;
2 invasion of perinephric fat;
3 invasion of renal vein and/or invasion of regional lymph nodes;
4 invasion of adjacent organs or distant metastases.

Renal pelvic transitional cell carcinoma

The surface of the renal pelvis is covered by transitional epithelium similar to that found in bladder and ureter.

Primary transitional cell carcinoma of the renal pelvis accounts for only 5% of renal tumours. It presents most frequently with haematuria and loin pain. The gross appearance of the tumour is of an exophytic papillary growth in the pelvis. A non-papillary lesion is rarer and appears as a rounded mass which invades the renal parenchyma and may on superficial examination be mistaken for a renal adenocarcinoma.

Histologically this tumour is identical to transitional cell neoplasms elsewhere in the urinary tract with layers of transitional cells covering a thin branching vascular fibrous connective tissue stroma. There is a variable degree of cellular pleomorphism and mitotic activity and four grades are described according to the degree of differentiation.

The prognosis depends on staging rather than grading. Four stages are described:

1 tumour confined to pelvic epithelium;
2 infiltration into the lamina propria of the epithelium;
3 infiltration into renal parenchyma;
4 invasion of adjacent structures or distant metastases.

CYSTIC DISEASES OF THE KIDNEY

Table 21.15 and Fig. 21.41 summarize the congenital and acquired cystic diseases of the kidney.

Infantile polycystic disease

This is a rare **autosomal recessive** disorder that presents in infancy with renal failure. The cut surface of the kidney shows radially arranged cysts without demonstrable normal renal parenchyma. There is an association with congenital hepatic fibrosis (see Chapter 19).

Adult polycystic kidney

The most important and commonest of these diseases is adult polycystic disease. This condition presents in adult life with loin pain, an abdominal mass and haematuria. Macroscopically, both kidneys are replaced by numerous thin-walled cysts derived from tubular epithelium (Fig. 21.42). Histologically there is normal renal tissue between these cysts.

An important cause of hypertension and of renal failure, this disease has an **autosomal dominant** inheritance. It affects 1 in 500 individuals and accounts for 5–10% of chronic dialysis patients and 5–10% of renal transplant procedures. It is associated with cysts in the liver (30%), pancreas and spleen and in 15% of patients there is an

Table 21.15 Cystic disease of the kidney.

Disease	Heredity	Age	Uni- or bilateral	Appearance	Histology	Associated malformation or disease
Simple cyst	None	Adults; rarely children	Usually unilateral	Single cyst or few cysts in the cortex	Nondescript lining	None
Dialysis cystic disease	None	Adults on long-term dialysis	Bilateral	Multiple cysts throughout cortex	Flattened tubular epithelial lining	Increased incidence of renal adenocarcinoma
Polycystic disease						
Adult polycystic disease	Autosomal dominant	Adults; rarely children	Bilateral	Large, bosselated, reniform; cysts in cortex and medulla	Glomerular cysts and cysts found anywhere along nephron	Cysts of liver, pancreas, lung; cerebral berry aneurysms
Infantile polycystic disease	Autosomal recessive	Infants, children	Bilateral	Large smooth kidney with radial fusiform cysts in cortext and medulla	Flat, cuboidal epithelium	Congenital hepatic fibrosis
Medullary cystic disease						
Medullary sponge kidney	None	Any age; usually adults	Unilateral or bilateral	Cysts at tip of papillae	Papillary cysts lined by flattened epithelium; medullary calcification	Renal stones
Uraemic medullary cystic disease	Variable	Children and adolescents	Bilateral	Small coarsely scarred kidneys with 1 to 20 mm cysts at co-medullary junction	Flat epithelial lining of cysts; glomerular sclerosis with interstitial fibrosis	None

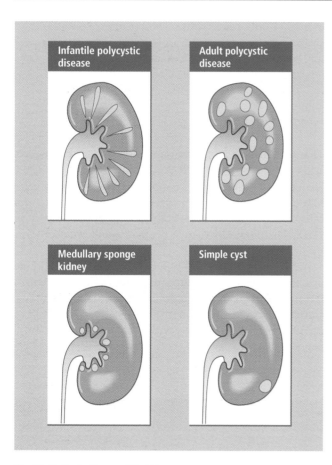

Fig. 21.41 Cystic disease of the kidney.

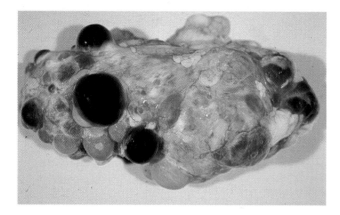

Fig. 21.42 Adult polycystic disease of the kidney. Note the enlarged kidney containing numerous thin-walled cysts, some of which contain blood.

association with congenital (berry) aneurysms of the cerebral arteries.

RENAL STONES (Table 21.16)

Renal calculi are important as they are a cause of urinary obstruction, are frequently complicated by infec-

tion and are often an indication of serious underlying metabolic disease. The most commonly encountered ones are:

- **struvite or triple phosphate stones** which contain magnesium, ammonium phosphate and carbonate apatite. These stones are found in alkaline urine and are often associated with infection. Characteristically they are large and take the form of the renal pelvis (Fig. 21.43), hence the name staghorn calculus. In cases associated with hypercalciuria it is important to exclude hyperparathyroidism, sarcoidosis and vitamin D intoxication, all conditions associated with excess calcium excretion;
- **calcium oxalate stones** are common and are very hard and black in colour due to the presence of altered blood caused by the sharp oxalate crystals injuring the renal pelvis;
- **uric acid stones** are found in some cases of gout (Fig. 21.44) but may also occur in the absence of hyperuricosuria;

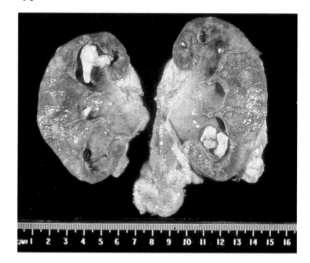

Fig. 21.43 Staghorn triple phosphate calculus of the renal pelvis.

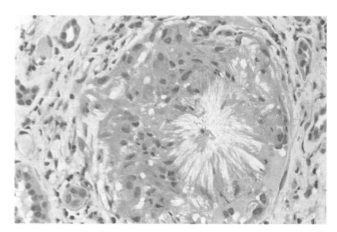

Fig. 21.44 Gout. Histology shows needle-like urate crystals in the renal parenchyma. (H&E.)

Table 21.16 Renal stones.

Type	Frequency	Predisposing factors	Urine pH	Morphology
Calcium oxalate	70%	*Hypercalcaemia* Primary hyperparathyroidism Metastatic tumours in bone Idiopathic hypercalciuria *Hyperoxaluria* Inherited Intestinal diseases High vitiamin C intake Ethylene glycol poisoning	Any pH	Hard, small (<5 mm), multiple stones; radiopaque
Phosphate calculi (mixture of calcium phosphate and magnesium ammonium phosphate)	15%	Urinary infections by urea-splitting bacteria, commonly *Proteus* spp.	Alkaline	Soft, grey-white; often large, filling the pelvicaliceal system (staghorn calculus); radiopaque
Uric acid (urates)	10%	Most cases occur in patients with normal serum uric acid levels Gout; frequency has decreased after allopurinol therapy	Acidic	Yellow-brown; small, hard, smooth; often multiple; radiolucent
Cystine and xanthine stones	Rare	Cystinuria, xanthinuria	Any pH	Yellowish; soft, waxy, small; multiple; cystine stones are slightly radiopaque; xanthine stones are radiolucent

- **cysteine stones** are found in the rare inborn error of metabolism, cystinuria, which is inherited as a Mendelian recessive. They may form staghorn calculi and are notable for not being radiopaque.

The lower urinary tract

THE URETERS

Abnormalities of the number and position of the ureters are seen in up to 2% of autopsies as incidental findings.

Idiopathic hydronephrosis involves functional obstruction at the **pelvic–ureteric junction (PUJ obstruction)**. This condition may result from congenitally abnormal ureteric innervation or muscle arrangement and its treatment is by surgical removal of the PUJ region. Long-term hydronephrosis leads to renal exstrophy.

Acquired hydronephrosis may arise from tumours of the renal pelvis or ureter, aberrant renal arteries causing compression of the ureters, impacted renal stones, fibrosis in the retroperitoneum, strictures, bladder tumour or urethral obstruction due to prostatic hyperplasia (Fig. 21.45).

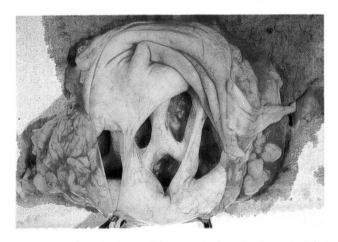

Fig. 21.45 Hydronephrosis secondary to ureteric obstruction due to renal stone. Note the grosssly dilated renal pelvis and calyceal system.

Strictures of the ureters may be the result of infection, tumour, trauma, radiation or endometriosis.

The commonest primary **tumour** of the urethra is transitional cell carcinoma, which is rare. The ureter is more commonly involved by invasion from carcinomas of the bladder, testicular germ cell tumours, carcinoma of the uterine cervix and by retroperitoneal tumours, including lymphoma.

THE BLADDER

The bladder is lined by transitional epithelium with the cells up to 7–8 cells thick. The underlying mucosa contains muscle and adventitia. Brunn's nests are invaginations of epithelium into the mucosa.

Congenital anomalies of the bladder include diverticula, exstrophy, urachus. Other rather unusual anomalies include endometriosis and amyloidosis.

FORMS OF CYSTITIS

Acute inflammation of the bladder, **acute cystitis**, may result from urinary tract infection (see below).

The bladder may be included in the field of pelvic irradiation and **radiation cystitis** will occur, probably secondary to ischaemia as a result of radiation vasculopathy.

Drugs, particularly cyclophosphamide, can cause an acute, **haemorrhagic** cystitis.

Chronic forms of **infective cystitis** are seen in tuberculosis and schistosomiasis. Chronic non-specific cystitis is characterized by epithelial hyperplasia and chronic inflammation with cystic dilatation of Brunn's nests in the submucosa, leading to **cystitis cystica**. Glandular metaplasia may occur in these nests, resulting in **cystitis glandularis**.

Hunner's interstitial cystitis is associated with ulceration, vasculitis and eosinophilia and its cause is unknown.

Malakoplakia is an unusual form of chronic inflammation that is found in the bladder, ureter, prostate, lungs, colon and renal pelvis. Macroscopically, the lesion features raised, yellow plaques or polyps in the bladder mucosa. The histology shows abundant macrophages containing round, laminated concretions containing iron and calcium called **Michaelis–Gutman bodies** (Fig. 21.46). The cause may be a defect in removal of phagocytosed microbes.

URINARY TRACT INFECTIONS

Urinary tract infections (UTIs) are very common in the community and hospital, the latter accounting for 30% of all hospital-acquired infections.

Infection may involve the **upper** (pyelitis and pyelonephritis, see above) or **lower** tract (cystitis), although both tracts are often involved. The bladder and ureters are normally sterile, whereas the anterior urethra is colonized with faecal and skin flora which cause the majority of UTIs. *Escherichia coli* is the commonest pathogen.

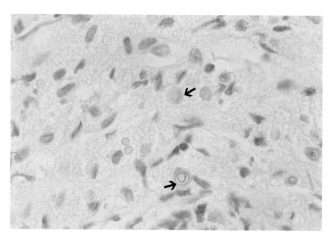

Fig. 21.46 Malakoplakia. Bladder biopsy shows the foamy macrophages and characteristic Michaelis–Gutmann bodies (arrowed). (PAS.)

Epidemiology

The incidence of UTI is related to age and sex; females are more susceptible because of a shorter urethra (Table 21.17). A proven UTI in children and males may indicate investigation for a specific underlying cause, such as underlying structural abnormalities or renal stones.

Pathogenesis

There are two main routes of infection – ascending (common) and haematogenous (rare).

Host defences include:
- regular flushing action and complete emptying of the bladder;
- antibacterial activity of secretions (e.g. prostatic secretions) and immunoglobulins (IgA).

Predisposing host factors include those in Table 21.17 and diabetes mellitus.

Uropathogenic organisms are selected from the faecal flora. For example, virulence factors for uropathogenic *E. coli* are:
- fimbriae to allow attachment to the uroepithelium;
- increased K capsule production;
- production of haemolysin.

In the presence of structural abnormalities of the bladder or catheterization, specific virulence factors are not required.

Table 21.17 Incidence of urinary tract infections.

Age	Female (%)	Male (%)	Comments
Infants (>1 year)	0.5	2.0	Congenital abnormalities, posterior urethral valves
Preschoolchildren	1.0	1.0	Structural abnormalities, vesicoureteric reflux
Schoolchildren	1.6	0.3	Structural abnormalities
Adults	4.0	0.1	Sexually active females, pregnancy
Elderly	15.0	3.5	Catheterization, neurogenic bladder, prostatism

Clinical findings

The classic symptoms of a UTI are **dysuria** and **frequency**, with or without fever. Involvement of the upper tract produces loin pain and tenderness. Exceptions to this are seen in infants and children where symptoms can be non-specific (fever, crying, feeding problems, diarrhoea and vomiting); in pregnancy and in the elderly where patients may be asymptomatic. Patients with renal tuberculosis or with renal abscesses may present with a pyrexia of unknown origin.

Investigations and interpretations

Methods of sampling urine for microbiology are given in Table 2.2, Chapter 2. Three main types of sample may be obtained:
- clean-catch (bag urine);
- midstream urine (MSU);
- catheter stream urine.

Wet preparations of urine are viewed for the presence of white cells, red blood cells, casts and organisms. For culture, 2 μl of urine is plated on to selective medium, cysteine lactose electrolyte-deficient **(CLED) agar**. The indicator in CLED is bromothymol blue and colonies of lactose fermenters are pink. The deficiency of electrolytes prevents *Proteus* sp. swarming all over the plate. The time taken for the specimen to reach the laboratory, the presence of contaminating squame cells, mixed cultures of organisms, the number of pus cells and clinical details are used in the interpretation of the results.

A significant bacteriuria is defined by an MSU containing $\geq 10^5$/ml of organisms in pure culture (Kass). Because the terminal urethra is not sterile and a background of bacterial contamination is inevitable, this number represents the presence of bacteria in voided urine that significantly exceeds numbers due to contamination. However, this figure is based on research on young women and in other patients lower numbers may be significant. Care must be taken in interpreting samples from urinary catheters as this may represent colonization only.

Organisms isolated (Figs 21.47 and 21.48)

- *Escherichia coli* accounts for 50% and 75% of community and hospital infections respectively. Other enteric

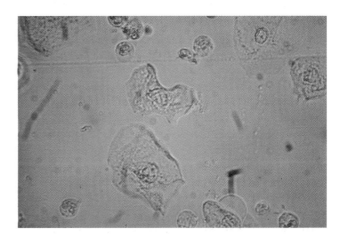

Fig. 21.47 Wet preparations of urine are viewed for the presence of white cells, casts and organisms. As in this slide, the presence of squamous cells suggest perineal contamination of the specimen (courtesy of M. Crow).

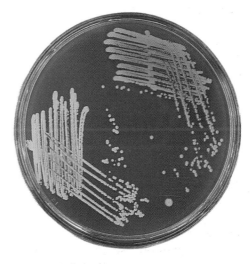

Fig. 21.48 Urine is cultured on selective medium CLED (cysteine lactose electrolyte deficient) agar. Colonies of lactose fermenters are pink and non-lactose fermenters are blue. The deficiency of electrolytes prevents *Proteus* sp. from swarming all over the plate.

Gram-negative bacilli and *Enterococcus* spp. account for most other infections.

- *Proteus* sp. are associated with stone formation.
- *Staphylococcus saphrophyticus* causes a large proportion of UTIs in young, sexually active females.
- The more resistant organisms (*Enterobacter, Klebsiella, Pseudomonas* spp.) tend to occur in hospitalized or long-term catheterized patients.
- *Staphylococcus epidermidis* and *Candida albicans* colonize catheters but do not often cause infections.

Management

Management includes **hydration** (intravenous if necessary), **antibiotics** and, in some cases, investigating underlying abnormalities. Drainage of pus may be indicated when an abscess is present.

Antibiotics are concentrated in urine and for most uncomplicated UTIs (cystitis) a 3-day oral course is appropiate. For hospitalized patients and those with complicated infections, longer courses and initial intravenous therapy are required, e.g. ampicillin plus gentamicin or cefuroxime. The choice of antibiotic depends on known sensitivities of the organisms (Chapter 2) and a local knowledge of antibiotic susceptibility (Tables 21.18 and 21.19).

NEOPLASMS

Benign tumours

Benign tumours of the bladder include inverted papilloma (Brunnian adenoma), adenomatoid tumour and extra-adrenal paraganglioma.

Malignant tumours

Ninety-five per cent of malignant bladder tumours are of urothelial origin. Of these, 90% are transitional cell carcinomas, 5% are squamous cell carcinomas, 2% are adenocarcinomas, mixed or undifferentiated.

Transitional cell carcinoma

This is an important tumour because it is common. It has a prodrome of hyperplasia and dysplasia which implies possible early detection and it may be multiple and recurrent, becoming worse with time and more difficult to manage.

Incidence. In the USA and Europe, bladder cancer accounts for 3% of deaths per year. Eighty per cent of patients are aged 50–80 years and there is a male to female ratio of 3:1. There is a marked geographic variability with urban dwellers having a much higher incidence and the disease being more common in Egypt, where it is associated with schistosomiasis (representing 40% of all malignancy) but rare in Japan.

Aetiology. Industrial carcinogens, particularly exposure to aniline dyes used in textile/rubber/plastics printing/cable industries (benzidine, β-naphthylamine) are implicated. There is a lag period of 20 years. Also implicated are tryptophan metabolism abnormalities; smoking; cyclophosphamide and analgesic abuse nephropathy.

Clinical presentation. Patients present with painless haematuria, symptoms related to concurrent UTI and dysuria.

Table 21.18 Percentage of community urinary isolates sensitive to antibiotics in the Oxford area in 1991.

	Antibiotic	% of organisms sensitive
First-line treatment	Amp-/amoxycillin	60*
	Trimethoprim	78
	Cephradine	88*
Second-line treatment	Co-amoxyclavanate	88
	Nitrofurantoin	88*
	Ciprofloxacin	92

* Useful in pregnancy.

Table 21.19 Urinary tract infections; whom to treat?

Symptomatic All age groups	Treat
Asymptomatic Infants/children (vesicoureteric reflux; danger of renal damage)	Rotating prophylaxic antibiotics
Pregnancy (occurs in 5%; if untreated, 30% of patients will go on to develop pyelonephritis in late pregnancy)	Treat Amoxycillin Cephalosporins safe
Elderly, common (often catheterized; resistant organisms more likely)	Antibiotics debatable

Pathology. Macroscopically these tumours may be solitary or multiple, papillary or non-papillary, pedunculated or sessile (Fig. 21.49). Seventy-five per cent occur in trigone of the bladder.

Microscopically, malignant transitional cells form papillary or solid tumours. Invasion depth is an important part of staging (Fig. 21.50). Three grades are seen. Glandular formation and mucin production may be seen in 25–30%. Inflammatory infiltrate is seen at the tumour base.

In transitional cell carcinoma, there is a progression from hyperplasia, to atypical hyperplasia, dysplasia, carcinoma-*in-situ* to carcinoma (Table 21.20).

Spread and metastasis. These tumours may spread locally. Lymph node metastasis is seen in 25% of invasive tumours. Distant metastases occur in regional and distant lymph nodes.

Table 21.20 Staging of transitional cell carcinoma of the bladder—single most reliable prognostic factor, the basis on which therapeutic decisions made.

pTis	Carcinoma-*in-situ*
pT1	Not extending beyond lamina propria
pT2	Invasion of superficial muscle
pT3	Invasion of deep muscle (outer half) or perivesical
pT4	Invasion of prostate, uterus or vagina

Prognosis. This tumour tends to recur. Five-year survival is closely related to tumour stage:
- T1 (>90%);
- T2 (30–80%);
- T3 (10–30%);
- T4 (10%).

Lymph node metastasis is associated with minimal long-term survival. Grade, age, location, vascular invasion and tumour margin are also important factors.

Squamous carcinoma

It is important to differentiate from squamous carcinoma of the bladder with focal squamous metaplasia. The cause is chronic cystitis associated with squamous metaplasia, most imortantly, infection with *Schistosoma haematobium* and cyclophosphamid therapy.

These tumours present as large, ulcerated, necrotic masses. Most are poorly differentiated and 60% of patients are dead within 1 year. Five-year survival is 40% with muscle invasion and 15% with perivesical invasion.

Adenocarcinoma

Cystitis glandularis forms the basis for this tumour. Microscopic variants are seen, such as clear cell and signet-ring adenocarcinoma. The 5-year survival is in the region of 20%.

THE URETHRA

Posterior urethral valve is a congenital abnormality occurring mainly in males which is composed of folds of mucous membrane. The condition leads to infection and hydronephrosis in childhood.

Urethral caruncle is a small, red inflammatory granulation tissue nodule seen at the external urethral orifice, mainly in women. The cause is unknown and treatment is by surgical excision.

Most cases of **infectious urethritis** are sexually trans-

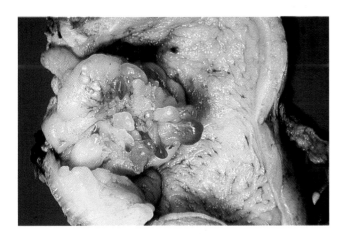

Fig. 21.49 Papillary transitional cell carcinoma of the bladder arising from the trigone.

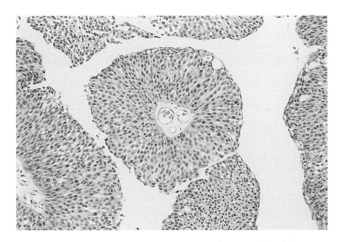

Fig. 21.50 Histology of papillary transitional cell carcinoma, Grade II. (H&E.)

mitted (see Chapter 22). They may result in the formation of urethral strictures.

Tumours of the urethra are rare. These may be transitional cell carcinoma (TCC) of the prostatic urethra in males or squamous or adenocarcinoma of the lower urethra.

FURTHER READING

Tisher C.C. & Brenner B.M. (1989) *Renal Pathology: with Clinical and Functional Correlations*. J.P. Lippincott, Philadelphia.

Diseases of the Male Reproductive System

The testis

NORMAL ANATOMY AND DEVELOPMENT

Normal gonadogenesis is described in Chapter 23. The early gonad is identical in both sexes and develops from the urogenital ridge in the posterior coelomic cavity. In the presence of a Y chromosome in the male, the gonads develop into testes; the Müllerian ducts regress and the Wolffian ducts develop to form the internal male reproductive organs, including the vasa deferentia and seminal vesicles. Normally, the testes descend from the abdominal cavity through the inguinal canal to the scrotum in the last trimester of pregnancy.

Before puberty, the testes are small and are composed of seminiferous tubules lined by inactive germ cells and Sertoli cells (Fig. 22.1). Following puberty, the testes enlarge and show active spermatogenesis with spermatogonia, spermatocytes, spermatids and spermatozoa (germ cells; Fig. 22.2). Sertoli cells regulate spermatogenesis;

Leydig cells are seen in the interstitium and produce testosterone (under luteinizing hormone control).

Abnormalities of sexual development

Absence of one or more testes is rare. In Klinefelter's disease, there is failure of testicular development at puberty. Table 22.1 lists the main congenital abnormalities of sexual development.

A number of abnormalities of testicular descent occur. Three per cent of full-term male infants may show **undescended testis**, or extrascrotal arrest of testicular descent along the normal path of migration; **ectopic testis** represents a location outside the normal route of descent and is rare. If the testis is located to the scrotum before the age of 8 years, normal spermatogenesis is likely. After puberty, an undescended testis undergoes atrophy (Fig. 22.3) and is at greater risk of developing a germ cell neoplasm; even if returned to the scrotum there is a moderately increased tumour risk.

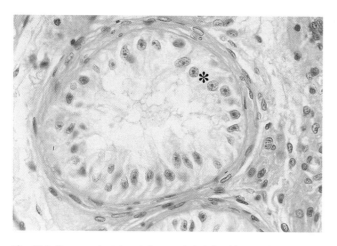

Fig. 22.1 The pre-pubertal seminiferous tubule is lined by Sertoli cells (✱) only without spermatogenesis. (H&E.)

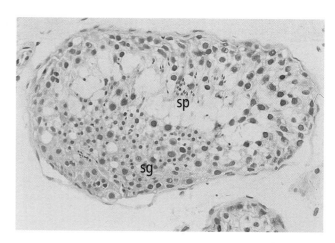

Fig. 22.2 The normal adult seminiferous tubule shows spermatogensis (sp); spermatogonia (sg); spermatocytes; spermatids and spermatozoa. (H&E.)

Table 22.1 Abnormalities of sexual development.

Syndrome	Karyotype	Gonads	External genitalia
True hermaphroditism	Variable 46XX,46XY mosaicism	Both ovarian and testicular tissue are present	Variable; male or female or both
Sex chromosome defects			
Klinefelter's syndrome	47,XXY	Gonadal dysgenesis (streak ovaries)	Female (poorly developed secondary sex characteristics; infertile; amenorrhoea)
Turner's syndrome	46,XY	Testes (immature)	Female; end-organ failure to androgen action; no uterus (infertile, amenorrhoea); secondary sex characteristics well-developed due to adrenal oestrogens
Failure of development of external genitalia	46,XY	Testes	Male; ambiguity caused by undescended testes, bifid scrotum, hypospadias and poor penile development
Bilateral cryptorchidism	46,XY	Testes	Failure of testicular development; infertillty
Female pseudohermaphroditism primary (idiopathic)	46,XX	Ovaries	Male (unknown cause)
Androgens *in utero*	46,XX	Ovaries	Female; variable masculinization at birth
Adrenogenital syndromes	46,XX	Ovaries	Female; masculinization at birth due to excess adrenal androgenic hormones

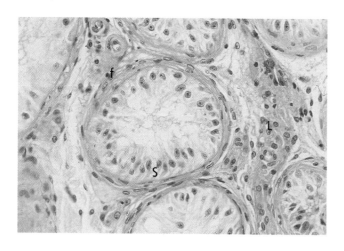

Fig. 22.3 Testicular biopsy from a patient with a history of undescended testis and infertility. There is testicular atrophy with fibrosis (f) around seminiferous tubules and prominent interstitial (Leydig) (L) cells. The tubules contain only Sertoli cells (S) and no spermatogenesis is seen. (H&E.)

Infertility

About 10% of couples experience difficulty in producing a child when they want to. Infertility may affect either partner. Male causes of infertility (approximately 40% of cases) result in a failure to produce sperm (azoospermia) or a decreased number of sperm in the semen (oligospermia) and results from three main causes—pretesticular, testicular and posttesticular.

Pretesticular causes of infertility
- Hypopituitarism (reduced pituitary gonadotrophins).
- Chromosomal abnormalities.
- Thyroid dysfunction.
- Adrenal dysfunction.

Testicular causes of infertility
- Testicular atrophy due to maldescent, exogenous oestrogens, radiation, alcoholic cirrhosis; infection.
- Germ cell aplasia; the seminiferous tubules are lined entirely by Sertoli cells ('Sertoli only' syndrome).
- Spermatocytic maturation arrest.

Post-testicular causes of infertility
- Obstruction to outflow of spermatozoa.
- Psychosexual problems.
  Clinical investigations should include:
- general physical examination and evaluation of alcohol intake;
- screens for syphilis and other infection;
- assessment of spermatogenesis by examination of semen sperm count;
- assessment of patency of the duct system with vasograms;
- testicular biopsy for assessment of spermatogenesis.
  Obstruction to outflow is the commonest cause of male infertility and may be amenable to surgery.

Causes of scrotal swelling (Fig. 22.4)

The presentation of a male patient with a mass or with enlargement of the scrotum is relatively common in surgical practice. Acute inflammatory conditions present with pain; chronic inflammatory disease and tumour are usually painless.

Scrotal swellings should be examined with care, with the possibility of tumour always being borne in mind. Causes of scrotal swelling are listed in Table 22.2.

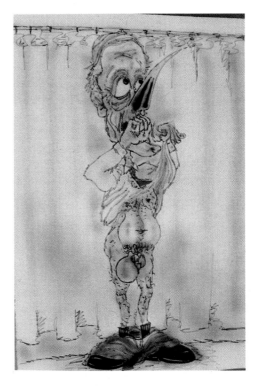

Fig. 22.4 Scrotal swelling is a common surgical outpatient occurrence. (From an original, courtesy of Dr Rachel Armstrong.)

Table 22.2 Causes of scrotal swelling.

Infection
Infection of the scrotal skin.
Acute epididymo-orchitis; acute bacterial infection, mumps
Chronic epididymo-orchitis; tuberculosis; syphilis, granulomatous orchitis
Trauma
Testicular torsion
Testicular tumour
Mass in the epididymis
Adenomatoid tumour
Spermatocoele (cyst in epididymal ducts – sometimes called an epididymal cyst)
Tumour of the scrotal skin
Varicocoele (in spermatic cord)
Inguinal hernia
Hydrocoele of the tunica vaginalis

INFECTION

Epididymo-orchitis

Infection of the epididymis and testis usually presents as testicular swelling and pain. Causes of epididymo-orchitis include the following.

Bacterial infections

Gram-negative enteric bacilli are the most frequent pathogens and are seen especially after manipulation of the genitourinary tract or in association with prostatitis. Tuberculosis is rare in western countries but is common wherever tuberculosis is prevalent. It is most likely to infect the epididymis. The *Mycobacterium* gains access to the epididymis from the urethra.

Sexually transmitted diseases

Sexually transmitted diseases (STDs) involving the testis include *Chlamydia trachomatis* and *Neisseria gonorrhoeae*. Only 50% of males have a uretheral discharge. Other STDs are listed in Table 22.3.

Viral infections

Mumps orchitis occurs in 20% of postpubertal males who acquire mumps parotitis. It usually causes an acute attack of testicular pain and swelling. Only in a small number of cases with mumps orchitis result in testicular atrophy and sterility.

Granulomatous orchitis

This is an uncommon inflammatory condition of unknown cause. The testis is enlarged and replaced by non-caseating granulomas. This may represent an autoimmune phenomenon and it is important to know of the condition as it may mimic tumour clinically.

TESTICULAR TUMOURS

Benign tumours

Benign **epidermoid cyst**, arising in the scrotal skin, represents 1–3% of all testicular tumours. Histopathological examination of the cyst is important in case it represents part of a mature cystic teratoma.

Adenomatoid tumour of the epididymis is thought to represent a benign mesothelioma of the tunica vaginalis. Microscopically, these tumours are composed of gland-like spaces lined by flattened mesothelial cells (Fig. 22.5).

Malignant tumours (Table 22.4)

Germ cell tumours

Germ cell tumours account for over 90% of testicular tumours.

Table 22.3 Sexually transmitted diseases.

Disease	Clinical features	Organism
Gonorrhoea	Urethritis, prostatitis, epididymitis, arthritis, cervicitis, pelvic inflammatory disease	*Neisseria gonorrhoeae*
Syphilis	Chancre	*Treponema pallidum*
Secondary syphilis	Fever, lymph node enlargement, skin rashes, mucosal patches and ulcers, condyloma latum	
Tertiary syphilis	Gumma, tabes dorsalis, general paresis (dementia paralytical), aortitis	
Herpes genitalis	Penile, vulvular or cervical ulcers	Herpes simplex type 2
Condyloma acuminatum	Cervical carcinoma, penile carcinoma	Human papillomavirus (HPV)
Chancroid	Chancres, lymphadenopathy	*Haemophilus ducreyi*
Chlamydia	Conjunctivitis urethritis, Reiter's syndrome, pelvic inflammatory disease, lymphogranuloma venereum, ulcers, lymphadenopathy	*Chlamydia trachomatis* (Serotypes A–K) (Serotypes L$_1$–L$_3$)
Granuloma inguinale	Ulcerating nodules, lymphadenopathy	*Calymmatobacterium donovani*
AIDS	Opportunistic infections, Kaposi's sarcoma	Human immunodeficiency virus (HIV)

AIDS, Acquired immune deficiency syndrome.

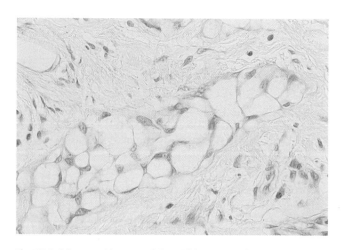

Fig. 22.5 Adenomatoid tumour of the epididymis. Note the gland-like spaces lined by flattened mesothelial cells. (H&E.)

Table 22.4 Classification of testicular tumours.

Tumour type	Frequency	Age (years)
Germ cell tumours		
Seminoma	30%	30–50
MTU (embryonal carcinoma)	20%	15–30
TD (teratoma)	10%	10–30
Endodermal sinus tumour (yolk sac tumour)	Rare	10–30
MTT (choriocarcinoma)	Rare	10–30
MTI (mixed germ cell tumour)	35%	10–50
Gonadal stromal tumours		
Undifferentiated	1%	Any age
Leydig cell	1%	Any age
Sertoli (granulosa–theca) cell	1%	Any age
Mixed stromal	Rare	Any age
Mixed germ cell/stromal	Rare	10–50
Lymphoma	2%	60–80

MTU, Malignant teratoma undifferentiated; TD, teratoma differentiated; MTT, malignant teratoma trophoblastic; MTI, malignant teratoma intermediate.

Epidemiology. The incidence of testicular germ cell tumours is increasing. In the UK there are now 5400 new cases per year, with an incidence of 2.3 per 100 000.

The age at presentation may be between 20 and 25 years but peaks at 30–45 years with a late rise over 80 years.

There is marked geographical and racial variation:
• in Denmark the incidence is 4.9 per 100 000;
• in Japan the incidence is 0.7 per 100 000;
• in San Francisco whites the incidence is 4 per 100 000;
• in San Francisco blacks the incidence is 1 per 100 000;

The incidence in rural males is greater than for urban males, as is the incidence in skilled or professional males compared to unskilled or manual male workers (ratio = 2:1).

Aetiology. Testicular germ cell tumours have recognized causative factors which include:
• cryptorchidism;
• genetics;
• hormonal;
• heat.

The role of trauma is controversial. Carcinogens, radiation and mumps infection are not implicated.

Classification. The classification of testicular germ cell tumours is confusing because more than one classification system is used. Attempts have been made to classify these tumours on histogenic grounds (see Chapter 11; Fig. 22.6).

Nevertheless, two main systems exist—the American and World Health Organization (WHO) and the British Testicular Tumour Panel classification which are often used interchangeably (Table 22.5).

Histogenesis. Markers may be useful in diagnosis of germ cell tumours and in monitoring treatment and include:
• human chorionic gonadotrophin (hCG) for malignant teratoma trophoblastic (MTT);
• α-fetoprotein (AFP) for yolk sac elements;
• placental-like alkaline phosphatase (PLAP) for seminoma (70–90%);
• ferritin for seminoma (Table 22.6).

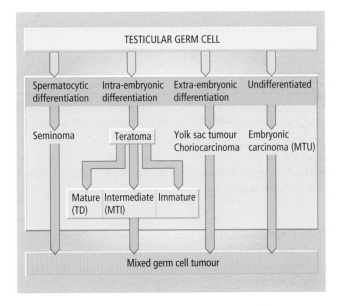

Fig. 22.6 The histogenetic classification of testicular germ-cell tumours.

Table 22.5 Classification of testicular germ cell tumours.

British classification	American/WHO classification
Seminoma	Seminoma
Teratoma differentiated (TD)	Mature teratoma
Malignant teratoma intermediate (MTI)	Immature teratoma
Malignant teratoma undifferentiated (MTU)	Embryonal carcinoma
Malignant teratoma trophoblastic (MTT)	Choriocarcinoma
Yolk sac tumour	
Others	

Table 22.6 Staging of testicular germ cell tumours.

Stage 1	Disease confined to testis
Stage 2	Regional node metastasis (infradiaphragmatic)
Stage 3	Distant node metastasis (supradiaphragmatic)
Stage 4	Extralymphatic metastasis

Behaviour and treatment. Before the advent of cisplatinum in the 1970s, teratoma differentiated (TD) and seminoma had a more favourable prognosis than malignant teratoma intermediate (MTI), malignant teratoma undifferentiated (MTU) and MTT. Now up to 95% of all testicular tumours are completely curable and the more undifferentiated ones respond better to chemotherapy. Eighty per cent of stage 1 differentiated teratomas are cured by surgery alone; 20% of patients will get recurrent disease and require chemotherapy.

Pathological features associated with relapse in undifferentiated teratoma include blood vessel and lymphatic invasion.

In situ germ cell tumour. **Microscopic appearances**: large cells with vesicular nuclei and clear cytoplasm may mix with or replace normal germ cells and Sertoli cells. PLAP is positive in over 90% of cases (normal germ cells are negative).

In situ seminoma is increased in cryptorchid testes and is a definite precursor for seminoma (50% have tumour after 5 years).

Seminoma. This tumour is virtually never seen in patients under 10 years of age; it occurs between 25 and 55 years of age with a peak at 35 years.

Presentation is with a testicular mass, with discomfort or pain in 50%. Macroscopically, these tumours are cream in colour, well-delineated and the tunica is usually intact. Microscopic features include large regular polygonal cells with thin fibrous septa and abundant lymphocytes admixed with the tumour cells. The cells have clear cytoplasm and prominent nucleoli and are often periodic acid–Schiff-positive, PLAP- and vimentin-positive and cytokeratin-negative.

These are rapidly growing tumours. Lymphatic metastases occur first, then haematogenous spread. Fatal cases are due to lung involvement with respirator insufficiency and sepsis.

Seminoma is extremely radiosensitive. The 5-year survival is good and is as follows:
- stage 1: 97–100%;
- stage 2: 86–98%;
- stages 3 and 4 (25%): 80%.

Special types of seminoma. Seminoma with **syncytiotrophoblast-like giant cells** is seen in up to 14% of cases and is associated with HCG-positive trophoblast cells.

Spermatocytic seminoma represents 4% of seminomas and is seen in an older age group. This tumour contains three cell types in tumour and is PLAP-negative. It acts in a benign fashion, and treatment is with surgery alone.

Anaplastic seminoma is the least differentiated variant.

Teratoma (TD and MTI). Thirty-two per cent of testicular germ cell tumours are teratomas. In the infant TD and MTI are most common.

1 Mature teratomas (infant). These represent 5% of all germ cell tumours and are seen exclusively in children.

2 Teratoma differentiated. These are seen from 12 years on (mean 30 years). They look mature but they may metastasize.

3 Malignant teratoma intermediate. This is much more common in adults than TD, and is histologically immature, containing immature elements.

Malignant teratoma undifferentiated (Fig. 22.7). MTU presents between 20 and 35 years of age and is seen only very rarely in patients under 12 years of age.

Macroscopically, it is soft and grey, with focal necrosis and haemorrhage. Histologically, it consists of sheets of pleomorphic cells with clefts and papillae. Early metastasis to retroperitoneal nodes occurs.

MTU had a poor prognosis prior to current therapeutic regimens. Now there is a 95–98% 2-year survival for stage 1 and 2 MTU.

Malignant teratoma trophoblastic. In its pure form, MTT represents 0.3% of germ cell tumours and may be seen as a small element in up to 15% of germ cell tumours. Macroscopically, careful sampling of haemorrhagic areas of the tumour is essential. Histology shows multinucleated syncytiotrophoblast cells and mononuclear cytotrophoblast cells.

MTT used to be rapidly lethal in its pure form, with early haematogenous spread and a 2-year survival of less than 20%. Prognosis is now much better with current chemotherapy regimens.

Yolk sac tumours. Yolk sac tumour may be seen in childhood as pure lesion where it represents the commonest testicular tumour in children up to 5 years; in adults it occurs as part of other germ cell tumours. In childhood, it is responsive to chemotherapy. AFP is a reliable tissue

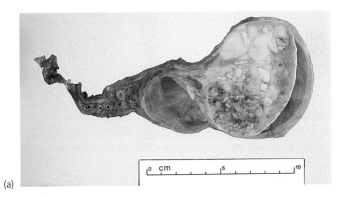

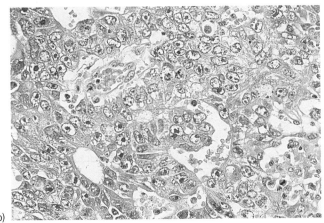

Fig. 22.7 Testicular germ cell tumour. Malignant teratoma undifferentiated (MTU) (embryonal carcinoma). (a) The testis is enlarged and contains soft grey tumour with areas of necrosis and haemorrhage. (b) Histology shows large pale cells arranged in a papillary and syncytial pattern. (H&E.)

and serum marker. In adults, it is always associated with other germ cell tumour elements.

Other tumours. These include mixed germ cell tumours, polyembryoma, carcinoid and rhabdomyosarcoma.

Gonadal stromal tumours

Gonadal stromal tumours represent 2–6% of all testicular tumours. Leydig cell tumours may be associated with oestradiol secretion. Sertoli cell tumour (non-metastasizing) is a common testicular tumour in dogs but is very rare in humans.

Leydig cell tumours. This is the most common gonadal stromal tumour. Occasionally, bilateral and familial cases are seen. The tumour is seen from 2 to 90 years but has a mean age at presentation of 45 years. Presentation may be with precocious puberty or gynaecomastia in adults, as the tumour produces testosterone, oestradiol and progesterone.

Macroscopically, these tumours are 2–3 cm in size with

a characteristic brown colour. Histology shows nests, trabeculae and sheets of polyhedral cells with eosinophilic cytoplasm containing lipid and Reinke crystalloids. Some 7–10% have a malignant course but most are benign.

Sertoli cell tumours. These tumours present between the ages of 20 and 50 years and may be associated wih Peutz–Jeghers syndrome. Macroscopically, they are yellow or white, well-delineated and may be gritty on sectioning. Histology shows tubular structures without lumina. Patients may present with gynaecomastia and loss of libido. Malignancy is rare (<10% cases).

Granulosa cell tumours. These are rare tumours of infants. They are grey or yellow, up to 5 cm in size, solid nodular or cystic. There may be a high mitotic rate, but are not malignant in behaviour. Only very rarely do they present in adults, where they may be associated with gynaecomastia. They may have nuclear grooves and Call–Exner bodies like their ovarian counterpart.

Gonadoblastoma. Gonadoblastoma is a mixed germ cell tumour/sex cord stromal tumour occurring in patients with gonadal dysgenesis (46,XY or 45,XO/46,XY–where only 20% are phenotypically male). They are smooth, lobulated yellow/brown tumours with focal calcification. Histology shows a characteristic nesting pattern with a peripheral palisade of stromal cells. They are regarded as premalignant but at diagnosis 50% will contain germ cell tumour.

Lymphoma

Lymphoma may cause an enlarged testis in men over 50 years of age. Lymphoma presents as a mass or with systemic signs (fever, weight loss). The epididymis is often involved. Macroscopically, the tumour is said to resemble fish flesh, and may be grey or white to brown. Testicular lymphoma is usually a diffuse, large cell, non-Hodgkin's lymphoma. The prognosis relates to the stage of disease but the disease is often bilateral.

Leukaemic involvement of the testis is common, especially in acute leukaemia of childhood.

The prostate gland

NORMAL ANATOMY

The normal prostate gland weighs up to 25 g. It is composed of two lateral lobes, a median lobe and an anterior and a posterior lobe. It encircles the prostatic urethra into which pass the ejaculatory ducts. Histologically, the normal prostate is composed of glandular elements (50%), smooth muscle (25%) and fibrous tissue (25%; Fig. 22.8). The prostatic secretion makes up most of the volume of the seminal fluid and is rich in acid phosphatase.

The prostate gland is closely related anatomically to the rectum, through which the prostate can be palpated. It is possible to sample the prostate via needle biopsy or fine-needle aspiration using a rectal approach.

INFECTION

Acute bacterial prostatitis is a common condition caused by Gram-negative coliform bacteria. Gonococcal prostatitis forms part of the spectrum of gonorrhoea in the male.

Chronic prostatitis may be bacterial in origin but in many cases no bacteria are isolated. Tuberculous prostatitis is rare and usually secondary to infection in some other part of the genitourinary tract.

Granulomatous prostatitis may be secondary to extravasated secretions or to previous surgery.

PROSTATIC NEOPLASMS

Benign prostatic hyperplasia

This is the commonest disease process involving the prostate gland. With increasing age, the prostate undergoes

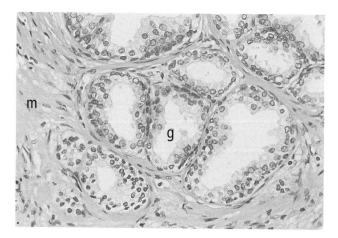

Fig. 22.8 The normal prostate consists of regular glands (g), muscle (m) and fibrous tissue. (H&E.)

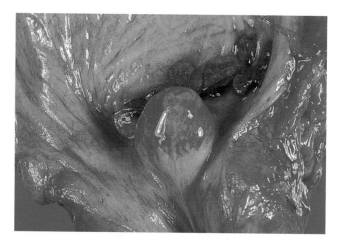

Fig. 22.9 Benign prostatic hyperplasia involving the median lobe. This patient presented with urinary retention; note the focal bladder ulcers representing the site of the urinary catheter tip.

hyperplasia of the glandular and fibromuscular elements. Symptoms of prostatic hyperplasia are common and include:
- poor urinary stream;
- slow urinary stream;
- urinary frequency;
- nocturesis;
- urinary retention (Fig. 22.9).

The long-term effects of obstruction to urinary flow is hypertrophy of the bladder wall which results in the formation of bladder trabeculae (Fig. 22.10). Chronic obstruction predisposes to chronic urinary infection, hydronephrosis and chronic pyelonephritis.

Carcinoma of the prostate

Epidemiology

Carcinoma of the prostate gland has an increasing incidence with age and is as common as lung carcinoma in men:
- 40–50 years: 4.8/100 000 per year;
- age 70–75 years: 513/100 000 per year.

'Latent' prostatic carcinoma is said to be present in 35% of males over 50 years of age and in 60% of males over 80 years of age.

There is a low incidence of prostatic carcinoma in the Far East. In the USA, it is a disease that is more common in blacks than whites. Endocrine factors are important in the aetiology. Tumour growth is androgen-dependent. Benign prostatic hyperplasia does not predispose to carcinoma.

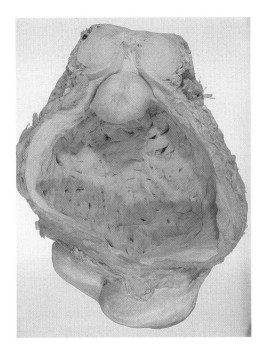

Fig. 22.10 Benign prostatic hyperplasia. This patient had chronic urinary retention; note the diffuse bladder diverticula which have developed in association with chronic outflow obstruction due to prostatic enlargement (top).

Diagnosis

Diagnosis of prostatic carcinoma is by a variety of methods:

- rectal examination;
- transrectal ultrasound—for staging;
- prostatic-specific acid phosphatase (PSAP) and prostate-specific antigen (PSA) in serum and in tissue are useful for monitoring response to treatment and recurrences;
- histological examination of tissue from transurethral prostatectomy (TURP).

Pathology

Carcinoma of the prostate may have a yellow appearance macroscopically due to the lipid content of the cells. The tumour arises in the peripheral or outer zone of the gland (classically posterior) and may be multifocal. Because of this lateral origin, clinical symptoms may occur late and histological examination of material obtained at TURP may only be positive if there is extensive tumour.

Microscopic examination shows variable differentiation of glands (Fig. 22.11). Perineural invasion is common. Immunohistochemistry shows positive staining for PSAP and PSA.

Subtypes of prostatic adenocarcinoma include:

- large duct;

- endometrial (endometrioid);
- transitional cell carcinoma;
- mixed adenocarcinoma and transitional cell carcinoma.

Grading

Five grades have been described (Gleason) and these are relevant to the staging, spread and prognosis of prostatic adenocarcinoma.

Staging

Staging of prostatic adenocarcinoma is done clinically:

- A—lesion not palpable or clinically apparent;
- B—palpable tumour, confined to prostate;
- C—tumour localized to the periprostatic area;
- D—distant metastasis (D1 pelvic, D2 distant).

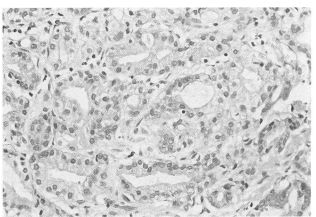

(a)

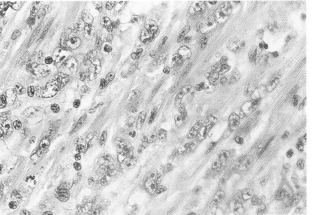

(b)

Fig. 22.11 Prostatic adenocarcinoma. (a) This is a well-differentiated tumour showing well-formed glands. (b) This is a poorly-differentiated tumour showing infiltration in to muscle. (H&E.)

Spread and metastasis

Capsular invasion is common (up to 90%), followed by pelvic spread. Metastases occur to bone and lymph nodes and will be present in 40% at the time of diagnosis.

Treatment and prognosis

Treatment of prostatic carcinoma involves hormonal manipulation, surgery and irradiation. More than 75% of patients present with stage C or D disease. Prognosis depends upon grade of the tumour and stage:

* stage A and B tumours have a 50–80% 10-year survival;
* stage C and D tumours (which require hormonal therapy) have a 10–40% 10-year survival.

Other tumours of the prostate are rare and include embryonal rhabdomyosarcoma in childhood.

The penis

NORMAL STRUCTURE

The penile urethra is lined in part by squamous and in part by transitional epithelium and is a component of the urinary tract.

The commonest congenital abnormalities relate to the position of the urethral opening on the penis. In **hypospadias** the opening is situated on the ventral aspect of the penis; **epispadias** is rare and the urethral opening is located on the dorsal aspect of the penis.

Phimosis is a condition where the foreskin is too tight to be retracted; it may be a congenital or acquired condition.

INFECTIONS/INFLAMMATIONS

Gonococcal urethritis and non-gonococcal urethritis (NGU) are described in Chapter 23 and other sexually transmitted diseases involving the penis are listed in Table 22.3. Inflammation of the glans penis is termed **balanitis**.

The skin of the penis is prone to develop a number of skin disorders including:

* viral warts;
* lichen planus;
* psoriasis;
* lichen sclerosis—termed **balanitis xerotica obliterans** in the penis;
* fungal infection.

TUMOURS

Benign

Benign squamous papillomas may occur in the penile skin.

Condyloma acuminatum is a common tumour caused by human papillomavirus (HPV). It is seen on the coronal sulcus of the glans or on the inner surface of the foreskin. They may be multiple and may become very large (giant condylomas). Histology shows koilocytic cell changes, similar to those seen in HPV-associated vulval warts and HPV infection of the uterine cervix.

Malignant

The most important malignant tumour of the penis is **squamous cell carcinoma**. It is an uncommon malignancy, representing less than 1% of all malignant tumours in men.

This tumour is thought to be associated with HPV infection. There may be an association between squamous carcinoma of the penis in men and carcinoma of the cervix in female partners of these men.

Carcinoma of the penis is rarely seen in circumcised males; it is more common in oriental populations. It occurs in the age group from 35 to 75 years.

The common sites for this tumour are the glans and the inner surface of the foreskin. The lesion may present as a

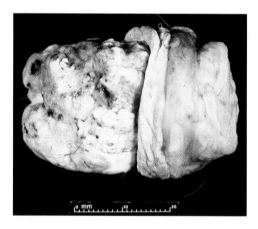

Fig. 22.12 Squamous carcinoma of the penis. This is a surgical pathology specimen. This patient had a painless, rapidly growing, ulcerating tumour originating beneath the foreskin.

white plaque, a pale papule, or as an ulcerated, painless tumour (Fig. 22.12).

The tumour locally infiltrates the corpora cavernosa before metastasizing to regional inguinal lymph nodes.

Treatment is surgical and the 5-year survival is in the region of 60%. Radiotherapy may be used to treat recurrences.

Diseases of the Female Reproductive System

CONTENTS

INTRODUCTION

The human female genital tract is composed of both the external genitalia (the vulva) and the internal organs (the vagina, cervix, uterus, fallopian tubes and ovaries) which combine the functions of reproduction with gender interaction. The genital organs are also in proximity to the lower portions and external orifices of both the gastrointestinal and urinary tracts. Disease processes involving these organ systems, as well as the skin of the vulva and perineal region, can have an effect on the genital tract organs (Fig. 23.1).

EMBRYOLOGY AND DEVELOPMENT

Development of the female reproductive organs is most easily understood by considering separately the organogenesis of the three functional regions of the genital tract. These are:

- the **gonads** (ovaries);
- the **genital ducts** (fallopian tubes, uterus, cervix and vagina);
- The **external genitalia** (the vulva).

The earliest stages of organogenesis of all three of these reproductive structures are **gender-indifferent**. Consequently they have the capacity to develop into either male or female reproductive organs, the final outcome pri-

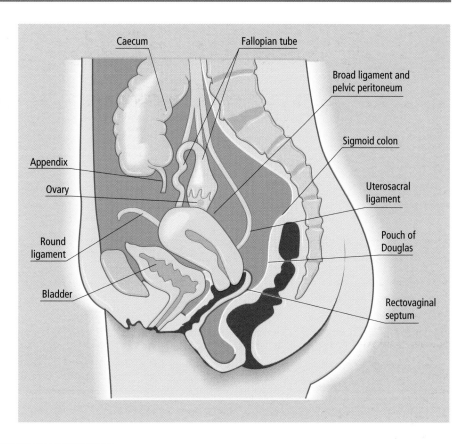

Fig. 23.1 The normal female genital tract.

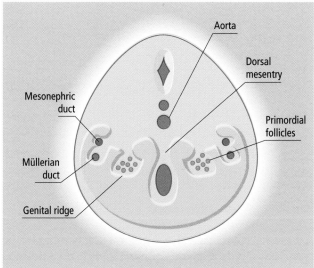

Fig. 23.2 The gonads develop from the genital ridge and underlying mesenchyme.

marily being determined by the **sex chromosome** composition at fertilization. Subsequent organ development is influenced by the expression of the **sex hormone receptors** and, the balance and circulating levels of **sex hormones** to which the developing reproductive organs are exposed *in utero* and postpartum.

A brief summary of embryological development is provided in order to clarify the origin of some embryological remnants occurring in the adult female genital tract as well as explaining the background to the histogenic classification of ovarian neoplasms (Fig. 23.2).

The ovaries

The gonads develop as paired gender-indifferent structures early in gestation from coelomic epithelium covering the medial surface of the **urogenital ridge** and the underlying mesenchyme. The surface epithelium forms cords of cells which extend into the mesenchyme (**primitive sex cords**), segregating the indifferent gonads into outer cortex and inner medulla. During the fifth week of development, **primordial germ cells** migrate from the **yolk sac**, along the hind-gut mesentery to the developing gonadal ridges, where they merge into the developing primitive sex cords. In the presence of a male XY karyotype there is preferential development of the medulla to from the functional components of the testis. In the absence of a Y chromosome and the presence of a female XX karyotype, the medulla degenerates and the cortex slowly develops over the next 5 weeks to form the

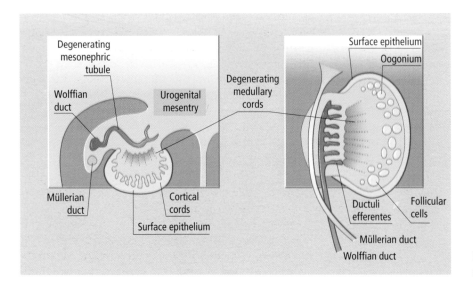

Fig. 23.3 Development of the male and female gonads.

ovaries. The sex cords separate from the surface forming the **primary follicles**, composed of a central **oögonia** derived from the primary germ cells surrounded by a **follicular cell layer** formed from the coelomic epithelium, which in adult ovaries forms the **granulosa cells**. The future steroid hormone-secreting **thecal cells** of the mature ovary develop around the primary follicle from mesenchymal cells of the gonad. By term, the female fetus has developed its full complement of primary follicles for release during ovulation in adult life (Fig. 23.3).

The female genital tract

The female genital ducts develop from the paired **paramesonephric (Müllerian) ducts**, as invaginations on the lateral surface of the urogenital ridges, during the sixth week of development. The caudal portions of the ducts migrate to the midline and fuse to form the epithelial and glandular lining of the fallopian tubes, uterus, cervix and upper third of the vagina (Fig. 23.3). The smooth muscle and connective tissue layers develop from the mesenchyme adjacent to the ducts.

Incomplete fusion of the caudal portions of the paramesonephric ducts may result in a range of congenital uterovaginal structural anomalies. The lower two-thirds of the vagina forms by canalization of an area of condensed endoderm, the **vaginal plate**, which forms on the posterior wall of the urogenital sinus. The endoderm-derived epithelium subsequently extends into the upper third of the vagina, replacing the glandular **Müllerian** mucosa.

Within the urogenital ridges, during the early indifferent stage of genital tract development, the male **mesonephric (Wolffian)** ducts also develop, irrespective

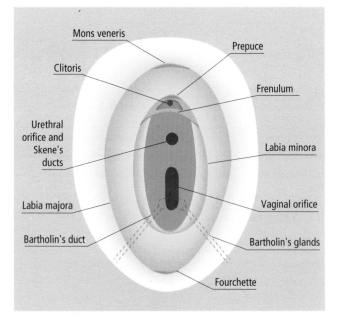

Fig. 23.4 The external female genitalia.

of the karyotypic gender. They then subsequently degenerate. Cystic remnants of mesonephric duct development may however persist in the adult female pelvis.

The female external genitalia (the vulva) develops on the surface of the embryo during the fourth week as the **genital tubercle** (from which the **clitoris** develops), the **urogenital membrane** and **folds** (which form the **hymen** and **labia minora** respectively) and the **labioscrotal swellings** (which form the **labia majora**; Fig. 23.4).

A full term female infant possesses reproductive organ structures which undergo further growth and development during adolescence prior to becoming functionally effective at the menarche.

A general principle that may be applied when considering the pathological disease processes involving the female genital tract is to localize the clinical symptoms and signs in relation to the three different regions of the tract outlined during embryological development. Thus the vulva can be affected by a variety of disease conditions involving the skin; the organs derived from the genital ducts are tubular structures which in cross-section are composed of three principal tissues, an inner layer of epithelium whose histological type differs at different levels according to the specialized function it is intended to fulfil. A middle layer of smooth muscle which is, in turn, surrounded by an outer connective tissue layer. The majority of disorders involving the tubular genital tract structures primarily affect the inner epithelial layer. Similarly, disorders of the ovaries can be related to embryogenesis; indeed, the histogenic classification of ovarian neoplasms attempts to ascribe patterns of histological differentiation according to the purported recapitulation in ovarian neoplasms of the embryonic cellular precursors.

Finally, consideration of the effects of other organ systems, particularly the hypothalamic–pituitary axis, as well as other endocrine organs in the pathogenesis of disease, should always be considered (see Chapter 14).

In this chapter, infectious diseases of the female reproductive tract will be considered first, followed by the pathology of the vulva, vagina, cervix, endometrium, myometrium, fallopian tubes, ovaries and placenta.

SEXUALLY TRANSMITTED DISEASE IN THE FEMALE AND MALE

Infectious diseases of the reproductive tract are common in males and females. The incidences of sexually transmitted diseases (STD) have increased by 20% over the last decade. The incidences of genital herpes and warts and *Chlamydia* have increased, whereas the incidences of syphilis and gonorrhoea have declined. Important aspects of management of STD include contact tracing and the treatment of partners. Extragenital sites such as anal and pharyngeal sites must be screened as eradication of infection from these sites is more difficult. Infection with more than one agent should be suspected (e.g. gonococcus and *Chlamydia*).

Table 22.3 in Chapter 22 lists the STDs seen in both males and females.

Presentation of sexually transmitted disease

STDs have a variety of presentations:

- as a lesion (genital warts and ulcers);
- with pain (genital herpes, especially in recurrent disease); other lesions can be typically painless (e.g. syphilitic chancre);
- pruritis – genital herpes; candidal infections; pubic lice and secondary syphilis;
- as a discharge – gonococcus and *Trichomonas* infection.

Urethritis

STDs in the male usually present as urethritis. There are two main types of infection:
- gonococcal urethritis (Fig. 23.5);
- non-gonococcal urethritis (NGU) in the male which in the female equates with the acute urethral syndrome (symptoms of dysuria and frequency with a sterile pyuria).

Chlamydia causes 50% of cases and the remainder are of unknown cause. Other causes of urethritis are herpes simplex virus (HSV; Fig. 23.6) and *Trichomonas* (Fig. 23.7; Table 23.1).

Skin and mucous membrane lesions

Males generally present earlier than females with the complaint of unsightly skin lesions in the genitoanal region. Lesions in the vagina or cervix may not be so obvious and females may be asymptomatic or present in the later stage of the disease.

Genital ulcers

Genital ulcers are found in:
- syphilis, typically a single chancre at the point of inoculation;

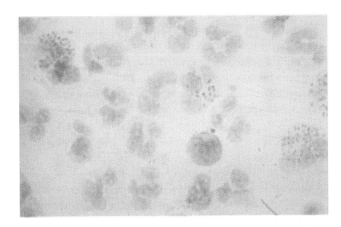

Fig. 23.5 Gonococcal urethritis. Diplococci are seen in a urethra smear within pus cells. (Gram stain.)

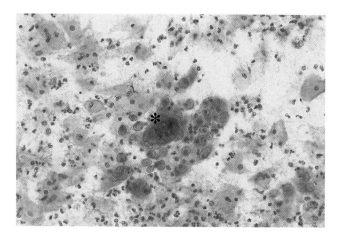

Fig. 23.6 Cervical smear. Herpes simplex infection. Note the multi-nucleated cells (✱) with glassy chromatin. (PAP.)

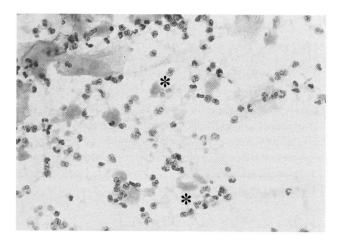

Fig. 23.7 Cervical smear. *Trichomonas vaginalis*. The flagellate organisms (✱) are pale-staining and slightly larger than pus cells. (PAP.)

- genital herpes (HSV2 is more common than HSV1); multiple vesicular lesions are seen; the virus remains latent and recurrent disease is common;
- lymphogranuloma venereum (LGV, *Chlamydia*), chancroid (*Haemophilus ducreyi*) and granuloma inguinale (*Calymmatobacterium granulomatis*) are rare causes, being more prevalant in Africa and the Far East.

Papular lesions

Molluscum contagiosum (pox virus) produces umbilicated pearly lesions. In children the lesions occur at other sites and are not venereally acquired.

Verrucous papules of condylomata lata are caused by human papillomaviruses (HPV; Fig. 23.8). Multiple large warts may appear and spread to other regions is common.

Candidal infections (e.g. vulvovaginitis in the female and balanitis in the male) produce a pruritic papular rash with erythematous areas and satellite lesions.

Scabies is associated with papular lesions with diagnostic burrows.

Pubic lice

Pubic lice or crab lice (*Pthirus pubis*) are observed as lice or nits (eggs) attached to hairs (Fig. 23.9).

Syphilis

Syphilis was formerly a common infection. It produces a wide range of clinical features which can mimic many different diseases. Its incidence is decreasing but it is still an important disease. It causes a latent infection with manifestations of the disease occurring many years after the inital infection. Not all untreated infections proceed

Table 23.1 Features of gonococcal and chlamydial infection in females and males.

	Gonococcus	*Chlamydia*
Typical features	Asymptomatic (males/females)	Asymptomatic (males/females)
	Combined dysuria and purulent urethral discharge (males)	Dysuria or a purulent urethral discharge (males)
	Cervicitis with vaginal discharge (females)	Cervicitis with vaginal discharge (females)
Complications	Disseminated gonococcaemia (septicaemia, skin rash, arthritis; males)	Reiter's syndrome (reactive arthritis, uveitis skin/mucous membrane dermatitis; males)
	Pelvic inflammatory disease (females)	Pelvic inflammatory disease (females)
Diagnosis	Urine/cervical swab	Urine/cervical swab
	Smear, intracellular Gram-negative diplococci	*Chlamydia* antigen test (ELISA/fluorescence test)
	Culture	

ELISA, Enzyme-linked immunosorbent assay.

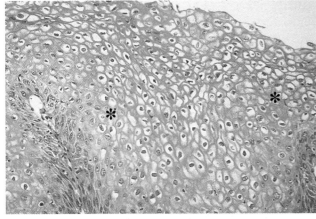

(a)

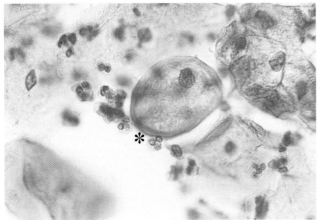

(b)

Fig. 23.8 Human papilloma virus (HPV). (a) Cervical biopsy showing the typical koilocytes (✱) with enlarged, irregular cell nuclei and peri-nuclear halos. (H&E.) (b) Cervical smear showing the typical koilocytes (✱) with enlarged, irregular cell nuclei and peri-nuclear halos. (PAP.)

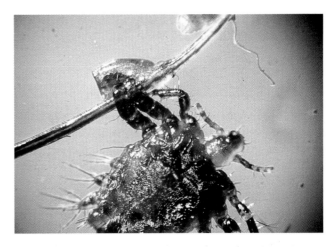

Fig. 23.9 Pubic louse, *Pthirus pubis.*

through the stages from primary to tertiary disease (Table 23.2). The organism is difficult to cultivate *in vitro* and serology is the mainstay of diagnosis. There are two types of test:

- non-specific tests based on a cross-reaction between the organism and cardiolipin, e.g. rapid plasma reagin (RPR) test. Biological false-positives are possible;
- specific tests using antigen, e.g. *Treponema pallidum* haemagglutination (TPHA) and the more sensitive and specific fluorescent antibody test, FTA.

Syphilis is easily treated with penicillin and tertiary syphilis is rarely seen.

Table 23.2 Clinical features of the various stages of syphilis.

	Primary disease	Secondary disease	Tertiary disease
Clinical features	Painless chancre	6–8 weeks later	3–30 years later
	May go unnoticed	Disseminated disease	Progressive disease
	Heals in about 6 weeks	Maculopapular, pustular rash; snail track mouth ulcers; condylomata lata; systemic features, fever, headaches	Any organ affected; neurosyphilis; cardiovascular; gummas of bone
Diagnosis	Dark-field microscopy of lesion aspirate	Dark-field microscopy of lesion aspirate	Biopsy and histology show gummas and plasma cells
Serology (% positive)			
RPR	80	100	0
TPHA	65	100	95
FTA	85	100	98

RPR, Rapid plasma reagin; TPHA, *Treponema pallidum* haemagglutination; FTA, fluorescent antibody.

INFECTIONS OF THE FEMALE REPRODUCTIVE SYSTEM

Vulvo-vaginitis

The acid pH of the vagina during the reproductive years is brought about by the action of *Lactobacillus* and other normal vaginal flora. In this environment, the vagina is relatively resistant to pathogens. There are two main causes of vaginitis.

- *Candida* (thrush) is very common and is usually endogenous in nature, rarely sexually acquired (Fig. 23.10). It arises as a result of an imbalance of the normal flora. Predisposing factors include:
  (a) high oestrogen levels (combined contraceptive pill and pregnancy);
  (b) diabetes;
  (c) steroids;
  (d) broad-spectrum antibiotics.
  Recurrent infections are common. Species other than *Candida albicans* are more difficult to treat.
- *Trichomonas* is a protozoal organism that is nearly always sexually acquired.
  Infection may be asymptomatic in 25% of females (Fig. 23.7).

Presentation
- Vaginal discharge; *Trichomonas vaginalis* produces copious watery frothy discharge which accumulates in the vaginal fornices; *Candida* spp. produce thick adherent plaques on the vaginal wall.
- Pruritis.
- Idour (fishy smell of *Trichomonas*).

Diagnosis
Diagnosis is made by obtaining a high vaginal swab (HVS) for microscopy and culture.

Anaerobic vaginosis (bacterial vaginosis)

This is not an inflammatory condition and pus cells are not seen. The presence of *Gardnerella vaginalis* as an indicator of anaerobic vaginosis is debatable as it can be found as part of the normal vaginal flora. What seems more likely is that this condition represents a shift from the normal flora to an overgrowth of the anaerobic component. It is successfully treated with metronidazole.

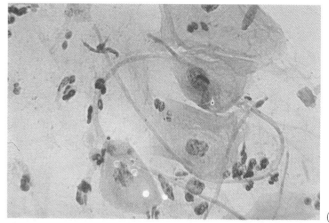
(a)

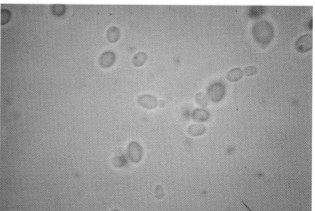
(b)

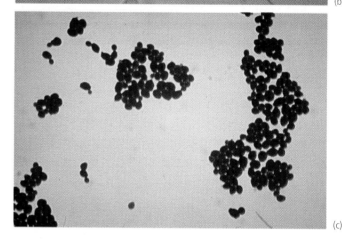
(c)

Fig. 23.10 Candida. (a) Hyphae seen in a cervical smear. (PAP.) (b) Seen to be budding in this unstained vulval swab specimen. (c) Stained with Gram stain.

Diagnosis
This is diagnosed by detecting the following:
- the presence of clue cells (epithelial cells covered with organisms);
- malodorous thin discharge;
- pH of discharge > 4.5.

Toxic shock syndrome

Two-thirds of toxic shock syndrome (TSS) cases are related to menstruating women and the use of tampons. *Staphylococcus aureus* is found as normal vaginal flora in only 5% of women. *Staph. aureus* is thought to be associated with the use of hyperabsorbable tampons which lead to a low [Mg^{2+}], encouraging increased production of TSS toxin 1. The toxin acts as a superantigen, resulting in multisystem failure.

Diagnosis and Management

The diagnosis is a clinical one and the clinical features include:
- a pyrexia > 38.9°C;
- a systolic blood pressure < 90 mmHg;
- a rash with subsequent desquamation, especially on the palms and soles;
- involvement of three or more organ sites, e.g. central nervous system, renal, liver and haematological abnormalities.

A vaginal discharge often accompanies this disease. Culture of this or the tampon may grow *Staph. aureus*. The management includes:
- aggressive fluid replacement and support of organ systems;
- flucloxacillin, not for treatment of the disease *per se* but to prevent relapses.

Cervicitis

The cervix is partly lined with columnar epithelium. A clear mucous discharge maintains the cervix at a neutral pH. The cervix is more susceptible to infections than the vagina.

Gonococcus and *Chlamydia* produce a cervicitis with purulent discharge. In the female the vaginal discharge may go unnoticed and females may act as reservoirs for the disease.

Presentation

Clinical overlap in symptoms occurs between gonococcal and chlamydial infection (see Table 23.1) and, in 30%, a dual infection occurs. Asymptomatic infections occur and these may present later as pelvic inflammatory disease in the female.

HSV and HPV infections occur on the cervix; HPV 16 and 18 are strongly associated with cervical intraepithelial neoplasia (CIN) and carcinoma of the cervix (Fig. 23.8).

Diagnosis and treatment

Diagnosis is made by obtaining a cervical swab. For uncomplicated gonococcal disease, treatment is with 3 g oral amoxycillin and probenicid; for resistant strains (increased penicillin resistance and strains producing β-lactamases), quinolones are used. Tetracycline is added to treat any associated chlamydial disease and may be used in combination with amoxycillin.

Bartholinitis

Causes of infection of the Bartholin's gland include gonococcus, *Chlamydia* and infections with normal flora (anaerobes and coliforms). Drainage and surgical marsupialization are important aspects of management.

Pelvic inflammatory disease

Pelvic inflammatory disease (PID) is not a strict definition and includes salpingo-oophoritis, endomyometritis and pelvic abscesses. Ascending infection from the cervix is important in the aetiology of this disease. There are two main types of ascending infection:
- STD; e.g. gonococcus and *Chlamydia*;
- infections from normal vaginal flora, e.g. anaerobes and coliforms.

Intrauterine contraceptive devices (IUCD) are associated with PID as they provide a vehicle for ascending infection. Actinomycetes often colonize these devices but endometritis is extremely rare. Tuberculosis of the female genital tract is also rare in the UK but is a common cause of female infertility in countries where tuberculosis is endemic.

Acute endometritis and salpingitis may present as acute pelvic pain with fever and may be confused with acute appendicitis.

Cervicitis due to gonococcal and chlamydial disease may be asymptomatic and, of these, at least 10% will develope PID. Salpingo-oophoritis may be recurrent and chronic, leading ultimately to bilateral fallopian tubal damage. This may cause tubal occlusion, ectopic pregnancies and chronic pelvic pain.

Chlamydial infections are the commonest identifiable infectious cause of infertility. The **Fitz-Hugh–Curtis syndrome** is a perihepatitis caused by primary spread of the organisms from the fallopian tubes to the liver capsule.

Postoperative and postpartum pelvic infections

The normal vaginal flora and, in particular, anaerobes cause the majority of these infections. *Staphylococcus aureus* and *Streptococcus pyogenes* have also to be considered. Confusion surrounds the role of mycoplasmas as a cause of a postpartum fever. For prevention of obstetric and gynaecological infections, perioperative prophylactic antibiotics are recommended.

Management of pelvic infections

Management strategies include:

- localization of the infection by imaging techniques;
- HVS, cervical swabs, aspirates and blood cultures;
- empiric treatment for STD and pelvic infections, including cefuroxime and tetracycline;
- empiric treatment for other pelvic infections, including cefuroxime and metronidazole (Table 23.3).

DISEASES OF THE VULVA

The external portion of the female genital tract, known as the **vulva**, comprises the labia majora and minora, the

Table 23.3 Diagnosis and treatment of sexually transmitted disease.

	Organism	Diseases	Diagnosis	Treatment
Bacteria	*Treponema pallidum*	Syphilis, congenital syphilis	Serology; RPR, TPHA, FTA	Penicillin
	Neisseria gonorrhoeae	Gonorrhoea, PID Disseminated GC	Culture; urethral, cervical swabs, BC	Penicillin Quinolones
	Chlamydia trachomatis	NGU, cervicitis, PID Reiter's syndrome	Antigen detection; cervical swabs	Tetracycline
		Lymphogranuloma venereum	Serology L1, 2 and 3	Tetracycline
	Mycoplasma sp.	? PID, postpartum fever	Culture, difficult	Erythromycin
	Ureaplasma sp.	NGU	Culture, difficult	Tetracycline
	Anaerobes	Anaerobic vaginosis	Culture; HVS	Metronidazole
	Calymmatobacterium granulomatis	Granuloma inguinale	Smear and biopsy (Donovan bodies)	Tetracycline
	Haemophilus ducreyi	Chancroid (soft sore)	Smear and culture	Erythromycin
Fungi	*Candida albicans Candida* sp.	Thrush, vaginitis	Culture; HVS	Clotrimazole, nystatin Fluconazole
Viruses	Herpes simplex virus 2 (1)	Genital herpes	EM Culture	Acyclovir
	Human papilloma virus (HPV 16, 18)	Genital warts CIN, carcinoma	Appearance (colposcopy)	Physical removal
	Molluscum contagiosum virus	Molluscum contagiosum	Appearance, EM	Self-limiting
	Hepatitis B virus	Hepatitis	HBsAg, HBeAg Anti-HBc	Prevention, vaccination
	HIV	AIDS	HIV antibody	AZT (not a cure)
Protozoa	*Trichomonas vaginalis*	Vaginitis	Microscopy or culture	Metronidazole
Arthropods	*Pthirus pubis*	Pubic or crab lice	Observation of nits or lice	Malathion Lindane
	Sarcoptes scabiei	Scabies	Observation of mite	Lindane

AIDS, acquired immunodeficiency virus; BC, blood culture; CIN, cervical intraepithelial neoplasia; EM, electronmicroscopy; FTA, flourescent antibody; HBc, hepatitis B core; HBeAg, hepatitis B e antigen; HBsAg, hepatitis B surface antigen; HIV, human immunodeficiency virus; HVS, high vaginal swab; NGU, non-gonococcal urethritis; PID, pelvic inflammatory disease; RPR, rapid plasma reagin; TPHA, treponema pallidum haemagglutination.

entrance to the vagina (the introitus) and the external urethral meatus (see Fig. 23.4).

Vulval dermatoses and inflammations

The vulval skin is susceptible to the same dermatological disorders that occur elsewhere on the skin. In addition, dermatological conditions confined to the vulval skin and mucosa may develop, usually presenting with pruritus and manifest as red (erythematous) or white (leukoplakic) areas of non-neoplastic epidermal thickening; these may be difficult to differentiate clinically from areas of neoplastic transformation. The conditions causing these changes are grouped together under the term **vulval dermatoses** (formerly referred to as vulval dystrophies); the current classification is summarized in Table 23.4.

The vulval mucosa is exposed to sexually related infections such as *Candida albicans* as well as viral warts due to HPV.

Vulval neoplasia

A form of preinvasive cancer known as intraepithelial neoplasia may occur on the vulval mucosa (**vulval intraepithelial neoplasia, VIN**). The condition is characterized by being a disorder in which architectural, nuclear and cytoplasmic changes are confined to the epithelium without extension beyond the basement menbrane. The process has the capacity to regress to normality or progress to invasive neoplasia.

The condition is increasingly being diagnosed in young sexually active women. A biopsy of the vulva may need

Table 23.5 The histopathological grading of vulval intraepithelial neoplasia (VIN).

VIN I	The normal cellular maturation and stratification are disturbed with the changes confined to the lower basal third of the epidermis
VIN II	Extension of atypical cells into the middle third of the epidermis
VIN III	Full-thickness involvement of the epidermis

to be undertaken in some circumstances in order to distinguish between vulval dermatoses and VIN. As with the other types of intraepithelial neoplasia, VIN is divided into three grades. The features are summarized in Table 23.5.

The coexistence of HPV infection in the epidermal cells may be manifest as **koilocytosis** (vacuolated squamous cells with irregular hyperchromatic nuclei). A high proportion of women in whom VIN is detected on further examination and investigation are found also to have intraepithelial or invasive neoplastic changes elsewhere in the genital tract, most commonly involving the cervix. Approximately 5% of cases of VIN progress to develop invasive squamous cell carcinoma of the vulva (Fig. 23.11). Individuals in whom VIN is detected therefore warrant further follow-up because of the multifocal character of the disease and to assist the early detection of other anogenital disease.

Invasive vulval carcinoma is most commonly of squamous cell type. It occurs in an older age group than VIN, having a peak incidence in postmenopausal women in the sixth to seventh decades of life. Vulval cancer constitutes about 5% of primary female genital tract malignancies. A higher than expected incidence of other intraepithelial and invasive neoplasias of other genital

Table 23.4 The histopathological classification of vulval dermatoses.

Disorder	Histopathology	Old terminology
Squamous hyperplasia	Hyperkeratosis Acanthosis Chronic demal infiltrate	Hypertrophic dystrophy
Lichen sclerosis	Hyperkeratosis Epidermal atrophy +/− subepidermal homogeneous zone Chronic dermal infiltrate	Atrophic dystrophy
Mixed dermatosis	Adjacent areas of squamous hyperplasia and lichen sclerosis	Mixed dystrophy

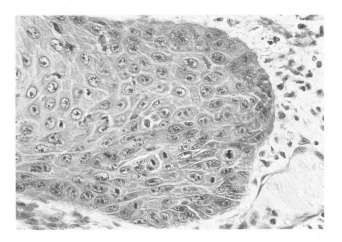

Fig. 23.11 Invasive squamous carcinoma of the vulva is arising from an area of vulval intra-epithelial neoplasia (VIN). (H&E.)

Table 23.6 The clinical staging of invasive vulval neoplasia (International Federation of Obstetrics and Gynaecology; FIGO).

Stage I	A neoplasm of less than 2 cm diameter, confined to the vulva, without identifiable inguinal lymphadenopathy
Stage II	A neoplasm of greater than 2 cm diameter, confined to the vulva, without identifiable inguinal lymphadenopathy
Stage III	A vulval neoplasm of any size accompanied by lymphadenopathy, or extension beyond the vulva without lymphadenopathy
Stage IV	Metastases to lymph nodes or any other sites are present

tract organs as well as the anogenital region is observed, most commonly involving the cervix.

A major principle in the management of female genital tract malignancies is that the prognosis is related to clinical staging; the most widely used staging classification in the management of gynaecological malignancies is that proposed by the International Federation of Obstetrics and Gynaecology (**FIGO**). The features used in the staging of vulval neoplasms are summarized in Table 23.6.

In the absence of identifiable lymph node metastases the 5-year survival after surgery or radiotherapy is in excess of 70%; this is reduced to 40% or less in the presence of lymph node metastases.

THE VAGINA

The commonest disorder of the vagina is infection. Infection commonly presents as a vaginal discharge which may be due to a variety of pathogens, including *Candida albicans, and Trichomonas vaginalis*.

Embryological remnants of the mesonephric duct may persist, clinically presenting as vaginal wall cysts.

In postmenopausal women, **uterovaginal prolapse** where the uterus and cervix herniate through the pelvic diaphragm due to laxity of the supporting ligaments may occur, particularly in those of high parity.

Vaginal adenosis is a rare condition in which there is ectopic persistence, most commonly in the upper third of the vagina, of glandular endocervical type epithelium. The condition is associated with *in utero* exposure to non-steroidal oestrogen, most commonly **diethylstilboestrol (DES)**, formerly used in North America in women with a history of recurrent spontaneous abortion.

Exposure to DES appears to inhibit the normal migration of endodermal sinus-formed squamous epithelium to replace the Müllerian mucosa lining the upper third of the vagina. Vaginal adenosis is a benign disorder but its persistence after the menarche can predispose the af-

fected individual to malignant transformation into either clear cell carcinoma or, less commonly, squamous cell carcinoma (arising from metaplastic transformation of the area of adenosis into squamous epithelium).

Vaginal neoplasia

Vaginal intraepithelial neoplasia (VAIN) is a rare condition most commonly occurring in the upper third of the vagina of perimenopausal women who have either concomitant CIN or, carcinoma or a past history of treatment of these diseases. The pathogenesis of VAIN appears to be similar to CIN and will be discussed in the section on cervical disorders.

Invasive vaginal neoplasia is a rare disease representing 1–2% of gynaecological malignancies; secondary neoplastic infiltration of the vagina, notably by cervical carcinoma, is commoner than primary neoplasia. Presentation is commonly with intermenstrual or post-menopausal bleeding. Squamous cell carcinoma is the commonest primary neoplasm.

In prepubescent females **sarcoma botryoides**, a rare neoplasm of mesodermal origin, derived from the lamina propria of the vaginal wall can occur. The enoplasm presents either as solitary or multiple polyps at the introitus and the appearance has been likened to 'a bunch of grapes'.

Prognosis of vaginal neoplasms is related to the FIGO clinical stage (Table 23.7).

THE CERVIX

The cervix comprises the non-keratinizing stratified

Table 23.7 The International Federation of Obstetrics and Gynaecology (FIGO) staging of primary vaginal neoplasms.

Stage	Extent	Percentage 5-year survival rate
Stage 0	Intraepithelial neoplasia	100 (if treated)
Stage I	Confined to the vaginal wall	85
Stage II	Extends beyond the vagina but not to involve the pelvic wall	85
Stage III	Extends to the pelvic wall and/or the pubic symphysis	40
Stage IV	Extension beyond the true pelvis or involvement of the bladder or rectum	0

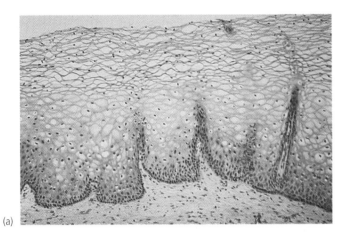

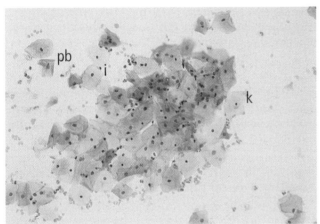

Fig. 23.12 (a) Histology of the normal ecto-cervix shows stratified squamous epithelium. (b) A normal cervical smear shows mature keratinizing (k) cells (orange), intermediate (i) and parabasal (pb) cells (blue). Note the small, regular nuclei. Papanicolau stain.

Cervical intraepithelial neoplasia

CIN is a condition involving the ectocervical epithelium where a portion of the epithelial thickness is replaced by cells showing varying degrees of nuclear and cytoplasmic abnormality. The changes most commonly arise at the **transformation zone** adjacent to the squamocolumnar junction of the cervix (Figs 23.13 and 23.14).

The term CIN is preferable to **preinvasive cervical disease** or other similar terms because in up to 70% of women affected, the epithelial changes regress back to normality over time. This statement is not, however, intended to instil a sense of complacency in the reader concerning the management of the condition because a high proportion of individuals developing high-grade intraepithelial changes do go on to develop invasive cervical carcinoma, causing in excess of 2000 deaths per year in England and Wales.

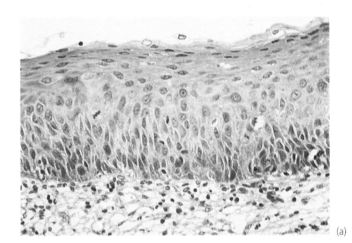

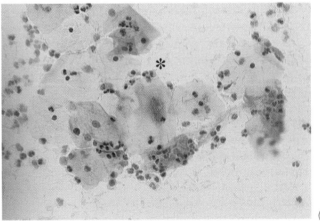

Fig. 23.13 (a) Histology of the transformation zone shows moderate dysplasia or Grade 2 CIN. (H&E.) (b) The cervical smear shows moderate dyskaryosis or CIN 2. Note the enlarged, hyperchromatic cell nucleus (✱). (PAP.)

squamous epithelium-covered **ectocervix** and the mucus-secreting glandular **endocervix** (Fig. 23.12). Although in continuity with the body of the uterus, the cervix is usually considered as a separate organ with regard to both its physiological function and the disease processes that affect it.

The cervix in the non-gravid female acts as a gated channel, permitting the flow of menstrual blood and shed endometrium externally during menstruation and the passage of spermatozoa deposited in the vagina into the uterine cavity. In the gravid female, cervical tone ensures cervical competence, preventing premature onset of labour.

The principal pathological conditions involving the cervix are **CIN** and **invasive cervical carcinoma**. These are diseases of currently or previously sexually active females.

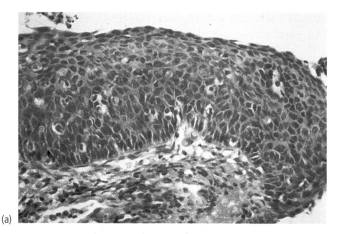

(a)

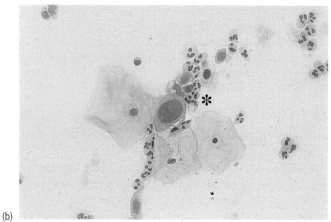

(b)

Fig. 23.14 (a) Histology of the transformation zone shows severe dysplasia or Grade 3 CIN. (H&E.) (b) The cervical smear shows severe dyskaryosis or CIN 3. Note the enlarged, hyperchromatic cell nucleus (✳). (PAP.)

Grading of intraepithelial neoplasia

The grading of CIN is usually based on the histological assessment of a cervical biopsy for the degree of cellular atypia and the proportion of the epithelial thickness occupied by the atypical cells. The disorder is divided into three grades, with the changes in grade I being mildest. The term **dysplasia** is also used by some clinicians. Cytologists apply the term **dyskaryosis** to the equivalent nuclear abnormalities observed in the exfoliated cells collected on the spatula during a cervical smear examination. The grading is summarized in Table 23.8.

Epidemiology

The age-specific prevalence of cervical epithelial disorders. If untreated, proportionately more high-grade cases of CIN will progress to invasive squamous cell carcinoma of the cervix than will low-grade cases within a given period of time (Fig. 23.15).

When the disorder does progress, there are certain generalizations that can be made concerning the peak ages at which the different grades occur (Table 23.8) and estimates of the time course for progression to occur (Table 23.9). From these estimates, and the known peak age prevalences, it would seem that there can be up to a 10-year interval between the development of CIN III and progression to invasive squamous cell carcinoma of the cervix.

As shown in Table 23.9, all grades of CIN show a peak prevalence during the years when females are most fertile, therefore treatment must aim whenever possible to preserve fertility.

Therapeutic methods used to treat CIN include direct ablation of CIN, removal of the transformation zone, cone biopsy and hysterectomy (for women who no longer wish to retain their fertility).

Risk factors implicated in the pathogenesis of cervical intraepithelial and invasive neoplasia. A large number of risk factors have been implicated in the causation of cervical intraepithelial and invasive neoplasms; these are summarized in Table 23.10.

Invasive cervical carcinoma

Invasive cervical carcinoma is a disease affecting currently or previously sexually active females with median age at diagnosis in the UK of 48 years. It causes about 2000 deaths per year in England and Wales.

The clinical presentation may be with:
- vaginal discharge;
- bleeding (intermenstrual, postcoital, postmenopausal);

Table 23.8 The grading of cervical intraepithelial neoplasia (CIN).

CIN I	(Mild dysplasia)	Cells of the entire epithelium thickness may show nuclear abnormalities, but those of the middle and upper thirds undergo normal cytoplasmic differentiation
CIN II	(Moderate dysplasia)	Full-thickness nuclear abnormalities with cell polarity loss extending beyond the basal third of the epithelium
		Stratification and cytoplasmic differentiation are preserved in the outer third
CIN III	(Severe dysplasia) (Includes carcinoma-*in-situ*)	Abnormal cells showing polarity loss occupy more than two-thirds of the epithelial thickness

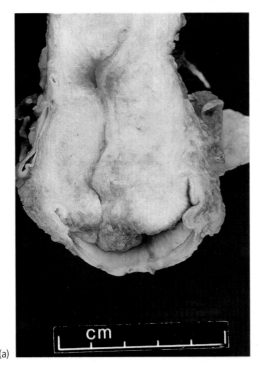

(a)

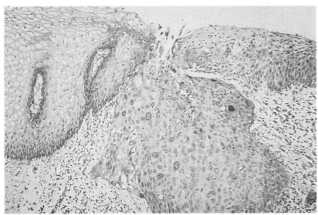

(b)

Fig. 23.15 (a) Hysterectomy specimen shows a stage I, invasive cervical carcinoma. (b) Histology of the cervix shows a moderately differentiated invasive squamous carcinoma. (H&E.)

Table 23.10 Risk factors for the development of cervical intraepithelial and invasive neoplasia.

Experience of intercourse at an early age	Occurrence of first pregnancy at an early age
Multiple sexual partners	High parity
Low socioeconomic status	Tobacco smoking
History of venereal disease	Use of oral contraception
Herpes simplex (type II) virus infection	Immune suppression – particularly cell-mediated
Human papillomavirus (HPV) HPV 6 and 11 – CIN HPV 16 and 18 – invasive neoplasia	African blacks c-*myc*/c-*ha-Ras* oncogene overexpression
Role of male factor – partners of uncircumcised males at higher risk	

CIN, Cervical intraepithelial neoplasia.

Table 23.9 Age-specific prevalence of cervical epithelial disorders.

All grades of CIN	20–29 years
Mean age when CIN III diagnosed	35 years
Invasive squamous carcinoma	50–59 years
Median estimates of the time course for progression through the grades of CIN:	
CIN I to CIN III	3–6 years
CIN II to CIN III	2 years
CIN III to invasive carcinoma	3–10 years

CIN, Cervical intraepithelial neoplasia.

- evidence of metastatic spread if the disease is already advanced.

Speculum examination usually reveals an ulcerated or exophytic neoplastic mass involving the cervix. Less commonly, the carcinoma may show an infiltrative pattern of proliferation when the cervix appears enlarged and on bimanual examination the cervix is firmer than usual. The uterus may be immobilized due to extension to involve neighbouring pelvic structures.

In excess of 90% of cervical carcinomas are of squamous cell type; the remainder are usually adenocarcinomas originating from the endocervical glandular mucosa.

Spread of invasive cervical carcinoma occurs by direct infiltration of neighbouring pelvic organs, initially by extension into the upper vagina, then the parametrium, bladder, rectum and pelvic bones. Lymphatic permeation may result in systemic dissemination. Blood-borne dissemination is rare in cervical carcinoma.

Staging of cervical neoplasia

Staging to assess the extent of the cervical carcinoma is performed using the FIGO criteria, as shown in Table 23.11.

The proportion of cases presenting at the different clinical stages in developed countries and their prognosis based on the 5-year survival after diagnosis are summarized in Table 23.12. In developing countries where the provision of cervical screening facilities are in their infancy, the proportion of women present with advanced cervical carcinoma is of the order of 75%.

Table 23.11 Clinical staging of cervical neoplasia (International Federation of Obstetricians and Gynaecologists; FIGO).

Stage 0	Intraepithelial neoplasia
Stage I	Invasion is confined to the cervix
Stage II	Invasion by the carcinoma beyond the cervix but confined to the upper two-thirds of the vagina or the parametrium, but without extension to the pelvic wall
Stage III	Invasion to involve the lower third of the vagina or extension to the pelvic wall
Stage IV	Extension to beyond the true pelvis or to involve the bladder or rectum

Table 23.12 Proportion of cases of cervical carcinoma according to International Federation of Obstetricians and Gynaecologists (FIGO) stage and their 5-year survival rate.

FIGO stage	Stage at clinical presentation (%)	5-year survival rate (%)
Stage I	50	85–90
Stage II	35	70–75
Stage III	10	30–35
Stage IV	5	10

THE UTERUS

The uterus functions as the site of implantation and development of the fertilized ovum after its passage along the fallopian tube to the endometrial cavity.

In the non-pregnant state, the uterus undergoes a cyclical proliferation of the endometrial lining in preparation for implantation of a fertilized ovum; in the absence of implantation occurring, the endometrium is shed during menstruation. The cyclical events are produced by changes in the circulating blood oestrogen and progesterone levels which are controlled by the hypothalamic–pituitary axis.

Pathological disorders affecting the uterus can most easily be discussed by considering separately the **myometrium** and the **endometrium**.

The myometrium

The myometrium is the site of development of probably the commonest benign neoplasm occurring in females, the **leiomyoma (uterine fibroid)**, a pale white, firm neoplasm with a whorled configuration, composed of

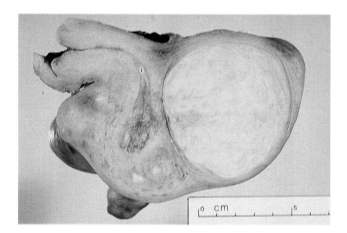

Fig. 23.16 This uterus contains a single large intramyometrial fibroid which causes distortion of the uterine cavity. Some smaller fibroids are seen in the lower and contralateral myometrium.

smooth-muscle fibres (Fig. 23.16). Leiomyomas are often multiple in number and can be located in subserosal, intramural or intramucosal sites. The peak age of incidence is 35–45 years; the majority are asymptomatic. When symptomatic, submucosal leiomyomas may:
- cause menorrhagia due to an increase in the endometrial surface area;
- cause subfertility;
- cause recurrent spontaneous abortion;
- impede delivery if located in the lower uterine segment or cervix.

Leiomyomas are responsive to circulating levels of sex hormones and may enlarge during the first trimester of pregnancy or undergo infarction ('red degeneration') during the mid-trimester of pregnancy.

Rarely, malignant transformation of a leiomyoma or *de novo* development of a **leiomyosarcoma** of the myometrium occurs. This malignant neoplasm has a peak prevalence in perimenopausal women after the age of 50, some 10 years later than the peak age for leiomyomas. The prognosis is determined by the site, extent and mitotic rate of the neoplasm.

The myometrium is also a common site for the development of endometriosis. In this location the condition is known as **adenomyosis**.

The endometrium

The commonest symptom of endometrial disease is a change in a woman's menstrual pattern, manifest as increased menstrual blood loss (menorrhagia), intermenstrual, postcoital or postmenopausal bleeding. This may be associated with abdominal discomfort referable to the uterus or, less frequently, systemic symptoms due to anaemia (usually hypochromic, microcytic) or spread of the disease beyond the uterus.

The commonest conditions affecting the endometrium are idiopathic conditions, hormonal dysfunctions and endometrial polyps. Less frequent causes are endometritis (acute and chronic), endometrial hyperplasia, **intraendometrial neoplasia (IEN)** and endometrial carcinoma (most commonly, adenocarcinoma).

Initial clinical assessment usually involves biopsy of the endometrium by dilatation and curettage or suction curettage. These procedures are primarily performed to provide a tissue diagnosis and, in the case of some of the benign conditions, such as endometrial polyps, they may also provide a therapeutic outcome.

Endometrial polyps (Fig. 23.17)
Endometrial polyps are composed of benign, sex hormone-unresponsive proliferations of endometrial glands and stroma. Two age groups of women are particularly prone to their development – in perimenopausal women the polyps are commonly multiple and may be an expression of benign endometrial hyperplasia (see below); in postmenopausal women a single polyp is more common. Ulceration at the tip of the polyp followed by non-menstrual bleeding is the major symptom.

Endometritis
Endometritis may be acute or chronic in terms of the chronology of symptoms and the histological pattern of inflammation.

Acute endometritis most commonly follows a septic abortion and the causation is usually bacterial. Actinomyces infection is associated with use of IUCDs but is a rare cause of endometritis. Polymorphonuclear neutrophils are present throughout the endometrial stroma as well as within the epithelium and lumen of the endometrial glands.

Chronic endometritis is characterized by the presence of **plasma cells** in the stromal inflammatory infiltrate. The condition is manifest as painful, irregular uterine bleeding; causes include retained placental tissue after abortion, stillbirth and live delivery. Because of the cyclical menstrual shedding of the endometrium, caseating granulomas are not formed in tuberculous endometritis.

Endometrial hyperplasia
Controversy surrounds the terminology and prognostic significance applied to hyperplasia of the endometrium and intraendometrial carcinoma (probably better termed intraendometrial neoplasia, IEN).

Endometrial hyperplasia is a term best applied to those histopathological conditions where there is architectural distortion of the endometrial glands **without** cytological atypia/dyskaryosis and the risk of progression to invasive endometrial carcinoma is low. The term includes **cystic glandular hyperplasia**, where cystic dilatation of endometrial glands occurs and **adenomatous hyperplasia**, where the density of glands per unit area/field examined is increased. These conditions are associated with:

- prolonged unopposed exposure to oestrogenic stimulation, due to anovular cycles;
- excess endogenous secretion by stromal ovarian neoplasms;
- obesity (due to the peripheral metabolism of adrenal androgenic steroids in adipose tissue);
- unopposed administration of exogenous oestrogen.

IEN refers to those cases where histological examination shows the presence of cellular atypia/dyskaryosis in association with glandular architectural abnormalities.

IEN can be graded using the degree of cellular atypia shown, extent of cellular multilayering in the glands and glandular architectural abnormality (Table 23.13).

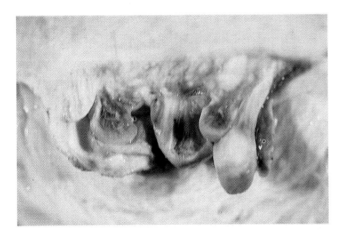

Fig. 23.17 Endometrial polyps can produce menorrhagia or intermenstrual bleeding.

Table 23.13 The histopathological features used to grade intraendometrial neoplasia (IEN).

IEN I	The glands show mild cellular atypia with increased nuclear to cytoplasmic ratio. The normal polar orientation of the nuclei is maintained
IEN II	The glands show multilayering of cells lining the endometrial glands. The individual cells show a moderate degree of atypia
IEN III	The glands are composed of cells showing loss of polarity, increased nuclear to cytoplasmic ratio with rounded nuclei containing coarsely clumped chromatin and enlarged nucleoli. (This grade equates with *in-situ* endometrial carcinoma)

Endometrial carcinoma

Endometrial carcinoma is a disease of perimenopausal and postmenopausal women (median age of presentation 56 years), typically obese (due to peripheral metabolism of adrenal androgens to oestrogens), nulliparous or of low parity. Previous pregnancies or the use of the combined oral contraceptive protect against the development of endometrial neoplasia. Clinical presentation is with either intermenstrual or postmenopausal bleeding. Risk factors associated with the development of endometrial carcinoma are summarized in Table 23.14.

Over 90% of endometrial carcinomas are adenocarcinomas and, at the time of initial diagnosis, in the region of 70% of cases the carcinoma is still confined to the uterine cavity (FIGO stage I; Fig. 23.18). The clinical staging is based on FIGO which incorporates assessment of the neoplasm extent, the size of the uterine cavity, histological differentiation and the depth of uterine wall invasion is shown in Table 23.15 and the prognosis of the stages is summarized in Table 23.16.

As the majority of endometrial carcinomas are well-differentiated adenocarcinomas (grade 1) and confined to the uterine body (stage I), total abdominal hysterectomy and bilateral salpingo-oophorectomy is the preferred treatment. Preoperative intracavity or postoperative

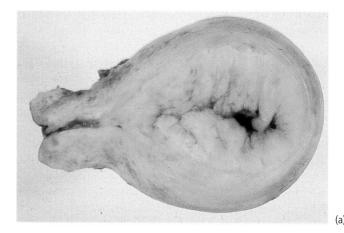

(a)

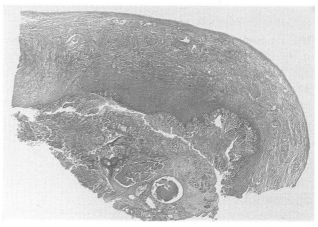

(b)

Fig. 23.18 Endometrial adenocarcinoma. (a) This tumour has almost filled the endometrial cavity. (b) Histology shows how the tumour has invaded into the myometrium. (H&E.)

Table 23.14 Risk factors implicated/associated with the development of endometrial carcinoma.

Nulliparity (two-to threefold increase in risk)	Diabetes mellitus
Unopposed peri- and postmenopausal oestrogenic stimulation	Hypertension High dietary fat consumption
Non-cyclical postmenopausal hormone replacement treatment	Gross obesity (increased peripheral steroid conversion)
Polycystic ovary syndrome	Intraendometrial neoplasia

Table 23.16 Prognosis of endometrial carcinoma based on initial clinical stage (International Federation of Obstetricians and Gynaecologists; FIGO (1989)).

FIGO stage	5-year survival rate (%)
Stage I	75–85
Stage II	55–65
Stage III	35–45
Stage IV	Less than 10

Table 23.15 The clinical staging of endometrial carcinoma (International Federation of Obstetricians and Gynaecologists; FIGO).

Stage 0	Intraendometrial neoplasia
Stage I	Carcinoma confined to the uterine body
Grade 1	Well-differentiated
Grade 2	Moderately differentiated (partially solid)
Grade 3	Poorly differentiated (predominantly solid)
Stage II	Extension to involve the cervix
Stage III	Extension outside the uterus but confined to the true pelvis
Stage IV	Extension beyond the true pelvis or invasion of the bladder or rectum

external beam radiotherapy in combination with surgery is used for stage II and poorly differentiated endometrial neoplasms. Progesterone may be administered when distant metastatic disease is present at initial staging or following disease relapse, to facilitate a reduction in neoplasm volume.

Endometriosis

Endometriosis is a condition typically affecting older

nulliparous or women of low parity who may experience a variety of symptoms referable to the sites of disease involvement accompanied by cyclical pain coinciding with the onset of menstruation. This is due to the localized bleeding from the site of the endometriosis causing pressure and irritation. Endometriosis is due to the presence of hormonally responsive benign endometrial glands and stroma in sites outside the mucosal lining of uterine the cavity.

Pathological and clinical terminology distinguishes between two main variants of endometriosis–**adenomyosis**, which is endometriosis confined to the myometrium of the uterus (this is in fact commoner in multiparous women) and **external endometriosis** which most commonly affects the other genital organs (Fig. 23.19) but can be located in extragenital sites. Table 23.17 summarizes those sites most frequently affected.

The pathogenesis of endometriosis is unknown. Various theories have been proposed, including retrograde menstruation (Sampson's theory) due to reflux into the peritoneum via the fallopian tubes and metaplasia of Müllerian-derived epithelium and mesenchyme (Novak's theory) accounting for all pelvic, abdominal wall and visceral sites. Implantation of endometrium during hysterectomy and, rarely, caesarean section may account for deposits in laparotomy scars. Lymphovascular dissemination of endometrial emboli may explain lymph node and pulmonary endometriosis.

THE FALLOPIAN TUBES

Acute or chronic salpingitis (often due to preceding sexually transmitted infection, with consequent risk of fibrosis leading to infertility) and ectopic pregnancy are the commonest conditions involving the fallopian tubes.

Acute salpingitis is associated with *Neisseria gonorrhoeae* and chlamydial infection secondary to sexual transmission and streptococcal infection following septic abortion or delivery. Ascending infections have been implicated in the pathogenesis of salpingitis in IUCD users. **Chronic salpingitis** is most commonly due to *Mycobacterium tuberculosis* infection, a rare disorder in developed countries.

Ectopic pregnancy is the implantation and development of the conceptus outside of the uterine cavity (Fig. 23.20). This condition complicates up to 1 in every 250 pregnancies. The commonest implantation site is the ampulla of the fallopian tube. The risk of developing an ectopic pregnancy is increased with a past history of IUCD use or PID.

Primary invasive neoplasia of the fallopian tube is very rare, accounting for less than 1% of genital tract neoplasms. The neoplasm occurs in women aged 40–60

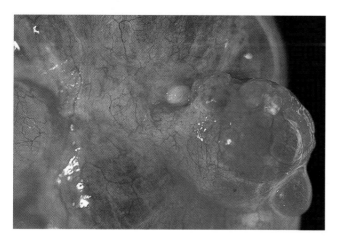

Fig. 23.19 Endometriosis involving the ovary produces multiple blood-filled 'chocolate cysts'. This patient presented with pelvic pain and infertility.

Table 23.17 Sites involved by endometriosis.

| Uterine wall (adenomyosis) |
| Fallopian tubes (infertility) |
| Ovaries ('chocolate cysts') |
| Cervix and vagina |
| Extragenital sites |
| Bladder |
| Intestines |
| Appendix |
| Umbilicus |
| Laparotomy scars |
| Lymph nodes |
| Lungs |

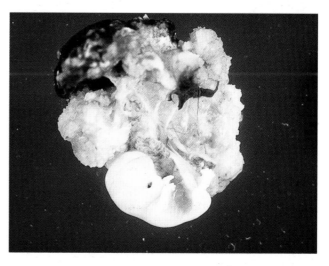

Fig. 23.20 A fallopian tubal ectopic pregnancy.

Table 23.18 The International Federation of Obstetricians and Gynaecologists (FIGO) clinical staging of fallopian tube neoplasia (1989).

Stage 0	Intraepithelial neoplasia
Stage I	Invasion is confined to the fallopian tube
Stage II	Invasion of one or both fallopian tubes with pelvic extension
Stage III	Invasion of one or both tubes with intraperitoneal dissemination
Stage IV	Invasion of one or both fallopian tubes with extraperitoneal metastases

years and the histopathological appearance is of a papillary adenocarcinoma which may contain **psammoma bodies**. The prognosis is generally poor, owing to the majority of cases presenting with advanced stage III disease. Staging using the FIGO recommendations is summarized in Table 23.18.

THE OVARIES

The ovaries are affected by a variety of pathological conditions including:

- anomalous gonad development, which is usually accompanied by disordered physical sexual development (such as in Turner's syndrome, XO genotype where the ovary is replaced by fibrous tissue, the external genitalia appear infantile and the uterus is of small size);
- exaggeration of the normal physiological function, for example benign functional retention cysts of the ovary;
- involvement secondary to other disease processes, for example ovarian endometriosis causing a 'chocolate cyst' and imbalances of the hypothalamic–pituitary axis or exogenous administration of sex hormones;
- ovarian neoplasms which represent a significant source of female mortality.

Benign functional ovarian cysts (Fig. 23.21)

The development of functional cysts is confined to the child-bearing years of a woman's life and their development often reflects either temporary disordered hypothalamic–pituitary–ovarian axis dysfunction or early regression of a pregnancy. Under the normal hormonal influence of the hypothalamic–pituitary axis, one ovary forms a fluid-filled follicular swelling on its surface, the **Graafian follicle**, rupture of which results in release of the ovum at ovulation. The ruptured follicle then normally forms the corpus luteum which soon de-

generates if fertilization and implantation of the ovum fail to occur. The development of ovarian distension cysts may be asymptomatic or cause pelvic pain, dyspareunia, subfertility or menstrual irregularity.

Two main types of cysts arise from derangement of the normal physiological activity.

1 Follicular ovarian cysts, single or multiple clear or yellow fluid-containing cysts, rarely of greater than 7 cm in diameter, resulting from failure of Graafian follicle rupture followed by further cyst enlargement. The cysts are lined by granulosa cells and tend to regress spontaneously.

2 Theca–lutein cyst, tend to be single, arising due to persistence of the corpus luteum or luteinization of the theca and granulosa cells of a follicular cyst. Histologically the cyst is lined by granulosa cells. Eventual rupture of the cyst may produce acute pelvic pain after a period of amenorrhoea, due to intra-abdominal bleeding from the cyst.

A rarer disorder, involving bilateral ovarian enlargement, is due to hyperplasia of the cortex by multiple enlarged Graafian follicle, at various stages of development, surrounded by a dense fibrous capsule, and is known as the **Stein–Leventhal (polycystic ovary) syndrome**. The syndrome presents with secondary amenorrhoea in obese young females with hirsutism and bilateral ovarian enlargement. Endometrial hyperplasia, intraendometrial neoplasia and endometrial carcinoma may subsequently develop if untreated by either medical treatment or wedge resection of the ovaries.

Ovarian neoplasms

Due to their complex development, the ovaries are cap-

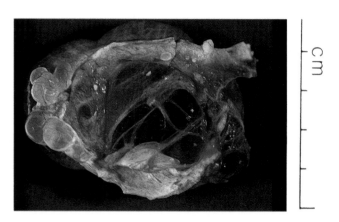

Fig. 23.21 Cut section of this ovary shows a range of functional ovarian cysts. The small yellow cysts represent the corpus luteum (cl) and the larger, blood-filled cysts are follicular (F) cysts.

able of differentiating into an extremely diverse range of neoplasms including benign, borderline/low malignant potential and frankly malignant.

Although malignant ovarian neoplasms account for about a quarter of all gynaecological malignancies, they cause nearly half the female genital tract malignancy deaths, owing to the clinical presentation occurring at an advanced stage. This is in part due to the deep abdominal location of the ovaries (Fig. 23.22).

Histogenesis of ovarian neoplasms (Fig. 23.23)

The classification of ovarian neoplasms is shown in Table 23.19. They can be categorized into three principal groups:

- **epithelial** (Figs 23.24 and 23.25);
- **germ cell** (Fig. 23.26);
- **sex cord–stromal** tumours (Fig. 23.27).

This classification is based upon the three primary

Table 23.19 Histological classification of ovarian neoplasms.

Histological category	Tissue differentiation
Epithelial (60%)	
Serous (cystadenoma/ cystadenocarcinoma)	Fallopian tube
Mucinous (cystadenoma/ cystadenocarcinoma)	Endocervix
Endometrioid	Endometrium
Brenner tumour	Urothelium
Clear cell	Mesonephroid
Mixed or unclassifiable	
Germ cell (20%)	
Mature (dermoid) cystic teratoma	Well-differentiated
Immature teratoma	Moderately differentiated
Dysgerminoma	Undifferentiated
Endodermal sinus (yolk sac) tumour	Poorly differentiated
Mixed malignant germ cell tumour	Moderate to poorly differentiated
Gonadal sex cord–stromal neoplasms (10%)	
Granulosa cell tumour	Granulosa cell
Thecoma and fibrothecoma	Thecal cells and stromal fibroblasts
Sertoli cell tumour	Sertoli cell
Leydig cell tumour	Leydig and interstitial cells
Secondary neoplasms (10%)	
Krukenberg tumour	Gastric signet-ring adenocarcinoma
Burkitt's lymphoma	Lymphoid

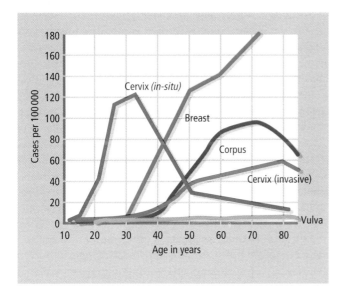

Fig. 23.22 The incidence of cancer in women according to age.

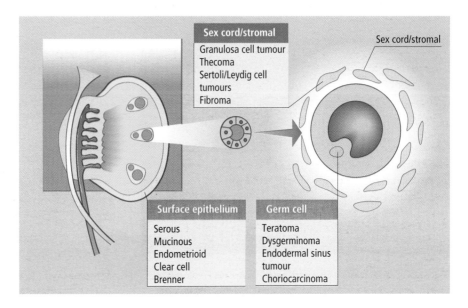

Fig. 23.23 The histogenesis of ovarian neoplasms.

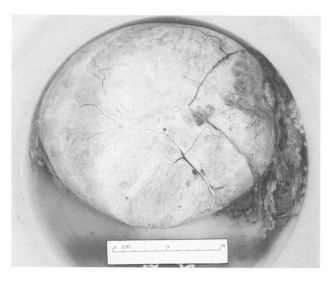

Fig. 23.24 Ovarian tumour of epithelial origin. Mucinous cystadenomas may reach a massive size. Rupture during surgical removal may lead to 'pseudomyxoma peritonei'.

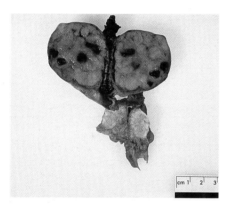

Fig. 23.25 Ovarian tumour of epithelial origin. An endometrioid carcinoma of the ovary is small in size but this patient already has disseminated metastases.

tissue components incorporated into the gonad during embryological development, becoming the pathological precursor of neoplasms in the developed ovary. The three primary tissue components appear to retain the capacity to differentiate into a variety of tissue types, accounting for the histological diversity of appearance. The surface epithelium of the adult ovary retains the potential to differentiate into epithelium, mimicking the mucosal lining of the different component organs of the female genital and urinary tract. Similarly, germ cell and sex cord–stromal neoplasms recapitulate yolk sac structures (from which the germ cell precursors originate) and urogenital ridge mesenchyme, at the indifferent stage, when capable of differentiation into male or female gonadal germ cells and stroma (see Chapter 11).

Although epithelial neoplasms represent 60% of ovarian tumours, they represent approximately 90% of malignant neoplasms. Epithelial neoplasms are classified according to the pattern and degree of epithelial differentiation.

Germ cell neoplasms occur most frequently in young women (Table 23.20) and may secrete detectable blood levels of α-fetoprotein (AFP; yolk sac tumours or malignant teratomas with yolk sac elements), human chorionic gonadotrophin (hCG) and placental alkaline phosphatase (PLAP; malignant teratomas with focal elements of choriocarcinoma). Biochemical measurement of these marker proteins may be used to monitor the response to therapy.

Sex cord–stromal neoplasms can occur at any age and may be steroid hormone-secreting, producing a variety of feminizing or virilizing effects dependent on whether oestrogenic or androgenic steroids predominate.

Metastatic ovarian tumours are commonly bilateral in their involvement. The commonest primary sites are the

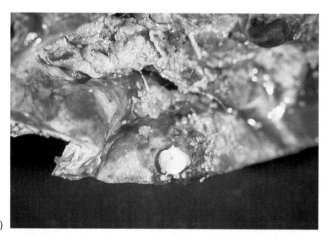

(a)

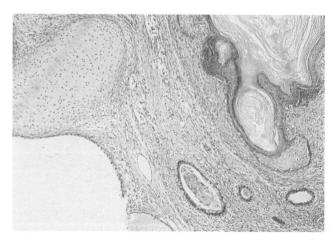

(b)

Fig. 23.26 Ovarian tumour of germ cell origin. (a) A mature cystic teratoma (ovarian dermoid) contains hair, sebaceous glands and teeth. (b) Histology of a mature cystic teratoma shows well differentiated epithelial and cartilaginous elements.

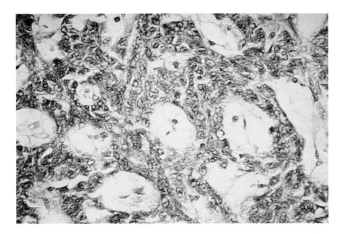

Fig. 23.27 Ovarian tumour of sex cord–stromal origin. Granulosa cell tumour. Histology shows cells with grooved nuclei and Call–Exner body formation. (H&E.)

stomach (Krukenberg tumour), colon, breast and from elsewhere in the genital tract.

The causation of the majority of ovarian neoplasms is unknown. Risk factors for their development are summarized in **Table 23.21**. A minority of individuals may have an autosomal dominant inheritance.

The management and prognosis of ovarian malignancy are dependent on the FIGO staging (Table 23.22) and the degree of differentiation of epithelial and germ cell neoplasms. The prognosis according to the FIGO stage is summarized in Table 23.23.

Table 23.24 provides a synopsis of terms that are applied to diseases involving the ovaries, some of which have already been discussed. The remainder have been summarized for brevity and to assist the reader in revision for examinations.

INFERTILITY

About 10% of couples experience difficulty in producing a child when they want to. More than 80% will conceive

Table 23.20 Age-specific prevalence of ovarian neoplasms.

Histological category	Prevalent age
Malignant germ cell neoplasms	Under 20 years
Epithelial neoplasms	Over 40 years
Sex cord–stromal neoplasms	Any age
Peak age incidence of benign neoplasms	40–49 years
Peak incidence of malignant neoplasms	50–59 years

Table 23.21 Risk and protective factors in the pathogenesis of ovarian neoplasms.

Risk factors	Protective factors
Nulliparous/low parity	Previous pregnancy
Aged over 40 years	Previous use of combined oral contraceptive
Domicile in Westernized cultural environment	
Family history of ovarian neoplasia	
Previous treatment for breast or colonic carcinoma	
Talcum powder (applied to vulva, contraceptive diaphragms and condoms)	
Ovarian endometriosis (endometrioid carcinoma)	

Table 23.22 Clinical staging of ovarian neoplasms.

Stage I	Disease is confined to the ovaries
Stage Ia	Unilateral
Stage Ib	Bilateral
Stage Ic	Ascites present or ovarian capsule breached
Stage II	Extension to involve other pelvic structures
Stage III	Abdominal peritoneum involved
Stage IV	Distant metastatic disease present

Table 23.23 Prognosis according to the International Federation of Obstetricians and Gynaecologists (FIGO) stage of ovarian neoplasms (1989).

FIGO stage	5-year survival rates (%)
Stage Ia	85
Stage Ib–II	40
Stage III	15
Stage IV	Less than 5

Less than a quarter of patients present with stage Ia or b disease, accounting for the poor prognosis associated with the disease.

within the first 2 years but 10% (i.e. 1% of the total) will remain infertile if no treatment is given.

Infertility may affect either partner. Female causes of infertility (approximately 60% of cases) include:
- ovulatory failure;
- PID or endometriosis and occluded fallopian tubes;
- hyperandrogenic syndromes;
- chromosomal abnormalities;

Table 23.24 A synopsis of terms used in describing ovarian disease.

Borderline/carcinoma of low malignant potential	A category of usually serous and mucinous ovarian neoplasms of intermediate prognosis, whose appearance is characterized by the presence of papillary excrescences within cystic areas. Microscopy shows the papillae to be composed of two or more cell layers with variable nuclear atypia. Stromal invasion is absent
Brenner tumour	A benign solid or cystic ovarian neoplasm formed from transitional-type epithelium. The neoplasm is often an incidental finding associated with mucinous epithelial neoplasms and cystic teratomas
Call–Exner bodies	Occur in granulosa cell tumours as microscopic spaces containing eosinophilic material (including cellular nuclear debris) surrounded by a rosette of cells
Dysgerminoma	Ovarian homologue of the testicular seminoma
Krukenberg tumour	Bilateral metastatic signet-ring cell carcinoma originating from a primary gastric adenocarcinoma
Mature teratoma	'Dermoid cyst' of the ovary. Constitutes 95% of germ cell neoplasms
Meig's syndrome	Ascites and hydrothorax (uni- or bilateral) occurring in association with a benign ovarian fibroma
Psammoma bodies	Microscopic concentrically laminated extracellular calcified structures. Occur in association with papillary neoplasms (ovarian serous cystadenocarcinoma, papillary carcinoma of the thyroid, mesothelioma, papillary adenocarcinoma of the fallopian tubes) and meningiomas
Pseudomyxoma peritonei	Copious mucin is formed within the peritoneal cavity, following implantation of mucin-secreting cells in the peritoneum following leakage from mucinous ovarian neoplasms or mucocoele of the appendix
Reinke crystals	Microtrabecular structures occurring in the cytoplasm or nucleus of cells in Leydig cell tumours
Schiller–Duval bodies	Pseudoglomerular adenopapillary structures with a central blood vessel. Occur in yolk sac tumours
Struma ovarii	A mature cystic teratoma in which over 80% of the volume is composed of thyroid tissue. The tissue is hormonally functional

- thyroid dysfunction;
- adrenal dysfunction;
- psychosexual problems.

Clinical investigations should include:

- general physical examination, including a pelvic examination and cervical smear;
- screens for syphilis and rubella antibody;
- assessment of ovulation with use of a temperature chart (a fall in temperature followed by a rise in 0.5°C indicates ovulation), endometrial biopsy, luteal-phase plasma progesterone and ultrasonic monitoring of ovarian follicles;
- assessment of patency of the fallopian tubes by laparoscopy and hysterosalpingography.

Ovulatory failure is treated with gonadotrophin (clomiphene); surgery may be performed on blocked fallopian tubes; gamete intrafallopian transfer (GIFT) or *in vitro* fertilization and embryo transfer (IVF and ET) may be offered if these measures are not effective.

THE PLACENTA AND GESTATIONAL TROPHOBLASTIC DISEASES

The **placenta** develops as a disc-shaped structure attached to the uterine wall from the **decidua** (a modified form of **maternal** uterine endometrium) and the **chorion** (a component of the **fetal** membranes).

The placenta functions as an **exchange organ** permitting diffusion and active transport of nutrients, fluid, electrolytes, metabolites and, to a limited extent, cells across the **maternofetal barrier**. To fulfil this function the placenta is richly vascularized and the cellular interface between the maternal and fetal circulations in the mature placenta is formed by the **chorionic villi** which facilitate anchorage to and exchange with the decidua. The chorionic villi are covered by an outer layer of **syncytiotrophoblast** and an inner layer of **cytotrophoblast** cells. The syncytiotrophoblast secretes hCG and human placental lactogen (hPL); both may be used to monitor trophoblast proliferation such as pregnancy testing and monitoring response to treatment of trophoblastic disorders.

Conditions that affect the placenta include the following.

- **Abnormal site of implantation**:
  (a) **ectopic pregnancy** – commonly in the fallopian tube;
  (b) **placenta praevia** – implantation in the lower uterine segment with the placenta partially or completely covering the internal cervical os;
- **Maternal conditions affecting the placenta** include abnormalities of uterine cavity architecture, either con-

genital or acquired following previous surgery. Maternal diseases include:

(a) systemic hypertension;

(b) pre-eclampsia;

(c) eclampsia;

(d) diabetes mellitus;

(e) renal and haematological disorders may affect the maternal vascular supply to the site of placentation and can result in placental abruption, infarction and degeneration in the placenta with resultant fetal compromise or even death;

• **multiple gestations** – examination of the placenta and fetal membranes by the pathologist may be requested to distinguish between monozygotic and dizygotic twins sharing a single fused placenta. Dizygotic gestations form two separate chorionic and amnionic sacs (Fig. 23.28).

Trophoblastic disease

The term trophoblastic disease encompasses both benign (**partial** and **complete hydatidiform mole** – 95%) and malignant (**choriocarcinoma** – 5%) proliferations of trophoblastic tissue.

Hydatidiform mole (Fig. 23.29)

Hydatidiform moles show widely differing incidences according to ethnic origin and geographic location, occurring at a frequency of about 1 in 2000 pregnancies in western European countries and the USA compared with 1 in 200 pregnancies in many developing countries, particularly in the Pacific basin. Risk factors include pregnancies in women of very young or old age groups, consanguineous partnerships, malnutrition and low

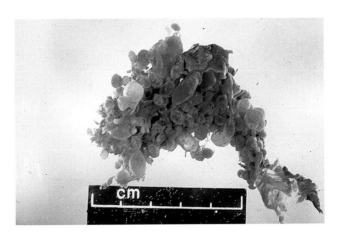

Fig. 23.29 Hydatidiform mole. The grape-like clusters consist of hydropic trophoblast villi associated with trophoblast proliferation.

socioeconomic circumstances and racial origin (Southeast Asia and Mexico).

Clinical features include irregular vaginal bleeding after an episode of amenorrhoea, excessive nausea and vomiting. Examination usually reveals a large-for-dates uterus with absent fetal heart sounds. A pregnancy test is very strongly positive and ultrasound scanning shows a characteristic pattern of echogenicity. A minority of cases are only detected on histological examination of uterine curettings from an apparently incomplete spontaneous abortion.

The macroscopic of the spontaneously aborted or curetted tissue is characterized by sheets of oedematous, hydropic villi – this appearance has been likened to a 'bunch of grapes' (see Fig. 23.29). Histologically the villi are composed of oedematous core of stroma from which blood vessels are absent. The surface of the villi is covered by hyperplastic syncytiotrophoblast and cytotrophoblast.

The hydatidiform mole can be divided into two groups according to the macroscopic and microscopic appearance of the placental villi, the presence or absence of the development of identifiable fetal tissue and the cytogenetic karyotype of the molar tissue.

The **complete hydatidiform mole** is composed entirely of hydropic chorionic villi and no fetal tissue is present; the karyotype has a 46,XX complement (both X chromosomes are of paternal origin; Fig. 23.30).

The **partial hydatidiform mole** has the appearance of a placenta in which hydropic villi occur focally and may intermingle with normal villi containing fetal vessels. An identifiable gestation sac or fetal tissue, usually of abnormal morphology, may be present. The karyotype is commonly triploid (69,XXX or 69,XXY); the additional haploid is of paternal origin (Fig. 23.31).

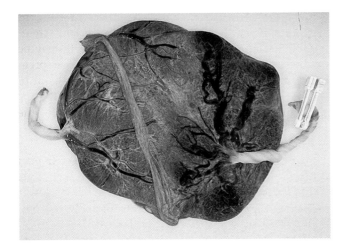

Fig. 23.28 A twin placenta.

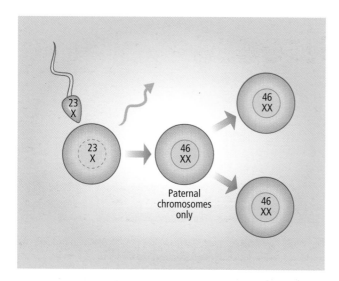

Fig. 23.30 The cytogenetics of a complete hydatidiform mole.

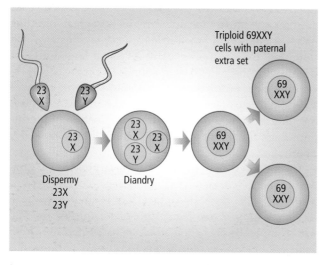

Fig. 23.31 The cytogenetics of a partial hydatidiform mole.

Choriocarcinoma

This is a malignant proliferation of trophoblastic tissue causing invasion of the maternal vasculature. Villus differentiation is absent in choriocarcinoma and the neoplasm forms either a single or multiple haemorrhagic nodule within the uterus.

Half of choriocarcinomas develop after a preceding hydatidiform mole, with the remainder arising after a normal pregnancy or abortion (both spontaneous and therapeutic).

Trophoblastic diseases are highly responsive to chemotherapy and the therapeutic response can be monitored by measurement of the β-subunit of hCG.

FURTHER READING

Fox H. (ed.) (1987) *Haines and Taylor Obstetrical Pathology*, 3rd edn. Churchill Livingstone, Edinburgh.

Kurman R.J. (ed.) (1994) *Blaustein's Pathology of the Female Genital Tract*, 4th. edn. Springer-Verlag, New York.

Peterson F. (1988) *Annual Report of the Results of the Treatment in Gynaecological Cancer*. FIGO, Stockholm.

Shepherd J.H. (1989) Revised FIGO staging for gynaecological cancer. *Br. J. Obstet. Gynaecol.* **96**: 889–892.

Breast Disease

THE NORMAL FEMALE BREAST (Fig. 24.1)

Introduction

Embryologically, breast ducts and lobules are derived from **ectoderm** as a modified form of sweat gland; breast stroma is derived from underlying **mesenchyme**.

The adult breast is composed of approximately **20 lobes** separated by fibrous septa. Each lobe comprises **lobular units** made up of **ducts** and **acini** which are lined by two layers of cells, **epithelial** and **myoepithelial** cells, to provide secretory and contractile function respectively. Ducts and acini are surrounded by intralobular loose connective tissue. Interlobular connective tissue is more dense and fibrous (Fig. 24.2).

The lobule, together with its terminal duct, is called the terminal duct lobular unit (TDLU) and most pathological lesions arise from this area (see Fig. 24.1).

Breast development, lactation and regression

Ductal structures proliferate slowly prepubertally, then more rapidly at puberty. Most of the increase in size is due to connective tissue deposition (principally fat). During pregnancy, the number and size of lobules increase markedly with a reversal of gland to stroma ratio and secretory activity begins with formation of secretory vacuoles. After cessation of lactation, these changes reverse, although not completely. After the menopause, the lobules involute.

Congenital and developmental abnormalities

Congenital anomalies of the breast are common but usually of little clinical significance. The following congenital abnormalities exist.

- **Abnormalities of the milk line.** Accessory nipples and accessory breast tissue are of no significance.
- **Development asymmetry** is very common and varies from minor differences to unilateral amastia, which may involve underlying pectoral muscle.
- **Congenital inversion of the nipples** is common and is clinically important because it may make nursing difficult and may be confused with the nipple retractions associated with breast cancer.

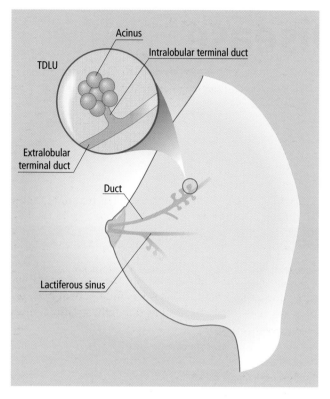

Fig. 24.1 The normal female breast including the terminal duct lobular unit (TDLU).

- 'Virginal hypertrophy' is the commonest reason for breast reduction.
- **Mammary hamartoma** consists of a well-defined mixture of lobules, elastotic tissue and fat and is benign.

CLINICAL EVALUATION OF BREAST DISEASE

Clinical presentation of breast disease

Breast disease may present with:
- a lump;
- pain;
- change in shape;
- nipple abnormality;
- nipple discharge.

A lump in the breast

Investigation of breast lumps includes:
- clinical examination;
- mammography;
- fine-needle aspiration (FNA);
- biopsy.

If the breast lump is cystic, FNA may be therapeutic, but any residual mass must be biopsied (Table 24.1).

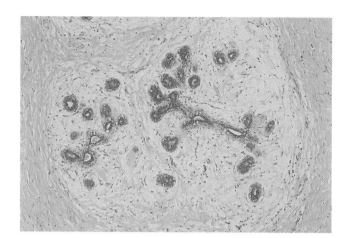

Fig. 24.2 The lobular acinus surrounded by loose connective tissue. (H&E.)

Pain in the breast

Diffuse, mild pain may occur during the premenstrual phase in most women. A painful mass may imply an inflammatory lesion and may also be present in advanced carcinoma.

Nipple discharge

A discharge of milk occurs in pregnancy and lactation but may occur at other times (galactorrhoea). In breasts showing fibrocystic change, there may be a non-haemorrhagic nipple discharge. **Bloody discharge** is seen in:
- fibrocystic change;
- intraductal papilloma;
- intraductal carcinoma.

Skin changes

Infiltration of the skin by malignant disease will produce **skin tethering**, followed by ulceration. Infiltration of dermal lymphatics results in **lymphoedema (peau d'orange)**. Acute inflammatory change may be seen overlying a breast abscess. **Paget's disease** of the nipple looks like eczema macroscopically, but is due to intraepidermal spread of carcinoma cells, usually from an underlying ductal carcinoma.

Table 24.1 Causes of a lump in the breast.

Congenital	
Acquired	
Infection	Abscess, acute mastitis
Neoplasm	
Benign	Fibroadenoma
Malignant	Carcinoma
Vascular	Vasculitis, arterial medial calcification
Inflammatory	Fibrocystic change, duct ectasia, chronic mastitis
Traumatic	Fat necrosis

Methods for evaluating breast disease

Physical examination

Physical examination of a breast mass, including self-examination, may be useful in detecting a carcinoma but only in advanced cases. **Features suggestive of malignancy** include:

- pain and tenderness on palpation;
- skin tethering;
- lymphoedema (*peau d'orange*);
- nipple retraction;
- blood-stained nipple discharge;
- fixation or non-mobility of the lump;
- a solitary lump in a non-lumpy breast.

Mammography

A mammograph is a soft-tissue radiograph of the breast. It will detect areas of **breast deformity**, increased breast **thickening** and **calcification**, all of which may be markers of malignancy or of carcinoma-*in-situ* or inflammatory or fibrocystic change. Mammography may detect the presence of a breast carcinoma which has not yet become palpable.

Biopsy

The definitive means of evaluating a breast mass is by **microscopic evaluation** of the breast tissue. This may be done in three main ways.

1 Fine-needle aspiration. This method provides a sample for cytological evaluation. Nipple aspiration may provide cells for cytological evaluation. This technique employs aspiration of fluid from the breast ducts (Table 24.2).

2 Tru-cut biopsy/core needle biopsy. This provides core of tissue for histology.

3 Incisional or excisional open biopsy. Part or all the mass may be removed for histology. This permits assessment of the cells and the architecture of the breast tissue. **Frozen section** evaluation of breast tissue removed as a biopsy may be evaluated quickly while the patient is under anaesthesia. This method is described in Chapter 1.

Table 24.2 Indications for fine-needle aspiration of the breast.

Investigation of any palpable lump
Preoperative confimation of carcinoma
Confirmation of inoperable carcinoma
Confirmation of recurrence/metastasis
Diagnosis/treatment of simple cysts
Supplement of mammography in screening
To obtain material for further analysis

Screening for breast disease

Screening involves applying a test to a large group of the population to identify a disease, preferably in an early stage. Factors influencing efficiency of a screening programme include:

- attendance;
- selection of target population;
- predictive value of the test;
- sensitivity of the test;
- screening interval.

Several large trials suggest benefits of mammographic screening for detection of early breast cancer. In the UK, the Forrest Report recommended:

- a target population aged 50–64 years;
- 3-yearly single-view mammography.

Many problems are found in the mammographic screening programme and these include patient bias, patient selection, lead time and lead length, so results must be assessed carefully.

BENIGN, NON-NEOPLASTIC BREAST DISEASE

Inflammation

Mastitis

Acute. Acute mastitis refers to bacterial infection of the breast, usually by staphylococci or, less commonly, streptococci. It is usually unilateral and is most often seen in conditions in which the skin is cracked or fissured, as in the first few weeks of nursing or in patients with eczema or other dermatological conditions of the nipples. Staphylococci tend to produce single or multiple breast abscesses; streptococci usually produce a diffuse spreading infection. Therapy is with antibiotics and surgical drainage if an abscess is present. Mastitis may heal with a dense scar and skin retraction that may later be confused with breast cancer.

Chronic. Chronic infections like tuberculosis are rare in the breast.

Fat necrosis

Fat necrosis is usually post-traumatic, whether accidental or surgically induced. Adipocyte death leads to a **foreign-body giant cell reaction** to extruded fat. This may be associated with fibrosis and calcification of the breast tissue. Clinically, **fat necrosis may mimic breast carcinoma**.

Mammary duct ectasia

Mammary duct ectasia consists of distended ducts filled with secretion, exciting a periductal inflammatory response (Fig. 24.3). There may be epithelial ulceration. Duct ectasia may cause **nipple discharge** which is occasionally bloody and this may create an impression of malignancy. Histology shows that a marked chronic inflammatory reaction is most prominent around ducts and may contain granulomas, neutrophils, lymphocytes and sometimes prominent plasma cells (**plasma cell mastitis**). Mammary duct ectasia is sometimes associated with pituitary adenomas, suggesting that prolactin secretion may contribute to its development. Mammary duct ectasia can resemble carcinoma by physical examination and by mammography.

Galactocoele

Galactocoele is observed during lactation when one or more ducts become cystically dilated with milk. A galactocoele may be secondarily infected, causing acute mastitis with or without abscess formation.

Fibrocystic change (benign proliferative breast disease, chronic mastitis or cystic mastopathy)

Fibrocystic change comprises a variety of changes which vary in their extent from case to case. In some patients fibrosis predominates and in others, cystic change predominates. A number of proliferative phenomena are also seen and when these predominate, the term **benign proliferative breast disease** is sometimes used.

The changes of fibrocystic change include:
- **fibrosis**;
- **macrocyst formation**, e.g. blue-domed cyst of Bloodgood;
- **microcyst formation** (Fig. 24.4);
- **apocrine metaplasia**;
- **epithelial hyperplasia** (or **epitheliosis**; Fig. 24.5) is seen as an increased number of epithelial cells within pre-existing glandular components, which may be mild, moderate or severe;
- **adenosis** (an increased number or enlargement of glandular components), may be **simple**, **blunt duct** or **sclerosing**.

The cyst lining is usually cuboidal or columnar in smaller cysts but may be flattened or atrophic in larger cysts. The usual lining epithelium has cells similar to normal duct epithelium. A variant, **apocrine metaplasia** of the epithelial lining, is characterized by large cells with strikingly eosinophilic cytoplasm and small deeply hyperchromatic nuclei. The epithelium in apocrine metaplasia may also show epithelial overgrowth with papillary projection formation (Fig. 24.6). The stroma around the cysts is characteristically compressed and may be in-

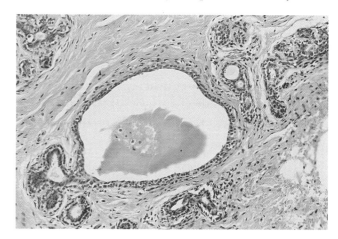

Fig. 24.4 Fibrocystic change. A microcyst contains protein secretion. (H&E.)

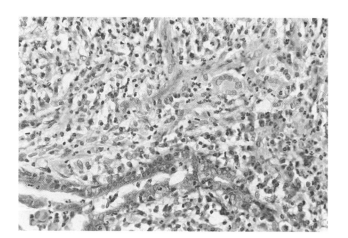

Fig. 24.3 Mammary duct ectasia. The duct epithelium may be ulcerated and is surrounded by inflammatory cells. (H&E.)

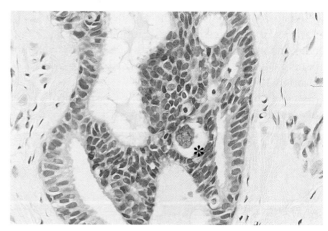

Fig. 24.5 Fibrocystic change. Usual epithelial hyperplasia (epitheliosis) with focal calcification (✱) which may be detected by mammography. (H&E.)

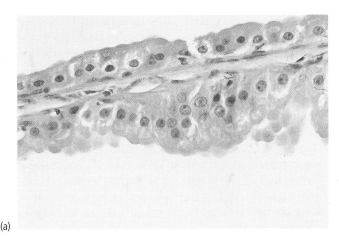

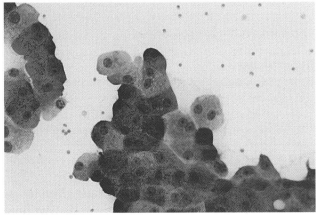

Fig. 24.6 Fibrocystic change. Apocrine metaplasia. (a) Note the pink, granular epithelial cell cytoplasm seen in this biopsy. (H&E.) (b) This fine needle aspirate (FNA) contains typical cells with granular cytoplasm. (MGG.)

Epithelial tumours

Intraduct papilloma. Benign neoplastic papillary growths can develop within a principal lactiferous duct (**intraductal papilloma**) and cause serous and bloody nipple discharge, a small, palpable, subareolar tumor or nipple retraction. Intraductal papillomas form delicate branching structures composed of fibrovascular cores covered by cuboidal or cylindrical epithelial cells that often fill a dilated duct (Fig. 24.8). Intraductal papillomas must be distinguished from papillary carcinoma.

Histological features favouring a diagnosis of intraductal papilloma include the presence of both epithelial and myoepithelial cells in the papillary fronds; the absence of cytological atypia or abnormal mitotic figures and the absence of abnormal growth patterns, apocrine metaplasia, or absence of a vascular connective tissue core. Solitary intraductal papillomas are not considered precursors of papillary carcinomas; multiple intraductal papillomas may be part of the **multiple intraduct**

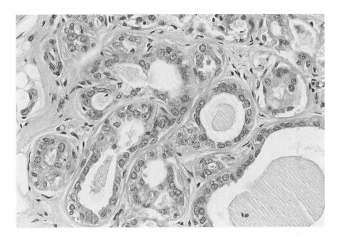

Fig. 24.7 Fibrocystic change. Sclerosing adenosis (or glandular hyperplasia) is seen. (H&E.)

filtrated by lymphocytes. Despite sometimes florid changes, the apocrine metaplasia is a benign change. Simple fibrocystic change is not associated with increased risk of carcinoma of the breast.

Sclerosing adenosis produces a complex histological appearance which may mimic malignancy (Fig. 24.7). Several entities are recognized, from a focus of sclerosing adenosis in otherwise typical cystic disease to the **radial scar** (< 1 cm) and **complex sclerosing lesion** (> 1 cm). The latter two form the whole lesion which is usually stellate: distinction from malignancy may be difficult, even histologically.

BREAST TUMOURS

Benign tumours

Benign breast tumours may be epithelial, mesenchymal or mixed.

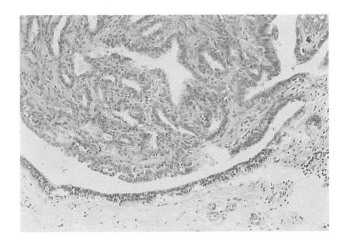

Fig. 24.8 A benign intraduct papilloma from a patient who presented with a breast cyst and nipple discharge. (H&E.)

papillomatosis syndrome which carries an increased risk of invasive malignancy.

Adenomas. These include nipple adenoma, which may mimic Paget's disease, tubular adenoma and lactating adenoma.

Mesenchymal tumours

Any connective tissue tumour may occur, including lipoma, fibroma and haemangioma.

Mixed tumours

Fibroadenoma. Fibroadenoma comprises a mixed epithelial and stromal proliferation (Fig. 24.9). There are two patterns, **intracanalicular** and **pericanalicular**.

Fibroadenomas are well-circumscribed and are often associated with sclerosed stroma. They are freely mobile within the breast adipose tissue and have been termed clinically as '**breast mice**'. They tend to be more common in women of younger age group. Fibroadenomas are clinically significant because they form palpable breast nodules that must be biopsied to prove their benign character. Fibroadenomas change in size through the menstrual cycle and in pregnancy; regression or calcification may occur postmenopausally. Uncommonly, carcinoma-*in-situ* or ductal carcinoma may arise in a fibroadenoma.

Lactating adenoma resembles tubular adenoma but shows epithelium with prominent secretory activity and is observed most often in lactating breasts. **Fibroadenomatosis** is a component of fibrocystic disease characterized by multiple small areas resembling fibroadenomas.

Premalignant breast disease

Hyperplasia

Hyperplasia is divided into usual and atypical types.

Usual hyperplasia. In usual hyperplasia, there is no atypia but there is a small increased risk of malignancy which is divided into mild (no increased risk), moderate and severe (1.5–2× increase).

Atypical hyperplasia. The recognition of these entities attempts to define the onset of neoplasia as distinct from hyperplasia. They represent a continuum from benign to malignant disease and hence precise categorization may be difficult.

The importance of atypical hyperplasia is twofold:
- it carries an increased risk of subsequent malignancy;
- it is being increasingly recognized since the advent of breast secreening.

Two basic types of atypical proliferation are recognized: ductal and lobular.
1 **Atypical ductal hyperplasia (ADH).** Both cytological and architectural features are used to identify this entity. The risk of developing malignancy is increased by four.
2 **Atypical lobular hyperplasia (ALH).** ALH involves replacement of part of a lobule by atypical cells. Any lesion with the appropriate cytological characteristics but lacking the precise features of lobular carcinoma-*in-situ* (see below) is termed ALH. The risk of developing malignancy is increased by four.

Carcinoma-*in-situ*

Four types of carcinoma-*in-situ* are recognized. The incidence of these is increasing due to mammography. In decreasing order of incidence, they are as follows.

Ductal carcinoma-in-situ (DCIS; Fig. 24.10). DCIS pro-

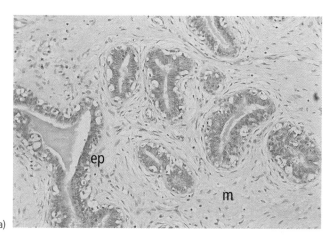

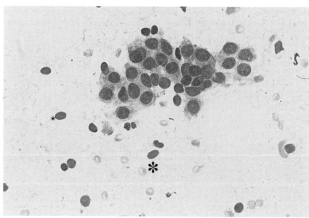

Fig. 24.9 A benign fibroadenoma of breast. (a) Note the epithelial (ep) and mesenchymal (m) elements. Myoepithelial cells surround the basement membrane of the ducts. (H&E.) (b) FNA cytology of the tumour contains cohesive sheets of benign epithelial cells with 'bare nuclei' (✳) of myoepithelial cells. (MGG.)

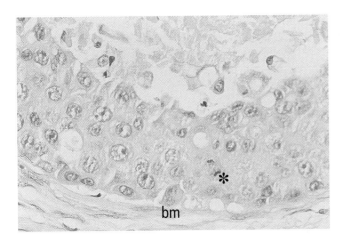

Fig. 24.10 Ductal carcinoma-*in-situ* (DCIS). The atypical ductal cells (note the mitosis (*)) are confined within the basement membrane (bm); there is no stromal invasion. (H&E.)

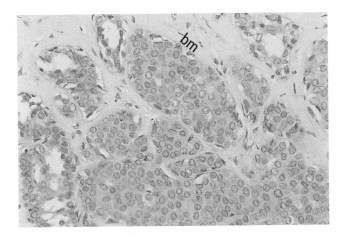

Fig. 24.11 Lobular carcinoma-*in-situ* (LCIS). The atypical lobular cells fill the lobules but are confined within the basement membrane (bm); there is no stromal invasion. (H&E.)

duces a breast mass or is detected by mammography. It is a multifocal disease and is bilateral in about 20%. This type of carcinoma is most often associated with **Paget's disease of the nipple**. There are two forms described in the most common classification.

1 Comedo type. Area of central necrosis is surrounded by solid malignant epithelium but confined to ducts: 50% develop invasive carcinoma in 3 years.

2 Non-comedo type. Includes cribriform and micropapillary types: 30% develop invasive cancer in 10–15 years.

Lobular carcinoma-in-situ (LCIS; Fig. 24.11). This involves expansion of the lobular unit by non-cohesive small malignant cells. This disease is often clinically and mammographically undetectable, frequently multifocal and bilateral, occurring in premenopausal women. There is a long *in situ* phase but the risk of developing malignancy is increased by 11 in the ipsilateral or contralateral breast.

Non-invasive papillary carcinoma. This condition comprises intraduct papilloma with superimposed changes of DCIS.

Paget's disease (Fig. 24.12). Paget's disease is a distinctive pattern of carcinoma-*in-situ* within the nipple skin. Paget's disease is associated with DCIS or invasive carcinoma within the underlying breast and classically presents as a unilateral eczematous eruption.

Phyllodes tumours (cystosarcoma phyllodes) (Fig. 24.13)

Phyllodes tumours (cystosarcoma phyllodes) is the malignant counterpart of the fibroadenoma. It is less well-circumscribed with an increased tendency to stromal proliferation, nuclear pleomorphism, mitoses and increased cellularity. These tumours can be graded on the basis of these features and tend to recur locally. They may, rarely, metastasize.

Malignant tumours

Although non-intrinsic tumours (e.g. lymphoma) and any tumour of connective tissue can occur, the vast majority of breast tumours are epithelial or mixed. Metastases to the breast are rare.

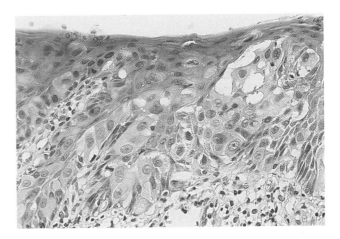

Fig. 24.12 Paget's disease of the breast is seen in the nipple skin, and represents skin invasion by ductal carcinoma cells from an underlying ductal carcinoma. (H&E.)

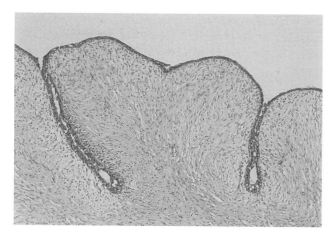

Fig. 24.13 Phyllodes tumour of the breast has typical 'leaf-like' architecture due to proliferation of the stromal cells beneath the epithelium. (H&E.)

Table 24.3 Risk factors for breast carcinoma.

	Increased risk
Family history of premenopausal bilateral breast cancer	⟩⟩ 4×
Age	⟩⟩ 4×
Country of residence	> 4×
Previous breast cancer	> 4×
Irradiation of chest	2–4×
Social class (V versus I)	2–4×
Family history (first-degree relative)	2–4×
Race (commoner in Caucasians)	< 2×
Previous ovarian cancer	< 2×
Previous endometrial cancer	< 2×
Early menarche	< 2×
Late menopause	< 2×

Epidemiology

Incidence. Carcinoma of the breast causes approximately one-fifth of cancer deaths in women. The incidence is 28.4 per 100 000 women in the UK (1984) and is increasing. Breast carcinoma is responsible for 15 000 deaths annually in the UK.

Age. The peak incidence is 45–75 years but breast cancer occurs at any age *postmenarche*.

Sex. This is a disease of predominantly women but it does occur in men (<1% of all breast carcinomas). The incidence in men with Kleinfelter's syndrome (XXY) is the same as that in women.

Geographical variation. Breast cancer is common in the West (particularly in the UK), but is uncommon in the east (Japan).

Risk factors. Factors associated with a higher risk of breast cancer include increasing age, increasing lifetime exposure to oestrogens (early menarche, late menopause, nulliparity, older age at birth of first child), obesity, exogenous oestrogens, fibrocystic breast disease (when associated with atypical epithelial hyperplasia), breast cancer in the other breast and breast cancer in first-degree relatives (Table 24.3). Breast feeding is protective.

Clinical presentation of breast carcinoma

Early disease (with an impalpable lesion) is usually asymptomatic but by the time a mass is detected and local symptoms are present, the disease may be widespread (Fig. 24.14).

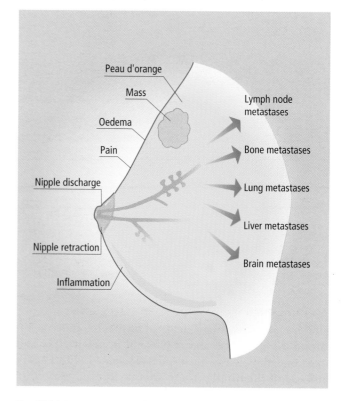

Fig. 24.14 Late presentation of breast cancer can include: a painful breast mass, nipple discharge; nipple retraction or crusting; peau d'orange; local oedema and inflammation; and metastatic disease in lymph nodes, bone, brain, lung or pleura.

Macroscopic features

Several types of breast carcinoma are recognized:
- scirrhous;
- atrophic scirrhous;
- encephaloid;
- diffuse;

Table 24.4 Classification of breast tumours.

Carcinoma-in-situ	
Lobular carcinoma-*in-situ*	40% bilateral/multifocal
Ductal carcinoma	
Invasive carcinoma	
Invasive lobular carcinoma	15% of breast cancers often have oestrogen receptor
Infiltrating ductal carcinoma	Commonest type
Invasive comedo type	
Invasive papillary carcinoma	65% 30-year survival
Adenoid cystic carcinoma	Good prognosis
Apocrine carcinoma	Oestrogen receptor-negative
Lipid-rich carcinoma	50% 2-year survival
Glycogen-rich carcinoma	Rare
Paget's disease of the nipple	With underlying ductal carcinoma
Inflammatory carcinoma	Clinical entity
Mixed carcinomas	Common (approximately 12%)
Special types of ductal carcinoma:	
Tubular	90–95% 10-year survival
Mucoid	58% 30-year survival
Medullary	58% 30-year survival
Other tumours	
Sarcomas	
Lymphomas	
Metastatic tumours	

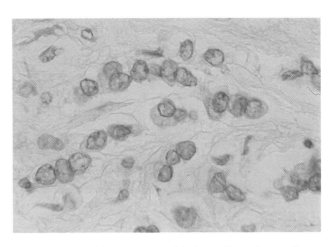

Fig. 24.15 Invasive lobular carcinoma of the breast. The malignant cells may be seen infiltrating in single file through a fibrotic stroma. (H&E.)

Table 24.5 Incidence of different types of ductal tumour.

Carcinoma of no special type (ductal)	60–70%
Carcinoma of special type	
Tubular carcinoma	1–5%
Medullary carcinoma	< 5%
Mucinous carcinoma	< 5%
Papillary carcinoma	1%
Infiltrating lobular carcinoma (may be bilateral)	10–20%
Mixed tumours (ductal and lobular) and rare types	10%

- mastitis carcinomatosa;
- mucoid.

The histological classification is more important.

Microscopic features

A variety of microscopic types of breast carcinoma are described (Table 24.4).

Pathological types of breast carcinoma

Invasive lobular carcinoma. Approximately **10%** of infiltrating breast carcinomas are **lobular carcinomas** which can be differentiated from infiltrating ductal carcinoma only by histological features (Fig. 24.15). Lobular carcinoma is more frequently bilateral than infiltrating ductal carcinoma and is more frequently oestrogen receptor-positive than ductal carcinoma. The low grade prognosis is similar to that of overall infiltrating ductal carcinoma.

Invasive ductal carcinoma. Approximately **85%** of infiltrating breast carcinomas are **ductal carcinomas** (lacking other specific features) (Fig. 24.16).

Histological variants exist with a **better prognosis** than regular infiltrating ductal carcinoma and these include:

- **medullary** carcinoma (Fig. 24.17);
- **tubular** carcinoma (Fig. 24.18);
- **mucinous** (**colloid**) carcinoma (Fig. 24.19);
- **papillary** carcinoma.

Histological variants exist with a **worse prognosis** than regular infiltrating ductal carcinoma and these include:

- inflammatory carcinoma (dermal lymphatic carcinomatosis);
- Paget's disease of the nipple;
- unclassifiable and anaplastic types;
- mixed lobular and ductal carcinoma (Table 24.5).

Histological grading

Histological grading provides the most powerful prognostic information and is from grade I (well-differentiated); grade II (moderately differentiated) and grade III (poorly differentiated) according to the following criteria:

- degree of tubule formation;
- nuclear pleomorphism;
- mitotic rate.

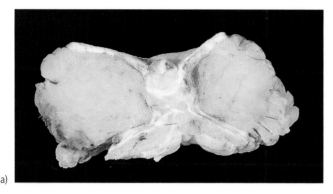

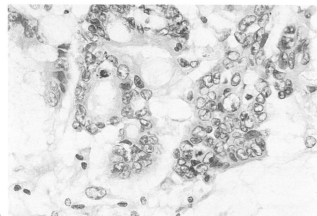

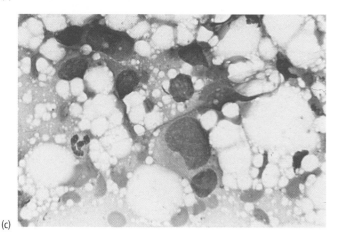

Fig. 24.16 Invasive ductal carcinoma of the breast. (a) The tumour has infiltrated the breast and the overlying nipple and has a firm, grey, gritty appearance on cut surface. (b) Malignant cells are infiltrating through the stroma. (H&E.) (c) FNA cytology shows poorly cohesive malignant cells with pleomorphic, enlarged nuclei. (MGG.)

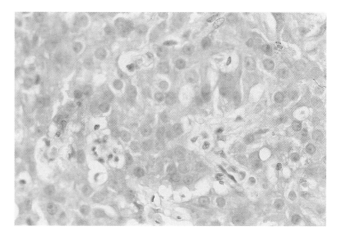

Fig. 24.17 Medullary carcinoma of the breast. This tumour has a good prognosis and is well circumscribed, consisting of cells forming a syncytial pattern admixed with lymphoid cells. (H&E.)

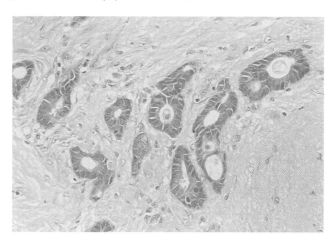

Fig. 24.18 Tubular carcinoma of the breast. This is a well differentiated tumour infiltrating in distinctive tubules. (H&E.)

Spread of breast carcinoma

Breast cancer spreads via **lymphatics**; axillary, supraclavicular and cervical lymph nodes or via the **blood stream**; to distant sites, particularly bone, pleura and lungs, liver, ovaries and brain.

Staging

Staging is done clinically and histopathologically (Table 24.6).

Prognosis

Overall 5-year survival is in the region of 80%, but depends on several parameters (Table 24.7).

Biological prognostic markers

A variety of prognostic markers may now be examined during histopathological examination of breast tumours.

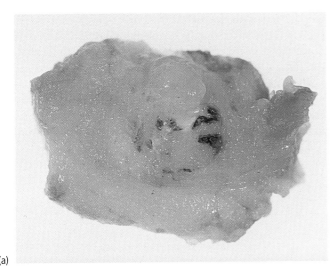

(a)

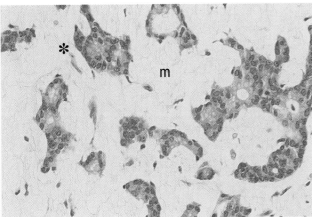

(b)

Fig. 24.19 Mucoid (colloid) carcinoma of the breast. (a) This tumour has a glistening, gelatinous appearance on cut surface. (b) Malignant cells (✱) 'float' in a sea of mucin (m). (H&E.)

- **Oestrogen receptor status.** Oestrogen receptor-positive tumours tend to be of lower grade and respond to anti-oestrogen therapy.
- **Epidermal growth factor receptor (EGFR) status.** EGFR-positive tumours do less well.
- **Cell kinetics and DNA ploidy.** Aneuploid tumours do worse than diploid.
- **Amplification of c-erb-B2.** Correlates with poor prognosis.

DISEASES OF THE MALE BREAST

Gynaecomastia

Gynaecomastia involves predominantly ductal proliferation with various degrees of epithelial hyperplasia.

Most cases are idiopathic (with no identifiable cause) but there may be the following associations:
- testicular atrophy (as in Klinefelter's syndrome, cirrhosis of the liver, lepromatous leprosy);
- conditions associated with increased oestrogen levels such as oestrogen-secreting tumour of the testis or adrenal;
- increased gonadotrophin levels, as in choriocarcinoma of the testis;
- increased prolactin levels, as in diseases of the hypothalamus and pituitary;

Table 24.6 Staging of breast carcinoma.

TNM classification: T(umour); N(odes); M(etastasis)	
T1	< 2 cm
T2	2–5 cm (or < 2 cm and tethered)
T3	> 5 cm (or < 5 cm with infiltration over the tumour)
T4	Any size with extension to the chest wall or skin, wider than the tumour
N0	No nodal involvement
N1	Mobile ipsilateral axillary nodes
N2	Fixed ipsilateral axillary nodes
N3	Supraclavicular or contralateral axillary nodes
M0	No distant metastases
M1	Distant metastases
Clinical classification	
Stage I	Mobile lump, no nodes
Stage II	Mobile lump, mobile nodes, or tethered lump
Stage III	Fixed lump ± mobile nodes
Stage IV	Distant metastases

Table 24.7 Features of prognostic significance.

Size, e.g. 5-year survival 96.3% if < 2 cm but 82.2% if > 5 cm if node negative
Type, e.g. good prognosis of medullary carcinoma despite high-grade features
Grade, e.g. high-grade tumours have worse prognosis
Stage, e.g. stage I 80%, stage II 68%, stage III 40% and sage IV 10% 5-year survival
Number of involved lymph **nodes**
Infiltrating border–irregular versus well-circumscribed
Perineural, lymphatic + vascular **invasion**
Spread to remote quadrants
Skin/nipple involvement
Presence of **hormone receptors**
Expression of **oncogenes**

- drugs, especially **digoxin**.

Gynaecomastia is a benign condition which is not considered to be premalignant.

Breast carcinoma

Carcinoma of the male breast has approximately 1% of the incidence of carcinoma of the female breast and is usually observed in the very elderly. These cancers resemble those of the female breast, but tend to disseminate more rapidly since the male breast is much smaller than the female breast and the tumours rapidly involve the axillary nodes, skin or chest wall. Distant metastases are also common. Histologically, these tumours are **ductal carcinomas**. Prognosis tends to be poor because of the delay in diagnosis in the male, despite the small amount of breast tissue present.

Perinatal and Paediatric Disease

INTRODUCTION

Probably the major difference between the pathology of the perinatal period and that of adult life is that the initiating event or primary disease process takes place in the context of the normal processes of development and maturation. Indeed, in order to make a specific diagnosis, the initial problem for both the clinician and the pathologist is often to disentangle the secondary effects of disturbed development from the primary disease. This is not to say that these secondary effects are unimportant as, frequently, they are not only the cause of presentation, but are the major determinants of eventual morbidity and mortality.

As an introduction to the terminology used in this chapter, the reader should note that:
- the **perinatal** period is from the 24th completed week of gestation to the end of the 7th day of age;

- the **neonatal** period is between day 0 and 28 days (with the late neonatal period between 7 days and 28 days of age);
- an **infant** is between 28 days and 1 year of age;
- a **child** is between 1 year of age and puberty.

PERINATAL AND PAEDIATRIC BIOCHEMISTRY

Introduction

Paediatric medicine provides the chemical pathologist with a range of clinical and analytical problems which are very different from those in adult clinical practice. Limited and often non-specific clinical signs and symptoms of metabolic problems, such as the observation of 'failure to thrive', leave the paediatrician much more in need of investigative support than colleagues in adult medicine and of these, chemical pathology probably makes the most valuable contribution to diagnosis in paediatric medicine. The rapid rate of change of physiological functions in paediatric patients requires rapid analysis, often in very small specimens, and requires rapid interpretation. The paediatrician needs to be well-tuned to the biochemical mechanisms of pathological processes and thus to be able to select the most valuable tests to request in these limited specimen volumes. Modern paediatric practice requires, particularly in neurology and endocrinology, the need for general screening protocols which, although expensive and often with low diagnostic yield, may make the diagnostic process more efficient and less invasive for the patient. In any clinical environment it is essential that the chemical pathologist works closely with the paediatrician to co-ordinate the whole process.

Blood samples and reference ranges

Limited supply of blood has been a major difficulty in biochemical investigations in childhood, although automated analysers are now very thrifty. Plasma samples have the advantage of yielding a larger volume than that from clotted samples. It is particularly important for the paediatrician to check with the local laboratory sample type and volume requirements prior to venepuncture.

Of particular note is the need to be aware of reference ranges for biochemical investigations, which vary widely in most analytes throughout the paediatric period (Table

Table 25.1 Common biochemical analytes that vary during the paediatric period.

Albumin
Alkaline phosphatase*
Aspartate transaminase
Bicarbonate
Bilirubin
Calcium†
Creatinine
Creatine kinase
Glucose†
γ-Glutamyltransferase†
Metadrenalines
Phosphate†
Potassium
Protein†
Total thyroxine†
Thyroid-stimulating hormone†
Uric acid

* Particularly in the first year of life and at puberty.
† Particularly in the neonatal period.

Table 25.2 Metabolic disturbances in the neonatal period.

Common
Birth asphyxia
Hypoglycaemia
Hyperbilirubinaemia
Respiratory distress syndrome
Convulsions
Endocrine
Sexual orientation
Growth disorders
Metabolic acidosis
Hypocalcaemia
Fluid balance disorders
Rare
Inborn errors of metabolism
Tumours

25.1). The variation is particularly acute in the neonatal period and gestational age at birth as well as postnatal age are important considerations. Of particular note are the ranges of blood glucose which are lower in the neonatal period; steroids which are lower with absent sex hormone levels and alkaline phosphatase and phosphate which are higher throughout childhood, largely reflecting the changes in bone growth and turnover. Puberty is the usual cut-off for the changeover to adult reference ranges.

During the first year of life, and particularly in the neonatal period, the clinician needs to work very closely with the chemical pathologist to detect and identify acute metabolic disease processes (Table 25.2). Amongst the most common biochemical abnormalities include:
- hypoglycaemia (Table 25.3);
- keto- and lactic acidosis (Table 25.4);
- hyperbilirubinaemia (see Chapter 19; Table 25.5);
- hypocalcaemia;
- electrolyte disturbances and hyperammonaemia (Table 25.6).

If no obvious mechanical or structural cause is found, a screen to detect an inborn error, particularly if the main feature is hypoglycaemia, metabolic acidosis or hyperammonaemia, should be instigated as soon as possible (Chapter 6).

These biochemical features act as pivotal markers of a wide range of disorders of carbohydrate, amino acid, organic acid and fatty acid metabolism and should be easy to investigate at any centre. This **initial screen** should include:
- plasma and urine amino acids;
- urine organic acids;
- blood lactate ± pyruvate;
- plasma glucose;
- plasma ammonia;

Table 25.3 Causes of hypoglycaemia in the neonatal period.

Newborn	
Transient neonatal hypoglycaemia	
Birth asphyxia and hypoxia	
Prematurity and small-for-dates—inadequate glycogen stores	
Infant of diabetic mother	
Hypothermia	
Cardiac disease	
Neonatal period	
Starvation	
Hyperinsulinaemia	Insulinoma
	Nesidioblastosis
Inborn errors of metabolism	Glycogen storage disease I, III, VI
	Galactosaemia
	Organic acidaemias
	Hereditary fructose intolerance
	Fatty acid oxidation defects
	Disorders of gluconeogenesis
	Amino acid disorders
Endocrine disorders	Hypopituitarism
	Hypoadrenalism
	Growth hormone deficiency
Liver disease	
Drugs	Sulphonylureas
	Salicylates
	Ethanol
	β-Blockers

Table 25.4 Causes of metabolic acidosis in neonatal period.

Overproduction of acid
Asphyxia/hypoxia
Inborn errors of metabolism
Carbohydrate metabolism
Pyruvate and lactate metabolism
Branched-chain amino acid metabolism
Infection
Cardiac failure
Underutilization or excretion
Liver failure
Disorders of gluconeogenesis
Renal disease
Glomerular disease
Tubular acidoses

Table 25.5 Biochemical investigations of neonate with prolonged jaundice.

Blood
Bilirubin—total and conjugated
Liver function tests, including γ-glutamyltransferase
Lipids, including ketones and free fatty acids
Glucose
Lactate
Electrolytes
Creatinine and urea
Calcium and phosphate
Immunoreactive trypsin
α_1-Antitrypsin
Clotting indices
Ammonia
Amino acids
Thyroid function tests
Galactose-1-phosphate uridyltransferase
Urine
Amino acids
Organic acids
Sugars (chromatography)

Table 25.6 Causes of hyperammonaemia in childhood.

Neonatal period
Urea cycle defects
Organic acidaemias
Asphyxia
Liver disease
Postictal
Transient neonatal hyperammonaemia
Generalized illness
Intravenous feeding
Postneonatal period
Urea cycle defects
Organic acidaemias
Amino acid disorders
Liver disease
Reye's syndrome
Valproate therapy
Infections

- routine biochemical tests;
- urine screen for reducing substances.

Further tests will be required in the presence of persistent symptoms and normal results. In many cases the abnormality may only be detectable after the institution of dynamic tests or prolonged starvation and these should be carefully supervised.

Aminoacidurias

Aminoacidurias may be generalized or specific. **Specific aminoacidurias** generally signify a specific **enzyme defect** in a metabolic pathway leading to an increased release into the circulation of the amino acid prior to the block. Occasionally, specific amino acidurias are caused by defective renal tubular reabsorption of that amino acid, the main example being cystine (often together with arginine, valine and ornithine) in **cystinuria**. Cystinuria presents with formation of cystine stones in the kidney or renal tract. Increased bone turnover will lead to increased excretion of **hydroxyproline**, which is an amino acid exclusive to **collagen**. In the neonatal period, and particularly if there is liver failure, there may be transient increases in excretion of specific amino acids (such as tyrosine or taurine) which are not of concern clinically but must be monitored.

Generalized aminoaciduria may be caused by acquired renal tubular damage (e.g. in heavy metal poisoning (cadmium or gold) and vitamin deficiencies) or in Fanconi syndrome where the finding is usually accompanied by glycosuria, phosphaturia and bicarbonate loss (proximal tubule defects) and by retarded growth.

Galactosaemia

This rare disease (incidence in UK of ~1 : 70 000 live births) usually presents in the early postnatal or neonatal period with prolonged jaundice, failure to thrive, hypoglycaemia, vomiting and gastrointestinal disturbances. The jaundice is typically a conjugated hyperbilirubinaemia and plasma liver transaminases are elevated. It is caused by deficiency in the liver of either galactose-1-phosphate uridyltransferase or, more rarely, of galactokinase. Diagnosis is suggested by a positive urine test for reducing substances (predominantly sugars) and a negative test for glucose and by clinical improvement when lactose- and galactose-containing milk is withdrawn. It is confirmed by chromatography of urine sugars. Although rare, it is an important life-threatening and treatable condition.

Biochemical screening for neonatal disease

Most of the inborn errors of metabolism present during childhood, often in the first few days of life, and although some may present with characteristic clinical features such as in alkaptonuria, albinism or some of the mucopolysaccharidoses, the majority will have only very subtle or non-specific signs which may not develop until infancy or later in childhood (Tables 25.7 and 25.8). Inheritance characteristics and degree of penetrance make a huge difference on the point at which inherited metabolic disorders present. Neonatal screening programmes are mandatory in the UK for phenylketonuria (PKU) and hypothyroidism (Chapter 6) and are proposed for many other inherited conditions, including cystic fibrosis and galactosaemia, but are not yet practical for national screening.

Table 25.7 Inherited disorders detectable antenatally by DNA analysis.

Adrenoleucodystrophy
α_1-Antitrypsin deficiency
Congenital adrenal hyperplasia (common form-21 hydroxylase deficiency)
Cystic fibrosis
Dihydropteridine reductase deficiency
Duchenne–Becker muscular dystrophy
Familial hypercholesterolaemia
Familial adenomatous polyposis coli
Familial isolated growth hormone deficiency
Fragile X syndrome
Haemophilia A and B
Hereditary retinoblastoma
Huntington's chorea
Lesch–Nyhan syndrome
Lowe's syndrome
Myotonic dystrophy
Norrie–Wiskott–Aldrich disease
Ornithine transcarbamylase deficiency
Osteogenesis imperfecta type IV
Phenylketonuria
Polycystic kidney disease (adult)
Sickle-cell anaemia
Thalassaemias α and β
Tuberous sclerosis
Wilson's disease
X-linked agammaglobulinaemia

Table 25.8 Treatable inborn errors of metabolism.

Glycogen storage disease types
Phenylketonuria
Biotinidase deficiency
Familial hypercholesterolaemia
Wilson's disease
Familial growth hormone deficiency
Haemophilias
Most of the amino acid disorders

Screening for phenylketonuria

In the UK the incidence of PKU is approximately 1 case per 10 000 live births. This autosomal recessive disorder of phenylalanine metabolism, due mainly to a deficiency of the hepatic enzyme phenylalanine hydroxylase, is a serious condition which, if untreated in the first weeks of life, results in severe mental retardation.

Diagnosis is made by estimation of phenylalanine concentrations in blood taken from neonates after 6 days of feeding when exposure to dietary phenylalanine should have stressed the metabolic pathway sufficiently to cause an elevation in levels in those affected. This procedure was the first national screening programme to be introduced and phenylalanine is measured by the **Guthrie test**, a microbiological bioassay, or by chromatography, which gives the advantage of assessing other blood amino acid levels semiquantitatively. A small quantity of blood is collected from the heel of the baby and blotted on to paper from which amino acids can be eluted and assayed.

Treatment of affected individuals is dietary phenylalanine restriction which should be continued rigorously until at least the age of 10 years and plasma phenylalanine levels should be monitored regularly. Problems can occur later in life when fetuses of women with uncontrolled PKU are at risk of severe malformation and brain damage. Screening for PKU is statutory in the UK and the programme has been highly successful.

Screening for neonatal hypothyroidism

Some years after the screening programme for PKU was established, methods became available to measure **thyroid-stimulating hormone (TSH)** in small volumes of blood by radioimmunoassay and thus a programme was set up for screening for neonatal hypothyroidism using the same sampling procedure as for PKU screening.

Hypothyroidism has an incidence of approximately 1 in 5000 live births and results in cretinism with mental and growth retardation if untreated. An alternative method for screening is by looking for **low plasma thyroxine levels**. Treatment is by replacement of thyroxine from the point of diagnostic confirmation but an unknown proportion of babies with elevated blood TSH have a transient defect and so current practice is to withdraw the thyroxine after approximately 5 years of age and to evaluate the biochemical response.

CONGENITAL MALFORMATIONS AND CHROMOSOMAL DISORDERS

This section will deal only with a general approach to congenital malformations, most examples being considered within specific organ or system chapters.

Definitions

- **Congenital malformation.** A macroscopic structural abnormality attributable to faulty development and present at birth.
- **Deformation.** An abnormality of form produced by external forces on an otherwise normally developing fetus.

- **Sequence.** A pattern of malformations, derived from a single cause.
- **Syndrome.** A pattern of malformations, directly related to a common pathogenesis. Where the relationship is less direct, two or more malformations may be described as being an association. The borderline between a syndrome and an association is often indistinct.

A good example of these interrelationships is provided by an examination of the causes and effects of lack of amniotic fluid (Fig. 25.1). Reduced amniotic fluid or oligohydramnios may result either from insufficient production or excessive loss of liquor. A significant component of amniotic fluid is fetal urine and any pathology which reduces production, such as renal agenesis or cystic disease, or impedes excretion, such as urethral valves, will cause oligohydramnios. Chronic amniotic fluid loss via ruptured membranes will produce a similar result.

As a consequence of the lack of amniotic fluid, the compressive effects on the fetus by the uterus produce deformations involving the facies – low-set ears, pinched nose, small hypoplastic mandible – and contractures of the feet (talipes). The cause of the lung hypoplasia is, however, less clear. Although it can be deformative in origin, the pathogenesis in oligohydramnios is more

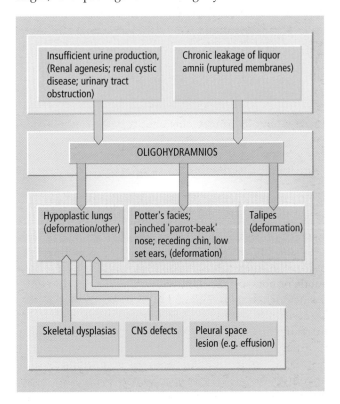

Fig. 25.1 Diagram showing the inter-relationships between the causes and effects of oligohydramnios.

complex and probably due more to abnormal loss of lung liquid from the developing lungs. The combination of renal agenesis, oligohydramnios, the abnormal facies, talipes and hypoplastic lungs is known as **Potter's syndrome**.

An understanding of these interrelationships ensures a more logical approach to any constellation of malformations. Once the facies and hypoplastic lungs are recognized as a consequence of oligohydramnios (oligohydramnios sequence), effort can be concentrated on the underlying problem and risks to future pregnancies be determined on that factor alone. Thus, infantile polycystic kidney is autosomal recessive and carries a 1 : 4 risk of recurrence (Fig. 25.2); renal dysplasia is multifactorial in origin and carries a low recurrence risk (2–3%).

Although lung hypoplasia is often the most important determinant of immediate neonatal outcome, its significance in terms of recurrence risk is entirely related to the underlying cause. It can be deformative in origin, where any cause of reduced pleural cavity may restrict normal lung growth; an effusion in rhesus disease; or poor rib growth associated with various skeletal dysplasias.

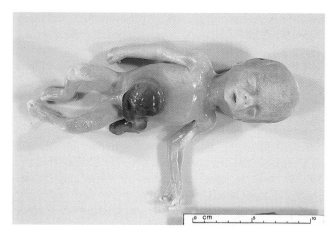

Fig. 25.3 Trisomy 18 (Edward's syndrome) in a 19 weeks gestation fetus. Usually characteristic even at this gestation, trisomy 18 is distinguished by typical round facies with small, often low-set ears. As seen here, exomphalos is common and inward curving with overlapping of the fingers characteristic. Internal abnormalities are variable but congenital heart disease and renal anomalies are frequent.

Aetiology

Congenital malformations may be genetic in origin, with an abnormality involving varying amounts of DNA, from whole chromosomes to single genes or less. Deletions of whole autosomes are rare in neonates, the loss of genetic material being incompatible with survival. The usual whole-chromosome disorders involve the presence of extra material (e.g. trisomy 21, Down syndrome; trisomy 18, Edward's syndrome; Fig. 25.3). More restricted genetic abnormalities may be associated with malformations or a syndrome inherited in an autosomal recessive or dominant pattern.

It is often difficult to ascribe a malformation to either a multifactorial or purely environmental aetiology on an individual basis. Where population-based studies have shown a malformation or syndrome to have a risk of recurrence which does not fit simple Mendelian inheritance patterns (e.g. renal cystic dysplasia has a 2–3% risk of recurrence), it is presumed that there is interaction between environmental factors and a genetically susceptible background. A pure environmental origin of malformation, such as teratogenic drugs, e.g. thalidomide, can occasionally be identified, although even in this circumstance, fetal outcome might be affected by genetically determined handling of the drug.

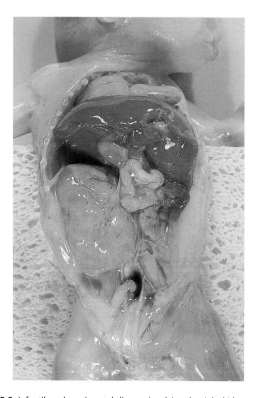

Fig. 25.2 Infantile polycystic renal disease involving the right kidney which is replaced by a large, multicystic mass. This condition is usually bilateral.

Incidence

The prevalence of congenital malformations largely depends on when, in development, it is measured. As a general rule, the earlier in gestation, the greater their incidence. Although figures are very imprecise, it is estimated that up to 50% of first-trimester spontaneous abortions have chromosomal disorders, particularly autosomal trisomies, sex chromosomal monosomies or triploidies, whereas only 5% of stillbirths show chromosomal abnormalities. At the end of the first week of life, 0.5% of infants will have chromosomal disorders, 1% a monogenic disorder and 2% malformations of multifactorial origin.

Investigation and diagnosis

Malformation can be diagnosed by a variety of techniques, each of which has its advantage and limitations.
- **Fetal ultrasound.** Can identify some major malformations, such as those affecting the central nervous system, kidney or heart. Some lesions, however, may not be detectable until relatively late in gestation when termination, if desired, becomes difficult.
- **Amniocentesis.** Samples of amniotic fluid obtained during this procedure contain fetal cells which can be cultured to diagnose chromosomal disorder. Biochemical analysis of fluid can occasionally be valuable. Very high levels of α-fetoprotein and acetylcholinesterase are associated with neural tube defects.
- **Chorionic villus sampling (CVS).** Provides a sample of fetal tissue much earlier in gestation than is possible with amniocentesis. Besides chromosomal disorder, the availability of specific DNA probes now permits diagnosis of some metabolic or other inheritable disorders such as muscular dystrophy or cystic fibrosis.

Short stature

Short stature is defined as height below the third centile for the child's age, based on a standard Tanner–Whitehouse growth chart. Short stature is commonly explained by familial, perinatal or social factors (Table 25.9). Organic disease may cause short stature and these causes may be treatable. It is important to make the diagnosis early to prevent dangerous complications of these disorders.

Table 25.9 Causes of short stature.

Common causes
Intrauterine growth retardation
Familial short stature (how tall are the parents?)
Familial delayed puberty
Social causes of short stature (diet)
Treatable organic causes
Endocrine
Growth hormone deficiency
Hypothyroidism
Cushing's disease
Renal
Renal tubular acidosis
Chronic renal failure
Gastrointestinal
Crohn's disease
Coeliac disease
Other causes of malabsorption
Respiratory
Cystic fibrosis
Chronic infections
Asthma
Bone disease
Achondroplasia
Dyschondroplasia
Neurological disease
Craniopharyngioma
Anorexia nervosa
Genetic
Turner's syndrome

CONGENITAL, PERINATAL AND NEONATAL INFECTIONS

Infections of the neonate may be congenital (acquired *in utero*), perinatal (acquired during birth) or postnatal (maternally or nosocomially acquired; Table 25.10).

Infections such as human immunodeficiency virus (HIV) and *Listeria* can be acquired at all stages, whereas *Toxoplasma* infections acquired *in utero* may present years later. The acronym **TORCH** (*Toxoplasma*, rubella, cytomegalovirus and herpes simplex virus (HSV)) is often used when screening for neonatal infection but this term is outdated because of the importance of other aetiological agents and in this cost-conscious era it does not help in targeting the most appropriate investigations.

Congenital infections

The fetal response to infection is basically the same for all pathogens. It is therefore difficult to differentiate

Table 25.10 Classification of obstetric and neonatal infections.

Organism	Congenital	Perinatal	Postnatal
Toxoplasma gondii	+		
Treponema pallidum	+		
Rubella	+		
Parvovirus B19	+		
Cytomegalovirus	+	+/–	+/–
*Neisseria gonorrhoeae**		+	
*Chlamydia trachomatis**		+	
Hepatitis B		+	
Herpes simplex	+/–	+	
Human immunodeficiency virus	+	+	+/–
Listeria monocytogenes	+/–	+/–	+
Group B streptococcus		+/–	+
Escherichia coli	+	+/–	+
Herpes zoster	+/–		+
Enterovirus (echo)	+		+

* Causes ophthalmia neonatorum.

clinically the different diseases. Common features are hepatosplenomegaly, eye defects, mental retardation, hearing defects and low birth weight. Infections may result in fetal hydrops or fetal death. National screening of antenatal sera is done for syphilis and rubella and in some regions hepatitis B.

Toxoplasmosis

Toxoplasma is a protozoal parasite transmitted to humans via contaminated cats' faeces or undercooked meat, especially lamb. Prevention includes avoidance of these sources. Only one-third of normal adults in the UK are seropositive, compared to two-thirds in France. Transmission rates are greatest in the third trimester, whereas the risk of severe fetal damage is greatest in the first trimester. The opposite is the case with rubella. Congenitally infected neonates may be normal at birth but may present years later with chorioretinitis (Fig. 25.4).

Diagnosis during pregnancy relies on a latex agglutination test followed by the dye test. Unlike France, routine screening of serum is not done in the UK because of the lower prevalence of the disease. At present screening is not thought to be cost-effective but this is under review.

Depending on whether the infection occurs early or late in pregnancy, the mother should be counselled on the risk to the fetus. The options are therapeutic abortion or drug therapy (spiramycin, pyrimethamine and sulphadiazine).

Syphilis (*Treponema pallidum*)

Congenital syphilis is rare but preventable by antenatal screening and treatment of infected mothers. Between 1988 and 1991 only 20 cases were reported in the UK. In untreated primary and secondary disease all infants will be infected and, of these, 50% will be symptomatic.

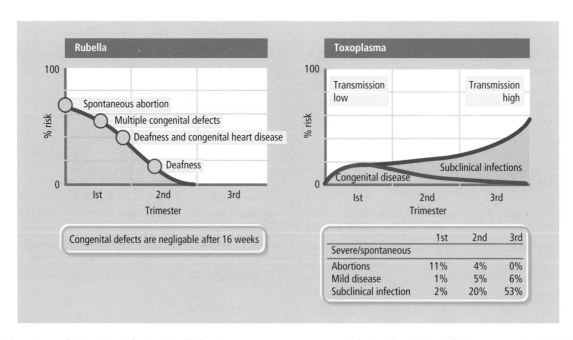

Fig. 25.4 The outcome of intra-uterine infection with rubella and toxoplasmosis. The earlier the fetus is infected, the more severe the disease. However, toxoplasma is more often transmitted to the fetus later in pregnancy. Infants with subclinical infection are normal at birth but develop CN involvement and chorioretinitis months to years later.

Special features of congenital disease include skin and mucosal lesions and abnormalities of bone and cartilage (saddle nose). Diagnosis is essentially serological and penicillin is used for treatment.

Rubella

Primary maternal infection during pregnancy may be mild or asymptomatic. In contrast, infection of the fetus during the first trimester results in fetal death or severe defects.

Maternal rubella infection can be diagnosed by detecting specific immunoglobulin M (IgM) or by evidence of seroconversion. Postnatal disgnosis of congenital rubella includes detection of specific IgM in cord blood (see Fig. 25.4) and IgG levels persisting beyond the normal 6-month period of maternal antibodies and isolation of virus from the throat or urine. Since the introduction of measles, mumps and rubella (MMR) vaccine for preschool children, the incidence of congenital rubella has decreased. Between 1991 and 1992 there were only 16 reported cases in the UK.

Prenatal testing is now being encouraged and those found to be seronegative are vaccinated.

Parvovirus B19

Parvovirus causes erythema infectiosum (fifth disease) in children and aplastic crises in patients with sickle-cell disease.

The infection is associated with hydrops fetalis and spontaneous abortions in congenital infections. There is little evidence for congenital malformation. Prevention is difficult and there are no specific guidelines. The virus causes characteristic inclusions in fetal red cells in bone marrow, liver, lung, heart and placental tissues (Fig. 25.5).

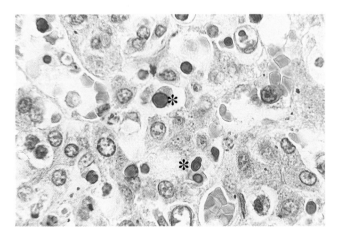

Fig. 25.5 Parvovirus B19 infection. This is a section of liver from a stillborn fetus with intrauterine fetal hydrops. Note the glassy purple nuclear inclusions (✲) in fetal red blood cells in the liver sinusoids. (H&E.)

Cytomegalovirus

At present, cytomegalovirus (CMV) is the commonest cause of congenital infections (approximately 250 cases in the UK). Infection in the mother may be primary or reactivation, both being generally subclinical.

About 40% of primary infections will involve transmission to the fetus. Of these, only a minority (about 10%) will eventually show features of infection; the rest will be unaffected.

Congenital infection from reactivation of infection is rare. The asymptomatic nature of CMV infection during pregnancy makes diagnosis difficult. CMV infection can be diagnosed in the neonate by viral culture or antigen detection from throat swabs and urine and by serology (IgM and IgG). Perinatal CMV infection acquired from the birth canal or breast-feeding may be confused with congenital infection. CMV is commonly spread around nurseries.

Prevention is difficult, although it is advised that pregnant women working with young infants should be aware of the risk and avoid secretions and institute regular hand-washing.

Human immunodeficiency virus

Mother-to-infant transmission of HIV can occur *in utero*, at delivery or as a consequence of breast-feeding. At 1 year approximately 50% of infants will be infected. At-risk mothers should be offered antenatal screening and counselling. In HIV-positive mothers, transmission can be reduced by taking azothiaprine (AZT), undergoing elective caesarean section and by not breast-feeding.

Diagnosis of infection in the neonate is difficult. Maternal antibodies may be present for up to 18 months, making regular monitoring of IgG levels essential. Alteratively, culture of the virus or detection of viral DNA by polymerase chain reaction may enable the diagnosis of neonatal HIV infection to be made. General preventive measures are as for the general population at risk.

Perinatal infections

Perinatal infections include organisms acquired from the birth canal (normal flora and sexually transmitted diseases (STDs)) and those transmitted via maternal blood at delivery (hepatitis B).

Listeria, group B streptococci and *Escherichia coli* cause sepsis and meningitis in the neonate either as an early-onset (perinatal) or as a late-onset disease (postnatal). Predisposing factors include prolonged rupture of membranes, prematurity, immunological immaturity, breaches of integument by cannulae and lack of normal flora.

Ophthalmia neonatorum

This is a purulent conjunctivitis occurring 2–5 days postpartum which is acquired via cervical infection with *Neisseria gonorrhoeae* or *Chlamydia trachomatis*. Untreated disease may lead to blindness. Gonococcus is diagnosed by culture and treated with topical antibiotics. Chlamydial disease is diagnosed by antigen detection and treated with topical antibiotics. An associated pneumonia may be present and this should be treated with oral or intravenous erythromycin.

Hepatitis B

Hepatitis B is transmitted from mothers acutely infected with the virus or who are carriers, especially hepatitis B e antigen (HBeAg)-positive carriers.

The majority of infants are asymptomatic but there is a higher incidence in later life of chronic liver disease and hepatoma.

Antenatal screening of high-risk groups is worthwhile, as up to 90% of perinatal infections can be prevented if the neonate is given both passive and active immunization. At delivery, the neonate of an hepatitis B surface antigen (HBsAg)-positive and HBeAg-positive mother should be given hepatitis B immunoglobulin (HBIg) and commenced on a course of hepatitis B vaccine.

A neonate of a mother who is HBsAg and anti-HBe does not require HBIg but requires immediate vaccination as above. All such infants should be followed at 1 year to check their immune status.

Herpes simplex virus

In the mother, HSV 2 (and, with increasing frequency, HSV 1) can cause primary or recurrent genital herpes. Primary infections within the first trimester can cause congenital defects and fetal death, but this is very rare.

Neonatal herpes acquired at birth is commoner but still rare, considering the prevalence of the disease in the UK (between 1986 and 1991 there were only 71 cases reported).

Infected infants may present with disseminated disease, encephalitis or mucocutaneous lesions. The morbidity and mortality are high.

Diagnosis is by culture of the virus from neonatal material. Prevention of infection is controversial and no guidelines exist. To screen at-risk mothers just before delivery and to perform Caesarean sections on those mothers found to be excreting virus is debatable and different practices exist throughout the country. Acyclovir is used for neonatal infections.

Varicella-zoster virus

This infection is a problem when chickenpox occurs in a seronegative mother towards the end of pregnancy or just after delivery; neonatal varicella is a severe disease.

In proven cases antivaricella-zoster immunoglobulin can be given to the mother to attenuate the illness and at birth to the neonate together with acyclovir.

Enteroviruses

Postnatal infections with enteroviruses may be acquired at birth from the mother or be acquired nosocomially from other neonates and staff in the nursery. The neonate may present with a viral meningitis but the majority of infections are subclinical.

Outbreaks in nurseries may be controlled by the use of human immunoglobulin and strict adherence to hospital infection control measures.

Bacterial sepsis and meningitis

In early-onset disease the neonate presents at birth, stillborn or with a septicaemic illness. In a previously healthy infant late-onset disease (occurring 7 days after birth) presents as a meningitis. This has a better prognosis than early-onset disease. The infant presents with subtle signs of a bulging fontanelle, irritability and poor feeding and handling.

Diagnosis is via culturing blood and cerebrospinal fluid (Fig. 25.6). Empiric treatment includes ampicillin and an aminoglycoside.

Group B *Streptococcus*

This infection accounts for 0.3 per 1000 live births in the UK. Prevention is difficult as there is no effective screening procedure for at risk infants. Group B streptococci are

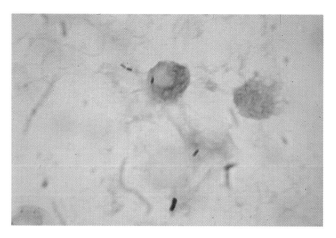

Fig. 25.6 *Listeria monocytogenes.* Gram stain of a specimen of cerebrospinal fluid shows scanty Gram positive bacteria. The microscopy of clinical specimens may be difficult to interpret as the organisms are often scanty, pleomorphic and may be Gram variable.

normal vaginal flora in up to 25% of women and irradiation of the organism is difficult.

Listeria monocytogenes

Granulomatosis infantisepticum results from transplacental infection and usually results in a stillborn infant.

Sepsis at birth characteristically causes meconium staining. Maternal infections may be subclinical or present as a flu-like febrile illness. Blood cultures are worth taking from the mother at this stage (Fig. 25.7). Because the infection is thought to be acquired from contaminated foodstuffs, guidelines exist for its prevention.

Pregnant women are advised to avoid, soft ripened cheeses and pâté and to heat thoroughly cook-chilled and poultry dishes. Since the introduction of these guidelines, the incidence of listeriosis has declined to the present rate of about 0.03 cases per 1000 live births.

Escherichia coli

The incidence of neonatal *E. coli* infections has declined in recent years. The majority of organisms carry the K1 antigen (a capsular antigen), which in this age group is related to virulence.

Prevention is difficult as this is a normal bowel organism.

PATHOLOGY OF ABORTION AND STILLBIRTH

The perinatal period is defined as extending from the 24th completed week of gestation to the end of the 7th day of neonatal life (although, following World Health Organization recommendations, data should now be collected for fetuses greater than 22 weeks of gestation or 500 g body weight). Fetal loss before 24 weeks is defined as an abortion.

Rather than consider the pathology of abortion and stillbirth separately, it is more convenient to classify fetal loss which occurs in the second and third trimester as either due to maternal factors, fetal factors or a combination of both.

Maternal factors

- **Uterine abnormalities.** Malformations such as a bifid uterus or acquired uterine lesions such as fibroids typically cause early loss by interfering with placentation.
- **Cervical incompetence.** It is unclear whether this is an acquired or congenital problem, but early silent dilatation of the uterine cervix, usually starting in the early second trimester, can result in abortion or predispose to ascending infection.
- **Endocrine.** Although a matter of some dispute, some pregnancies may fail early because of insufficient production of progesterone by the corpus luteum.
- **Immunological.** There is good evidence that, for a successful pregnancy, the mother has to mount an appropriate immunological response to fetal tissues. Where this fails or is incomplete, spontaneous abortion may result. Interestingly, couples with shared human leucocyte antigens (HLA) are more likely to abort.
- **Impairment of uteroplacental blood flow.** This is probably one of the major identifiable causes of loss in later gestation. It is particularly associated with pre-eclamptic toxaemia (PET), a specific condition of pregnancy presenting clinically with raised blood pressure, proteinuria and oedema. PET leads to reduced uteroplacental blood flow, causing fetal growth retardation and sometimes death.

A pathological manifestation of the disease is the failure of normal invasion of the uterine spiral arteries by trophoblast in early pregnancy, a physiological event which results in destruction of uterine vessel walls with dilatation and increased uterine blood flow. In PET, uterine vessels remain of relatively small diameter, acquire lipid in the intima which has some resemblance to atheroma, and the normal increase in blood flow fails to occur.

Pathological examination of the fetus in the above circumstances rarely provides a specific diagnosis, although indications of the primary pathology may be obtained.

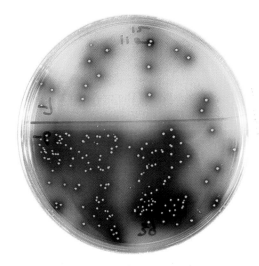

Fig. 25.7 Plate of *Listeria monocytogenes* isolated on selective Oxford agar. The medium contains aesculin which when hydrolysed turns the surrounding medium black (courtesy of M. Crow and G. Curtis).

Thus, a growth-retarded fetus with a placenta showing ischaemic changes would be a sign of impaired uteroplacental blood flow.

Fetal factors

- **Chromosomal.** As discussed above, chromosomal abnormality is most commonly associated with early fetal loss.

Both maternal and fetal factors

- Infection. This results from either maternal blood-borne disease affecting the placenta and fetus or an ascending infection through the uterine os, this latter event occurring in up to 30% of abortuses less than 24 weeks of gestation.

  A wide variety of infective agents may be transmitted across the placenta, but include viral, e.g. rubella, CMV or herpes, bacterial, e.g. listeriosis or syphilis, or protozoal, such as toxoplasmosis.

NEONATAL PATHOLOGY

Neonatal pathology can be subdivided broadly into those problems associated with prematurity and those more typically associated with delivery at term.

Birth, significantly before the normal 37–42 weeks of gestation, creates problems due to immaturity of organs or systems. Some consideration of their normal function is often important if the pathology is to be fully understood.

Lungs

Besides the change from fetal to adult circulation, one of the most critical events of birth is the rapid establishment of respiration during which the lungs must convert from fluid-filled organs into air-filled tissues capable of supporting respiration almost within seconds. For successful transition, the lung must be of sufficient size and airway epithelium differentiated into pneumocyte subtypes:
- type 1 pneumocytes in association with the development of blood–air barriers for gaseous exchange;
- type 2 pneumocytes to produce surfactant.

Hyaline membrane disease
(Figs 25.8 and 25.9)
The most common pulmonary association of very

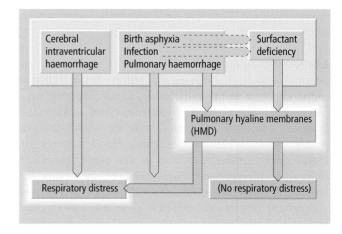

Fig. 25.8 Diagram of the pathogenesis of hyaline membrane disease (HMD).

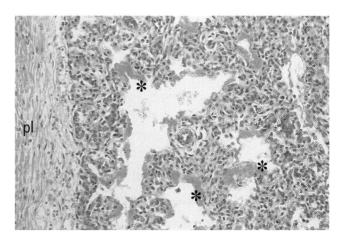

Fig. 25.9 Hyaline membrane disease (HMD) in the lung of a 27 week's gestation infant. The eosinophilic membranes (✳) line the more distended terminal airways. Note that they do not involve the terminal air sacs adjacent to the pleural surface (pl).

preterm birth, hyaline membrane disease (HMD) is a pathological term describing the presence of eosinophilic 'membranes' lining the respiratory airways and alveoli. Clinically it presents as respiratory distress syndrome (RDS) in which the infant demonstrates cyanosis, tachypnoea, sternal recession and grunting. The two terms HMD and RDS are often used synonymously but, whilst overlap is common, RDS in particular may be caused by other pathological conditions than HMD.

Surfactant deficiency. This is by far the commonest cause of HMD and hence RDS in the very preterm infant. Surfactant is produced by the type 2 pneumocyte from about 20 weeks of gestation, although adequate levels of surfactant are not usually produced until much later in gestation. Surfactant is necessary to reduce surface tension forces generated at the alveolar air–liquid interface and which promote lung collapse, particularly when alveoli are small (end of expiration). During the considerable respiratory effort required to expand the collapsed terminal air saccules, damage to pulmonary epithelium and vasculature occurs, with consequent leakage of protein-rich fluid into the airways. The hyaline membranes themselves comprise necrotic debris from airway epithlium and precipitated protein of the transudate (Fig. 25.9). Management usually involves the administration of exogenous, often artificial surfactant to maintain alveolar expansion and ventilatory support, including increased inspired oxygen concentrations.

Sequelae of hyaline membrane disease

• **Resolution.** For most infants, regenerative activity after acute damage leads to restoration of airway epithelium accompanied by a resurgence in surfactant levels. Hyaline membranes are removed by macrophages and there is minimal or no fibroblastic activity to produce permanent damage.

• **Air leaks.** The major acute respiratory complication of HMD and therapy results from the abnormal pressures generated in the airways or alveoli. Physical disruption to tissues may lead to air leakage either into the interstitium (pulmonary interstitial emphysema–PIE) or into the pleural space, resulting in a pneumothorax. Both may lead to further respiratory embarrassment.

• **Bronchopulmonary dysplasia (BPD).** For a small proportion of infants, the acute lung injury associated with HMD passes into a phase of more chronic damage and continuing ventilator dependence. Probably the most important cause of continuing damage is toxic free radicals generated in association with high inspired oxygen concentrations. In a few cases, physical trauma from high ventilator pressures may also contribute. The major pathological feature of this chronic lung disease is interstitial fibrosis, but if damage is severe, an obliterative bronchiolitis may also occur (Figs 25.10 and 25.11).

• **Meconium aspiration.** Primarily a feature of term birth, this occurs as a consequence of birth asphyxia. Fetal hypoxia produces reflex anal dilatation and release of meconium. Deep gasping breathing movements also precipitated by hypoxia may cause meconium to be aspirated during delivery. Its thick sticky nature leads to obstruction of fetal airways and further adds to the fetal asphyxia.

Brain

If the lungs are the major determinant of survival, then

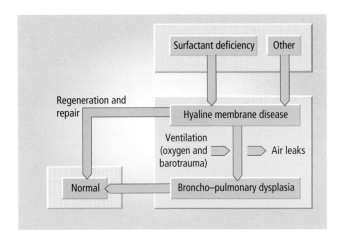

Fig. 25.10 Diagram of the pathogenesis of bronchopulmonary dysplasia (BPD).

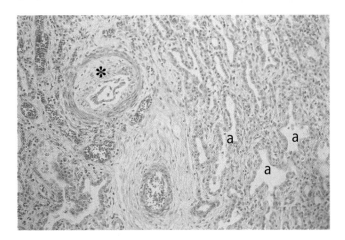

Fig. 25.11 Acute bronchopulmonary dysplasia in the lung of a preterm infant dying at 2 weeks of age. The lung parenchyma shows thickening of interstitium and alveoli (a) are lined by cuboidal epithelium of type 2 pneumocytes. To the top and left, an airway shows incomplete obliteration by fibrous tissue (✳). The adventitia around the small pulmonary artery is still prominent although the vessel lumen is within normal limits.

the brain is usually the main determinant of quality of survival. With modern technology, very preterm infants are not dependent on normal cerebral function to survive. Although many aspects of normal respiratory control are dependent on brainstem activity, the ventilator can take over these functions adequately.

Germinal layer haemorrhage/intraventricular haemorrhage

Before 34 weeks of gestation the lateral wall of the cerebral lateral ventricle is lined by a mass of immature cells–the germinal layer (GL). These gradually migrate away from the ventricle and mature into various glial subtypes, but whilst it persists, the fragile vasculature of the GL makes it vulnerable to haemorrhage (Fig. 25.12).

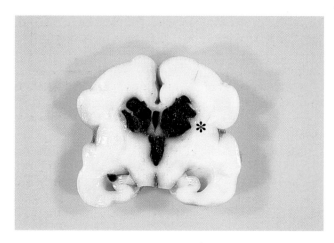

Fig. 25.12 Germinal layer and bilateral intraventricular haemorrhage in the brain of a 25 week's gestation baby. The germinal layer origin is more easily seen on the left although there is some involvement of the per-ventricular tissues at the angle of the ventricle on the right (∗). In survivors, there is a greatly increased risk of neurodevelopmental handicap from damage to the long fibres of the internal capsule.

The main precipitating factor appears to be rapid changes in cerebral blood flow which occur because of poor autoregulatory control in the preterm infant. Intraventricular haemorrhage may follow and may cause death if severe. Lateral spread into the cerebral tissues may cause neurological deficits in survivors.

Hypoxic–ischaemic brain injury

Because of the cardiorespiratory complications associated with preterm birth, the immature neonate is particularly vulnerable to hypoxic–ischaemic brain damage. It may also occur secondarily to the GL haemorrhages discussed above. In the full term neonate, however, cerebral damage is more likely to follow intrapartum asphyxia when blood flow and oxygen delivery to the placenta are impaired during the uterine contractions of labour.

The region of the brain susceptible to hypoxic–ischaemic injury alters with gestation and the nature of the insult. Thus, the periventricular white matter is more vulnerable in the immature infant where necrosis (periventricular leukomalacia) may damage the long fibres of the internal capsule and cause spastic motor deficits. Grey matter such as basal ganglia or cerebral cortex is more susceptible to injury in term infants subject to birth asphyxia, although severe acute hypoxia may cause injury at any gestation.

Trauma

The other major mechanism of cerebral damage may occur during traumatic delivery. It is most commonly seen in term infants, often following the use of obstetric forceps, when rapid delivery is needed because of fetal distress. Physical distortion of the head may tear the tentorium cerebelli or (less commonly) the falx cerebri, giving rise to intracranial haemorrhage.

Gut

Necrotizing enterocolitis (Fig. 25.13)

Although more characteristic of preterm infants, it may be found at any gestation. Clinically presenting with abdominal distension, blood in stools and pneumatosis coli (air in bowel wall) visible radiologically, necrotizing enterocolitis (NEC) is a patchy necrosis of the bowel, most typically the terminal ileum. Perforation and peritonitis may result, although the relatively sterile bowel content makes the peritonitis less catastrophic than might be supposed. The perforation in the bowel wall can often be left to heal without surgical intervention. The pathogenesis is not entirely clear, but it most likely results from bowel ischaemia and secondary overgrowth of various gas-forming pathogenic bacteria in the gut wall, giving rise to the pneumatosis.

Other organs

Although many other organs can demonstrate specific pathology, most are rare and beyond the scope of this chapter. However, clinical problems are not uncommon and usually are attributable to functional immaturity.

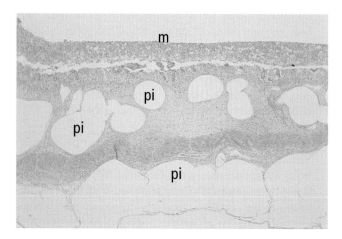

Fig. 25.13 Photomicrograph of typical necrotizing enterocolitis. At the top, the mucosa (m) is necrotic and normal architecture has been all but lost an occasional residual gland. The submucosa contains one of the more typical features observed clinically but sometimes not remaining in specimens coming to pathological examination – pneumatosis intestinalis (pi). Histologically it is represented by round empty spaces but with time may become lined by a macrophage giant-cell reaction.

Thus the skin and subcutaneous tissues of the premature infant are poor both in retaining water and heat production. The immune system is poorly developed and the neonate is vulnerable to infections, many of them opportunistic. In this regard, the neonate can be considered to be in an immunocompromised state. The immature tubular epithelium of the kidneys may not concentrate glomerular filtrate very efficiently and may compound the problems of water balance.

PAEDIATRIC PATHOLOGY

As with topics such as malformation, many conditions which typically present in the paediatric age group are dealt with in the context of the the specific organ or system rather than under paediatric pathology. This section will confine itself therefore to two areas: sudden death in infancy and paediatric neoplasia.

Sudden unexpected death in infancy– sudden infant death syndrome

Figure 25.14 illustrates an approach to considering the problem of infant death but the percentages are only approximate. In just under a half of cases of infants who die suddenly, the infants die outside of hospital unexpectedly and in only some 10–20% of these will a full autopsy reveal a cause of death. It is the 90% of unexpected infant deaths in whom post mortem fails to reveal significant pathology that constitute what is currently known as sudden infant death syndrome (SIDS).

Definition
'The sudden death of an infant or young child which is unexpected by history and in which thorough postmortem examination fails to reveal an adequate cause of death'.

This is a pathological diagnosis but one which is often far less clear-cut than it appears. It is sometimes problematic as to what constitutes a sudden death, what constitutes a thorough post mortem, and what pathological findings can be considered a sufficient cause of death.

Epidemiology (Fig. 25.15)
The incidence of SIDS in the UK has fallen sharply in recent years from a mean of 2–3/1000 infants to approximately 1/1000 infants. This would appear to be related to the current advice to place infants **on their back** rather than their front **for sleeping**. The most common age is from 2–4 months but may occur from 1 week to up to a year, although greater than 6 months is unusual. Winter is more common than summer and SIDS has been associated with viral epidemics, particularly influenza. Death typically occurs at night, in the early hours, although collapse in the mother's arms is recorded. **Risk factors** include:
- a poor socioeconomic condition;
- parental smoking;
- high maternal parity;
- premature birth.

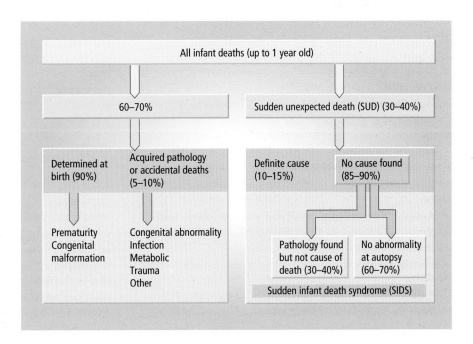

Fig. 25.14 Diagram of the approach to considering sudden infant death (SID).

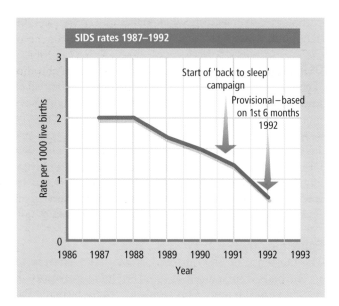

Fig. 25.15 The sudden infant death rates (SIDs). Note the difficulty in fully interpreting the change in recommendations as SID rates were already falling.

'Causes' of sudden infant death syndrome

By definition, the death of any infant in whom a diagnosis of SIDS is made cannot be explained or attributed to specific cause. However, innumerable hypotheses have been generated to account for these deaths, the most prominent of which are outlined below.

- **Infection.** Infant deaths occur in an age group when infection is common. The problem is deciding on the significance of histological changes or viral and bacteriological isolates that may be obtained. It has been suggested that death might result from overwhelming infection or some form of anaphylaxis to common bacteria.
- **Asphyxia.** Accidental or deliberate asphyxia can never be entirely excluded by autopsy and always remains a possibility, however unlikely.
- **Hyperpyrexia.** The observation of elevated rectal temperatures in SIDS cases, sometimes many hours after death, suggests that pyrexia may have caused or contributed to death. Some babies may be overwrapped in cold weather and have difficulty in losing excess heat, particularly at the peak risk age when mobility is limited.
- **Apnoea.** Cessation of breathing may be due to failure of central control or precipitated by some airway obstructive event.
- **Metabolic disease.** Defects in medium-chain fatty acid metabolism due to acyl-coenzyme A dehydrogenase deficiency have been detected in some cases. Other disorders involving carbohydrate or amino acid metabolism have also occasionally been found. Studies of

lung surfactant have suggested that SIDS may be associated with abnormal surfactant production leading to sudden lung collapse. Results however have been conflicting and many observations may be post-mortem artefact.

Conclusion

In making any assessment of the various hypotheses, a number of difficulties which are a particular problem in the study of SIDS need to be borne in mind.

First, it is often difficult to identify an adequate control population and therefore to be sure that the abnormalities or changes found in cases of SIDS are peculiar to that group. For instance, histological changes within the respiratory tract which might suggest infection as a cause of death can also be found in infants in whom this is not the diagnosis.

Second, caution has to be exercised in ensuring that apparently abnormal results are not due to post-mortem artefact. This aspect is particularly true in the study of metabolic defects such as surfactant abnormalities or enzyme defects.

Third, and perhaps most importantly, each proposed theory of sudden infant death may only be a partial or, in a few cases, complete explanation of some deaths. Claims that the cause of SIDS has been identified should be regarded with suspicion. Further, many of these theories are not mutually exclusive and it is likely that the interaction of a number of elements culminates in infant death. For instance, the peak incidence of SIDS is at 3 months of age, when the infant respiratory drive may be relatively poor.

Vulnerability to infection may be increased in premature babies because of reduced numbers of maternally derived antibodies normally acquired before birth. Infection in combination with overwrapping might lead to problems of heat loss. Hyperpyrexia in the presence of poor respiratory drive could lead to respiratory arrest and death.

Paediatric tumours

After the first year of life, malignant neoplasms are a major cause of death in childhood, having taken over from infection due to improvements in therapy. The incidence is approximately 100/million per year and about one-third of this number die from their tumour, although, in isolation, this latter statistic hides a considerable variation in the malignancy of different tumours. Some aspects of congenital and childhood tumours have been discussed in Chapter 11. An indication of the main proportion of childhood malignancies is given in Table 25.11.

Table 25.11 Paediatric neoplasms.

Leukaemias	35 (%)
Central nervous system	25 (%)
Lymphoma	11 (%)
Neuroblastoma	6 (%)
Wilms (nephroblastoma)	6 (%)
Rhabdomyosarcoma	5 (%)
Other (bone, retinoblastoma, hepatoblastoma)	17 (%)

Aetiology

Environment. Compared with adult neoplasms, the influence of environment on childhood tumour induction and production is relatively limited, with hereditable factors being more important. Study of atomic fall-out survivors indicates that radiation is undoubtedly associated with induction of leukaemia, neoplasia usually developing within 5 years of exposure.

Solar radiation may stimulate solid tumorigenesis in hereditable defects of DNA repair such as xeroderma pigmentosa. Drugs have rarely been implicated but the association of childhood vaginal adenocarcinoma with the administration of diethylstilboestrol to the mother and consequent fetal exposure is well-established. Some studies suggest that maternal smoking increases the risk of childhood cancers in exposed fetuses. Viruses are constantly sought, but perhaps the only major well-established association is between endemic Burkitt's lymphoma and Epstein–Barr virus.

Genetic. The best studied link between genes and tumour production, and an important one in illustrating possible relationships, is that of retinoblastoma.

Retinoblastoma

This is an uncommon tumour of childhood (< 2.5%) but, when it occurs, is often bilateral. Bilateral tumours usually develop at an earlier age than unilateral tumours (8 versus 26 months) and are often familial (18% bilateral; 6.5% unilateral).

Advances in molecular biology have allowed a specific gene deletion to be identified on the long arm of chromosome 13 (13q14). The deleted gene appears to code for a protein of approximately 800 amino acids in size, which is capable of binding to DNA and probably has a regulatory function. Gene deletion in both chromosomes is necessary for the tumour to occur. In familial or bilateral tumours, one gene is deleted in the germ cell, thus requiring only one somatic mutation to occur to produce a homozygous deletion. In sporadic retinoblastoma it is the presence of a homozygous mutant allele requiring two genetic events which leads to tumour occurrence.

Other recognized chromosomal abnormalites in childhood solid tumours include a specific translocation associated with neuroblastoma (see below). A small portion of chromosome 2 is translocated to the short arm of chromosome 1, this portion containing an oncogene (n-*myc*), amplification of which may be associated with aggressive tumour behaviour.

Deletions of the p13 region of chromosome 11 may also be found in some Wilms tumours, although in some syndromes in which Wilms tumours form a significant component the deletion may be found more frequently.

Some tumour subtypes are discussed elsewhere in organ or system chapters, and so only the briefest details relevant to childhood are listed here.

Leukaemia

Constituting about a third of all childhood neoplasia, its incidence in this age group appears to be declining (Table 25.12).

Lymphomas

In childhood, non-Hodgkin's lymphoma is more common than Hodgkin's disease and is almost confined to three high-grade subtypes, slightly more than a half of which are of T-cell origin. The low-grade, often B-cell tumours seen in adults are rare in the paediatric age group (Table 25.13).

Central nervous system tumours

Central nervous system (CNS) tumours are the commonest solid tumour of childhood and comprise approximately 20% of all neoplasia. Compared with adults, meningeal tumours are very rare, whereas more primitive neuroepithelial tumours exemplified by medulloblastomas are a more important subgroup.

Table 25.12 Paediatric leukaemias.

Acute lymphoblastic	80%
Acute non-lymphoid	15%
Chronic lymphocytic	< 1%
Chronic myeloid	1–5%

Table 25.13 Childhood lymphoma.

Hodgkin's disease (45%)		Non-Hodgkin's lymphoma (55%)
Lymphocyte-predominant	15–30%	
Nodular sclerosing	40–60%	Lymphoblastic
Mixed cellularity	20–40%	Burkitt/Burkitt-like
Lymphocyte-depleted	<5%	Immunoblastic/large cell

Table 25.14 Central nervous system tumours.

Gliomas	40–50%	Mainly astrocytic; 20% are highly anaplastic but most behave in a benign manner
Primitive neuroepithelial	20%	
Ependymomas	10–15%	
(Craniopharyngiomas)	10%	
Other	5–10%	Germ cell tumours, dysgerminoma, teratoma

Infratentorial tumours are relatively more common than in an older age group (see Chapter 27; Table 25.14).

Neuroblastoma

Age and presentation. Neuroblastoma presents as a mass or with symptoms related to the secretory activity of the tumour cells. Neuroblastoma is a tumour seen primarily in children up to 3 years of age. Fifty per cent present within the first year.

Site. The sites of neuroblastoma are adrenal medulla and paravertebral sympathetic ganglia. Occasionally they arise elsewhere.

Diagnosis. Diagnosis is by biopsy and diagnostic histology or by detection of catecholamine metabolites vanillylmandelic acid and homovanillylmandelic acid in the urine.

Histology. Histology shows sheets of small round cells with little cytoplasm. Evidence of ganglion differentiation may be present.

Prognosis. Early presentation implies a better prognosis. Two-year survival is 70% when the tumour presents neonatally; survival is 5% if it presents after 2 years of age. Evidence of differentiation is a good prognostic feature.

Wilms tumour (nephroblastoma) (Fig. 25.16)

Age and presentation. Nephroblastoma presents with abdominal pain and mass or haematuria. Up to 40% present within the first 2 years of life and 85% by the age of 5 years. They may be bilateral and may be associated with abnormalities such as aniridia, other genitourinary malformations and hemihypertrophy.

Site. Nephroblastoma may arise from persistent blastematous elements within the kidney (nephrogenic rests).

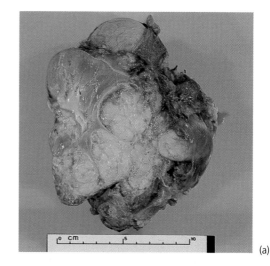

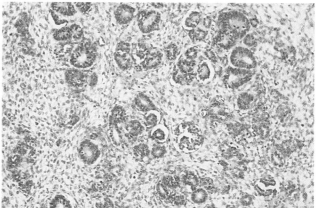

Fig. 25.16 (a) Nephroblastoma (Wilms tumour) in a kidney of a 5-year-old child. In this case the tumour has extended beyond the renal capsule of the kidney. A typical 'pushing' margin is present at the junction with the normal renal tissue near the upper pole. (b) Photomicrograph of nephroblastoma in which the tumour is forming epithelial tubules and glomeruli.

Histology. Three elements are present in varying proportions—blastema, stroma and epithelial differentiation with tubule and primitive glomerulus formation.

Prognosis. Survival is greater than 90%. Foci of anaplastic change confer poor prognosis.

Other tumours

• **Rhabdomyosarcoma.** This is the commonest malignant soft-tissue tumour, which can present as a mass in almost any site but the main locations are the head and neck and genitourinary tract. Prognosis is poor in deeper sites but survival may be up to 90% in more superficially presenting tumours. Various histological subtypes also affect the prognosis.

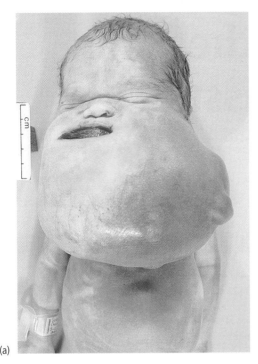

(a)

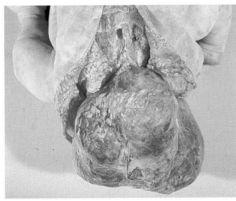

(b)

Fig. 25.17 (a) Cervical teratoma in an infant of near term gestation. Although the tumour is 'benign' histologically, this less common site for tumour neoplasm may cause death shortly after birth due to airway obstruction. (b) Sacrococcygeal teratoma in a newborn infant. This is a more common site of presentation.

- **Hepatoblastoma.** These include < 1% of childhood tumours, usually presenting before the age of 3 years as a palpable upper abdominal mass in the liver. Histologically, the tumour may show cords of cells resembling fetal hepatocytes, although a mesenchymal component may be prominent. Spread may be direct, to local lymph nodes or lungs.
- **Teratomas.** Sacrococcygeal teratomas are the commonest congenital tumours readily apparent at birth (Fig. 25.17). Despite their often large presenting size, they usually have a very good prognosis. Like other germ cell tumours, gonads and midline, paraspinal locations are other favoured sites.

Complications of treatment

In addition to the acute complications of radiation- or drug-based tumour therapy, the young age and often successful result make the potential long-term sequelae of therapy more significant. Sterility may result from gonadal irradiation, particularly in females. Radiation may also impair normal growth where bones and joints are affected. Deformities may also occur. In the CNS, radiation may produce frank infarction, although more subtle effects are more usual. A reduction in intelligence may result from treatment of medulloblastoma, although the precise mechanism is not clear.

Second malignancies are also a problem, some of which may take years to become manifest. Bone irradiation may lead to osteosarcoma or fibrosarcoma development, often after 10 or more years, whereas treatment of a primary tumour in the head and neck may lead to thyroid carcinoma arising more than 30 years later.

FURTHER READING

Keeling J.W. (ed.) (1987) *Fetal and Neonatal Pathology*. Springer Verlag, London.

Bergman A.B., Beckwith J.B. & Ray C.G. (eds.) (1990) *Proceedings of the Second International Conference of Causes of Sudden Death in Infants*. University of Washington Press, Seattle. pp. 83–102.

Clayton B. & Round J. (1994) *Clinical Biochemistry and the Sick Child*, 2nd edn. Blackwell Scientific Publications, Oxford.

Pathology of the Skin and Soft Tissue

C O N T E N T S

INTRODUCTION

The skin is the largest organ of the body and that most immediately exposed to the environment. Consequently, it is liable to infection and to physical and chemical damage, both directly from this environment as well as from internal agencies. Further modifications in the basic structure will also be produced by the site the skin occupies and by ageing.

NORMAL APPEARANCE OF THE SKIN

The skin is divisible into three main areas.

Epidermis (Fig. 26.1)

This comprises four layers.

1 **Horny layer/keratin layer.** The anuclear surface layer.
2 **Granular layer.** Consists of flattened cells filled with keratohyaline granules which are rich in sulphur.
3 **Squamous cell layer.** Cells are flattening as they approach the surface and are united by intercellular bridges formed from desmosomes and tonofilaments and separated by intercellular spaces.
4 **Basal layer.** Cuboidal cells are found resting on the basement membrane and providing the site of epidermal proliferation.

Dermoepidermal junction

This area binds the epidermis and the dermis together and is the site of several antigens. These can be identified by immunocytochemical techniques and provide markers for some skin disorders (Fig. 26.2).

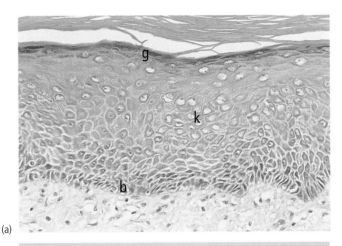

(a)

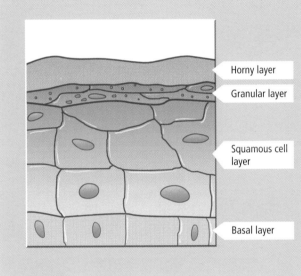

(b)

Fig. 26.1 Normal skin. (a) High power view showing the components of the epidermis. g, granular layer; b, basal layer; k, keratinocytes. (H&E.) (b) The epidermis.

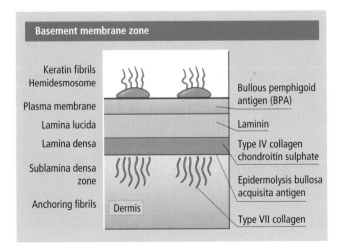

Fig. 26.2 The location of antigens in the basement membrane zone.

Dermis

Developing from mesenchymal cells, this is the site of the appendages, blood vessels and nerves which contribute to the functions and integrity of the skin. Hair, sebaceous glands and apocrine glands have a common developmental pathway while eccrine glands develop separately.

HISTOLOGY OF THE SKIN

Epidermis

Keratinocytes (Fig. 26.3)

These squamous cells are the fundamental cells of the epidermis, developing from basal cells and distinguished at electronmicroscopy by the **keratohyaline** bundles in their cytoplasm and at light microscopy by antibodies to **cytokeratins**. There are 5–10 layers of keratinocytes in the squamous layer of the epidermis, varying with the site and affecting proportionally the thickness of the keratin

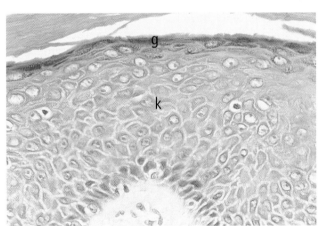

(a)

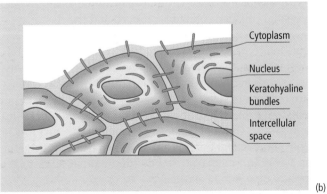

(b)

Fig. 26.3 Normal skin. (a) High power view showing keratinocytes (k) and granular layer (g). (b) Keratinocytes.

layer. The skin of the palms and soles has the thickest squamous layer and has the thickest keratin layer.

Melanocytes (Fig. 26.4)

Seen in haematoxylin and eosin sections as round cells with clear cytoplasm, they lie in the basal layer of the epidermis. They are recognized at electronmicroscopy by the **melanosomes** in their cytoplasm in the absence of keratohyaline bundles and at light microscopy by antibody markers. The cells include dendritic processes linking them as units with keratinocytes, roughly one melanocyte to 10 keratinocytes, and via which melanosomes are passed to the keratinocytes. Melanosomes are the source of pigmentation, often more conspicuous in basal cells than melanocytes, and are stimulated by ultraviolet light. Blacks have the same number of melanocytes as whites but these are more active, larger and include more melanosomes. The melanosomes in blacks are also more plentiful in keratinocytes in all parts of the epidermis than amongst whites.

Langerhans cells (Fig. 26.5)

These cells are not distinguishable in haematoxylin and eosin-stained sections and can only be identified at electronmicroscopy or by immunocytochemical techniques. The identifying feature at electronmicroscopy is the **Birbeck** or 'tennis racket' granule seen in the cytoplasm. Immunohistochemistry shows positive immunostaining for **S100**. Langerhans cells are scattered throughout the epidermis and to a lesser extent in the dermis and contribute to the immune responses of the skin.

Dermis

Types I and III collagen are the main constituents of the dermis, with type III collagen appearing in equal amounts in the fetus but as less than 20% in the adult. With increasing age the number of fibroblasts falls and the total collagen content is reduced and the elastin component altered. In some exposed areas such as the face, elastin is more prominent due to thickening and tangling of the fibres associated with coincident loss of elasticity. In regions not exposed to the sun the fibres in the elderly are reduced in size and number but similarly inelastic, an effect contributing to apparent thinning of the skin in this age group. Thinning is, however, mainly due to a loss of subcutaneous fat but it is also contributed to by a change in the ground substance of the dermis that adds to the progressive loss in elasticity.

The **sebaceous, apocrine and eccrine** glands are distinguished by their epithelial cells. Those of the sebaceous glands are relatively large with basophilic, often vacuolated or reticulated cytoplasm representing loss of

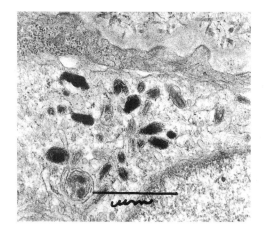

Fig. 26.4 Skin. Electronmicrograph of melanocytes showing melanosomes.

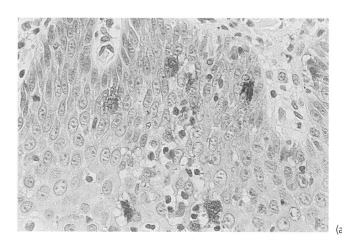

(a)

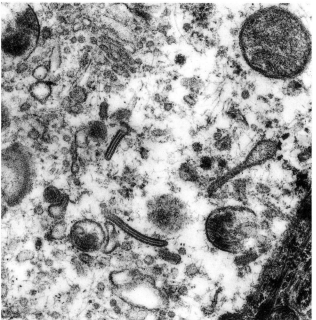

(b)

Fig. 26.5 Skin. (a) Langerhans cells stained positively (brown) for S100 using immunohistochemistry. (b) Electronmicrograph of Langerhans cells showing 'tennis racket' inclusions.

fat following tissue processing. Sebaceous glands generally accompany hair follicles but, particularly in the genital regions, can occur alone. Apocrine or scent glands are normally confined to the axilla and genital areas and are identified by minute blebs of cytoplasm issuing from their luminal surfaces. These cells are tall or cuboidal with a slightly granular eosinophilic cytoplasm and are supported by **myoepithelial cells**. The eccrine or sweat glands, in contrast, include none of the cytoplasmic features of the other glands and are formed from small cuboidal cells which stain either lightly or darkly and rest upon myoepithelial cells. **Ducts** are associated with all three types of glands and provide a pathway to the skin surface for their secretions.

DISEASES OF THE SKIN

Introduction

Skin diseases initially present to the student a confusing array of clinical and histological changes. These include infectious diseases largely confined to the skin, primary skin disorders and cutaneous manifestations of a variety of systemic disorders, as well as a range of skin and soft-tissue tumours. Where a cause can be identified, as is mainly the case with infective conditions, such as the mite producing scabies or the virus of chickenpox, the clinical and histological features can be confidently categorized but all too often the cause of a particular skin disease is unclear. Drugs, for example, produce a wide range of changes virtually mimicking all other dermatological conditions and labelling a rash as arising from drugs often depends upon the exclusion of other possible causes and the reaction resolving or reappearing with withdrawal or re-exposure to the drug. This lack of specificity of a reaction either clinically or histologically reflects the limited responses available within the skin, to which is invariably added an absence of any known specific marker for the cause, in this example a drug, but a restriction equally applicable for other common skin diseases, including some forms of eczema. Contributing to these dilemmas and providing diagnostic difficulties is also a potential changing pattern of reaction depending upon the time of examination. Dermatologists have inadvertently aggravated matters further by adherence to Latin terminology, the use of eponyms and a passion for subdividing conditions that is all too often based on small numbers of examples. Since the reader is unlikely or even needs at this stage to master these innumerable conditions, no attempt is made to provide a comprehensive description of skin disorders. For this reason, more specialized texts and atlases have been recommended at the end of this chapter for those who wish to pursue skin and soft-tissue pathology at a more advanced level or who wish to consult a reference source when reading up any specific clinical cases they may encounter.

The reader is, however, probably aware from experience of a range of dermatological descriptions and using this knowledge, aspects of some of the commoner primary non-infectious skin disorders (Table 26.1) will be presented as well as some cutaneous manifestations of systemic disorders and common skin tumours. Infective skin disorders arise from cutaneous or systemic infections and include bacterial, viral, fungal and protozoal causes

Table 26.1 Some descriptive terms used in clinical dermatology.

Macular–papular
Erythematous–vesicular
Erythematous–desquamative
Follicular–pustular
Purpuric
Urticarial
Blistering
Nodular

Each term may be appropriate to more than one skin disorder and any skin disorder may manifest more than one of these appearances.

Table 26.2 Examples of micro-organisms producing skin disorders.

BACTERIAL	
Staphylococcus aureus	Boils; impetigo; secondary to many skin disorders
Streptococcus *pyogenes*	Impetigo; cellulitis; scarlet fever
Mycobacterium sp.	Lupus vulgaris; swimming pool granuloma; fishtank granuloma; leprosy
Treponema	Syphilis; yaws; pinta
VIRAL	
Papilloma	Warts
Pox	Chickenpox
Coxsackie	Hand, foot and mouth disease
Herpes	Cold sores; shingles
FUNGAL	
Dermatophytes	Athlete's foot; ringworm
Candida	Thrush; vaginitis
PROTOZOAL	
Leishmania	Leishmaniasis
HELMINTHS	
Schistosoma	Swimmer's itch
Filarial worms	Elephantiasis
PARASITES	
Sarcoptes	Scabies

(Table 26.2). Recognition or isolation of these organisms or their antigenic characterization, serologically or within the skin by immunocytochemical or molecular biological techniques, provides the ultimate proof that the skin changes arise from such infections.

INFECTIONS OF SKIN AND SOFT TISSUES

The skin's commensal flora and other factors (natural acidity and inhibitory subtances such as fatty acids) combine to form an effective barrier against infection. However, several pathogens are able to breach this barrier and cause infection (Table 26.3). Other mechanisms include secondary invasion of the skin or toxin-mediated disease. Bacteria, viruses, fungi and parasites can all cause skin and soft-tissue infections. Fungi tend to be of low pathogenicity, invade keratinized tissue only and produce superficial infections, whereas some *Streptococcus* spp. are highly pathogenic and penetrate the deeper tissues, to devastating effect.

Bacterial infections

Relatively few bacterial species are responsible for the large variety of primary pyodermas. For instance, *Streptococcus pyogenes* can cause erysipelas, cellulitis and necrotizing fasciitis depending on how far the infection penetrates the layers of skin or soft tissue (Fig. 26.6).

Table 26.3 Examples of microbial pathogens causing skin and soft-tissue infections.

Mode of infection	Examples of pathogens	
Breach of intact skin	Bacteria	*Staphylococcus aureus*, *Streptococcus pyogenes*, *Clostridium* spp., *Mycobacterium* spp., *M. leprae*
	Viruses	Papilloma, molluscum contagiosum, Orf
	Fungi	Dermatophytes, *Candida* spp.
	Parasites	Scabies (arthropod), *Leishmania* (protozoa)
Systemic infections with secondary skin manifestations	Bacteria	*Neisseria gonorrhoeae* and *N. meningitidis*, *Treponema pallidum*, *Rickettsia* spp.
	Viruses	Herpesviruses, measles, rubella
	Fungi	Dimorphic fungi, *Candida* spp.
Toxin-mediated bacteria		*Staphylococcus aureus* (scalded skin syndrome, toxic shock syndrome)
		Streptococcus pyogenes (Scarlet fever)

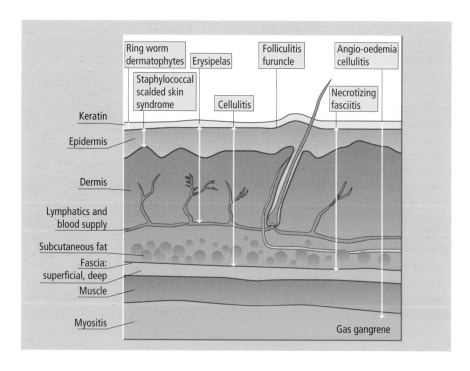

Fig. 26.6 Bacterial infection of the skin and soft tissue.

Names for infections of the subcutaneous tissue, fascia and muscle tend to be confusing due to the fact that similar disease processes are given different names depending on the aetiology of the infection, e.g. necrotizing fasciitis and streptococcal gangrene are one and the same.

Impetigo

In 80% of cases, infection is due to *Strep. pyogenes*, 10% mixed with *Staphylococcus aureus*. Ten per cent of cases of bullous impetigo are caused by *Staph. aureus* phage type 71. This is highly communicable amongst children and in conditions of poor hygiene and overcrowding. Skin acquisition of *Strep. pyogenes* leads to infection via traumatized skin. Secondary nasopharyngeal carriage follows, being different serotypes to the strains normally causing pharyngitis. Skin strains are potentially **nephritogenic**. Infection produces vesicular and crusted yellow lesions mainly on the face. The lesion heals without scarring and is treated with penicillin.

Staphylococcal scalded skin syndrome

This is a toxin-mediated disease as a result of the reaction of exfoliative toxin. Bullous impetigo is a mild form of this disease that affects infants and may cause epidemics in special care baby units. It produces flaccid bullae with fever. **Nikolsky sign** may be positive (separation of layers within epidermis on rupture of bullae). It affects all of the epidermis and scarring is possible on healing. Large areas of exposed skin (compare burns) often require fluid replacement and flucloxacillin.

Folliculitis, furuncles and carbuncles

Infection of the hair follicle is commonly caused by *Staph. aureus*. A **furuncle (boil)** develops from **folliculitis** but penetrates deeper into the dermis. A **carbuncle** extends into the subcutaneous fat and results in a large lesion, forming multiple abscesses. The latter are commoner in diabetics. Spontaneous drainage usually occurs but a particular problem is recurrent furuncles. Prophylaxis includes antibiotic treatment, general skin hygiene, often cleansing with chlorhexidine soap and irradication of staphylococcal nasal carriage with topical Naseptin or mupirocin.

Erysipelas and cellulitis

These conditions are very similar and are compared in Table 26.4. Another similar infection is **erythrasma**. This is a superficial bacterial infection characterized by brown maculopapular rashes in the genital area, caused by *Corynebacterium minutissimum*. *Erysipelothrix rhusiopathiae* and *Vibrio vulnificus* are rarer causes of cellulitis, being associated with workers handling meat and fish and infections acquired in marine waters, respectively.

Table 26.4 Comparison of erysipelas and cellulitis.

	Erysipelas	Cellulitis
Aetiology	*Streptococcus pyogenes*	*Streptococcus pyogenes* and *Staphylococcus aureus*
Age	Children and young adults	Any age, especially elderly and diabetics
Location of infection	Superfical cellulitis with lymphatic involvement	Spreading infection into subcutaneous tissue and lymph nodes
Appearance	Sharp demarcation of lesion	Erythematous diffuse oedematous lesion
Diagnosis	Clinical	Bacteraemia rare Surface swabs often not helpful
Recurrences	Common	Common
Treatment	Intravenous benyzlpenicillin	Intravenous benzylpenicillin and flucloxacillin

Chronic ulcerations

Diabetes and peripheral vascular disease predispose to chronic, superficial ulcers. These ulcers are colonized by coliforms, *Pseudomonas*, *Enterococcus* and anaerobes which on occasions cause infection. *Staph. aureus*, *Strep. pyogenes* and anaerobes are primary pathogens and the finding of coliforms from low-quality specimens such as superficial swabs can be misleading. Chronic ulcers are often overtreated with antibiotics, providing a breeding ground for resistant organisms. Treatment should include:

- simple cleansing routines with appropriate dressings;
- antibiotics in selected cases (not topical antibiotics).

Chronic ulcerations may also occur with some mycobacterial species, e.g. *Mycobacterium marinum* is a cause of **fishtank granuloma**. Ulcerative cutaneous diphtheria occurs in the tropics.

Infectious gangrene and gangrenous cellulitis

Deeper layers of the skin, subcutaneous fat and muscle are affected to various degrees. Gas gangrene is a myositis and is at the end of a disease spectrum in which wounds contaminated by *Clostridium perfringens* progress rapidly to a life-threatening disease. However *C. perfringens* more commonly produces an anaerobic cellulitis where there is no associated myonecrosis. The distinction between other types of soft-tissue infections is blurred and a summary of other infections is provided in Table 26.5. In general, anaerobes and facultative anaerobes predominate. Features of these infections include foul-smell-

Table 26.5 Infectious gangrene and gangrenous cellulitis.

Condition	Progressive bacterial synergistic gangrene	Synergistic necrotizing cellulitis	Streptococcal gangrene, necrotizing fasciitis	Clostridial (anaerobic) cellulitis	Gas gangrene
Infection involves	Subcutaneous tissue	Subcutaneous tissue	Fascia → Muscle	Subcutaneous tissue → fascia	Muscle
Precipitating factors	Abdominal surgery	Diabetes	Diabetes, abdominal surgery	Trauma, wound contamination	Trauma, devitalized tissue
Pathogens	Microaerophilic streptococci (*Streptococcus milleri*) and *Staphylococcus aureus*	Mixed anaerobes and Coliforms	β-Haemolytic streptococci, coliforms	*Clostridium perfringens* (other spp.)	*C. perfringens* (other spp.)

ing discharge, gas in the tissues (**crepitus**) and necrosis of overlying tissue with blackened skin. Extensive surgical debridement is required to stop the spread of these diseases followed by appropriate antibiotics.

Anthrax

This rare infection is caused by *Bacillus anthracis*, a Gram-positive, spore-bearing bacillus associated with farm animals, particularly cattle. Ninety-five per cent of cases are cutaneous as a result of skin inoculation. The remaining are pulmonary due to inhalation of spores.

Infection with *B. anthracis* tends to produce a vasculitis and results in a necrotizing, haemorrhagic inflammation of skin. The disease has a variable clinical course but death can occur rapidly if the disease is not diagnosed and treated.

Mycobacterial infection

Mycobacterium tuberculosis. This rarely infects the skin but may do so in the form of **lupus vulgaris**, causing red patches over the face. **Scrofuloderma** is skin involvement over a tuberculous lymph node, usually in the neck.

Mycobacterium leprae. This a common infection in tropical countries. The clinicopathological features of leprosy (**Hansen's disease**) are dependent on the immunological activity of the host, with a spectrum of disease ranging from **tuberculoid** to **lepromatous** forms (Table 26.6).
1 **Tuberculoid leprosy** occurs in patients who have developed a **T-cell (delayed) hypersensitivity** reaction to the organism. Bacteraemia is rare and the organism is localized focally within the skin, producing a hypopigmented patch. If there is nerve involvement, a **peripheral nerve palsy** may develop. The disease has a slow progression.
2 **Lepromatous leprosy** occurs in patients who have a low level of cellular immunity. Thus the organisms spread via multiplication in skin macrophages, producing nodular skin lesions. Bacteraemia occurs to peripheral

Table 26.6 Clinicopathological forms of leprosy.

	Lepromatous	Tuberculoid
Cell-mediated immunity	Negative	Strong
Lepromin test	Negative	Positive
Visceral lesions	Common	Absent
Skin lesions	Numerous	Few
	Nodular	Macular
Number of treponemes	Numerous	Few
Number of lymphocytes	Few	Numerous
Macrophages	Diffuse	Granulomas
Hypoaesthesia of skin	Rare	Common

sites as the organism grows preferentially at temperatures less than 37°C. Extensive destruction of tissue leads to **disfigurement**.

Spirochaete infections

Syphilis. This is caused by *Treponema pallidum* and is associated with skin lesions at the early and advanced stages. In the **primary stage**, a **primary chancre**, an indurated painless skin ulcer, is seen, usually on the genitalia which may exude fluid rich in organisms. In the **secondary stage**, a variety of skin rashes may occur with a specific lesion, **condyloma latum**, occurring in the anogenital region as a moist papule containing treponemes. In **late** and **tertiary syphilis**, **gummas** are seen in the skin. These are nodular masses of granulomatous inflammation with central necrosis without demonstrable treponemes.

Pinta. This disease is endemic in Central America and is caused by *Treponema carateum*. It is transmitted by direct contact. The early lesions present as red scaly skin nodules.

Yaws. This disease is caused by a *Treponema pertenue*. Yaws is found in tropical countries, particularly in children and is transmitted by direct contact.

Fungal infections

Dermatophytes (Fig. 26.7)

The dermatophytes are a group of fungi that produce **superficial mycoses** by invading keratin. They commonly infect the hair, nails and skin. Collectively they are termed **ringworm** but comprise three main genera:

- *Trichophyton*, e.g. *T. rubrum*, *T. mentagrophytes*;
- *Microsporum*, e.g. *M. canis*;
- *Epidermophyton*—*E. floccosum* is a single species.

The term **tinea** is used with the anatomical site to describe any dermatophyte infection, e.g. **tinea capitis** (scalp ringworm) and **tinea pedis** (athlete's foot). The fungi differ in their predilection for different body sites and may be exclusive to humans (**anthropophilic**) or zoonotic (**zoophilic**; Table 26.7). Clinical features are:

- skin—produces a round scaly lesion with raised margins and may be intensely itchy;
- hair—produces brittle hair shafts, scarring of the scalp and hair loss;
- nails—produces thickening and discoloration (**onychomycosis**).

Treatment includes:

- keratolytic agents, e.g. **Whitfield's ointment**;
- topical antifungals, the azoles, e.g. miconazole, clotrimazole;
- oral antifungals, especially for hair and nail infections where long courses are required, e.g. azoles (ketoconazole), griseofulvin, Terbinafine.

Yeast infections

Candida spp. (Fig. 26.8) can cause intertrigo, paronychia and onychomycosis and in conditions of specific immunological abnormalities, chronic mucocutaneous candidosis. Lipophilic yeasts are responsible for pityriasis versicolor (*Malassezia furfur*) and seborrhoeic dermatitis (*Pitysporum* spp.). Pityriasis versicolor is characterized by hypo- or hyperpigmented lesions on the trunk. Treatment of both conditions is with topical azoles.

Viral infections

Papillomaviruses cause warts, usually on the hands and feet and in the genital area. Apart from those viruses causing primary skin lesions, the majority of viruses cause skin lesions secondary to a viraemia. Lesions are either **vesicular** or **maculopapular**. Vesicular lesions are caused by **herpes simplex**, **varicella-zoster** and some enteroviruses (hand, foot and mouth disease, Coxsackie A viruses). Maculopapular lesions are produced by

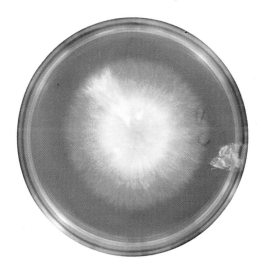

Fig. 26.7 *Trichophyton rubrum* forms large, grey colonies when grown on a culture dish.

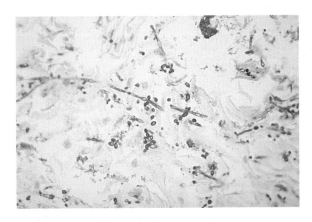

Fig. 26.8 Candida spores and hyphae. (PAS.)

Table 26.7 Dermatophyte infections in humans.

	Anthrophilic dermatophytes	Zoophilic dermatophytes
Tinea capitis	Trichophyton tonsurans	Trichophyton verrucosum (cattle) Microsporum canis
Tinea unguium	Trichophyton rubrum Trichophyton mentagrophytes	
Tinea corporis	Trichophyton rubrum	Microsporum canis
Tinea cruris	Trichophyton rubrum Epidermophyton floccosum	
Tinea pedis	Trichophyton rubrum Trichophyton mentagrophytes Epidermophyton floccosum	

human parvovirus (**B19**), **measles**, **rubella** and many arboviruses.

Parasitic infections

Leishmaniasis

Leishmania trophozoites multiply in macrophages in the skin without granuloma formation. Massive enlargement of affected organs may occur. The diagnosis depends upon finding the organisms in biopsy material or smears. There are three types of *Leishmania*.

Cutaneous leishmania. This is caused by *Leishmania tropica* and is confined to the skin. A papule is seen which progresses to a chronic ulcer, termed **oriental sore**. Distribution of this disease is seen throughout the tropics.

Mucocutaneous leishmania. This is caused by *L. braziliensis*, found in Central and South America and affects the face, nose and oral cavity.

Visceral leishmania (kala-azar). This is caused by *L. donovani*, endemic in the Mediterranean region and South and East Asia. It involves the reticuloendothelial system with skin involvement being rare.

Cutaneous larva migrans

This is a rare disorder caused be larval forms of animal nematode from **hookworm** and **roundworms** of dogs and cats.

Filariasis

Onchocerciasis. Due to *Onchocerca volvulus*, this is a common cause of skin and eye infection in Africa. It is transmitted by the bite of the *Simulium* **fly** and is characterized by the formation of subcutaneous nodules (**onchocercomas**) composed of tangled masses of worms surrounded by fibrosis.

Lymphatic filariasis. Causing obstruction to lymphatics and **elephantiasis**, this disease is caused by infection with *Wuchereria bancrofti* and *Brugia malayi*. Transmitted by mosquitoes, it is seen in South and South East Asia.

Scabies

Scabies represents an infestation of the skin by *Sarcoptes scabiei*. The scabies mite burrows into the skin and the female lays eggs in these burrows. The typical site of infection is the wrists but infection may spread to any site, especially in the immunocompromised patient or where poor hygiene is a problem. Clinical features include a characteristic rash and intense itching.

PRIMARY SKIN DISEASES

Introduction—the skin's response to injury

The skin responds in a limited number of ways to injury. Acute inflammation may involve the epidermis and dermis and will manifest clinically as redness, heat, pain and swelling. Fluid accumulation in the epidermis is seen between keratinocytes and is termed **spongiosis**. If severe, this will lead to **vesicle** formation. Dermal oedema may cause epidemal elevation, resulting in **wheal** formation. Severe injuries lead to necrosis and possible ulceration. Chronic injury and inflammation lead to thickening of the epidermis (**acanthosis**), thickening of the stratum corneum (**hyperkeratosis**) or dermal fibrosis. The range of general and specific skin reponses to injury are given in Table 26.8.

Inherited skin diseases

Ichthyosis

This group of disorders have dominant, sex-linked and recessive variants, some presenting at birth and others later in life. Uniform body involvement is seen in some of

Table 26.8 Responses of the skin to injury.

Terminology	Histology	Clinical appearance
Acanthosis	Hyperplasia of keratinocytes; thickening of epidermis	Plaque/papule
Acantholysis	Separation of epidermal cells	Intraepidermal vesicle
Atrophy	Thinning of the epidermis	Thinning of the skin
Dyskeratosis	Abnormal keratinization	None
Dysplasia	Dysplasia of keratinocytes	Papule
Exocytosis	Inflammatory cells in epidermis	None
Hyperkeratosis	Increased rate of maturation of keratinocytes with thickening of the stratum corneum	Silvery surface scales
Parakeratosis	Increased rate of maturation of keratinocytes with premature shedding giving nucleated cells in the stratum corneum	None
Pustule	Epidermal abscess	Pus-filled abscess
Spongiosis	Epidermal oedema	Intraepidermal vesicle

the neonatal forms, producing a **collodion baby**, and a more restricted distribution in older patients.

Epidermolysis bullosa

Epidermolysis bullosa includes several inherited variants with clinical onset in infancy. Vesicles form as a result of minor trauma. Defective intercellular attachment or defective anchoring of basal cells results in vesicle formation at various levels of the epidermis. Epidermolysis bullosa simplex is a mild disease that is dominantly inherited. In the **recessive–dystrophic** form of epidermolysis bullosa there is extensive ulceration and scarring and oral lesions are seen.

Darier's disease

Also known as **keratosis follicularis**, this is inherited as an autosomal dominant trait. Suprabasal clefts form in the epidermis as a result of acantholysis.

Hailey–Hailey disease (benign familial pemphigus)

This is inherited as an autosomal dominant trait and is characterized by localized eruptions of vesicles in the skin of the axillae and groins.

Pseudoxanthoma elasticum

This rare, recessively inherited disorder of elastic fibres produces soft yellow plaques in the skin. Histologically, there is accumulation of abnormal elastic fibres in the dermis. Other sites involved include the ocular fundi and arteries.

Classification of skin disease based on clinical appearances

Macular–papular (Fig. 26.9)

A **macule** is a round, generally reddened and flat area of skin, while a **papule** is similar but elevated. The two lesions often coexist and each may enlarge and become confluent. If the latter change is diffuse the entire skin is reddened and a substantial loss of heat may result. Drugs are often responsible for these reaction patterns but they are also seen in some examples of **lichen planus** and **lupus erythematosus**.

The most striking histological finding is an infiltrate of mononuclear cells either at the base of the epidermis (lichen planus) or around appendages (lupus erythematosus). If **eosinophil polymorphs** are also evident, the possibility of a **drug reaction** must be considered and the infiltrate may then be mainly perivascular. The cellular infiltrate may involve the epidermis and here be associated with focal destruction of basal cells and ultimately separation of the epidermis and the dermis. The dermal

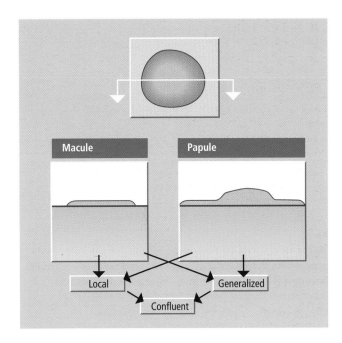

Fig. 26.9 Skin. Macular–papular disorder.

infiltrate is principally responsible for the colour change in the skin and will also, if substantial, produce in part the papular changes. Other factors contributing to these are thickening of the epidermis, oedema and increased vascularity but the oval nature of the lesions and their distribution are not easily accounted for. The changes, clinically and histologically, are not exclusive to all examples of macular–papular rashes nor found in all biopsies of lichen planus or lupus erythematosus but other histological features are often apparent that help to distinguish the specific skin disorder.

Lichen planus (Fig. 26.10). This is extremely irritant and involves both the **skin** and the **mucosa**. Clinical variants occur, one affecting the **scalp** and producing focal hair loss, **alopecia**, and spontaneous remission occurs in most patients between 9 and 18 months. The disorder occurs worldwide with adults mainly affected and is a fairly common condition in dermatology clinics.

Lupus erythematosus. This may either be restricted to the skin (**discoid lupus**) or form part of a systemic disorder (**systemic lupus erythematosus**) which in 80% of patients involves the skin. Both types of disorder are commoner in women than men and both have immunological abnormalities (see Chapters 7 and 9). Discoid lupus is almost confined to the face and exacerbated by many factors but particularly sunlight. The disorder is persistent and can produce scarring and depigmentation but only rarely does systemic involvement supervene. Systemic lupus

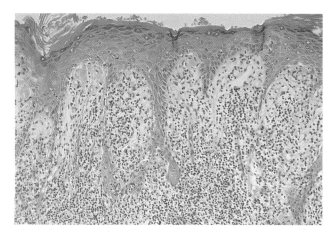

Fig. 26.10 Lichen planus. The epidermis is thickenend with patchy loss of parts of the granular layer. At the base of the epidermis there is irregularity amounting to a 'saw tooth' pattern associated with a band of chronic inflammatory cells lying almost entirely in the dermis. (H&E.)

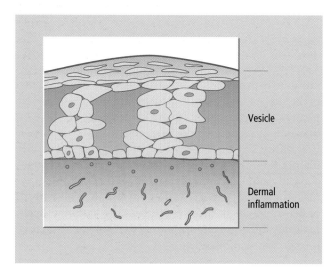

Fig. 26.11 Skin. Erythematous–vesicular disorder.

erythematosus, while often involving the face, is not restricted to this area and may affect the mucosa. In the scalp alopecia results. The tempo of the disorder is variable and this as well as therapy modifies the appearances and leads to a wide spectrum of clinical and histopathological features in the skin manifestations.

Erythematous–vesicular (Fig. 26.11)

Reddening or **erythema** is a common part of many skin disorders. **Vesicles** are small, often pinpoint accumulations of fluid in the epidermis and are usually found with variable inflammation of the surrounding skin. If the vesicles rupture the skin will weep, secondary infection may supervene and fluid loss occur. These changes when in flexures can produce splits and cracks as well as surface

crusting and in the longer term thickening. The appearances and their sequelae are characteristic of **eczema** which has many associations and clinical types but both may also arise from drugs, contact sensitivity (allergic dermatitis) and many other causes labelled by the histopathologist as **dermatitis**. Amongst these, dandruff (seborrhoeic dermatitis of the scalp), varicose eczema, washing detergent eczema, cradle cap and nappy rash are common examples. Specific skin disorders such as **erythema multiforme** may manifest similar features at some period in their course.

The epidermis is oedematous which is evident as widening of the intercellular spaces and with further increase in this fluid content localized keratinocyte loss and vesicle formation develop. Moderate numbers of inflammatory cells, principally mononuclear, accumulate in the papillary dermis, often around vessels and a few infiltrate into the epidermis. Thickening of the skin clinically correlates additionally with a thickened epidermis in all its layers, including elongation of the rete pegs.

Eczema. This term is most usually associated with the **atopic variant** which is a **familial** disorder, often combined with **asthma** and **hayfever** and associated with raised levels of **immunoglobulin E (IgE)**. The disorder starts in infancy and in the majority of patients resolves before adolescence. The face, flexures of the limbs and neck are sites of predilection. Nevertheless, there are many other forms of eczema and a useful division is into those with external and those with internal causes (Table 26.9).

Erythema multiforme. This is a skin disorder occasionally induced by **infection** or **drugs** but most usually of unknown cause. It can have a variety of appearances including eczematous but the most characteristic lesions are likened to shooting targets (**targetoid**) because of their raised oval configuration and central vesicle. Any part of the body can be involved, including mucosal sites, and in

Table 26.9 Forms of eczema.

Exogenous
Irritants
Allergic contact
Infective
Endogenous
Atopic
Seborrhoeic
Nummular
Pompholyx

most patients the condition is self-limiting in a few days and does not recur.

Erythematous–desquamative

The epidermis is continuously being replaced and as a part of this process the keratin layer is regularly shed. Certain skin disorders involve an increased cell turnover in the epidermis and consequent desquamation but abnormalities within the keratin and increased adhesiveness of the upper epidermis may be other contributory factors. Typical disorders are **psoriasis** and **ichthyosis**, both of which are **inherited** and both of which are of unknown cause. A similar change may appear in the course of other disorders, including reactions to drugs.

The involved epidermis is thickened, which may also be reflected in an increase in the granular layer and this is covered by a thick layer of **keratin**. Within the keratin there may be **parakeratosis** which is the presence of nuclei within this layer, often combined with an absence of the granular layer. The dermis may include inflammatory changes.

Psoriasis (Fig. 26.12). A disorder affecting 21% of the population in the UK, it is recognized in males more than females, often with an onset in adolescence, and it invariably has **lifelong** persistence. Any part of the body may be affected, with lesions developing and regressing, but new lesions do not always recur at the same sites. Several clinical forms are described and systemic features, particularly an **arthritis** resembling rheumatoid arthritis, can complicate the disorder. The typical lesion is distinct, reddened and covered by **silvery scales** and a wide variation in size and number can be encountered.

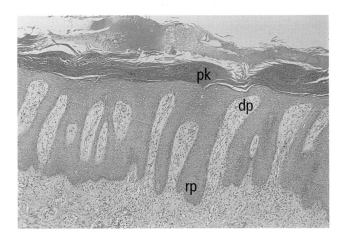

Fig. 26.12 Psoriasis. There is substantial parakeratosis (pk) and some keratosis on the epidermal surface. The epidermis is thickened with marked elongation of the rete pegs (rp) which have rounded ends. Within the dermal papillae (dp) vessels are dilated and acute and chronic inflammatory cells are evident.

Ichthyosis. This term implies a resemblance to **fish skin** which describes the clinical features of this group of disorders (see page 618).

Follicular–pustular

Many skin disorders have a follicular distribution but only in some is this indicative of their site of origin. **Folliculitis** is a term describing inflammation around hair follicles which may be a component of many other skin disorders but can occasionally arise from bacterial infection and if persistent result in small pustules. Skin pustules are experienced by many people at some time, rarely with symptoms other than cosmetic, but for a few are a significant component of acne. The **blackhead** or **comedone** characteristic of **acne** is a combination of sebum and keratin blocking a follicle and accompanied by a mild folliculitis. Only in a few patients is there substantial inflammation in the surrounding tissues or bacterial infection. Such phenomena do, however, form part of **acne rosacea**, the disorder that gives the sufferer a rubicund facial appearance and in some a bulbous reddened nose (**rhinophyma**). In these circumstances the follicles have ruptured and there is a focal granulomatous response in the dermis.

Acne vulgaris. This is common in **puberty** and affects at least 80% of the population at that time. Although in most individuals the disorder is self-limiting and leaves no residue, for a minority lesions persist, nodules of inflammation and cysts develop and gross scarring follows. The face and upper part of the trunk are principally involved. Apart from a hormonal effect, principally from androgens, other causative factors include active sebaceous glands, heat and humidity.

Purpuric

Bleeding into the dermis is the histological change underlying purpura. The effect can clinically extend from millimetre lesions (**petechiae**) to large areas of bruising (**ecchymoses**), and is distinct from inflammation in that in this the vascular change is predominantly one of **vasodilatation**. The causes of purpura are legion and include primary skin disorders, platelet disorders and systemic diseases with cutaneous involvement (Table 26.10).

Urticarial

Alternatively known as **nettle rash** or **hives**, these rashes may be localized or diffuse and produce swelling of the involved area from **oedema**. The change is associated mainly with **histamine** release which provokes dilatation and altered permeability in capillaries and small venules. The source of the histamine and other mediators is **mast cells** which are found with **eosinophil polymorphs** in

Table 26.10 Examples of causes of purpuric skin disorders.

Confined to the skin
Senile purpura
Scurvy
Vasculitis

Platelet abnormality
Idiopathic thrombocytopenic purpura
Thrombotic thrombocytopenic purpura

Systemic disorder component
Henoch–Schönlein purpura
Meningococcal septicaemia
Vasculitis
Drug-related

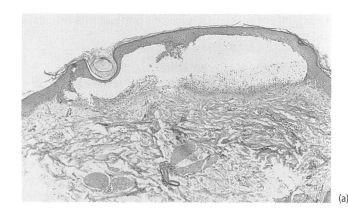

(a)

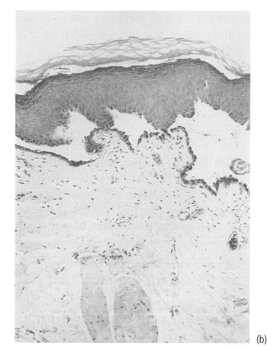

(b)

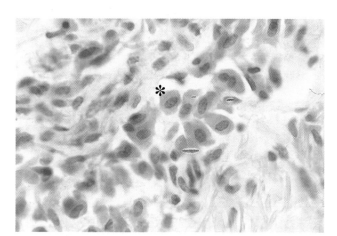

Fig. 26.13 Mast cells (✱). Dermal mastocytosis.

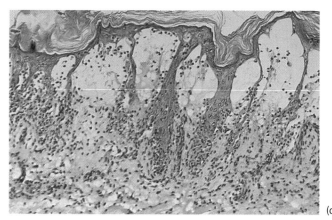

(c)

these lesions. The cause of the release of these mediators includes a wide range of local and systemic stimuli, physical and chemical, although in a fair proportion of long-term sufferers, particularly, no cause is identified. A very rare group of patients may be affected by a form of **mastocytosis**.

Mastocytoses (Fig. 26.13). These represent a group of disorders associated with accumulations of **mast cells** which are generally confined to the skin. The localized type is **urticaria pigmentosa** which is self-limiting and predominantly a disorder of **infancy**. Adults are more likely to have diffuse and systemic patterns of involvement which, although persistent, have an undeserved reputation for becoming malignant.

Blistering (Fig. 26.14)

Blistering or **bullous lesions** are caused by a wide variety of agents including burns and drugs and are associated

Fig. 26.14 Blistering disorders. (a) A subepidermal blister associated with bullous pemphigoid. (b) An intraepidermal blister associated with pemphigus vulgaris. (c) A subepidermal blister forming part of erythema multiforme. This disorder is not a primary blistering disorder, but usually presents as an erythematous–vesicular disorder. (H&E.)

with immunological changes and, very rarely, pregnancy and childhood. They can also develop in the course of many other skin disorders such as erythema multiforme, urticaria, lichen planus and psoriasis.

The title **bullous disorders** is invariably confined to those with immunological changes, although it remains unsettled as to whether these precede or antedate the skin lesions (Table 26.11).

At a diagnostic level the histopathologist needs to decide where in the epidermis the bulla is – **intraepidermal** or **subepidermal** – and where in the tissue immunoglobulins and complement are localized (Table 26.12). Knowledge of any circulating antiepithelial or antibasement membrane antibodies may also assist in distinguishing the pemphigus disorders from bullous pemphigoid.

Dermatitis herpetiformis. This extremely irritant disorder presents in young adults, many of whom will have or will develop **intestinal villous atrophy**. Blisters are confined to the skin and, in untreated patients, appear in crops over many years.

Bullous pemphigoid. A skin disease of the **elderly**, this affects mucous membranes and includes a variant causing substantial scarring. Without corticosteroids death from infection and fluid loss results but treatment has to be continued for many years.

Linear IgA disease. This shares many of the features of dermatitis herpetiformis and bullous pemphigoid and also merges with the bullous disorders of childhood.

Pemphigus disorders. The **middle-aged** are affected and lesions may first involve the mucosa. The **vulgaris** form is the commonest and differs from the **foliaceus** type in that the blistering is immediately above the basal layer rather than in the region of the granular layer and in that it has a more persistent and, if untreated, invariably fatal course. Both forms may need distinguishing from **benign familial pemphigus** or **Hailey–Hailey disease** which is a rare hereditary disorder virtually confined to the groins and axillae and unrelated to immunoglobulin deposition.

Nodular

Skin and soft-tissue tumours produce nodular lesions but nodularity associated with skin disorders is less common. The lesions may be in the dermis or subcutaneous tissues and are typified by **panniculitis**. Panniculitis is a histopathological term rather than a clinical diagnosis that implies inflammation and necrosis of fat, often associated with vascular changes. The overlying skin is often discoloured, reflecting the underlying nodule and also vasodilatation and congestion in response to this. The inflammation may be acute, chronic or granulomatous and is found either in the septa around the fat lobules, or confined within the lobules or affecting both septa and lobules. For each pattern of distribution there are multiple causes (Table 26.13), although histologically overlap occurs, which can produce some confusion.

Erythema nodosum. The title implies **red nodules** and these are usually painful, multiple and on the lower legs of young adult women. With time the nodules enlarge and alter in colour to that compared to 'apple jelly' but, ultimately, regression occurs. The importance of the disorder is that it is a marker of other diseases, most importantly streptococcal infections, tuberculosis and sarcoid.

Table 26.11 Bullous disorders of the skin.

Dermatitis herpetiformis
Bullous pemphigoid
Cicatricial pemphigoid
Linear immunoglobulin A disease
Pemphigus vulgaris
Pemphigus foliaceus

Table 26.12 Localization of immune deposits in bullous disorders.

Dermatitis herpetiformis	IgA	Papillary dermis (granular)
Linear immunoglobulin A (IgA) disease	IgA	Dermoepidermal junction (linear)
Bullous pemphigoid	IgG, C3	Dermoepidermal junction (linear)
Pemphigus disorders	IgG, C3	Intraepithelial

Table 26.13 Types of panniculitis.

Septal
Erythema nodosum
Infection
Insect bite
Lymphoma
Eosinophilic panniculitis

Lobular
Nodular vasculitis
α_1-Antitrypsin deficiency
Pancreatitis

Mixed
Infection
Connective tissue disorders

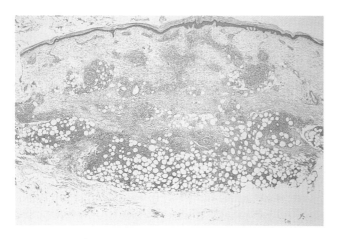

Fig. 26.15 Nodular vasculitis. The inflammatory changes involve the dermis and the underlying fat. They present around vessels as well as within the fat lobules and septae. (H&E.)

Drugs, notably sulphonamides, were also incriminated and clearly all of these associations raise the possibility of an underlying immunological cause.

Nodular vasculitis (Fig. 26.15). This is a term describing nodules, primarily on the legs, which are associated with a vasculitis, usually localized rather than systemic. The vessel involvement ranges from an inflammatory cell infiltrate to vessel wall destruction and secondary thrombosis. Middle-aged women are the main sufferers and, although individual lesions may ulcerate due to infarction, healing and recrudescence over a period of years is the usual course.

Disorders of skin pigmentation

Localized areas of skin may be darker or paler than normal. **Vitiligo** is patchy light skin most visible in tanned individuals or those with dark skin. This condition is associated with a partial or complete loss of melanocytes. Vitiligo is thought to have an **autoimmune** basis and is associated with other autoimmune diseases, in particular Addison's disease, thyroiditis and pernicious anaemia.

In **albinism**, the number of melanocytes is normal but there is a genetic inability to produce melanin.

Freckles (ephelis) are tan/brown macules that appear after sun exposure. Histologically, melanocytes are present in normal number but basal cells contain increased amounts of melanin.

Lentigo is a small brown macule that, unlike freckles, does not darken after sun exposure. Histologically, the dark pigmentation is due to melanocytic hyperplasia. Other benign and malignant hyperpigmented skin elevations are described in Chapter 27.

Cutaneous manifestations of systemic disease

A substantial number of systemic disorders include skin changes (Table 26.14). These changes range from the expected (e.g. jaundice with liver disease) to peculiar non-specific rashes such as **pyoderma gangrenosum** associated with **ulcerative colitis**. It is also true that for any organ, more than one skin manifestation exists and often more than one skin change may accompany any specific organ disorder. Examples of erythema multiforme, aphthous mouth ulcers, erythema nodosum and epidermolysis bullosa acquisita are all found in about 5% of patients with **Crohn's disease**. Many similar findings are documented elsewhere as well as in clinical texts and their histological aspects have no unique features but two groups of skin disorders do warrant further mention.

First, there are disorders that are truly **multiorgan**, such as lupus erythematosus, sarcoidosis and amyloid, which also have cutaneous involvement (see Chapter 7).

Second, there are skin manifestations that may herald **malignancy** (Table 26.15).

Dermatomyositis. This is rarer than the other connective tissue disorders and it affects the muscles and vessels as

Table 26.14 Selected examples of systemic disease with dermatological manifestations.

Organ	Systemic disease	Skin feature
Brain	Tuberous sclerosis	Sebaceous adenoma
Heart	Bacterial endocarditis	Osler's nodes
	Rheumatic fever	Erythema nodosum
Lungs	Tuberculosis	Erythema nodosum
Liver	Cirrhosis	Spider angiomas, hyperpigmentation and telangiectasia
	Obstructive jaundice	Pigmentation and pruritus
Pancreas	Pancreatitis	Panniculitis
Kidney	Renal failure	Calcinosis cutis and pruritus
Stomach	Carcinoma	Migratory thrombophlebitis
Small intestine	Coeliac disease	Dermatitis herpetiformis
Large intestine	Polyposis	Cysts, pigmentation, alopecia and nail dystrophy
	Ulcerative colitis	Pyoderma gangrenosum
Thyroid	Hyperthyroidism	Pretibial or localized myxoedema
	Hypothyroidism	Hair loss
Adrenal	Addison's disease	Pigmentation
	Cushing's disease	Hirsutism and bruising
Joints	Rheumatoid arthritis	Rheumatoid nodules and pyoderma gangrenosum
Lymph node	Hodgkin's disease	Pruritus
Skin	Neurofibromatosis	Pigmented spots and nodules

Table 26.15 Examples of skin markers of internal malignancy.

Dermatomyositis	Underlying malignancy in 25% Mainly carcinomas
Acanthosis nigricans	Mainly abdominal carcinomas Especially stomach
Necrolytic migratory erythema	Pancreatic glucagonoma
Bullous pemphigoid Erythema multiforme Generalized pruritis Erythroderma	Carcinomas: any association may only reflect the age of the patient Lymphomas and leukaemias in 15%
Paget's disease	Breast carcinoma

well as the skin. The skin, particularly of the face and less often the limbs, is oedematous with a purplish-red erythema. If there is an associated tumour, removal can produce a remission but otherwise the disorder can prove rapidly fatal.

Acanthosis nigricans. Thickening and pigmentation of the epidermis result. This change is localized and apart from malignancy can be found with a range of endocrine disorders (see Chapter 14) and some drugs.

Necrolytic migratory erythema. This condition is particularly associated with **pancreatic malignancy**. The skin of the abdomen and lower legs is involved in a cyclic eruption. Initially there is a macule with a central bulla which is succeeded by a healed central pigmented zone encircled by an encrusted red margin. These lesions coalesce and enlarge, producing a geographical pattern and do not entirely regress if the underlying pancreatic tumour is resected.

SKIN TUMOURS

Benign

Everyone has a skin tumour at some time in their lives and most usually more than one. Such tumours are hence common but the majority are benign. Perhaps because of this the exact incidence of benign skin tumours is unknown. Equally unknown is the cause of these neoplasms in contrast to the malignant forms, particularly the commonest types.

The benign tumours recognized at birth are called **naevi**. They should be distinguished by a prefix such as **epidermal**, **melanocytic** or **vascular**, but this is not al-

ways done. It is now realized that lesions clinically and histologically indentical with naevi can develop after birth and are hence indistinguishable from naevi.

Naevi will have similar growth patterns to their host, generally enlarging until after puberty, in contrast to other benign lesions which potentially enlarge continuously. Skin tumours can arise from any of the cells contributing to the epidermis or the dermis and for each benign example there is potentially a malignant variant (Table 26.16), although in the dermis malignant primary tumours are rare. Amongst the epidermal tumours there are variants which histologically are malignant but clinically do not usually behave as such (Table 26.17). The epidermal tumours clinically are infinitely easier to recognize than the dermal types which usually present as a subcutaneous mass, only rarely associated with any pigmentation, melanin or haemosiderin. The diagnosis of dermal tumours is thus more reliant upon histological examination than epidermal tumours, some of which are curetted and never submitted for histological examination.

Epidermal cysts (Fig. 26.16)

These are lined by a stratified squamous epithelium and envelope keratin which grossly is cheesy, yellow-white and greasy.

Some cysts (**pilar** or **tricholemmal** cysts) differ in that their lining is a low-set cubical type and similar to that of the **hair root sheath**. This observation has given rise to the suggestion that these cysts develop from the hair follicles and is in keeping with a punctum on the surface of the overlying skin that provides a potential pathway between

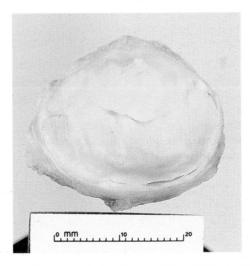

Fig. 26.16 Epidermal cyst. The lesion has been bisected. There is a thin capsule enclosing soft yellow-white, cheesy material which is keratin.

Table 26.16 Common benign tumours and their malignant counterparts.

Benign	Malignant
EPIDERMIS	
Keratinocytes	
Epidermal cyst	
Epidermal naevus	
Squamous cell papilloma (Wart)	Squamous cell carcinoma
Clear cell acanthoma	
Basal cell papilloma (Seborrhoeic wart)	Basal cell carcinoma
Melanocytes	
Junctional naevus	
Compound naevus	Melanoma
Intradermal naevus	
Spitz naevus	
DERMIS	
Fibroblasts	
Keloid/hyperplastic scar	
Dermatofibroma	Fibrosarcoma
Angiofibroma	
Vascular	
Pyogenic granuloma	
Haemangioma	
Angiokeratoma	Angiosarcoma
Angioleiomyoma	
Glomus tumour	
Lymphangioma	Lymphangiosarcoma
Nerve	
Neuroma	
Neurofibroma	Neurofibrosarcoma
Neurilemmoma	
Appendageal	
Sebaceous adenoma	Carcinoma
Hidradenoma	Carcinoma
Fat	
Lipoma	Liposarcoma

Table 26.17 *In situ* epidermal changes with the potential for malignancy.

Keratinocytes	
Bowen's disease	SCC 3–5%
Actinic/solar keratosis	SCC less than 1%
Chondrodermatitis nodularis helicis	SCC rarely
Keratoacanthoma	SCC rarely
Sebaceous naevus	BCC less than 10%
Melanocytes	
Lentigo maligna	Melanoma
Dysplastic naevus	Melanoma
Melanocytic naevus	Melanoma 25–30%

SCC, Squamous cell carcinoma; BCC, basal cell carcinoma.

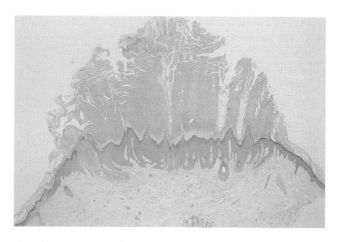

Fig. 26.17 Squamous papilloma or viral wart. There is marked increase in the surface keratin which is forming columns. The epidermis is thickened with elongated rete pegs that have a centripetal pattern. (H&E.)

the cyst lumen and the environment. The high incidence of these tumours on the **scalp** where they may reach an enormous size is further support for an origin from the follicular apparatus.

Epidermal naevi

Such naevi are evident either at birth or during early infancy. They can involve large areas of skin and then are prone to infection and a cause of substantial cosmetic disfigurement. The areas include irregular thickening of the epidermis, usually with increased keratinization and pigmentation of the keratinocytes.

Squamous cell papilloma (Fig. 26.17)

Most probably the commonest form of benign skin tumour, the tumour is usually, but not invariably, papillomatous with a thickened epithelium covered in keratin protruding from the skin surface. Many of these tumours are attributed to **papillomavirus** infection and recognized as **warts**.

Clear cell acanthoma

A further example of a localized thickening in the epidermis, the involved cells are distinct from those around them because they are cubical and more uniform, and because their cytoplasm is clear and filled with **glycogen**.

Basal cell papilloma

This provides another example of a **wart**, although not due to papillomavirus infection. Patients are usually over 40 years of age and a wide variation in size is encountered. The thickened area lies above that of the surrounding epidermis and encloses small cysts filled with keratin. Histologically variants occur but the predominant cell type is similar to the basal cell. Excessive **pigmentation** can cause confusion with a melanoma.

Melanocytic naevi (Fig. 26.18)

These develop from melanocyte precursor cells (naevus cells) that are arrested during the terminal phase of their migration from the neural crest to the epidermis. Naevi develop in childhood but persist into adult life. A number of different forms of these tumours occur, commonly referred to as **moles**, some apparent at birth and others developing later, although regressing in adulthood (Table 26.18). The different types are separated according to the location of the melanocytes in the epidermis and dermis: when melanocytes are confined to the dermo-epidermal junction or dermis, naevi are **junctional** or **intradermal** respectively, while those with melanocytes in both areas form **compound naevi**.

Histologically the distinction between **congenital** and **acquired** is now acknowledged as not as clear-cut as was once believed and even the association with hairs is not a reliable indicator of congenital naevi. Naevi that are recognized after birth are usually evident between 12 and 30 years of age and since junctional naevi occur mainly in children, compound naevi in young adults and intradermal ones in adults, the possibility of a maturation process is clearly raised. A further reason for believing in such a progression is that in the intradermal naevi the melanocytes can be associated with a change involving loss of some of their epithelial characteristics and their ability to form melanin, and the assumption of neural characteristics. This change is also supportive evidence for the origin of melanocytes from neural tissue and may explain the histological differences between these **melanocytic naevi** and the **blue naevi** which also differ in that they are confined to the dermis.

Table 26.18 Melanocytic naevi.

Congenital		
Giant (bathing trunk)		> 20 cm diameter
Intermediate		< 20 cm diameter
Small		< 1.5 cm diameter
Acquired		
Epidermal melanocytes	Junctional	mm–< 1 cm diameter
	Compound	3–5 mm diameter
	Intradermal	mm–cm
Dermal melanocytes	Blue naevus	5 mm diameter
	Cellular blue naevus	5 mm diameter

Spitz naevus

A very important form of a **compound naevus**, this grows very rapidly and is invariably restricted to children and young adults. The growth pattern is clearly alarming and some of the histological features similarly raise the suspicion of malignancy.

Dermal benign tumours

These often escape categorization until after histological examination and, while some are restricted to one cell type or dermal component, others include more than one cell type or dermal component and a few merge with the epidermis.

Keloids, for example, which in reality are areas of gross scarring, involve solely fibroblasts and develop particularly amongst blacks following either trivial or substantial injury to the skin.

Angiomas, of which there are several different clinical variants, are restricted to aggregates of blood vessels often present from birth.

Angiofibromas and **dermatofibromas** are tumours involving both excessive fibrous tissue formation and increased numbers of vessels while **angioleiomyomas**, also involving two dermal components, differ in that smooth muscle replaces fibrosis as the principal tumour constituent. **Angiokeratomas** are tumours with numerous enlarged blood vessels that lie so close to the epidermis that in sections the reactive hyperplasia of the epidermis appears to envelop these vessels.

Tumours of skin appendages

These are usually benign and are identified by their distinctive histological features and classified according to their differentiation (Table 26.19). They present as **painless skin nodules** and are **rarely malignant**.

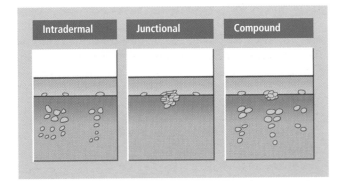

Fig. 26.18 Types of melanocytic naevi.

Table 26.19 Tumours of skin appendages.

Tumour	Differentiation	Sites
Eccrine poroma	Eccrine	Feet, hands (mainly in elderly)
Eccrine spiradenoma	Eccrine	All over
Clear cell hidradenoma	Eccrine	All over
Syringocystadenoma papilliferum	Eccrine	Face, scalp
Syringoma	Eccrine	Lower eyelids
Trichofolliculoma	Hair	Face, solitary
Trichoepithelioma	Hair	Face, may be multiple
Pilomatrixoma	Hair	All over (mainly children)
Cylindroma	Apocrine	Scalp (may be multiple)
Hidradenoma papilliferum	Apocrine	Vulva in females
Naevus sebaceous	Sebaceous	Scalp, face (from birth)
Sebaceous adenoma	Sebaceous	Rare

Malignant

While there is potentially a very large number of malignant skin tumours, in practice only three are commonly encountered – **squamous cell carcinomas, basal cell carcinomas and melanomas**.

The common denominators for these three tumours are:
- they arise in the epidermis;
- if recognized early they can be cured;
- the appearance of one tumour carries a substantial risk of a further similar tumour;
- they are all increasing in frequency;
- inherited and environmentally induced precursors occur;
- they affect whites rather than blacks and mainly adults in both races;
- they are related to sun exposure;
- immunosuppression increases their incidence.

There is a bulk of circumstantial evidence relating these skin tumours and **sun exposure**. Nevertheless, it must not be forgotten that other environmental agents can be involved, including **chemicals**, both industrial and therapeutic (Table 26.20) and **inherited conditions** (Table 26.21).

The **human papillomavirus** may play a role in **squamous cell carcinomas**, especially in the immunosuppressed patients, and long-standing **scars**, including those from vaccination, in basal cell carcinomas.

Sun exposure via ultraviolet light has a cumulative effect upon the skin; the **Ultraviolet A** waves damage the **dermis** and the **Ultraviolet B** waves damage the **epidermis**, although the two augment one another and exactly

how the damage is produced is unknown. These effects are also aggravated by other environmental factors such as wind, heat and even washing. A cumulative effect is probably necessary for skin tumour induction and is the reason why doubts are expressed about holes and thinning in the ozone layer contributing to skin cancer since these changes are, relative to the increase in skin cancer, new events and have not been present for a sufficient time to effect any change. Nevertheless, there is fully justified concern that in the future the ozone changes may precipitate an even greater increase amongst skin cancers.

The increase in the numbers of skin cancers is believed to have arisen from a very marked change in social attitudes. 'Pale and interesting' was formerly the ideal of the upper white social classes and tanning a mark of the outdoor manual labourer. Increasingly during the last few decades these concepts have been replaced by the view that 'brown is beautiful' amongst all white classes and none more so than those in Australia. The common skin cancers have reached epidemic proportions in Australia amongst the white population and particularly those of Celtic origin.

The evidence indicates that sun damage initiated in childhood is the most important factor, although short intensive exposure in the adult can certainly contribute to melanoma in those unused to sunbathing. Similar obser-

Table 26.20 Chemicals associated with some forms of skin cancer.

Chemical	Therapeutic indications
Polycyclic aromatic hydrocarbons (tars)	Psoriasis
Anthralin	Psoriasis
Benzoyl peroxide	Acne
Arsenic	Asthma/tonics
Nitrogen mustard	Lymphomas

Table 26.21 Inherited conditions that predispose to common malignant skin tumours.

Celtic origin	Basal cell carcinoma Squamous cell carcinoma Melanoma
Xeroderma pigmentosa	Squamous cell carcinoma Melanoma
Naevoid basal cell carcinoma	Basal cell carcinomsa
Familial dysplastic naevus syndrome (atypical mole syndrome)	Melanoma
Self-healing epithelioma of Ferguson–Smith	Squamous cell carcinoma

vations have been made in other countries and there is worldwide a **doubling incidence** amongst the common skin tumours with every **10° decrease in latitude** and a direct linear increase amongst whites as they approach the equator.

The observed effects of ultraviolet light on skin components (Table 26.22) support the notion that the sun harms the skin, as does the occurrence of skin tumours in patients exposed to ultraviolet light for therapeutic reasons, e.g. acne and psoriasis.

Basal cell carcinoma (Fig. 26.19)

Alternatively known as **rodent ulcer**, because of its ability persistently to erode into the supporting tissues and so destroy them, this tumour only very rarely metastasizes. **Metastases** occur in 0.002% of patients or, more meaningfully, in 1 in 50 000 patients.

Basal cell carcinomas are the commonest malignant skin tumours in whites with a ratio of 4:1 with squamous cell carcinomas but an equal incidence in blacks. Men are more affected than women. The tumour appears in elderly patients and on dry rather than greasy skin in sun-exposed areas as well as in skin folds on the face.

Approximately 70% occur as single lesions but only 60% are correctly diagnosed clinically. At least a third of the patients will have a further tumour within 5 years. The tumour is thought to arise from the basal cells of the hair follicles rather than from potentially all basal cells of the epidermis—a view supported by the restriction of basal cell carcinomas to hair-bearing skin and their histological similarity very often to hair follicles.

Basal cell carcinomas vary in size depending upon the stage at which the patient presents but the majority are under 2 cm in diameter. They may be flat, papular, nodular and ulcerated or form an area of thickening. The cell type is similar to the basal cell of the epidermis and almost all tumours are attached to the basal layer. The cells are uniform with easily evident mitoses and a distinctive arrangement to the peripheral cells compared to a **palisade**. The palisade separates the irregular and variably sized islands of basal cells from the stroma and there may be an artificial separation of the cells and the stroma due to loss of some of the mucopolysaccharides in the stroma during tissue fixation. The stroma has a bluish appearance and is generally infiltrated by mononuclear cells and in two-thirds of tumours includes small amounts of amyloid derived from keratinocytes.

Variants from these appearances that can cause confusion are evidence of **keratin** raising the possibility of a squamous cell carcinoma; excessive **melanin** or **iron** pigmentation raising the possibility of a melanoma and cystic degeneration, which may be sufficient to imitate an adenocystic carcinoma. A number of descriptive terms are used to describe different variants of the tumour but the only one possibly of significance is the **morphoeic basal cell carcinoma**. This variant includes a substantial amount of stroma and the tumour cells are in infiltrating strands rather than as islands. Many authorities believe this variant is more likely to recur after therapy than the other forms of basal cell carcinoma.

Table 26.22 Effects of sunlight on the skin.

Physiological	Pathological
Increase in size and number of melanocytes	Activation of herpes simplex, SLE etc.
Decrease in Langerhans cells	Sunburn (solar erythema)
Inhibition of fibroblast repair	Suntan
Premature ageing	Solar keratosis (and acceleration of their growth)
	Epidermal tumours

SLE, Systemic lupus erythematosus.

Squamous cell carcinoma (Fig. 26.20)

Epidemiology. This is the second commonest malignant skin tumour and is principally a tumour of **elderly males**. It occurs on sun-exposed areas and in slightly less than half of the patients presents as a single tumour. Metastases do occur and when the lip is involved these may affect as many as 10% of the patients but for most examples spread from the skin is unusual.

The majority of these tumours have no precursors but a minority arise from solar keratoses and Bowen's disease (Table 26.17) and even smaller numbers from inherited disorders (Table 26.21).

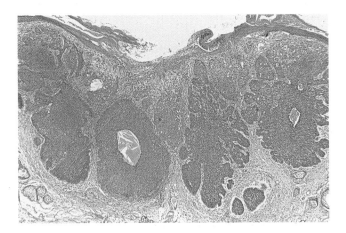

Fig. 26.19 Basal cell carcinoma. Islands of uniform basal cells arise from the epidermis and fill the dermis. There is degeneration of cells in the centre of some islands with cyst formation. (H&E.)

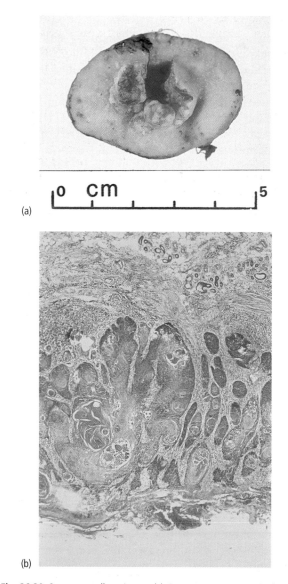

(a)

(b)

Fig. 26.20 Squamous cell carcinoma. (a) Gross appearance. A raised irregular ulcer projects from the skin surface and has also infiltrated into the underlying tissues. (b) Microscopic appearance. Tongues of squamous cells, some investing keratin, are spreading into the underlying dermis.

Macroscopic features. Grossly the lesion may be indistinguishable from a basal cell carcinoma but a few are papillary and others covered with flakes of keratin.

Microscopic features. The squamous cells vary from easily recognizable squamous cells to highly undifferentiated cells and in any part of this spectrum there may be keratin within the cell cytoplasm or seen as extracellular collections, keratin pearls, surrounded by tumour cells. A variable fibrous change is found in the stroma and within this a mononuclear cell infiltrate.

The tumour invades irregularly into the dermis and

ultimately into the supporting tissues. If the lesion is exceptionally well-differentiated or if it has a smooth rounded invading edge it may be difficult to decide if the tumour is malignant. To resolve these dilemmas any spread below the level of the sweat glands is designated as malignant. Some tumours, particularly in the very old, may be totally undifferentiated and entirely formed of spindle-shaped cells and will then need distinguishing from spindle cell melanomas and spindle cell sarcomas, a distinction aided by labelled antibodies.

Other confusing tumour variants are those that include sufficient apoptotic cells, often here referred to as acantholytic cells, to result in bullous formation and those that are papillary, hyperplastic and largely exophytic, **verrucous carcinomas**, which mimic **viral warts**.

Solar keratoses

These **dysplastic lesions** combine an increase in keratin, parakeratosis, dysplasia amongst the keratinocytes of the lower third of the epidermis and **solar elastosis** in the dermis.

Bowen's disease

This is **carcinoma-*in-situ*** of the epidermis. The change may develop in a solar keratosis and the two conditions are then histologically inseparable unless there is an absence of elastosis in the dermis, an observation favouring some examples of Bowen's disease.

Melanoma (Fig. 26.21)

Epidemiology. At one time referred to as **malignant melanoma**, these tumours have doubled in incidence every 10 years in Scandinavia and quadrupled in incidence in the USA during the same period. They continue to increase in number and affect annually 10 people per 100 000 in **Wales** but over 40 people per 100 000 in **Queensland** and have their highest incidence worldwide in **Australia**.

Adults are particularly affected and the age of the affected groups is falling. Amongst children the tumour is not found before puberty but in rare examples of transplacental spread of malignancy to the newborn, melanoma is disproportionately commoner than other malignancies.

In the UK there is a 2:1 incidence between female and male patients but in Australia more men are affected. Lesions in women are more often on the lower limbs than elsewhere and in men the upper back is the site of predilection. Although **sun exposure** is seen as the principal cause, 25–30% of melanomas arise in relation to a **melanocytic naevus** and a much higher number from **dysplastic naevi**, especially if the patient can be categorized as a member of the **familial dysplastic naevus syn-**

histologically are not always possible. Amongst all melanoma patients there is an 80% 5-year survival. Important prognostic information is provided histologically from the depth of invasion of the tumour into the dermis either as observed–Clark's levels–or as measured–Breslow's thickness (Table 26.25; Fig. 26.22).

These observations also differentiate different phases in the growth of a melanoma with an initial **radial** or *in situ* growth phase and a later *vertical* growth phase. Other features such as ulceration, high mitotic rate or vascular invasion, although regarded as bad prognostic indicators, do not provide such clear-cut implications for patients.

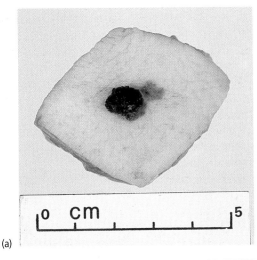

(a)

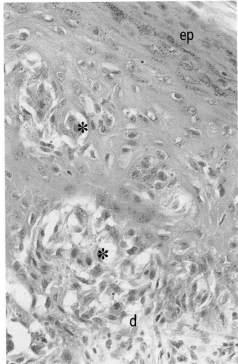

(b)

Fig. 26.21 Melanoma. (a) Gross appearance. A dark brown to black lesion arising from the skin surface which, on section, is seen to spread into the underlying tissues. Microscopic appearance. Many pleomorphic melanocytes (✳) are seen within the epidermis (ep) and the dermis (d) associated with a mononuclear inflammatory cell response. Brown melanin pigment is seen within melanocytes and lying free within the dermis. (H&E.)

drome (Table 26.23). A total of 6–18% of patients give a family history of melanoma.

Classification and staging. Clinically four main types of melanoma have been described (Table 26.24), although prognostically these distinctions have no significance and

Table 26.23 National Institutes of Health categorization of familial dysplastic naevus syndrome.

A	Few dysplastic naevi; no personal or family history of melanoma
B	Personal and family dysplastic naevi; no personal or family history of melanoma
C	Personal dysplastic naevi and melanoma; no family history of melanoma
D	Personal history of dysplastic naevi and melanoma; family history of melanoma

The risk of melanoma ranges from no risk in A to 100% in D.

Table 26.24 Clinical types of melanoma with their percentage incidence.

7%	Lentigo maligna melanoma	90% of melanomas in the head and neck areas
64%	Superficial spreading melanoma	50% history of preceding melanocytic naevus
28%	Nodular melanoma	May appear spontaneously or within superficial spreading melanoma
1%	Acral lentiginous melanoma	40% incidence in Japanese and the main melanoma in Africans. Found on the palms, soles and bed of nails

Table 26.25 Five-year prognosis for melanoma.

Clark's levels	5-year survival (%)	Breslow thickness
Level 1 Intraepidermal	100	
Level 2 Papillary dermis	90	> 0.75 mm
Level 3 Junction of the reticular dermis but not entering this	67	
Level 4 Reticular dermis	40	> 3.5 mm
Level 5 Subcutaneous fat		

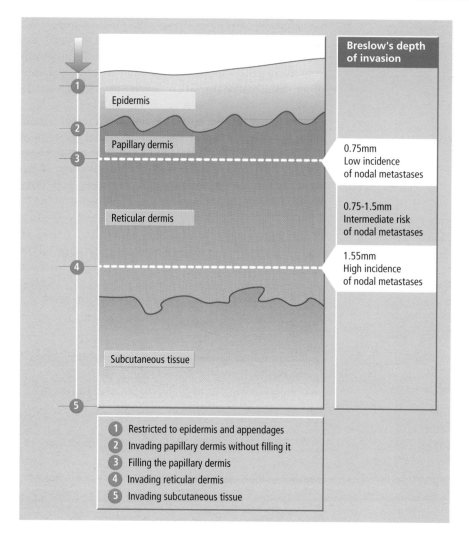

Fig. 26.22 Staging of melanoma.

Clearly the clinician's aim is to diagnose melanoma in its earliest phases as well as to recognize changes in naevi that may herald the onset of melanoma, basically any type of change.

Macroscopic features. The tumours range from flat pigmented areas to variably sized nodules and may in some examples be devoid of pigment.

Microscopic features. Tumour cells are large and include cuboidal and spindle forms with conspicuous nucleoli and fairly abundant cytoplasm. The cytoplasm may be clear or eosinophilic and any melanin is generally finely dispersed. The melanocytes lie individually, in groups and in infiltrating strands and infiltrate the epidermis and the dermis. Vascular invasion occurs but is generally difficult to recognize. The principal change in the dermis is a mononuclear infiltrate aligned along the base of the tumour.

Those melanomas classified as **lentigo maligna** generally include increased numbers of dysplastic melanocytes at the dermoepidermal junction and lower part of the epidermis, associated with elongation of the rete pegs and elastosis in the dermis – changes that can precede a melanoma by 10–20 years. Metastases are often recognizable grossly and microscopically because of their pigmentation and occur in draining lymph nodes as well as throughout the body, including the brain.

Dysplastic naevi

These are diagnosed clinically and histologically, although the two diagnoses do not always match. Any cytological atypia of melanocytes combined with architectural abnormalities such as bridging of melanocytes between rete pegs and some papillary fibrosis suggest the diagnosis which most often complicates a compound naevus. Most dysplastic naevi do not progress to melanoma.

Other malignant tumours including metastases

All of these tumours (Table 26.26), relative to squamous cell carcinoma, basal cell carcinoma and melanoma are uncommon. Most are not clinically recognized and need histological examination for identification, although **angiosarcomas** are a possible exception. These present particularly on the forehead and scalp as a fairly rapidly expanding area similar to a bruise. Most of the other tumours appear as cutaneous nodules associated with some overlying discoloration of the skin. The commonest sources of **metastatic carcinoma** are breast and lung, reflecting the high incidence of these tumours, but any primary carcinoma may produce skin metastases and these can be the first evidence of the tumour. Melanoma metastases may not be associated with pigment and hence present a diagnostic dilemma and may also be the first and only evidence that the patient has a melanoma.

Cutaneous malignant lymphoma

Cutaneous malignant lymphoma may occur primarily in the skin, or in the course of disseminated disease (5–10% with Hodgkin's lymphoma; 15–20% of patients with non-Hodgkin's lymphoma). T-cell lymphoma has a particular predilection for skin.

Mycosis fungoides (*cutaneous T-cell lymphoma*; Fig. 26.23). This T-cell lymphoma primarily affects the skin, with dissemination to lymph nodes and viscera occurring later in the disease's history. It is characterized by large, malignant mycosis cells (or **Lutzner** cells) with hyperchromatic, irregularly lobated, **cerebriform** nuclei and a **helper T-cell** (CD4) phenotype. Clinically, the disease can be divided into three stages: **erythematous, plaque** and **tumour**. In the plaque stage, invasion of the epidermis is seen with the formation of groups of mycosis cells forming so-called **Pautrier microabscesses** which are pathognomonic for the disease. By the tumour stage of the disease, lymph node and visceral involvement is seen in 70% and, when this occurs, 5-year survival rate is less than 10%. When fatal, this disease terminates as immunoblastic T-cell lymphoma (see Chapter 16).

Sézary syndrome. This may be regarded as a leukaemic variant of mycosis fungoides. It is characterized clinically by generalized erythroderma with intense itching. Sézary cells (indistinguishable from mycosis cells) are seen in the peripheral blood.

Cutaneous B-cell lymphoma. The commonest forms of cutaneous B-cell lymphoma are immunoblastic and lymphoplasmacytoid (Chapter 16). Unlike T-cell lymphomas, they rarely involve the epidermis but present as a dermal infiltrate or nodular mass. Primary B-cell lymphoma of the skin is rare, but up to 25% of B-cell lymphomas will present with skin involvement.

Merkel cell carcinoma (Fig. 26.24)

Merkel cells are found in the epidermis. They are **neuroendocrine cells** derived from the neural crest. They have a role in tactile sensation in some animals and are found in particularly high concentrations at the base of rodent whiskers. Rarely, they can undergo malignant change in humans and are seen as solitary nodules in the extremities, head or neck in elderly individuals. They are **aggressive** malignant tumours.

Histologically they resemble **small cell/oat cell carcinomas** and must be distinguished from metastases of such tumours. Immunohistochemical studies show both neuroendocrine and epithelial cell markers. Electronmicroscopy shows the presence of cytoplasmic neurosecretory granules.

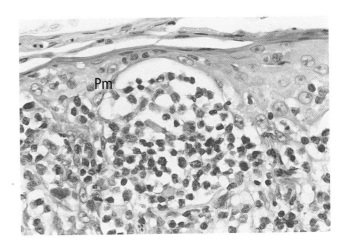

Fig. 26.23 Mycosis fungoides. Plaque stage with Pautrier microabscesses (Pm) in the epidermis. (H&E.)

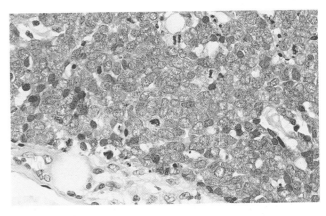

Fig. 26.24 Merkel cell carcinoma. Note the round, small, blue cells with abundant mitoses. (H&E.)

Table 26.26 Examples of uncommon malignant skin tumours.

Metastatic	Carcinoma, sarcoma and melanoma
Lymphomas	T-cell—mycosis fungoides
	B-cell—rarely primary and more often part of a systemic process
	Hodgkin's disease
	Langerhan's cell histiocytosis (histiocytosis X)
Appendage	Carcinomas of sweat, apocrine and eccrine glands
Vascular	Angiosarcoma
	Kaposi's sarcoma
Other	Merkel-cell tumour (neuroendocrine carcinoma of the skin)
	Dermatofibrosarcoma protuberans
	Spindle cell sarcomas

SOFT-TISSUE TUMOURS

Introduction—histogenesis of soft-tissue tumours

The dermis is a complex tissue composed of smooth muscle, nerve, fibroblasts, vessels and fat. Benign and malignant tumours may arise from these elements (Table 26.27). These are similar to soft-tissue tumours at other sites.

In this chapter, tumours of fibrous tissue, fat and vascular tissue will be discussed. Tumours of muscle are covered in Chapter 20 and tumours of peripheral nerve are discussed in Chapter 27.

Tumours of fibrous tissue

Benign
Dermatofibroma (fibrous histiocytoma; Fig. 26.25). This is a common neoplasm presenting as a slow-growing nodular dermal lesion composed of fibroblasts, histiocytes and variable amounts of collagen.

Xanthomas (Fig. 26.26). These are tumour-like collections of dermal foamy histiocytes, often with characteristic multinucleate giant cells (**Touton giant cells**). Subtypes are associated with certain **hyperlipidaemias**.

Eruptive xanthomas are found on buttocks, thighs, knees and elbows and appear and disappear with chang-

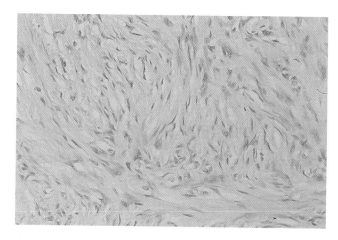

Fig. 26.25 Dermatofibroma of skin. Note the plump and spindle cells with pale nuclei. (H&E.)

Table 26.27 Soft-tissue tumours.

Histogenesis	Benign tumour	Malignant tumour
Mesenchymal cells		
Fibroblast	Fibroma	Fibrosarcoma
Nerve		
Schwann cell	Schwannoma	Malignant peripheral nerve sheath tumour
Neural fibroblast	Neurofibroma	Malignant peripheral nerve sheath tumour
Fat		
Lipocyte	Lipoma	Liposarcoma
Vessels		
Endothelial cells	Haemangioma	Haemangiosarcoma
	Lymphangioma	Kaposi's sarcoma
		Lymphangiosarcoma
Muscle		
Smooth-muscle cells	Leiomyoma	Leiomyosarcoma
Striated muscle cells	Rhabdomyoma	Rhabdomyosarcoma

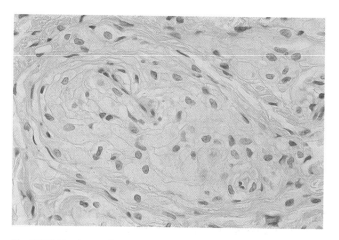

Fig. 26.26 Xanthoma of skin. Note the collections of foamy, lipid-filled cells. (H&E.)

ing plasma triglyceride levels. They may occur in types I, IIB, III, IV and V hyperlipoproteinaemia. **Tuberous xanthomas** are yellow nodules most commonly associated with types II and III. **Tendinous xanthomas** have a similar association and are seen in Achilles tendons and extensor tendons of the fingers. **Plane xanthomas** occur in skin folds most commonly in association with types II and IIA. **Xanthelasmas** are soft yellow plaques that occur on eyelids either idiopathically or assocated with types II and III hyperlipidaemia.

Atypical fibroxanthoma. This is a nodular lesion, commonly occurring on sun-exposed sites, often the head and neck, of elderly patients. Histologically, it is characterized by proliferation of fibroblasts and histiocytes showing atypia, pleomorphisms and mitoses. The lesion is poorly circumscribed with extension into fat. The lesion may recur if inadequately excised but does not metastasize.

Malignant

Dermatofibrosarcoma protruberans (Fig. 26.27). This is a slow-growing, locally invasive spindle cell tumour that may metastasize over many years if left unexcised. It may also ulcerate. Histologically it is composed of pleomorphic spindle cells arranged in a storiform pattern. These tumours tend to occur on the trunk.

Tumours of fat

Benign

Lipoma. Lipomas are very common subcutaneous tumours arising in older adulthood. Histologically they are composed of mature adipose tissue. They may contain areas of fibrous tissue (**fibrolipoma**), proliferating vessels (**angiolipoma**) or bone marrow elements (**myelolipoma**).

Malignant

Liposarcoma. Although uncommon in terms of malignant tumours as a whole, liposarcomas are amongst the more common of all the sarcomas. They may grow to reach a large size. Four histological types are recognized (well-differentiated, myxoid, round cell, pleomorphic) but in all the histological hallmark is the presence of **lipoblasts** (Fig. 26.28).

Vascular neoplasms

Benign and malignant tumours may be derived from endothelial cells, pericytes or glomus cells. In Chapter 15, congenital and hereditary vascular diseases are discussed.

Benign

Haemangiomas. Haemangiomas are commonly present at birth and are probably hamartomatous rather than neoplastic in origin. Two forms exist – **capillary** and **cavernous**.

Lymphangiomas. Cavernous lymphangioma or **cystic hygroma** is a benign tumour that occurs in the neck of infants. It can cause considerable enlargement of the neck and may lead to obstruction during birth. It is commonly seen in Turner's syndrome. Lymphangiomas may also occur in the mediastinum and retroperitoneum in adults. These are probably hamartomatous rather than neoplastic.

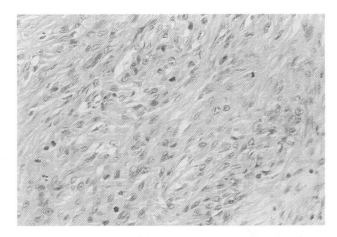

Fig. 26.27 Dermatofibrosarcoma protruberans. Note the cellular pleomorphism, the cells organized in fascicles and the mitoses. (H&E.)

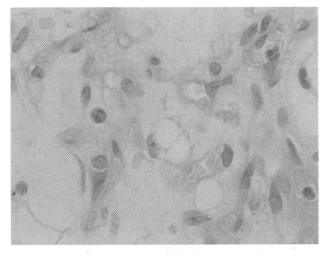

Fig. 26.28 The lipoblast (centre). The hallmark of liposarcoma. (H&E.)

Pyogenic granuloma. This lesion is probably a nodule of inflamed granulation tissue but is classified as an inflamed angioma by many. It may appear as a rapidly growing polyp, reaching 1–2 cm in a few weeks and then rapidly regressing. It is found in the skin or mouth following trauma and is particularly common in pregnancy.

Glomus tumour (glomangioma). These tumours occur in the skin, most commonly in the nailbeds of the fingers and toes. They occur in adults, forming small firm, red-blue lesions that are extremely painful. They vary in size from 1 mm to 1 cm. The histology shows solid nests of round pale cells with glassy round nuclei. The cells show distinct cell borders giving the so-called 'chicken-wire' appearance (Fig. 26.29). There is a rare malignant form of this tumour.

Haemangiopericytoma. These are rare tumours derived from pericytes that surround blood vessels. Histolo-

gically, these tumours consist of dense sheets of dark cells containing slit-like vascular channels ('stag horn' vessels; Fig. 26.30). There is a rare malignant form of this tumour.

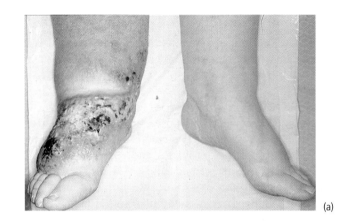

(a)

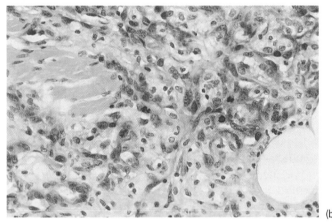

(b)

Fig. 26.31 Angiosarcoma of the skin. (a) Skin of the right lower leg. Note the limb oedema and ulceration and haemorrhage of the tumour. (b) Note the cellular pleomorphism, vascular channels and mitoses. (H&E.)

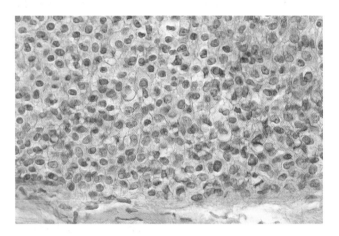

Fig. 26.29 Glomus tumour. Note the 'chicken wire' appearance of the cells. (H&E.)

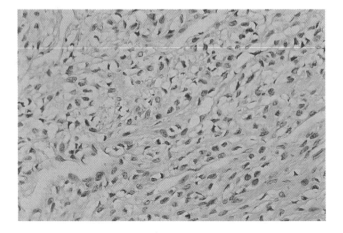

Fig. 26.30 Haemangiopericytoma. These cells are concentrated around vascular channels. (H&E.)

Malignant

Angiosarcoma. Angiosarcoma is a rare malignant neoplasm of **endothelial cells**. It is a tumour of adults. It may occur at any site in the body but is found most commonly in the skin, bone, soft tissue, liver and breast. The endothelial cells show cytological atypia. The better differentiated tumours show well-formed vascular spaces (Fig. 26.31). The prognosis is poor as vascular metastases occur early on.

Hepatic angiosarcoma is associated with **thorium dioxide (Thorotrast)** and **vinyl chloride** exposure. Angiosarcoma is associated with **radiation** exposure and may occur in mastectomy scars or in lymphoedematous arms after radical mastectomy for breast cancer (Stewart–Treves syndrome).

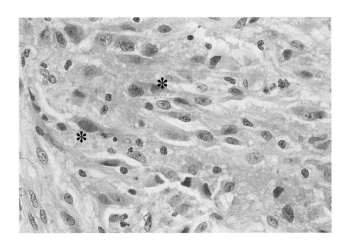

Fig. 26.32 Kaposi's sarcoma. Plaque stage. Slit-like vascular channels are seen surrounded by extravasated red cells and spindle cells with pleomorphic nuclei (✳).

Kaposi's sarcoma (Fig. 26.32). The tumour in the skin or viscera ranges from a small area of telangectasia to fairly large purple lesions. Lesions of Kaposi's sarcoma appear as purple **patches**, **plaques** or **nodules** in the skin which may ulcerate. In the viscera, they may occur as haemorrhagic masses. Haemorrhage is apparent on sectioning and this may cause death if the neoplasm involves the lung or gastrointestinal tract. The tumour is formed from spindle-shaped endothelial cells and is assumed to be vascular in origin. Multiple thin-walled vessels form the tumour with free red cells amongst a supporting stroma of spindle cells. With time and therapy, particularly irradiation, the lesion becomes fibrotic, often nodular and iron pigment is widely deposited.

Epithelioid haemangioendothelioma. This tumour consists of sheets of epithelioid or epithelial-shaped endothelial cells containing intracytoplasmic lumina in which red blood cells are found (Fig. 26.33). This tumour is considered by some to be of borderline malignancy. They do recur and metastases have been documented. They are found in the skin and soft tissues and variants are seen in the **liver** and **lung** (**intravascular bronchioloalveolar tumour**).

Lymphangiosarcoma. Lymphangiosarcoma is a rare malignant neoplasm of lymphatic endothelium. It is associated with radiation therapy, particularly at sites or lymphoedema. The prognosis is poor with early metastases.

Tumours of uncertain histogenesis

Synovial sarcoma
This is a sarcoma of young adults arising not from synovium but from sites near tendon sheaths. They have a biphasic histological pattern with epithelial and spindle cell elements.

Granular cell tumour (Fig. 26.34)
These are small (usually <3 cm), firm, poorly encapsulated benign tumours found in the tongue and subcutanous tissues of young to middle-aged adults. The tumours have a characteristic histological morphology, they have granular pink cytoplasm, and they may be derived from **Schwann cells**.

Tumour-like conditions

Some non-neoplastic processes can mimic tumours in their behaviour and clinical presentation.

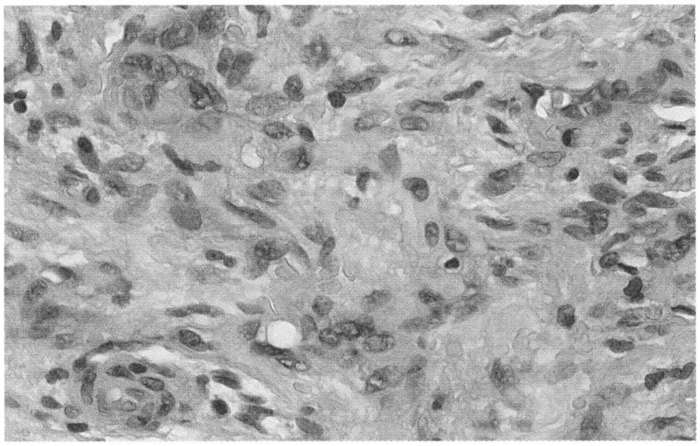

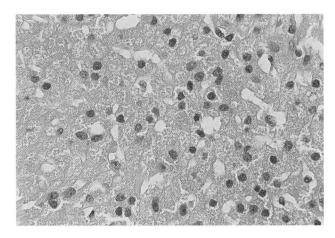

Fig. 26.33 Haemangioendothelioma. Note the epithelioid cells, some with intracytoplasmic vacuoles. (H&E.)

Fig. 26.34 Granular cell tumour. Note the pink cells with round nuclei and granular cytoplasm. (H&E.)

Fibromatosis

These are non-neoplastic aggregates of fibroblasts with infiltrative properties, classified according to site (**palmar**, **plantar** and **penile fibromatosis/Peyronie's disease**). **Desmoid** represents aggressive fibromatosis which can reach a massive size and are highly infiltrative but non-metastasizing. Intra-abdominal desmoids may be associated with **Gardner's syndrome**.

Myositis ossificans

This is a tumour-like lesion occurring in either skeletal muscle or subcutaneous fat. The lesion may form by fibrous replacement and ossification of a haematoma.

Nodular fasciitis

This is a reactive fibroproliferative lesion that affects young to middle-aged adults of both sexes and consists of fibroblasts similar to those seen in granulation tissue.

FURTHER READING

Enzinger F.M. & Weiss S.W. (1988) *Soft Tissue Tumours*, 2nd edn. Mosby, St. Louis.

Fry L., Wojnarowska F.T. & Shahrad P. (1985) *Illustrated Encyclopaedia of Dermatology*, 2nd edn. MTP Press, Lancaster.

McKee P.H. (1989) *Pathology of the Skin*. Gower Medical, London.

Diseases of the Nervous System, Including the Eye

Introduction

The primary objective of the clinician examining the nervous system is to determine the site of a lesion and identify the underlying pathological process. In order to arrive at this goal, an understanding of embryogenesis and functional anatomy of the nervous system is required. A brief review of development is provided in order to assist the reader in understanding the types of congenital malformations, the histogenesis and classification of nervous system neoplasms.

DEVELOPMENT

Neural tube development

Nervous system development commences with condensation of surface ectoderm on the dorsal aspect of the embryo, forming the **neural plate** (Fig. 27.1). The neural plate develops a central longitudinal groove forming neural folds, the outer margins of which proceed to migrate medially, fusing with the opposite fold, forming the **neural tube**.

The lumen of the neural tube is lined by pseudostratified **germinal matrix** neuroepithelium which functions as a stem cell population from which develop neuronal and glial cells (the term **glial** refers to cells showing **astrocyte**, **oligodendrocyte** or **ependymal** differentiation).

Cells remaining as the lining layer of the neural tube differentiate into ependymal cells, whilst the remainder undergo neuronal, astrocytic and oligodendrocytic differentiation with peripherally migration and organization, referred to as the period of neuroblast migration. At the cranial pole of the neural tube the migrating neurones become organized into a series of vertically oriented columns formed from successive horizontal neurone layers, an appearance akin to a stack of coins. This forms the functional units of the cerebral cortex grey matter. A

proportion of astrocytes and oligodendrocytes migrate into the grey matter to provide structural and metabolic support to the neurones. The remainder align themselves with axons, forming the white matter (Fig. 27.2).

The cranial pole of the neural tube subsequently undergoes accelerated growth with flexion and dilatation of the lumen, forming rudimentary brain and ventricles, referred to as the period of prosencephalic diverticulation. Compartmentation of the cranial pole follows, forming the paired cerebral hemispheres. A further increase in the surface area of the cerebrum is accomplished by the formation of the interhemispheric and Sylvian fissures. Later, during the fifth and sixth months of gestation sulci develop, further increasing cortical surface area without the need to increase significantly the cranial cavity volume.

A minority of migrating neurones remain in proximity to the developing ventricular cavities of the brain, forming the deep grey nuclei of the basal ganglia and diencephalon.

Following migration and differentiation, neurones attain an end-stage of differentiation, becoming mitotically inactive, whilst the glial cell population retains the capacity for replication. This feature is of significance in respect to the age of development, site and histogenic category of nervous system neoplasms.

The coverings of the central nervous system

The developing neuraxis is invested in concentric layers of fibrous membranes derived from the neural crest.

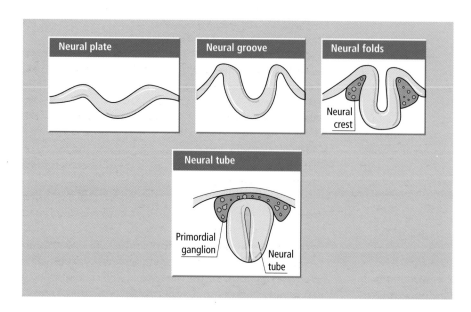

Fig. 27.1 Neural tube development.

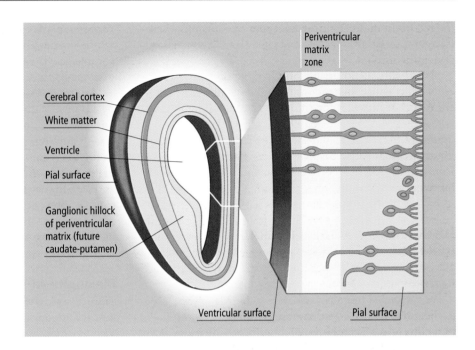

Fig. 27.2 The structure of the cerebral cortex.

Between these membranes circulates cerebrospinal fluid (CSF), providing metabolic and physical support to the brain and spinal cord. The potential spaces available between the concentric layers are of clinical significance as sites within which haemorrhage can occur and routes for the dissemination of infection and metastatic spread of neoplasms.

Diseases of the central nervous system

CONGENITAL ABNORMALITIES

Nervous system developmental abnormalities represent a relatively common form of malformation, an increasing proportion of which can now be detected *in utero* using biochemical assays and ultrasonography. The aetiology of these defects is variable, including genetic, chromosomal (trisomies and deletions) and environmental factors.

The majority of malformations follow disruption of one of the following developmental stages:
- neural tube closure;
- neuroblast migration;
- prosencephalic diverticulation.

The commonest group of disorders are **neural tube defects** (with a prevalence of 4–5 per 1000 total births in the UK) which arise during the third and fourth weeks of development, resulting in a range of malformations of mainly the lumbosacral spinal cord and defective closure of the overlying tissues.

The types of neural tube defects in order of increasing severity are.
- **Spina bifida occulta.** A common condition, usually clinically silent, arising from defective fusion of the vertebral arches and investing membranes. The overlying skin is intact.
- **Spina bifida cystica.** A defect of vertebral arch and skin fusion with protrusion of a meningeal sac containing either CSF alone (spina bifida with meningocoele) or in association with spinal cord and nerve roots (spina bifida with meningomyelocoele).
- **Spina bifida with myeloschisis.** Complete failure of closure of a segment of neural tube and its coverings, resulting in exposure on the body surface of the unfused spinal cord and nerve roots.

Fusion malformations at the cranial pole of the neuraxis include the following.
- **Encephalocoele.** Defective cranial cavity closure, most commonly in the occipital region, with herniation of brain and meninges.
- **Anencephaly.** A disorder incompatible with sustained life; there is an absence of skull vault development together with defective neural fold fusion.
- **Holoprosencephaly** is a failure of forebrain evagination preventing formation of the paired hemispheres and their lateral ventricles. The condition may coexist with **cyclopia** and is most commonly associated

with abnormalities of chromosome 13, causing severe mental retardation, facial abnormalities and premature death.

Malformations occurring later in development, principally affect neuroblast migration and development of cerebral gyri. A range of conditions occur, including **agyria**, where there is failure of neuroblast migration with consequent absence of gyral and sulcal development, except for interhemispheric and Sylvian fissures. **Pachygyria** results from disruption of gyral development, forming a small number of broad gyri.

INFECTIONS OF THE CENTRAL NERVOUS SYTSTEM

Infections of the nervous system involve;
- the meninges (**meningitis**);
- the pía arachnoid (**leptomeningitis**);
- the dura (**pachymeningitis**);
- the cerebral and spinal parenchyma (**encephalitis**);
- both the meninges and the brain parenchyma (**meningoencephalitis**).

Meningitis

The term meningitis is generally accepted to mean leptomeningitis, that is, inflammation of the pia mater and arachnoid. Infectious organisms may reach the meninges via the blood stream, skin or gastrointestinal tract. Infection may result from:
- direct spread from the middle ear or sinuses;
- skull fractures;
- surgical procedures;
- lumbar puncture.

Clinical presentation of meningitis is with fever, neck pain, headache, vomiting and photophobia. Physical examination may reveal evidence of meningeal irritation, including neck stiffness and a positive Kernig sign (the inability to straighten a raised bent leg).

Meningitis is classsified according to the type of inflammatory response seen.

Neonatal meningitis
Infection may be acquired during passage of the fetus through the birth canal and thus will include organisms found at this site including group B streptococci, *Escherichia coli* and *Listeria monocytogenes*.

Infantile, childhood and adolescent meningitis
In infants, the most common pathogen was *Haemophilus influenzae* before the introduction of *H. influenzae* b (Hib)

vaccine. In early adolescence the meningococcus *Neisseria meningitidis* is the most common organism. *Streptococcus pneumoniae*, the pneumococcus, causes meningitis at the extremes of life.

Meningitis due to meningococcus may be accompanied by a purpuric rash. The mortality rate is high, being in the order of 10% in the UK. This rate can be reduced by giving intravenous benzyl penicillin to the patient as soon as the diagnosis is suspected by the general practitioner. In 1994, 70% of cases in the UK were due to serogroup B and 26% to serogroup C. A vaccine exists for group A and C but at present there is no effective vaccine for group B.

Clusters of infections do occur during the winter months, necessitating antibiotic prophylaxis with rifampicin of close ('kissing') contacts.

Meningitis in immunocompromised patients
The causes include *Cryptococcus neoformans*, *Candida albicans* and *Histoplasma*.

Acute lymphocytis meningitis
The commonest causes of a lymphocytic meningitis are infections with enterovirus and mumps virus. In 30% of cases of acute 'viral meningitis' no virus can be identified.

Tuberculous meningitis
Tuberculous meningitis tends to be a chronic infection and is seen in association with miliary tuberculosis in young children and the immune suppressed.

Chronic meningitis
Tuberculosis, fungal infection or meningovascular syphilis may produce chronic meningitis. Complications of chronic meningitis include:
- fibrosis around cranial nerves resulting in cranial nerve palsies;
- fibrosis around the fourth ventricle causing obliterative hydrocephalus;
- obliterative vasculitis causing cerebral ischaemia and infarction.

Diagnosis of meningitis
Examination of the CSF will show lymphocytes in viral menigitis; there may be neutrophil polymorphs, raised protein and lowered glucose in bacterial meningitis. Culture and Gram staining may identify the infectious organism. Where the infectious organism or where antibiotics have already been given, antigen or PCR techniques may be employed. Meningococcal serology may also be helpful.

Treatment
Viral meningitis requires supportive treatment. In cases

of suspected bacterial meningitis, urgent antibiotic treatment must be implemented, often before obtaining CSF, with combined antibiotics for a range of likely organisms.

Cerebral abscess

Cerebral abscesses are localized areas of suppurative infection within the brain parenchyma. They are more commonly due to infection with anaerobic organisms. Disease associations include:

- infective endocarditis;
- chronic, suppurative lung disease, e.g. bronchiectasis;
- chronic middle ear infection;
- chronic sinusitis;
- right-to-left cardiac shunts.

Clinically, patients with cerebral abscess present with the symptoms of a space-occupying lesion. Diagnosis is by brain computed tomographic scan or magnetic resonance imaging. The CSF may be normal or show neutrophils, increased protein and reduced glucose levels. CSF cultures may or may not be positive. Treatment is by surgical drainage of the abscess with antibiotic therapy.

Encephalitis

Viral encephalitis

Virus reaches the brain via the blood and infection results in neuronal necrosis, oedema and perivascular inflammatory infiltrates. Clinically, patients present with fever, headaches, cerebral dysfunction and sometimes with fits. Lumbar puncture will show a lymphocytosis. Treatment is supportive and cerebral oedema may be managed with steroids.

Table 27.1 lists the most common causes of viral encephalitis. These diseases tend to occur in epidemics and many are due to arthropod-borne viruses (arboviruses). Of particular importance are the following.

- **Herpes simplex virus** (HSV) is a cause of encephalitis in the young, the old and the immune-suppressed. HSV 2 is associated with neonates and may be acquired from the birth canal. HSV 1 is more common in adults and may be acquired from the mouth (cold sores). Diagnosis may be made by culture of CSF, ploymerase chain reaction methods, serology, or definitively by brain biopsy. Cowdry A viral inclusions may be seen and viral protein may be identified by immunohistochemistry or *in situ* hybridization tests.
- **Poliomyelitis** is acquired via the faecal–oral route, the infection being caused by an enterovirus. The virus selectively infects the meninges and lower

Table 27.1 Causes of viral encephalitis.

Epidemic (arbovirus) encephalitis
Eastern equine encephalitis
Western equine encephalitis
Venezuelan equine encephalitis
St Louis encephalitis
California encephalitis
Japanese B encephalitis
Herpes simplex virus (types I and II)
Enterovirus encephalitis
Measles
Varicella (chickenpox)
Herpes simplex
Progressive multifocal leukoencephalopathy
Cytomegalovirus
HIV (AIDS encephalitis)
Subacute sclerosing panencephalitis

HIV, Human immunodeficiency virus; AIDS, acquired immune deficiency syndrome.

motor neurones in the anterior horn of the spinal cord and medulla oblongata. Loss of motor neurones results in paralysis of affected muscles which, in time, atrophy and undergo fibrotic contracture. The disease is now rare in developed countries due to immunization in childhood.

- **Rabies** infects humans via the bites of dogs, cats or wild animals. The virus has an incubation period of 1–3 months. It passes along peripheral nerves at the site of the bite to affect the basal ganglia, hippocampus and brainstem of the central nervous system (CNS).

Infected neurones feature intracytoplasmic inclusions (Negri bodies). Rabies produces a necrotizing encephalitis that is ultimately fatal. Patients present with fever, convulsions and hydrophobia (fear of water). Antirabies vaccine treatment immediately after exposure is effective in many cases.

- **Progressive multifocal leucoencephalopathy (PML)** is caused by papovavirus SV40 and affects immune-deficient patients. It results in demyelination of cerebral white matter with rapid cerebral dysfunction and a high mortality rate.
- **Subacute sclerosing panencephalitis (SSPE)** affects children several years following a measles infection and is thought to be due to a chronic measles virus infection. It is characterized by progressive neuronal degeneration and death within a year or two after onset.
- **Slow virus infections** include Creutzfeldt–Jakob disease, scrapie and kuru (see below). These diseases are characterized by viral infection with a long latent period between infection and onset of a slowly progressive disease.

Protozoal infection

Toxoplasma infection may be congenital or acquired. It is a particularly important infection in immune-suppressed patients and is seen in acquired immunodeficiency syndrome (AIDS).

Cerebral malaria is caused by infection with *Plasmodium falciparum*. Infected erythrocytes clog small capillaries, resulting in cerebral ischaemia and oedema, followed by convulsions and coma.

African trypanosomiasis (sleeping sickness) is caused by *Trypanosoma rhodesiense* and *T. gambiense*, transmitted by the bite of the tsetse fly. Cerebral involvement follows blood-borne dissemination of the organism and is characterized by diffuse neuronal degeneration.

Other parasites which may infect the brain include trichinosis, cysticercosis, schistosomiasis, hydatid disease and *Entamoeba histolytica*.

Examination of the cerebrosopinal fluid

The biochemical and cellular constituents of the CSF will aid in the diagnosis of a variety of diseases and some of these are listed in Tables 27.2 and 27.3. Apart from infectious processes, cytopathology of the CSF may be of value in the diagnosis of a variety of tumours of the brain.

TUMOURS OF THE CENTRAL NERVOUS SYSTEM

Primary neoplasms of the brain, spinal cord, peripheral nervous system and their coverings have an annual incidence of approximately 6 per 100 000, accounting for 1% of deaths. In children, 20% of neoplasms arise within the nervous system.

For simplicity, the neuraxis can be likened to a tube attached to a hollow sphere, with the lumen formed by the ventricles and central spinal canal; the wall is composed of the white and grey matter and the outer surface is covered by protective fibrous membranes and bone. Neoplasms and other expansile processes (both intrinsic (arachnoid cysts) and extrinsic (disc protrusions)) commonly produce symptoms referable to their site and layer of origin, speed and pattern of growth.

The majority of childhood nervous system neoplasms occur within the **infratentorial** compartment, whilst in adults the **supratentorial** compartment is the commonest site (Fig. 27.3). Neuroepithelial neoplasms have a worse prognosis and occur most commonly in males; meningiomas are more frequent in females. In some sites, notably the frontal and parietal lobes, neoplasms may attain a considerable size before becoming clinically apparent, whilst in other locations, comparatively small tumours, which in histological terms are considered benign, such as third ventricle colloid cysts producing obstructive hydrocephalus by impeding CSF flow through the interventricular foramina, can result in sudden death.

The different tissue layers give rise to different categories of neoplasms:
- the bone and cartilage encasing the nervous system may infrequently give rise to benign and malignant cartilagnous and osseous tumours (Fig. 27.4);
- meningiomas arise from the arachnoid layer of the leptomeninges;

Table 27.2 Cerebrospinal fluid (CSF) changes in infections of the central nervous system.

	Encephalitis	Bacterial meningitis	Viral meningitis	Brain abscess
CSF pressure	Raised	Raised	Raised	May be very high
Gross appearance	Clear	Turbid	Clear	Clear
Protein	Slightly elevated	High	Slightly elevated	Elevated
Glucose	Normal	Very low	Normal	Normal
Inflammatory cells	Lymphocytes	Neutrophils	Lymphocytes	Neutrophils + lymphocytes
Gram stain	Negative	Positive	Negative	Occasionally positive
Ziehl–Neelsen stain	Negative	Negative	Negative	Negative
Bacterial culture	Negative	Positive	Negative	Occasionally positive
Viral culture	Positive in 30% or less	Negative	Positive	Negative

Table 27.3 The examination of the cerebrospinal fluid.

	Normal	Abnormalities
Colour	Clear, colourless	Yellow (xanthochromic): indicates old haemorrhage Red: subarachnoid haemorrhage or traumatic lumbar puncture Purulent: bacterial meningitis Clear with clot on standing: high protein, common in tuberculous meningitis
Protein	20–50 mg/dl	Marked increase: infection, haemorrhage, tumour Moderate increase: many causes
Oligoclonal protein bands		Multiple sclerosis, syphilis
Serology		VDRL positive in neurosyphilis
Glucose	50–80 mg/dl (75% of blood glucose)	↑ Bacterial meningitis ↑ Hyperglycaemia
Cells	0–5 (mostly lymphocytes)	↑ Neutrophils: bacterial infection ↑ Lymphocytes: viral, fungal, tuberculous meningitis, syphilis, degenerative diseases
Organisms		Identify by culture and Gram stain

VDRL, Venereal Disease Research Laboratory.

- astrocytomas and oligodendrogliomas arise within the white matter;
- ependymomas and choroid plexus papillomas develop from tissue within the ventricular cavities.

The sites, modes and rates of growth largely determine the onset of symptoms:

- meningiomas often present when already a considerable size, their initial expansion being compensated for by demyelination of the underlying white matter;
- gliomas proliferate by infiltration and commonly are beyond the scope of curative resection by the time of presentation;
- ependymomas and choroid plexus papillomas commonly present early, when still small in terms of volume, owing to acute obstructive hydrocephalus.

In the adult nervous system the neural supportive cells, namely those of astrocytic and oligodendrocyte lineage, retain the capacity of cellular division, unlike nerve cells which forgo this function as a consequence of specialization occurring with attainment of developmental maturity. As a consequence, neuronal neoplasms in adults occur rarely, whilst tumours of glial tissue are the commonest group in adults and children. The term glioma is frequently applied by pathologists and clinicians to neoplasms of astrocyte, oligodendrocyte or ependymal cell origin.

In general, consideration of the above features in combination with neuroradiology permits a clinician to apply a pathological sieve to identify the category of neoplasm causing clinical symptoms, although ultimate confirmation is by biopsy or removal and histopathological assessment.

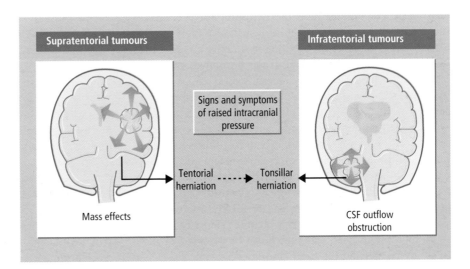

Fig. 27.3 Signs and symptoms of raised intracranial pressure.

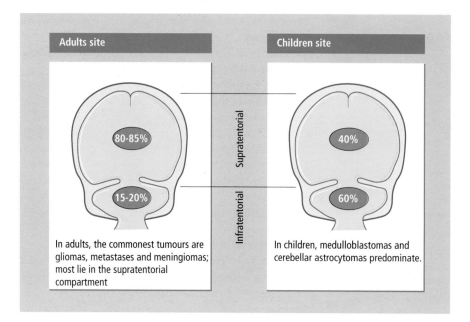

Fig. 27.4 The sites for central nervous system tumours.

The effects of nervous tissue expansion

The human CNS tissues are compartmentalized and surrounded by protective layers of connective tissue and bone which protect the nervous system from mechanical injury. The rigidity of the compartments also imposes a constraint to the expansile effect of proliferating neoplasms. Several mechanisms attempt to compensate against the harmful effects of nervous tissue swelling, at least during the early stages.

The compressive effects of a slowly growing extrinsic neoplasm such as a meningioma are initially compensated for by demyelination of the underlying white matter, then by indentation of the cortex. Collapse of the adjacent ventricle followed by brain herniation into a neighbouring compartment more commonly accompanies a rapidly expanding neoplasm such as a high-grade astrocytoma, acute brain swelling secondary to cerebral bleeding or trauma (Fig. 27.5). If left untreated, the volume changes and shift in tissues ultimately cause death by irreversible compression of the vital cardiorespiratory centres in the brainstem.

The cerebral hemispheres and cerebellum can compensate for the compressive and expansive effects of neoplasms more satisfactorily than the brainstem and spinal cord. In children, the cranial fontanelles remain functionally patent until 18 months of age; this permits expansion of the cranial cavity to compensate for the increase in volume due to a neoplasm. This change will be manifest as an increase in head size which can be assessed objectively by measuring the head circumference.

Clinical features of central nervous system neoplasms

The clinical presentation of neoplasms is commonly insidious with onset over months in slowly growing or extrinsic lesions, eventually causing raised intracranial pressure–particularly infratentorial and extrinsic neoplasms. More rapid proliferation causes focal signs such as local compression of cranial nerves or epileptic seizures, the pattern being dependent on the neoplasm location (Fig. 27.6).

Neoplasms arising within the ventricular cavities cause obstruction of CSF flow causing a rise in intracranial pressure, hydrocephalus and, if acute in onset, headache and even sudden death.

Classification

The classification of nervous system neoplasms is based on the appearance of the neoplastic cell component recapitulating the morphological appearance of the embryogenic cellular precursors (see Fig. 27.4; Tables 27.4 and 27.5).

Theories of oncogenesis

Theories abound concerning the aetiology of nervous system neoplasms. Those currently showing the strongest correlation are:

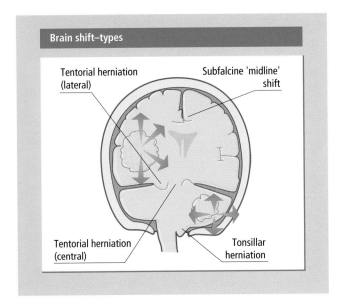

Fig. 27.5 The types of brain shift resulting from intracranial tumours.

Table 27.4 Classification of central nervous system neoplasms.

Neoplasm	Incidence (%)
Primary neoplasms	70–75
Gliomas Glioblastoma Astrocytoma Ependymoma Oligodendroglioma Choroid plexus papilloma	45
Medulloblastoma	3
Meningioma	15
Acoustic nerve sheath (schwannoma/neurilemmoma)	5
Pituitary	5
Neuronal	0.5
Metastatic secondaries Bronchus Breast Renal Gastrointestinal tract Melanoma	20–25

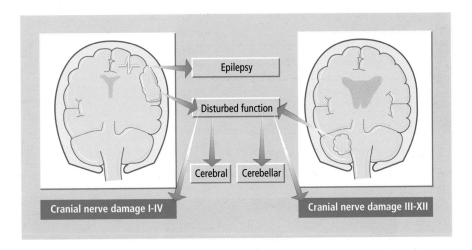

Fig. 27.6 The effects of intracranial tumours.

- **previous cranial irradiation** (radiation was previously used to treat tinea capitis, a scalp condition), shows an increased risk of developing astrocytomas and meningiomas;
- **immune suppression** (including AIDS) predisposes to primary CNS lymphoma (usually B cell);
- **oncogene** deletion, inactivation or overexpression; in some instances this can be shown to be associated with hereditary predisposition to the development of CNS neoplasms (Table 27.6).

Control of **growth factor** expression, particularly epithelial and platelet-derived growth factor.

Primary nervous system neoplasms will be considered in more detail based on their location and tissue of origin (Fig. 27.7).

Neoplasms arising from white and grey matter

Astrocytoma

A neoplasm of astrocyte lineage represents 40% of CNS neoplasms. The clinical presentation is usually with

Table 27.5 Disorders associated with the development of central nervous system neoplasms.

Disease	CNS 'tumour'
AIDS	B-cell lymphoma
Sturge–Weber syndrome	Excessive vascularity of the meninges
Tuberous sclerosis (epiloia, Bourneville disease)	Giant cell astrocytoma
Von Hippel–Lindau disease	Haemangioblastoma
Von Recklinghausen's disease (neurofibromatosis)	Neurofibroma, neurofibrosarcoma, schwannoma, meningioma

AIDS, Acquired immune deficiency syndrome.

Table 27.6 Chromosomal abnormalities associated with central nervous system neoplasms.

Neoplasm	Chromosomal locus or oncogenes	
	Deleted	Overexpressed
Acoustic schwannoma	17, 22	
Low-grade astrocytoma	10, 17	c-cis, c-erb B, n-ras, c-myc, EGFR, 53 (bss)
High-grade astrocytoma	9, 10, 17	(gain on chromosome 7)
Haemangioblastoma (in von Hippel–Lindau syndrome)	3p	
Medulloblastoma	1, 17q	c-myc
Meningioma	22	

EGFR, Epithelial growth factor receptor.

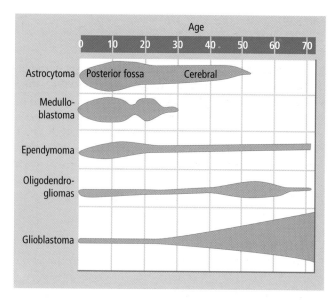

Fig. 27.7 The pattern of incidence of neuroepithelial tumours related to age.

protracted headache due to raised intracranial pressure, focal seizures or progressive neurological deficit.

Astrocytomas (Fig. 27.8) can be categorized according to:

- their site of origin;
- cellular appearance and density;
- the presence of necrosis;
- hyperplasia of endothelial cells lining blood vessels penetrating the neoplasm.

These features permit pathological grading which correlates with prognosis.

Generally astrocytomas arise within the white matter and proliferate by infiltration of the surrounding tissue. Their deep location and ill-defined margins frequently prevent complete resection (an exception is childhood

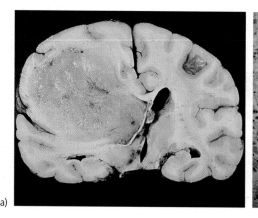
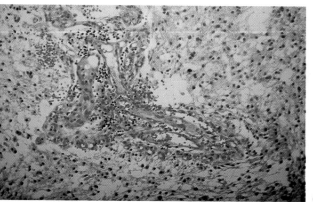

Fig. 27.8 Grade IV (glioblastoma multiforme) (a) The tumour is solitary and located in the cerebral cortex. (b) The tumour is cellular and associated with endothelial cell hyperplasia in the blood vessels.

cerebellar astrocytomas, which are often peripherally located and amenable to resection).

Terminology and grading. Much confusion exists in the literature concerning the terminology applied to the different grades of astrocytic neoplasm, with some authors preferring to apply the terms anaplastic and malignant astrocytoma or glioblastoma multiforme to high-grade tumours. Other authors find it is preferable to use the term astrocytoma with the grade as postscript (either descriptive—low/high, or a numerical value from I to IV). The site and grade are the most significant prognostic parameters.

Oligodendroglioma (Fig. 27.9)

Oligodendrogliomas are neoplasms arising in the white matter of the cerebral hemispheres from cells forming the myelin sheath and represent 3% of nervous system tumours. Clinical presentation is typically with headache

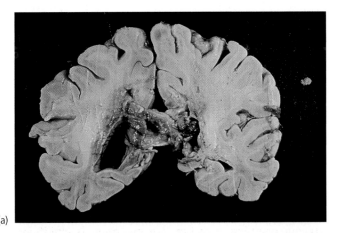

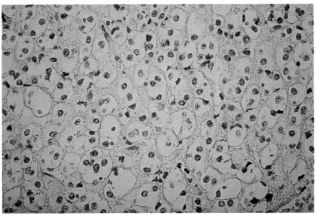

Fig. 27.9 Oligodendroglioma. (a) This tumour is located in the deep periventricular white matter. These tumours are associated with calcification and may be detected on X-ray. (b) Histology shows round cells with an eccentric nucleus, giving a 'fried egg' appearance. (H&E.)

due to increased intracranial pressure or with focal seizures. They are characterized by forming sheets of relatively uniform rounded cells with an eccentrically located nucleus surrounded by clear cytoplasm—an appearance likened to that of a fried egg (Fig. 27.9(b)). Focal granules of extracellular calcification are often present and can be detected radiologically. Oligodendrogliomas tend to be less aggressive in their growth pattern than astrocytomas.

Neoplasms of neuronal origin

Following migration and maturation the neuronal cell population become 'permanent' cells, losing the capacity to replicate and regenerate. Because of these maturational changes, neoplasms of the neuronal cell population are rare in adults, but do occur in childhood and adolescence, probably arising from remnants of the germinal primordium.

The terminology applied to describe neuronal neoplasms arising in childhood may, on first inspection, appear complex; the commonest neoplasm is the **medulloblastoma** which usually arises in the midline of the cerebellum in proximity to the fourth ventricle, causing raised intracranial pressure and hydrocephalus (Fig. 27.10. The medulloblastoma arises from primitive germinal matrix cells in the external granular cell layer of the cerebellum, forming densely cellular sheets of small hyperchromatic 'carrot-shaped' cells, which in places become arranged around blood vessels forming rosettes. Mitoses are usually frequent.

Histologically similar neoplasms arising elsewhere in the CNS, most commonly in the supratentorial compartment, are termed **primitive neuroectodermal tumours**

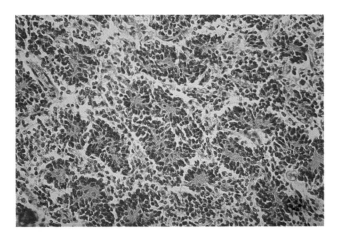

Fig. 27.10 Medulloblastoma. These blue cells are arranged in rosettes. The cells are elongated or 'carrot-shaped' on longitudinal section. (H&E.)

(PNET). Similar neoplasms also occur in the eye, termed **retinoblastoma**, and in association with peripheral nervous system sympathetic ganglia and the adrenal medulla, termed **neuroblastoma**. One other rare site, in this case occurring in adults, is the vault of the nose, the **olfactory neuroblastoma**.

Neuronal neoplasms rarely arise in adults; those occurring include the **gangliocytoma**, a hamartomatous collection of well-differentiated ganglion cells and the **ganglioglioma**, a mixed proliferation of ganglion cells and astrocytes. These neoplasms can occur in both the CNS and peripheral nervous system. They are characterized by slow growth and usually present with seizures, with symptoms localizing to the frontal and temporal lobes.

Neoplasms arising from ependyma and ventricular cavities

Ependymoma (Fig. 27.11)

This is a neoplasm arising from the ependymal lining of the ventricle, most commonly within the fourth ventricle of children and young adults. Clinical presentation is usually with headache due to blockage of CSF flow, causing raised intracranial pressure and hydrocephalus.

The histological appearance is characterized by the epithelial appearance of the neoplastic cells, arranged in sheets or forming pseudorosettes around blood vessels, where intracytoplasmic **blepharoplasts**, derived from the ciliary apparatus, may be observed near the luminal aspect. Variants of the ependymoma include papillary, myxopapillary and subependymoma.

Choroid plexus papilloma

This is usually a well-differentiated neoplasm of the choroid plexus arising in the ventricular cavities of chil-

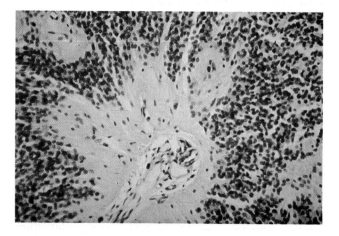

Fig. 27.11 Ependymoma of the fourth ventricle. The tumour cells form pseudorosettes around blood vessels. (H&E.)

dren and young adults, causing headache due to raised intracranial pressure secondary to increased CSF secretion and obstruction to CSF flow by desquamated neoplastic cells.

Colloid cyst

This is a cuboidal or pseudostratified epithelium-lined thin-walled cyst arising in the fourth ventricle which causes obstruction of CSF flow.

Neoplasms of vascular tissue

Haemangioblastoma

Haemangioblastoma is a benign, often partially cystic, neoplastic proliferation of blood vessels most commonly arising in the cerebellum of young adults. The clinical presentation includes headache secondary to obstructive hydrocephalus, gait disturbance or symptoms secondary to complications of polycythaemia due to ectopic secretion of erythropoietin. The neoplasm occurs in association with von Hippel-Lindau disease.

Neoplasms of central nervous system coverings

Meningioma (Fig. 27.12)

Meningioma is a firm, white, lobulated, usually benign neoplasm arising from the arachnoid cells of the leptomeninges. It presents most commonly parasagittally, overlying the convexities of the hemispheres, but may also occur in the ventricles and in the spinal canal. Clinical symptoms are usually referable to the site of local compression. Meningiomas may attain a significant size before becoming clinically apparant. They may also be multifocal and there is a 30% risk of recurrence after surgical resection. The neoplasm is commoner in females and appears to be hormonally responsive as rapid enlargement may occur during pregnancy.

Histologically the neoplasm is composed of ovoid or spindleform cells which may form whorls with or without a central focus of calcification, known as a **psammoma body**.

Central nervous system nerve sheath tumours

Schwannoma (neurilemmoma)

Schwannoma is a benign neoplastic proliferation of Schwann cells arising from cranial or posterior spinal nerve roots, producing clinical symptoms referable to the nerve affected. The neoplasms may be sporadic, unilat-

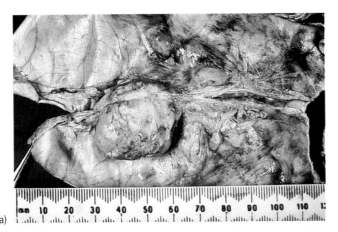

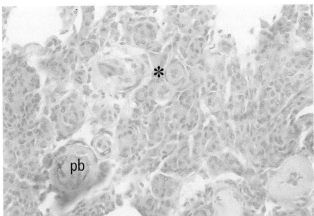

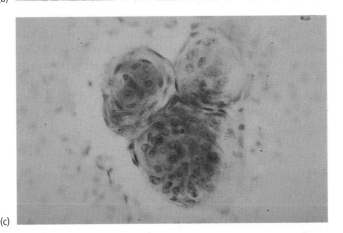

Fig. 27.12 Meningioma. (a) This firm, well circumscribed tumour is attached to the dura. It was an incidental finding at post mortem. (b) Histology shows cellular whorls (✲) and calcific psammoma bodies (pb). (H&B.) (c) A brain smear shows the cohesive whorled arrangement of the meningothelial cells. (PAP.)

eral or bilateral and may or may not occur in association with neurofibromatosis.

The commonest site is on the eighth cranial nerve within the cerebellar pontine angle, causing nerve deafness secondary to compression.

The schwannoma is composed of interlacing bundles

of spindle-shaped cells (known as Antoni A areas) alternating with less well-defined areas (known as Antoni B areas). Schwannomas, unlike neurofibromas (a nerve sheath tumour usually occurring in the peripheral nervous system), usually develop at the periphery of the nerve sheath causing nerve compression without disruption of the architecture, permitting complete removal (Fig. 27.13).

Primary lymphoma of the central nervous system

Primary CNS lymphoma is almost always of diffuse B-cell non-Hodgkins lymphoma presenting with headache, seizures or disordered mentation. The condition occurs *de novo* in individuals in the sixth and seventh decade. It is seen with increasing frequency in younger individuals who have been subjected to immune suppression following organ transplantation, chemotherapy for other malignant disease and in victims of AIDS. Epstein–Barr virus is increasingly being implicated in the pathogenesis of this category of lymphoma.

Histologically the lymphoma is characterized by perivascular and subarachnoid infiltration of CNS tissue.

Neoplasms arising at other sites

Pineal gland neoplasms
Pineal gland neoplasms are most commonly of germ cell type, similar in appearance to that occurring in the ovary and testis. Less frequently encountered neoplasms include astrocytomas and pineoblastoma (a variant of PNET). The clinical presentation is as a result of raised intracranial pressure secondary to aqueduct and third ventricle obstruction.

Neoplasms of the sellar region
Craniopharyngioma. Craniopharyngioma is a multicystic, partially calcified neoplasm of childhood and young adults arising from epithelial remnants of **Rathke's pouch**. It is present in the pituitary stalk, producing a suprasellar mass which causes visual loss by chiasmatic compression and growth retardation. The cystic spaces contain dark viscous fluid which has been likened to **engine oil** in appearance.

Histologically the neoplasm is composed of sheets of well-differentiated squamous epithelium surrounding cystic spaces and associated with cholesterol crystal clefts and multinucleate giant cells.

Pituitary adenoma. This is benign neoplastic proliferation of subpopulations of cells within the anterior pituitary lobe which may be either functionally active, usually

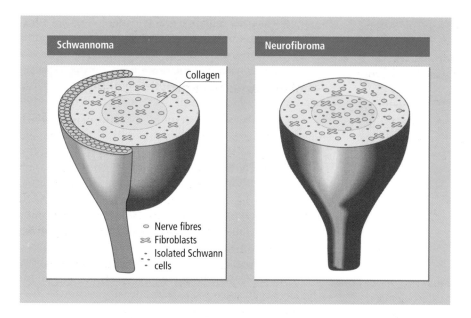

Fig. 27.13 The respective structures of schwannoma and neurofibroma.

resulting in excess secretion of trophic hormones, or inactive, producing hormonal deficits or clinically silent (see Chapter 14). Clinical presentation may be due to endocrine end-organ dysfunction, visual failure with bitemporal hemianopia due to chiasmatic compression or headaches.

In addition to biochemical measurement of blood levels of trophic hormones, functional assesment of surgically resected pituitary adenoma tissue is possible using immunohistochemistry.

Neoplasms of the spinal cord

Spinal cord neoplasms can be classified according to the vertebral level and the tissue plane affected.

Extradural and intradural neoplasms most commonly produce spinal cord compression with consequent nerve root pain and neurological deficit below the level of the tumour. Extradural tumours are commonly due to either metastatic carcinoma infiltrating vertebral bone or infiltration and expansion of bone marrow by myeloma or lymphoma.

Intradural neoplasms are commonly of nerve sheath origin – either schwannomas arising from the posterior nerve root within the spinal canal or neurofibroma arising outside the spinal canal, but extending through the intervertebral foramina, the so-called 'dumb bell' tumour. Meningiomas and myxopapillary ependymomas also develop within the intradural compartment, the latter most commonly arising from the filum terminale.

Intramedullary neoplasms arising within the spinal cord parenchyma include ependymomas, astrocytomas and metastatic neoplasms.

Metastatic central nervous system disease

Approximately a quarter of clinically symptomatic CNS neoplasms are metastatic in origin. The commonest primary sites are bronchus, breast, bowel, kidney and melanoma (Fig. 27.14).

The metastases most commonly develop as circumscribed solitary or multifocal deposits within superficial white matter of the cerebrum adjacent to the junction between grey and white matter. The metastases produce clinical symptoms referable to the mass effect at their site of implantation. Extensive haemorrhage in association with brain metastases is particularly associated with melanoma, renal cell carcinoma and choriocarcinoma.

Bone metastases may cause spinal cord compression by

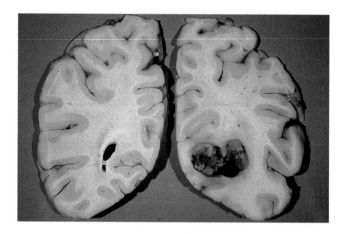

Fig. 27.14 Metastatic malignant melanoma to the cerebral cortex.

extradural expansion causing back pain, paraplegia and incontinence. Metastases to bone presenting in this manner include bronchus, breast, kidney and prostatic carcinoma. Myeloma and lymphoma arising in the marrow also cause extradural cord compression.

Diffuse meningeal infiltration by metastatic carcinoma occurs in up to 5% of victims of carcinomatosis, most commonly of breast, bronchus, bowel, melanoma or childhood leukaemia origin (Table 27.7). The condition often causes intractable head and neck pain, cranial nerve deficits, limb weakness, hydrocephalus with optic nerve infiltration and papilloedema.

Paraneoplastic syndromes

The occurrence of peripheral neuropathy and progressive cerebellar ataxia in the absence of identifiable metastatic involvement of the nervous system may precede the presentation of the primary malignancy.

The disorder appears, at least in a proportion of cases, to be an autoimmune-mediated condition in which the participating antibodies recognize antigenic determinants common to both the nervous system and the primary neoplasm. The paraneoplastic syndrome most commonly occurs in association with small cell bronchial carcinomas.

Phakomatoses (neurocristinopathies)

The phakomatoses are a group of syndromes in which multiple abnormalities of the eyes, nervous system and visceral organs occur. These anomalies take the form of hamartomatous, hyperplastic or neoplastic proliferation of neuroectodermal derived tissue, most commonly that formed from the neural crest. The syndromes considered in this category for the most part show a genetic, usually **autosomal dominant** linkage. Syndromes categorized under this heading include:

- von Recklinghausen's disease (neurofibromatosis);
- tuberous sclerosis (Bourneville–Pringle disease);
- Sturge–Weber syndrome;
- ataxia telangiectasia (Louis-Bar syndrome);
- von Hippel–Lindau's syndrome;
- Turcot's syndrome;
- Li–Fraumeni syndrome;
- Tourraine syndrome.

CEREBROVASCULAR DISEASE

Introduction

Approximately 10% of deaths in developed countries are due to cerebrovascular disease; this represents the third commonest cause of adult deaths (after cardiovascular disease and cancer).

One-third of acute strokes are fatal. Survival of the remaining two-thirds of patients is determined by the age, the anatomical location, the extent of cerebral flow impairment and the underlying cause.

The major causes are infarction (50% are due to arterial thrombosis, 30% are embolic) and haemorrhage (two-thirds occur within the brain parenchyma; one-third occur in the subarachnoid space due to rupture of a berry aneurysm).

Half of stroke survivors sustain significant long-term disability. Cerebrovascular disease therefore is a significant cause of morbidity and mortality; a large proportion of these cases are preventable by the identification of risk factors and appropriate treatment.

A variety of risk factors have been identified; the most epidemiologically significantly are shown in Table 27.8.

Table 27.7 Neoplasms that commonly metastasize to the central nervous system.

Bronchus
Melanoma
Breast
Kidney
Bowel
Choriocarcinoma
Kidney
Melanoma
Metastases causing diffuse meningeal infiltration
Bronchus
Breast
Melanoma
Leukaemia (childhood)
Bowel
Metastases causing extradural cord compression
Bronchus
Breast
Kidney
Prostate
Myeloma
Lymphoma

Table 27.8 Risk factors in the development of cerebrovascular disease.

Hypertension
Cerebral artery atherosclerosis
Ischaemic heart disease
Valvular heart disease
Diabetes mellitus

The cerebral circulation

The blood supply to the brain is derived from:
• the paired vertebral arteries, which merge forming the basilar artery; this in turn bifurcates to supply the posterior cerebral arteries;
• the paired internal carotid arteries, supplying the middle and anterior cerebral arteries and anastomosing with the posterior cerebral arteries via the posterior communicating arteries.

The blood supply to the brain is summarized in Fig. 27.15.

Clinical effects of cerebrovascular disease

Impairment of cerebral circulation causes irreversible

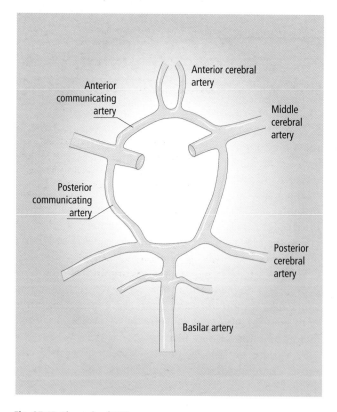

Fig. 27.15 The circle of Willis.

parenchymal damage by infarction or haemorrhage, resulting in clinical symptoms which are determined by the site and size of the structural damage, as opposed to transient disruption of physiological function, such as is observed in transient ischaemic episodes. The major clinical symptoms based on the area of circulation effected are summarized in Table 27.9.

Haemorrhagic cerebrovascular disease

Haemorrhagic cerebrovascular disease most commonly arises from the arterial circulation with high-pressure leakage of blood; the exception is subdural haemorrhage which arises from venous bleeding. Intracranial haemorrhage is classified according to the compartmental or layer within which haemorrhage occurs.

• **Extradural haemorrhage.** This is due to arterial pressure bleeding into the extradural space, most commonly following a fracture of the petrous temporal bone of the skull overlying the course of the middle meningeal artery.
• **Subdural haemorrhage.** This is haemorrhage occurring at venous pressure secondary to tearing of the cortical veins close to their point of drainage into the superior sagittal sinus. The condition is commonest in the elderly due to the combination of age-related brain volume shrinkage and minor head trauma, causing shearing of the cortical veins as they traverse the subdural space (Fig. 27.16).
• **Subarachnoid haemorrhage.** This occurs due to bleeding at arterial pressure into the subarachnoid space, usually following spontaneous rupture of a small saccular aneurysmal dilatation at the bifurcation of arteries, referred to as **berry aneurysm** (Fig. 27.17).

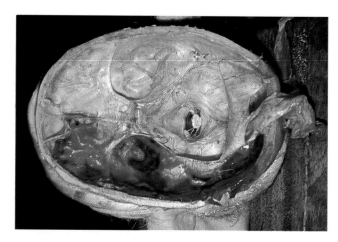

Fig. 27.16 A subdural haematoma found at post mortem in an elderly woman who fell downstairs.

Table 27.9 Clinical effects of cerebrovascular disease.

Arterial territory	Area of supply	Clinical deficit
Anterior cerebral (internal carotid)	*Cortical*—Medial frontal/ parietal lobes	Contralateral leg weakness; cortical sensory loss
	Deep branches—anterior communicating, choroidal, basal ganglia and anterior limb of the internal capsule	Incontinence, confusion Akinetic mutism (in bilateral frontal disease)
Middle cerebral (internal carotid)	*Cortical*—External cortical surface of frontal, temporal and parietal lobes	Contralateral hemiparesis; hemianopia; hemiplegia with relative leg sparing
	Deep (lenticulostriate)—basal ganglia and internal capsule	Aphasia/dysphasia (dominant hemisphere) Contralateral limb neglect; dressing apraxia (non-dominant hemisphere)
Posterior cerebral (vertebrobasilar circulation)	*Cortical*—inferior surface, temporal and occipital lobes (including visual cortex)	*Cortical branches* Homonymous hemianopia Macular sparing (the macula is supplied by the middle cerebral arteries) Amnesia (with bitemporal disease) Nominal and colour aphasia in dominant hemisphere Cortical blindness (if bilateral)
	Deep branches—midbrain, posterior thalamus and choroid plexus	*Deep branches* Hemiballismus and hemisensory disturbance ('thalamic syndrome') Third cranial nerve palsy, contralateral hemiplegia (Weber's midbrain syndrome)
Basilar artery (vertebral arteries)	Medulla, pons and cerebellum (and posterior cerebral artery territories)	Variable pattern depending on the level involved, producing a combination of motor, sensory, cranial nerve and cerebellar signs
Vertebral arteries	Medulla, inferior cerebellar surface	*Cerebellum*—dysarthria, severe vertigo, ipsilateral ataxia, nystagmus to the occluded side, hypotonia
		Medulla—contralateral limb and truncal pain and temperature loss. Ipsilateral fifth—eighth nerve palsy. Ipsilateral sympathetic paralysis (due to occlusion of the posterior inferior cerebellar artery)
Spinal arteries Anterior spinal artery	Spinal cord (anterior two-thirds of spinal cord)	Leg weakness Bladder and bowel dysfunction Pinprick and temperature lost (vibration and proprioception preserved)
Posterior spinal artery (rarely involved by vascular disease due to rich collateral radicular arterial supply)	Spinal cord (posterior one-third spinal cord; dorsal columns)	Vibration and proprioception

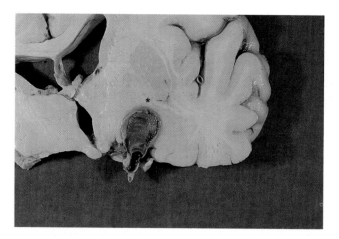

Fig. 27.17 A berry aneurysm containing thrombus from a patient who died from a subarachnoid haemorrhage.

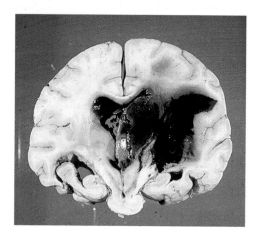

Fig. 27.18 An intracerebral haematoma from a patient with hypertension.

- **Intracerebral haemorrhage.** This represents haemorrhage into the basal ganglia and thalamus of hypertensive middle aged individuals due to rupture of microscopic **Charcot–Bouchard aneurysm** (Fig. 27.18).

Thrombotic cerebral venous disease

Causes of thrombotic occlusion of cortical veins, sagittal and sigmoid sinuses are summarized in Table 27.10.

Clinically, cortical and venous sinus thrombosis are manifest as headache with subsequent seizure. A proportion of cases then progress to coma with papilloedema.

Ischaemic brain damage

The brain has a high metabolic requirement, utilizing 20% of the resting cardiac output to maintain normal function.

Table 27.10 Ischaemic brain damage.

Causes of cerebral venous occlusion	Causes of ischaemic brain damage

Primary
Dehydration
Haematological disorder
   (polycythaemia, sickle-cell disease)
Exogenous oestrogen
Pregnancy
 	
Secondary
Infection of mastoid and frontal
   sinuses
	Prolonged cardiac arrest
	Systemic hypotension
	Respiratory failure
	Severe anaemia
	Carbon monoxide poisoning
	Altitude sickness

Within the brain there are areas of the grey matter which show selective vulnerability to ischaemia, notably:
- the hippocampus;
- the cerebellar Purkinje cells;
- the small pyramidal neurones of the amygdala, frontal and occipital cortex.

The first two regions are also susceptible to damage secondary to status epilepticus and hypoglycaemia.

Additionally the so-called **watershed areas** of the brain lying at the overlapping margins of the arterial territories, already described, are vulnerable to **hypotensive** damage (Table 27.10).

DISORDERS OF MYELIN

The myelin sheath within the white matter of the CNS is formed by oligodendrocytes. Myelin disorders are primarily a disorder of oligodendrocyte function. The disorder may arise from an inherited defect of myelination such as occurs in the leukodystrophies, a group of metabolic disorders in which normal myelin fails to form, with consequent accumulation of intermediary metabolites. Acquired myelination disorders occur when normal myelin is formed but subsequently undergoes destruction, either acutely or subacutely, accompanied by perivenous inflammation, suggesting an immune component in the pathogenesis.

The ensuing white matter 'scar' is filled by proliferating astrocytes after microglial phagocytosis of the damaged myelin. The disorders of myelin involving the different CNS regions are summarized in Table 27.11.

TRAUMA

Trauma is the principal cause of young adult deaths in

Table 27.11 Disorders of myelin.

Condition	Age	Pathology	Associated condition	Course
Acute disseminated perivenous encephalomyelitis (postinfectious encephalitis)	Adolescence and young adults	Perivenular demyelination and chronic inflammatory infiltrate in deeper layers of cortex, thalamus and pons Axons preserved	Postviral infections—measles, mumps, rubella, varicella-zoster Delayed hypersensitivity reaction to rabies vaccine	Develops 4–5 days post exanthema 10–20% mortality after measles and rubella Remainder recover
Acute haemorrhagic leucoencephalopathy	Any	Widespread petechial, larger haemorrhages and infarcts in white matter. Necrosis of vein walls Perivascular demyelination. Acute-on-chronic inflammation Brain swelling	Disseminated intravascular coagulopathy (DIC) Immune complexes Complement activation	High mortality
Multiple sclerosis	Third to fourth decade	Demyelinating plaques in deep and periventricular white matter of cerebrum, optic nerves, brainstem, cerebellar peduncles and dorsal columns of cord. In acute phase, acute myelin destruction with axonal preservation and perivascular cuffing by T cells and lipid-laden macrophages. Later heals forming an astroglial scar often centred on a venule	CSF IgG oligoclonal band Aetiology unknown Probable interaction between genetic susceptibility and environmental factors, as evidenced by the wide geographic difference in prevalence	Variable, the majority experience relapsing course with progressive neurological deficit
Progressive multifocal leucoencephalopathy (PML)	Adults	Multifocal deep white matter and basal ganglia demyelination with cyst formation	JC virus (a papovavirus) infection in immune-suppressed individuals	Rapidly fatal
Central pontine myelinolysis	Adults (fourth–fifth decade)	Symmetrical demyelination of central region of the pons	Malnourishment Hyponatraemia Immune suppression	High mortality

CSF, Cerebrospinal fluid; IgG, immunoglobulin G.

most developed countries, with the severity of injury to the brain being a major determinant of mortality. Injuries to the spine and peripheral nervous system are associated with significant morbidity.

Evolution within the animal kingdom ensured that the delicate neuraxis became surrounded by a protective layer of bone. The presence of the bone and rigid fibrous compartmental membranes in the skull has become a double-edged sword to modern-day humans, especially when subjected to high-velocity transportation injuries.

Injuries to the nervous system can best be classified by considering their effects on the brain separately from those to the spinal cord and peripheral nervous system.

Brain trauma can be considered to occur due either to a **penetrating injury** in which the head receives a direct blow or is hit by a missile, causing disruption to the skull and underlying brain, or a **closed injury** in which the head experiences a rapid change in velocity, such as following a road traffic accident. In this situation there is

movement of the brain within the skull, with the ensuing damage being due to the brain making contact with roughened surfaces within the skull. The brain areas most susceptible are the poles and inferior surfaces of the frontal lobes, the temporal poles and surrounding the Sylvian fissure.

There is also often accompanying diffuse white matter damage due to torsional injury secondary to brain rotation around the axis of the corpus callosum and brainstem. This causes shearing of the axons within the corpus callosum, cerebral peduncles and upper brainstem.

In practical terms, it can be difficult to distinguish completely between open and closed brain injuries, as the impact of a blow to the head (known as the **coup injury**) causes displacement of the brain, with resultant collision with the skull surface opposite (the **contrecoup injury**) causing contusion or actual disruption of the brain at the point of impact.

Events subsequent to a head injury include extradural, subdural and intracerebral haemorrhage; cerebral oedema with raised intracranial pressure and brain herniation due to impaired vasomotor autoregulation. Hypoxic brain damage due to arterial hypoperfusion may then follow, affecting the **watershed** boundary zones.

Trauma to the spinal column

Penetrating injuries cause partial or complete transection of the cord with consequent neurological deficit distal to the level of the injury. Non-penetrating injuries to the vertebral column cause spinal cord injuries by compression or displacement of the vertebrae.

DEGENERATIVE DISEASES OF THE NERVOUS SYSTEM

The term neurodegenerative diseases refers to a diverse group of nervous system disorders with varying ages of onset, characterized by the progressive degeneration of neurones following completion of their normal development. There may be (clinical) involvement of the motor or sensory system, the cortex, subcortical nuclei, cerebellum and spinal cord, alone or in combination. The pathogenesis of the conditions is unknown, but may show a genetic pattern of transmission and a proportion of the disorders result in the development of **inclusion bodies** within the perikaryon of degenerating neurones (Table 27.13), formed from the abnormal accumulation of neuronal cytoskeletal proteins.

Table 27.12 The cytoskeleton of nucleated cells of neurones and muscle fibres.

Cytoskeletal element	Constituent molecule	Molecular weight (kDa)	Subunit diameter (nm)	Ultrastructure
Microtubule	α and β tubulin monomers	55	25	Tubes of indefinite length
Intermediate filaments	Neurofilaments	68, 145, 220	10	Helical rods of indefinite length
Microfilaments	Actin and myosin	45	5 360–650	Rods of indefinite length
Microtrabecular (cross-linking and anchorage proteins)	τ and microtubule-associated proteins (MAPs)	55–65		

Table 27.13 Neurodegenerative disorders associated with inclusion bodies.

Disease	Clinical symptom	Macroscopic features	Intracellular inclusion	Distribution	Cytoskeletal composition
Alzheimer's	Dementia	Global cerebral atrophy	Neurofibrillary tangle (NFT)	Amygdala, hippocampus, basal forebrain cortical layer III and IV neurones	Neurofilaments τ MAP-2
			Hirano body	Hippocampus	Actin Myosin
Parkinson's	Voluntary movement disorder Dementia*	Substantia nigra depigmentation	Lewy body	Dopaminergic cells of the substantia nigra, locus coeruleus, vagal nucleus Cortex*	Neurofilaments (some are phosphorylated)
Pick's	Dementia	Frontal and temporal lobe atrophy	Pick body	Hippocampus, frontal and temporal lobes	Neurofilaments Microtubule τ

MAP, Microtubule-associated protein.

*The presence of cortical Lewy bodies is associated with dementia in Parkinson's disease.

The neuronal cytoskeleton

Nerves, like all other cells, have an **intracellular cytoskeleton** which is responsible for providing the structural framework that determines the size and shape of the cell as well as facilitating intracellular transport and intercellular communication, the specialized process for which nerves have evolved.

The principal components of the nucleated cell cytoskeleton are shown in Table 27.12 and a selection of the commoner neurodegenerative conditions with their intracellular inclusions are shown in Table 27.13.

Ageing in the human brain

The brains of cognitively normal eldely individuals show an age-related generalized reduction in brain volume and weight, with associated gyral atrophy, sulcal widening and dilatation of the brain ventricles. These changes are due in part to nerve cell loss.

The brains of elderly non-demented individuals may accumulate small numbers of **neurofibrillary tangles** (Fig. 27.19), that are confined to the hippocampus together with sparse numbers of **senile plaques** (Fig. 27.20).

Senile plaques are extracellular spheroidal accumulations of nerve cell processes (neurites) up to 200nm diameter forming a corona surrounding a central amyloid core. The principal protein constituent of the core material has been identified as a 4kDa protein whose gene is located on chromosome 21, known as β/A_4 amyloid.

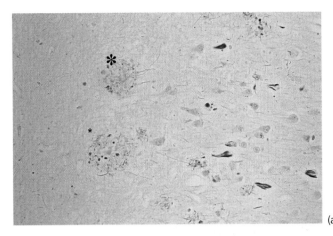
(a)

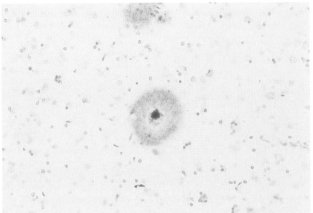
(b)

Fig. 27.20 Alzheimer's disease. (a) Senile (argyrophilic) plaques (✱). These are extracellular collections of degenerated cellular processes around a central mass of amyloid material (measuring between 150 and 200 µm). (Silver stain.) (b) Congo red staining of a senile plaque shows the central amyloid deposit.

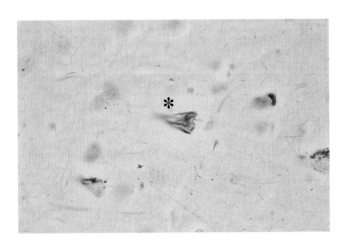

Fig. 27.19 Alzheimer's disease. Neurofibrillary tangles (✱) are seen in the cytoplasm of affected cells, demonstrated here using a silver stain.

Alzheimer's disease (Fig. 27.21)

Alzheimer's disease is the commonest cause of adult-onset dementia, with in excess of 750000 sufferers in the UK. The disease is characterized by generalized cerebral atrophy, often accompanied by more pronounced changes in the parahippocampal gyrus, temporal lobe and frontal/parietal association cortex. This is accompanied by cortical neuronal degeneration as well as neuronal loss from discrete subcortical nuclei which project to the cortex. There are accumulations of modified cytoskeletal elements in some neurones (Table 27.13), accompanied by the deposition of β/A_4 amyloid in senile plaques and arterial blood vessel walls of meningeal and cortical blood vessels (known as **congophilic angiopathy**).

Senile plaques, neurofibrillary tangles and cere-

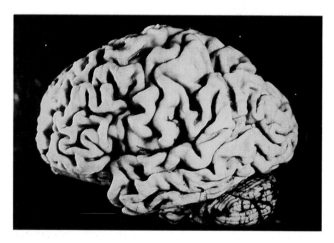

Fig. 27.21 Alzheimer's disease. Cerebral atrophy is present with widening of the sulci and thinning of the gyri. The lateral ventricles (not seen) are dilated.

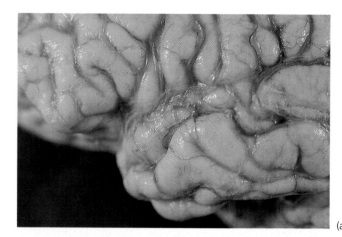

(a)

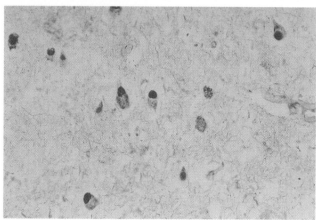

(b)

Fig. 27.22 Pick's disease (pre-senile dementia). (a) The brain shows selective temporal lobe atrophy. (b) Affected neurons contain Pick bodies (eosinophilic cytoplasmic inclusions), shown here using a silver stain.

brovascular amyloid are also present in abundance in a similar distribution to that seen in Alzheimer's disease, in the brains of Down syndrome individuals living beyond the mid third decade. Recent advances in the molecular biology of Alzheimer's disease point to a mutation in the gene coding for the β-amyloid/A_4 protein, present on chromosome 21, in some familial forms of Alzheimer's disease. Further genes for familial forms of Alzheimer's disease have been identified on chromosomes 14 and 19.

Parkinson's disease

Parkinson's disease is a progressive disorder affecting voluntary movements controlled by the dopaminergic neurones that project to the corpus striatum and cortex. The disease is characterized by the loss of dopamine-producing neurones from the pigmented nuclei after having initially developed Lewy inclusion bodies. A minority of Parkinson disease sufferers become demented due to the development of Alzheimer disease cortical changes or by developing Lewy bodies in cortical neurones.

Pick's disease

Pick's disease is a rare dementing disorder of late middle-aged individuals, sometimes showing a familial tendency. Pathologically the disease is characterized by severe atrophy of the frontal and temporal lobes resulting from nerve cell loss and secondary gliosis. Diseased cells either become swollen, **Pick cells**, or develop intracellular **Pick body** inclusions (Fig. 27.22).

Creutzfeldt–Jakob disease

This is a rare, rapidly progressive dementing disorder with accompanying myoclonus which most frequently occurs during the sixth decade of life. Pathologically the condition is characterized by widespread neuronal loss, astrocyte proliferation and **spongiform** vacuolar change in the cortex, subcortical nuclei and cerebellum.

The disease is **transmissible**. Controversy exists over its relationship to a range of spongiform encephalopathies that occur in animals, including scrapie, a disease of sheep and bovine spongiform encephalopathy (BSE).

Huntington's disease

Huntington's disease is an autosomally dominant inherited disease with onset of involuntary choreiform movements and dementia between 25 and 40 years of age; there is progression over a period up to 15 years leading to death.

The disease primarily affects the corpus striatum (formed by the caudate nucleus and putamen) causing atrophy due to loss of cortical projecting GABAergic neurones, involved in positive feedback circuits in the control of movement.

Motor neurone disease

Motor neurone disease is a progressive degenerative disease of both cranial nerve and spinal motor neurones with onset commonly during the fifth decade of life. The disorder causes increasing muscle weakness and wasting, commencing in the small muscles of the hand and resulting in death within 3 years of onset. There is progressive loss of anterior horn cells and atrophy of the ventral nerve roots, particularly in the cervical cord.

Human immunodeficiency virus-induced encephalopathy

Neurological illness is the presenting feature in 10% of AIDS cases and some 30–40% of infected individuals develop neurological symptoms at some stage in the evolution of the illness. Autopsy data have shown pathological changes in the nervous system in up to 90% of cases. The pathological changes observed are summarized in Table 27.14.

Table 27.14 Pathological changes seen in human immunodeficiency virus (HIV) encephalopathy.

Brain		
Adults	Macroscopic	Cerebral atrophy with ventricular dilatation
	Microscopic	Pallor of the white matter due to demyelination and gliosis
		A perivascular infiltrate and multinucleate giant cells are a variable feature
Children	Macroscopic	Retarded brain growth and development
	Microscopic	White matter pallor. Perivascular inflammation and multinucleate giant cells. Calcification of the basal ganglia
Spinal cord	Microscopic	Vacuolar myelopathy—mid-thoracic cord in the lateral and dorsal columns. Arises within the myelin sheath

Opportunistic infections associated with HIV encephalopathy include:
  Toxoplasma gondii
  Cryptococcus neoformans
  Cytomegalovirus

Diseases of the peripheral nervous system

DEVELOPMENT OF THE PERIPHERAL NERVOUS SYSTEM

The peripheral nervous system comprises the nerves and ganglia of the cranial, spinal and autonomic (sympathetic and parasympathetic) nervous system. These are derived from the cells of the **neural crest** which is neuro-ectodermal-derived tissue that migrates away from the neural folds at about the time when the folds are starting to fuse, to form neuronal and satellite elements of the neuroendocrine system and pigmentary melanocytes.

Disorders of the peripheral nervous system can affect **motor**, **sensory** or **autonomic** function or a combination of these systems. Signs of peripheral nervous system dysfunction are summarized in Table 27.15. Causes of nervous system pathology are best considered based on their anatomical location, illustrated in Fig. 27.23.

PERIPHERAL NERVOUS SYSTEM NEOPLASMS

The commonest peripheral nervous system primary neoplasms are of nerve sheath origin, comprising benign schwanommas (neurilemmoma) and neurofibroma. They are both of Schwann cell origin, the former type distinguished by its paraneural location causing displacement and compression of nerve fibres without infiltration (Fig. 27.13).

Neurofibromas are composed of a benign proliferation of Schwann cells and fibroblasts, with the latter producing a variable amount of intercellular substance. The mixed cell proliferation arises within the nerve matrix, causing expansion and distortion, making dissection without a degree of nerve fibre destruction technically difficult.

Neurofibromas rarely develop on cranial nerves, even in von Recklinghausen's disease, which is characterized by the presence of multiple peripheral neurofibromas, *café au lait* skin discoloration, a high risk of sarcomatous transformation in the neurofibromas and the development of intracranial meningiomas.

TRAUMA TO THE PERIPHERAL NERVOUS SYSTEM

Both penetrating and avulsion injuries to the nerve plexuses cause the severed ends initially to retract and

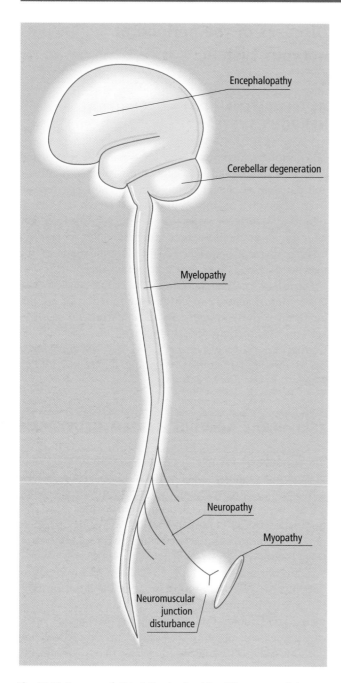

Fig. 27.23 Summary of clinical disorders involving different areas of the nervous system.

then to undergo **Wallerian degeneration**, forming a traumatic neuroma. Subsequently, the proximal portion of the nerve develops neuritic sprouts which, if sited in proximity to the severed distal nerve segment, may reinnervate by regrowth along the nerve sheath. Crush injuries to the peripheral nerves usually cause a period of paraesthesia, following which nerve function returns.

Diseases of the eye

DEVELOPMENT OF THE EYE

The eyes develop from neuroectoderm as paired **optic grooves** during the fourth week of gestation at the cranial pole of the neuraxis. The optic grooves dilate, forming paired **vesicles** which invaginate forming the **optic cups**, within which are trapped mesoderm and surface ectoderm. The mesoderm forms the connective tissue of the cornea, iris, choroid, sclera as well as the ciliary muscles. The surface ectoderm forms the lens and the corneal epithelium. The neuroectoderm develops into the optic nerve fibres, the retina, pupillary sphincter muscles and surface epithelium of the iris and ciliary body.

The eyes are paired sensory exteroreceptors, formed from developmental outgrowths of the brain. Their proximity to the brain together with their capacity to be inspected by ophthalmoscopic examination permits the clinician to observe at close hand primary diseases of the inner layers of the eye, changes secondary to brain disease, such as papilloedema secondary to raised intracranial pressure and stigmata due to systemic disease such as hypertension and diabetes mellitus. The anatomy of the eye is summarized in Fig. 27.24.

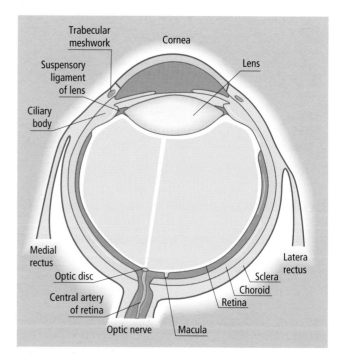

Fig. 27.24 The structure of the eye.

Table 27.15 Signs of peripheral nervous system disease.

Signs of lower motor neurone neuropathy	Signs of upper motor neurone neuropathy	Signs of autonomic neuropathy
Weakness	Weakness	Postural hypotension
Wasting	Spasticity	Incontinence
Fasciculation	Hyperreflexia with clonus	Impotence
Hypotonicity	Extensor plantar response	Altered perspiration
Diminished reflexes	Loss of abdominal reflexes	

INFLAMMATORY DISEASES OF THE EYE

The intraocular tissues of the eye have a privileged immune surveillance status in health. However, this status may be breached by disease with any structure or layer of the eye becoming inflamed by a variety of pathogenic processes:

- conjunctivitis;
- inflammation of the cornea (keratitis);
- iritis;
- inflammation of the ciliary body (cyclitis);
- uveitis;
- scleritis;
- choroiditis;
- optic neuritis;
- inflammation of the interior of the eye (endophthalmitis);
- inflammation of the eyelid (blepharitis).

These include infective (pyogenic bacterial, syphilis, gonorrhoea) and autoimmune systemic disorders (rheumatoid arthritis, sarcoidosis, Reiter's syndrome).

The uveal tract within the eye is particularly prone to inflammatory involvement, especially following penetration of the globe, thereby breaching the ocular–blood barrier, exposing ocular tissue antigens, with a risk of autoimmune-directed inflammation arising in the opposite eye. This condition is known as **sympathetic endophthalmitis**.

OCULAR NEOPLASMS

The eye can be considered as a sphere composed of successive tissue layers from which different categories of neoplasm can arise (Fig. 27.24).

The majority of primary ocular neoplasms arise within the posterior segment from either the retina, usually in childhood as **retinoblastoma** (Fig. 27.25), or from the choroid, including the retinal pigment epithelium layer (Fig. 27.26). In adults they usually arise as choroidal melanoma.

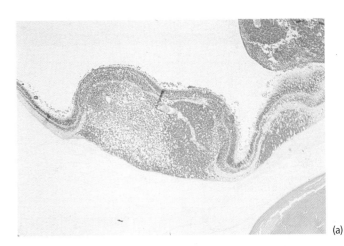

(a)

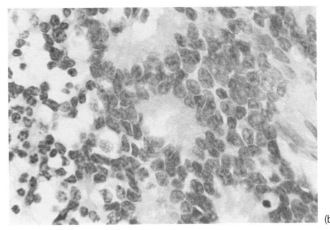

(b)

Fig. 27.25 Retinoblastoma of the eye. (a) This low power view shows the origin from the retina. (b) Histology shows a cellular tumour consisting of round, blue cells arranged in rosettes. (H&E.)

Secondary neoplastic metastases most commonly develop within the highly vascular choroid. Neoplasms may also arise from the optic nerve, its nerve sheath or from other structures within the orbit.

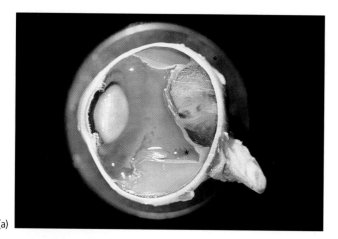

(a)

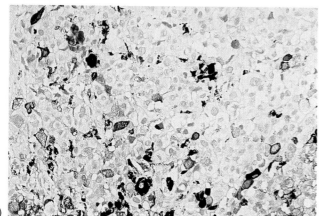

(b)

Fig. 27.26 The eye. Choroidal melanoma. (a) This is a sagittal section through the fixed eye specimen showing the tumour in the choroid. (b) A melanin stain (Masson Fontana) shows that some of these cells contain melanin.

RETINAL VASCULAR DISEASE

Disease of the retinal blood vessels are a common cause of adult-onset, acquired visual impairment and blindness affecting both the arterial and venous vasculature. The causes include:

- diabetic retinopathy;
- hypertensive retinopathy;
- arteritis, particularly giant cell arteritis;
- retinal artery emboli (atheromatous, septic in septicaemia and endocarditis, and thrombotic).

TRAUMA TO THE EYE

The eyes, with their external location in contact with the environment, are at risk from trauma, mainly of a mechanical and chemical form. Since the eye is spherical, the forms of trauma it can be subjected to can be classified similarly to the CNS as non-perforating and perforating forms.

GLAUCOMA

The term glaucoma refers to a group or category of ocular conditions characterized by the development of an increase in intraocular pressure sufficient to disrupt optic nerve function by causing cupping of the nerve head and impairment of the visual fields.

Glaucoma results from an inbalance of the mechanisms controlling the rates of secretion and absorption of the aqueous humour by the ciliary body and the trabecular meshwork, respectively (see Fig. 27.24). A variety of congenital and acquired disorders can cause glaucoma:

- congenital defects of the canal of Schlemm;
- in association with congenital aniridia;
- familial (wide-angle) glaucoma;
- closed-angle glaucoma;
- dislocation of the lens;
- adhesions from uveitis;
- secondary to retinal artery narrowing in diabetes or hypertension;
- secondary to arteriovenous fistulas.

CATARACTS

A cataract is an opacity of the lens of the eye. The lens is derived from ectoderm and consists of modified epithelial cells. It does not receive a blood supply and derives its oxygen from the aqueous humour of the anterior chamber of the eye. Cataracts develop as the epithelial cells break down and fragment.

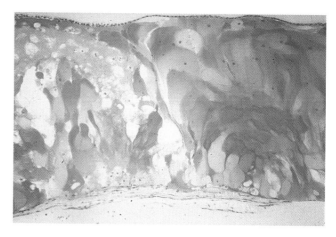

Fig. 27.27 The degenerative changes seen in a congenital cataract.

Senile cataract is an age-related phenomenon whose mechanism is not understood. Cataracts are associated with diabetes mellitus where sorbitol deposition secondary to high blood glucose exerts an osmotic effect accelerating this degeneration. Other causes include:

- trauma;
- radiation;
- long-term use of steroids;
- congenital infection (rubella) (Fig. 27.27);
- hypoparathyroidism.

Treatment is by extraction of the diseased tissue and replacement with a prosthetic lens.

FURTHER READING

Esiri M.M. (1996) *Oppenheimer's Diagnostic Neuropathology*. Blackwell Science, Oxford.

Weller, R.O. (1984) *Colour Atlas of Neuropathology*. Oxford University Press, New York.

Glossary

Abortion Fetal loss before 24 weeks gestation.

Abrasion Injury to epithelium involving scraping away of the superficial layers of the epithelium.

Abscess Localized collection of pus resulting from an inflammatory reaction, bacterial infection.

Abruptio placentae Premature separation of the placenta from the uterine wall before the onset of labour.

Acanthocyte An erythrocyte characterized by irregular spike-like projections of the cell membrane.

Acantholysis Separation of individual cells of the epidermis, often resulting in bulla (blister) formation.

Acanthosis Increased thickness of the stratum spinosum of the epidermis.

Achalasia Failure of a sphincter of a viscus to relax causing dilatation proximally.

Achlorhydria Lack of gastric acid secretion.

Acidosis Disturbance of acid–base balance characterized by acidity (decreased pH) of body fluids.

Activated lymphocyte A lymphocyte that has reacted immunologically on exposure to an antigen.

Acquired Due to an event after birth.

Acute Appearing rapidly (e.g. acute inflammation).

Addiction A state of strong dependence on a chemical substance to an extent that an abnormal clinical state results following abrupt abstention.

Adenocarcinoma Malignant neoplasm of glandular or secretory epithelium.

Adenoma Benign glandular neoplasm.

Adenosis Glandular proliferation (e.g. sclerosing adenosis).

Adhesion Abnormal band or layer of connective tissue fixing two or more normally separate structures.

-aemia Suffix–'of the blood'.

Aetiology Cause of a disease.

Agenesis Failure of a tissue or organ to form during embryogenesis.

Aging The gradual changes that occur in an organism with the passage of time (that do not result from injury or disease).

Agranulocytosis Absence of mature granulocytes in the peripheral blood.

Agonal Terminal event, immediately prior to death

Albinism A congenital absence of melanin pigment in the skin, hair and eyes, resulting from a failure of synthesis.

Alcoholism Abuse of alcohol beverages to an extent that interferes with the drinker's health, social interactions, or performance.

Alkalosis Disturbance of acid base balance characterized by alkalinity (increased pH) of body fluids.

Allele One copy of a paired gene.

Allergy Excessive and/or inappropriate immunological reaction to an environmental antigen (allergen) (see hypersensitivity).

Allergen An antigen that evokes a type I hypersensitivity response.

Allograft Tissue transplanted between two individuals of the same species.

Amenorrhoea Absence of menstruation. **Primary amenorrhoea** if no menstrual periods have occurred by age 16 years; **secondary amenorrhoea** if there is cessation of normally established menstruation.

Amniocentesis Withdrawal of fluid from the amniotic sac.

Amphophilic Having an affinity for both basic and acid dyes.

Amyloid Insoluble extracellular material of variable composition (e.g. immunoglobulin light chains, amyloid protein A) causing enlargement and malfunction of the organs in which it is deposited.

Amyloidosis Deposition of amyloid in the interstitial space.

Ana- Prefix–absent.

Anaemia Abnormally low blood haemoglobin concentration.

Anaerobe A micro-organism that can multiply only in the absence of oxygen.

Anamnestic (response) Immunological response enhanced by pervious exposure to the same agent.

Anaphylaxis Excessive and/or inappropriate type I immunological reaction.

Anaplasia Lack of differentiated features, usually in a tumour.

Anasarca Massive generalized oedema associated with fluid accumulation in body cavities.

Anergy A state of diminished immunologic reactivity to antigens.

Aneuploid Abnormal chromosome numbers other than in exact multiples of the haploid state (i.e. not diploid, tetraploid, etc.).

Aneurysm Abnormal permanent dilation of a blood vessel wall or part of a heart chamber.

Angina pectoris Ischaemic retrosternal myocardial pain that typically occurs on exertion and is relieved by rest.

Angiitis See 'arteritis' and 'vasculitis'. Inflammation and structural damage of the vessel wall.

Anisocytosis Abnormal variation in size of red blood cells.

Ankylosis Fusion of a joint, resulting in its impaired mobility.

Anlage (primordium) The earliest grouping of primitive embryonic cells from which an organ or tissue develops.

Annular Encircling the circumference of a hollow tube.

Annulus The circumference of a cardiac valve ring.

Anomaly A deviation from normal of the form, shape or position of a structure, tissue or organ.

Anoxia Lack of oxygen.

Antibody Immunoglobulin with antigen specificity.

Antidote Agent countering the harmful effects of a poison.

Antigen A substance binding specifically to an antibody or T-cell antigen receptor.

Antigenic determinant The structural component of an antigen molecule that is responsible for specific interaction with the antibody it induces.

Antiserum Serum containing specific antibody.

Antitoxin Antibody capable of neutralizing a bacterial toxin.

Aplasia Failure of growth of a tissue.

Apoptosis A form of normal or pathological individual cell death characterized by activation of endogenous endonucleases.

APUDoma Neoplasm of APUD cells (APUD is amine precursor uptake and decarboxylation) (e.g. carcinoid tumour).

Arteriosclerosis Any pathological condition causing thickening of a vessel wall and stenosis of the lumen.

Arthus reaction A hypersensitivity reaction characterized by necrosis and acute inflammation at the site of antigen entry caused by the formation and deposition of local immune complexes (in antibody excess).

Arteritis See 'vasculitis' and 'angiitis'. Inflammation and structural damage of the vessel wall.

Ascites Abnormal accumulation of fluid in the peritoneal cavity.

Aseptic 1 Performed in such a way as to avoid infection (e.g. by using sterile instruments); 2 inflammatory illness not due to any identifiable bacterium (e.g. aseptic meningitis).

Asphyxia Consequence of suffocation or mechanically impaired respiration.

Asthma A reversible condition caused by narrowing of the respiratory airways due to bronchial smooth muscle contraction.

Atelectasis Failure to expand.

Atheroma A focal, intimal accumulation of lipid, calcium, degraded collagen and macrophages in the intima of arteries.

Atherosclerosis The pathological process involving atheroma formation.

Atopy Condition characterized by predisposition to allergies.

Atresia Embryological failure of formation of the lumen of a normally hollow viscus or duct (e.g. biliary atresia).

Atrophy Pathological or physiological cellular or organ shrinkage.

Attenuation Reduction in the virulence of a microorganism.

Atypia Departure from the typical normal appearance, usually histological.

Auto-antibody Antibody reactive with the body's own tissues or constituents.

Autograft Tissue transplanted in the same individual from which it is taken.

Autoimmune disease A disease resulting from a specific immune response directed against the body's own tissues.

Autoimmunity Abnormal state in which the body's immune system reacts against its own tissues or constituents.

Autolysis Digestion of tissue by the enzymes contained within it.

Autopsy Synonymous with necropsy or postmortem examination.

Autosomal (gene) Residing on any autosome (autosomes are chromosomes other than sex chromosomes).

Azoospermia Absence of speramatozoa in the semen.

Azotemia Elevation in blood levels of nonprotein nitrogenous compounds, mainly urea, uric acid and creatinine.

B lymphocyte A lymphocyte that is primed in the bursa of Fabricius (in bird) or the bursa equivalent (foetal liver or bone marrow) in mammals. The B cell gives rise to plasma cells and is responsible for humoral immunity.

Bacteraemia Presence of bacteria in the blood.

Bacteriuria Presence of bacteria in the urine.

Band cell A neutrophil recently released from the bone marrow and characterized by an unsegmented nucleus that forms a continuous band.

Barr body A small, darkly staining mass of chromatin seen adjacent to the inner surface of the nuclear membrane in female cells during interphase.

Barrett's oesophagus The presence of gastrointestinal columnar epithelium in the oesophagus.

Basophilic Staining preferentially with basic dyes.

BCG (bacille Calmette–Guérin) An attenuated strain of mycobacterium bovis that is used to actively immunize against tuberculosis (and as a nonspecific immune stimulant).

Bence-Jones protein Monoclonal immunoglobulin light chains detectable in the urine of some patients with B lymphocyte and plasma cell neoplasms.

Benign Relatively harmless (contrast with malignant).

Beta particle A particle emitted in radioactive decay consisting of either an electron or a positron.

Biopsy The process of removing tissue for diagnosis, or a piece of tissue removed during life for diagnostic purposes.

'Blast' cell Any primitive cell but especially a primitive haemopoietic cell.

Blastema The primitive cells from which tissues are formed.

Blastocyst The ball of cells constituting the early embryo at the time of implantation in the uterus.

-blastoma Suffix – tumour histologically resembling the embryonic state of the organ in which it arises and more commonly seen in young children (e.g. retinoblastoma).

Blood coagulation The sequential process by which multiple plasma coagulation factors interact to finally cause the conversion of fibrinogen to fibrin.

Bronchiectasis Permanent abnormal dilatation of bronchi.

Bruit (murmur) An abnormal sound caused by turbulent blood flow in the cardiovascular system.

Bursa of Fabricius A small lymphoepithelial sac near the cloaca in birds that is critical to inducing B lymphocyte differentiation.

Bulla A thin-walled fluid-filled cavity (e.g. bulla of skin > 5 mm) or gas (e.g. emphysematous bulla of lung).

Cachexia Extreme wasting of the body often associated with a malignant neoplasm.

Calcification Process occurring naturally in bone and teeth, but abnormally in some diseased tissues ('dystrophic' calcification) or as a result of hypercalcaemia ('metastatic' calcification).

Calculus Stone.

Callus 1 New bone formed within and around a bone fracture; 2 patch of hard skin formed at the site of repeated trauma.

Cancer A general term, in the public domain, usually implying any malignant tumour or neoplasm.

Carbuncle Large pus-filled swelling, usually on the skin, often discharging through several openings and invariably due to a staphylococcal infection.

Carcinogen An agent that causes malignant neoplasms.

Carcinogenesis Mechanisms of the causation of malignant neoplasms.

Carcinoid Tumour of usually low-grade malignancy arising from APUD cells but not characterized by the production of a peptide hormone from which an alternative name might be derived.

Carcinoma A malignant epithelial neoplasm.

Carcinoma-*in-situ* A malignant epithelial neoplasm that has not yet invaded through the original basement membrane; synonymous with intra-epithelial neoplasia.

Carcinomatosis The presence in the body of widely disseminated cancer.

Cardiac tamponade A restriction of cardiac filling caused by accumulation of fluid in the pericardial sac.

Cardiomyopathy A primary myocardial disease of unknown cause in the absence of congenital, hypertensive, valvular, or ischaemic heart disease.

CD Cluster differentiation (or designation); a standard numerical coding scheme for antigens borne by different types and sub-types of leucocytes and some other cells; used for identification of these cells by immunological methods.

Caseation Type of necrosis, characteristically associated with tuberculosis, in which the dead tissue has a cheesy, structureless consistency.

Cell degeneration A reversible abnormality in cell structure.

Cellular (Cell-mediated) **immunity**. The specific type of immune response that is mediated by T lymphocytes.

Cellular oncogene (c-*onc*) Intrinsic cellular gene corresponding to a viral nucleic acid sequence (v-*onc*) that is believed to play a role in cell growth regulation. Inappropriate expression may cause cancer.

Cellulitis Diffuse acute inflammation of the skin and subcutis caused by streptococcal infection.

Cerebrovascular accident (CVA) Cerebral infarction, or haemorrhage within or around the brain; synonymous wth 'stroke'.

Ceroid Insoluble, intracellular lipopigment found in cardiac myocytes and in atheroma.

Cestode A tapeworm.

Chalone A chemical substance, released by a cell, that inhibits cellular proliferation.

Chemotaxis Migration of cells induced by some chemical influence such as complement components, and accounting for the accumulation of leucocytes in inflamed tissues.

Child Term used to describe the period of time between 1 year of age and puberty.

Cholestasis Reduced or absent bile flow, thus leading to jaundice (cholestatic jaundice).

Choristoma A developmental abnormality in which tissues not normally present in an organ grow in a disorganized fashion to produce a tumour. Not a true neoplasm (contrast with hamartoma).

Chromatin A complex of nucleic acids and histones that constitute chromosomes.

Chromatolysis (of nucleus) Dissolution of the nucleus evident from the loss of its staining characteristics.

Chronic Persisting for a long time (contrast with acute).

Chronic inflammatory cells Cells commonly present in the tissues in chronic inflammation, representing the effector cells of the immune response, phagocytosis and repair (lymphocytes, plasma cells, macrophages and fibroblasts).

Chronic periaortitis A local complication of advanced aortic atherosclerosis featuring medial thinning and a variable adventitial chronic inflammatory cell infiltrate. May be associated with dilated and undilated aortas (*see* chronic periarteritis).

Chronic periarteritis A local complication of advanced arterial atherosclerosis featuring medial thinning and a variable adventitial chronic inflammatory cell infiltrate (*see* chronic periaortitis).

CIN Cervical intraepithelial neoplasia, a precursor of invasive squamous cell carcinoma of the cervix uteri; graded I to III depending on the degree of severity.

Cirrhosis (liver) Irreversible architectural disturbance characterized by nodules of regenerating hepatocytes with intervening fibrosis; a consequence of many forms of chronic liver injury.

Clonal deletion theory A theory advanced to explain natural tolerance to self-antigens which states that clones of lymphoid cells which react against self-antigens are permanently deleted on contact with the antigen during fetal life.

Clonal selection theory The hypothesis that a specific immune response is the rusult of selection, by reaction of the antigen with surface receptors on lymphocytes, of one or more clones of lymphocytes from a pre-existing mass of many millions of lymphocyte clones.

Clone A number of identical cells (or nucleic acid sequences) derived from a single precursor.

Clot (blood) Coagulated blood *outside* the cardiovascular system (contrast with thrombosus)

Cloudy swelling Early reversible cell degeneration in states of injury, characterized by increased intracellular water, affected cells are swollen, and the cytoplasm appears cloudy.

Coagulative necrosis Cell death in which the cell becomes a homogeneous eosinophilic anuclear mass with retention of the basic cell outline.

Cold agglutinin An antibody that induces erythrocyte agglutination at temperatures below normal body temperature.

Collagen The fibrous protein formed in interstitial tissue from tropocollagen units secreted by fibroblasts.

Comedo(ne) Plug of material (e.g. in some intraduct breast carcinomas, and in the lesions of acne vulgaris).

Commensalism A natural state in which two organisms live together with benefit to one and no harm to the other, or with benefit to both (symbiosis).

Comminuted (fracture) Bone broken into fragments at fracture site.

Complement Collective noun for a set of blood proteins which when activated by, for example, antigen–antibody reactions forms an amplifiation cascade with various effects including leucocyte chemotaxis and cell lysis.

Complications Events secondary to the primary disorder (e.g. cerebral haemorrhage is a complication of hypertension).

Compound Involving more than one structure (e.g. compound naevus involves dermis and epidermis).

c-*onc* See cellular oncogene.

Concussion Transient loss of consciousness immediately following a head injury in the absence of detectable structural abnormality in the brain.

Condyloma Warty lesion, often on genitalia.

Congenital Condition attributable to events prior to birth, not necessarily genetic or inherited, giving rise to conditions present at birth.

Congestion Engorgement with blood.

Consolidation Solidification of lung tissue, usually be an inflammatory exudate; a feature of pneumonia.

Consumption coagulopathy An acute reduction in blood coagulation factors resulting from their utilization in patients developing extensive intravascular coagulation.

Contact inhibition Cessation of cell proliferation that occurs when cells come into contact with one another.

Contraction Shortening or reduction in size.

Contusion (Bruise). An injury characterized by extravasation of blood into the tissues without significant tissue disruption.

Coombs' test (Antiglobulin test). A method of detecting the presence of antibody fixed on the surface of erythrocytes.

Cowdry A inclusion body A large, round eosinophilic intranuclear inclusion body surrounded by a halo and occurring in cells infected by many viruses (most commonly herpes viruses).

Crepitus Gas in the subcutaneous tissues.

Curling's ulcer Acute peptic ulceration of the stomach or duodenum following a severe burn on the surface of the body.

Cushing's disease The clinical picture resulting from the overactivity of the adrenal cortex due to a functional disorder in the hypothalamus or a pituitary tumour.

Cushing's syndrome The term used to describe the above set of clinical signs and symptoms resulting from an excess of glucocorticoids in the circulation but includes that involving a pathological process in the adrenal itself, from ectopic or inappropriate production of adrenocorticotrophic hormone (ACTH) or from excessive administration of glucocorticoids.

Cyanosis Bluish discoloration of the skin and mucous membranes owing to an increased concentration of reduced haemoglobin in the blood.

Cyst Cavity with an epithelial lining and containing fluid or other material (contrast with pseudocyst).

Cytokines Substances produced by one cell which influence the behaviour of another.

Cytopathic (virus effect) Causing cell injury, not necessarily lethal.

Cytotoxic Causing cell injury, not necessarily lethal.

Death The irreversible cessation of normal life processes. From a legal standpoint, death is usually defined as cessation of detectable electrical activity in the brain along with cardiac and respiratory arrest.

Debridement The surgical removal of devitalized tissue and foreign material from an area of injury until surrounding or underlying healthy tissue is exposed.

Deformation An abnormality of form produced by external forces on previously normal structures.

Degeneration Disorder characterized by loss of structural and functional integrity of an organ or tissue.

Definitive host In infectious disease, the host in which a parasite has its adult and sexual existence.

Degranulation The process in which cells lose their cytoplasmic granules.

Delayed hypersensitivity A type of immunologic hypersensitivity reaction that is manifested several hours (usually 24–72 hours) after exposure to the inciting antigen. The term is restricted in current usage to type IV hypersensitivity.

Deletion In genetics, a chromosomal abnormality characterized by loss of part of the chromosome.

Dementia An organic brain disorder characterized by progressive loss of cognitive functions and failure of memory.

Demyelination Loss of myelin from around nerve fibres.

Denudation Exposure of subepithelial tissues due to removal of the surface epithelium.

Desmoplasia Induction of connective tissue growth, usually in the stroma of tumours.

Diagnosis Determination of the nature of disease.

Diapedesis Passage of blood cells between endothelial cells into the perivascular tissue; characteristic of inflammation.

Diarrhoea An increase in the fluidity of bowel movements beyond what is usual for the individual.

Differentiation 1 Embryological–process by which a tissue develops special characteristics; 2 pathological–degree of morphological resemblance of a neoplasm to its parent tissue.

Diffuse Affecting the tissue in a continuous or widespread distribution.

Diploid Twice the haploid chromosome number or DNA content.

Disease Abnormal state capable of causing ill health.

Disseminated intravascular coagulation (DIC) Formation of widespread thrombi in the microcirculation with uncontrolled haemorrhage.

Diverticulum Abnormal hollow pouch communicating with the lumen of the structure from which it has arisen.

Dominant Characteristic of a gene of which only one copy is necessary for it to be expressed.

Doubling time (Generation time) The time required for all components of a cell culture to multiply by 2. In neoplasms, the time taken for the constituent number of cells to multiply by 2.

Drug Any chemical with therapeutic properties.

Drug abuse Excessive non-therapeutic use of a drug to the extent of developing dependence to the drug.

Drug dependence A state in which an established level of dosage or increasing doses of the drug are needed to prevent symptoms of withdrawal.

Dysentery Acute inflammation of the colon characterized by passage of liquid stools containing blood and mucus.

Dysfunctional uterine bleeding Excessive, disorderly menstrual bleeding resulting from hormonal imbalance.

Dysgenesis Defective development of an organ or tissue giving rise to an organ that is structurally abnormal.

Dyskaryosis Abnormal growth and differentiation of a cell; in exfoliated epithelial cells, often preneoplastic and graded as mild, moderate or severe.

Dyskeratosis The abnormal, often premature keratinization of squamous epithelial cells during maturation.

Dysmenorrhoea Painful menstruation.

Dysphagia Difficulty in swallowing, usually manifested as a sensation of food becoming obstructed.

Dysplasia Abnormal growth and differentiation of a tissue; in epithelia this is graded as mild, moderate or severe and may be pre-neoplastic.

Dyspnoea Any alteration in breathing associated with awareness of respiratory effort.

Dystrophic calcification See calcification.

Dystrophy Abnormal development or degeneration of a tissue.

Dysuria Pain or difficulty with urination.

Ecchymoses Any bruise or haemorrhagic spot, larger than petechiae, on the skin (may be spontaneous in the elderly, usually due more to vascular fragility than to coagulation defects).

Ectasia Abnormal dilatation.

Ectoderm The outer germ layer of the embryo that gives rise mainly to the skin and neural tissue.

Ectopic Tissue or substance in or from an inappropriate site (but not by metastasis).

Eczema An acute or chronic non-contagious inflammatory condition of the skin.

Effector cells In immunology, lymphocytes that have been activated by antigen exposure which are the direct mediators of the immune response.

Effusions Abnormal collection of fluid in body cavity (e.g. pleura, peritoneum, synovial joint).

Elastosis Increase in elastin in a tissue.

Elephantiasis A clinical state caused by chronic lymphatic obstruction and characterized by lymphoedema and hyperplasia of the skin.

Elliptocyte (Ovalocyte) An oval-shaped erythrocyte.

Embolus Fluid (e.g. gas, fat) or solid (e.g. thrombus) mass mobile within a blood vessel and capable of blocking its lumen.

Emigration of leucocytes The active outward passage of leucocytes through the intact walls of the microcirculation.

Emperipolesis The penetration of and movement through a cell by another cell (usually a lymphocyte within a macrophage). Should be distinguished from phagocytosis.

Emphysema Characterized by the formation of abnormal thin-walled gas-filled cavities; pulmonary emphysema—in lungs, surgical emphysema—in connective tissues.

Empyema Cavity filled with pus (e.g. empyema of the gallbaldder).

Endoderm The inner germ layer of the embryo that gives rise to the gastrointestinal tract, liver, pancreas and respiratory tract.

Endometriosis The occurrence of endometrial glands and stroma in a location other than the endometrium.

Endophytic Tumour growing inwards from a surface; usually by invasion and thus malignant (contrast with exophytic).

Endotoxin A lipopolysaccharide component of the cell walls of Gram-negative bacteria that has cytotoxic properties.

End-stage kidney A chronically damaged kidney in which the original underlying renal disease cannot be determined.

Enterotoxin An exotoxin produced by bacteria that has an adverse effect on the epithelial cells of the gastrointestinal tract.

Eosinophilic Having an affinity for the acidic dye eosin.

Epidemic Affecting a large number of persons in one geographic region at the same time.

Epidemiology The science concerned with the factors that determine the incidence and distribution of disease in a population.

Epilepsy A disorder characterized by recurrent seizuers due to paroxysmal abnormal electrical discharges in the brain.

Epithelioid Histologically resembling epithelium. Epithelioid cells may be derived from macrophages and are a distinctive feature of granulomas.

Epitope An antigenic determinant, or that part of a molecule that reacts with the binding site of an antibody.

Eponym Name of a disease derived from its association with a place or person (e.g. Cushing's disease).

Erosion Loss of superficial layer (not full-thickness) of a surface (e.g. gastric erosion).

Erythema Abnormal redness of skin due to increased blood flow.

Erythrocyte rouleaux Aggregation of erythrocytes in the blood in a stack-like configuration resembling a pile of coins.

Essential (disease type) Without evident antecedent cause; synonymous with primary and idiopathic.

Exophytic Tumour growing outwards from a surface, usually because it lacks invasive properties (contrast with endophytic).

Exotoxin A protein complex secreted by bacteria into the environment that has the potential for causing changes in cells at a location different from the site of infection.

Expressivity In genetics, the degree to which a heritable trait is manifested by an individual carrying the gene for the trait.

Extrinsic 1 Outside the structure and, for example, compressing it; 2 Cause external to the body (e.g. extrinsic allergic alveolitis);

(contrast with intrinsic).

Exudate Extravascular accumulation of protein-rich fluid due to increased vascular permeability (contrast with transudate).

Facultative intracellular organisms Microorganisms that can multiply both extracellularly and intracellularly.

Fatty change The accumulation of lipid in the cytoplasm of cells.

Fc receptor A cell surface receptor present on some leucocytes that binds with the Fc (fragment, crystallizable) end of some immunoglobulin molecules.

Fibrillation The uncoordinated and ineffective contraction of single muscle fibres.

Fibrinoid Resembling fibrin (e.g. fibrinoid necrosis).

Fibrinolysis Dissolution of fibrin by enzymatic action resulting from activation of the enzyme plasmin in the bloodstream.

Fibrinous Rich in fibrin (e.g. fibrinous exudate).

Fibroid Benign smooth-muscle tumour (leiomyoma) commonly arising from uterine myometrium.

Fibromatosis A tumour-like, but non-metastasizing, infiltrative proliferation of fibroblasts and myofibroblasts.

Fibrosis Process of depositing excessive collagen in a tissue.

Fistula Abnormal connection between one hollow viscus and another or with the skin surface.

Fluke A trematode (flatworm).

Focal Localized abnormality (contrast with diffuse).

Follicular Forming a circumscribed structure resembling a follicle.

Fomite (Fomes) An object harmless in itself that harbours infectious agents and may thus serve to transmit an infection.

Forme fruste Early stage of a disease before it has developed a complete set of characteristics.

Foreign body giant cell A multinucleated macrophage that has its nuclei dispersed haphazardly throughout the cytoplasm.

Foreign body granuloma A localized aggregate of macrophages around an inert foreign body.

Fracture An injury characterized by a break in the tissue.

Free radicals Chemical radicals characterized by unpaired electrons in the outer shell and therefore highly reactive.

Friable Easily crumbled or broken.

Frostbite Tissue injury resulting from exposure of the tissue to freezing temperatures.

Fungating Forming an elevated growth, usually neoplastic (and usually malignant).

Furuncle A boil.

Galactorrhoea Flow of milk unrelated to lactation, usually caused by abnormally increased levels of prolactin.

Gamete A haploid germ cell—either an ovum or a spermatozoon.

Gamma ray A photon emitted by a radionuclide.

Ganglion Cystic lesion containing mucin-rich fluid associated with a joint or tendon sheath.

Gangrene Necrosis of tissues; 'dry' gangrene—sterile; 'wet' gangrene—with bacterial putrefaction.

Gene The fundamental unit of heredity that carries a single Mendelian trait.

Genome The normal complement of chromosomes with the genes they contain.

Genotype The genetic make-up of an individual.

Germ layers The 3 fundamental embryonic divisions of cells—ectoderm, endoderm, and mesoderm—from which the organs and tissues are derived.

Giant cell Abnormally large cell, often multinucleated.

Gliosis Increase in glial fibres, within the central nervous system; analogous to fibrosis elsewhere in the body.

Goitre Enlarged thyroid gland.

Goblet cell A mucin-secreting cell characterized by a large cytoplasmic vacuole filled with mucin.

Grade Degree of malignancy of a neoplasm usually judged from its histological features (e.g. nuclear size and shape, mitotic frequency).

Graft Any tissue that is transplanted from one site to another.

Graft-versus-host (GVD) disease A disease in which foreign immunocompetent cells introduced into a host react immunologically against host tissues.

Granulocytopaenia (Neutropaenia.) A decrease in the number of neutrophil leucocytes in peripheral blood below 1500/μl.

Granulation tissue Newly formed connective tissue comprising capillaries, fibroblasts, myofibroblasts and inflammatory cells embedded in mucin-rich ground substance (see healing).

Granuloma An aggregate of epithelioid macrophages, often including giant multinucleate cells also derived from macrophages (histiocytes).

Ground substance The acellular amorphous matrix of connective tissue, composed mainly of proteoglycans and water, in which cells are embedded.

Gumma Focal necrotic lesion in tertiary stage of syphilis.

Gynaecomastia Enlargement of the male breast.

Haematin The crystalline product of oxidation of haeme from the ferrous to the ferric state.

Haematocrit Volume fraction of blood consisting of cells.

Haematoidin A golden-yellow crystalline material deposited in tissues as a result of breakdown of haemoglobin.

Haematoma Localized collection of blood or blood clot, usually within a solid tissue.

Haematopoiesis The production and development of blood cells.

Haemochromatosis A disorder characterized by iron overload and deposition of iron in parenchymal cells of various organs, resulting in cell necrosis.

Haemoconcentration An increase in the cell concentration of blood caused by a decrease in its fluid content.

Haemoglobinopathy A disorder caused by an alteration in the molecular structure of haemoglobin.

Haemolysis The liberation of haemoglobin from erythrocytes.

Haemolytic anaemia Anaemia characterizecd by a shortened lifespan of erythrocytes.

Haemorrhage Escape of blood from the vascular system.

Haemosiderosis The presence of increased amounts of stored iron in a tissue; differs from haemochromatosis in that there is no parenchymal cell necrosis.

Haemostasis The arrest of bleeding from a damaged blood vessel.

Half-life The time taken for a substance to be reduced to half its original concentration by a process of natural decay or elimination.

Hamartoma Congenital tumour-like malformation comprising two or more mature tissue elements normally present in the organ in which it arises.

Haploid Single allocation of unpaired chromosomes, as found in ova and spermatozoa.

Haptens Small molecules that are not antigenic by themselves but can act as antigens when complexed with larger molecules.

Healing The process of restoration of integrity to injured tissue by organization of granulation tissue.

Hernia Abnormal protrusion of an organ, or part of it, outside its usual compartment.

Heterotopia Presence of normal tissue in an abnormal location, usually due to an error in embryogenesis.

Histiocyte Macrophage within tissue.

Histogenesis In the context of neoplasms, a term meaning the putative cell of origin.

Homograft Transplantation from one individual to another of the same species.

Hyaline Amorphous texture, sometimes due to the deposition or accumulation of intra- or extracellular material.

Hydrocoele Fluid-filled cavity, especially surrounding a testis.

Hyperaemia Increased blood flow, usually through a capillary bed as in acute inflammation.

Hyperchromatic Increased histological staining, usually of nucleus.

Hyperkeratosis Formation of excess keratin on the surface of stratified squamous epithelium (e.g. epidermis).

Hyperplasia Enlargement of an organ, or a tissue within it, due to an increase in the number of cells.

Hypersensitivity Excessive or inappropriate reaction to an environmental agent, often mediated immunologically (see allergy).

Hypertrophy Enlargement of an organ, or part of it, due to an increase in the size of cells.

Hypervariable The four or more segments in the heavy and light chains of the immunoglobulin molecule that display marked variation in amino acid sequence and are responsible for conferring specificity to the antibody.

Hypoplasia Incomplete development of an organ from its anlage; the hypoplastic organ is smaller but structurally normal.

Hypovolaemia An abnormal decrease in intravascular blood volume.

Hypoxaemia A reduction in the amount of oxygen in arterial blood.

Hypoxia Reduction in available oxygen.

Iatrogenic Caused by medical intervention.

Icterus (Jaundice) A yellow discoloration of tissues caused by an increase in the plasma bilirubin level.

Idiopathic Unknown cause; synonymous with primary, essential and cryptogenic.

Idiotype An antigenic determinant present on and characteristic of a particular antibody molecule, located in the variable region (i.e.; the site of antigen-binding).

Immediate hypersensitivity A type of hypersensitivity response that is manifested within minutes after exposure to the inciting antigen. The term is currently restricted in usage to type 1 hypersensitivity responses.

Immersion syndrome (Trench foot) Tissue injury caused by prolonged exposure of the tissue to non-freezing cold water.

Immune complex The product of interaction between an antigen and an antibody; small, soluble immune complexes may be carried in the circulation to be deposited in tissues, leading to immune complex disease.

Immune response The specific host response mediated by lymphocytes against a molecule that is recognized as foreign (the antigen).

Immune surveillance theory The theory that one major function of the immune system is to recognize and destroy neoplastic cells at their inception.

Immunity The ability of the host to defend against foreign antigens.

Immunization Production of a protective immune response by the deliberate introduction of foreign antigens into the host.

Immunoblast A large, actively proliferating lymphoid cell that is formed as a result of antigen-induced transformation of a lymphocyte (both B and T lymphocytes); it is the immediate precursor of the effector cells.

Immunoglobulin (Antibody) A protein synthesized by plasma cells that functions as a specific antibody, reactive against the antigen that stimulated transformation from a B lymphocyte into that plasma cell.

Immunologic memory The capacity of the immune system to respond more rapidly and strongly to a subsequent challenge by an antigen to which the host has been previously exposed.

Inborn error of metabolism A congenital biochemical abnormality resulting from the failure of synthesis of a protein (usually an enzyme) due to a specific genetic defect.

Incision An injury produced by a sharp instrument characterized by cutting of tissue.

Inclusion body A microscopically visible intracellular mass associated with intracellular viral or chlamydial replication.

Incompetence (valvular) Allowing regurgitation when valve is closed.

Incubation period The time between exposure to an infectious agent and the first appearance of clinical symptoms due to that infection.

Induration The process of becoming hard.

Inert Not causing a reaction when introduced into the body.

Infant Term used to describe the period between 28 days and 1 year of age.

Infarction Death of tissue (an infarct) due to insufficient blood supply.

Infection Multiplication of a microorganism in tissues.

Infectious disease A disease caused by infection.

Infectivity The ability to produce infection.

Infiltrate Abnormal accumulation of cells (e.g. leucocytes, neoplastic cells) or acellular material (e.g. amyloid) in a tissue.

Inflammation The response of living tissue to an injurious agent. It may be acute or chronic.

Initiation In carcinogenesis, the transformation of a cell into a neoplastic cell by a carcinogenic agent.

Inspissation The process of thickening of a fluid resulting from evaporation of water.

Interferon A group of proteins that inhibit viral replication and have a wide variety of effects on cells.

Interleukins Cytokines produced by leucocytes.

Intermediate host The host in which a parasite has its larval or nonsexual existence.

Intrinsic 1 Within a structure rather than compressing it from without; 2 defect without obvious external cause (e.g. intrinsic asthma); (contrast with extrinsic).

Intussusception Invagination or telescoping of a tubular structure, especially bowel.

Invasion Property of malignant neoplastic cells enabling them to infiltrate normal tissues and enter blood vessels and lymphatics.

Involution Reduction in size of an organ or part of it; may be physiological (e.g. shrinkage of thymus gland before adulthood).

Ischaemia An inadequate blood supply to an organ or part of it.

-itis Suffix–'inflammatory'.

Jaundice (Icterus) Yellow discoloration of tissues caused by elevation of plasma bilirubin level.

Junctional At the interface between two structures (e.g. junctional naevus is characterized by naevus cells at the dermo–epidermal junction).

Karyolysis Disintegration of the nucleus.

Karyorrhexis Nuclear fragmentation seen in necrotic cells.

Karyotype Description of the number and shape of chromosomes within a cell, normally characteristic of a species.

Keloid A nodular, enlarging scar resulting from excessive collagen deposition during healing of a skin wound.

Keratinization Production of keratin by normal or neoplastic stratified squamous epithelium.

Kernicterus A disorder characterized by deposition of bilirubin in the brain in neonates resulting in diffuse neuronal damage.

K (killer) cell A lymphocyte that does not mark as either a T or a B cell and is the effector cell in antibody dependent cell-mediated cytotoxicity.

Kinins A group of chemical mediators derived from activation of precursor proteins in the plasma that act on blood vessels, smooth muscle, and pain-sensitive nerve endings (e.g. bradykinin).

Koilocytosis Vacuolation of the cells of stratified squamous epithelium (e.g. skin, cervix) often characteristic of human papillomavirus infection.

Kwashiorkor A form of protein–calorie malnutrition, usually in children, characterized by growth retardation, oedema, and abnormal synthesis of plasma proteins and structural proteins.

Labile cell A cell that is continually dividing throughout life to replace cells that are being continuously lost from the body.

Laceration An injury characterized by tearing of tissue.

Langerhans' cell A specialized dendritic macrophage in the skin, capable of presenting antigen.

Langhans' giant cells Multinucleated macrophages that have their nuclei arranged in a ring or horseshoe pattern at the periphery of the cell, typically seen in epithelioid cell granulomas (e.g. tuberculosis).

Latent (interval) Period between exposure to the cause of a disease and the appearance of the disease itself (e.g. incubation period).

Leiomyo- Prefix–of smooth muscle (e.g. leiomyosarcoma–malignant neoplasm of smooth muscle).

Lesion Any abnormality associated with injury or disease.

Leucocytosis Excessive number of white blood cells (leucocytes).

Leucopaenia Lack of white blood cells.

Leucoplakia A clinical condition characterized by the development of thickened white patches on a mucosal surface.

Leukaemia Neoplastic proliferation of white blood cells; classified into acute and chronic types, according to onset and likely behaviour, and from the cell type (e.g. lymphocytic, granulocytic).

Leukemoid reaction A severe reactive proliferation of neutrophil leucocytes that resembles leukaemia.

Leukotrienes Vasoactive metabolites or arachidonic acid.

Lipo- Prefix–of adipose tissue (e.g. lipoma–benign adipose tumour).

Lipofuscin A granular, brown pigment present in parenchymal cells of elderly individuals.

Liquefactive necrosis A type of necrosis characterized by enzymatic liquefaction of necrotic cells.

Lithiasis Formation of calculi (stones) (e.g. cholelithiasis–gallstones).

Lobar Affecting a lobe, especially of lung as in lobar pneumonia.

Lobular Affecting or arising from a lobule (e.g. lobular carcinoma of the breast).

Locus The site of a gene on the chromosome.

Lymphadenopathy A general term used to denote enlargement of a lymph node due to any cause.

Lymphoedema Progressive non-pitting oedema of subcutaneous tissue caused by lymphatic obstruction.

Lymphokine Cytokine produced by lymphoctyes.

Lymphoma Primary malignant neoplasm of lymphoid tissue classified according to cell type.

Lysis Dissolution or disintegration of a cell, usually as a result of chemical effects.

Macrocyte An erythrocyte with an increased corpuscular volume.

Macrophage A large cell derived from monocyte precursors in the bone marrow that functions in phagocytosis and the immune response.

Major histocompatibility complex (MHC) The chromosomal region containing the genes that control the histocompatibility antigens.

Malabsorption syndrome A group of diseases characterized by failure of absorption of dietary nutrients from the intestine.

Malformation Structural abnormality of the body.

Malignant Condition characterized by relatively high risk of morbidity and mortality.

Malnutrition Any disorder of nutrition.

Marantic (thrombus) Occurring in association with severe wasting (marasmus), usually in infants.

Marasmus A form of protein–calorie malnutrition, usually in children characterized by growth retardation and wasting but usually with retention of appetite and mental alertness.

Margination Gathering of leucocytes on endothelial surface of capillaries and venules in acute inflammation.

Maturation The process whereby a primitive cell reaches its final structure and functional capacity.

Megaloblast A large abnormal erythrocyte precursor characterized by asynchrony of nuclear and cytoplasmic maturation.

Melanoma Malignant neoplasm of melanocytes (except 'juvenile' melanoma which is benign).

Melaena Darkening of stools due to the presence of blood.

Menarche The onset of cyclic menstruation in the adolescent female.

Menopause The period of life during which normal cyclic menstruation ceases.

Menorrhagia Excessive uterine bleeding coupled with normal cycle length.

Mesenchyme The embryonic tissue derived from the mesoderm that becomes the connective tissue of the body.

Mesoderm The middle germ layer of the embryo that gives rise mainly to the connective tissues.

Metachromatic A staining pattern in which tissue takes on a colour different from that of the stain.

Metaplasia Reversible change in the character of a tissue from one specialized cell type to another.

Metastasis Process by which a primary malignant neoplasm forms secondary tumours (metastases) at other sites, most commonly by lymphatic, vascular or transcoelomic spread.

Metastatic calcification See 'calcification'.

Microangiopathy Any disorder affecting the microcirculation.

Microcyte An erythrocyte with a decreased corpuscular volume.

Microinvasion Limited invasion of the tissue through the basement membrane by the cells of a carcinoma.

Mitotic figure A cell undergoing mitotic division as identified by microscopic examination.

Mole 1 Common benign skin lesion composed of melanocytes and/or melanocytic naevus cells; 2 Hydatidiform mole–rare benign disorder of pregnancy characterized by swollen chorionic villi and hyperplastic trophoblast.

Monoclonal Attributable to a single clone of cells and thus more characteristic of a neoplasm than of a reactive process (contrast with polyclonal).

Monoclonal gammopathy A disease characterized by the presence of a large amount of one immunoglobulin type produced by a single clone of B lymphocytes.

Mononuclear cells Histological name for leucocytes other than polymorphonuclear leucocytes and not otherwise identifiable precisely.

Monosomy The absence of one of a pair of homologous chromosomes in an otherwise diploid cell.

M protein A term often used for the monoclonal immunoglobulin in plasma associated with B lymphocyte and plasma cells.

Mucin A viscous fluid composed of glycoproteins that is secreted by mucous glands.

Mucocoele Mucus-filled cyst or hollow organ (e.g. mucocele of the gallbladder).

Mural On the wall of a hollow structure (e.g. mural thrombus on the inner wall of the left ventricle).

Murmur (Bruit) An abnormal sound produced by turbulent blood flow in the cardiovascular system.

Mutation Alteration in the base sequence of DNA, possibly resulting in the synthesis of an abnormal protein product; often an early stage in carcinogenesis.

Mycosis 1 Mycosis–fungal infection; 2 mycosis fungoides–cutaneous T-cell lymphoma entirely unrelated to any fungal infection.

Mycotic aneurysm An aneurysm resulting from infection of the arterial wall. (Note: The term mycotic covers all infections in this context and is not restricted to fungal infections; it is therefore a misnomer.)

Myeloid pertaining to the granulocyte series of cells.

Myeloproliferative disorder A neoplastic proliferation of one or more cell lines of the bone marrow, including granulocytic, erythrocytic and megakaryocytic precursors.

Myopathy A general term used to denote a muscle disorder.

Myxoedema A condition associated with swelling of a tissue caused by accumulation of hydrated mucopolysaccharides.

Myxoid Having a mucin-rich consistency.

Naevus Coloured lesion on skin, often congenital.

Natural killer (NK) cells Lymphocytes that do not mark as either B or T lymphocytes which are cytotoxic without being specifically sensitized against the target cell.

Necrosis Cellular or tissue death in a living organism, irrespective of cause (compare with apoptosis, gangrene and infarction).

Nematode A roundworm.

Neonatal Term used to describe the period between day 0 and 28 days after birth.

Neoplasm Abnormal and uncoordinated tissue growth persisting after withdrawal of the initiating cause (synonymous in modern usage with 'tumour' and 'new growth').

Nephritic syndrome A condition characterized by oliguria, haematuria, proteinuria, hypertension, oedema and azotemia.

Nephritogenic Causing renal disease (more specifically, the nephron).

Neuroendocrine system (formally APUD system) A system of cells scattered throughout the body that secrete biologically active peptide hormones and amines.

Neurogenic Disorder attributable to interruption of nerve supply (e.g. neurogenic atrophy of muscle).

Neutropaenia A decrease in the absolute neutrophil count of peripheral blood below 1500/µl.

Nondisjunction The failure of homologous chromosomes or sister chromatids to separate during meiotic or mitotic cell division.

Normal 1 Statistical–distribution of a numerical variable in which the mode, median and mean are equal; 2 biological—natural state, free of disease.

Normoblast Nucleated precursor cells of the erythroid series.

Nosocomial Originating in a hospital.

Nuclear cytoplasmic ratio The ratio of the diameter of the nucleus of the cell to the diameter of the cytoplasm.

Null cell A lymphocyte that does not have surface immunoglobulin and does not produce E rosettes when incubated with sheep red blood cells.

Obligate intracellular organisms An organism that can grow and multiply only inside living cells.

Occult Abnormality present, but not observable.

Oedema Abnormal collection of fluid within or, more usually, between cells.

Oligoclonal bands In cerebrospinal fluid protein electrophoresis, the presence of 2–5 distinct immunoglobulin bands.

Oliguria A decrease in urine output—in an adult, to less than 400 ml/24 hours.

-oma Suffix—'tumour' (except 'granul*oma*', 'ather*oma*', 'st*oma*', etc.).

Oncofetal Fetal characteristics expressed by tumours (e.g. carcinoembryonic antigen).

Oncogene A gene inappropriately, abnormally, or excessively expressed in tumours and responsible for their autonomous growth.

Oncogenesis The process by which neoplasms are produced.

Oncotic pressure The osmotic pressure exerted by colloids in a solution.

Opportunist (microorganism) Usually harmless, but causing disease in an individual with impaired immunity or some other susceptibility.

Opsonization Enhancement of phagocytosis by factors (opsonins) in plasma.

Organization Natural process of tissue repair involving granulation tissue formation.

-osis Suffix—'state' or 'condition', usually pathological (e.g. osteoarthrosis, acidosis).

Osmotic pressure The force needed to counterbalance the force of osmotic flow across a semipermeable membrane.

Osteomalacia A condition in adults resulting from failure of mineralization of bone, leading to bone-softening and excessive accumulation of uncalcified osteoid.

Osteoporosis A condition characterized by a reduction in total bone mass, usually manifested as thinning of trabecular bone.

Pandemic An epidemic disease that has an unusually wide distribution, usually involving more than one continent.

Pannus An abnormal mass of inflamed granulation tissue. The term is usually used in relation to the cornea and synovial membrane.

Papillary Surface of a lesion characterized by numerous folds, fronds or villous projections.

Papilloedema Swelling of the optic disk.

Papilloma Benign neoplasm of non-glandular epithelium (e.g. squamous cell papilloma).

Pap smear A cytologic preparation made from a scraping of the uterine cervix and stained with Papanicolaou stain.

Parakeratosis Excessive keratin in which nuclear remnants persist within the stratum corneum (a histological sign of increased epidermal growth).

Paraneoplastic syndrome Any complex of symptoms in a patient with cancer that cannot be directly attributed to the physical presence of either the primary tumour or its metastases.

Paraprotein Abnormal plasma protein, usually a monoclonal immunoglobulin in multiple myeloma.

Parasite Organism living on or in the body (the host) and dependant on it for nutrition.

Pathergy Florid, non-specific inflammatory response following minor trauma.

Pathogen A disease-producing microorganism.

Pathogenesis Mechanism through which the cause (aetiology) of a disease produces the clinicopathological manifestations.

Pathogenicity Ability (high, low, etc.) of a microorganism to cause a disease.

Pathognomonic Pathological feature characteristic of a particular disease.

Pavementing Adhesion of marginated leucocytes to the vascular endothelium as a prelude to their emigration out of the vessel.

Pedunculated On a stalk (contrast with sessile).

Pellagra The disease resulting from niacin deficiency, characterized by dermatitis, dementia, and diarrhoea.

Penetrance The frequency with which a heritable trait is manifested in individuals carrying the gene for the trait.

-penia Suffix—'deficiency' (e.g. leucopenia—abnormally low white blood cell count).

Perinatal Occurring between the 24th completed week of gestation and the end of the 7th day after birth.

Peptic (ulcer) Due to the digestive action of gastric secretions.

Petechiae Minute haemorrhagic lesions.

Permanent cell A cell that has no capacity for mitotic division in postnatal life.

Phagocytosis Ingestion of microorganisms or other particles by a cell, especially neutrophil polymorphonuclear leucocytes and macrophages.

Phenotype The morphologic characteristics of an individual that result from interaction of genetic and environmental factors.

Phlebitis Inflammation of a vein.

Phlebothrombosis Venous thrombosis.

Pinocytosis A method of active transport across the cell membrane characterized by formation of invaginations of membrane around extracellular fluid with the formation of pinocytic vesicles (pinosomes).

Plasma cell The effector cell resulting from antigen-induced transformation of B lymphocytes that produces specific antibody against the antigen that induced its formation.

Plasmid In bacteria, an extrachromosomal genetic element that contains autonomously replicating DNA distinct from the bacterial chromosome.

Pleiomorphism Variation in size and shape, usually of nuclei and characteristic of malignant neoplasms.

Pleurisy Inflammation of the pleura.

Pluripotent Capable of differentiating into more than one cell type of one or two germ cell layers.

Pneumoconiosis Fibrotic lung disease due to dust inhalation.

Pneumonia Inflammation of the lung.

Poikilocytosis Abnormal erythrocyte shape.

Polyclonal Indicative of more than one cell clone; feature of reactive rather than neoplastic proliferations (contrast with monoclonal).

Polycythaemia Excessive number of red blood cells.

Polymorphic Consisting of more than one cell type.

Polyp Sessile or pedunculated protrusion from a body surface.

Polyploidy An increase in the number of chromosomes by exact multiples of the number of chromosomes present in diploid cells.

Polyposis Numerous polyps.

Premalignant A pathologic process other than cancer that has an increased tendency to become a malignant neoplasm.

Premature baby A baby that weighs less than 2500 g at birth.

Preterm delivery The birth of a fetus before 34 weeks of gestation.

Primary 1 Initial event without apparent antecedent cause, synonymous with essential or idiopathic (e.g. primary hypertension); 2 a neoplasm arising in the organ in which it is situated; (contrast with secondary).

Primordium *See* 'anlage'.

Prodromal Any feature heralding the appearance of a disease.

Prognosis Probable length of survival or disease-free state, especially after diagnosis and treatment of malignant neoplasms (e.g. 60% 5-year survival).

Prolapse Protrusion or descent of an organ or part of it from its normal location.

Promoter In neoplasia, a chemical substance that has no carcinogenic activity but is capable of increasing the incidence and rate of development of a neoplasm in a tissue previously exposed to a carcinogen.

Protein–calorie malnutrition Disease resulting from insufficient supply of protein and calories to the body.

Psammoma body A discrete, round, concentrically laminated, mineralized body seen in certain neoplasms (e.g. thyroid and ovary).

Pseudocyst Cavity with a distinct wall but lacking an epithelial lining (contrast with cyst).

Pseudohermaphroditism The presence of gonads of one sex but internal and external reproductive organs that are either ambiguous or of the sex different from gonadal sex.

Pseudomembrane 'False' membrane consisting of inflammatory exudate rather than epithelium.

Pseudopolyp In the intestine, a polypoid structure composed of inflammatory tissue and not neoplasm.

Punctum Small orifice, especially where an epidermal cyst communicates with the skin surface.

Purpura Small haemorrhages into the skin.

Pus Creamy material consisting of neutrophil polymorphs, in various stages of disintegration, and tissue debris.

Pustule Small abscess on skin.

Putrefaction Decomposition or rotting of dead tissue due to bacterial action.

Pyaemia Pus-inducing organisms in the blood.

Pyknosis Shrinkage of nucleus in a necrotic cell.

Pyogenic Inducing or forming pus (e.g. pyogenic bacteria).

Pyrogen A chemical substance that acts on the temperature-regulating mechanism of the body and results in fever.

Radiation Emission of waves or particles from a source. Ionizing radiation has enough energy to displace electrons from atoms and lead to formation of unstable ions on interaction with tissues. Nonionizing radiation does not have an adequate energy to cause ionization in tissues.

Radioactivity A phenomenon exhibited by unstable isotopes of chemical elements that undergo spontaneous decay, emitting various high-energy particles.

Radioresistant In tissues and neoplasms, indicating a relative resistance to the harmful effects of radiation in therapeutic dosage ranges.

Radiosensitive In tissues and neoplasms, indicating a relative sensitivity to the harmful effects of radiation in therapeutic dosage ranges.

Radiotherapy The use of ionizing radiation in the treatment of disease, usually cancer.

Raynaud's phenomenon Presents as a secondary manifestation of many diseases in which small vessel vasculitis occurs. Characterized by numbness, pallor or cyanosis of the hands and feet in response to cold.

Raynaud's disease A process of unknown cause charcterized by small vessel spasm without structural vascular abnormality. Characterized by numbness, pallor or cyanosis of the hands and feet in response to cold.

Reactive (process) Reversible response to an external stimulus.

Recanalization One end result of healing of a thrombus, characterized by organization and the formation of new vascular channels that serve to re-establish the circulation.

Recessive Characteristic of a gene of which both copies are necessary for it to be expressed.

Recurrence Neoplasm growing at, or close to, site of previously treated primary neoplasm of identical type.

Reflux Backward flow of the contents of one hollow viscus to another.

Regeneration Formation of new cells identical to those lost.

Rejection Damage to or failure of a tissue or organ transplant due to an immunological host-versus-graft reaction.

Relapse Reappearance of the clinicopathological manifestations of a disease after a period of good health.

Remission Period of good health prior to possible relapse.

Repair Healing with replacement of lost tissue, but not necessarily by similar tissue (usually results in fibrosis).

Reservoir of infection An alternative host of passive carrier of a pathogenic microorganism.

Resolution Restoration of normality.

Reticulocyte An erythrocyte soon after its release from the bone marrow; it differs from other erythrocytes in being slightly larger and containing cytoplasmic RNA.

Reverse transcriptase An RNA-dependant polymerase possessed by retroviruses that permits synthesis of a DNA copy of viral RNA.

Rhabdomyo- Prefix – 'of striated muscle' (e.g. rhabdomyosarcoma – malignant neoplasm of straited muscle).

Rickets A condition in children resulting from the failure of mineralization of bone (causing growth retardation and abnormal ossification).

Rouleaux *See* 'erythrocyte rouleaux'.

Saprophyte Organism deriving its nutrition from dead cells or tissue.

Sarcoma Malignant connective tissue neoplasm.

Scar A mass of collagen that is the end result of repair of an injury.

Schistocyte (Schizocyte) A deformed erythrocyte resulting from apposition of adjacent parts of the cell membrane.

Scirrhous Scar-like (e.g. scirrhous carcinoma of the breast).

Sclerosis Hardening of a tissue often due to deposition of excess collagen.

Scurvy The disease resulting from vitamin C (ascorbic acid) deficiency, characterized by abnormal collagen synthesis and vascular fragility.

Secondary 1 Attributable to some known cause (e.g. secondary hypertension); 2 neoplasm formed by metastasis from a primary neoplasm; (contrast with primary).

Sensitivity In diagnostic pathology, the portion of time a diagnostic test is positive in patients who have the disease or condition. A sensitive test has a low false-negative rate.

Sensitization The first exposure of an individual to an antigen leading to a primary immune response in cases where subsequent exposure to the antigen causes a hypersensitivity reaction.

Septic Infected.

Septum Membrane or boundary dividing a normal or abnormal structure into separate parts.

Serology In infectious diseases, the detection of serum antibodies as evidence of a specific infection.

Serous 1 Serous exudate or effusion – containing fluid resembling serum; 2 Serous cyst containing fluid resembling serum.

Sessile (polyp) With a broad base rather than a discrete stalk (contrast with pedunculated).

Sexually transmitted disease (STD) An infectious disease acquired through sexual contact.

Shock State of cardiovascular collapse characterized by low blood pressure (e.g. due to severe haemorrhage).

Sideroblast An erythroid precursor in the bone marrow that contains stainable iron in the form of ferritin in the cytoplasm.

Signet-ring cell Neoplastic cell (adenocarcinoma) in which the nucleus shows crescentric deformation by a large globule of mucin within its cytoplasm.

Signs Observable manifestations of disease (e.g. swelling, fever, abnormal heart sounds).

Sinus (pathological) Abnormal track (tract) leading from an abscess to the skin surface and often discharging pus.

Specificity In diagnostic pathology, the proportion of the time a diagnostic test is negative in patients who do not have the disease or condition. A specific test has a low false-positive rate.

Spherocyte An erythrocyte of decreased diameter recognizable on smears by the absence of the usual central area of pallor.

Spongiosis Epidermal oedema causing partial separation of cells.

Sprue A disorder of the small intestine characterized by abnormal structure of villi and malabsorption.

Stable cell A cell that has a long lifespan and does not undergo mitotic division unless stimulated to regenerate.

Stage A recognized phase in the development or progression of a disease (usually a neoplasm); (compare with grade).

Stasis Stagnation of fluid often due to obstruction.

Steatorrhoea Excess fat in the faeces, a manifestation of intestinal malabsorption.

Steatosis Fatty change, especially in liver.

Stellate granuloma A specific morphologic type of epithelioid granuloma which has a central stellate zone of neutrophils.

Stenosis Narrowing of a lumen.

Stoma Any normal, pathological or surgically constructed opening between one hollow structure and another or the skin.

Strangulation Obstruction of blood flow by external compression (e.g. strangulated hernia).

Stricture Narrowing of the lumen of a hollow viscus by fibrous thickening of the wall or surrounding tissue, leading to obstruction of flow of luminal contents.

Stroma Non-neoplastic reactive connective tissue within a neoplasm.

Suppuration Formation of pus; a feature of acute inflammation.

Symptoms The patient's complaints attributable to the presence of a disease (e.g. pain, malaise, nausea).

Syndrome Combination of signs and symptoms characteristic of a particular disease, no one feature alone being diagnostic.

Systematic Concerning each body system separately.

Systemic Concerning all body systems as a whole.

Tamponade (cardiac) Compression of heart, and therefore restriction of its movement, by excess pericardial fluid or by pericardial fibrosis.

Telangiectasia Dilated small blood vessels.

Tensile strength The ability to withstand stretching force.

Teratogen An agent acting on the fetus *in utero* during organogenesis that causes congenital structural anomalies.

Teratoma Germ-cell neoplasm in which there are representatives of endoderm, ectoderm and mesoderm; usually benign in the ovary, and malignant in the testis.

Thalassaemia A group of disorders characterized by quantitatively decreased or absent synthesis of one of the globin chains of the haemoglobin molecule.

Thrombocytopenia Decreased number of platelets in peripheral blood.

Thrombocytosis Increased number of platelets in peripheral blood.

Thromboembolism The transport of detached fragments of a thrombus in the circulation from its point of formation to another blood vessel.

Thrombophlebitis Venous inflammation associated with a thrombus.

Thrombus Solid mass of coagulated blood formed within the circulation (contrast with clot).

T lymphocyte A lymphocyte that is primed by the thymus during its development in fetal life.

Tolerance The decreasing effect on the body of the same dose of a drug in response to continued use of the drug.

Tophus A mass formed by the deposition of urate crystals in connective tissues.

Torsion Abnormality resulting when an object is twisted either upon itself or on a pedicle.

Totipotent Capable of differentiating into all the different types of tissues in the organism.

Toxaemia Presence of a toxin in the blood.

Toxin Substance having harmful effects, usually of bacterial origin by common usage.

Toxoid A bacterial exotoxin that has been altered in such a way as to lose its toxicity while retaining its antigenicity.

Trabeculation Abnormal appearance of a surface characterized by ridges.

Transformation Process in which cells are converted from normal to neoplastic.

Transfusion Introduction of blood or blood components directly into the bloodstream.

Transfusion reaction Any adverse clinical effect that results from transfusion of blood or blood components.

Translocation Exchange of chromosomal segments between one chromosome and another.

Transplantation The grafting of tissues from one site to another or from one individual to another.

Transudate Abnormal collection of fluid of low protein content due to either hypoproteinaemia or increased intravascular pressure in capillary beds (contrast with exudate).

Trauma Injury.

Trematode A flatworm.

Trisomy Presence of three copies of a particular chromosome in otherwise diploid cells (e.g. trisomy 21 is a feature of Down's syndrome).

Tropocollagen The molecular unit of collagen as it is secreted by the fibroblast.

Tumour Abnormal swelling, now synonymous with neoplasm and 'new growth'.

Tumour markers Secretory products of neoplasms that are released into the blood or other body fluids, detection of which aids diagnosis of the tumour.

Type (neoplasm) Identity of a neoplasm determined from its differentiated features or assumed origin (histogenesis).

Ulcer Full-thickness defect in a surface epithelium or mucosa.

Vaccination Administration of an antigenic preparation for the purpose of establishing immunity to an infectious disease in the recipient.

Varicose Distended and tortuous, especially referring to a blood vessel (e.g. varicose vein).

Vasculitis See 'arteritis' and 'angiitis'. Inflammation and structural damage of the vessel wall.

Vasoconstriction Narrowing of a blood vessel resulting from contraction of medial smooth muscle.

Vasodilatation Increase in luminal diameter of a blood vessel resulting from relaxation of medial smooth muscle.

VDRL Venereal Diseases Research Laboratory (test for syphilis).

Vector An animal, usually an arthropod, that carries and transfers an infective agent from one host to another.

Vegetation A polypoid mass of thrombus formed on the endocardial surface of the heart, usually on a cardiac valve.

Venereal Transmitted by sexual intercourse or intimate foreplay.

Vesicle (skin) Small fluid-filled blister < 5 mm diameter.

Villous Characterized by numerous finger-like projections (villi).

Viraemia (microorganism) Presence of a virus in the blood.

Viral oncogene (v-*onc.*) A nucleotide sequence carried by a virus that corresponds to a similar sequence in the DNA of mammalian cells.

Virilization The abnormal development of secondary male sexual characteristics in a female.

Virulence The degree to which a microorganism is capable of causing pathologic changes in tissues after infection.

Viscid Having a high viscosity, rendering the substance thick and sticky.

Viscus A hollow organ.

Vitamins A group of organic essential nutrients that are necessary in trace amounts for normal metabolism.

Volvulus Loop of twisted intestine.

Warthin–Finkeldey cell A multinucleated giant cell seen in tissues infected with the measles virus.

Wheal A localized, raised skin lesion produced by dermal and epidermal oedema.

Withdrawal syndrome The clinical state caused by abstention from a drug an individual is addicted to.

Xanthoma A yellow skin lesion caused by deposition of lipids in dermal macrophages.

Xenograft Transplantation from one species to another.

Xerophthalmia A disorder characterized by dryness of the cornea, frequently associated with denudation and thickening.

Xerostomia Dryness of the mouth resulting from decreased secretion of saliva.

Zygote The diploid totipotent cell that results from union of the haploid male and female gametes.

Further Reading

General pathology

Bancroft J.D. & Cook H.C. (1984) *Manual of Histological Techniques*. Churchill Livingstone, London.

Connor J.M. & Ferguson-Smith M.A. (1993) *Essential Medical Genetics*, 4th edn. Blackwell Scientific Publications, Oxford.

Cotran R.S., Kumar V. & Robbins S.L. (1989) *Pathologic Basis of Disease*, 4th edn. WB Saunders, Philadelphia.

Gresham, G.A., Turner, A.F. (1979) *Postmortem Procedures (an illustrated textbook)*, Wolf Medical Publications Limited, London.

Knight, B. (1983) *The Coroner's Autopsy*. Churchill Livingstone, Edinburgh.

Knight, B. (1987) *Legal Aspects of Medical Practice*, 4th edn. Churchill Livingstone, Edinburgh.

Mitchinson M.J. *et al.* (1996) *Essentials of Pathology*. Blackwell Science, Oxford.

Polak, J. & Van Noorden S. (eds) (1986) *Immunocytochemistry. Practical Applications in Pathology and Biology*, 2nd edn. Wright PSG, Bristol.

Rubin, E. & Farber J.L. (eds) (1988) *Pathology*. JB Lippincott, Philadelphia.

Rosai J. (1989) *Ackerman's Surgical Pathology*, 7th edn. CV Mosby, St Louis.

Sternberg S.S. (1992) *Histology for Pathologists*. Raven Press, New York.

Underwood J.C.E. (1992) *General and Systemic Pathology*. Churchill Livingstone, Edinburgh.

Underwood J.C.E. (1987) *Introduction to Biopsy Interpretation and Surgical Pathology*. Springer-Verlag Amsterdam.

Systemic pathology

Bloodworth J.M. (ed) (1982) *Endocrine Pathology*, 2nd edn. Williams and Wilkins, New York.

Esiri M.M. (1996) *Oppenheimer's Diagnostic Neuropathology*. Blackwell Science, Oxford.

Kurman R.J. (ed) (1987) *Blaustein's Pathology of the Female Genital Tract*. Springer-Verlag, New York.

Miller A.B. (1985) *Screening for Cancer*. Academic Press, New York.

Page D.L. & Anderson T.J. (1987) *Diagnostic Histopathology of the Breast*. Churchill Livingstone, Edinburgh.

Ruddon R.W. (1987) *Cancer Biology*, 2nd edn. Oxford University Press, Oxford.

Sherlock S. (1989) *Diseases of the Liver and Biliary System*, 6th edn. Lippincott, London.

Stehbens W.E. & Lie J.T. (1995) *Vascular Pathology*. Chapman and Hall, London.

Tisher C.C. & Brenner B.M. (1989) *Renal Pathology: with Clinical and Functional Correlations*. Lippincott, Philadelphia.

Unni K.K. (ed). (1988) *Bone Tumours*. Churchill Livingstone, New York.

Wigglesworth J. & Singer D. (eds) (1990) *Textbook of Fetal and Perinatal Pathology*. Blackwell Scientific Publications, Oxford.

Pathology atlases

Atkinson B.F. (1992) *Atlas of Diagnostic Cytopathology*. WB Saunders, Philadelphia.

Becker A.E. & Anderson R.H. (1983) *Cardiac Pathology*. Churchill Livingstone, Edinburgh.

Begemann H. & Rasketter J. (1989) *Atlas of Clinical Haematology*. Springer-Verlag, New York.

Curran R.C. (1985) *Color Atlas of Histopathology*, 3rd edn. Oxford University Press, New York.

Dunnill M.S. (1987) *Pulmonary Pathology*. Churchill Livingstone, London.

Gresham G.A. (1992) *A Colour Atlas of General Pathology*, 2nd edn. Mosby Year Book, St Louis.

Hoffbrand A.V. & Pettit J.E. (1987) *Clinical Haematology Illustrated: An Integrated Text and Colour Atlas*. Saunders, London.

McKee P.H. (Ed) (1996) *Pathology of the Skin*, 2nd edn. Gower, London.

Marcove R.C. & Arlen M. (1992) *Atlas of Bone Pathology*. JB Lippincott, Philadelphia.

Mirra J.M. (ed.) (1989) *Bone Tumours: Clinical, Radiological and Pathological Correlations*. Lea and Febiger, New York.

Mitros F.A. (1988) *Atlas of Gastrointestinal Pathology*. JB Lippincott, Philadelphia.

Netter F.H. (1970s and 1980s) *The Ciba Collection of Medical Illustra-*

tions (12 books). Ciba Medical, New Jersey.

Olsen E.G. (1987) *Atlas of Cardiovascular Pathology.* Kluwer Academic, Massachussetts.

Risdon R.A. & Turner D.R. (1980) *Atlas of Renal Pathology.* Lippincott, London.

Royal College of Surgeons of Edinburgh. (1983) *Color Atlas of Demonstrations in Surgical Pathology.* Williams & Wilkins, Baltimore.

Sandritter T. (1979) *Macropathology: Text and Color Atlas,* 5th edn. Mosby Year Book, St Louis.

Weller R.O. (1984) *Color Atlas of Neuropathology.* Oxford University Press, New York.

Wenig B.M. (1993) *Atlas of Head and Neck Pathology.* WB Saunders, Philadelphia.

Wheater P.R. (1985) *Basic Histopathology: A Colour Atlas and Text.* Churchill Livingstone, London.

Woodruff J.D. & Parmley T.H. (1988) *Atlas of Gynaecologic Pathology.* Lippincott, New York.

Clinical Chemistry

Clayton B. & Round J. (1994) *Clinical Biochemistry and the Sick Child,* 2nd edn. Blackwell Science, Oxford.

Brook C.G.D. & Marshall N. (1995) *Essentials of Endocrinology,* 3rd edn. Blackwell Science, Oxford.

Bryson P.D. (1989) *Comprehensive Review in Toxicology,* 2nd edn. Aspen Publishers Inc., Rockville.

Walmsley R.N. & White G.H. (1994) *A Guide to Diagnostic Clinical Chemistry,* 3rd edn. Blackwell Science, Oxford.

Haematology

Bloom A.L. & Thomas D.P. (1987) *Haemostasis and Thrombosis,* 2nd edn. Churchill Livingstone, London.

Habeshaw J.A. & Lauder I. (eds) (1988) *Malignant Lymphomas.* Churchill Livingstone, Edinburgh.

Hoffbrand A.V. & Pettit J.E. (1992) *Essential Haematology,* 3rd edn. Blackwell Scientific Publications, Oxford.

Immunology

Chapel H.M. & Haeney M. (1993) *Essentials of Clinical Immunology,* 3rd edn. Blackwell Scientific Publications, Oxford.

Roitt I.M. (1994) *Essential Immunology,* 8th edn. Blackwell Science, Oxford.

Microbiology

Bell D., Gilks C., Molyneux M., Smith D. & Wyatt G. (1995) *Lecture Notes on Tropical Medicine,* 4th edn. Blackwell Science, Oxford.

Elliott T.S.E. & Hastings J.G.M. (1996) *Lecture Notes on Medical Microbiology,* 3rd edn. Blackwell Science, Oxford.

Mandell G.L., Douglas R.G. & Bennett J.H. (eds) (1990) *Principles and Practice of Infectious Disease,* 3rd edn. Wiley, New York.

Manson-Bahr P.E. & Bell D.R. (eds) (1987) *Manson's Tropical Disease,* 19th edn. Balliére-Tindall, London.

Rubin R.H. & Young L.S. (eds) (1988) *Clinical Approach to Infection in the Compromised Host,* 2nd edn. Plenum Press, New York.

Woods G.L. & Gutierrez Y. (1993) *Diagnostic Pathology of Infectious Diseases.* Lea & Febiger, Philadelphia.

Index